Newer Trends in ART

Editors

Nandita Palshetkar
MD FCPS FICOG
Medical Director, Bloom IVF
Mumbai, Maharashtra, India
Professor of Gynecology
DY Patil Medical College
Navi Mumbai, Maharashtra, India
President, FOGSI (2019–2020)
Past President, MOGS (2016–2017)
Past President, IAGE (2017–2018)

Hrishikesh D Pai
MD FCPS FICOG MSc (USA)
Gynecologist and Head of IVF Unit
Lilavati Hospital
Scientific Director, Bloom IVF
Mumbai, Maharashtra, India

Rishma Dhillon Pai
MD DNB FCPS DGO FICOG FRCOG
Consultant Gynecologist
Jaslok, Hinduja and Lilavati Hospitals
Mumbai, Maharashtra, India

Sunita Tandulwadkar
MD FICS FICOG
Head, Department of Obstetrics and Gynecology
Chief, Department of IVF and Endoscopy
Ruby Hall Clinic, Pune, Maharashtra, India

Kinjal R Shah
DFP DNB FNB DNB
Obstetrics and Gynecology
Central Railway Hospital
Mumbai, Maharashtra, India

Manisha T Kundnani
MD FNB FNUS
Scientific Director, Consultant Fertility and
Reproductive Medicine Specialist
Fertility Square, IVF Clinic
Mumbai, Maharashtra, India

JAYPEE

JAYPEE BROTHERS MEDICAL PUBLISHERS
The Health Sciences Publisher
New Delhi | London | Panama

Jaypee Brothers Medical Publishers (P) Ltd

Headquarters
Jaypee Brothers Medical Publishers (P) Ltd
4838/24, Ansari Road, Daryaganj
New Delhi 110 002, India
Phone: +91-11-43574357
Fax: +91-11-43574314
Email: jaypee@jaypeebrothers.com

Overseas Offices
J.P. Medical Ltd
83 Victoria Street, London
SW1H 0HW (UK)
Phone: +44 20 3170 8910
Fax: +44 (0)20 3008 6180
Email: info@jpmedpub.com

Jaypee-Highlights Medical Publishers Inc
City of Knowledge, Bld. 235, 2nd Floor
Clayton, Panama City, Panama
Phone: +1 507-301-0496
Fax: +1 507-301-0499
Email: cservice@jphmedical.com

Jaypee Brothers Medical Publishers (P) Ltd
Bhotahity, Kathmandu, Nepal
Phone: +977-9741283608
Email: kathmandu@jaypeebrothers.com

Website: www.jaypeebrothers.com
Website: www.jaypeedigital.com

Inquiries for bulk sales may be solicited at: jaypee@jaypeebrothers.com

Newer Trends in ART

First Edition: **2019**

ISBN: 978-93-88958-83-7

Printed at: Samrat Offset Pvt. Ltd.

Indian Society for Assisted Reproduction (ISAR) Internal Publication Board

24th Annual ISAR Mumbai Organising Team

ORGANISING CHAIRPERSONS

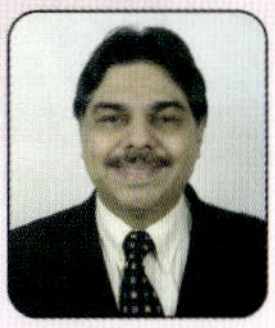
Hrishikesh D Pai

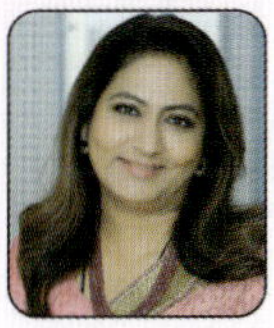
Nandita Palshetkar

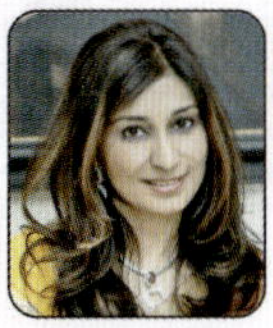
Rishma Dhillon Pai

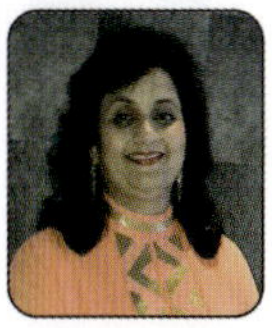
Sunita Tandulwadkar

ORGANISING VICE CHAIRPERSONS

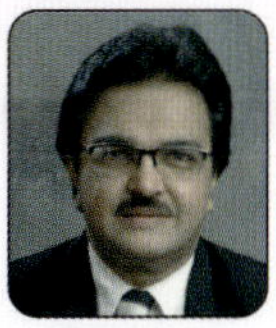
Prakash Trivedi

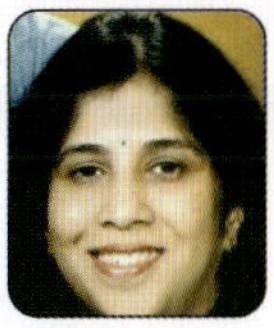
Padmarekha Jirge

ORGANISING SECRETARIES

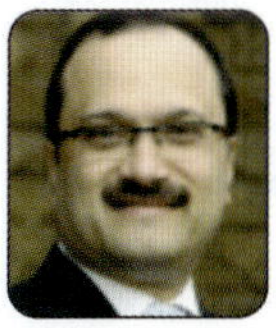
Ameet Patki

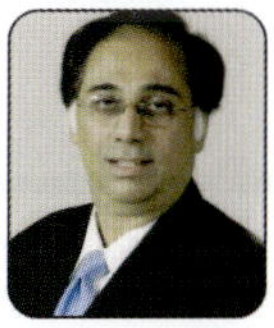
Bipin Pandit

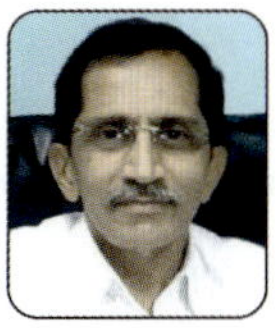
S. Krishnakumar

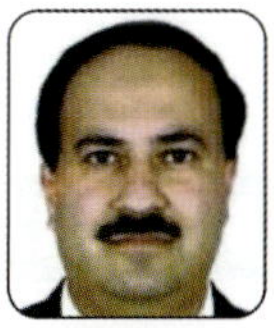
Sudesh Kamat

JOINT ORGANISING SECRETARIES

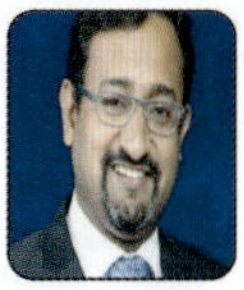
Kundan Ingale

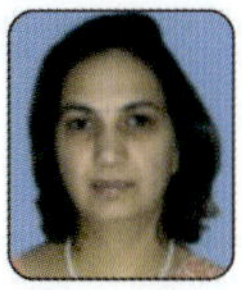
Sarita Bhalerao

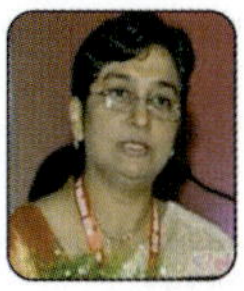
Sadhana Patwardhan

TREASURERS

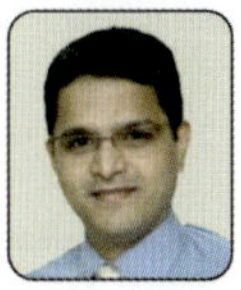
Kedar Ganla

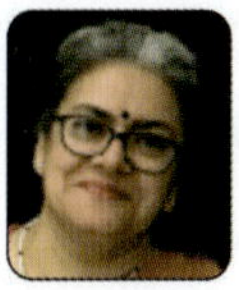
Anahita Chauhan

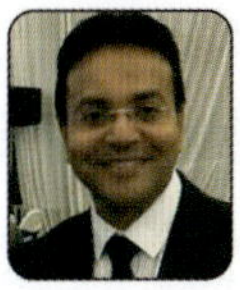
Ashish Kale

MSR COMMITTEE 2016 - 2018

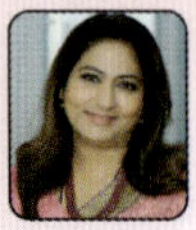

Nandita Palshetkar
Chairperson

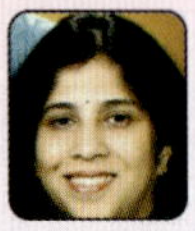

Padmarekha Jirge
Gen. Secretary

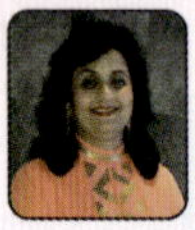

Sunita Tandulwadkar
Senior Chairman

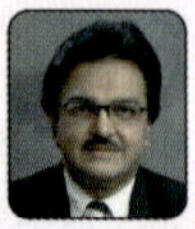

Prakash Trivedi
Executive Vice Chairperson

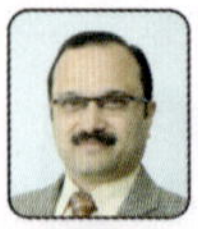

Ameet Patki
Clinical Secretary

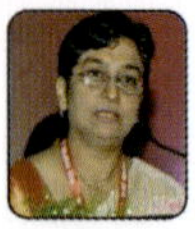

Sadhana Patwardhan
Librarian

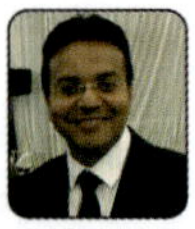

Ashish Kale
Treasurer

MANAGING COMMITTEE MEMBERS

Kundan Ingle, Kedar Ganla, Chaitanya Shembekar, Sudhesh Kamat, Pradeep Chitre, Shashikant Umbardand, Varsh Baste, Kalyan Baramade, Laxmi Shrikhande, Mamta Dighe, Manjushree Boob

MSR COMMITTEE 2018 - 2020

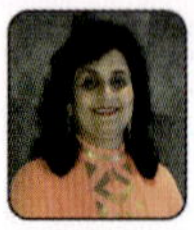

Sunita Tandulwadkar
Chairperson

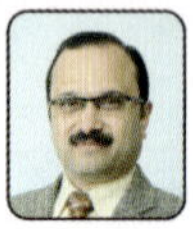

Ameet Patki
General Secretary

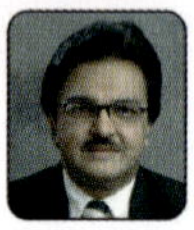

Prakash Trivedi
Senior Chairperson

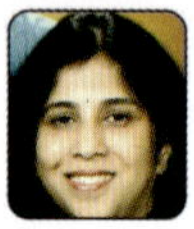

Padmarekha Jirge
Executive Vice Chairperson

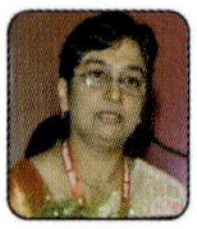

Sadhana Patwardhan
Clinical Secretary

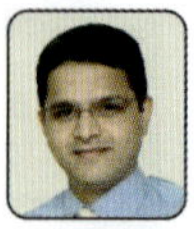

Kedar Ganla
Librarian

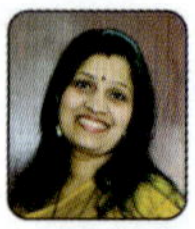

Ashwini Kale
Treasurer

MANAGING COMMITTEE MEMBERS

Ashish Kale, Chaitanya Shembekar, Kundan Ingale, Rohan Palshetkar Sudesh Kamat, Kalyan Barmade, Prerna Shinde, Varsha Baste, Manjushree Boob, Prakash Patil, Rachana Deshpande, Shashikanth Umard and, Manjiri Valsangkar

PAST CHAIRMANS

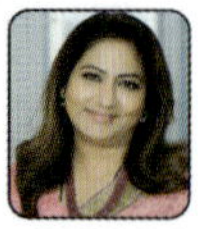

Nandita Palshetkar

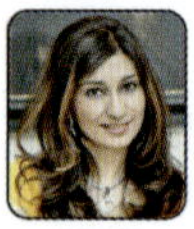

Rishma Dhillon Pai

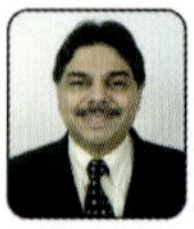

Hrishikesh Pai
Founder Chairperson

MOGS COMMITTEE 2018 - 2019

MOGS Office Bearers 2018-2019

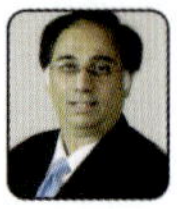

Bipin Pandit
President

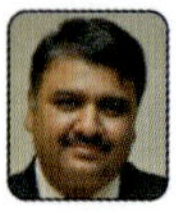

Jaydeep Tank
Vice President

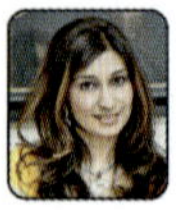

Rishma Dhillon Pai
Vice President

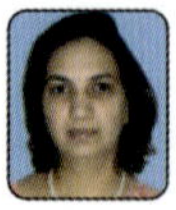

Sarita Bhalerao
Secretary

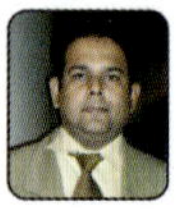

Niranjan Chavan
Joint Secretary

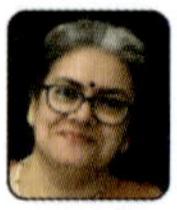

Anahita Chauhan
Treasurer

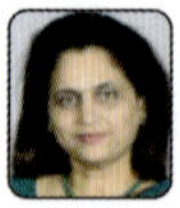

Suvarna Khadilkar
Librarian

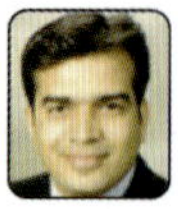

Rajendra Sankpal
Clinical Secretary

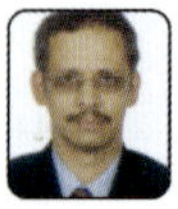

Shailesh Kore
Jt. Cilinical Secretary

MOGS Managing Council Members 2018-2019

Ameya Purandare
Atul Ganatra
Ganpat Sawant
Geetha Balsarkar
Kedar Ganla
Komal Chavan
Madhuri Mehendale
Mandakini Megh
Mansi Medhekar
Nagendra Sardeshpande
Parikshit Tank
Pratik Tambe
Priti Vyas
Priya Vora
Punit Bhojani
Purnima Satoskar
Rajendra Nagarkatti
Raju Sahetya
Reena Wani
Sanket Pisat
Sudha Tandon
Sujata Dalvi
Vandana Bansal
Vijaya Babre

MOGS Past Presidents

Vinita Raut (2017-18) **Nandita Palshetkar** (2016-17) **Arun Nayak** (2015-16) **Ameet Patki** (2014-15) **Suchitra N Pandit** (2013-14)

ISAR MANAGING COMMITTEE 2018-2019

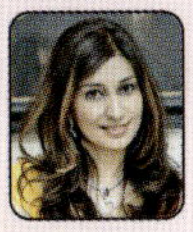

Rishma Dhillon Pai
President

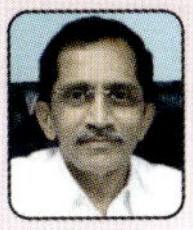

S. Krishnakumar
Hon. Secretary General

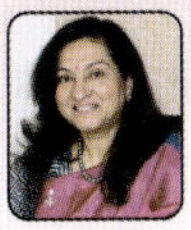

Jaideep Malhotra
President Elect 2019

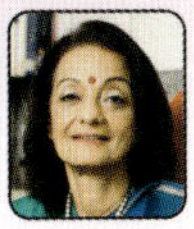

Duru Shah
Immediate Past President

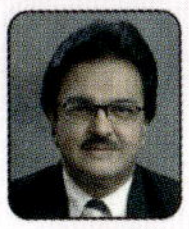

Prakash Trivedi
Vice President

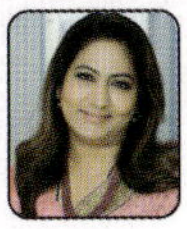

Nandita Palshetkar
Second Vice President

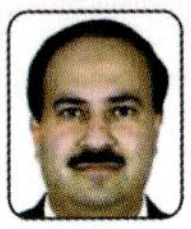

Sudesh Kamat
Chairman - Embryology

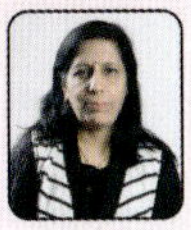

R. B. Agarawal
Vice Chairman - Embryology

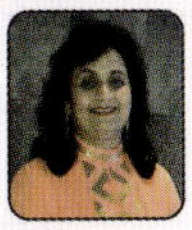

Sunita Tandulwadkar
Hon. Joint Secretary

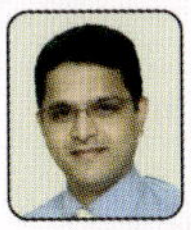

Kedar Ganla
Hon. Treasurer

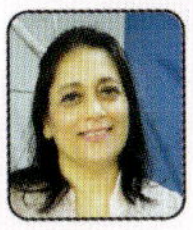

Sujata Kar
Hon. Joint Treasurer

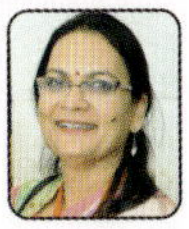

Asha Baxi
Hon. Clinical Secretary

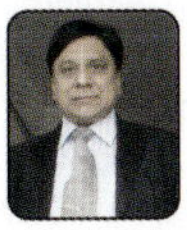

A. Suresh Kumar
Hon. Librarian

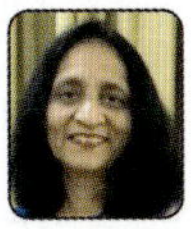

Madhuri Patil
Editor of JHRS

PAST PRESIDENTS

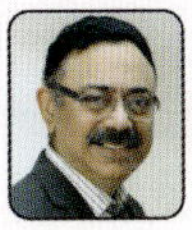

Narendra Malhotra

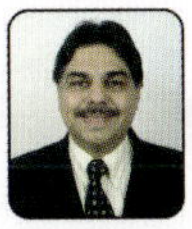

Hrishikesh Pai

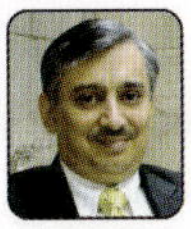

Manish Banker

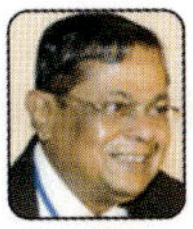

Dhiraj Gada

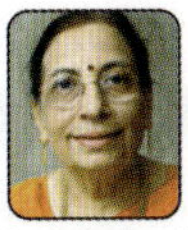

Sadhana Desai

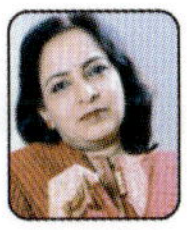

Kamini Rao

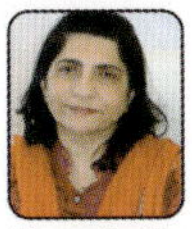

Firuza Parikh

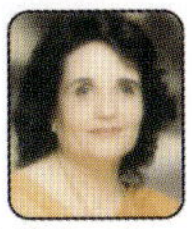

Late Mehroo Hansotia

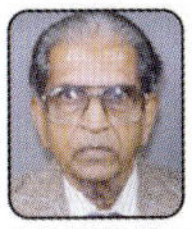

Mahendra N. Parikh
Founder President

MEMBERS

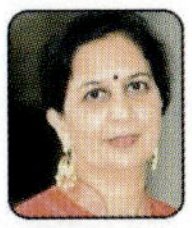

Archana Baser

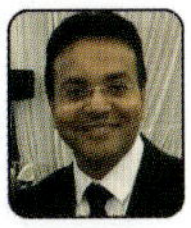

Ashish Kale

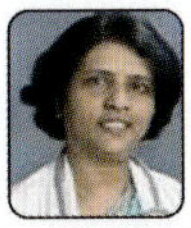

Mangala Kawade

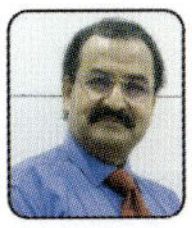

Prakash S. Patil

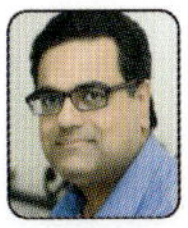

Rajesh Modi

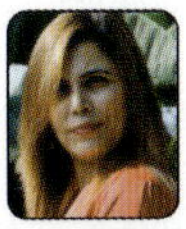

Seema Pandey

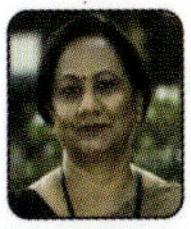

Shobhana Patted

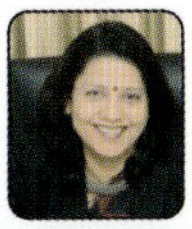

Laxmi Shrikhande

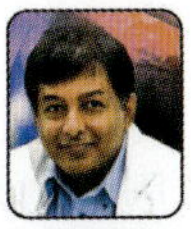

M S Shrinivas

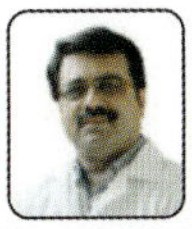

Himanshu Patel

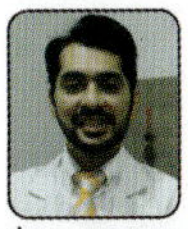

Keshav Malhotra

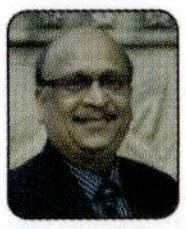

Natchandra Chimote

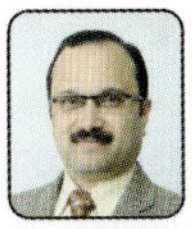

Ameet Patki

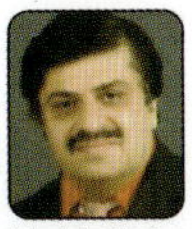

Nimish Shelat

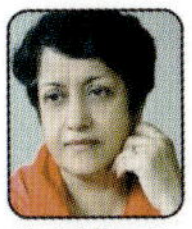

Tarini Taneja

ISAR STATE CHAPTERS 2018-2019

No.	STATE CHAPTERS	CHAIR PERSON	HON. GEN. SECRETARY
1	Andhra Pradesh Chapter	Padmaja V	Chandana V
2	Bihar Chapter	Shanti Roy	Pragya Mishra
3	Chandigarh Chapter	G K Bedi	Pooja Mehta
4	Chhattisgarh Chapter	A. Suresh Kumar	Tripti Nagaria
5	Delhi Chapter	G K Tripathi	Shivani Sachdev Gaur
6	Goa Chapter	Kedarnath Padte	Abhijit Kamat
7	Gujarat Chapter	Kanthi Bansal	R G Patel
8	Haryana Chapter	Maninder Ahuja	Jyoti Malik
9	Himachal Pradesh Chapter	Bishan Dhiman	Sandeep Rathod
10	Jammu & Kashmir Chapter	Sunil Chaudhary	Indu kaul
11	Jharkhand Chapter	S K Gupta	Neha Priyadarshini
12	Karnataka Chapter	M S Srinivas	Shobhana Patted
13	Kerala Chapter	Sathy M Pillai	Fessy Louis
14	Madhya Pradesh Chapter	Virendra Shah	Gajendra Tomar
15	Maharashtra Chapter	Nandita Palshetkar	Padmarekha Jirge
16	North East Chapter*	Arun Madhab Baruah	Vijay Nahata
17	Odisha Chapter	Jayshree Pattnayak	Babita Panda
18	Punjab Chapter	P S Bakshi	Jasmine Kaur Dahiya
19	Rajasthan Chapter	Sanjay Makwana	Renu Makwana
20	Tamilnadu & Pondicherry Chapter	Kamala Selvaraj	Sanjeeva N Reddy
21	Telangana Chapter	Mamata Deendayal	Shanthakumari
22	UP Chapter	Sadhna Gupta	Rajul Tyagi
23	Uttarakhand Chapter	Aarti Luthra	Ritu Prasad
24	West Bengal Chapter	Gita Ganguly	Gautam Khastgir

*** North East Chapter Consist 8 States:** Arunachal Pradesh, Assam, Meghalaya, Manipur, Mirzoram, Nagaland, Sikkim & Tripura

2019 ISAR

INTERNATIONAL FACULTY

isar

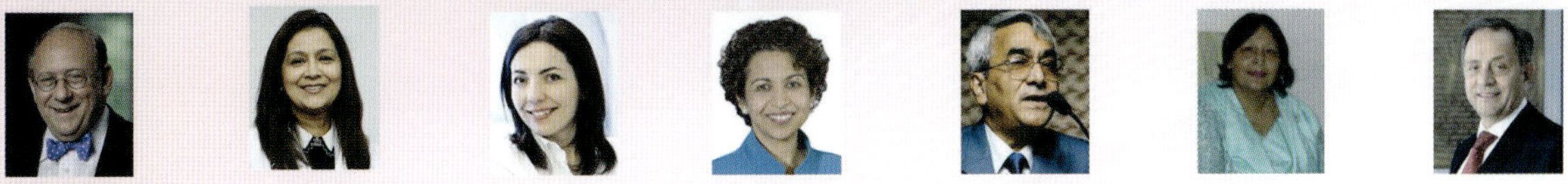

Alan Decherney
USA

Alka Goyal
Canada

Alexia Chatziparasidou
Greece

Anuja Dokras
USA

Bhola Risal
Nepal

Ashma Rana
Bangladesh

Basil Tarlatzis
Greece

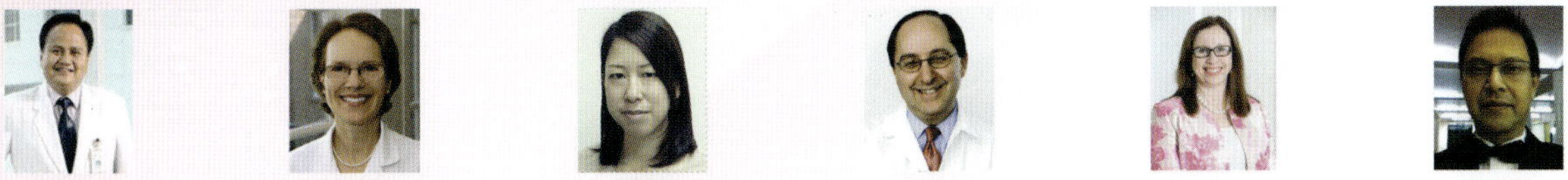

Budi Wiwecko
Indonesia

Catherine Racowsky
USA

Cheimi Toyama
Japan

Christos Coutifaris
USA

Clare Boothroyd
Australia

Dib Dutta
UK

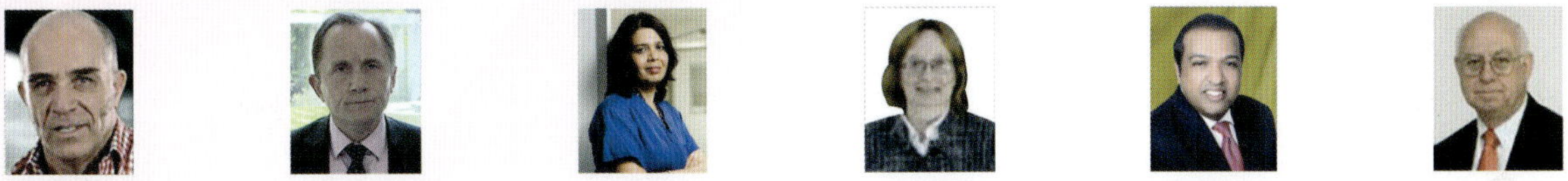

Diego Ezcurra
Spain

Edward Morris
UK

Geeta Nargund
UK

Helene Russel
USA

Ishwaran K K
Malaysia

Joe Leigh Simpson
USA

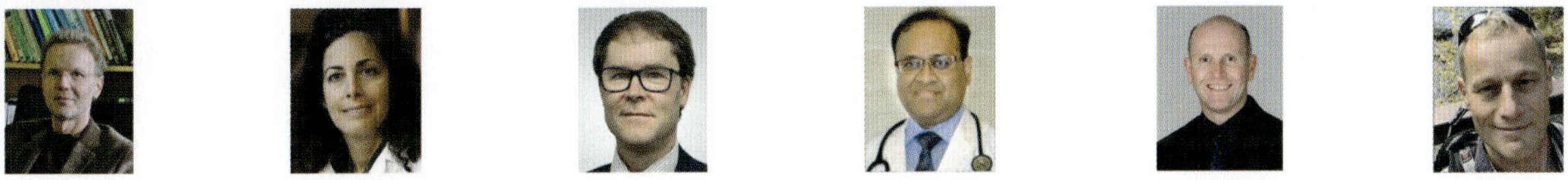

Keith Ray
USA

Laurel Stadtmauer
USA

Luk Rombauts
Australia

Maruf Siddiqui
Bangladesh

Neil Johnson
New Zealand

Neils Ramsing
Denmark

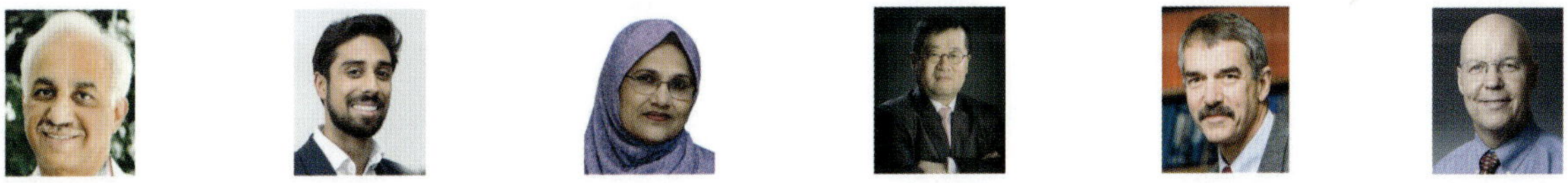

Pankaj Srivastava
Dubai

Prafulla Nargund
UK

Rashida Begum
Bangladesh

Ri-Cheng Chian
Canada

Richard Paulson
USA

Richard Reindollar
USA

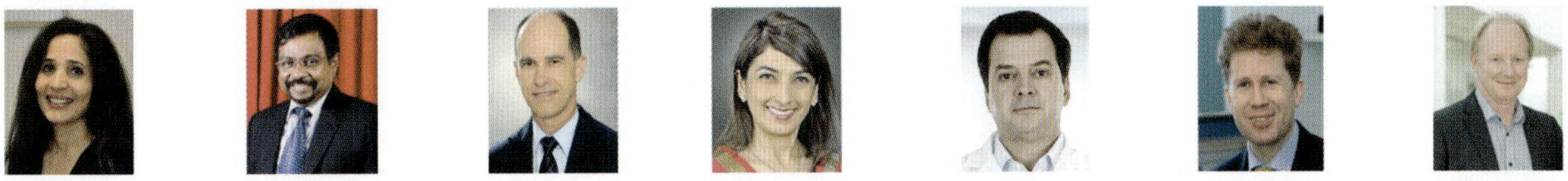

Reena Agarwal
UK

Rohana Nalin Haththotuwa
Sri Lanka

Sandro Esteves
Canada

Sapna Bajaj
UK

Dr Sergio Soares
Portugal

Stephen Keay
UK

Steven D Fleming
Australia

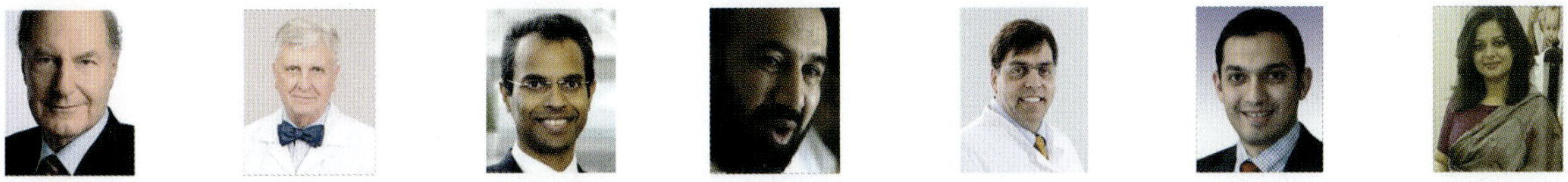

Stuart Campbell
USA

Vladislav Korsak
Russia

V P Singh
New Zealand

Mohammad Hashim Wahaaj
Afghanistan

Arvind Chandra
Germany

Nikhil Purandare
UK

Anu Chawla
UK

Contributors

A Suresh Kumar MBBS MD (Obs & Gyn) PhD (DHUM) MAIGE FACS
Senior Infertility Specialist
Ashoka's Advanced IVF Centre
Ashoka Superspecialty Women Hospital and IMSI, ICSI Test Tube Baby Centre
Raipur, Chhattisgarh, India

Aarti Deenadayal Tolani MS Diploma in Endoscopy (Germany) Trained in embryology (Singapore)
Shenoy Hospital
Hyderabad, Telangana, India

Abarajda V Fellow in Reproductive Medicine
Rao Hospital
Coimbatore, Tamil Nadu, India

Abha Khurana MBBS DNB (Obs & Gyn) Fellowship in Reproductive Medicine
Wing Commander Classified Specialist (Obs & Gyn)
Specialist in Reproductive Medicine
Command Hospital Air Force
Bengaluru, Karnataka, India

Aditi Joshi

Akanksha Mishra
Chief Embryologist
Janini IVF, New Delhi, India

Alan DeCherney

Alex C Varghese PhD
Scientific Director
Astra Fertility Clinic
4303, Village Centre Court, Mississauga, ON L4Z 1S2, Canada
Lab Director
CRAFT Hospital and Research Centre
Kodungallur, Kerala, India

Alexia Chatziparasidou MSc
Senior Clinical Embryologist
Director of Embryolab IVF Unit
Co-founder of Embryolab Academy
Greece

Alka Kriplani MD FRCOG FAMS FICOG FIMSA FICMCH FCLS
Professor and Head
All India Institute of Medical Sciences
New Delhi, India

Ameet Patki MD DNB FCPS DGO FRCOG
Scientific Director
Fertility Associates, Khar
Mumbai, Maharashtra, India
Gen. Secretary ISAR

Amiti Agrawal MBBS MS FMIS FRM Masters in Reproductive Medicine (London)
Associate Fertility Consultant
Bloom IVF & Babies and US IVF Centre
Opera House, Mumbai, Maharashtra, India

Amruta DS Pathare PhD
Research Fellow
PD Hinduja Hospital and Medical Research Centre
Jaslok Hospital and Research Centre
Mumbai, Maharashtra, India

Anagha Deshpande MSc (Biotechnology)
Embryologist
Ramnarain Ruia College
Mumbai, Maharashtra, India

Anne Martini

Anupam Gupta MBBS MS (Obs & Gyn) FICMU FICMCH
Consultant
Aakanksha Test Tube Baby Centre
Dr Kusum Gupta Nursing Home
Agra, Uttar Pradesh, India
Vice President, FOGSI 2015
Chairperson International Academic Exchange Committee of FOGSI (2010–2012)
Joint Secy FOGSI 2008
Vice Chairman, UP Chapter of ISAR

Anupama Deenadayal Mettler
Embryologist IIRC
Shenoy Hospital
Hyderabad, Telangana, India
Certified ESHRE Embryologist

Anver Kuliev

Apoorva Pallam Reddy MS DNB
Reproductive Endocrinologist
Medical Director
Phoenix Speciality Clinic
Bengaluru, Karnataka, India

Arun Baruah MD PhD FICOG FICMCH
Consultant
Sampreeti Hospital
Sivasagar, Assam, India

Arya Salaskar MSc (Biochemistry)
Senior Embryologist
DY Patil IVF Centre
Bloom IVF Centre
Mumbai, Maharashtra, India

Asha Baxi MS FRCOG
Director
Disha Fertility & Surgical Center
Indore, Madhya Pradesh, India

Asha R Rao MD DGO FICOG
Medical Director
ART Specialist
Rao Hospital
Coimbatore, Tamil Nadu, India

Ashwini M MBBS MS Fellow in Reproductive Medicine (RGUHS)
Senior Consultant
Gunasheela Surgical and Maternity Hospital
Bengaluru, Karnataka, India

Bharti Dhorepatil DNB DGO FICS Dip Endoscopy
Director and Chief IVF Consultant
Shree Hospital, Ssmile IVF RM Unit
Pune, Maharashtra, India

Biswanath Ghosh Dastidar MBBS (Hon; Cal) MSc (Oxon)
Scientific Director
Ghosh Dastidar Institute for Fertility Research
Kolkata, West Bengal, India

BN Chakravarty
Founder Reproductive Medicine
Director Institute of Reproductive Medicine
Kolkata, West Bengal, India

C Mohamed Ashraf MD DGO DPS (Germany)
Chairman and Medical Director
CRAFT Academy of Reproductive Sciences
Thrissur, Kerala, India

CB Nagori MD DGO
Director and Infertility Consultant
Dr Nagori's Institute for Infertility and IVF
Ahmedabad, Gujarat, India

Charumati Pekhale MBBS DGO DNB
Consultant
Lilavati Hospital IVF Centre
Mumbai, Maharashtra, India

Damodar R Rao MD Fellowship in Endocrinology, Fellowship in Reproductive Medicine
Associate Director and ART Specialist
Consultant in Infertility & Endoscopy
Rao Hospital
Coimbatore, Tamil Nadu, India

Deepa Talreja MS DNB FNB
Reproductive Medicine

Devika Gunasheela MBBS MRCOG (Lond) Fellow in Reproductive Medicine (RGUHS)
Director
Gunasheela Surgical and Maternity Hospital
Bengaluru, Karnataka, India

Dhanashri Natu MS DNB (Obstetrics & Gynaecology) FNB Fellow in Reproductive Medicine
Lilavati Hospital and Research Centre
Mumbai, Maharashtra, India

Dhiraj Gada MD DGO DFP FICMCH
Director
Shalby Gada Life ART Centre
Indore, Madhya Pradesh, India

Diksha Goswami MD FNB (Rep Med) MRCOG FICOG DNB
Director
Pushpanjali IVF
Pushpanjali Multispecialty Hospital
Agra, Uttar Pradesh, India

Elizabeth Burt

Erika Desai MBBS MS (Obs & Gyn) MCh (Rep Med & Surgery)
Consultant
NOVA IVI Fertility
Chennai, Tamil Nadu, India

Fessy Louis MBBS DGO DNB
Senior Consultant and Assistant Professor
Department of Reproductive Medicine
Amrita Fertility Centre, AIMS,
Kochi, Kerala, India

Gajendrakant Tripathi
Chairperson
Delhi State Chapter of ISAR
Delhi State Chapter of ISPAT
Org Secretary
55th AICOG 2012 Varanasi

Gaurav Majumdar

Gautam Khastgir MD FRCS (Edin) FRCOG (Lon) FICOG
Medical Director
Bengal Infertility and Reproductive Therapy Hospital (Birth)
Kolkata, West Bengal, India

Geetha Haripriya MD DGO FRCOG (Lon)
CHAIRPERSON
Prashanth Fertility Research Centre
Chennai, Tamil Nadu, India

Hetal Patolia MD
Well Women Clinic
Asian Bariatrics
Ahmedabad, Gujarat, India

Hima Shah MSc (Stem Cells and Regenerative Medicine)
Embryologist
Mumbai Fertility Clinic & IVF Center
Mumbai, Maharashtra, India

Himanshu Patel MSc (Clinical Embryology) PhD (Stem Cell Biology)
Director
Stem Cure
Ahmedabad, Gujarat, India

Hrishikesh D Pai MD FCPS FICOG MSc (USA)
Gynecologist and Head of IVF Unit
Lilavati Hospital
Scientific Director, Bloom IVF
Mumbai, Maharashtra, India

Indira Hinduja MD PhD DGO DFP
Honorary Gynecologist and Obstetrician, IVF Specialist
PD Hinduja Hospital and Medical Research Centre and Jaslok Hospital and Research Centre
Mumbai, Maharashtra, India

Ishwaran

Jaideep Malhotra MD FICMCH FICOG FICS FMAS FIAJAGO FRCOG FRCPI
Managing Director (ART)
Rainbow IVF Hospital
Agra, Uttar Pradesh, India
Professor
Dubrovnik International University, Croatia
Imm Past President, IMS
President Elect, SAFOMS, 2019–2021
President Elect, ISPAT
Editor-in-Chief, SAFOMS and SAFOG Journal
Member, FIGO, Reproductive Endocrinology and Infertility
Member, FIGO, RDEH
Regional Director of South Asia Ian Donald School of Ultrasound Vice President, ISARM

Jatin P Shah MD DGO
Director
Mumbai Fertility Clinic and IVF Centre
Mumbai, Maharashtra, India

Jayamangala Gogate
Senior Consultant
Obstetrician and Gynaecologist and Infertility Specialist
BLOOM IVF
Lilavati Hospital
Mumbai, Maharashtra, India

Jayshree Pattnaik
Consulting Gynecologist
SCB Medical College
Cuttack, Odisha, India

JB Sharma
Professor
Department of Obstetrics and Gynecology
All India Institute of Medical Sciences
New Delhi, India

Jignasha Chauhan BSc (Microbiology) DMLT
Senior Embryologist
Babies and US Fertility and IVF centre
Lilavati Hospital
Mumbai, Maharashtra, India

Jiteeka Thakkar MBBS DGO DFP
Consultant Obstetrician and Gynecologist and Infertility Specialist
Kedia Nursing Home
Junior Consultant
BLOOM IVF
Lilavati Hospital
Mumbai, Maharashtra, India

Joe Leigh Simpson

Julia Szeptycki
Senior Embryologist
Astra Fertility Clinic
4303, Village Centre Court, Mississauga
ON L4Z 1S2, Canada

Jyoti Gupta

Jyoti Malik MBBS DGO DNB MNAMS FICS
Laparoscopic Surgeon and Infertility Specialist and Medical Superintendent
JJ Institute of Medical Sciences and Roots IVF fertility Institute,
Bahadurgarh, Haryana, India

Kalyani Bade MSc Biotechnology
Embryologist
Lilavati Hospital
Mumbai, Maharashtra, India

Kamala Selvaraj MD DHO PhD
GG Fertility and Women's Specialty Hospital
Chennai, Tamil Nadu, India

Kamini A Rao DGO DORCP DCh MRCOG FRCOG (UK) MCh (UK) FICOG PGDMLE (Law) FNAMS
Medical Director
Milann (A Unit of BACC Healthcare Pvt Ltd)
Bengaluru, Karnataka, India

Kanthi Bansal MD DGO FICOG
Director
Safal Fertility Foundation
Ahmedabad, Gujarat, India

KD Nayar MD DGO Dip Obs(Ireland) FICOG
Chief Consultant and Director
Fertility and IVF
Akanksha IVF Centre
Mata Chanan Devi Hospital
New Delhi, India

Kedar Ganla MD DNB FCPS DGO DFP
Consultant Fertility Physician, Scientific Director
Ankoor Fertility Clinic
Mumbai, Maharashtra, India
Managing Committee Member, ISAR

Keshav Malhotra MBBS MCE
Director
Rainbow IVF & Global Rainbow Healthcare
Agra, Uttar Pradesh, India

Kinjal R Shah DFP DNB FNB DNB
Obstetrics and Gynecology
Central Railway Hospital
Mumbai, Maharashtra, India

KK Gopinath MBBS MD DGO
Executive Director
Edappal Hospitals Pvt Ltd
Kerala, India

Korsak Vladislav Stanislavovich
Professor
General Director ICRM
Russia

Korula George MD DGO MRACOG
Head of Reproductive Medicine
Baptist Hospital
Bengaluru, Karnataka, India

KU Kunjumoideen MD DNB
Consultant IVF Specialist
ARMC AEGIS Hospital
Kerala, India

Kuldeep Jain MD FART (Singapore)
Director
KJIVF and Laparoscopy Centre
New Delhi, India

Kundan Ingale
Consultant and Director
Nirmiti Clinic, Centre for Assisted Reproduction and Endoscopy
Pune, Maharashtra, India

Kusum Zaveri MD DGO DFP
Honorary Gynecologist and Obstetrician, IVF Specialist
PD Hinduja Hospital and Medical Research Centre and Jaslok Hospital and Research Centre
Mumbai, Maharashtra, India

Laurel Stadtmauer MD PhD
Jones Institute of Reproductive Medicine
Eastern Virginia Medical School
Norfolk, USA

Laxmi Goel MBBS MD
Consultant
Bloom Fertility centre
Fortis Escorts Hospital
Faridabad, Haryana, India

Laxmi Shrikhande MBBS MD (Obs/Gyn) FICOG FICMU FICMCH
Consultant
Shrikhande Fertility clinic
Shrikhande Hospital and Research Centre Pvt Ltd
Nagpur, Maharashtra, India

Madhoo Loomba MS DGO Diploma in Pelviscopy & ART
Chairperson and Medical Director
Madhuraj Advanced Infertility & IVF Centre
Madhuraj Hospital (P) Ltd
Kanpur, Uttar Pradesh, India

Poonam Loomba MD
Loomba Hospital and IVF Centre
Haryana, India

Madhuprita Agrawal MD (Obs & Gyn)
Infertility Specialist
Ashoka Superspecialty Women Hospital and IMSI, ICSI Test Tube Baby Centre
Raipur, Chhattisgarh, India

Madhuri Patel B Pharm
Director
Stem Cure
Ahmedabad, Gujarat, India

Mala Arora FRCOG FICOG D Obst (UK)
Director
Noble IVF Center
Faridabad, Haryana, India
Past Chairperson ICOG

Mala Raj MBBS DGO FICOG Dip Endoscopic Surgery (Germany) Dip Reproductive Medicine (Germany)
Laparoscopy and Infertility Specialist
Aesthetic Gynecologist
Managing Director
Firm Hospitals
Chennai, Tamil Nadu, India

Mamata Deenadayal MD DGO
Founder and Chief Medical Director
Mamata Fertility Hospital
Secunderabad, Telangana, India

Mangala Ketkar MBBS DGO
Director and Consultant
Nagpur Test Tube Centre and Ketkar Hospital
Nagpur, Maharashtra, India

Maninder Ahuja MBBS DGO FICOG CIMP FIAOG
Consultant Gynecologist and IVF Specialist
Director
Ahuja Health care services
Faridabad, Haryana, India

Manish Banker MD
Medical Director
Nova IVI Fertility
Director,
Pulse Women's Hospital
Ahmedabad, Gujarat, India
Past President, Indian Society for Assisted Reproduction (ISAR)
Chairperson, Scientific Committee, IFFS 2016

Manisha Bhagat MBBS, MS(Obs & Gyn) FNB (Reproductive Medicine)
Consultant IVF and Gynecologist
Jammu, Jammu & Kashmir

Manisha Takhtani Kundnani MD FNB FNUS
Consultant Fertility Specialist
Reproductive Medicine Specialist
Fertility Square, IVF Clinic
Mumbai, Maharashtra, India

Meenu Handa MS DNB MRCOG (I) Fellow Reproductive Medicine
Senior IVF Consultant
Fortis Bloom IVF Center
Fortis Memorial Research Institute
Gurugram, Haryana, India

Milind Shah MD DGO DFP FICOG FIAOG
Professor and Head
Department of Obstetrics and Gynecology
Gandhi Natha Rangaji Homoeopathic Medical College
Solapur, Maharashtra, India
Naval Maternity & Nursing Home,
Ashakiran Sperm Bank and Infertility Center, Solapur
President of ISOPARB (2016–18), Vice President (2014–16)
Deputy Secretary General, FAOPS (Asia Oceania Federation of Perinataology Societies)
Vice President of FOGSI (2011)
Past Chairman, Rural Obstetrics Committee of FOGSI (2004–008)
President Solapur OBGY Society (2001-2002)
Joint Treasurer, ISPAT
Managing Committee Member, ISAR & IAGE
Steering Committee Member, Asia Safe Abortion Partnership

Mirudhubashini Govindarajan FRCS (C)
Clinical Director
Womens Center and Hospitals
Coimbatore, Tamil Nadu, India

Mohit Saraogi MD DNB DGO FCPS MNAMS ICOG
Director
Iris IVF Centre
Sarogi Hospital
Mumbai, Maharashtra, India

Monica Singh MD DNB FMAS FICOG
Infertility Specialist and Endoscopist
Bhopal Test Tube Baby and Endoscopy Centre
Secretary, Bhopal Obstetric & Gynaec Society (2015–16)
Secretary, MP Chapter IFS, Vice President Bhopal OBGYN Society

Muralidhar V Pai

N Sanjeeva Reddy
Professor and Head
Department of Reproductive Medicine and Surgery
Sri Ramachandra Medical College and Research Institute
Chennai, Tamil Nadu, India

Nandita Palshetkar MD FCPS FICOG
Medical Director, Bloom IVF
Mumbai, Maharashtra, India
Professor of Gynecology
DY Patil Medical College
Navi Mumbai, Maharashtra, India
President, FOGSI (2019–2020)
Past President, MOGS (2016–2017)
Past President, IAGE (2017–2018)

Nayana H Patel MD (Obs & Gyn)
Director
Akanksha Hospital and Research Institute
Anand, Gujarat, India

Nikhil Datar MD DNB FCPS FICOG DGO LLB
Medical Director
Cloudnine Hospital
Mumbai, Maharashtra, India

Nikita Lad MD DGO FCPS FRM (Homerton UK)
IVF Specialist
DY Patil Fertility Center
Mumbai, Maharashtra, India

Nilam Ghamne MSc (Biotechnology)
Embryologist
Bloom IVF
DY Patil Fertility Centre
Mumbai, Maharashtra, India

Nimish R Shelat MBBS MD FCPS
Consultant Fertility Specialist
Shree Nandan Hospital and Shelat General Hospital
Surat, Gujarat, India

Nupur Agarwal MBBS DGO DNB FNB-IVF MNAMS
Consultant Fertility and IVF
Akanksha IVF Centre
Mata Chanan Devi Hospital
New Delhi, India

Pankaj Talwar MBBS MD (Gyn & Obs)
Head
Assisted Reproductive Technologies (ART) Center
Army Hospital (Research & Referral)
New Delhi, India

Parul Kotdawala MD (Gyn)
Consultant Gynecologist & Endoscopy Surgeon
VS Hospital & NHL Municipal Medical College
Ahmedbabd, Gujarat, India

Parzan Mistry MS DNB FMAS MAMS
Fellowship in Reproductive Medicine
Consulting Obstetrician–Gynecologist and Infertility Specialist
Bloom IVF, Masina Hospital
Mumbai, Maharashtra, India

Pawan Dhir MS (Obs & Gyn) FRSH (London) Diploma Ian Donald USG
Director
Siddharth IVF—Endoscopy Center
Rashmi Nursing Home
Bharuch, Gujarat, India

Pinky Shah DGO DNB FNB
Core Fertility Specialist
Morpheus IVF, Morpheus Life Sciences
Mumbai, Maharashtra, India

PM Gopinath MD DGO FMMC FICS FICOG MBA (HSM)
Director and Senior Consultant
Department of Obs and Gyne & IVF
SIMS Hospitals
Chennai, Tamil Nadu, India

Pooja Awasthi MSc (Applied Biochemistry)
Head and Clinical Embryologist
Origin IVF and Fertility Centre
Meenakshi Hospital
Ghaziabad, Uttar Pradesh, India

Pooja Mehta MBBS MD (Obs & Gyne)
Infertility Specialist and Head
Fortis Bloom IVF Centre
Mohali, Punjab, India

Poornima Nadkarni MD DGO FCPS
Director
Nadkarni Hospital & Test Tube Baby Centre
Valsad, Gujarat, India

Pragya Mishra MBBS MRCOG FRCOG PhD DFFP FICOG Dip in Gyn Endoscopy
Consultant (Infertility Specialist)
NuLife Test Tube Baby Centre, Patna
MGM Hospital and Research Centre Pvt Ltd
Patna, Bihar, India

Prakash Trivedi MD DGO FCPS DNB
Consultant Gynecologist, Endoscopist, ART Consultant, Sonologist and Urogynecologist
Dr Trivedi's Total Health Care Pvt. Ltd., & Aakar IVF Centre
Mumbai, Maharashtra, India

Prashant Patil DGO DNB FNB in Rep Med
IVF Consultant
Adesh IVF
Bathinda, Punjab, India

Pratap Kumar MD DGO FICS FICOG
Professor
Kasturba Medical College
Manipal Assisted Reproductive Centre (MARC)
Manipal Academy of Higher Education (MAHE)
Manipal, Karnataka, India

Pritimala Gangnurde MBBS DNB (Obs & Gyn) PG training in Reproductive Medicine & Endocrinology
Masters in Reproductive Medicine (UK)
Fellowship in Obs & Gyn USG
Consultant Fertility Specialist
Bloom IVF
Cloudnine Hospital
Medical Director, Pearl Fertility & IVF
Medical Director, Pearl Diagnostics
Mumbai, Maharashtra, India

Rachana Kaveri

Rajnikant Contractor
Member of Ex CSB (Central Supervisoy Board)
PCPNDT Act (Government of India)
Member of NIMC (National Inspection Monitoring Committee)PCPNDTACT
Government of India
Ex Member of SSB
PCPNDT Act (Government of Gujarat)
Member, MTP Act Committee Government of Gujarat
Member, FOGSI CORE
Committee PCPNDT Cell
Medicolegal Chairperson, ISAR ART
PCPNDT Act

Rajul Tyagi MBBS DGO FICMCH
Director
Javitri Hospital & Test Tube Baby Centre
Lucknow, Uttar Pradesh, India

Rana Choudhary DNB FCPS DGO DFP MNAMS FICMCH
Associate Consultant
Ankoor Fertility Clinic, Mumbai
Mumbai, Maharashtra, India

Randhir Singh MD MIAP LLB
President APMP
Bhopal, Madhya Pradesh, India
Vice President
MP-NHA and Founder Secretary, MP Chapter IFS

RB Agrawal MSc (Clinical Embryology) LEADS UK
Senior Embryologist
Ashoka's Advanced IVF Centre
Ashoka Superspecialty Women Hospital and IMSI, ICSI Test Tube Baby Centre
Raipur, Chhattisgarh, India

Reem Sabouni

Reeta Mahey MD DNB MICOG
Associate Professor
All India Institute of Medical Sciences
New Delhi, India

Renu Makwana MBBS MS FICOG
Senior Gynecologist and Obstetrician and Fetal Medicine Specialist
Vasundhara Hospital
Jodhpur, Rajasthan, India

Rina Agrawal

Rishma Dhillon Pai MD DNB FCPS DGO FICOG FRCOG
Consultant Gynecologist
Jaslok, Hinduja and Lilavati Hospitals
Mumbai, Maharashtra, India

Ritu Hari MSc Human Genetics MS (UK) PhD
Medical Geneticist
CRAFT Hospital and Research Centre
Thrissur, Kerala, India

Rohan Krishnakumar

Rohan Palshetkar MS (Obs & Gyn)
Assistant Professor
DY Patil Medical College
Mumbai, Maharashtra, India

Roya Rozati MD (AIIMS) FRCOG (London)
Head and Professor
Department of Obstetrics and Gynaecology
Owaisi Hospital and Research Center
Deccan College of Medical Sciences
Hyderabad, Telangana, India
Medical and Research Director
Maternal Health Research Trust

RS Sharma PhD
Head
Scientist G and Senior Deputy Director General
Division of Reproductive Biology
Maternal & Child Health
Indian Council of Medical Research
New Delhi, India

Rushika Mistry MSc Life Science (Applied Medicine)
Senior Embryologist
Bloom IVF Lilavati Hospital
Mumbai, Maharashtra, India

Rutvij Dalal MBBS DGO (GOLD MEDALIST) DNB FNB (REPRODUCTIVE MEDICINE)
IVF AND INFERTILITY SPECIALIST
Gurugram, Haryana, India

S Krishnakumar MD DGO ECRES
JK Women Hospital
Mumbai, Maharashtra, India
SEC General, IAGE, ISAR

Sadhana Patwardhan MD (Ped) MD (Obs and Gyn)
Director and Consultant
Nagpur Test Tube Centre and Ketkar Hospital
Nagpur, Maharashtra, India

Samoylovich Yanina Andreevna

Sandros C Estevas

Sanjay Makwana MBBS MS FIAGES FICOG
Senior ART Specialist and Endoscopic Surgeon
Vasundhara Hospital
Jodhpur, Rajasthan, India

Sarita Sukhija MD (Obs & Gyn) FICOG FICRS Masters in Biotechnology of Human Reproduction and Embryology
Sr Consultant IVF
IVF Course Director
World Laproscopy Hospital
Artemis Hospitals
Gurugram, Haryana, India

Sathy M Pillai MBBS DGO MD
Chief Infertility Specialist
Samad IVF Hospitals
Thiruvananthapuram, Kerala, India

Sejal Naik MS (Obs & Gyn)(Gold Medalist) FMAS FRM
Consultant Gynec Endoscopist and Infertility Specialist
Rahul Hospital and Well Women Clinic
Surat, Gujarat, India
Managing Committee Member, Indian Association of Gynec Endoscopists (2018–19)
Hon Secretary Surat Obs & Gynec Society (2018–19)

Selvapriya Saravanan MD (Obs & Gyn) FICOG DRM(Kiel) Fellow Fetal Medicine (MGR Uni)
Director
Spring Fertility And Fetocare Centre
Kanyakumari

Shailaja Gada Saxena MBBS MSc Genetics (UK) PhD
Head (Molecular Medicine)
Reliance Life Sciences (RLS), Dhirubhai Ambani Life Sciences Centre
Navi Mumbai, Maharashtra, India

Shailendra Mahimkar MD DNB FCPS DGO DFP DICOG
Interventional Gynaecologist
Bloom IVF
Lilavati Hospital and Research Centre,
Mumbai, Maharashtra, India

Shamim Khandaker MS (Obs & Gyn) FNB (High-risk Pregnancy and Perinatology)
Assistant Professor
North Bengal Medical College
Darjeeling, West Bengal, India
Fellow of National Board in Reproductive Medicine
Lilavati Hospital, Mumbai, Maharashtra, India

Shanti Roy MBBS (Hon) Gold Medalist DGO MS MNAMS FICOG FICS FICMC
Consultant Obstetrician and Gynecologist
Shivam Hospital and Research Institute
Patna, Bihar, India

Shashank Joshi MD DM FRCP FACE FICP FACP
Consultant Endocrinologist
Lilavati Hospital
Mumbai, Maharashtra, India

Shashidhar B

Shefali Agarwal

Shilpa Damodar MSc
Safal Fertility Foundation
Ahmedabad, Gujarat, India

Shivanand Sakhare MS (Obs & Gyn) (Gold Medalist) DNB FCPS
Fellow of National Board in Reproductive Medicine
Director
Fertility Experts Clinic
Mumbai, Maharashtra, India

Shivani Sachdev MD DNB MRCOG (UK)
Director
SCI Healthcare
New Delhi, India

Shobhana Patted MD DGO DNB FICOG
Director
Patteds Fertility and Research Centre
Belgaum, Karnataka, India

Singh VP

Skand Shekhar MD
Clinical Endocrinology Fellow
National Institutes of Health
10 CRC, Rm 5-2741
Bethesda, Maryland, USA

Sona Dharmendra PhD Scholar
All India Institute of Medical Sciences
New Delhi, India

Sonal Panchal MD
Consultant Sonography Specialist
Dr Nagori's Institute for Infertility and IVF
Ahmedbabd, Gujarat, India

Soumil Trivedi DNB MBBS Fellowship in Minimal Access Surgery (MUHS)
Consultant Gynecologist, Endoscopist, Sonologist & Fertility Specialist
Dr Trivedi's Total Health Care Pvt Ltd and Aakar IVF Centre
Mumbai, Maharashtra, India

Steven D Fleming
Director Embryology
Cooper Surgical, Fertility and Genomic Solutions
Australia

Sudarsan Ghosh Dastidar MD
Director
GD Institute for Fertility Research
Kolkata, West Bengal, India

Sudesh A Kamat MSc
Consultant Embryologist
Bloom IVF Centre, Lilavati Hospital
Mumbai, Maharashtra, India

Sudha Prasad MD (Obs and Gyn) FICOG FICMCH
Director Professor and IVF Coordinator
IVF and Reproductive Biology Centre
Departemnt of Obstetrics and Gynecology
Maulana Azad Medical College
New Delhi, India

Sugandha Goel MBBS MS (Obs and Gyn) Fellowship in Infertility and Laparoscopy
Associate
Safal Fertility foundation and Bansal Hospital
Ahmedbabd, Gujarat, India

Sulbha Arora MD DNB
Clinical Director
Consultant Reproductive Medicine
Nova IVI Fertility

Suneeta Mittal MD FRCOG (ae) FICOG FAMS FICMCH FIMSA FICLS
Director and Head (Obs and Gyn)
Fortis Memorial Research Institute
Gurugram, Haryana, India
Formerly Head (Obs and Gyn)
All India Institute of Medical Sciences (AIIMS), New Delhi, India

Sunita Arora MBBS MD FICS FICOG
Senior Consultant Infertility and IVF
Bloom IVF
Fortis Lafemme Hospital
New Delhi, India

Sunita Sharma

Sunita Tandulwadkar MD FICS FICOG
Head
Department of Obstetrics and Gynecology
Chief, Department of IVF and Endoscopy
Ruby Hall Clinic, Pune, Maharashtra, India

Surekha Kadam DNB DGO FCPS
Clinical Associate
Bloom IVF, Lilavati Hospital
Mumbai, Maharashtra, India

Surendra Pal Singh Virk MSc PhD
Laboratory Director
Virk Center for Human Reproduction
Jalandhar, Punjab, India

Svetlana Rechitsky

Taswin Kaur

Trupti Nagaria MD FICOG
Professor and Head
Department of Obstetrics and Gynecology
Pt. JNM Medical College
Raipur, Chhattisgarh, India

Unnati Mamtora MBBS DGO DNB
Consultant Fertility Specialist
Bloom IVF
Mumbai, Maharashtra, India

Vanie Thapar MBBS MD (Obs and Gyn)
Consultant
New Life Infertility Research Centre
Suman Hospital
Ludhiana, Punjab, India

Varsha Baste
Consultant Gynecologist, Obstretician & Infertility Specialist
Director
Baste Maternity Hospital & Pushpa Fertility Center
Nashik, Maharashtra, India

Vasan SS DNB (Surg) DNB (Uro) Fellowship in Andrology & Incontinence
Uro-Andrologist, Chairman and Head
Department of Andrology
Manipal Fertility
Bengaluru, Karnataka, India

Vidisha Bhatt MSc (Biotechnology)
Research Associate
Stem Cure
Ahmedabad, Gujarat, India

Vineet Mishra MD PhD
Professor and Head
Department of Obstetrics and Gynecology
Institute of Kidney Diseases and Research Centre
BJ Medical College Campus
Civil Hospital
Ahmedabad, Gujarat, India

Virendra Shah MSc (Biotechnology)
Senior Embryologist
Shalby Gada Life ART Centre
Indore, Madhya Pradesh, India

Vrunda Kuchekar MSc (Life Sciences)
Chief Embryologist
Bloom IVF
Mumbai, Maharashtra, India

Walker P

Preface

Good communication is a bridge between confusion and clarity.

–Nat Turner

This book has been launched to commemorate the 24th Annual Conference of Indian Society for Assisted Reproduction.

The field of assisted reproduction has seen dramatic advancements over the last few decades. Multiple new techniques have been introduced in this ever-growing versatile field to improve the success rates and provide efficient management to infertile patients. The field demands a multidisciplinary approach involving reproductive medicine specialists, reproductive endocrinologists, clinical embryologists, urologists, genetic counselors, researchers, ethicists, and other clinical and paraclinical support staff.

This book titled, *Newer Trends in ART* is a unique effort to gather experiences from experts from all over the world—all of whom are authorities in their respective field, to provide concise and updated information and integrated management approach to deal with different situations.

The book is divided into various sections focusing on every aspect of infertility treatment, ranging from general evaluation, diagnosis, management of various gynecological conditions pertaining to infertility, to specific topics related to ART treatments including induction protocols, laboratory management, cryopreservation, preimplantation genetic testing; with a separate section focused on the latest advances in this field. The chapters have been drafted in a manner that it will serve as a reference for the novice consultant as well as the "seasoned experts".

We thank and appreciate all our authors for their fine contributions. We really hope that the readers get a comprehensive overview of the subject and a ready reference for practicing evidence-based reproductive medicine.

Nandita Palshetkar
Hrishikesh D Pai
Rishma Dhillon Pai
Sunita Tandulwadkar
Kinjal R Shah
Manisha T Kundnani

Contents

SECTION 1: Historical Aspects of ART

1. **The Development of In Vitro Fertilization in India** 1
   Rina Agrawal, Elizabeth Burt

SECTION 2: General Principles in Managing Infertile Couples

2. **Understanding Reproductive Physiology in ART** 5
   Pratap Kumar
3. **Evaluation of Female in ART** 9
   Varsha Baste, Shobhana Patted, Shamim Khandaker
4. **Evaluation of the Infertile Male** 16
   Vasan SS, Shashidhar B, Pragya Mishra, Shanti Roy
5. **Thyroid and Infertility** 25
   Jayamangala Gogate, Shashank Joshi, Dhanashri Natu
6. **Prolactin and Infertility** 35
   Manisha Takhtani Kundnani, Vanie Thapar
7. **Obesity and Infertility** 40
   Sanjay Makwana, Renu Makwana

SECTION 3: Common Gynecological Disorders and Infertility

8. **Female Genital Tuberculosis** 45
   JB Sharma, Sona Dharmendra, Shefali Agarwal, Poonam Loomba, Jyoti Gupta
9. **Pelvic Inflammatory Disease** 54
   Sudha Prasad
10. **Endometriosis: Infertility and ART** 58
    Prakash Trivedi, S Krishnakumar, Soumil Trivedi, Rohan Krishnakumar
11. **Adenomyosis: Newer Trends in Assisted Reproductive Technology** 66
    KD Nayar, Kuldeep Jain, Amiti Agrawal, Nupur Agarwal
12. **New Trends in Fibroids and Infertility** 75
    Parul Kotdawala, Mala Raj, Ishwaran, Parzan Mistry

13. **Polycystic Ovary Syndrome** 80
Shivanand Sakhare, Manisha Bhagat, Kundan Ingale

14. **Tubal Factor in Infertility** 88
Muralidhar V Pai

15. **ART in Seropositive Couples** 91
Nandita Palshetkar, Hrishikesh D Pai, Deepa Talreja, Nikita Lad, Shamim Khandaker

16. **Isthmocele: An Under Diagnosed Cause of Infertility** 96
Singh VP, Walker P

SECTION 4: Fertility Enhancing Endoscopic Surgeries

17. **Hysteroscopy: Instrumentation** 101
S Krishnakumar, Aditi Joshi, Rachana Kaveri

18. **Fertility Enhancing Hysteroscopic Surgery** 108
Asha Baxi, Apoorva Pallam Reddy

19. **Fertility Enhancing Laparoscopic Surgeries** 113
Alka Kriplani, Bharti Dhorepatil, Reeta Mahey

20. **Medicolegal Aspects of Endoscopy** 121
Nikhil Datar

SECTION 5: Current Concepts in Male Infertility

21. **Genetic, Lifestyle, and Environmental Factors in Male Infertility** 125
Skand Shekhar, Anne Martini, Alan DeCherney

22. **Medical Management of Male Infertility** 130
Kedar Ganla, Rana Choudhary

23. **Azoospermia** 136
Mohit Saraogi, HD Pai

24. **Oligozoospermia** 140
Vineet Mishra, Pawan Dhir

25. **Sperm DNA Fragmentation: Methods to Determine, Clinical Implications and Approaches of its Reduction** 145
Himanshu Patel, Vidisha Bhatt, Madhuri Patel

SECTION 6: Radiology in Infertility

26. **Ultrasound and Color Doppler in Infertility** 154
Narendra Malhotra, Diksha Goswami, Jaideep Malhotra

27. **Ultrasound Mapping of Fibroids** 164
Mamata Deenadayal, Aarti Deenadayal Tolani, Anupama Deenadayal Mettler

SECTION 7: Ovarian Stimulation

28. Ovulation Induction and Superovulation 173
Rishma Dhillon Pai, Madhoo Loomba, Rutvij Dalal

29. Ultrasonography in Follicular Monitoring 185
Sonal Panchal, CB Nagori

30. Intrauterine Insemination 197
Ameet Patki, Kedar Ganla, Rana Choudhary

31. Individualization of Controlled Ovarian Stimulation 204
Damodar R Rao, Abarajda V, Asha R Rao

32. Mild Ovarian Stimulation Protocol 211
Korula George, Abha Khurana

33. Stimulation Protocols in Cancer Patients 216
N Sanjeeva Reddy, Kamala Selvaraj, Erika Desai

34. Management of Poor Responders in ART 221
Nimish R Shelat

SECTION 8: The Endometrium

35. Endometrium and ART 229
Korsak Vladislav Stanislavovich, Samoylovich Yanina Andreevna

36. Thin Endometrium 234
Sathy M Pillai, KK Gopinath, Fessy Louis, KU Kunjumoideen

37. Endometrial Receptivity Analysis 243
Manish Banker, Poornima Nadkarni

38. Recurrent Implantation Failure 248
Sulbha Arora, Mirudhubashini Govindarajan, Laxmi Shrikhande

SECTION 9: The IVF Lab: Establishing and Maintenance; and Technical Aspects

39. Setting of an ART Laboratory 261
Rajul Tyagi, Meenu Handa, Sunita Arora, Kalyani Bade

40. Quality Control and Quality Assurance 264
Alex C Varghese, Julia Szeptycki

41. Accreditation of the Assisted Reproductive Technique Laboratory 277
Surendra Pal Singh Virk, Arya Salaskar, Nilam Ghamne

42. Culture Media 283
Prashant Patil, Jignasha Chauhan

43. Gamete and Embryo Morphology 291
Pinky Shah, Hima Shah

44. **Sperm Preparation Techniques** 304
Virendra Shah, Randhir Singh, Monica Singh, Anagha Deshpande

45. **General Principles of Micromanipulation** 311
Steven D Fleming

46. **IVF/ICSI/IMSI/PICSI** 315
Sudesh A Kamat, Vrunda Kuchekar, Akanksha Mishra

47. **Assisted Hatching** 330
Kanthi Bansal, Sugandha Goel, Hetal Patolia, Shilpa Damodar

48. **Day 3 versus Day 5 Embryo Transfer** 337
Biswanath Ghosh Dastidar, Sudarsan Ghosh Dastidar, Geetha Haripriya

49. **Time-lapse Monitoring** 345
Hrishikesh D Pai, Nandita Palshetkar, Rushika Mistry, Rohan Palshetkar

50. **Newer Technologies in the IVF Laboratory** 351
RB Agrawal, A Suresh Kumar, Madhuprita Agrawal

51. **Troubleshooting in the IVF Laboratory** 360
Keshav Malhotra, Gaurav Majumdar

52. **Preventing Mix Up in In Vitro Fertilization Laboratory** 368
PM Gopinath, Parzan Mistry

SECTION 10: Clinical Procedures and Protocols

53. **Oocyte Retrieval** 372
Shailendra Mahimkar, Suresh Kumar, Trupti Nagaria

54. **Embryo Transfer** 377
Sadhana Patwardhan, Mangala Ketkar

55. **Frozen Embryo Transfer** 388
Jatin P Shah

56. **Elective Single Embryo Transfer** 394
Gautam Khastgir

57. **Luteal Phase Support** 402
BN Chakravarty, Sunita Sharma

58. **Ovarian Hyperstimulation Syndrome** 409
Anupam Gupta, Pooja Mehta

59. **Adjuvant Therapies in ART** 416
Surekha Kadam, Kinjal R Shah

60. **Optimize Oocyte Yield to Maximize Live Birth in Assisted Reproductive Technology** 422
Sandros C Estevas

SECTION 11: Beyond ART

61. **Pregnancy after Assisted Reproductive Technology** 428
Vijay Nahata, Arun Baruah

62. **First and Second Trimester Screening** 431
Selvapriya Saravanan

63. **Recurrent Miscarriage** 438
Mala Arora

64. **Ectopic Pregnancy** 444
Suneeta Mittal, Sarita Sukhija, Laxmi Goel

65. **Fetal Reduction** 453
Devika Gunasheela, Ashwini M

SECTION 12: Cryopreservation

66. **Cryopreservation in ART** 459
Hrishikesh D Pai, Nandita Palshetkar, Kinjal R Shah, Arnav Pai

67. **Semen Banking** 470
Milind Shah, Jayshree Pattnaik, Unnati Mamtora, Charumati Pekhale

68. **Oocyte Banking** 476
Nandita Palshetkar, Hrishikesh D Pai, Rohan Palshetkar, Jiteeka Thakkar

69. **Ovarian Tissue Freezing** 481
Pankaj Talwar, Pooja Awasthi

SECTION 13: Third Party Reproduction

70. **Oocyte and Embryo Donation** 490
Maninder Ahuja, Jyoti Malik, Pritimala Gangnurde

71. **Surrogacy** 496
Nayana H Patel, Shivani Sachdev, Gajendrakant Tripathi

72. **Uterus Transplantation** 501
Taswin Kaur, Kamini A Rao

SECTION 14: Preimplantation Genetic Testing

73. **Preimplantation Genetic Testing: A Pivotal Component of ART** 513
Joe Leigh Simpson, Svetlana Rechitsky, Anver Kuliev

74. **Preimplantation Genetic Testing** 520
Ritu Hari, C Mohamed Ashraf, Shailaja Gada Saxena, Dhiraj Gada, Alexia Chatziparasidou

75. **PGT: Technical Aspects, Biopsy, and Analysis** 530
Ritu Hari, C Mohamed Ashraf

76. **Genetic Analysis: FISH/CGH/Microarray/NGS** 535
Alexia Chatziparasidou

SECTION 15: Regulations of ART in India

77. **Guidelines of Assisted Reproductive Technologies and Surrogacy** 540
Roya Rozati, RS Sharma

78. **PCPNDT Act versus IVF/ART: Medicolegal Problems in ART** 549
Rajnikant Contractor

SECTION 16: Miscellaneous and Future Directions

79. **Application of Stem Cells in Infertility** 554
Sunita Tandulwadkar, Sejal Naik

80. **CatSper Channel** 559
Indira Hinduja, Amruta DS Pathare, Kusum Zaveri

81. **What is new in Assisted Reproductive Technology?** 566
Reeta Mahey, Hrishikesh D Pai, Arnav Pai

82. **Robotics in Infertility: Technical Aspects and its Present Day Relevance** 570
Reem Sabouni, Laurel Stadtmauer

Index *575*

ERRATA

- In Chapter 13, the correct spelling of author is Shivanand Sakhare.
- In Chapter 81, Dibajyoti is not author of this chapter.

The Development of In Vitro Fertilization in India

1

Rina Agrawal, Elizabeth Burt

INTRODUCTION

Subfertility is not a condition unique to the developed world, and difficulties in conceiving affect couples worldwide. Treatment options for subfertility tend to lend themselves to controversy and ethical debate; however, this is with good reason, given the sensitive nature of the work and responsibilities that clinicians hold. This is true even in highly regulated countries where public consultation, government legalization, and regular audit of clinical work occur. The licensing and legislation infrastructure is only beginning to catch up with the advance of fertility treatment in several countries.

India is a prime example where a developing country has a rapid pace of expansion, globalization, and opportunity. It has achieved one of the fastest market growths within this sector. If regulations significantly lag behind clinical practice, then we can expect some degree of professional misconduct and commercial exploitation. This is having a significant impact on the framework of fertility practice in India.

In this chapter, we examine the incidence of subfertility in India, the origins of fertility treatment, and the legalization and current regulatory landscape in this rapidly developing and populous country, which is tipped to complete 2,60,000 assisted reproductive technology (ART) cycles per year by 2020.

SUBFERTILITY IN INDIA

It is estimated that subfertility of various etiologies affects 27.5 million couples in India. The nation faces comparable environmental and lifestyle challenges to other countries and an increasing prevalence of both female and male subfertility across a diverse population (Kumar et al. 2014). This includes factors such as delayed marriages, delayed childbearing, an increasing female work force, a higher prevalence of the use of contraception, and lifestyle factors such as obesity, smoking, and alcohol use. Furthermore, there is now an increased incidence of sexually transmitted infections (Bhilhar et al. 2015) and polycystic ovarian syndrome (Balaji et al. 2015) affecting female fecundity. Many couples therefore require fertility treatment (15%), although only approximately 1% of them currently seek help. The barriers to treatment are multifactorial, including the balance between social tradition driving the wish for treatment and parenthood and the stigma of infertility exposed by those seeking treatment. This is compounded further by the prohibitive costs for treatment and the disruption to daily living the treatment necessitates. Gender inequality is more pronounced in India and subfertility increases the social pressures on women, especially in the most rural areas. Not being able to conceive, generates relationship and extended family tensions, and subfertility increases the incidence of violence against women and divorce rates.

REPRODUCTIVE MEDICINE IN INDIA

India quickly followed the United Kingdom with the second baby born via in vitro fertilization (IVF) in 1978, but the news was shrouded in contention and debate. After the birth of Louise Brown in the UK on July 25, 1978, baby Durga was born a few months later in India on October 3 of the same year. The parents of the Indian baby forbade publication of their clinical care and the birth of their daughter, which led to the integrity of the work being challenged. This had substantial repercussions for Dr Subhas Mukerji who led the pioneering work and established a scientific landmark in Indian reproductive medicine. The news of the baby was told in the media, but not documented in medical journals or shared with the scientific community in the conventional manner, which denied Dr Subhas Mukerji the credit for his successful endeavor. Following news of the baby and the claims that she was born via IVF technology, the Indian government set up an enquiry to investigate, but concluded that the claims were fabricated and false.

The Indian government then prevented Dr Mukerji from further publication or attending scientific conferences to present and defend his work. He was barred from reproductive medicine and transferred to an insignificant role in ophthalmology in a smaller subdistrict of India. Surrounded by dishonor, disbelief, and humiliation, sadly, Dr Subhas Mukerji committed suicide on June 19, 1981.

Dr Anand Kumar played two pivotal roles in the history of IVF in India. Firstly, his scientific team in Mumbai, along with the clinical lead, Dr Indira Hinduja, took the credit for the first Indian baby born with IVF on August 6, 1986. Secondly, and somewhat ironically, years later, Dr Kumar also led a noble campaign supporting Dr Mukerji's claim for precedence. Dr Kumar reviewed the steps and process of Dr Mukerji's work through detailed analysis and revision of his presentations and publications, and published a paper documenting Dr Mukerji's work chronologically. His aim was to provide the evidence for restoring Dr Mukerji's professional reputation and substantiating his rightful place as the creator of the second baby born through IVF technology in the world. The Indian Council of Medical Research (ICMR) added its poignant acknowledgement in 2002, 21 years after Dr Mukerji's death.

India is a heterogeneous country with old traditions and social constructs nestling alongside "new" western ideology and technology. This has inevitably led to conflict in acceptability and apparent contradictions in moral conduct. On one hand, there is a conservative and private approach to reproductive medicine and, on the other hand, there is the overt fertility "tourism" trade that is occurring in India. Owing to the concentration of fertility clinics in major Indian cities (55%), coupled with the high price of treatment, many Indian couples are unable to access services; this exemplifies the inequalities in awareness and provision of treatment. However, the comparatively lower price of treatment than in many other parts of the world makes India a very attractive destination for many foreign patients. Thus, finding the balance between medicine and commercialism is a challenge for the Indian government and the regulatory bodies of the fertility practices in India.

India has hit the headlines over several issues related to IVF treatment, some welcome and some less so. Compared with other countries, India has a greater degree of moral autonomy, which has led to some practices and outcomes drawing criticism from around the world. There have been cases which have emphasized the distinction between what is "possible" and what is "right". With new regulations being put in place, standardized procedures will start to harmonize concepts for professional practice, but currently there is no official code of practice.

In some clinics, the opportunity to be a mother is offered to older postmenopausal women, and in other clinics multiple embryos are placed in the uterus. This raises serious ethical dilemmas. India was the focus of attention in May 2016 with news of the birth of baby to a 72-year-old woman. This may be a record, but it was not an isolated event, as pregnancies in women long past menopausal age are reported to be relatively common in some clinics. This case, however, provoked worldwide attention, and caused questions about the appropriate use of reproductive technology and potentially exposed Indian clinics to public criticism. The motives of such parents varied, but the stigma of being "barren" was often cited as a justification for treatment, thus completely overruling responsible medical care and the interests of any children. A new Bill (*see* below) intends to ban the use of treatment for females over the age of 50, in line with policy in many other countries.

India is keeping pace with other countries in all aspects of reproductive medicine. In 2002, it was the second country to perform a complete orthotopic ovarian transplant for a female with Turner Syndrome (Mhatri et al. 2005). On May 18, 2017, it completed its first uterine transplant at the Pune Galaxy Care Laparoscopy Institute. India has also been at the forefront of surrogacy practice, which is discussed further below.

NATIONAL REGISTRY

In vitro fertilization and reproductive treatment is commercially very appealing. This has led to a massive expansion within the women's health care sector, but the organization of clinics and their regulation is on an *ad hoc* basis. By 2020, it is predicted that India's clinics will be performing 2,60,000 cycles per year. Worryingly, clinics can be opened with minimal scrutiny of the treatments on offer or the qualifications and skill of those providing care.

The ICMR and Indian Society for Assisted Reproduction (ISAR) have appreciated that this may compromise patient's safety; success rates and procedures are therefore being put in place to rectify this weakness. They have advocated the adoption of an accreditation and licensing system similar to that of the UK.

Previously there has been no official central data collection for assisted reproductive treatments and, as a consequence, keeping track of the number of cycles, success rates, and treatments offered by the clinics in India is suboptimal. This lack of surveillance motivated the implementation of a national registry to aid data sharing and clinical transparency, not only nationally but also internationally [e.g. International Federation of Fertility Societies (IFFS)]. Recognition of variations in practice globally, appreciating the diversity in pathologies affecting effectiveness, analyzing the incidence of complications, and gaining exact figures on pregnancy outcomes will benefit both the reproductive medicine community and especially the patients. There have been concerns regarding issues such as the number of embryos transferred, inappropriate handling of gametes and misuse of technology for sex selection. With registration, practices can be held accountable, treatment can be monitored to ensure that only ethically sound treatment is carried out and that there is adequate safety with treatment carried out to the highest quality. With the aim of formal information sharing, the National ART Registry of India (NARI) was founded in 2001 by the ISAR. This in turn supplies information to the global registries such as International Committee for Monitoring Assisted Reproductive Technology (ICMART) (Malhotra et al. 2013). Engagement with the registry is advantageous for both the clinic and the patients. There is an ongoing concern that not all fertility centers are registered, with only about 30% in compliance, as there is no enforcement, and participation is voluntary. The awaited Assisted Reproductive Technology (Regulation) Bill will, however, make it compulsory for ART clinics to register.

Following the creation of the registry, there has also been the publication of several important documents, including the *National Guidelines for Accreditation, Supervision and Regulation of ART Clinics in India and Ethical Guidelines for Biomedical Research on Human Subjects* published in 2005 and 2006 respectively by ICMR.

CURRENT LEGALIZATION

In vitro fertilization and fertility treatment present many ethical and legal challenges. Respect for the law is paramount, but also to the sensitivities of native culture and society in reproductive medicine. Although the fundamentals are universal, the permutations and interpretations vary in different countries. Understanding how fertility treatment may affect issues such as legitimacy, parentage, and inheritance is of great cultural significance.

When donor eggs or sperm are used as part of treatment, it is vital that the prospective parents and the donor understand the legal situation in order to give informed consent. Donors have no parental rights over the child and their information is kept confidential. Under Indian law, insemination using donor sperm does not constitute adultery because sexual intercourse does not occur, and if an Indian married couple has artificial insemination and conceives a child, she or he is considered legitimate. The act of insemination itself though, is not considered sufficient to consummate the marriage and therefore there is still the possibility of the marriage being subject to annulment. If this were to occur after successful treatment resulting in pregnancy, the child would be considered illegitimate with the associated adverse societal consequences.

REPRODUCTIVE MEDICINE BILLS

There are two parliamentary Bills within India concerning reproductive medicine. The Assisted Reproductive Technology (Regulation) Bill has had various editions from 2009 until 2015 and the current draft is awaiting government approval, as in 2017. The vision of the Bill is to transform the current fragmented provision into cohesive care, with sustainable practice and standardized organization, protocols, and pricing. Care should be provided by competent practitioners, following evidence based medicine. There is a clear exclusion of preimplantation genetic diagnosis for nonmedical sex selection, which is currently reported to be carried out, and provides clear guidance for the use of embryos for research purposes. Ultimately, the aims of the Bill are to provide comprehensive monitoring and supervision for all aspects of reproductive medicine.

Initially incorporated into the Assisted Reproductive Technology (Regulation) Bill, but subsequently separated, was the Surrogacy Bill, which was expedited and released in November 2016. Since surrogacy was first legalized in India in 2002, there was increasing awareness and anxiety over the development of the surrogacy "industry". This has accelerated the need for strict rules and expectations for this niche of reproductive medicine. Amid significant international press coverage, nonaltruistic surrogacy has been banned, and now only family members can act as surrogates for relatives. Surrogacy will be available only for Indian couples who are childless, have proven subfertility, and have been married for more than 5 years. They must have certificates both of essentiality and eligibility issued to prove this. There is no provision for couples in same-sex relationships or for single individuals. Surrogates must be married, already have their own children and can be reimbursed only for medical costs and insurance. They can act as a surrogate only once and they must have a medical certificate ensuring physical and psychological well-being. The clinics need to be fully registered and clinical details must be archived for at least 25 years. Failure to comply with this jurisdiction will incur a custodial sentence and a significant fine.

This is welcome news for many, and sets to eliminate the corporate edge from this very beneficial medical intervention. The objectives of the Bill are to remove the financial incentive and replace it with responsible medical care. Not all, however, view the policy favorably.

The original surrogacy arrangement had benefits for both the surrogate and the intended parents, and although not perhaps viewed as an ideal situation, it provided advantages for many families. This is a situation where it should be questioned if it is appropriate to impose Western idealistic ideas in a heterogeneous culture and on potentially vulnerable patients. It has been voiced that the intention of doing good and preventing perceived harm may, in fact, cause harm. For many Indian women, paid surrogacy has provided an avenue and opportunity to provide a better life for their own family. Equally, for many visiting couples the option of surrogacy in India has given them hope of having a child, which is denied in their own country. Any practice of surrogacy that may adversely affect the health of women or the welfare of children should not, of course, be condoned, but it has been suggested that banning "commercial" surrogacy may, in fact, open up more illicit activity and its well-known risks.

CONCLUSION

India has maintained a fast tempo of growth and technological advancement in IVF, comparable to its peers in other countries. It is apparent that the current state of practice has not been achieved without significant dedication, turmoil, and collaboration. The moral compass of IVF can, at times, be hard to navigate but India has strived to provide reputable, world-class fertility treatment.

ACKNOWLEDGMENTS

I am grateful to Professor Roger Gosden (Virginia, USA) and Professor Duru Shah (President of Indian Society for Assisted Reproduction) for their valuable help during the preparation of this manuscript.

I would also like to thank my colleagues in India, Professor CN Purandhare, Dr Hrishikesh Pai, Dr Nandita Palshetkar, Dr Narendra and Dr Jaideep Malhotra, Dr Rishma Pai, and Dr Shanta Kumari for their helpful advice.

SUGGESTED READING

1. Balaji S, Amadi C, Prasad S, et al. Urban rural comparisons of polycystic ovary syndrome burden among adolescent girls in a hospital setting in India. Biomed Res Int. 2015;2015:158951.
2. Bhilwar M, Lal P, Sharma N, et al. Prevalence of reproductive tract infections and their determinants in married women residing in an urban slum of North-East Delhi, India. J Nat Sci Biol Med. 2015;6(Suppl. 1):S29-34.
3. Kumar S, Murarka S, Mishra VV, et al. Environmental & lifestyle factors in deterioration of male reproductive health. Indian J Med Res. 2014;140 Suppl:S29-35.
4. Malhotra N, Shah D, Pai R, et al. Assisted reproductive technology in India: A 3 year retrospective data analysis. J Hum Reprod Sci. 2013;6(4):235-40.
5. Mhatre P, Mhatre J, Magotra R. Ovarian transplant: a new frontier. Transplant Proc. 2005;37(2):1396-8.

Understanding Reproductive Physiology in ART

2

Pratap Kumar

OVARIAN CYCLE

The main roles of ovary are gametogenesis and hormonogenesis. The fetal gonads have 6–7 million oogonia, which is reduced to 1–2 million at birth and later 300,000–500,000 at puberty. However, only about 500 will ultimately ovulate in a woman's reproductive years.

During the reproductive years, there is a continuous atresia of oocytes. The follicles are either in resting, growing, atretic, or ready to ovulate. It takes nearly 85 days for a primordial follicle to grow to preantral stage and another 14 days for mature folliculogenesis. The first part of development before antral follicles is hormone independent, whereas the next part from antral to maturity is hormone dependent.

This hormonogenesis has two parts, and it is called "two cell gonadotropin system" **(Fig. 1)**. The theca cells have luteinizing hormone (LH) receptor and granulosa cells follicle-stimulating hormone (FSH) receptors. Stimulation of theca cells produces androgen. FSH induces aromatization in the granulosa cells, which converts androgens into estrogen.

Thus, androgen production influences estrogen production. If androgen is high, it inhibits aromatization and produces follicular atresia. The ideal situation for the initial stage of follicular development is low LH level and high FSH level, as seen in the early menstrual phase.

Follicular phase: Follicular phase is an orderly sequence, which results in development of a mature follicle. This usually takes 10–14 days. It involves four phases **(Fig. 2)**:

1. Recruitment
2. Selection
3. Dominance
4. Ovulation.

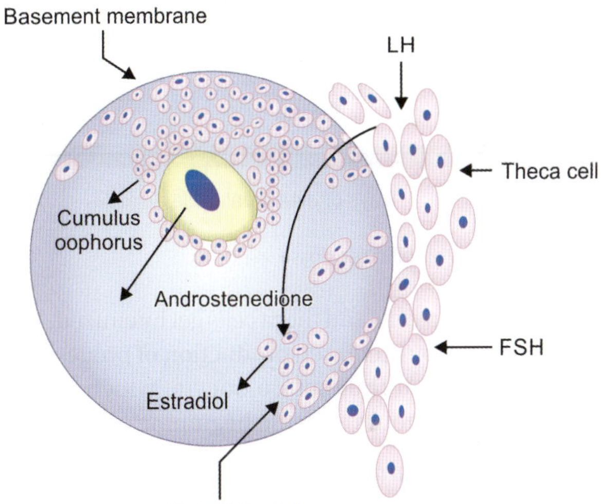

Fig. 1: Two cell gonadotropin system.

1. *Recruitment:* The process of recruitment begins at the end of corpus luteal development of the cycle preceding. During recruitment, follicles in both ovaries actively grow and secrete estrogen.
2. *Selection:* Between day 5 and 7 of the current cycle, a single follicle becomes destined to mature and ovulate. This process is termed as selection, wherein the dominant follicle is formed.
3. *Dominance:* The interval of growth preceding ovulation but following selection is called dominance. The dominant follicle controls the endocrine milieu as it prepares itself, the reproductive tract, and hypothalamic-pituitary axis for ovulation.
4. *Ovulation:* One of the paramount events at the mid cycle is the LH surge, which stimulates three major events.
   i. Resumption of meiosis.

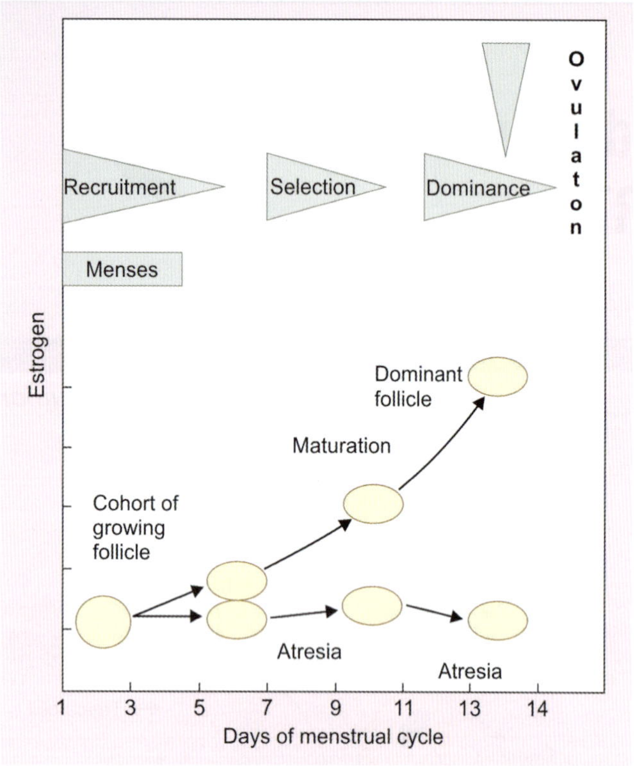

Fig. 2: Four phases of follicular phase.

ii. Granulosa cells and theca cells get luteinized. This is followed by increased production of progesterone.
iii. Extrusion of the mature oocyte, which happens usually 36 hours after the beginning of LH surge.

Mechanism of ovulation: This involves proteolytic digestion of follicular wall (mediated by prostaglandins) leading to rupture of the follicle and oocyte release. The ovum survives only 12–24 hours and then disintegrates.[1,2]

FSH Threshold and Window

Due to the increased pulsatility frequency of gonadotropin-releasing hormone (GnRH) secretion, there is an increased perimenstrual FSH secretion. The other reasons for increase in FSH are declining estrogen, inhibin A, and progesterone in the late luteal phase as the corpus luteum deteriorates.

After this perimenstrual rise, FSH remains at the same level for several days. Subsequently, its level declines under the negative feedback of inhibin B and E2 is produced by the growing pool of recruited follicles. During this decline in FSH, the most mature follicle is rescued from atresia and continues to grow. This follicle then becomes the dominant Graafian follicle. This grows faster than the others and produces higher amounts of E2 and inhibins. Hence, in the human species decremental follicular phase, FSH concentrations are fundamental for single dominant follicle selection.

Luteal Phase

After the expulsion of oocyte, granulosa and theca cells within the follicle shift from production of estrogen and follicular peptides to the production of estrogen and progesterone. This process termed as "luteinization", actually begins prior to ovulation, but requires LH surge for completion. The luteal function depends both qualitatively and quantitatively on normal development of the granulosa and theca cells during the preceding follicular phase. Inadequate proliferation of gonadal stromal cells in the follicular phase results in decreased secretion of estrogen and progesterone. This in turn may cause altered function of the fallopian tube and endometrium, possibly resulting in abnormal gamete or embryo transport and decreased opportunities for implantation. It is interesting to note that the lifespan of corpus luteum is fixed being around 14 days, irrespective of the follicular stage duration. Toward the end of luteal phase, the corpus luteum regresses unless rescued by human chorionic gonadotropin (hCG) from the implanting embryo. This is known as luteolysis.

ENDOMETRIAL CYCLE

Every month, the uterus prepares for a pregnancy by generating a thick bed of secretory endometrium for implantation. Due to failure of fertilization of the oocyte or implantation, menstruation starts. The endometrium has two principle components: (1) the glandular epithelium and (2) supporting stromal cells.

During the menstrual cycle, the epithelium differentiates to form three functional zones. The basalis, spongiosum, and stratum compactum. The endometrial events can be divided into three phases **(Fig. 3):**

1. Menstrual phase
2. Proliferative phase
3. Secretory phase.

Menstrual Phase

The beginning of each endometrial cycle is characterized by complete shedding of the spongiosum and stratum compactum layers during menstruation, which lasts for 3–5 days. The fall in plasma progesterone and estrogen levels due to degeneration of corpus luteum leads to withdrawal of hormonal support of the endometrium, which causes the withdrawal bleed.

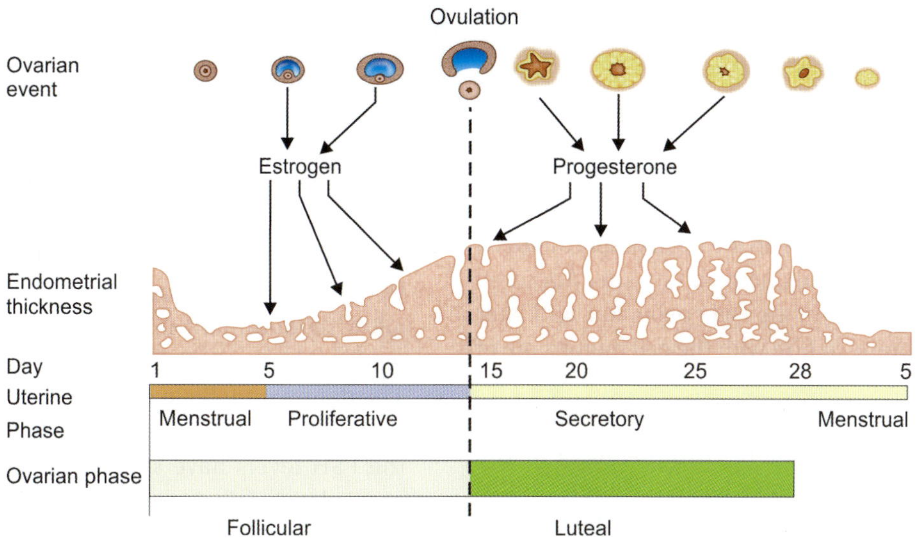

Fig. 3: Phases of endometrial events.

Due to profound vasoconstriction of uterine vessels, oxygen and nutrition are less to the endometrium and hence except the basalis layer of endometrium, rest of it is shed. After initial vasoconstriction, there is dilatation resulting in hemorrhage.

Proliferative Phase

When menstrual flow ceases, endometrium begins to thicken. It regenerates from the basalis layer. This takes 10 days or so. The ovarian follicular phase corresponds to menstrual proliferative phase of endometrial cycle. Changes in plasma concentration of estrogen and progesterone cause proliferative phase and growth of endometrium. The growth of the endometrium during this phase increases from approximately 0.5 mm to 3.5 mm in height.

Secretory Phase

Progesterone, which is secreted by the corpus luteum after ovulation will act upon the estrogen primed endometrium. This converts the endometrium to actively secreting tissue. The glands have more glycogen with numerous and densely coiled blood vessels. These changes are essential to make the endometrium helps in implantation.

FEEDBACK OSCILLATION OF THE HYPOTHALAMOPITUITARY OVARIAN SYSTEM

Hypothalamus produces intermittent pulsatile secretion of GnRH and is transported to the pituitary gland. Release of the pituitary gonadotropin (FSH and LH) secretion.

PREOVULATORY SURGE OF LH AND FSH CAUSES OVULATION

High level of estrogen around the time of ovulation causes positive feedback stimulatory effect on the anterior pituitary, which leads to big surge of secretion of LH and to a lesser extent of FSH surge. This excess LH surge leads to ovulation and subsequent development of corpus luteum. Hence in assisted reproductive technology (ART) cycle, there is need to suppress the LH surge (which will be discussed in other chapters).

MALE REPRODUCTIVE SYSTEM

Each testis has about 1,000 seminiferous tubules, which produces spermatogenesis. Testosterone is produced by specialized glandular cells called interstitial cells (or Leydig's cells) between the tubules. Sertoli cells support and nourish the sperm.

Spermatogenesis

Spermatogonia, which contains 46 chromosomes. Deoxyribonucleic acid (DNA) replication occurs to produce primary spermatocytes. By undergo meiosis, secondary spermatocytes II produce spermatids (with 23 unique chromosomes). These later change to the mature spermatozoa (also containing 23 unique chromosomes). This is the final event called spermatogenesis.

Each spermatozoa has a head (which contains the 23 chromosomes), a mid piece (where mitochondria is present for energy production), and a tail. The head is enclosed by an acrosome having enzyme acrosin. This is needed for breaking down the outer layer and entering the oocyte during fertilization.

Fertilization

Following sexual intercourse, sperms travels from the vaginal toward the mature oocyte in the fallopian tube. During this process, acrosome on the head of spermatozoa would be removed, releasing acrosin enzyme. About 50 spermatozoa are attached to the zona pellucida, and later allow its cell membrane to fuse with the cell membrane of ovum.

The process of meiosis II is reactivated in the cytoplasm of ovum, dividing the 46 chromosomes in the nucleus getting 23 chromosomes for fertilization (unites with another 23 chromosomes from sperm). The other 23 chromosomes are eliminated along with the second polar body.

Once sperm penetration occurs, its head gets detached from its mid piece and tail. Later there is union of chromosomes from sperm and ovum to form a complete set of genetic makeup for the offspring—two haploid cells (sperm and ovum) will become a single diploid-celled zygote.

To understand the basics we need to understand the summary of the physiology in reproduction as discussed below.

HYPOTHALAMUS–PITUITARY–OVARY AXIS

The basics endocrine principles of functional hypothalamus-pituitary-ovary (HPO) axis are:

- Hypothalamus produces GnRH
- The GnRH stimulates pituitary to secrete FSH and LH
- The LH acts:
  - On theca cells in follicular phase and produce androgens and
  - On theca and granulosa cells in luteal phase producing androgens, estrogens and progesterone.
- The FSH acts on granulosa cells producing estrogens in the follicular and luteal phases
- Increasing estrogen and progesterone levels can suppress the hypothalamus and pituitary hormone production
- Sustained high levels of estrogen can result in a gonadotropin predominantly LH surge from the pituitary.

OVARIAN CYCLE PHYSIOLOGY

- In late luteal phase of previous cycle, because of the increasing FSH (due to CL regression and fall in estrogen and progesterone levels), recruit a cohort of antral ovarian follicles.[3,4]
- When there is a rise of the estradiol levels from the developing follicles—cause long feedback inhibition of GnRH and FSH production—fall in FSH levels—allowing dominant follicle selection (FSH selection window) by day 5-6 of the menstrual cycle.
- The dominant follicle develops further as it has more sensitivity and more receptors to FSH even though the FSH levels have started to fall and become the preovulatory follicle.
- The other follicles with lesser responding and fewer FSH receptor regress due the falling FSH levels.
- The sustained high levels of estradiol produced by the preovulatory follicle cause a positive feedback on highly purified (HP) resulting in LH and small FSH surge.
- The surge brings about final oocyte maturation, and triggers the cascade leading to ovulation.
- Following ovulation, progesterone and estrogen production from corpus luteum decreases.
- In the absence of rescue of corpus luteum by hCG from an implanting embryo, it starts regressing by the 8th postovulatory day.
- The consequently falling progesterone and estradiol levels remove the HP negative feedback allowing the GnRH to preferentially cause FSH increase. This allows the next cohort of FSH sensitive antral follicles to recruit.
- Activins, inhibins, and follistatin are hormones that aid and abet the above physiological sequence where GnRH, FSH, LH, estradiol, and progesterone are the major role players.

REFERENCES

1. Irianni F, Hodgen GD. Mechanism of ovulation. Endocrinol Metabol Clin North Am. 1992;21:19-38.
2. Speroff L, Glass RH, Kase NG. Clinical gynecologic endocrinology and infertility, 6th edition. Philadelphia: Lippincott Williams and Wilkins; 1999. pp. 201-46.
3. McGee EA, Hsueh AJ. Initial and cyclic recruitment of ovarian follicles. Endocr Rev. 2000;21:200-14.
4. Adhikari D, Liu K. Molecular mechanisms underlying the activation of mammalian primordial follicles. Endocr Rev. 2009;30:438-64.

Evaluation of Female in ART

3

Varsha Baste, Shobhana Patted, Shamim Khandaker

INTRODUCTION

Infertility is seen in one in every six couples. It affects 15% couple in reproductive age group. Female factor is responsible for 40% of cases, male factor for 40% and, combined for 20% of infertility **(Fig. 1)**.[1] Evaluation in cases of couples presenting with infertility is necessary when the couple fails to achieve successful pregnancy even after 12 months of appropriate and timely unprotected intercourse.[1,2] Both partners need to be evaluated at the same time. Earlier evaluation may be required in women more than age 35 years and in those presenting with history of oligomenorrhea or amenorrhea, or, there is likelihood of uterine/tubal/peritoneal disease or stage III–IV endometriosis and male subfertility **(Box 1)**. In such couples, evaluation can be started after 6 months of trial.

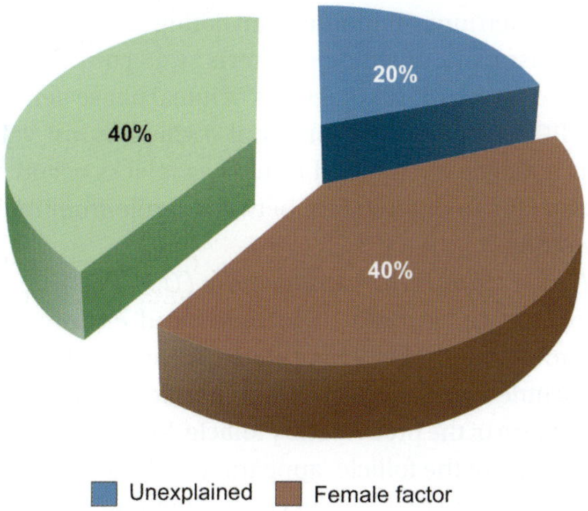

Fig. 1

HISTORY AND PHYSICAL EXAMINATION (BOXES 2 AND 3)

As these couples are undergoing tremendous stress, sufficient time should be given during first consultation. One needs to take a detailed medical and reproductive history along with family history. Importance should be given to physical examination along with general examination, e.g. height, weight, and body mass index (BMI) measurement.

Box 1

Earlier evaluation:
- Women over age 35 years
- History of oligomenorrhea or amenorrhea
- Known or suspected uterine/tubal/peritoneal disease or stage III–IV endometriosis
- Known or suspected male subfertility

Box 2

Relevant history:
- Duration of infertility
  - Past treatment history
  - Menstrual history
- Previous any pregnancy history
  - Past contraception use
  - History of sexual dysfunction
- Previous surgical history
  - Hospitalizations history
  - Pelvic inflammatory disease
  - Medical History like thyroid disease, galactorrhea, and hirsutism
- History of abnormal Pap smears
  - Family history of congenital defect
- History of occupation
  - Addiction to any substances.

Box 3

Physical examination:
- Body mass index (BMI)
- Blood pressure and pulse:
  - Thyroid examination
  - Breast examination
  - Signs of androgen excess
  - Vaginal or cervical abnormality or discharge
  - Uterine size, shape and mobility.
- Any adnexal masses or tenderness, nodularity at pouch of Douglas.[2]

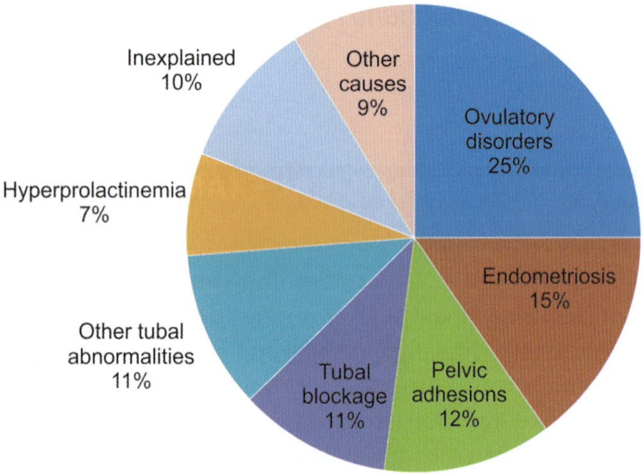

Fig. 2: Causes of female infertility.

Diagnostic Evaluation

Based on the history and physical examination, next diagnostic evaluations to be carried out in a systematic way, which should be also cost-effective to come to a definite cause of infertility **(Fig. 2)**.

Ovulatory Function

Around 15% of all infertile couples and in 40% of infertile women have anovulation.[3] Common causes of anovulation include polycystic ovarian syndrome (PCOS), thyroid disorders, hyperprolactinemia, weight gain or loss, obesity, and vigorous exercise.

The ovulatory function can be evaluated using the following methods, which are discussed below.

Menstrual History

Menstrual history is very important which always gives an initial assessment of ovulation. Women with regular menstrual cycles of 25–35 days with premenstrual symptoms are mostly ovulatory cycles in more than 95% of the cases. There are several tests, which can be used to document ovulation.

Tests of Ovulation

- *Serial basal body temperature (BBT):* BBT is a one of the oldest and simple method to detect ovulation. Biphasic BBT recordings are seen in an ovulatory cycles, while anovulatory cycles are usually monophasic. The 7 days prior to the mid-cycle rise in BBT is the most fertile period.[4] But some ovulatory women cannot document clearly biphasic BBT patterns. BBT monitoring would not indicate the exact time of ovulation. Also daily monitoring also becomes tedious. So the BBT test is no longer recommended nowadays.
- *Serum progesterone:* It value gives an objective confirmation of ovulation. It is preferably measured approximately 1 week before the expected period. In a woman with regular menstrual cycle, D21 measurement of serum progesterone value greater than 3 ng/mL gives an indication toward recent ovulation. Mid-luteal serum progesterone value greater than 10 ng/mL indicates adequate luteal support.[5]
- *Urinary luteinizing hormone (LH):* Urinary LH surge is an indirect evidence of ovulation. LH surge occurs 1–2 days prior to ovulation. Nowadays various commercial "ovulation predictor kits" are available in the market. These can be used to detect mid-cycle LH surge. However, sometimes LH kit may give false-positive and false-negative results.[6]
- *Endometrial biopsy (EMB) and histology*: A secretory endometrial on EMB implies ovulation, as it denotes the action of progesterone on the estrogen-primed endometrium. "Endometrium dating", which was done in past using histologic criteria, was considered the "gold standard" for diagnosis of luteal phase deficiency (LPD). Histologic endometrial dating has lost validity as a diagnostic method of LPD as it lacks accuracy. It also fails to differentiate between fertile from infertile women.[7]
- *Transvaginal ultrasonography (USG)* can be used to monitor growth of follicles and endometrium throughout the follicular phase. It can also be used to document ovulation by certain specific signs like sudden collapse of the preovulatory follicle, loss of well-defined margins of the follicle, appearance of fluid in pouch of Douglas, and presence of corpus luteum.
- *Other evaluations* aimed at to define cause of anovulation and its best possible management. Evaluation of serum

thyroid-stimulating hormone (TSH) and prolactin should be done in anovulatory women as thyroid disorders and/or hyperprolactinemia can cause anovulation.

Similarly, in women with amenorrhea, serum follicle-stimulating hormone (FSH), and estradiol should be measured. Amenorrhoeic women with high FSH, low estradiol can have ovarian failure, while those with low or normal FSH and low estradiol can have hypothalamic amenorrhea. As the management is completely different in both the cases, ovarian failure women may benefit from oocyte donation and hypothalamic amenorrhea women from exogenous gonadotropins for ovulation induction.

Ovarian Reserve Tests (Box 4 and Flowchart 1)

Ovarian reserve is a function of quantity and quality of oocytes. Ovarian reserve testing can be used to screen women at risk for diminished ovarian response to gonadotropin stimulation (poor responder). These women are less likely to become pregnant using ovulation induction agents and in vitro fertilization or intracytoplasmic sperm injection (IVF or ICSI).[8]

Box 4: Ideal ovarian reserve test.

- Affordable, noninvasive, and rapidly interpretable.
- Reproducible with minimal variability within the menstrual cycle and between cycles.
- Able to detect the decline in ovarian reserve at an early stage such that timely interventions could be pursued if desired.
- Valid, i.e. with good sensitivity and specificity

Flowchart 1

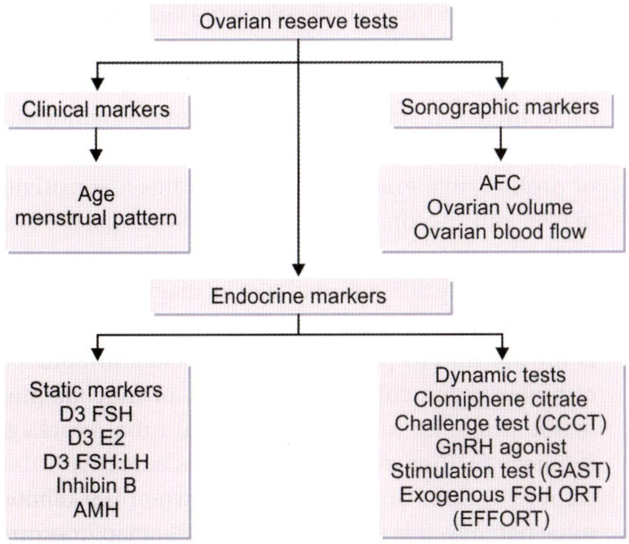

D3 FSH and Serum E2

A cycle-day 2–4 value of high serum FSH (>10–20 IU/L) is seen in women with poor response to ovarian stimulation and failure to conceive. Some limitation can be overcome by combining FSH with basal serum estradiol as an aid to interpret a "normal" basal serum FSH value (Box 5). Elevated serum estradiol level (>60–80 pg/mL), in the early follicular phase along with normal FSH value, has evidence for an association with diminished ovarian reserve; therefore, it helps to decrease the incidence of false negative testing.[8]

Clomiphene Citrate Challenge Test

Clomiphene citrate challenge test (CCCT) is done by giving 100 mg of clomiphene citrate daily for 5 days, from days 5–9 of the menstrual cycle. The levels of serum FSH are measured on day 3 and day 10. If the serum FSH levels are raised after clomiphene stimulation, it indicates decreased ovarian reserve. Elevated value of serum FSH on D10 has a higher sensitivity but lower specificity.[9]

Antral Follicle Count

Antral follicle count (AFC) is observed during transvaginal USG done in the early follicular phase (D2 or D3). It is the total of the small antral follicles measured in both ovaries. All follicles measuring 2–10 mm in mean diameter in the greatest two-dimensional plane are included in the AFC. An AFC less than 3-6 is suggestive of poor response to ovarian stimulation with gonadotropins during ART. However, it has a very poor predictive value for successful pregnancy.[10] AFC is easy to measure and gives immediate result. It also has good intercycle reliability. Error in measuring AFC can occur in women who are overweight and or when USG is performed by different sonographers leading to interobserver variability (Table 1).[8]

Serum Anti-Müllerian Hormone Level

Anti-Müllerian hormone (AMH) is secreted by granulosa cells of preantral and small antral follicles in the ovary.

Box 5: Limitations of D3 FSH.

- Low sensitivity and low negative predictive value
- Dependent on functional HPO axis
- Intercycle and intracycle variability: low precision
- Could not predict OHSS

(HPO: hypothalamus-pituitary-ovarian; OHSS: ovarian hyperstimulation syndrome)

Table 1: Comparison of ovarian reserve markers FSH, AFC and AMH hormone.

Tests	*Basal FSH*	*AFC*	*AMH*
Sensitivity for poor response	11–86%	9–73%	44–97%
Specificity for poor response	45–100%	73–97%	41–100%
AUC for poor response	0.68	0.76	0.78
Sensitivity for nonpregnancy	3–65%	7–34%	19–66%

(AFC: antral follicle count; AMH: anti-Müllerian hormone; AUC: area under the curve; FSH: follicle-stimulating hormone)

The secretion of AMH is gonadotropin-independent and is cycle-independent. Low serum AMH levels (<1 ng/mL) are associated with poor responses to controlled ovarian hyperstimulation in ART. AMH is earliest marker whose value starts decreasing in women predisposed to premature ovarian insufficiency, much earlier than other markers including AFC; so that they can take help of different management strategies like fertility preservation by oocyte or embryo freezing or to consider assisted reproduction procedures at much earlier age. AMH is also found to be very useful in measuring the residual ovarian reserve in young female treated for malignancy with chemotherapy or radiotherapy. Recent evidence suggests that AMH levels may be diminished in women taking prolonged oral contraceptive pills. Also its value may be diminished with women using gonadotropin-releasing hormone agonist and those who are obese.[11] On the other hand, AMH level is found to be two to three times more in women with PCOS.

The *POSEIDON group (Patient-Oriented Strategies Encompassing IndividualizeD Oocyte Number)* has proposed a classification for "low prognosis patients in ART"; shifting from poor ovarian response of Bologna criteria **(Fig. 3)**.[12]

The "low prognosis patients" in assisted reproductive technology according to the POSEIDON's are divided into four groups depending on oocyte quantity and quality.

Poseidon group 1

Young patients <35 years with adequate ovarian reserve parameters (AFC≥5; AMH ≥1.2 ng/mL) and with and unexpected poor or suboptimal ovarian response.

Subgroup 1a: <4 oocytes*
Subgroup 1b: 4–9 oocytes retrieved*

*after standard ovarian stimulation

Poseidon group 2

Older patients ≥35 years with adequate ovarian reserve parameters (AFC≥5; AMH≥1.2 ng/mL) and with an unexpected poor or suboptimal ovarian response.

Subgroup 2a: <4 oocytes*
Subgroup 2b: 4–9 oocytes retrieved*

*after standard ovarian stimulation

Poseidon group 3

Young patients (<35 years) with poor ovarian reserve pre-stimulation parameters (AFC<5; AMH<1.2 ng/mL)

Poseidon group 4

Older patients (≥35 years) with poor ovarian reserve prestimulation parameters (AFC<5; AMH<1.2 ng/mL)

Fig. 3

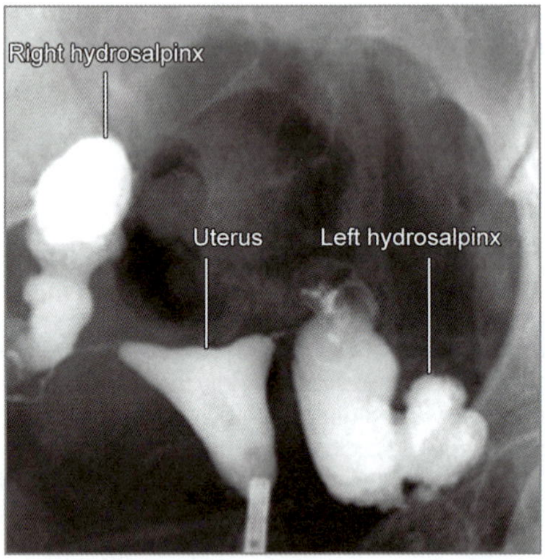

Fig. 4

Tubal Evaluation

The different tubal patency tests are complementary to each other. Sometimes accurate diagnosis of tubal obstruction requires more than one test.

- *Hysterosalpingography (HSG)* is radiographic investigation to evaluate the fallopian tubes **(Fig. 4)**. It is performed by injecting radio contrast of either oil-based or water-soluble media via the cervix into the uterine cavity. Contraindications to HSG is pregnancy, acute pelvic infection, and contrast allergy. HSG is done in the early follicular phase because during this time of cycle, there is no chance of inadvertent pregnancy and also maximum uterine visibility is possible because of proliferative endometrium. HSG has a sensitivity of 65% and specificity of 83%. Radiation exposure and high false negative rates are its major disadvantages. However, only 38% of tubal blocks diagnosed by HSG are confirmed by laparoscopy.[13] This high false positivity is mostly due to proximal tubal occlusion because of tubal spasm, collection of debris, or mucous plug inside proximal tubes. So, proximal tubal blockage requires further evaluation such as selective tubal catheterization. On the other hand, when HSG shows tubal patency, it is true positive in 94% at laparoscopy.

HSG is more specific for detecting distal tubal occlusion and has a high correlation with laparoscopic findings.[14]

- *Hysterosalpingo-contrast sonography (HyCoSy)* **(Fig. 5)**: Tubal patency is demonstrated with USG by visualizing intratubal flow of hyperechogenic contrast medium; thus, it allows detection of tubal patency, both by B mode and color Doppler ultrasound. Echovist is a suspension of soluble galactose microparticles in 20% (w/v) aqueous galactose solution and it can stand for 5–10 min. Hydroxyethyl cellulose and glycerol containing nonembryo-toxic gel (ExEm-ge) can also be used.
- As compared to Saline infusion sonography (SIS), HyCoSy with contrast is more efficient. It can also be used instead of HSG for screening for tubal patency. Also, both HSG and HyCoSy have comparable result with gold standard laparoscopy, 86.7% and 86.7%, respectively.[13] Sometimes, HyCoSy might be considered inferior to HSG because of tortuous fallopian tubes and difficulty to image the tubes as the tubes are not present at single plane. Moreover, bowel gas sometime reduces visibility of distal portion of the tube. HyCoSy with automated 3D-coded contrast imaging technology can overcome the disadvantages. With automated 3D volume acquisition, the tubes can be seen in coronal view. One can also visualize the full length of the fallopian tubes in 3D space. It is less operator dependent. The color-coded 3D-power Doppler imaging (PDI) with surface rendering allows the flow of contrast through the entire tube and the free spill from the fimbrial ends can be appreciated easily.
- *Laparoscopy with chromopertubation* is performed by passing a dilute solution of methylene blue or indigo carmine (preferred) through the cervix during laparoscopy. Laparoscopic dye test can be used to document tubal patency and identify distal as well as proximal tubal block. It is regarded as the "gold standard" for evaluating tubal patency. However, it is an invasive procedure and requires general anesthesia. The risk of major complication is low (<1%).
- *Chlamydia antibody test (CAT)* detects serum antibodies to *Chlamydia trachomatis*. It can be used as screening test if there is no history suggestive of tubal pathology; however, its clinical utility is questionable. CAT has moderate sensitivity (40–50%) and positive predictive value (60%). However, as compared to laparoscopy, CAT has a high negative predictive value (80–90%) for detection of distal tubal pathology **(Table 2)**.[15]

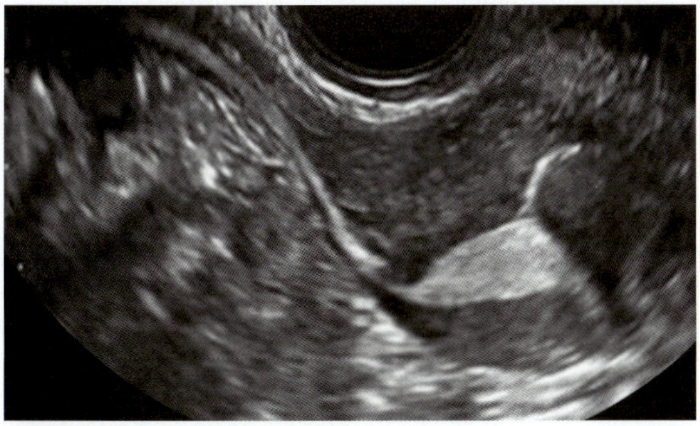

Fig. 5

RCOG RECOMMENDATION FOR TUBAL ASSESSMENT

Women who do not have comorbidities like pelvic inflammatory disease, previous ectopic pregnancy, or endometriosis; HSG is still the preferred tool for screening for tubal block. The advantages of HSG are its reliability, less invasiveness, and cost-effectiveness. Screening for tubal disease could be done with hysterosalpingo-contrast USG if necessary expertise is available in infertile women having no comorbidities. Laparoscopy and chromopertubation should be performed in women having comorbidities, so that pelvic pathologies can be assessed at the same time.

EVALUATION OF UTERUS

Abnormalities in the uterus are relatively uncommon causes of infertility. There are various methods to diagnose these:

- *Hysterosalpingography:* It can be used to determine the shape and size of the uterine cavity. It helps to diagnose various congenital anomalies like unicornuate, septate, bicornuate uterus, or acquired abnormalities in the uterine cavity like endometrial polyps, submucous fibroid, or synechiae. HSG has relatively lower sensitivity (50%) and low positive predictive value (30%) as compared to hysteroscopy. In such cases, further

Table 2: Tests for tubal evaluation

Tests	*Sensitivity*	*Specificity*
HSG	53%	87%
HyCoSy	93%	89%
CAT	40–50%	29–100%

(HSG: hysterosalpingography; HyCoSy: hysterosalpingo-contrast sonography; CAT: chlamydia antibody test)

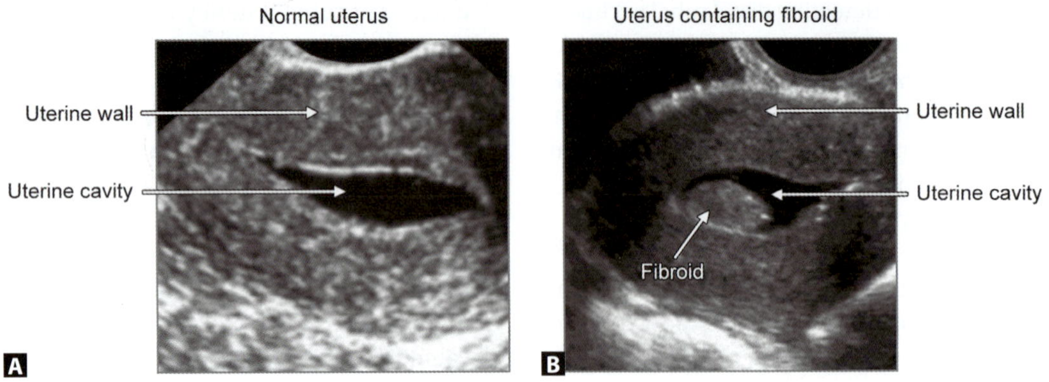

Figs. 6A and B: Images of sonohysterography. The uterine wall and saline in the uterine cavity are seen as black or "empty" space. A fibroid (benign tumor) is seen in the uterine cavity in the image on the right.

evaluation with pelvic MRI or 3D USG may help to differentiate between septate and bicornuate uterus.[14]

- *Sonohysterography* is a procedure in which normal saline is instilled into the uterine cavity during transvagianl USG. It is therefore better than normal transvaginal sonography (TVS) in delineation of the uterine cavity and intrauterine abnormalities like adhesions. Sonohysterography can diagnose various intrauterine pathology like endometrial polyps, submucous fibroid, and intrauterine synechiae with 90% accuracy **(Figs. 6A and B)**.[16]
- *Three-dimensional (3-D) ultrasound and magnetic resonance imaging (MRI):* These can be used for further assessment of the findings of with suspected pathology in TVS or HSG.
  - *Hysteroscopy* is the *gold standard* to diagnose and treat intrauterine pathologies. However, one should remembered that abnormal hysteroscopy findings are seen in 10–35% in normal HSG and 13.5% patient with normal USG.[17]
  - There is very low-quality evidence suggesting that routine pre-IVF hysteroscopy increases live birth rate (relative risk 1.48) and moderate quality evidence that it increases pregnancy rate (RR 1.45) in infertile women without any intrauterine abnormalities.

PERITONEAL FACTORS

Pelvic or adnexal adhesions and endometriosis are most common peritoneal causes leading to infertility. Laparoscopy is not recommended as routine during evaluation of an infertile woman; unless history and/or physical examination findings may raise suspicion of pelvic pathology or USG/HSG has revealed pelvic pathology such as an endometrioma or tubal disease.[18] Possibility of peritoneal factor leading to infertility should be kept in mind in women with unexplained infertility. Diagnostic laparoscopy will be of value in young infertile women presenting with long duration (>3 years) of infertility without any identifiable causative factor.

CONCLUSION

Evaluation of both the partners should be done systematically and in a cost-effective manner. Female should be evaluated for ovarian reserve followed by uterine pathology and then tubal status. The evaluation should help clinician to individualize the treatment plan.

REFERENCES

1. Practice Committee of American Society for Reproductive Medicine. Definitions of infertility and recurrent pregnancy loss: a committee opinion. Fertil Steril. 2013;99:63.
2. Practice Committee of the American Society for Reproductive Medicine. Diagnostic evaluation of the infertile female: a committee opinion. Fertil Steril. 2015;103(6):44-50.
3. Mosher WD, Pratt WF. Fecundity and infertility in the United States: incidence and trends. Fertil Steril. 1991;56:192-3.
4. Luciano AA, Peluso J, Koch EI, et al. Temporal relationship and reliability of the clinical, hormonal, and ultrasonographic indices of ovulation in infertile women. Obstet Gynecol. 1990;75:412-6.
5. The Practice Committee of the American Society for Reproductive Medicine. The clinical relevance of luteal phase deficiency: a committee opinion. Fertil Steril. 2012;98(5):1112-7.
6. Practice Committee of American Society for Reproductive Medicine in collaboration with Society for Reproductive Endocrinology and Infertility. Optimizing natural fertility: a committee opinion. Fertil Steril. 2013;100:631-7.

7. Coutifaris C, Myers ER, Guzick DS, et al. Histological dating of timed endometrial biopsy tissue is not related to fertility status. Fertil Steril. 2004;82:1264-72.
8. Practice Committee of the American Society for Reproductive Medicine. Testing and interpreting measures of ovarian reserve. Fertil Steril. 2015;103:e9-17.
9. Hendriks DJ, Mol BW, Bancsi LF, et al. The clomiphene citrate challenge test for the prediction of poor ovarian response and nonpregnancy in patients undergoing in vitro fertilization: a systematic review. Fertil Steril. 2006;86:807-18.
10. Hsu A, Arny M, Knee AB, et al. Antral follicle count in clinical practice: analyzing clinical relevance. Fertil Steril. 2011;95:474-9.
11. Kallio S, Puurunen J, Ruokonen A, et al. Antimullerian hormone levels decrease in women using combined contraception independently of administration route. Fertil Steril. 2013;99:1305-10.
12. Soares SR, Barbosa dos Reis MM, Camargos AF. Diagnostic accuracy of sonohysterography, transvaginal sonography, and hysterosalpingography in patients with uterine cavity diseases. Fertil Steril. 2000;73:406-11.
13. den Hartog JE, Morre SA, Land JA. Chlamydia trachomatis-associated tubal factor subfertility: immunogenetic aspects and serological screening. Hum Reprod Update 2006;12: 719-30.
14. Hamilton JA, Larson AJ, Lower AM, et al. Routine use of saline hysterosonography in 500 consecutive, unselected, infertile women. Hum Reprod. 1998;13:2463-73.
15. Jacobson TZ, Duffy JM, Barlow D, et al. Laparoscopic surgery for subfertility associated with endometriosis. Cochrane Database Syst Rev. 2010:CD001398.
16. Poseidon Group, Alviggi C, Andersen CY, et al. A new more detailed stratification of low responders to ovarian stimulation: from a poor ovarian response to a low prognosis concept. Fertil Steril. 2016;105(6):1452-3
17. Panchal S, Nagori C. Imaging techniques for assessment of tubal status. J Hum Reprod Sci. 2014;7(1):2-12.
18. Sardo A, Carlo C, Minozzi S, et al. Efficacy of hysteroscopy in improving reproductive outcomes of infertile couples: a systematic review and meta-analysis. Hum Reprod Update. 2016;22(4):479-96.

Evaluation of the Infertile Male

4

Vasan SS, Shashidhar B, Pragya Mishra, Shanti Roy

INTRODUCTION

Evaluation of infertile or subfertile male begins with even his physical appearance giving some clue to the clinician when the patient enters the clinicians' office. Male infertility may happen due to problems with sperm production, transport, or sexual dysfunction. Patient evaluation is directed toward identifying the above problems, which can be idiopathic many times. Male infertility is estimated to be around 7%[1] of all men around the world. According to World Health Organization (WHO) guidelines, infertility is defined as the inability to conceive after at least 12 months of unprotected intercourse. The incidence of which is approximately 16% or one in six to seven couples are infertile and 30–50%[2] of these cases are estimated to be due to male factor. Demographic data worldwide shows that male infertility is rising; however, it may reflect an increasing willingness on the part of couples to seek treatment and also as a consequence of large-scale publicity of available treatments apart from factors such as delayed parenthood, epigenetics, and genetics. Testicular dysgenesis syndrome, which comprises of increased rates of testicular cancer, undescended testis and congenital malformations, has been linked to declining sperm counts and environmental factors may also contribute.

CLINICAL EVALUATION GOALS

- To ascertain if the male is contributory or solely responsible for the couple's infertility. *This has a sociocultural importance in India.*
- To identify potentially correctable conditions.
- To identify irreversible conditions that may be amenable to assisted reproduction. This would include conditions that require additional genetic testing and counseling.
- To identify irreversible conditions those are not amenable to assisted reproduction and counsel for donor insemination or adoption.
- To identify significant underlying medical conditions that may have manifest as infertility.

BASIC CLINICAL EVALUATION OF THE MALE

- An urologist or a specialist in male reproduction should do reproductive evaluation of the male. *This is a specialized field and requires in-depth knowledge of anatomy and physiology of the reproductive system.*
- The first evaluation should include a detailed history and physical examination as outlined below.

Patient History

The history reviews medical problems including recent fevers, illnesses, cancer, and infections. These factors primarily affect the hypothalamic-pituitary-gonadal (HPG) axis, which results in hormonal imbalance and testicular damage causing reproductive failure and infertility.[3,4]

History should include consideration of the following:

- Reproductive history should include:
  - Duration of infertility
  - Age of partners
  - Previous fertility with same or different partner
  - Previous evaluation and treatment for infertility
  - Knowledge of reproductive cycle
  - Coital frequency and timing
  - Use of contraceptives and lubricants
  - Sexual dysfunction, nature and volume of ejaculate *[low volume and clear water like suggest ejaculatory*

duct obstruction (EDO) and failure to liquefy suggests prostatic dysfunction]
- ♦ Ejaculatory dysfunction *(difficulty in ejaculating during intercourse; difficulty in collecting semen sample).*

- Medical history should include:
  - ♦ Congenital anomalies, cryptorchidism *(50% of men with unilateral and 90% with bilateral cryptorchidism are subfertile)*
  - ♦ Chemotherapy or radiation exposure
  - ♦ Chronic medical illnesses
  - ♦ Chronic bronchitis *(may be related to Young's or Kartagener's syndrome or motility disorders)*
  - ♦ Postpubescent mumps *(30% risk of orchitis)*
  - ♦ Onset of puberty *(precocious in congenital adrenal hyperplasia and delayed in Kallmann's and Klinefelter's syndromes)*
  - ♦ Testicular torsion or trauma
  - ♦ Past surgeries and injuries
  - ♦ Medication or drug use.
- General history should include:
  - ♦ Occupation
  - ♦ Exposure to heat (at work or recreational sauna or steam) or environmental toxins such as pesticides
  - ♦ Family reproductive history.

Physical Examination

The examination consists of general body habitus examination, gynecomastia, penis, scrotal, and prostate evaluation.

Examination of Testes—Key Points

- Small soft testes indicate poor spermatogenesis.
- Small hard testes suggest postorchitis or post-torsion atrophy or Klinefelter's syndrome.
- Focal irregularities in consistency raise the suspicion of malignancy.
- Smooth firm nodules palpated on the surface of the testis usually represent tunica albuginea cysts.
- Mobile small hard bodies, corpora amylacea, may be palpated floating within the tunica vaginalis.
- Transillumination of the scrotum in a darkened room differentiates solid from cystic masses **(Fig. 1)**.

The testes that are normal in size and consistency generally have normal sperm production. However, testes with soft and small in volume are associated with impaired spermatogenesis.

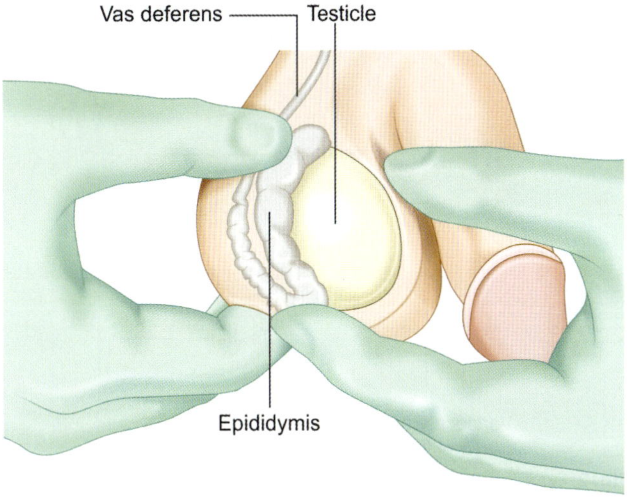

Fig. 1: Clinical examination of the scrotum.

Examination of Epididymis—Key Points

The normal epididymis is soft and barely palpable and is posterolateral to the testes. Epididymal pathology is often associated with irregularities or modularity. A full, firm, easily outlined epididymis that is nontender suggests epididymal obstruction. Epididymal cysts are generally located in the caput and are firm, smooth, and transilluminate.

Examination of Varicocele—Key Points

Subclinical or questionable varicoceles are of limited clinical interest. Examination should be done in standing position **(Fig. 2)**.

Examination of Prostate

In patient with azoospermia digital rectal examination is recommended to confirm the, size and consistency of the prostate, midline prostatic cyst, irregularities, tenderness, and palpable seminal vesicle, is noted.

When should the male be evaluated?

- Evaluation of the male should occur simultaneously with that of the female partner when there is no pregnancy after 1 year of regular unprotected intercourse. This should include both primary and secondary infertility.
- Evaluation should also be done at any time (postpuberty) if:
  - ♦ Known male risk factor for infertility like cryptorchidism
  - ♦ Female risk factor for infertility such as age more than 35 years

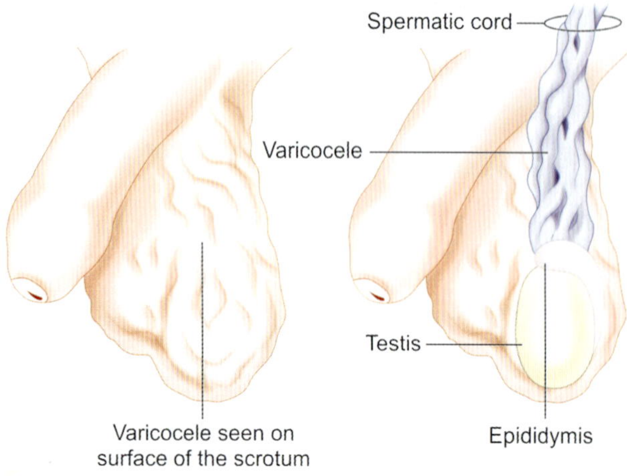

Fig. 2: Examination of varicocele.

- The male is desirous of knowing his fertility potential. *This should be accompanied by an explanation of the limitations of current investigations in identifying the fertility potential, e.g. 5% men with sperm concentration below 15 million/mL are normally fertile.*

Diagnosis

In most of the cases, diagnosis of causes for male infertility and corresponding treatment is possible. Treatment of male infertility has often yielded successful pregnancies also, cost-effective and less invasive than intracytoplasmic sperm injection (ICSI) or other assisted reproductive technology (ART) treatments.

SEMEN ANALYSIS

Semen analysis forms the cornerstone of evaluating male factor infertility. It is critical to obtain a representative sample, analyzed at a laboratory that routinely performs semen analysis in order to decide further management.[5-7]

- At least two semen samples must be obtained, preferably about a month apart with a 3–5 day abstinence period prior to each sample. *No decision should be based on a single report since semen parameters fluctuate with time. Surgical intervention in particular must never be based on fewer than two consistent reports. The best of various recent reports is taken to be indicative of the fertility potential of the man and should guide therapy.*
- In the 3-month-period prior to the sample, the patient should ideally have been free from any febrile or systemic illness and should not have been on medications known to affect spermatogenesis, particularly steroids, androgens, and antibiotics. *Febrile illnesses may even result in azoospermia in an otherwise fertile male.*
- The sample should be collected through masturbation in a wide-mouthed, clean container without spillage. The container should not have residue of any spermicidal detergents. Collection in a nonspermicidal condom is also acceptable, particularly for men who fail to produce a sample through masturbation.
- A man reporting difficulty in semen collection who produces "yellow semen" or scanty ejaculate should be asked to provide a semen sample by vibratory stimulation. *5% of Indian men have difficulty collecting a semen sample by masturbation. Sometimes they give a pseudoejaculate (urethral secretions or urine), which is misleadingly reported as showing azoospermia.*
- Sample should be maintained at room or body temperature till evaluation.
- Samples must be examined within one hour of collection. *This is particularly relevant in India since a large number of laboratories serve as collection centers for larger laboratories and there may be a delay in transport of sample to the central laboratory.*
- Samples must be reported by individuals qualified to evaluate them and who perform such tests routinely.
- The reports must mention the WHO criteria for a normal semen analysis since no Indian criteria on normal semen sample exist. *It is common to see reports from reputed laboratories quoting incorrect normal or reference ranges. This is detrimental to the patient's perception of his problem and is often the basis for prescribing unnecessary therapies.*
- It is important to understand that these are reference ranges and are neither necessary nor sufficient to produce a pregnancy. They are used to guide therapy and prognosticate outcome.
- *Computer-assisted semen analysis (CASA):* Routine use is controversial because of lack of understanding of specifications and limitations. In the majority, it does not offer any clinical advantage over a routine semen analysis.

Classification Based on Semen Analysis

The normal semen analysis parameters defined by the WHO 5th Manual are **(Table 1)**:

On at least two occasions:

Based on the semen analysis, patients should be classified into the following:

- *Oligoasthenoteratozoospermia (OAT):* Most semen analysis will lead to a diagnosis of this abnormality.

Table 1: The normal semen analysis parameters.	
Ejaculate volume	> 1.6 mL
pH	> 7.2
Sperm concentration (x 10^6/mL)	>15
% Motility	>39 type A + B or >32% type A
% Normal morphology	>4% by Kruger's criteria
WBC	<1 × 10^6/ mL
Agglutination	<20%

Abnormalities may be present in only one parameter. However, two or more of the following parameters—sperm density, motility, or morphology—are usually abnormal leading to the diagnosis of OAT.

- *Azoospermia:* The diagnosis of azoospermia is made with extreme caution because of its specific causes and management.
  - Complete absence of sperm in the ejaculate sample refers to azoospermia. Even a single mature sperm in the ejaculate can change the diagnosis to extreme oligospermia or cryptozoospermia. This differentiation is *critical* to the management of azoospermia
  - The semen specimen must be centrifuged at 3,000 g for at least 15 minutes and the pellet examined for sperms
  - Azoospermia should be confirmed in a second semen analysis.

The azoospermia can be categorized in to three etiological conditions such as (1) pretesticular, (2) testicular, and (3) post testicular. Men with abnormal hormonal profiles are considered under pretesticular azoospermia and are uncommon. Testicular azoospermia results in poor spermatogenesis. These conditions often require ART since they are not amenable to corrective therapy. The ductal obstruction or ejaculatory dysfunction is responsible for post-testicular azoospermia and often correctable. Hence, this is the principle objective of evaluating azoospermic men.

- Volume of ejaculate should be carefully documented. Low-volume ejaculate (<1 mL) has specific causes and management, different from other causes of azoospermia. In such cases, a properly done test for semen fructose is helpful.
- Low-volume ejaculate should be confirmed with the patient's impression of his ejaculate volume. *Most such men will state that they ejaculate only a few drops rather than a teaspoonful.*
- Common causes of low-volume ejaculate such as small period of abstinence or spillage during collection must be ruled out before diagnosing low-volume azoospermia.

Oligoasthenoteratospermia

The OAT evaluation is aimed at identifying causes, which are amenable to specific therapy before employing empiric therapy for the remaining idiopathic cases. Specific causes include varicoceles, hormonal abnormalities, infection, and genetic aberrations. Age, noninflammatory functional alterations in post-testicular organs, mitochondrial alterations, environmental pollutants, and "subtle" hormonal alterations are all considered possible causes of idiopathic OAT. Additionally, increase of reactive oxygen species (ROS) in tubules and seminal plasma and consequent apoptosis are shown to affect sperm concentration, motility, and morphology. The causal link between these pathologies and OAT is not always evident; nevertheless, the common final result is the impairment of spermatogenesis.

Semen fructose:

- Semen fructose is relevant in men with low-volume ejaculate. Low-volume ejaculate with absence of fructose indicates congenital bilateral absence of the vas deferens (CBAVD) or EDO *(laboratories often report difficulty in doing a fructose test in these patients because of insufficient quantity of semen. They should use proportionately less reagent and semen, and incorporate positive and negative controls).*

Antisperm Antibodies

Disruption of the epithelial-blood barrier elicits antisperm antibody (ASA). ASA may develop in patients with a vasectomy, vas obstruction, testicular trauma, torsion, malignancy, and infection of the urogenital tract. ASAs are found in 26–55% of infertile couples, in up to 19% of fertile men, and in 43% of fertile women, which means that not all ASA cause infertility. On the other hand, ASA may affect the following—cervical mucus penetration, acrosome reaction, zona binding, zona penetration, oolemma binding, and pronucleus formation. The effects of ASA on motility and on in vitro fertilization (IVF) are questionable.

- The ASA testing is a primary choice of when there is sperm agglutination, an abnormal postcoital test or isolated asthenospermia
- The ASA testing is advisable for couples with unexplained infertility

- The ASA found in the serum or seminal plasma by indirect testing is rather less significant than the ASA found on the surface of sperm by direct testing. Immunobead or the mixed antiglobulin reaction (MAR) is the gold standard test to assay the ASA. *Most laboratories test only the serum or seminal plasma by indirect testing. Such tests in isolation do not guide therapy*
- If sperms are to be used for ICSI, ASA testing is usually not needed.

EVALUATION OF RETROGRADE EJACULATION

Postejaculate Urine Examination

The presence of sperm in the postejaculate urine sample of a man with azoospermia or aspermia signifies retrograde ejaculation.

Low-volume ejaculate less than 1 mL associated with positive orgasm may be a clue for a retrograde ejaculation. Retrograde ejaculation is evaluated by observing sperm in postejaculatory urine. Conditions associated with retrograde ejaculation include surgery, such as bladder neck surgery, retroperitoneal lymph node dissection surgery for testicular cancer or prostate surgery, diabetes, multiple sclerosis, Parkinson's disease, or a spinal cord injury.

- During low-volume azoospermia or absent ejaculation Postejaculate urine should be checked for sperms in men
- In men suspected to have partial retrograde ejaculation (low-volume ejaculate with OAT), the urine should be collected in two containers. If the second sample of urine has a large number of sperm then this indicates partial retrograde flow of the ejaculate.

Semen Culture

Both leukocytes and immature germ cells appear similar and both are properly termed "round cells" in under wet mount microscopy. Often the round cells are improperly reported as "white blood cells (WBCs)" by many of the laboratories. There are various assays are available to discriminate leukocytes from immature germ cells. The traditional cytologic staining and immunohistochemical techniques are important among them.

- The clinician must make sure that the two types of cells are differentiated.
- More than 1 million/mL WBC is an indicator of true infection and merits treatment. We kept the figure of 10/hPF since most laboratories do not give quantitative measures and actually confuse WBCs with round sperms. A value of 10/hPF which roughly corresponds to 2–3 mill/mL may be discriminatory enough to generate suspicion of an infection. The WHO criteria of 1 mill/mL are mentioned in the table on semen analysis.
  Initial treatment may be given without a semen culture. *The infecting organisms such as Chlamydia and Mycoplasma cannot be grown on routine bacterial cultures hence cultures are often negative. Routine cultures tend to grow urethral organisms or commensals.*
- Persistent pyospermia despite an initial course of empirical antibiotics is an indication for seminal culture.

Specialized Test of Sperm Function and Semen

- These tests are not routinely indicated. *They will rarely detect treatable conditions. There is limited expertise in performing them.*
- Sperm vitality assays may differentiate viable nonmotile sperms from dead sperms. This is required in men with isolated, total asthenospermia. *Non-motile but viable sperms can be used in assisted reproduction (ART).*

SPERM DNA FRAGMENTATION AND ITS DIAGNOSTIC VALUE

Viable fertility prospects are independently associated with sperm DNA damage. These include defective fertilization, slow early embryo development, reduced implantation, and miscarriage, also birth defects in the offspring were noticed in animal studies. The oxidative damage to sperm DNA due to paternal smoking has also been associated childhood cancers. DNA fragmentation has proven to be a helpful technique in predicting the outcomes of couples undergoing IVF/ICSI.

REACTIVE OXYGEN SPECIES ESTIMATION

Physiological function of spermatozoa at the molecular level is altered by oxidative stress and it may significantly alter male fertility prospects. It is accurately determined by chemiluminescent assay. Nevertheless, the antioxidant counter mechanism of balancing the ROS in semen is difficult to investigate and so far not clearly understood.

Hormonal Evaluation

- An endocrine evaluation has to be performed under following conditions:
  - When the sperm concentration is below 10 million/mL

Table 2: The findings on hormone analysis.

Clinical status	*FSH*	*LH*	*Testosterone*
Normal men	Normal	Normal	Normal
Germinal aplasia	Elevated	Normal	Normal or decreased
Testicular failure	Elevated	Elevated	Normal or decreased
Hypogonadotropic hypogonadism	Decreased	Decreased	Decreased
Hypergonadotropic hypogonadism	Elevated	Elevated	Low-normal or decreased

- Whenever there is an impaired sexual function such as decreased volume of ejaculate and libido
- Clinical findings suggestive of a specific endocrinopathy

- The serum follicle-stimulating hormone (FSH) and serum testosterone levels should be the primary choice of hormonal evaluation.
- A repeat measurement of total testosterone, serum luteinizing hormone (LH) and prolactin levels should be obtained when the testosterone level is low *[free testosterone should not be obtained as most radioimmunoassay (RIA) for free testosterone are unreliable]*
- Serum estrogen and adrenal steroids should be measured only if clinically indicated. In hypogonadotropic hypogonadism, other pituitary hormones like adrenocorticotropic hormone (ACTH), thyroid-stimulating hormone (TSH), and growth hormone (GH) are assayed.
- A single measurement is usually sufficient to determine a patient's clinical endocrine status.

Many men with abnormal spermatogenesis have a normal serum FSH, but a marked elevation of serum FSH is clearly indicative of an abnormality in spermatogenesis.[8] The findings on hormone analysis should be interpreted according to the **Table 2**.

Clinical Pathway

- In case of bilaterally small testis serum, FSH and testosterone will be evaluated along with sexual dysfunction, loss of libido, or poor secondary sexual characteristics. Consensually small testis along with increased FSH, generally two times more than the normal reference range is indication for testicular impairment and these individuals do not need a diagnostics testicular biopsy or fine needle aspiration cytology (FNAC).
- However, in case of obstructive azoospermia serum FSH estimation is optional. *Normal FSH supports the diagnosis of obstructive azoospermia, but is not diagnostic. FSH may be normal even in men with testicular impairment. FSH may also be marginally raised in men with normal spermatogenesis.*
- Testosterone should also be evaluated in men with low-volume ejaculate and a palpable vas deferens. *Hypogonadism may be responsible for low-volume ejaculate. Palpable vas rules out CBAVD, a common cause of low-volume ejaculate.*

INHIBIN B

Inhibin B is a dimer molecule with alpha and beta B subunits. This molecule is widely synthesized in testis, predominantly by the Sertoli cells in the prepubertal testis. The inhibin B through a negative feedback mechanism controls the secretion of FSH. Hence, Inhibin B acts as a serum marker of spermatogenesis and it is used to assess the spermatogenesis of infertile men.

Inhibin B levels are crucial in understanding the outcome of testicular sperm extraction in men with nonobstructive azoospermia, and to assess the damage to spermatogenesis in men after radiotherapy or chemotherapy.[9,10]

Genetic Testing

It is estimated to be around 10% of the men with OAT have the genetic abnormalities. Among these genetic abnormalities, karyotypic abnormalities such as Klinefelter's syndrome or its variants, or deletions in the long arm of the Y chromosome (Yq microdeletions) are common. Identification of these abnormalities is crucial in understanding the etiology of the infertility. If patients choose to undergo ART, detection of genetic abnormalities helps in their counseling since a most of these abnormalities are genetically transmissible to the offspring.

- For men with persistent severe oligospermia who are considering ICSI (< 1 million sperm/mL). Karyotyping and Y chromosome microdeletion screening are must.
- Karyotyping is also indicated, if clinical features suggest a chromosomal abnormality such as Klinefelter's syndrome.
- Cystic fibrosis transmembrane conductance regulator (CFTR) gene mutation testing should be done in men with

CBAVD and their partners, only if they are considering IVF. However, mutations in Indian population appear to be different from the western populations and are not picked up by the commonly done tests.

ROLE OF IMAGING IN THE EVALUATION OF MALE INFERTILITY

Scrotal Color Doppler (Fig. 3)

More than confirmation of varicocele, it may also help in diagnosis of conditions like bilateral small testes, unilateral small testis, epididymal, testicular microlithiasis, testicular tumor, and thickened epididymis suggestive of previous orchitis, which may not be apparently diagnosed by clinical examination. Also by studying the vascular intratesticular patterns active foci of spermatogenesis may be identified which may help in successful sperm retrieval in case of obstructive azoospermia.

Detection of Varicoceles

- A clinical examination, performed in a warm room in the supine and standing position, before and after Valsalva maneuver should be used to diagnose varicoceles[11]
- Doppler ultrasound should be asked for only to confirm a clinical suspicion or in men with a short, scarred, or indurated scrotum that is difficult to evaluate
- Doppler may also be used to detect subclinical varicoceles on the right side of a patient with a clinical left sided varicocele that is planned for surgical correction. *There is some evidence to suggest that correction of such subclinical varicoceles may improve outcomes.*
- No additional imaging studies are required.

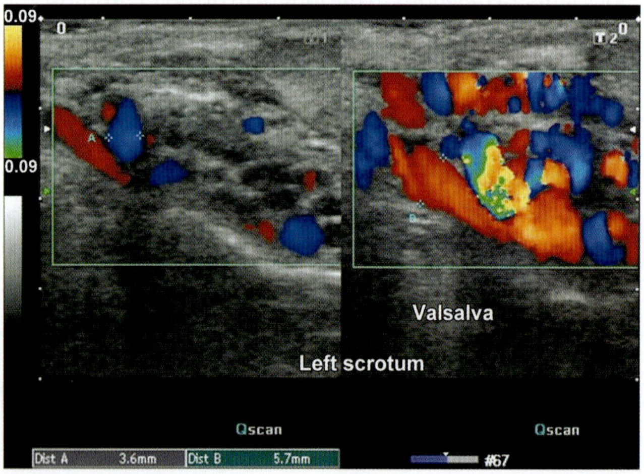

Fig. 3: Scrotal color Doppler.

Scrotal ultrasound and Doppler:

- Routine Doppler testing to detect varicoceles is not recommended. *Subclinical varicoceles detected only on Doppler tests do not result in improvement in semen parameters or pregnancy rates. See section on varicocele.*
- Doppler may be done to confirm a clinical diagnosis of varicocele and to evaluate the opposite side when there is a unilateral clinical varicocele.
- Scrotal ultrasound should be done in case a suspicious mass lesion is found on clinical examination or the scrotum is difficult to evaluate clinically due to previous trauma/surgery/infection.

Abdominal ultrasound:

- In men with CBAVD *have a higher incidence of congenital renal anomalies* hence, abdominal ultrasound should be done, particularly the kidneys.

Transrectal Ultrasound

Transrectal Ultrasonography

- The transrectal ultrasonography (TRUS) is indicated in men with low-volume ejaculate and a palpable vas deferens. *It may identify EDO as the etiology.*
- The TRUS may also be performed for medicolegal confirmation of a clinical CBAVD. *It may show an absent or hypoplastic seminal vesicle that usually accompanies CBAVD.*
- Presence of seminal vesicles on TRUS does not exclude the diagnosis of CBAVD. *Seminal vesicles may be normally present or present but hypofunctional in a subset of men with absent vas deferens. The diagnosis in such men will be clinical (Fig. 4).*
- The TRUS-guided injection of dye into the seminal vesicles may be performed immediately prior to a transurethral resection of ejaculatory ducts (TURED) in men with EDO. *This guides placement of the incision and allows confirmation of an adequate incision during surgery.*

Invasive Imaging Techniques

Vasography

- Formal vasography is almost never required in the diagnosis or management of azoospermia. *Rare indications are men with pelvic surgery or inguinal surgery or low-volume ejaculate where the site of block is unclear.*

- Saline infusion or the tests that do not result in inflammation of the vas are used for confirming vas patency. Usually, this is done during reconstructive procedure and this should not be performed as the separate diagnostic test.
    - Approximately 40–50% of all infertility cases are due to male factor and 2% of all them will show up suboptimal sperm parameters.
    - Though, the semen analysis is considered imperfect too for treating male infertility but remains corner stone in investigating male infertility.

Testicular Biopsy

- Before diagnosing obstructive azoospermia in men with a normal ejaculate volume, testicular biopsy is usually essential.

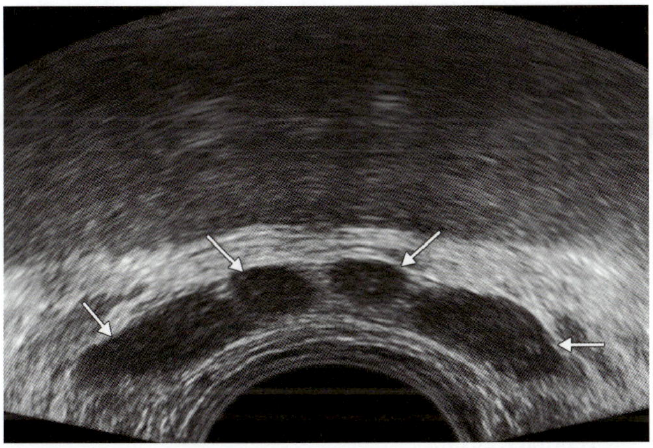

Fig. 4: Normal ultrasound anatomy of the seminal vesicles and vasa deferentia.

- Testicular needle biopsy gives information on par with open biopsy. Where reasonable, needle biopsy should be the choice against open biopsy.
- *This minimizes scarring and decreases problems during a subsequent reconstruction.*
- If an open biopsy is performed, it should be closed using nonabsorbable fine sutures to minimize inflammation.
- In men with small testis and FSH raised above 2X normal, testicular biopsy is done only to assess presence focal spermatogenesis prior to ICSI. In such cases, the biopsy should also be studied for evidence of carcinoma in situ.
- Multiple biopsies may be required to retrieve sperm in men with testicular impairment. These should be carried out in an IVF center with the facility to either immediately utilize or cryopreserve retrieved sperms.
- Evaluation of testicular biopsy requires considerable experience and pathologists must be aware of the requirements of the treating physician. **Flowchart 1** shows diagnostic algorithm.

CONCLUSION

Male infertility is influenced by various conditions. Among these, ductal obstruction and hypogonadotropic hypogonadism are reversible. However, conditions such as bilateral testicular atrophy secondary to viral orchitis are identifiable but irreversible. In case of many patients, the condition is termed idiopathic when the etiology of the abnormal semen analysis is not identifiable. On the other hand, even though patient has normal semen analysis and partner evaluation if the reason for infertility if not

Flowchart 1: Diagnostic algorithm

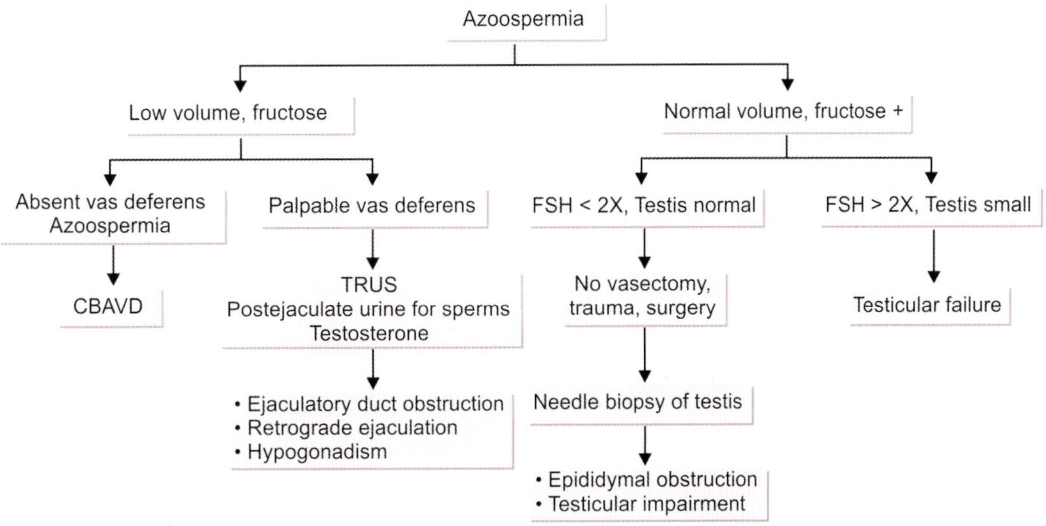

clear then the condition is termed "unexplained". Rarely, there are situations with normal semen analysis and still the infertility is due to male factor. The purpose of the male evaluation is to identify conditions and treat them for reversible conditions thereby it can improve the male fertility and allow them for the pregnancy through natural intercourse. There are conditions such as even azoospermic patients also may have active sperm production or could have sperm production induced with treatment.

ACKNOWLEDGMENT

The authors acknowledge that the above chapter has many of the guidelines published by the AUA (American Urology association), EAU (European Urology Association), and ASRM (American society for Reproductive Medicine)[12-14] and they are reproduced here.

REFERENCES

1. Boivin J, Bunting L, Collins JA, et al. International estimates of infertility prevalence and treatment-seeking: potential need and demand for infertility medical care. Hum Reprod. 2007;22:1506-12.
2. Brugh VM, Lipshultz LI. (2004). Male factor infertility: evaluation and management. Medical Clinics of North America. 2004;88(2):367-85.
3. Phillips KP, Tanphaichitr N. Human exposure to endocrine disrupters and semen quality. J Toxicol Environ Health B Crit Rev. 2008;11:188-220.
4. Omu AE. Sperm parameters: paradigmatic index of good health and longevity. Med Princ Pract. 2013;22(Suppl 1):30-42.
5. Eliasson Rune. Analysis of Semen. In Burger H, de Kretser D (Eds). The Testis. New York: Raven Press; 1981. pp. 381-99
6. Esteves SC. Clinical relevance of routine semen analysis and controversies surrounding the 2010 World Health Organization criteria for semen examination. Int Braz J Urol. 2014;40:443-53.
7. WHO. WHO Laboratory Manual for the Examination of Human Semen and Sperm-cervical Mucus Interaction, 4th edition. Cambridge, UK: Cambridge University Press; 1999.
8. Mortimer D. The essential partnership between diagnostic andrology and modern assisted reproductive technologies. Hum Reprod. 1994;9:1209-13.
9. Meachem SJ, Nieschlag E, Simoni M. Inhibin B in male reproduction: pathophysiology and clinical relevance. Eur J Endocrinol. 2001;145(5):561-71.
10. Jue JS, Ramasamy R. Significance of positive semen culture in relation to male infertility and the assisted reproductive technology process. Transl Androl Urol. 2017;6(5):916-22.
11. Tomasz Lorenc, Leszek Krupniewski, Piotr Palczewski, et al. The value of ultrasound in diagnosis of varicocele. J Ultraso. 2016;16(67):359-70.
12. ASRM. (2015). Diagnostic evaluation of the infertile male: a committee opinion. [online] Available from: https://www.asrm.org/globalassets/asrm/asrm-content/news-and-publications/practice-guidelines/for-non-members/diagnostic_evaluation_of_the_infertile_male_a_committee_opinion-noprint.pdf [Last Accessed February, 2019].
13. European Association of Urology. (2015). Guidelines on Male Infertility. [online] Available from: https://uroweb.org/wp-content/uploads/17-Male-Infertility_LR1.pdf [Last Accessed February, 2019].
14. American Urological Association. (2011). Optimal Evaluation of the Infertile Male. [online] Available from: http://www.auanet.org/guidelines/male-infertility-optimal-evaluation-(reviewed-and-validity-confirmed-2011) [Last Accessed February, 2019].

Thyroid and Infertility

5

Jayamangala Gogate, Shashank Joshi, Dhanashri Natu

INTRODUCTION

The thyroid gland plays a prime role in regulating our physiology. Secretion of various hormones like thyronines, triiodothyronine (T3), and thyroxine (T4) is under its control. Dietary iodide is their main component. Sodium/iodide symporter (NIS) transports these into the thyroid follicular cell against electrochemical gradient (active transport) stimulated by thyroid-stimulating hormone (TSH) or thyrotropin. Monoiodotyrosine (MIT) and diiodotyrosine (DIT) are formed by the oxidation of iodide at cell-colloid surface by enzyme thyroid peroxidase (TPO). Secondary coupling of MIT and DIT catalyzed by TPO leads to incorporation of tyrosyl residues in thyroglobulin molecule forming T3 and T4. Although the amount of T4 produced is greater than T3, biologically T3 is the more functionally active form **(Fig. 1)**.[1]

Thyroid disorders can either be due to overproduction of thyroid hormones (hyperthyroidism) or its deficiency (hypothyroidism) and these are known to have profound effect on reproduction.

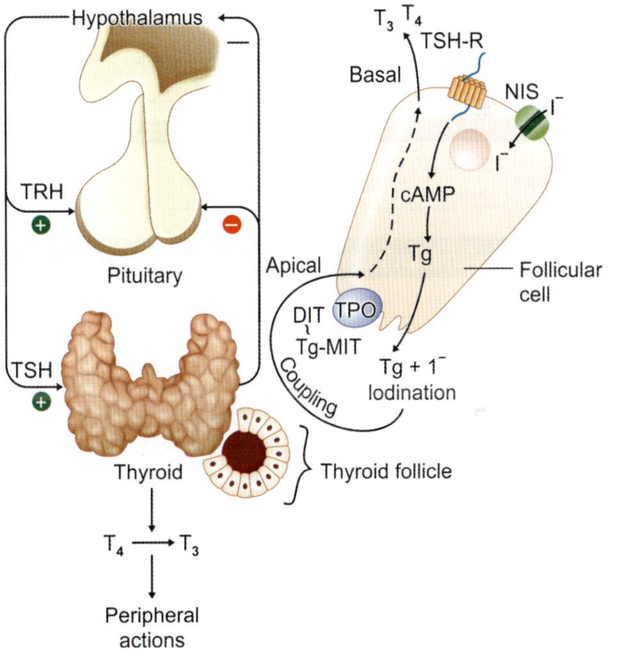

Fig. 1: Formation of thyroid hormones. (DIT: diiodotyrosine; MIT: monoiodotyrosine; T3: triiodothyronine; T4: thyroxine; TSH: thyroid-stimulating hormone; TPO: thyroid peroxidase)

HYPOTHYROIDISM

Hypothyroidism can be triggered off by an autoimmune process (autoimmune or Hashimoto's thyroiditis) or after a thyroid surgery or radioactive iodine (I-131) treatment. Subclinical hypothyroidism is characterized by raised serum TSH concentration in the presence of a normal free T4 level.[2] A few important causes of hypothyroidism are mentioned in **Table 1**.[3]

The common signs and symptoms of hypothyroidism are enumerated in the **Table 2.**[3]

The hormonal changes due to hypothyroidism are enumerated in the **Table 3.**[4]

Hypothyroidism and Female Fertility

Introduction

Subclinical hypothyroidism (SCH): It is defined as any serum TSH level greater than 4.5–5.0 mIU/L with normal free thyroxine (FT4) levels. The incidence in reproductive

Table 1: Causes of hypothyroidism.

Primary: Thyroid gland failure	***Secondary***
Congenital: ▪ Agenesis ▪ Ectopic thyroid remnants	*Hypothalamic disease*: Idiopathic, trauma, infiltrative disorders, tumors, and trauma
Defect in synthesis: Iodine deficiency	Isolated thyroid-stimulating hormone (TSH deficiency) or inactivity
Dyshormonogenesis	*Hypopituitarism*: Trauma, tumors, Sheehan's syndrome, infiltrative disorders, pituitary surgery or irradiation, genetic forms of combined pituitary
Antithyroid drugs	Hormone deficiency
Autoimmune: Hashimoto's thyroiditis	
Atrophic	
Infective	
Postsurgery	
Postradiotherapy	
Peripheral resistance to thyroid hormones	

Table 2: Signs and symptoms of hypothyroidism.

Symptoms	***Signs***
Tiredness, malaise	Dry coarse skin, cool peripheral extremities
Difficulty in concentrating	Myxedema
Impaired hearing	Diffuse alopecia
Dyspnea	Bradycardia
Weight gain, poor appetite	Tardy tendon reflexes
Constipation	Carpal tunnel syndrome
Dry skin, paresthesia	Serous cavity effusions
Hair loss	–
Feeling cold	–
Hoarse voice	–
Menorrhagia (followed by oligomenorrhea or amenorrhea)	–

age females is around 4–8%.[5,6] Menstrual irregularities are seen in approximately 23–25%. Oligomenorrhea is the most common clinical presentation. Menorrhagia is sometimes seen due to anovulation, poor uterine muscle tone, and platelet dysfunction. When undiagnosed, this can cause infertility, abortions, and adverse obstetrical and affect fetal neurodevelopment.[7-9]

Table 3: Hormonal changes in males and females in hypothyroidism

	Hypothyroidism	
	Males	***Females***
SHBG	Decreases or normal	Decreases
E_2	Normal	Decreases
Estrone		Decreases
Production rate of estrogen		No change or decreases
Metabolic clearance of estrogen or androgen	Decreases	Decreases
Free E_2		Normal
Testosterone	Decreases	Decreases
Delta 4-androstenedione	Decreases	Decreases
DHEA	Decreases	
Free testosterone	Decreases	Normal
Conversion of testosterone to delta 4-androstenedione	Decreases	Increases
Progesterone		Decreases or no change
LH	Normal	Normal
FSH	Normal	Normal
After GnRH		
LH	Decreases	Decreases
FSH	Decreases	Decreases

(DHEA: dehydroepiandrosterone; E_2: estrogen; FSH: follicle-stimulating hormone; GnRH: gonadotropin-releasing hormone; LH: luteinizing hormone; SHBG: sex hormone-binding globulin)

Incidence and Prevalence

It is commonly seen in women with ovulatory disturbances.[10-12] Literature review shows correlation between SCH and unexplained infertility.[10,13]

Thyroid autoimmunity and infertility: Infertile women are more likely to be TPO antibody-positive in spite of being euthyroid. Further, polycystic ovarian syndrome (PCOS) women have higher antithyroid antibodies. These women have decreased chances of developing ovarian follicles after induction with clomiphene citrate.[14]

Ovarian hyperstimulation and thyroid function:
Controlled ovarian hyperstimulation is the central process in IVF.[14] Serum estradiol levels in these patients may increase and reach supraphysiologic levels (approximately 4,000–6,000 ng/L). This high-estrogen causes rise of TBG (thyroglobulin), which reduces free thyroid hormone causing positive feedback mechanism to further increase TSH levels. Human chorionic gonadotropin (hCG) also has direct stimulatory effect on thyroid receptors, leading to increase in thyroid hormone and decreasing TSH.

American Thyroid Association (ATA) 2017 guidelines recommend:

- As the interpretation of the TSH reports during controlled ovarian hyperstimulation is difficult, perform thyroid function testing before or 1–2 weeks after the stimulation.
- Thyroid function testing should be done in all pregnancies following COH.
    - Ideally, the reference range/values of thyroid function tests should be population and trimester-specific. This can be defined by the laboratory and should represent typical population of that region. This reference range should be defined in healthy TPO antibody-negative pregnant women with optimal iodine intake and without thyroid illness.
    - If the reference range is not available, TSH assays performed in similar pregnant patient population can be used as reference.
    - If this is also not available then generally an upper reference limit of TSH of 4.0 mU/L may be used. For most assays, this limit represents a reduction in the nonpregnant TSH upper reference limit of 0.5 mU/L.
- In women who are not pregnant, but have slightly raised TSH levels due to controlled ovarian stimulation, values should be repeated after 2–4 weeks. This is the time required for the hormones to reach baseline levels.

Hypothyroidism in Males

As compared to females, fewer men have hypothyroidism with incidence of only 0.1%.[15,16] This has a distinct effect on their reproductive system.[17]

Hormonal Effects

In males with hypothyroidism, LH responses to GnRH are dampened.[18] This mimics a picture of hypogonadotropic, hypergonadotropic with sometimes a normal serum LH and FSH levels.[19-21] These men have low or normal serum-free testosterone and sex hormone-binding globulin (SHBG)[19,20] along with diminished levels of metabolites of androsterone and androstenedione.[22] Further serum prolactin levels may be raised. However, T4 replacement can correct this abnormality.[21] These men have reduced sexual desire and may suffer from erectile dysfunction or delay in ejaculation.[22] Men with postpubertal hypothyroidism may present with reduction in semen volume and motility of sperms. Hypothyroidism may affect the development and differentiation of Leydig and Sertoli cells and negatively affecting spermatogenesis.[23]

A study conducted by Krassas et al. (2008) in which semen samples were collected from hypothyroid males followed by treatment, demonstrated a decrease in sperm motility although statistically insignificant. After the euthyroid status was achieved following treatment, sperm morphology remained abnormal, but motility improved **(Flowchart 1)**.[24-26]

Management

The Endocrine Society, American Thyroid Association (ATA), and the American Association of Clinical Endocrinologists (AACE) have established guidelines on whether and when to treat thyroid dysfunction.[21]

- *Nonpregnant women:* Treatment of nonpregnant women for subtle thyroid abnormalities (TSH <5 mIU/L) is currently not recommended.[27] For a given laboratory, reference range should be determined by upper limit of normal for third-generation TSH assay. If this age-based upper limit is not available in an iodine sufficient area, an upper limit of normal of 4.12 mIU/L can be used.[28,29]
- *Pregnant women*—reference range of TSH in pregnancy depends on the trimester:
    - Recommended upper limit of normal in the first trimester—2.5
    - Recommended upper limit of normal in the second and third trimester—3.[14]
- *Women attempting pregnancy:* As the reference values of TSH change when a woman becomes pregnant, using pregnancy thresholds for the treatment of women attempting conception in order to minimize the potential risks associated with SCH in pregnancy has been advocated.[30] However, this is not accepted by all as the data is still insufficient.

Prevention of Overt or Subclinical Hypothyroidism

Women planning pregnancy or already pregnant women are advised to include at least 150 µg of iodine (potassium

Flowchart 1: Clinical evaluation in hypothyroidism.

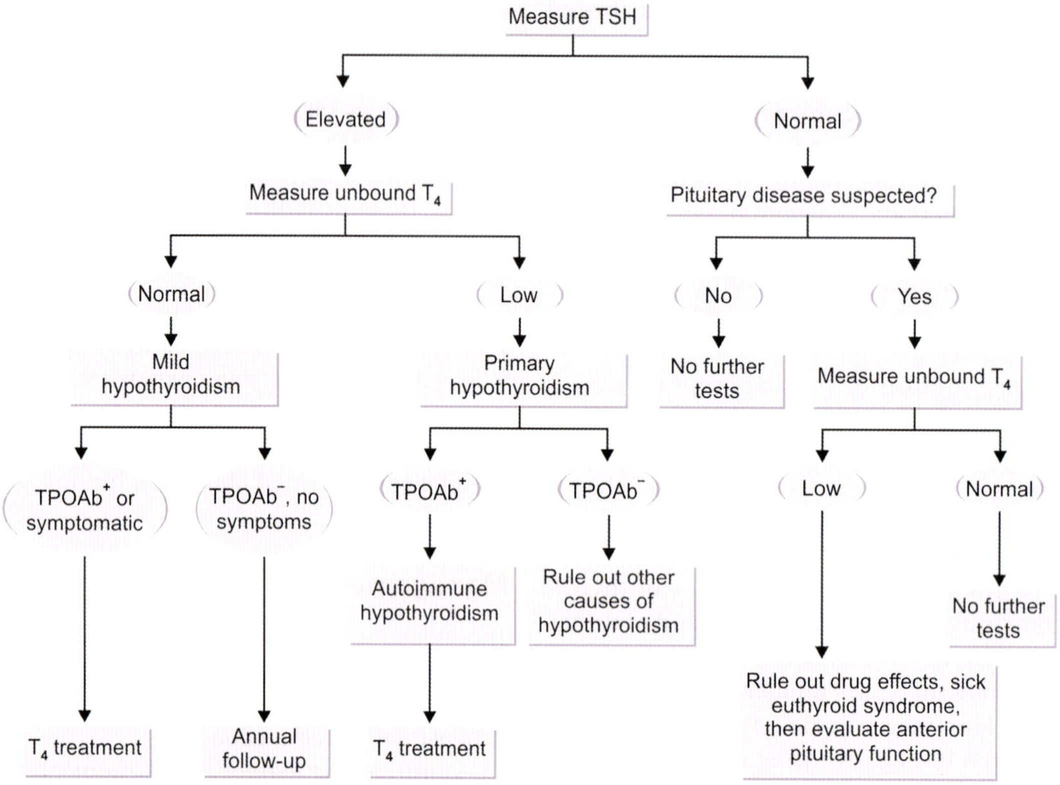

(TPOAb: thyroid peroxidase antibody; TSH: thyroid-stimulating hormone)

iodine), orally 3 months preconception.[14] All women suffering from subfertility and infertility should be evaluated for thyroid status.[14] Further, infertile women with overt hypothyroidism should take LT4 treatment.[14]

- *Limited evidence suggests that SCH (defined as TSH >2.5 mIU/L with a normal FT4) is correlated with infertility.*
- *There is fair evidence that SCH (defined as TSH levels >4 mIU/L) is associated with miscarriage.*
- *Treatment of SCH when TSH levels are more than 4.0 mIU/L is associated with improved pregnancy rates and decreased miscarriage rates.*[27]

Women with SCH undergoing IVF or intracytoplasmic sperm injection (ICSI) should be treated with LT4 with an aim to achieve a TSH concentration below 2.5 mU/L.[14] If there is no residual thyroid function, daily replacement dose of levothyroxine is 1.6 µg/kg/body weight (100–150 µg) to be taken empty stomach.[3] TSH response is gradual and measured at 2 -4 weeks, adjustments to the levothyroxine dose can be made by either increments or decrements of 12.5–25 µg on the basis of TSH levels. Preconceptionally it is crucial to achieve euthyroid status, preferable less than 2.5 TSH. For euthyroid pregnant women who are TPO antibody or thyroglobulin antibody positive, serum TSH measurements should be repeated on confirmation of pregnancy and repeated every month till midpregnancy.[14]

There is no sufficient evidence to say that LT4 therapy improves fertility in subclinically hypothyroid or thyroid autoantibody-negative women who are trying to get pregnant naturally (not undergoing ART). However, LT4 may be considered as it prevents progression of disorder to more significant hypothyroidism once the women gets pregnant as low-dose LT4 therapy (25–50 µg/day) hardly has any disadvantages.[14] The studies supporting LT4 therapy to improve fertility in nonpregnant and thyroid autoantibody-positive euthyroid women seeking natural conception (not undergoing ART) are inadequate, no recommendation can be made for LT4 therapy. Though limited evidence exists to determine advantages of LT4 therapy in improving success rates in TPO antibody-positive euthyroid women undergoing ART, LT4 supplementation (25–50 µg) may be considered.[14]

Thyroid autoantibody-positive euthyroid women undergoing ART—glucocorticoid is not recommended.[14] Euthyroid women with a history of recurrent pregnancy loss—intravenous immunoglobulin treatment is not recommended.[14] Pregnancy loss risk in TPO antibody-positive euthyroid women—insufficient data regarding benefit of LT4. TPO antibody-positive euthyroid pregnant women with a prior history of loss—LT4 (25–50 µg) may be considered given its potential benefits in comparison with its minimal risk.[14]

Thyroid autoimmunity is associated with miscarriage and it is associated with infertility. Levothyroxine treatment may improve pregnancy outcomes in women with positive thyroid antibodies, especially if the TSH level is above 2.5 mIU/L. (ASRM Guidelines)

HYPERTHYROIDISM (BOXES 1 AND 2; TABLE 4)

Definition: It is defined as increase in FT4, FT3, or both with subsequent suppression of pituitary TSH.

Subclinical hyperthyroidism: Normal serum thyroxine (T4) and triiodothyronine (T3), but decreased TSH levels.

In general population, the prevalence of hyperthyroidism is approximately 1.5%.

Hyperthyroidism in Females

Hyperthyroidism in females with infertility as studies by Poppe et al. was 2.3%.[31] In 1993, Joshi et al. described 5.8% infertility in 53 hyperthyroid patients.[32] Thyrotoxicosis leads to increase in serum levels of SHBG. This is seen during all phases of the menstrual cycle, the levels of estrogen are two- to threefold higher in hyperthyroid females as compared to euthyroid.[33] Increased binding of E2 to SHBG results in decreased metabolic clearance rate of estrogen.[34] Mean plasma levels of androstenedione and testosterone also rise. In hyperthyroid women, conversion ratio of androstenedione to estrone, as well as of testosterone to E2, is increased.[35-37] The mid-cycle LH peak is blunted as the baseline LH is frequently elevated, which affects ovulation.

Amenorrhea is associated with hyperthyroidism.[38] Hyperthyroidism may also cause irregular menses.[14] A study by Krassas et al. demonstrated around 22% of hyperthyroid women suffer from menstrual irregularities as compared to 8% in euthyroid controls.[14] A higher total T4 levels were seen in these females. Total T4 levels are a significant factor related to the development of menstrual abnormalities.[39]

Fertility in Subclinical and Overt Hyperthyroidism

Quintino-Moro et al. demonstrated, in a cross-sectional study in infertile women between 18 years and 50 years, that the prevalence of Graves disease was 52.3% and Hashimoto's thyroiditis 47%.[14]

Hyperthyroidism in Males

Thyrotoxic males display elevated SHBG levels,[40] and increased total and bound testosterone (T). Free T is transiently reduced or normal[41] with mean basal

Box 1: Causes of hyperthyroidism.

- Grave's disease
- Solitary toxic nodule
- Toxic multinodular goiter
- *Acute thyroiditis:*
  - Viral
  - Autoimmune
  - Postradiotherapy
- Thyrotoxicosis factitia
- Exogenous iodine administration
- Metastatic differentiated thyroid carcinoma
- Thyroid-stimulating hormone secreting tumors
- Human chorionic gonadotropin secreting tumors
- Hyperfunctioning ovarian teratomas

Box 2: Signs and symptoms in hyperthyroidism.

Signs:
- Psychosis
- Hyperkinesis
- Exophthalmos
- Lid lag
- Conjunctival edema
- Ophthalmoplegia
- Goiter
- Systolic hypertension
- Tachycardia
- Atrial fibrillation
- Fine tremors
- Warm peripheries
- Proximal muscle wasting
- Proximal myopathy
- Palmar erythema
- Pretibial myxedema

Symptoms:
- *Generalized*: Weight loss, increased appetite, irritability, malaise, heat intolerance
- *Musculoskeletal system*: Muscle weakness, tremors, choreoathetosis, myolysis
- *Respiratory and cardiovascular symptom*: Breathlessness, palpitations
- *Gastrointestinal*: Vomiting/diarrhea
- *Reproductive system*: Oligomenorrhea, loss of libido, gynecomastia
- *Miscellaneous*: Eye complaints, tall stature

Table 4: Hormonal changes in hyperthyroidism.

	Thyrotoxicosis	
	Males	***Females***
SHBG	Increases	Increases
E_2	Normal or increases	Increases
Estrone	–	Increases
Production rate of estrogen	–	No change
Metabolic clearance of estrogen or androgen	Decreases	Decreases
Free E_2	Increases	No change
Testosterone	Increases	Increases
Delta 4-androstenedione	–	Increases
DHEA	Increases	Increases
Free testosterone	No change	–
Bioavailable testosterone	Increases	–
Conversion of testosterone to delta 4-androstenedione	Increases	Increases or no change
Androgen conversion to estrone	Increases	Increases
Progesterone	Increases	Decreases or no change
LH	Increases or no change	Increases or no change
FSH	Increases or no change	Increases or no change
After GnRH:		
LH	Increases	Increases
FSH	Increases	Increases

(DHEA: dehydroepiandrosterone; E_2: estrogen; FSH: follicle-stimulating hormone; GnRH: gonadotropin-releasing hormone; LH: luteinizing hormone; SHBG: sex hormone-binding globulin)

bioavailable T decreased.[42] A few hyperthyroid males had high estrogen and enhanced peripheral conversion of androgen to estrogen.[43] These hormonal changes result in various symptoms and signs of estrogen excess leading to gynecomastia (24%),[44] decreased libido (70%),[9] erectile dysfunction (56%),[45] spider angiomas, and spermatogenetic dysfunction.[43,45] There may be minor elevations in basal serum LH and FSH in these men.[46] Rectification of thyrotoxicosis to euthyroid levels reverses these hormonal changes (Flowchart 2). Hyperthyroidism also leads to premature cessation of Sertoli cell proliferation.[1] Hyperthyroid males have 50% less differentiated Sertoli cells as compared to euthyroid males.[44]

Changes in Spermatogenesis

Hudson and Edwards proposed that hyperthyroidism affects sperm density, which is lower than the control, but can be reversed with correction of hyperthyroidism.[47] A prospective study by Krassas et al. in 2002[17] shows diminished sperm density and sperm morphology along with low motility. These were normalized after 5 months of therapy. However, the semen fructose, zinc, and magnesium were unaltered. Thus, hyperthyroidism leading to abnormal seminal parameters can be easily rectified with therapy.[24]

Treatment

If hyperthyroidism is diagnosed in an infertile couple, it warrants a euthyroid condition. Treatment of subclinical hyperthyroidism is unproven, but in face of hyperthyroidism with ovulatory dysfunction empirically treatment with anti-thyroid drugs is recommended.

- *Hyperthyroidism*: Treatment includes use of anti-thyroid drugs or reducing thyroid tissue by radioiodine therapy or thyroidectomy. Thioamides such as propylthiouracil, carbimazole, and methimazole are the main anti-thyroid drugs. They inhibit function of TPO and reduce oxidation and organification of iodide. They also decrease thyroid antibodies.
- *Propylthiouracil*: US Food and Drug Administration (FDA) approved in 1st trimester of pregnancy, thyroid storm, and adverse reactions to methimazole. Starting doses can be gradually reduced by titration. Alternatively, high doses with levothyroxine can be given (block replace regime) to avoid drug-induced hypothyroidism.

Thyroid function tests and clinical indications are evaluated in 4–6 weeks after starting the treatment and the dose is titrated based on unbound T4. 6–8 weeks of treatment is required. Careful control of thyrotoxicosis with antithyroid drugs, followed by potassium iodide therapy, is needed prior to surgery to reduce risk of thyrotoxicosis and reduce vascularity of the gland.

Complications of surgery:

- Bleeding
- Laryngeal edema
- Hypothyroidism

Flowchart 2: Evaluation of thyrotoxicosis.

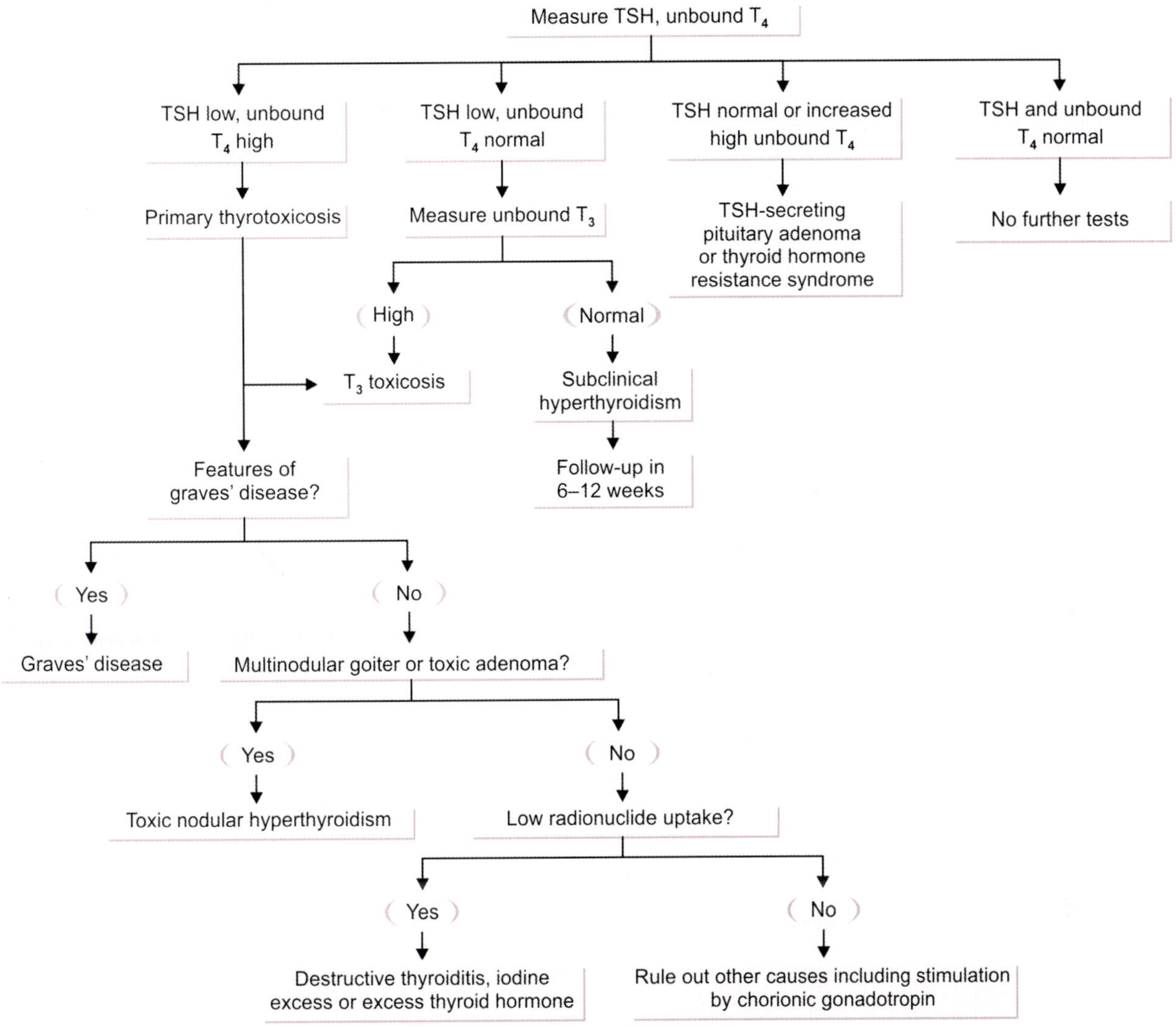

(TSH: thyroid-stimulating hormone)

- Hypoparathyroidism
- Recurrent laryngeal nerve injury.

Radioiodine [dosage: 370 MBq (10 mCi) and 555MBq (15mCi)] causes gradual destruction of thyroid tissue and may be used as initial treatment or for relapses after anti-thyroid drugs.

Radioactive iodine (I-131) therapy and infertility:

- Hyperthyroidism—I131, 10 mCi (370 MBq).
- The radiation effects of I-131 are more distinct in males as testis (highly radiosensitive).
- *Outcomes*: Transient suppression of spermatogenesis to azoospermia.
- Transient FSH elevations and inhibin B suppression can occur, starting at 3–6 months post–I-131 and lasting up to 18 months.[48-50]
- All young males need to be offered option of sperm cryopreservation before I-131 for fertility preservation,[51,52] especially in whom higher or cumulative doses of I-131 are indicated.
- Genetic risk in thyrotoxic women treated with 10 mCi of I-131 is negligible.[53]
- Conception is recommended after 1 year from I-131 treatment due to increased risk of miscarriage (40%) in first 12 months.[54]
- The offspring of men and women treated with ablative doses of I-131 neither showed increased in genetic risk

Table 5: Guidelines of international societies regarding investigation approaches in infertile women before or during pregnancy.

Society	Before ovarian stimulation	During ovarian stimulation	During (early) pregnancy
ASRM	It is rational to test TSH in infertile women planning conception.	No recommendation	No recommendation
ATA	Women with infertility should have screening with TSH, as part of their infertility workup.	There is insufficient evidence to recommend for or against screening for thyroid antibodies in women undergoing IVF.	Serum TSH values should be obtained early in pregnancy in women at high risk for overt hypothyroidism (including those with infertility)
ES	Individuals at high risk for thyroid illness (including infertile women or those with a known thyroid disease) should be identified before pregnancy and TSH should be measured. Universal screening for anti-TPO antibodies before pregnancy is not recommended.	No recommendation.	No agreement regarding screening recommendations for all newly pregnant women Universal screening for anti-TPO antibodies during pregnancy is not recommended.
ETA	No recommendation.	No recommendation.	▪ Evidence for screening for SCH in pregnancy is equivocal. ▪ Trimester-specific reference ranges for TSH and T4 (total or free) should be established in each antenatal hospital setting. If not available, the following reference range upper limits are recommended: First trimester 2.5 mIU/mL, second trimester 3.0 mIU/mL, and third trimester 3.5 mIU/mL. In hypothyroid women already treated with LT4 before conception, TSH should be checked every 4–6 weeks during the first trimester and once during the second and third trimesters.

(Anti-TPO: thyroid peroxidase antibodies; ASRM: American Society of Reproductive Medicine; ATA: American Thyroid Association; ES: Endocrine Society (US); ETA: European Thyroid Association; IVF: in-vitro fertilization; LT4: levothyroxine; SCH: subclinical hypothyroidism; T4: thyroxine; TSH: thyroid-stimulating hormone)

nor increased in incidence of thyroid dysfunction or malignancy.

REFERENCES

1. Wagner MS, Wajner SM, Maia AL. Is there a role for thyroid hormone on spermatogenesis? Microsc Res Tech. 2009;72:796-808.
2. Nussey S, Whitehead S. Endocrinology: An Intergrated Approach. BIOS Scientific. Oxford: Publishers; 2001.
3. Maia AL, Kim BW, Huang SA, et al. Type 2 iodothyronine deiodinase is the major source of plasma T3 in euthyroid humans. J Clin Invest. 2005;115:2524-33.
4. Krassas GE, Poppe K, Glinoer D. Thyroid Function and Human Reproductive Health. Endocr Rev. 2010;31:702-55.
5. Department of Endocrinology, Diabetes, and Metabolism (G.E.K.), Panagia General Hospital, 55132 Thessaloniki, Greece; Department of Endocrinology (K.P.), University Hospital Brugmann, 1020 Brussels, Belgium; and Division of Endocrinology (D.G.), Department of Internal Medicine, University Hospital Saint-Pierre, 1000 Brussels, Belgium 5. HARRISON
6. Ross DS. Serum thyroid-stimulating hormone measurement for assessment of thyroid function and disease. Endocrinol Metab Clin North Am. 2001;30:245-64.
7. Hollowell JG, Staehling NW, Flanders WD, et al. Serum TSH, T(4), and thyroid antibodies in the United States population (1988 to 1994): National Health and Nutrition Examination Survey (NHANES III). J Clin Endocrinol Metab. 2002;87:489-99.
8. Canaris GJ, Manowitz NR, Mayor G, et al. The Colorado thyroid disease prevalence study. Arch Intern Med. 2000;160:526-34.
9. Davis SL. Environmental modulation of the immune system via the endocrine system. Domest Anim Endocrinol. 1998;15:283-9.
10. Stagnaro-Green A, Chen X, Bogden JD, et al. The thyroid and pregnancy: a novel risk factor for very preterm delivery. Thyroid. 2005;15:351-7.

11. Haddow JE, Palomaki GE, Allan WC, et al. Maternal thyroid deficiency during pregnancy and subsequent neuropsychological development of the child. N Engl J Med. 1999;341:549-55.
12. Arojoki M, Jokimaa V, Juuti A, et al. Hypothyroidism among infertile women in Finland. Gynecol Endocrinol. 2000;14: 127-31.
13. Lincoln SR, Ke RW, Kutteh WH. Screening for hypothyroidism in infertile women. J Reprod Med. 1999;44:455-7.
14. Strickland DM, Whitted WA, Wians FH Jr. Screening infertile women for subclinical hypothyroidism. Am J Obstet Gynecol. 1990;163:262-3.
15. Abalovich M, Amino N, Barbour LA, et al. Management of thyroid dysfunction during pregnancy and postpartum: an Endocrine Society Clinical Practice Guideline. J Clin Endocrinol Metab. 2007;92:S1-47.
16. Garber JR, Cobin RH, Gharib H, et al. Clinical practice guidelines for hypothyroidism in adults: cosponsored by the American Association of Clinical Endocrinologists and the American Thyroid Association. Endocr Pract. 2012;18:988-1028.
17. Surks MI, Ortiz E, Daniels GH, Sawin CT, et al. Subclinical thyroid disease: scientific review and guidelines for diagnosis and management. JAMA. 2004;291:228-38.
18. Michalakis KG, Mesen TB, Brayboy LM, et al. Subclinical elevations of thyroid-stimulating hormone and assisted reproductive technology outcomes. Fertil Steril. 2011;95:2634-7.
19. Haddow JE, Knight GJ, Palomaki GE, et al. The reference range and within-person variability of thyroid stimulating hormone during the first and second trimesters of pregnancy. J Med Screen. 2004;11:170-4.
20. Bjoro T, Holmen J, Kruger O, et al. Prevalence of thyroid disease, thyroid dysfunction and thyroid peroxidase antibodies in a large, unselected population. The Health Study of Nord-Trondelag (HUNT). Eur J Endocrinol. 2000;143:639-47.
21. Meier C, Christ-Crain M, Guglielmetti M, et al. Prolactin dysregulation in women with subclinical hypothyroidism: effect of levothyroxine replacement therapy. Thyroid. 2003;13:979-85.
22. Hanna CE, LaFranchi SH. Adolescent thyroid disorders. Adolesc Med. 2002;13:13-35.
23. Velazquez EM, Bellabarba Arata G. Effects of thyroid status on pituitary gonadotropin and testicular reserve in men. Arch Androl. 1997;38:85-92.
24. Wortsman J, Rosner W, Dufau ML. Abnormal testicular function in men with primary hypothyroidism. Am J Med. 1987;82:207-12.
25. Jaya Kumar B, Khurana ML, Ammini AC, et al. Reproductive endocrine functions in men with primary hypothyroidism: effect of thyroxine replacement. Horm Res. 1990;34:215-8.
26. Corrales Hernandez JJ, Miralles Garcia JM, Garcia Diez LC. Primary hypothyroidism and human spermatogenesis. Arch Androl. 1990;25:21-7.
27. Gallagher TF, Fukushima DK, Noguchi S, et al. Recent studies in steroid hormone metabolism in man. Recent Prog Horm Res. 1966;22:283-303.
28. Carani C, Isidori AM, Granata A, et al. Multicenter study on the prevalence of sexual symptoms in male hypo- and hyperthyroid patients. J Clin Endocrinol Metab. 2005;90: 6472-9.
29. Krassas GE, Pontikides N. Male reproductive function in relation with thyroid alterations. Best Pract Res Clin Endocrinol Metab. 2004;18:183-95.
30. Wajner SM, Wagner MS, Maia AL. Clinical implications of altered thyroid status in male testicular function. Arq Bras Endocrinol Metabol. 2009;53:976-82.
31. Anbalagan J, Sashi AM, Vengatesh G, et al. Mechanism underlying transient gestational-onset hypothyroidism-induced impairment of posttesticular sperm maturation in adult rats. Fertil Steril. 2010;93:2491-7.
32. Wang C, Crapo LM. The epidemiology of thyroid disease and implications for screening. Endocrinol Metab Clin North Am. 1997;26:189-218.
33. Poppe K, Glinoer D, Van Steirteghem A, et al. Thyroid dysfunction and autoimmunity in infertile women. Thyroid. 2002;12:997-1001.
34. Joshi JV, Bhandarkar SD, Chadha M, et al. Menstrual irregularities and lactation failure may precede thyroid dysfunction or goitre. J Postgrad Med. 1993;39:137-41.
35. Akande EO, Hockaday TD. Plasma oestrogen and luteinizing hormone concentrations in thyrotoxic menstrual disturbance. Proc R Soc Med. 1972;65:789-90.
36. Ridgway EC, Longcope C, Maloof F. Metabolic clearance and blood production rates of estradiol in hyperthyroidism. J Clin Endocrinol Metab. 1975;41:491-7.
37. Southren AL, Olivo J, Gordon GG, et al. The conversion of androgens to estrogens in hyperthyroidism. J Clin Endocrinol Metab. 1974;38:207-14.
38. Burrow GN. The thyroid gland and reproduction. In: Yen SS, Jaffe RB (Eds). Reproductive endocrinology. Philadelphia: WB Saunders; 1986. pp. 424-40.
39. KrassasGE. The male and female reproductive system in thyrotoxicosis. In: Braverman LE, Utiger RD (Eds). Werner and Ingbar's the thyroid—a fundamental and clinical text, 9th edition. Philadelphia: Lippincott Williams &Wilkins; 2005. pp. 621-8.
40. Tanaka T, Tamai H, Kuma K, et al. Gonadotropin response to luteinizing hormone releasing hormone in hyperthyroid patients with menstrual disturbances. Metabolism. 1981;30:323-26.
41. von Basedow CA. Exophthalmus durch Hypertrophiedes Zellgewebes in der Augenhoehle. Wochenschriftfuer die Gesamte Heilkunde. 1840;6:197-204; 220-8.
42. Krassas GE, Pontikides N, Kaltsas T, et al. Menstrual disturbances in thyrotoxicosis. Clin Endocrinol (Oxford). 1994;40:641-4.
43. Goldsmith RE, Sturgis SH, Lerman J, et al. The menstrual pattern in thyroid disease. J Clin Endocrinol Metab. 1952;12:846-55.
44. Abalovich M, Levalle O, Hermes R, et al. Hypothalamic-pituitary-testicular axis and seminal parameters in hyperthyroid males. Thyroid. 1999;9:857-63.

45. Ruder H, Corvol P, Mahoudeau JA, et al. Effects of induced hyperthyroidism on steroid metabolism in man. J Clin Endocrinol Metab. 1971;33:382-7.
46. Kidd GS, Glass AR, Vigersky RA. The hypothalamic-pituitary-testicular axis in thyrotoxicosis. J Clin Endocrinol Metab. 1979;48:798-80.
47. Ridgway EC, Maloof F, Longcope C. Androgen and oestrogen dynamics in hyperthyroidism. J Endocrinol. 1982;95:105-15.
48. Krassas GE, Perros P. Thyroid disease and male reproductive function. J Endocrinol Invest. 2003;26:372-80.
49. Zahringer S, Tomova A, von Werder K, et al. The influence of hyperthyroidism on the hypothalamic-pituitary-gonadal axis. Exp Clin Endocrinol Diabetes. 2000;108:282-9.
50. Rijntjes E, Wientjes AT, Swarts HJ, et al. Dietary-induced hyperthyroidism marginally affects neonatal testicular development. J Androl. 2008;29:643-53.
51. Hudson RW, Edwards AL. Testicular function in hyperthyroidism. J Androl. 1992;73:117-24.
52. Meikle AW. The interrelationships between thyroid dysfunction and hypogonadism in men and boys. Thyroid. 2004;14:S17-25.
53. Carani C, Isidori AM, Granata A, et al. Multicenter study on the prevalence of sexual symptoms in male hypo- and hyperthyroid patients. J Clin Endocrinol Metab. 2005;90:6472-9.
54. Wichers M, Benz E, Palmedo H, et al. Testicular function after radioiodine therapy for thyroid carcinoma. Eur J Nucl Med. 2000;27:503-7.

Prolactin and Infertility

6

Manisha Takhtani Kundnani, Vanie Thapar

INTRODUCTION

Prolactin: The Hormone

Prolactin (PRL) is a hormone secreted by the lactotrophs in the anterior pituitary gland and is chemically similar to growth hormone (GH) and human placental lactogen. A single gene located on chromosome 5 encodes its synthesis and function. Various variants like little prolactin, big prolactin, and big big prolactin (macroprolactin) have been identified based on the size and structural modifications.

The secretion of prolactin is under hypothalamic control, predominantly by the tonic inhibition of Dopamine [also known as prolactin-release-inhibiting factor (PIF)], while the stimulatory signal is mediated by the hypothalamic thyrotropin-releasing hormone (TRH). The balance between Dopamine and TRH determines the amount of PRL released.[1] Estrogen on the other hand increases prolactin synthesis, while serotonin stimulates prolactin release. Several other extrapituitary sources such as placental lactogens, mammary glands, or PRL variants of immune cell origin may contribute to PRL-like substances in the periphery. Prolactin secretion follows a circadian rhythm, with the maximum secretion 5–8 hours after the onset of sleep. The release is pulsatile, and the frequency of pulses is maximum at midcycle and then it declines in the luteal phase.

PROLACTIN: FUNCTIONS AND ROLE IN REPRODUCTIVE PHYSIOLOGY

Prolactin plays many different roles in the body. The crucial one is the preparation of mammary glands for breastfeeding and stimulation of milk production in the postpartum period. Persistently high levels of prolactin in the initial a few months of breastfeeding suppress ovulation, mainly by suppression of LH. Breastfeeding women are thus amenorrheic and do not get pregnant. It also plays a significant role on fertility, immunity, and liver functions.

Prolactin also plays a role in regulation of reproductive function. It negatively modulates the secretion of luteinizing hormone (LH) and follicle-stimulating hormone (FSH) from the pituitary thereby affecting the gonadal functions. It has also been shown essential to maintain regular estrous cycles[2] and also to stimulate ovarian production of progesterone.[3]

Prolactin: Role in Male Reproductive Physiology

As in women, prolactin significantly affects the male reproductive systems. It acts on the hypothalamopituitary axis and affects the gonads, accessory reproductive glands, and sexual behavior. Hyperprolactinemia in males inhibits the pulsatile release of LH and inhibits the 5alpha-reductase activity, thus resulting in decreased testosterone levels and affecting spermatogenesis.[4,5] Many structural changes at microscopic levels like increased tubule wall thickness, germ cell exfoliation, disorganization of seminiferous tubules have been seen in hyperprolactinemic males.

HYPERPROLACTINEMIA AND INFERTILITY

High-prolactin levels or hyperprolactinemia can be associated with infertility in several ways. It is considered as the most common cause of anovulatory sterility. In women with reproductive disorders, the prevalence of hyperprolactinemia has been reported to be as high as 17%.[6]

High prolactin affects fertility by causing disruption of normal follicular development and atresia of the dominant follicle. It also suppresses LH activity thereby causing anovulation. It can also inhibit ovulation by inhibiting the activity of human chorionic gonadotropin (hCG).[7] Women with less severe hyperprolactinemia have intermittent disruption of ovulation. These women usually complain of irregular menstruation. Those with mild elevation of prolactin can have regular cycles, but usually have defective progesterone secretion resulting in luteal phase defect.[8] Elevated prolactin levels have also shown to induce adenomyosis in animal studies, which can also affect the fertility.[9]

Causes of Hyperprolactinemia

Hyperprolactinemia is one of the most common endocrine disorders of hypothalamopituitary axis. It can either be due to certain physiological conditions like pregnancy, breast stimulation, stress or coitus; or pathological conditions like pituitary tumors, hypothalamic pituitary lesions, hypothyroidism, polycystic ovarian syndrome (PCOS), drugs (dopamine analogs), or other conditions like chest wall injury, liver or renal failure.

Pituitary Tumors

Prolactin-secreting pituitary adenoma is the most common pituitary gland tumor. However, only two-thirds of pituitary-secreting adenomas are associated with hypersecretion of hormones. The rest are either asymptomatic or associated with symptoms of intracranial space-occupying lesions like headaches, nausea, vomiting, or visual field disturbances.

Magnetic resonance imaging (MRI) is the investigation of choice to diagnose adenomas. Adenomas are divided into microadenomas (less than 10 mm) or macroadenomas (more than 10 mm) depending upon their size. Microadenomas can also be seen in healthy people with normal prolactin levels. These usually do not grow large and can be treated with medications. Macroadenomas, however, need to be treated as these have the potential of growing further and compressing the neighboring vital structures and tissues.

Hypothyroidism

There is increased secretion of TRH from the hypothalamus in hypothyroid patients. TRH, in addition to stimulating the release of TSH, also increases the release of prolactin from the lactotrophs. Correction of hypothyroidism by thyroid supplements usually results in correction of both.

Polycystic Ovarian Syndrome

Many women with PCOS have increased prolactin levels. However, the relationship between PCOS and hyperprolactinemia is still controversial and it has been suggested that these pathologies have independent origins. According to the current guidelines, hyperprolactinemic women with PCOS should be evaluated for all other causes of hyperprolactinemia. Filho et al. studied 82 PCOS women and found that 16% have raised prolactin levels. These women with increased prolactin had different pathologies like pituitary adenoma, drug-induced hyperprolactinemia or macroprolactinemia. The authors thus concluded that hyperprolactinemia is not a manifestation of PCOS.[10]

Drug-induced Hyperprolactinemia

Many medications are known to cause increased prolactin levels. These medicines act as dopaminergic receptor blockers leading to inhibition of inhibitory control of hypothalamus on the pituitary. Most common of these are the antipsychotics. Other medicines that can cause raised prolactin include **(Flowchart 1)**:
- *Antidepressants*: Selective serotonin reuptake inhibitors (SSRIs) and serotonin reuptake inhibitors (SRIs) (fluvoxamine, fluoxetine, and paroxetine)
- Sedatives
- Anticonvulsants
- Opiates/opiate antagonists
- Estrogen/oral contraceptives
- Antacids (cimetidine)
- Metoclopramide
- *Antihypertensives*: Methyldopa and verapamil.

Clinical Manifestations of Hyperprolactinemia

The manifestations of hyperprolactinemia can either be due to excess prolactin; or could be because of the pressure effects of the adenomas on the neighboring structures. Increased prolactin levels can directly lead to induction of galactorrhea or hypogonadism.[11] Patients can otherwise present with headaches, visual field defects, or external ophthalmoplegia, which are caused by the pressure effect of the adenoma on neighboring vital structures.

Approximately, 50% of women with hyperprolactinemia have galactorrhea. However, many women with normal prolactin levels can present with galactorrhea. Menstrual abnormalities like amenorrhea or oligomenorrhea, or regular cycles with infertility are another common symptom in hyperprolactinemic women. Sometimes, patients may present with menorrhagia.

Sexual dysfunction, decreased libido, impotence, gynecomastia, and infertility are common symptoms in men with increased prolactin levels.[12] In contrast to women, men often present late in the course of the disease with symptoms of expansion of their pituitary tumor (i.e. headaches, visual defects, and external ophthalmoplegia) or symptoms from secondary adrenal or thyroid failure.

Young girls with hyperprolactinemia can present pubertal disorders, primary or secondary amenorrhea, hypogonadotropic hypogonadism, and galactorrhea.[13]

Diagnosis

A definitive diagnosis of hyperprolactinemia can only be made with laboratory test. It should ideally be measured in morning, after at least 8–10 hours of fasting, as food intake can affect the values. Stimulation of breast and nipples and sexual contact from a day prior should be avoided as this may cause prolonged alteration in the prolactin values.[14] The test is ideally conducted in the first half of the menstrual cycle.

Normal serum prolactin levels are generally in the range of 5-20 ng/mL in both sexes, though there can be individual laboratory variations. A value of more than 20 ng/mL on two successive measurements is defined as hyperprolactinemia. Patients with modest serum prolactin elevations should have multiple serum assays to rule out transient or physiological elevation. History of drug intake, thyroid or renal or hepatic dysfunction should be elicited.

The MRI of pituitary gland is recommended in all cases of increased prolactin to diagnose any pituitary tumor. PRL levels of more than 250 ng/mL usually indicate presence of prolactinoma; whereas, levels more than 500 ng/mL are considered diagnostic of macroprolactinoma.[15]

Patients with asymptomatic hyperprolactinemia should be evaluated for presence of macroprolactins. Serial dilutions of semen samples are recommended to rule out "hook effect" when there is discrepancy between a large pituitary tumor and a mild elevation in prolactin level.

In spite of thorough investigations, in many cases, no cause can be determined and these are considered idiopathic **(Flowchart 2)**.

Management of Hyperprolactinemia

First step in the management of hyperprolactinemia is the critical diagnosis. Specific tests should be conducted to rule out hypothyroidism, drug-induced hyperprolactinemia, renal or hepatic failure; and these should be treated accordingly.

Patients with *drug-induced hyperprolactinemia* need not be treated, if they are asymptomatic. The drug should either be discontinued or an alternative drug be substituted in symptomatic patients. However, if it is not possible to stop or substitute the drug, dopamine agonist should be prescribed with caution.

In patients with *hypothyroidism*, supplementation with thyroid supplements usually restores the normal prolactin levels.

Pituitary tumors can be managed by observation, medical therapy, surgery, or radiation. Asymptomatic patients with microprolactinomas need no treatment and are kept under observation.

Flowchart 1: Control of prolactin release from the hypothalamus.

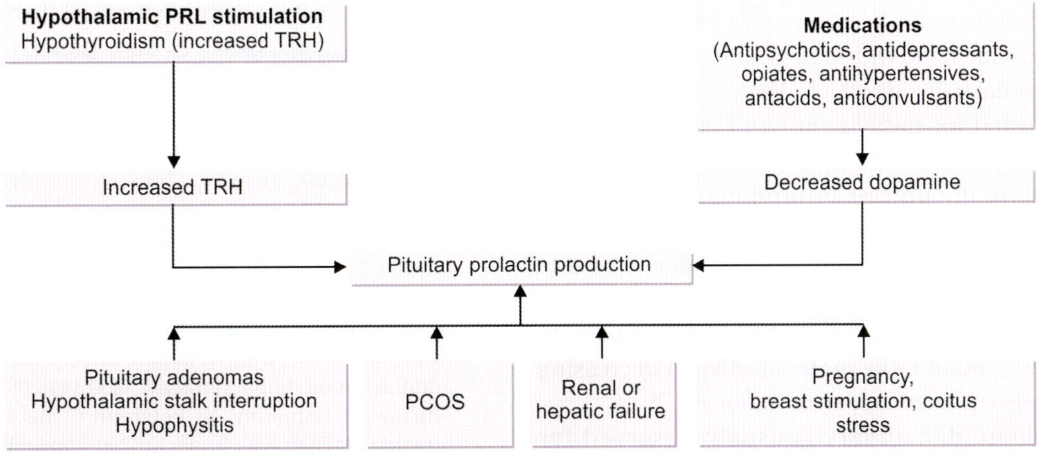

(PRL: prolactin; PCOS: polycystic ovarian syndrome; TRH: thyrotropin-releasing hormone).

Flowchart 2: Diagnosis and management of hyperprolactinemia.

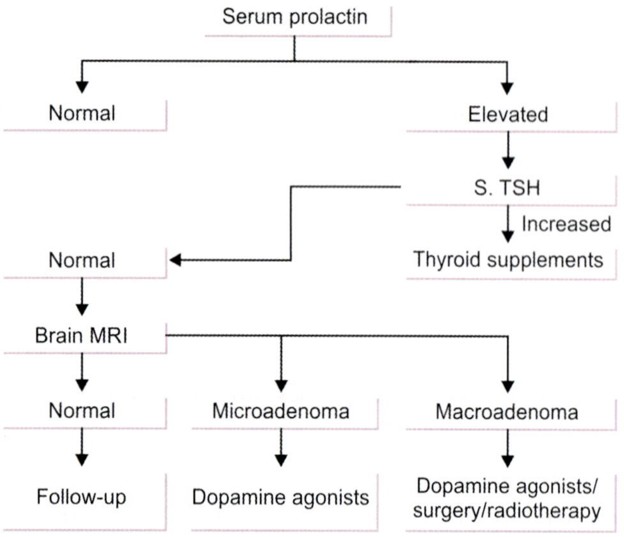

(MRI: magnetic resonance imaging; TSH: thyroid-stimulating hormone)

Dopamine agonists are the drug of choice in patients with symptomatic prolactin-secreting microadenomas or macroadenomas. These drugs effectively reduce prolactin levels and tumor size; and also help to restore gonadal functions. Cabergoline (0.5 mg once or twice a week) and bromocriptine (2.5 mg once or twice a day) are the two commonly used drugs. While on medical therapy, serum prolactin levels should be assessed in 3–4 weeks to see the efficacy and also titrate the dosages. Once the prolactin levels have normalized, evaluation can be done once in 6–12 months.

Bromocriptine is usually initiated at doses of 1.25–2.5 mg once daily at bedtime and gradually increased by 1.25 mg every week till desirable serum prolactin levels are obtained. The common side effects observed are nausea, diarrhea, abdominal pain, headache, dizziness, and fatigue. It is usually administered with food to reduce the incidence of gastrointestinal (GI) side effects. Vaginal administration is recommended for patients not able to tolerate oral bromocriptine.

Cabergoline in contrast to bromocriptine has the advantage of once or twice weekly dosages thereby increasing patients' compliance. The incidence of side effects also is much lower than bromocriptine. The usual dose is 1–2 mg/week. When compared to other dopamine agonists, it was found to be more effective in decreasing prolactin levels and in reduction of tumor size.[16]

Transsphenoidal surgery is usually reserved for symptomatic patients who are unable to tolerate or who do not respond to dopamine agonist therapy or those who have persistent visual symptoms despite adequate medical treatment. Patients with persistent disease following surgery or those with aggressive or malignant prolactinomas are advised radiation therapy. The main disadvantage of radiation therapy is delayed and inconsistent results along with the fear of damaging surrounding structures and the risk of hypopituitarism.

Pregnant Women with Prolactinomas

Women with invasive macroadenomas or adenomas close to optic chiasm are advised to continue dopamine agonist therapy during pregnancy. Serum prolactin levels should not be performed during pregnancy. MRI during pregnancy is recommended only if there is evidence of tumor growth such as visual field impairment. Bromocriptine therapy is recommended for women who experience symptomatic growth of prolactinomas during pregnancy.

SUMMARY

Prolactin is a hormone secreted by the anterior pituitary with the classic role of preparation of breast and stimulation of milk production. An increased serum prolactin levels can be observed in a variety of physiological and pathological conditions.

Hyperprolactinemia is a common cause of amenorrhea and infertility. The goals of the therapy are to normalize prolactin, restore gonadal function and fertility, and to reduce the tumor size. Dopamine agonists are effective in normalization of prolactin levels and restoration of fertility in most patients. Cabergoline is found to be more effective with less side effects. Surgery is recommended for resistant cases or for those not tolerating medical therapy.

REFERENCES

1. Verhelst J, Abs R. Hyperprolactinemia. Pathophysiology and management. Treat Endocrinol. 2003;2:23-32.
2. Horseman ND, Zhao W, Montecino-Rodriguez E, et al. Defective mammopoiesis, but normal hematopoiesis, in mice with a targeted disruption of the prolactin gene. EMBO Journal. 1997;16:6926-35.
3. Binart N, Helloco C, Ormandy CJ, et al. Rescue of preimplantatory egg development and embryo implantation in prolactin receptor-deficient mice after progesterone administration. Endocrinology. 2000;141:2691-7.
4. Murray FT, Cameron DF, Ketchum C. Return of gonadal functions in men with prolactin-secreting pituitary tumors. J Clin Endocrinol Metab. 1984;59:79.

5. Bartke A, Lloyd CW. Influence of prolactin and pituitary isografts on spermatogenesis in dwarf mice and hypophysectomised rats. J Endocrinol. 1982;46:321.
6. Crosignani PG. Management of hyperprolactinemia in infertility. J Reprod Med. 1999;44:1116-20.
7. Yoshimura Y, Tada S, Oda T, et al. Direct inhibitory ovarian effects of prolactin in the process of ovulation. Nihon Sanka Fujinka Gakkai Zasshi. 1989;41:83-9.
8. Shibli-Rahhal A, Schlechte J. Hyperprolactinemia and infertility. Endocrinol Metab Clin North Am. 2011;40:837-46.
9. Mori T, Singtripop T, Kawashima S. Animal model of uterine adenomyosis: is prolactin a potent inducer of adenomyosis in mice? Am J Obstet Gynecol. 1991;165:232.
10. Filho RB, Domingues L, Naves L, et al. Polycystic ovary syndrome and hyperprolactinemia are distinct entities. Gynecol Endocrinol. 2007;23:267-72.
11. Klibanski A. Clinical practice. Prolactinomas. N Engl J Med. 2010;362:1219-26.
12. Colao A, Vitale G, Di Sarno A, et al. Prolactin and prostate hypertrophy: a pilot observational, prospective, case-control study in men with prolactinoma. J Clin Endocrinol Metabol. 2004;89:2770-5.
13. Fideleff HL, Boquete HR, Sequera A, et al. Peripubertal prolactinomas: clinical presentation and long-term outcome with different therapeutic approaches. J Pediatr Endocrinol Metab. 2000;13:261-7.
14. Kruger TH, Leeners B, Naegeli E, et al. Prolactin secretory rhythm in women: immediate and long-term alterations after sexual contact. Hum Reprod. 2012;27:1139-43.
15. Melmed S, Casanueva FF, Hoffman AR, et al.; Endocrine Society. Diagnosis and treatment of hyperprolactinemia: an Endocrine Society clinical practice guideline. J Clin Endocrinol Metab. 2011;96:273-88.
16. Wang AT, Mullan RJ, Lane MA, et al. Treatment of hyperprolactinemia: a systematic review and meta-analysis. Syst Rev. 2012;24:33.

Obesity and Infertility

7

Sanjay Makwana, Renu Makwana

INTRODUCTION

Obesity is a common problem among women of reproductive age nowadays. Obesity and overweight involves an abnormal fat accumulation creating a new endocrine organ (adipose tissue) in the body that negatively affects the health of the body via noncommunicable disease risks. It is associated with health risks due to hyperinsulinemia and hyperleptinemia with significant adverse impact on fertility. It affects both males and females by affecting hypothalamic-pituitary-gonadal axis influencing spermatogenesis and ovulation. Due to increased body mass index (BMI), unpredictable response to ovulation induction drugs is noted resulting in decreased fecundity. High BMI carries increased chances of miscarriages, congenital anomalies and pregnancy complications. Couples should be advised for a modification in lifestyle to achieve normal BMI before planning for conception. Even moderate change of 5–10% of weight can do wonders by improving metabolic markers and fertility restoration.

Obesity is an undesirable product of modern era. It has been associated with decreased fecundity. Women with high BMI usually have irregular menstrual cycles, subfertility, polycystic ovarian syndrome (PCOS) and miscarriages. Even when they get pregnant, pregnancy is a roller coaster ride for them as chances of pre-eclampsia, gestational diabetes mellitus, intranatal and postnatal complications are more frequently encountered due to disturbed metabolic milieu and mechanical problems. Due to increased BMI, unpredictable response to ovulation induction drugs is noted along with decreased oocyte retrieval. Poor pregnancy rates are seen as there is decrease in embryo quality. Mechanical hindrance in these patients may affect safety of anesthesia, under dosing of drug, sonographic visualization of ovaries during ovum pick-up. Suboptimal sonographic visualization may miss some anomalies during antenatal period.

CLASSIFICATION OF OBESITY

According to World Health Organization (WHO), obesity is classified as class I for a BMI between 30 kg/m^2 and 34.9 kg/m^2, class II for a BMI between 35 kg/m^2 and 39.9 kg/m^2, and class III for a BMI greater than or equal to 40 kg/m^2. In turn, class I obesity is associated with (hence, labeled as) a "moderate risk", class II with a "high risk", and class III with a "very high risk" of mortality **(Table 1)**.

Table 1: Classification of obesity.

WHO definitions		***Surgical literature***	
BMI	***Classification***	***BMI***	***Classification***
<18.5	Underweight	<18.5	Underweight
18.5–24.9	Normal weight	18.5–24.9	Normal weight
25.0–29.9	Overweight	25.0–29.9	Overweight
30.0–34.9	Class I obesity	30.0–34.9	Obesity
35.0–39.9	Class II obesity	≥35 to 40	Severe obesity
≥40.0	Class III obesity	40–44.9	Morbid obesity
		≥45 to 50	*Super obesity*
BMI = Body weight/square of height		Metric: BMI = Kilograms/meters^2	

(BMI: body mass index)

Lifestyle changes, lack of exercise, and changes in dietary habits (Lawlor et al., 2003) leading to an excess of calorie intake over expenditure are major culprits. There is a fivefold rise in obesity in children's having obese parents. The distribution of body fat defines type of obesity which is more important than actual body weight. The Waist-hip ratio is better correlated with metabolic risks. The waist-hip ratio is inversely associated with metabolic risks (cardiovascular, diabetes and hypertension), waist circumference is difficult to measure in obese individuals and is variable, while BMI is easy to measure with less interobserver variability. Insulin resistance is an important marker of the metabolic effect of obesity.

ANATOMIC OBESITY

The anatomic obesity can be defined as per the distribution of fat **(Fig. 1)**.

- *Android obesity*: The fat is mostly distributed in the abdominal wall and in visceral mesentery, also known as central obesity or apple-shaped obesity. This fat is more active metabolically and easily delivers triglycerides to other tissues. This location of fat makes it less sensitive to insulin and more sensitive to catecholamines. Android obesity is associated with hyperinsulinemia, impaired glucose tolerance, diabetes mellitus, an increase in androgen production rates, decreased levels of sex hormone-binding globulin, and increased levels of free testosterone and estradiol (E2). Women with central obesity have decreased cortisol levels, which is consistent with increased leptin levels. Significant improvement can be observed in metabolic parameters with weight loss.

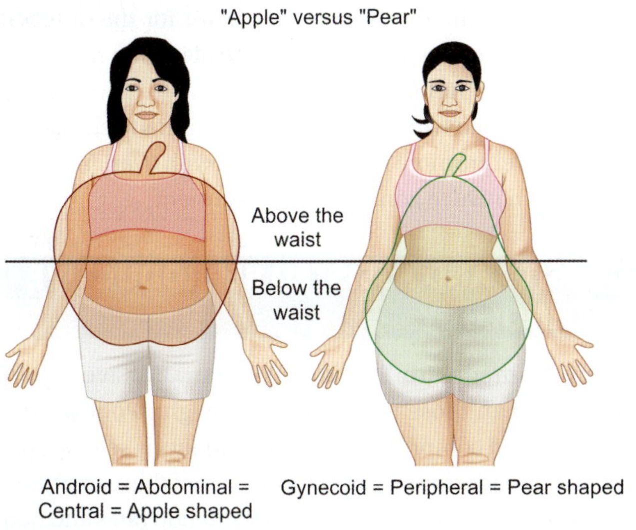

Fig. 1: Types of obesity, apple and pear-shaped person's body.

- *Gynecoid obesity*: Fat distribution in the lower body (femoral and gluteal regions) is known as gynoid type obesity (the pear shape). This type of obesity is more resistant to catecholamine and more sensitive to insulin than abdominal fat.

Fat is accumulated more in the lower body especially thighs and buttocks making a pear shape.

ENDOCRINE CHANGES IN OBESITY

The most important endocrine change in obesity is hyperinsulinemia/insulin resistance which is proportional to body fat. The reduced glucose response to a given amount of insulin is defined as the insulin resistance and may occur secondary to receptor resistance or decreased hepatic clearance of insulin and/or increased pancreatic sensitivity.

The other factors that affect insulin resistance are the amount of adipose tissue in the body, food habits and energy expenditures. Insulin receptors are downregulated by increase in insulin secretion. The insulin resistance affects the metabolism of carbohydrate, fat, and protein. Circulating levels of free fatty acids increase as a result of inadequate insulin suppression of the fat cell. Insulin resistance results in decreased catabolism of triglycerides, resulting in decrease in high-density lipoprotein (HDL) cholesterol and an increase in low-density lipoprotein (LDL) cholesterol, which is a major mechanism for the development of atherosclerosis. Although insulin resistance may occur irrespective of BMI, the common association of PCOS and obesity has a synergistic deleterious impact on glucose metabolism and can affect both hyperandrogenism and anovulation. Obese women who are not PCOS are in relative hypogonadotropic hypogonadism state with an unknown exact physiology. Obese people have hyperleptinemia that causes central leptin resistance and hypogonadism. These women have reduced luteinizing hormone (LH) levels, but follicle-stimulating hormone (FSH), anti-Müllerian hormone (AMH), and E2 levels and total antral follicle counts are normal. The reduced LH levels can be explained by an aromatization of androgens to estrogens resulting in decreased LH secretion from the pituitary. A significant improvement in these metabolic parameters is achieved with a modest weight loss of 5–10% of body weight.

The obesity is associated with high risk of diabetes and cardiovascular disease. The individual with three abnormal findings out of five clinical findings are labeled as persons with metabolic syndrome.

- Abdominal obesity: greater than 35 inches (40 inches in men) waist circumference
- Fasting glucose: 110 mg/dL or higher
- Hypertension: 130/85 or higher
- Triglyceride levels: 150 mg/dL or higher
- HDL cholesterol levels: less than 50 mg/dL.

Due to variability associated with measurements of insulin, the fasting glucose to fasting insulin ratio is no longer recommended to establish the presence of insulin resistance; a 2-hour oral glucose tolerance test is now the preferred method.

Interpretation of the 2-hour glucose response:

- Normal: less than 140 mg/dL
- Impaired: 140 = 199 mg/dL
- Noninsulin-dependent diabetes mellitus: 200 mg/dL and higher.

Interpretation of the 2-hour insulin response:

- Insulin resistance very likely: 100–150 U/mL
- Insulin resistance: 151–300 U/mL
- Severe insulin resistance: greater than 300 U/mL.

NATURAL FERTILITY AND OBESITY

Significant impact of body weight is seen at pubarche and natural fecundity in females. An increase in waist circumference and moderate obesity has significant impact over the spontaneous conception rates in otherwise ovulating women.

Insulin Sensitizers and Polycystic Ovarian Syndrome

Polycystic ovarian syndrome is a heterogeneous endocrine disorder with genetic predispositions and presents itself differently in each women of childbearing age. At fertility clinics, 90% of women with anovulation are PCOS, the prevalence appears to be correlated with the trend of obesity. The oligomenorrhea and anovulation with insulin resistance is associated with abdominal obesity. Active lifestyle is a secret for the betterment of reproductive outcome. It is clearly found that weight loss is associated with improved endocrine profile, restoration of ovulation and favorable fertility outcome. Loss of 6–8% of total weight leads to favorable outcome. A prior weight loss is found to have better fertility results.

A good workout schedule with insulin sensitizing drugs can help in creating negative caloric balance and this has created major turn round in PCOS management, though women with extreme obesity has not reflected the same benefit with insulin sensitizing drugs.

A recently published, placebo-controlled multicenter study has evaluated the combined effect of lifestyle modification and metformin on obese anovulatory women (BMI 43 $kg/m^{2)}$ with PCOS (Tang et al., 2006). It has been found that response to metformin in obese women was less than nonobese PCOS and this might be because of resistance to the standard metformin doses.

OBESITY AND ANOVULATORY INFERTILITY

Infertility with anovulation is seen more commonly in those with higher BMI. Higher doses of clomiphene and gonadotropins are required in obese women. Monitoring by transvaginal ultrasound scan is difficult and these women are at higher risk of poor response. Patients with BMI greater than 30 are found to have poor follicular growth in spite of higher antral follicle count. While those with a BMI of less than 25 had a monofollicular response. A higher BMI is associated with high gonadotropic threshold and extended FSH window. A positive association between obesity, amount of gonadotropins required along with higher cycle cancellation is found in many studies. In a meta-analysis of 13 studies, a strong correlation was found in reduction in ovulation rates, while there was no difference in pregnancy rates associated with obesity. This meta-analysis concluded that the combination of obesity and insulin resistance appears to be the most significant factor for the outcome of ovulogen treatment with the degree of insulin resistance being more important.

Slim women with resistance to clomiphene citrate and high LH level are more likely to respond with ovarian drilling as an alternative to gonadotropin treatment.

OBESITY AND ASSISTED REPRODUCTIVE TECHNOLOGY

Obese women with BMI greater than 35 have a poor outcome than those with a normal weight. Poor ovarian response and compromised embryo quality is seen in spite of more gonadotropin usage. It is seen that these treatment cycles are associated with lower implantation rates and poor pregnancy outcome (Brannian et al., 2001).

Possible explanations for poor assisted reproductive technology (ART) outcome:

- Poor absorption and distribution of ovulation induction drugs
- Hyperinsulinemia
- Hyperandrogenic hormonal milieu and endocrine abnormalities
- Leptin resistance leading to attenuated LH surge.

The above-mentioned findings were endorsed in a recent meta-analysis. Miscarriage incidences were usually found higher although a significant correlation of extreme weight on obstetric outcome could not be established.

PREGNANCY AND OBESITY

Obese pregnant patients carry significant risks for congenital anomalies (neural tube, omphalocele and cardiac defects). The risk of congenital anomalies appears real, because of undetected diabetes along with technical difficulty in ultrasound detection of anomalies. There is also increased risk of abortion in obese women who conceived spontaneously.

Obesity is also associated with increased risk of antepartum and intrapartum complications. They are at higher risk of pre-eclampsia, gestational diabetes and thromboembolic disorders, dysfunctional labor, increased cesarean sections and postpartum hemorrhage (PPH). Neonates born to these mothers are more prone for newborn intensive care unit (NICU) admissions, hypoglycemia, and birth defects and perinatal deaths. These mothers need special attention during antenatal, intranatal and postnatal period and therefore pregnancy costs much higher than their nonobese counterparts.

DELETERIOUS EFFECTS OF OBESITY UPON MALE FERTILITY

Obesity affects male infertility by influencing the hypothalamic-pituitary-gonadal axis, thus causing detrimental effects upon spermatogenesis and subsequent fertility. In particular, evidence indicates that excess adipose tissue can alter the relative ratio of testosterone and estrogen. Additional effects involve the homeostatic disruption of insulin, sex hormone-binding globulin, leptin and inhibin B, leading to diminished testosterone production and impairment to spermatogenesis. Aberrant spermatogenesis arising from obesity is associated with downstream changes in key semen parameters, defective sperm capacitation and binding, and deleterious effects on sperm chromatin structure.

EXERCISE IN OBESITY

"Though the genes load the gun: your lifestyle pulls the trigger."

"Food is the most abusive drug and exercise is the most underutilized medicine."

A supportive weight loss program in addition to diet helps to reduce weight. A better ovulation induction outcome and pregnancy is found with well-executed exercise and diet plan. A multidisciplinary approach can help in achieving early results. Surgical options like bariatric surgery can be considered an important tool but it is advisable not to conceive during rapid weight reduction as metabolic instability may have adverse pregnancy outcome.

CONCLUSION

- Body mass index is useful in clinical practice as it is a reliable, reproducible measurement. Arm circumference and waist-hip ratio should be considered in patients with high BMI.
- Couples should be counseled about the relation of obesity and its impact on fertility outcome. Before starting ART they should make aware of possibility of increased requirement of gonadotropins, decreased oocyte collection or poor ovarian response in spite of high doses and good antral follicle count.
- Even after conception there is increased risk of antepartum, intrapartum and postpartum complications, neonates also need increase medical attention. Couple needs to be motivated before starting the fertility management to bring BMI close to normal. Even weight loss of 6–8% of total body weight can bring favorable fertility outcome.
- Obesity has its negative impact on male fertility too. Usually couple share common lifestyle, so they should be counseled about the lifetime opportunity to change their lifestyle which not only will bring positive outcome in fertility but general health will also be improved.

SUGGESTED READING

1. Al-Azemi M, Omu FE, Omu AE. The effect of obesity on the outcome of infertility management in women with polycystic ovary syndrome. Arch Gynecol Obstet. 2004;270(4):205-10.
2. Ashton WD, Nanchahal K, Wood DA. Body mass index and metabolic risk factors for coronary heart disease in women. Eur Heart J. 2001;22:46-55.
3. Azziz R, Legro R, Giudice L. A twenty-first century research agenda for polycystic ovary syndrome. Best Pract Res Clin Endocrinol Metab. 2006;20(2):331-6.

4. Balen AH, Dresner M, Scott EM, et al. Should obese women with polycystic ovary syndrome receive treatment for infertility? BMJ. 2006;332:434-5.
5. Balen AH. Surgical management of PCOS. Best Pract Res Clin Endocrinol Metab. 2006;20:271-80.
6. Bellver J, Rossal LP, Bosch E, et al. Obesity and the risk of spontaneous abortion after oocyte donation. Fertil Steril. 2003;79:1136-40.
7. Chou SH, Mantzoros C. 20 years of leptin: role of leptin in human reproductive disorders. J Endocrinol. 2014;223(1):T49-62.
8. Conn JJ, Jacobs HS, Conway GS. The prevalence of polycystic ovaries in women with type 2 diabetes mellitus. Clin Endocrinol (Oxf). 2000;52:81-6.
9. Davidson LM, Millar K, Jones C, et al. Deleterious effects of obesity upon the hormonal and molecular mechanisms controlling spermatogenesis and male fertility. Hum Fertil (Camb). 2015;18(3):184-93.
10. ESHRE Capri Workshop Group. Nutrition and reproduction in women. Hum Reprod Update. 2006;12:193-207.
11. Falsetti L, Pasinetti E, Mazzani MD, et al. Weight loss and menstrual cycle: clinical and endocrinological evaluation. Gynecol Endocrinol. 1992;6(1):49-56.
12. Fleming R, Hopkinson ZE, Wallace AM, et al. Ovarian function and metabolic factors in women with oligomenorrhea treated with metformin in a randomized double-blind placebo-controlled trial. J Clin Endocrinol Metab. 2002;87:569-74.
13. Grenman S, Rönnemaa T, Irjala K, et al. Sex steroid, gonadotropin, cortisol, and prolactin levels in healthy, massively obese women: correlation with abdominal fat cell size and effect of weight reduction. J Clin Endocrinol Metab. 1986;63(6):1257-61.
14. Handelsman DJ, Swerdloff RS. Male gonadal dysfunction. Clin Endocrinol Metab. 1985;14:89-124.
15. Homburg R, Orvieto R, Bar-Hava I, et al. Serum levels of insulin-like growth factor-1, IGF binding protein-1 and insulin and the response to human menopausal gonadotrophins in women with polycystic ovary syndrome. Hum Reprod. 1996;11(4):716-9.
16. Maheshwari A, Stofberg L, Bhattacharya S. Effect of overweight and obesity on assisted reproductive technology—a systematic review. Hum Reprod Update. 2007;13:433-44.
17. National Institute for Health and Clinical Excellence (NICE). Fertility: assessment and treatment for people with fertility problems. A clinical guideline. London (UK): RCOG Press; 2004.
18. Pasquali R, Antenucci D, Casimirri F, et al. Clinical and hormonal characteristics of obese amenorrheic hyperandrogenic women before and after weight loss. J Clin Endocrinol Metab. 1989;68:173-9.
19. Tang T, Glanville J, Hayden CJ, et al. Combined lifestyle modification and metformin in obese patients with polycystic ovary syndrome. A randomized, placebo-controlled, double-blind multicentre study. Hum Reprod. 2006;21:80-9.
20. Wijeyaratne CN, Balen AH, Barth JH, et al. Clinical manifestations and insulin resistance (IR) in polycystic ovary syndrome (PCOS) among South Asians and Caucasians: is there a difference? Clin Endocrinol (Oxf). 2002;57:343-50.
21. Wild S, Pierpoint T, Jacobs H, et al. Long-term consequences of polycystic ovary syndrome: results of a 31-year follow-up study. Hum Fertil (Camb). 2000;3(2):101-5.
22. Sources:
    a. Obesity and Infertility. [online] Available from http://www.med.hku.hk/healthedu/issue77/e-issue77.pdf. [Last accessed February, 2019].
    b. [online] Available from cmebyplaza.com/.../Santoro%20Obesity%20and%20Infertility.pdf. [Last accessed February, 2019].
    c. [online] Available from d1l9wtg77iuzz5.cloudfront.net/.../original_USA_Weekend.pdf?1329693332. [Last accessed February, 2019].
    d. [online] Available from http://www.bjdvd.com/content/9/5/237.full.pdf. [Last accessed February, 2019].
    e. [online] Available from http://www.infertilitydoc.net/pdf/OBESITY_article.pdf. [Last accessed February, 2019].

Female Genital Tuberculosis 8

JB Sharma, Sona Dharmendra, Shefali Agarwal, Poonam Loomba, Jyoti Gupta

INTRODUCTION

Tuberculosis (TB) is global disease with 10.4 million new TB cases annually out of which about 2 million die.[1] Most cases occur in developing countries especially Asia and Africa.[1,2] Human immunodeficiency virus (HIV) infection, liberal immigration and due to globalization have fueled the epidemic of TB. Multidrug-resistant (MDR) TB and extensively drug-resistant (XDR) TB are serious forms of disease causing significant morbidity and mortality.[1,2]

Although pulmonary TB (PTB) is the most frequent form of TB, extrapulmonary TB (EPTB) and female genital tuberculosis (FGTB) are becoming more common.[1-3] Genital TB (FGTB) is responsible for causing significant morbidity, especially menstrual dysfunction and infertility, for the affected patients.[4-7] Early diagnosis and treatment may improve fertility outcome.[4,5]

EPIDEMIOLOGY OF FEMALE GENITAL TUBERCULOSIS

It is usually caused by *Mycobacterium tuberculosis* but rarely caused by *Mycobacterium bovis* or typical Mycobacteria. The incidence of FGTB varies being 1% in the United States of America, 5–23% in Pakistan, 0.8–2% in Italy, 4.2% in Saudi Arabia, 16.7% in Nigeria and 6.15–21.1% in South Africa, and 1–19% in India.[7-20] In India, the incidence is more in apex hospitals like All India Institute of Medical Sciences (AIIMS), New Delhi (26%) due to referral of cases from states like Bihar.[4,7] Incidence is very high (24.5% overall as 48.5% with tubal factor infertility)[20] in assisted reproduction seekers.

Mean age is 20–30 years in developing countries in contrast to 40 years in developed nations.[4,10,21] Incidence of TB has increased significantly due to HIV due to impaired immunity of depletion and dysfunction of macrophages especially CD4+ T cells.[21]

PATHOGENESIS

Female genital tuberculosis usually occurs due to spread of TB from lungs and other sites usually by hematogenous or lymphatic route or direct spread from intestines or lymph nodes. The fallopian tubes are affected in 90–100% cases followed by uterus (about 50–70%), ovary (15%), and cervix (5–10%).

PATHOLOGY

Fallopian Tubes

Fallopian tubes are affected in most (>90%) women with genital TB and the disease is usually bilateral. Various types of TB salpingitis can be TB endosalpingitis (infection starts from endosalpinx), TB exosalpingitis (spread of disease from intestinal), interstitial TB salpingitis, and salpingitis isthmica nodosa.[4-7,21] There may be blockade of both ends of fallopian tubes due to fibrosis.[4-7] Dense pelvic adhesions may be formed.[4-7,21]

There is hyperemia, miliary tubercles, caseous nodules and shaggy areas on tubes with adhesions and hydrosalpinx and pyosalpinx.[22,23]

Uterus

Endometrium is affected in 70% cases of FGTB with caseation and ulceration, but later distortion of cavity and destruction of endometrium occur causing Asherman's syndrome with amenorrhea.[24] There occurs implantation failure in TB endometritis.[25,26]

Ovaries

They are involved in 20–35% cases with TB oophoritis. With tubercles on the ovary, adhesions, caseation, tubo-ovarian cyst or mass formation or rarely complete destruction of ovaries.[4,21,25,27]

Peritoneum

Tuberculous peritonitis can occur with caseous nodules and tubercles on peritoneum and bowel with ascites and abdominal mass and may simulate as ovarian cancer with moderate rise in CA-125 levels. Often laparotomy is needed for diagnosis for suspected ovarian cancer.[28,29] Ascitic fluid tapping for biochemical analysis with adenosine deaminase levels[30] may confirm the diagnosis of TB and thus avoiding a needless laparotomy.

Cervix

Cervix is affected an about 5% cases with cervical growth or ulcer necessitating biopsy to diagnose TB and rule out cancer.[31]

Vagina and Vulva

They are rarely affected and may cause ulceration or hypertrophic lesions and may resemble cancer requiring biopsy to confirm diagnosis.[4,21]

ENDOMETRIAL FACTORS[24,32-34]

- There is decreased endometrial receptivity in FGTB.
    - Adverse effect on markers which are essential to make the endometrium receptive for embryonic implantation.[30]
    - Defective vascularization of the endometrium in FGTB with reduced subendometrial blood flow
    - Defective implantation due to harmful cytokines, genetic factors, natural killer cells and activated killer cells.[25,33] Antigonadotropic effect of *M. tuberculosis* requiring more ampules of gonadotropins in in vitro fertilization (IVF) cycle.
    - Destruction of endometrium with Asherman's syndrome.[24]
    - Poor oocyte development.

GENITAL TUBERCULOSIS AND INFERTILITY

Both primary and secondary infertility are quite common in FGTB (40–80%). Various causes of infertility in FGTB are as follows:

- *Tubal factors:*
    - Blockage of fallopian tubes
    - Loss of tubal function due to ciliary damage.
    - Perisalpingitis with adhesions and tubo-ovarian masses
    - Tubercular hydrosalpinx with or without obstruction occurs which has an adverse effect on embryonic implantation and ovarian function with very low pregnancy rate possibly due to harmful cytokines and growth factors which adversely affect the development of the oocyte.[32]
- *Defective ovarian factors:*[26,27,33]
    - Endocrine disruption due to FGTB
    - Chronic anovulation.

CLINICAL FEATURES

Various symptoms and signs of FGTB are given in **Box 1**. FGTB may be asymptomatic disease.

DIAGNOSIS

- *History taking*: Family or past history of TB or antituberculosis therapy (ATT) is very important.
- *Clinical examination*: Complete general physical examination for any TB elsewhere like lymphadenopathy (TB lymph nodes), skeleton TB (bones, joints, skin, etc.), cutaneous TB, chest examination (PTB), and abdominal examination (abdominal TB).
- *Gynecological examination*: Examination is done of external genitalia (vulvar or vaginal TB), speculum examination (cervical TB), bimanual examination (endometrial or fallopian tube TB) to diagnose of FGTB.
- *Investigations*:
    - Blood test for anemia, leukocytosis with lymphocytosis and raised erythrocyte sedimentation rate (ESR) may be there in TB.
    - *Serological tests:* They are not sensitive and specific and the World Health Organization (WHO) and Government of India have banned their use.
    - X-ray chest to exclude or confirm coexisting respiratory TB or old-healed lesions of post TB.
    - Mantoux (tuberculin) test and interferon-gamma release assays: They have limited utility with sensitivity of 55% and specificity of 80% and alone cannot be used for diagnosis of FGTB.
    - *Blood markers:* CA-125 is a marker for epithelial ovarian cancer (normal levels < 35 U/mL). Its levels are only moderately raised (usually < 200 U/ml) as

Box 1: Clinical features in female genital tuberculosis (FGTB).[4,5,9,10,21]

A. *Symptoms:*
- Asymptomatic (up to 10%)
- *General symptoms:*
  - Low-grade fever
  - Loss of weight
  - Loss anorexia
  - Malaise, heavy menstrual bleeding
- *Menstrual symptoms:*
  - Menorrhagia (in early stages due to ulcerative lesions)
  - Oligomenorrhea (in late stage)
  - Hypomenorrhea (in late stage)
  - Amenorrhea (primary and secondary due to endometrial atrophy)
- Primary and secondary infertility
- Abdominal lump
- Dyspareunia (painful colors)
- Abdominal pain
- Chronic pelvic pain
- Acute abdomen (due to in rupture of tubo-ovarian abscess or flare-up of TB after HSG or other gynecological procedures)
- Unhealthy vaginal discharge

B. *Signs:*
- No physical sign (common)
- *Systemic examination:*
  - Raised temperature
  - Lymphadenopathy (in TB lymphadenitis)
  - Crackles on chest auscultation (PTB)
  - Other systemic signs depending on site of EPTB (abdominal distention in abdominal TB)
- *Abdominal examination:*
  - Mass abdomen (vague or definite)
  - Doughy feel of abdomen
  - Ascites
- *Vaginal examination:*
  - Uterine enlargement (pyometra)
  - Tenderness and induration in forices
  - Adnexal masses (tubo-ovarian masses)
  - Fullness and tenderness in pouch of Douglas
  - Small-sized uterus (shrunken cavity in endometrial TB)
- Cervical lesion (hypertrophy or ulcer)
- Vulval hypertrophic lesion
- Vulval or vaginal ulcer.

compared to high rise (in 1,000 in cancer ovary) in FGTB. However, CA-125 is not a very reliable marker for diagnosis of FGTB.

- *Imaging methods:* They are of use only in tubo-ovarian masses.
  - *Ultrasonography (USG):* It may demonstrate unilateral or bilateral solid adnexal masses with scattered small calcifications with free fluid in pouch of Douglas in FGTB.

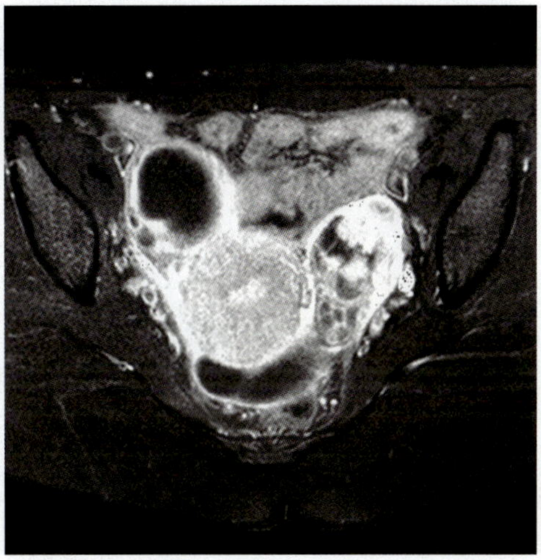

Fig. 1: Magnetic resonance imaging (MRI) with bilateral tubo-ovarian masses.

  - *Computerized axial tomography (CAT scan):* It may also demonstrate pelvic and abdominal masses with ascites, multiple pelvic, abdominal lesions with or without lymphadenopathy.[4,21]
  - *Magnetic resonance imaging (MRI):* It is useful in presence of abdominal and pelvic masses with better resolution than computed tomography (CT) scan. There were hypodense masses with rim enhancement abutting the pelvic walls in FGTB. We observed tubo-ovarian masses, unilateral or bilateral hydrosalpinx, adnexal cysts or tuberculous deposits on peritoneum or liver in our study of MRI in tubercular tubo-ovarian masses **(Fig. 1)**.[35]
    It may help in differentiating between carcinoma ovary and abdominopelvic TB but is nonspecific.
  - *Positron emission tomography (PET) scan:* An active TB lesion shows increase glucose uptake as observed by us in our study on 17 women of tubercular tubo-ovarian masses **(Fig. 2)**.[36] It also helps in differentiating between carcinoma ovary and abdominopelvic TB.
  - *Hysterosalpingography (HSG):* HSG is contraindicated in FGTB due to flare up subclinical infection. However, it is often performed as a part of infertility in suspected cases. It shows internal architecture of the female genital tract and helps in the diagnosis of genital TB **(Figs. 3 to 5)**.

We found tubal calcification, irregularity of tubal wall, unilateral or bilateral cornual block, unilateral or bilateral

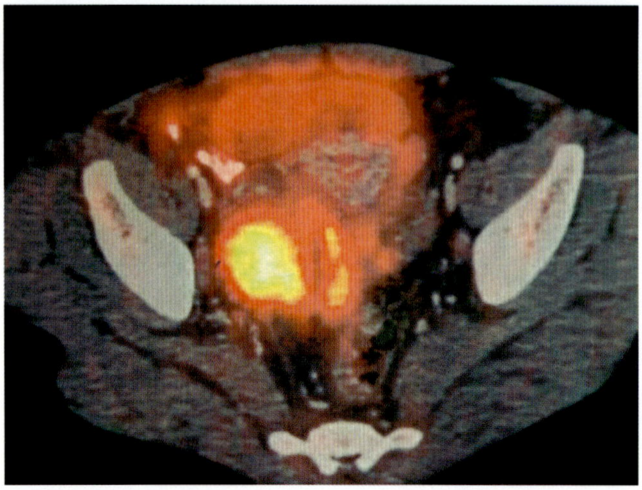

Fig. 2: Positron emission tomography-computed tomography (PET-CT) scan showing unilateral increased glucose uptake in tubo-ovarian masses due to genital tuberculosis.

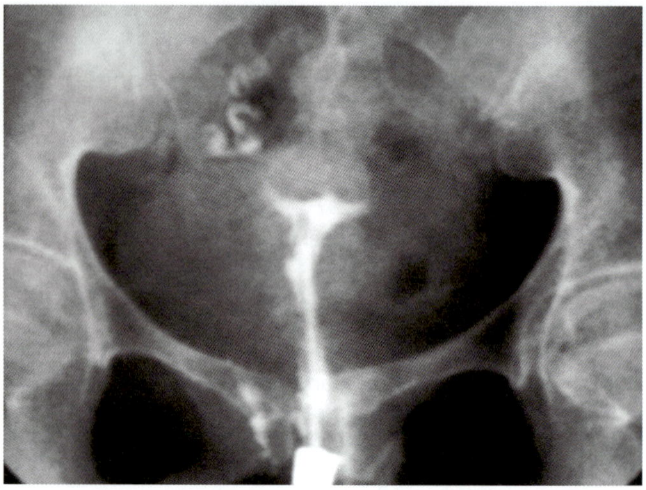

Fig. 4: Hysterosalpingography in genital tuberculosis contracted irregular uterine cavity with bilateral tubal block marked intravasation with bilateral pelvic venous system.

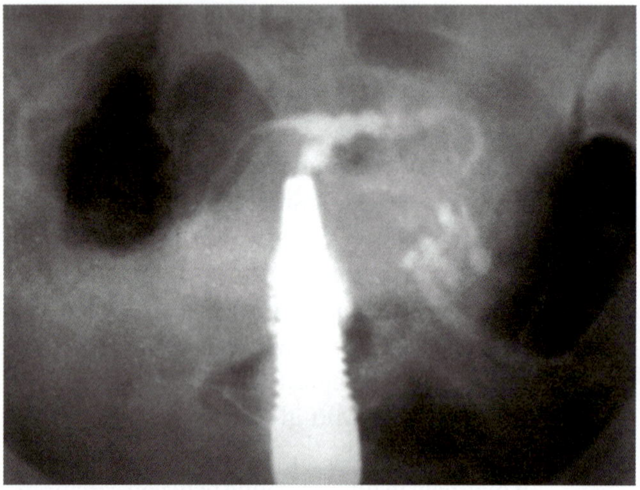

Fig. 3: Hysterosalpingography.

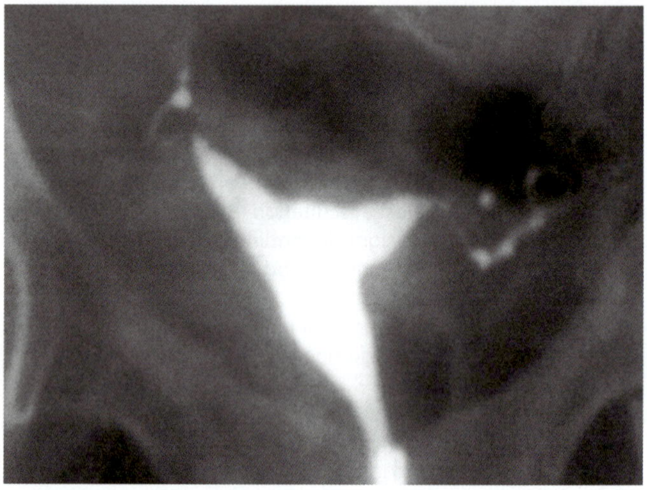

Fig. 5: *Hysterosalpingography in genital tuberculosis:* left tubal block and beaded pattern in right fallopian tube in a proven case of genital tuberculosis.

hydrosalpinx, vascular intravasation of dye in cases of genital TB in our study.[37]

- *Endometrial biopsy, curettage or aspirate (day 21)*: In the premenstrual phase, it is the most important test for the diagnosis of genital TB. A part of specimen is sent in formalin solution for histopathological testing for epithelioid granuloma.
- *Mycobacterial smear and culture*: Endometrial biopsy, aspirate, menstrual blood (in unmarried girls), are subjected to smear examination for acid-fast bacilli (AFB), Ziehl-Neelsen staining or fluorescent (auramine) staining is usually used for microscopic examination. It needs 104–105 mycobacteria/mL in the specimen to give a positive result. Culture is performed on Löwenstein-Jensen (LJ) medium. AFB smear. Solid and liquid mycobacterial cultures are very useful in picking up 100 µg/mL but need at least 14 days for the isolation of *M. tuberculosis*.[31] While LJ culture has a low sensitivity (30–35%), the radiometric culture BACTEC 460 developed by Becton Dickinson has a higher sensitivity (80–90%) with quicker results (5–10 days) and is particularly useful for drug susceptibility testing and for genital TB and MDR-TB.[38-40] Other rapid diagnostic methods are Mycobacteria growth indicator tube

(MGIT), modified Middlebrook 7H9 Broth, and specific gene probes contributing to more rapid identification and diagnosis.[39,40]

- *Polymerase chain reaction (PCR)*: It is a rapid (1–2 days), sensitive and specific molecular test for 65 kDa protein and MPT-64 gene in both PTB and EPTB samples. It targets encoding gene, the IS6110 element. Bhanu et al.[41] demonstrated *M. tuberculosis* DNA on PCR in 56% cases compared to 1.6% smear positive and 3.2% culture positive cases in genital TB. Jindal et al.[42] found endometrial TB PCR to have high sensitivity and specificity and may be positive in presence of as low as 1–10 organisms/mL. Rana et al.[43] used DNA PCR for better results. However, PCR can be false negative or there is a risk of false positive and should not be used for rapid diagnosis of TB nor to stop ATT.[44] It is our policy not to start ATT only for positive PCR on clinical in absence of disease of her tests.[4]
- GeneXpert can also be used for diagnosis of FGTB on endometrial aspirate or biopsies. It has low sensitivity but very high specificity.[45]

Endoscopy

- *Hysteroscopy:* Endoscopic visualization of the uterine cavity in genital TB may show a pale endometrium with varying grades (grade 1 to grade 4) of adhesions often involving ostia as observed by us **(Fig. 6)**.[45,46] There may be a small shrunken cavity. Hysteroscopy is difficult with more chances of complications like excessive bleeding, perforation and flare-up of genital TB as observed by us.[47]
- *Laparoscopy **(Figs. 7 to 9)**:* A laparoscopy with hysteroscopy is best method to see FGTB.[48,49]
  Various laparoscopic findings of FGTB include tubercles, shaggy areas, fimbrial block, beaded tubes, peritubal and periovarian adhesions, tubo-ovarian mass, hydrosalpinx and pyosalpinx.[48,49]

Baxi et al.[49] observed 85.7% sensitivity, 22.2% specificity and 77.7% negative predictive value of diagnostic laparoscopy in diagnosis of FGTB.

Adhesions: Various types of adhesions on omentum (48%), intestines, uterus and tubes are common especially perihepatic adhesions on laparoscopy in FGTB cases. In a laparoscopic study on 85 women with FGTB, we found tubercles, tubo-ovarian masses, caseous nodules, encysted ascites, pelvic adhesions, hydrosalpinx, pyosalpinx, beaded tubes, and tobacco pouch appearance. There were more complications and difficulty in laparoscopy in FGTB cases.[50]

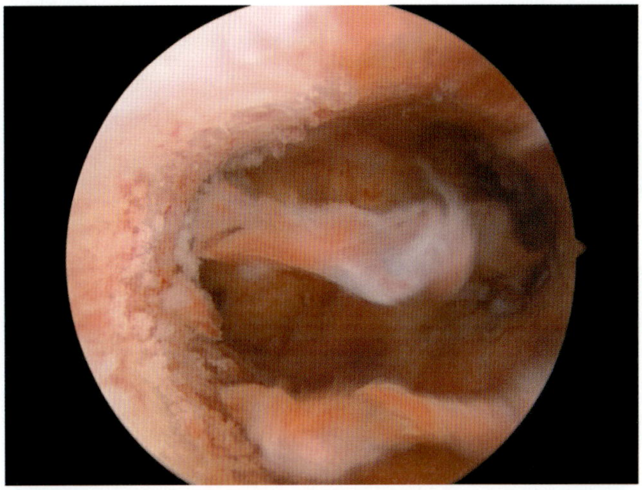

Fig. 6: Hysteroscopic findings in genital tuberculosis showing grade 2 adhesions.

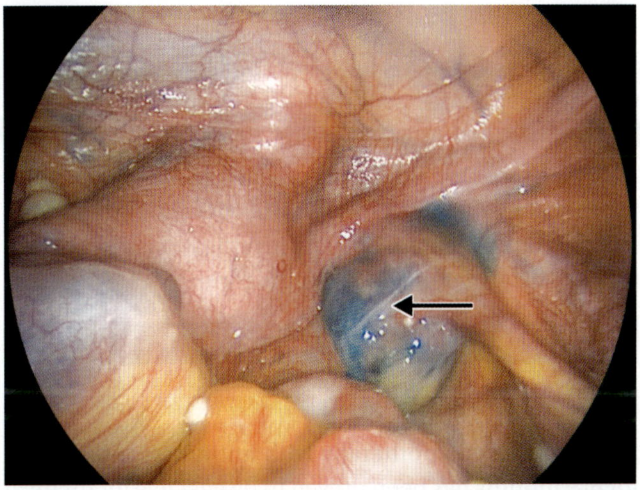

Fig. 7: Laparoscopic findings showing caseous nodule and adhesions near right fimbria and right-sided hydrosalpinx in proven case of genital tuberculosis.

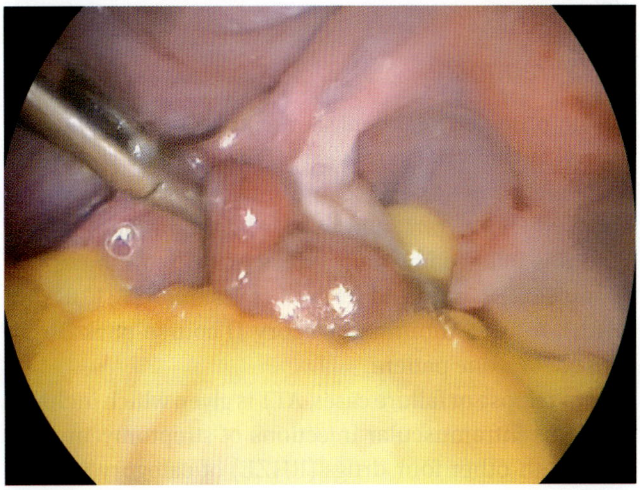

Fig. 8: Laparoscopic findings showing congested, dilated and inflamed right fallopian tube with tubercles in a female genital tuberculosis.

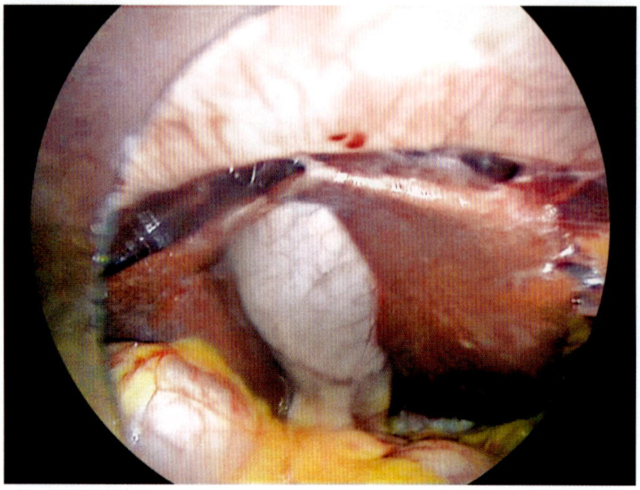

Fig. 9: Laparoscopic findings showing perihepatic adhesions (Fitz-Hugh-Curtis syndrome) in female genital tuberculosis.

We also observed new laparoscopic signs in abdominopelvic TB such as hanging gallbladder sign (due to perihepatic adhesions), ascending colonic adhesions, blue python sign (fallopian tubes are alternatively dilated and combined) and kissing fallopian tube sign in FGTB in our various studies.[51-54] History taking, examination and investigations can be used to make diagnosis of FGTB using algorithm.[55]

TREATMENT

Medical Treatment

Short-course chemotherapy with antituberculous drugs for 6–9 months has been proven to be effective for medical treatment of FGTB. We observed equal efficacy of 6 months and 9 months ATT in FGTB patients in our randomized trial.[56,57]

DOTS Treatment

Directly observed treatment short-course (DOTS) strategy is favored by the WHO to prevent MDR and for better results. WHO recommends DOTS and intake of rifampicin (R), isoniazid (H), pyrazinamide (Z) and ethambutol (E) for 2 months followed by daily intake of 4-month therapy of rifampicin (R), isoniazid (H) and ethambutol (E) (2RHZE-4HRE). A full 6 months (category I) course pack box is booked for a one patient.

For relapse or failure cases, ATT is given which includes 2 months intramuscular injections of streptomycin daily along with other four drugs (RHZE) of category I under direct supervision for first 2 months followed by four drugs (RHZE) daily for another month (intensive phase) followed by continuation phase with three drugs isoniazid (H), rifampicin (R) and ethambutol (E) daily for another 5 months (total 8 months).[4,21]

Non-DOTS Treatment

Patients not opting for DOTS treatment must take daily therapy of RHZE for 2 months (intensive phase) followed by RHE for 4 months (continuation phase). Convenient and economic combipacks are available in market. MDR FGTB is treated like pulmonary MDR with second-line drugs and is shown in Table 1 and is needed for long duration (18–24 months).

Monitoring

The women are counseled to adhere to treatment and consume proper diet and should report of any side effects of the drugs like hepatitis, loss of appetite, neuritis or vestibule cochlea toxicity.

Medical therapy is highly effective. Surgery in form of drainage of abscess can be done.[58] Various surgeries like hysteroscopy, laparoscopy, laparotomy and vaginal hysterectomy on FGTB are associated with higher complication rates.[4,21,47,50] Tuboplasty is avoided due to risk of flare-up of disease and ectopic gestation.[59]

In Vitro Fertilization

In spite of ATT, tubes remain blocked but endometrium is receptive, IVF-embryo transfer (ET) is recommended with pregnancy rate of 16.6% per transfer.[57] However, endometrial TB with shrunken small uterine cavity with Asherman's syndrome. Adoption or gestational surrogacy is advised to them.[60, 61]

New Tuberculosis Research

Newer drugs (bedaquiline) and newer vaccines and stem cell therapy are being investigated for treatment.

CONCLUSION

Female genital tuberculosis is a common disease causing infertility. It is diagnosed from history, examination, endometrial biopsy, laparoscopy and hysteroscopy. It is treated by 6 months of ATT with isoniazid, pyrazinamide, rifampicin and ethambutol. IVF-ET is indicated for tubal blockage and surrogacy for Asherman's syndrome.

Table 1: Category-wise treatment regimens for female genital tuberculosis (FGTB).[2-4,21]

TB diagnostic category	*TB patients*	*TB treatment regimens*			
		Initial phase (daily)	*Continuation phase (daily)*		
I	New FGTB case	2 HRZE dose INH 600 mg Rifampicin 450 (600 mg if >50 kg) Pyrazinamide 1,500 mg Ethambutol 1,200 mg for 2 months	4 HRE INH 600 mg Rifampicin 450 (600 mg if >50 kg) Ethambutol 1,200 mg dose for 4 months		
II	TB: relapse, treatment after default and treatment failure in FGTB	2 HRZES/IHRZE dose RHZE as in category I above. Injection streptomycin 0.75 g daily (DOTS) for 2 months followed by 1 month of RHZE	5 HRE dose INH 600 mg Rifampicin 450 (600 mg if >50 kg) Ethambutol 1,200 mg for 5 months		
III	Chronic and MDR-TB cases (still sputum-positive after supervised retreatment/ or culture positive or histopathologically proven FGTB)	*Drug*	*Dose (mg) if weight <45 kg*	*Dose (mg) if weight >45 kg*	
		Kanamycin (IM)			6–9 months intensive phase
		Ofloxacin (O)	500	750	
		Ethionamide (O)	600	800	
		Ethambutol (O)	500	750	
		Pyrazinamide (O)	1250	1,500	
		Ethambutol (O)	800	1,000	
		Cycloserine (O)	500	750	
		Ofloxacin (O)	600	800	18 months continuation phase
		Ethionamide (O)	500	750	
		Ethambutol (O)	800	1,000	
		Cycloserine (O)	500	750	

REFERENCES

1. World Health Organization. Global TB report 2017. Geneva: WHO; 2017.
2. World Health Organization. Global tuberculosis control: surveillance, planning, financing: WHO report 2006. Geneva: WHO; 2006.
3. TB India. Revised National Tuberculosis Control Programme (RNTCP). Annual status report 2017. Central TB Division, Directorate General of Health Services. Nirman Bhawan, New Delhi, India: Ministry of Health and Family Welfare; 2017.
4. Sharma JB. Tuberculosis and gynecological practice. In: Studd J, Tan SL, Chervenak FA (Eds). Current Progress in Obstetrics and Gynecology, 1st edition. Mumbai: Tree Life India; 2012. pp. 304-27.
5. Sutherland AM. Genital tuberculosis. Tubercle. 1980;79:66.
6. Parikh FR, Nadkarni S. Genital tuberculosis: a major pelvic factor causing infertility in Indian women. Fertil Steril. 1997;67:497-500.
7. Gupta N, Sharma JB, Mittal S, et al. Genital tuberculosis in Indian infertility patients. Int J Gynaecol Obstet. 2007;97: 135-8.
8. Sharma JB, Sneha J, Singh UB, et al. Comparative study of laparoscopic abdominopelvic and fallopian tube findings before and after antitubercular therapy in female genital tuberculosis with infertility. J Minim Invasive Gynecol. 2016;23:215-22.
9. Schaefer G. Female genital tuberculosis. Clin Obstet Gynecol. 1976;19:223-39.
10. Neonakis IK, Spandidos DA, Petinaki E. Female genital tuberculosis: a review. Scand J Infect Dis. 2011;43:564-72.
11. Khan SM. Incidence of genital tuberculosis in infertile women. J Pak Med Assoc. 1985;35:280-1.
12. Shahzad S. Investigation of the prevalence of female genital tract tuberculosis and its relation to female infertility: an observational analytical study. Iran J Reprod Med. 2012;10:581-8.
13. Marana R, Muzil L, Lucisano A, et al. Incidence of genital tuberculosis in infertile patients submitted to diagnostic laparoscopy: recent experience in an Italian University Hospital. Int J Fertil. 1991:36;104-7.
14. Chattopadhyay SK, Sengupta BS, Edrees YB, et al. The pattern of female genital tuberculosis in Riyadh, Saudi Arabia. Br J Obstet Gynaecol. 1986;93:367-71.
15. Emembolu JO, Anyanwu DO, Ewa B. Genital tuberculosis in infertile women in northern Nigeria. West Afr J Med. 1993;12:211-2.
16. Margolis K, Wranz PA, Kruger TF, et al. Genital tuberculosis at Tygerberg Hospital: prevalence, clinical presentation and diagnosis. S Afr Med J. 1992;81:12-5.

17. Oosthuizen AP, Wessels PH, Hefer JN. Tuberculosis of the female genital tract in patients attending an infertility clinic. S Afr Med J. 1990;77:562-4.
18. Malkani PK, Rajani CK. Pelvic tuberculosis. Obstet Gynecol. 1959;14:600-11.
19. Tripathy SN, Tripathy SN. Infertility and pregnancy outcome in female genital tuberculosis. Int J Gynaecol Obstet. 2002;76:159-63.
20. Singh N, Sumana G, Mittal S. Genital tuberculosis: a leading cause for infertility in women seeking assisted conception in North India. Arch Gynecol Obstet. 2008;278:325-7.
21. Kumar S, Sharma JB. Female genital tuberculosis. In: Sharma SK, Mohan A (Eds). Tuberculosis, 3rd edition. New Delhi: Jaypee Brothers Medical Publishers (P) Ltd.; 2016. pp. 311-24.
22. Duggal S, Duggal N, Hans C, et al. Female genital TB and HIV co-infection. Indian J Med Microbiol. 2009;27:361-3.
23. Sharma JB, Roy KK, Gupta N, et al. High prevalence of Fitz-Hugh-Curtis syndrome in genital tuberculosis. Int J Gynecol Obstet. 2007;99:62-3.
24. Sharma JB, Roy KK, Pushparaj M, et al. Genital tuberculosis: an important cause of Asherman's syndrome in India. Arch Obstet Gynecol. 2008;277:37-41.
25. Dam P, Shirazee HH, Goswami SK, et al. Role of latent genital tuberculosis in repeated IVF failure in Indian clinical settings. Gynecol Obstet Invest. 2006;61:223-7.
26. Malhotra N, Sharma V, Bahadur A, et al. The effect of tuberculosis on ovarian reserve among women undergoing IVF in India. Int J Gynaecol Obstet. 2012;117(1):40-4.
27. Sharma JB, Sneha J, Singh UB, et al. Effect of antitubercular, treatment on ovarian function in female genital tuberculosis with infertility. J Hum Reprod Sci. 2016;9:145-50.
28. Sharma JB, Jain SK, Pushparaj M, et al. Abdomino-peritoneal tuberculosis masquerading as ovarian cancer: a retrospective study of 26 cases. Arch Gynecol Obstet. 2010;282:643-8.
29. Koc S, Beydilli G, Tulunay G, et al. Peritoneal tuberculosis mimicking advanced ovarian cancer: a retrospective review of 22 cases. Gynecol Oncol. 2006;103:565-9.
30. Dwivedi M, Misra SP, Misra V, et al. Value of adenosine deaminase estimation in the diagnosis of tuberculous ascites. Am J Gastroenterol. 1990;85:1123-5.
31. Sharma JB, Malhotra M, Pundir P, et al. Cervical tuberculosis masquerading as cervical carcinoma: a rare case. J Obstet Gynaecol India. 2001;51:184.
32. Chen CD, Yang JH, Lin KC, et al. The significance of cytokines, chemical composition, and murine embryo development in hydrosalpinx fluid for predicting the IVF outcome in women with hydrosalpinx. Hum Reprod. 2002;17(1):128-33.
33. Chakravarty BN, Genital tuberculosis-ovarian function and endometrial receptivity. In: Mukherjee GG, Tripathy SN, Tripathy SN (Eds). Genital Tuberculosis, 1st edition. New Delhi: Jaypee Brothers Medical Publishers (P) Ltd.; 2010. pp. 27-42.
34. Sharma JB, Sneha J, Singh UB, et al. Effect of antitubercular therapy on endometrial function in infertile women with female genital tuberculosis. Infect disord Drug Targets. 2016;16:101-8
35. Sharma JB, Karmakar D, Hari S, et al. Magnetic resonance imaging findings among women with tubercular tubo-ovarian masses. Int J Gynecol Obstet. 2011;113:76-80.
36. Sharma JB, Karmakar D, Kumar R, et al. Comparison of PET/CT with other imaging modalities in women with genital tuberculosis. Int J Gynaecol Obstet. 2012;118:123-8.
37. Sharma JB, Pushparaj M, Roy KK, et al. Hysterosalpingographic findings in infertile women with genital tuberculosis. Int J Gynecol Obstet. 2008;101:150-5.
38. Grace GA, Devaleenal DB, Natrajan M. Genital tuberculosis in females. Indian J Med Res. 2017;145:425-36.
39. Neonakis IK, Gitti Z, Krambovitis E, et al. Molecular diagnostic tools in mycobacteriology. J Microbiol Methods. 2008;75:1-11.
40. Katoch VM. Newer diagnostic techniques for tuberculosis. Indian J Med Res. 2004;120:418-28.
41. Bhanu NV, Singh UB, Chakraborty M, et al. Improved diagnostic value of PCR in diagnosis of female genital tuberculosis leading to infertility. J Med Microbiol. 2005;54:927-31.
42. Jindal UN, Bala Y, Sodhi S, et al. Female genital tuberculosis: early diagnosis by laparoscopy and endometrial polymerase chain reaction. Int J Tuberc Lung Dis. 2010;14:1629-34.
43. Rana T, Singh UB, Kulshrestha V, et al. Utility of reverse transcriptase PCR and DNA-PCR in the diagnosis of female genital tuberculosis. J Med Microbiol. 2011;60(Pt 4):486-91.
44. Grosset J, Mouton Y. Is PCR a useful tool for the diagnosis of tuberculosis in 1995? Tuberc Lung Dis. 1995;76:183-4.
45. Sharma JB, Kriplani A, Dharmendra S, et al. Role of GeneXpert in diagnosis of female genital tuberculosis: a preliminary report. Eur J Obstet Gynecol Reprod Biol. 2016;207:237-8.
46. Sharma JB, Roy KK, Pushparaj M, et al. Hysteroscopic findings in women with primary and secondary infertility due to genital tuberculosis. Int J Gynecol Obstet. 2009;104:49-52.
47. Sharma JB, Roy KK, Pushparaj M, et al. Increased difficulties and complications encountered during hysteroscopy in women with genital tuberculosis. J Minim Invasive Gynecol. 2011;18:660-5.
48. Sharma JB, Roy KK, Pushparaj M, et al. Laparoscopic finding in female genital tuberculosis. Arch Gynecol Obstet. 2008;278:359-64.
49. Baxi A, Neema H, Kaushal M, et al. Genital tuberculosis in infertile women: assessment of endometrial TB PCR results with laparoscopic and hysteroscopic features. J Obstet Gynecol India. 2011;61:301-6.
50. Sharma JB, Mohanraj P, Roy KK, et al. Increased complication rates associated with laparoscopic surgery among patients with genital tuberculosis. Int J Gynecol Obstet. 2010;109:242-4.
51. Sharma JB. Sharma's hanging gallbladder sign: a new sign for abdominopelvic tuberculosis: an observational study. IVF Lite. 2015;2(3):94-8.
52. Sharma JB. Sharma's ascending colonic adhesion: a new sign in abdominopelvic tuberculosis with infertility. IVF Lite. 2016;3(1):18-22.
53. Sharma JB. Sharma's python sign: a new tubal sign in female genital tuberculosis. J Lab Physicians. 2016;8(2):120-2.

54. Sharma JB. Sharma's kissing fallopian tubes sign: a new tubal sign in female genital tuberculosis. J Obstet Gynaecol India. 2017;67(3):227-9.
55. Ministry of Health and Family Welfare, Government of India and World Health Organization. Index-TB guidelines for diagnosis and management of extrapulmonary tuberculosis (EPTB) in India. 2016. [online] Available from http//www.tbcindia.nic.in/showfile.php.lid=3245. [Last accessed February, 2019].
56. Arora R, Rajaram P, Oumachigui A, et al. Prospective analysis of short course chemotherapy in female genital tuberculosis. Int J Gynecol Obstet. 1992;38:31-4.
57. Sharma JB, Singh N, Dharmendra S, et al. Six months versus nine months anti-tuberculous therapy for female genital tuberculosis: a randomized controlled trial. Eur J Obstet Gynecol Reprod Biol. 2016;203:264-73.
58. American Thoracic Society/Centers for Disease Control and Prevention/Infectious Diseases Society of America: controlling tuberculosis in the United States. Am J Respir Crit Care Med. 2005;172:1169-227.
59. Sharma JB, Naha M, Kumar S, et al. Genital tuberculosis: an important cause of ectopic pregnancy in India. Indian J Tuberc. 2014;61(4):312-7.
60. Tripathy SN, Sapkal R. Tuberculosis Manual for Obstetricians and Gynecologists, 1st edition. New Delhi: Jaypee Brothers Medical Publishers (P) Ltd.; 2015.
61. Samantha J, Goswami SK, Mukherjee GG, et al. Gestational surrogacy in genital tuberculosis. In: Mukherjee GG, Tripathy SN, Tripathy SN (Eds). Genital Tuberculosis, 1st edition. New Delhi: Jaypee Brothers Medical Publishers (P) Ltd.; 2010. pp. 141-54.

Pelvic Inflammatory Disease

9

Sudha Prasad

INTRODUCTION

Inflammation of upper genital tract or commonly known as pelvic inflammatory disease (PID) occurs mostly due to genital tract infection. It may show involvement right from cervix up to the peritoneal cavity leading to conditions such as endocervicitis, endometritis, salpingitis, and peritonitis. Due to its asymptomatic behavior, actual incidence of PID is difficult to be assessed. According to literature, more than 8 lakhs women annually are affected by PID in the United States whereas in India, the average prevalence of PID was 11.55% with a prevalence of 12.5% in rural and 10.6% in urban areas.[1]

The disease has significant sequel and can cause tubal blockage leading to infertility, ectopic pregnancy, or chronic pelvic pain. Most of the women are less than 25 years old and among those at highest risk are sexually active adolescents.

Historically, PID was considered as a monoetiologic infection, mainly due to *Neisseria gonorrhoeae,* however, it is now well documented that it is polymicrobial in origin. Among approximately 70% of women suffering from PID, the upper genital tract cultures demonstrate anaerobic and facultative aerobic bacteria, usually associated with or without *N. gonorrhoeae* and *Chlamydia trachomatis.*

The inflammation induced by infection causes epithelial degeneration and loss of cilia of the mucosa of the fallopian tube along with an inflammatory cell infiltrate in the submucosa. Endosalpingitis occurs because of the edema of the fallopian tube which causes intraluminal agglutination, causing clubbing of the tube, or formation of hydrosalpinx. The tubes are thus partially or completely obstructed and dysfunctional, and this can cause ectopic pregnancies or infertility.

RISK FACTORS

Pelvic inflammatory disease can be seen as a consequence or complication of sexually transmitted disease (STD). Young women in the reproductive age group between 25 year and 29 years are at high risk. Young age at marriage, multiple sexual partners, intrauterine devices, illiteracy, and low socioeconomic status are other factors associated with increased risk of PID. In some studies, douching has been observed to double a woman's risk of infection upper genital tract.

ETIOLOGY

The most commonly isolated pathogen in early studies was *N. Gonorrhoeae.*[2-4] However, now its importance as a causative agent for PID is reduced, due to decrease in the prevalence of gonorrhea.[5] In up to 60% of women with confirmed salpingitis or endometritis, *C. trachomatis* is main organism detected and is a significant pathogen associated with PID.[6,7]

Approximately 60–70% women with PID have bacterial vaginosis. An increase in the anaerobic microflora in the vagina (*Gardnerella vaginalis* and genital mycoplasma), favors bacterial vaginosis. *Mycoplasma genitalium* may also cause PID occasionally.[8] In about 9–23% cases of PID, the etiology remains nongonococcal and nonchlamydial infection. These cases may be also associated with anaerobes like *Peptostreptococcus species* and *Prevotella* species.[9] Anaerobic invasion of the upper genital tract enhances the severity of the disease.[6]

PATHOGENESIS

The mucus barrier as well as the physical barrier of the cervix prevents the bacterial ascent. Hormones affect the function of the endocervical glands. The thin water mucus in the follicular phase allows the spermatozoa and microorganisms to penetrate easily. However, the thick cervical secretions in the luteal phase cause a hindrance for the sperms and other microorganisms to penetrate.

Immunology also plays a vital role in the cervical barrier; genetic polymorphism in toll-like receptor genes and certain human leukocyte antigen (HLA) class II alleles also possibly increase the risk of infection of the upper genital tract. Cervical infection differs in different individuals depending on their immune function and this can affect the risk of developing PID.

In women with bacterial vaginosis, mucolytic enzymes released by the organisms degrade the mucous plug and facilitate the ascent of cervical and vaginal microorganisms to the upper genital tract, which can cause endometritis and salpingitis. Endometrial organisms can spread to fallopian tubes due to retrograde bleeding during menstruation.

Tubal Inflammation

In cases of salpingitis, bacterial species isolated from the fallopian tubes fall into two main categories:

1. *Sexually transmitted disease organisms*—coinfections with *N. gonorrhoeae* and *C. trachomatis* are seen commonly leading to acute salpingitis, cervicitis, or urethritis. Cervicitis is usually self-limiting although chlamydial cervicitis may last for months.
   During PID, *C. trachomatis* bacteria attach to the epithelial surface of the fallopian tube and enter the cytoplasm by endocytosis. These cytoplasmic inclusions release elementary bodies into the lumen of the fallopian tubes. This causes damage to the ciliated cells of the fallopian tubes or they may become retort shaped. High quantities of various inflammatory markers like Interferon-gamma (IFN-gamma), interleukin-1 (IL-1), and IL-6 are released in the cervical secretions in women with cervicitis. These monokines accumulate in the tubes and might induce scarring and tissue damage.
   Gonococcal strains selective attack the nonciliated cells of the tubal mucosa. However, the ciliated cells show sloughing and ciliostasis. Once inside the nonciliated cells, gonococci are protected from immune defense factors, they traverse the cells, and are eventually released from their basal surfaces by exocytosis.
2. *"Endogenous" organisms*—many facultative and anaerobic bacterial species have been isolated-alone, or together with STD organisms from abscess material and/or cul-de-sac fluid. This gave rise to the concept of "polymicrobial PID". In anecdotal cases, viruses (viz. Coxsackie B5, ECHO 6, and herpes simplex virus-2) have being isolated from the upper genital tract in women with salpingitis.

Tubo-ovarian Abscess

Abscess formation is usually a late manifestation of PID and is seen with mixed facultative and anaerobic bacterial infections. An environment with low oxygen tension is created due to tissue destruction and bacterial metabolism, which favors anaerobic bacterial growth and these may eventually be the dominating isolate in abscess.

CLINICAL MANIFESTATION (CENTERS FOR DISEASE CONTROL AND PREVENTION GUIDELINES, 2015)[10,11]

Patient with PID can present with a spectrum of nonspecific clinical symptoms. These usually appear around the time of menstruation.

- Bilateral, dull lower abdominal and pelvic painisusually the most common symptom. The onset of pain is more rapid in gonococcal infection (3 days) than in chlamydial infection.
- Fever, fatigue, and headache
- Copious or purulent vaginal discharge
- Patients with endometritis can experience irregular, excessive vaginal bleeding.
- Dyspareunia
- About 5–10% women with acute salpingitis can have concomitant perihepatitis (Fitz-Hugh-Curtis Syndrome) due to transperitoneal or vascular dissemination of either gonococcal or chlamydial infection. These women can experience pain and discomfort in the right hypochondrium.

SIGNS

- *General examination reveals:*
  - High temperature, usually beyond 38.3°C
  - Tenderness on both quadrants of lower abdomen. Patients with perihepatitis (*Fitz-Hugh-Curtis* syndrome) have right upper quadrant tenderness due to inflammation of the liver capsule and *"violin string"* scar tissue formation.
- *Vaginal examination reveals:*
  - Abnormal vaginal discharge

- Congested urethral meatus or inflamed Bartholin's ducts through which pus may escape on pressure
  - *Speculum examination:* It shows congested cervix with purulent discharge coming out from the cervical canal
  - *Bimanual examination:* Tender uterus, tenderness of the fornices, which increases with movement of the cervix. A thickening or mass may be felt through the fornices.

DIAGNOSTIC PROCEDURES

Diagnosing of acute PID is quite difficult because of the wide variations in signs and symptoms. Laparoscopy can provide more accurate diagnosis of salpingitis. However, for acute cases and in vague and milder symptoms, this is nonjustifiable. Endometritis cannot be detected by laparoscopy along with the subtle inflammation of the fallopian tubes.

Consequently, vague clinical findings form the basis of diagnosis of PID.

Laboratory Examination

- Vaginal discharge may reveal ample numbers of white blood cell (WBC) on saline microscopy
- High erythrocyte sedimentation rate and increased CRP (C-reactive protein)
- Cervical swab culture will show growth of *N. Gonorrhoeae* or *C. Trachomatis.*

The most specific criteria for diagnosing PID include:

- Histopathologic evidence of endometritis on endometrial biopsy
- Thickened tubes, filled with fluid, with or without free fluid in pelvis; tubo-ovarian (TO) masses detected by transvaginal ultrasound or on magnetic resonance imaging (MRI); or tubal hyperemia suggested by Doppler studies.
- Laparoscopic findings consistent with PID.

TREATMENT

Women with acute PID should be treated with antibiotics. Injectable cephalosporins [ceftriaxone 250 mg intramuscular (IM) in a single dose or injection cefoxitin 2 g with tablet probenecid 1 g] along with tetracyclines (doxycycline 100 mg orally BD for 2 weeks) and metronidazole 500 mg orally twice a day for 2 weeks is usually the recommended treatment.

Other parenteral third-generation cephalosporins like ceftizoxime or cefotaxime can also be used along with doxycycline and metronidazole.

Women with tubo-ovarian abscesses (TOAs) should be admitted for monitoring. *Recommended treatment is:*

- Cefotetan 2 g intravenous (IV) every 12 hourly with doxycycline 100 mg IV every 12 hourly OR
- Cefoxitin 2 g IV every 6 hourly with clindamycin 900 mg IV every 8 hourly with gentamicin loading dose IV or IM (2 mg/kg), followed by maintenance dose (1.5 mg/kg) every 8 hours. Single daily dosing (3–5 mg/kg) can be given
- However, clindamycin (450 mg orally four times daily) with injection metronidazole IV 100 mg or tab 500 mg twice daily along with doxycycline provides a more effective anaerobic coverage in women with TOA.

Pelvic Inflammatory Disease and Assisted Reproductive Technology

Chronic inflammation after chlamydial infection leads to subsequent endosalpingitis leading to hydrosalpinx formation, which has been associated with poor fertility prognosis.

Inflammatory exudates may cause microvascular permeability leading to abnormal fluid collection inside the fallopian tubes. The disruption of secretion or absorption balance leads to formation of hydrosalpinx. Essential embryotropic substances are diluted by the low glycoprotein production and are enhanced cystic fibrosis transmembrane conductance regulator (CFTR)-mediated water permeability. This leads to low implantation rate following *in vitro* fertilization or embryo transfer (IVF/ET) procedures in women with hydrosalpinges. Therefore, salpingectomy, cornual clipping, or cauterization of the proximal part of tube with bipolar forceps is indicated in the presence of hydrosalpinx. IVF or intracystoplasmic sperm injection (ICSI) is the treatment of choice in these infertile women.

PREVENTION

- Preventative measures should focus on the detection and treatment of lower genital tract infection in women at high-risk.
- Safer sex practices, sexual health education, and counseling remain the cornerstone in STD prevention.
- Quick diagnosis, counseling, and treatment of partner are important.

- Early management can prevent long-term chronic sequel.

CONCLUSION

The PID can be treated with success, if it is diagnosed early. If not treated promptly, the infection may cause permanent damage of fallopian tubes, long-term problems, especially in respect to future fertility.

REFERENCES

1. Khan S, Ansari MA, Vasenwala SM, et al. A Community Based Study on Pelvic Inflammatory Disease in Postmenopausal Females: Microbiological Spectrum and Socio-Demographic Correlates. J Clin Diagn Res. 2017;11:LC05-LC10.
2. Ness RB, Keder LM, Soper DE, et al. Oral contraception and the recognition of endometritis. Am J Obstet Gynecol. 1997;176:580-5
3. Eschenbach DA, Buchanan TM, Pollock HM, et al. Polymicrobial etiology of acute pelvic inflammatory disease. N Engl J Med. 1975;293:166-71.
4. Taylor BD, Ness RB, Darville T, et al. Microbial correlates of delayed care for pelvic inflammatory disease. Sex Transm Dis. 2011;38:434-8.
5. Haggerty CL, Totten PA, Astete SG, et al. Mycoplasma genitalium among women with nongonococcal, nonchlamydial pelvic inflammatory disease. Infect Dis Obstet Gynecol. 2006;2006:30184.
6. Ness RB, Hillier SL, Kip KE, et al. Bacterial vaginosis and risk of pelvic inflammatory disease. Obstet Gynecol. 2004;104:761-9.
7. Taylor-Robinson D, Jensen JS, Svenstrup H, et al. Difficulties experienced in defining the microbial cause of pelvic inflammatory disease. Int J STD AIDS. 2012;23:18-24.
8. Ness RB, Hillier SL, Kip KE, et al. Bacterial vaginosis and risk of pelvic inflammatory disease. Obstet Gynecol. 2004;104:761-9.
9. Bjartling C, Osser S, Persson K. Mycoplasma genitalium in cervicitis and pelvic inflammatory disease among women at a gynecologic outpatient service. Am J Obstet Gynecol. 2012;206:476.
10. Soper DE, Brockwell NJ, Dalton HP, et al. Observations concerning the microbial etiology of acute salpingitis. Am J Obstet Gynecol. 1994;170:1008-14.
11. Workowski KA, Bolan GA; Centers for Disease Control and Prevention. Sexually Transmitted Diseases Treatment CDC Guidelines, 2015. MMWR: 2015:64:1-137.

Endometriosis: Infertility and ART

10

Prakash Trivedi, S Krishnakumar, Soumil Trivedi, Rohan Krishnakumar

INTRODUCTION

Endometriosis, a chronic condition, perhaps is the disease of the millennium, a sticky, perplexing, and unconquerable pathology, which though described by Rokitansky a century ago, has remained an enigma and its etiology is not clearly defined. Although women with endometriosis may be asymptomatic, they mostly present with pelvic pain, infertility, or pelvic mass.[1]

DEFINITION

Endometriosis is commonly defined by the presence of endometrial tissue growing outside the uterus, most commonly on the ovary and in the peritoneum, resulting in inflammation, adhesions, distortions of the pelvic anatomy, and infertility **(Fig. 1)**.

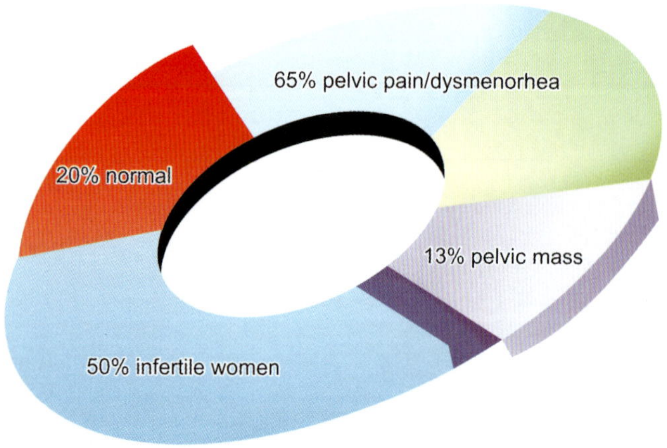

Fig. 1: Evidence of endometriosis using laparoscopic diagnosis.

POSSIBLE SITES OF ENDOMETRIOSIS

The disease is usually limited to the pelvis and lower abdominal organs.

- Reproductive tract
- Urinary tract
- Gastrointestinal (GI) tract
- Surgical scars and umbilicus
- Lungs
- Rarely, pericardium, pleura, central nervous system (CNS), nose, and eye

Susceptible tissues and organs are ovaries, uterosacral ligament, broad ligament, cardinal ligament, peritoneum of lower anterior abdominal wall, urinary bladder, round ligament, rectovaginal pouch, rectum, sigmoid colon, ureters, appendix, caecum, ascending colon, posterior vaginal fornix, vagina, peritoneum, and site of episiotomy.

INCIDENCE

Though true prevalence is difficult to quantify, it is reported that infertile women are six to eight times more likely to have endometriosis than fertile women.[2] Classical studies in literature suggest that 25–50% of infertile women have endometriosis and that 30–50% of women with endometriosis are infertile.[3] The prevalence of endometriosis in women undergoing a laparoscopy for evaluation of infertility is 10–50%, and for those with pelvic pain the reported prevalence ranges from 30% to 80%. The exact risk factors for endometriosis have not been established but the apparent factors include a low body mass index (BMI), alcohol use, and smoking.[4] In our country the incidence of endometriosis is reported more from Kerala and West Bengal.

SYMPTOMS

The classical triad of dysmenorrhea, dyspareunia, and infertility is the characteristic of the disease; the pain is often referred to rectum or lower sacral and coccygeal regions. Dysmenorrhea is progressive and not relieved by NSAIDs. The symptoms are often cyclical meaning that the pain is worse right before or during the period and then improves. Spotting or bleeding between periods.

Bowel and urinary problems including pain, diarrhea, constipation, and bloating may be seen in few.

SIGNS

Bimanual pelvic examination may reveal tender uterosacral ligaments, cul de sac nodularity, induration of rectovaginal septum, fixed uterus, adnexal masses, and generalized or localized pelvic tenderness.

INFERTILITY AND ENDOMETRIOSIS

Though a reasonable body of evidence demonstrates an association between endometriosis and infertility, a causal relationship has not been established, and whether endometriosis causes infertility or decrease in fecundity remains controversial. It is a known fact that endometriosis results in pelvic adhesions altering the pelvic anatomy, which is essential for fertility. Similarly, the result of treatment of endometriosis, for improving fertility is difficult to quantify as suppression of endometriosis by medical therapy has not been shown to improve fecundity rates and surgery for endometrioma is known to reduce ovarian reserve. Surgery for stage III and IV endometriosis can be useful to treat pelvic adhesions that may impact reproductive function with frozen pelvis and obliterated pod). Pregnancy rates (PRs) among patients with endometriosis seem to be related to the severity of endometriosis. Patents with stage I endometriosis have been reported to have PRs up to 55% and those with stage III and stage IV had 43% and 32%, respectively.

Though exactly not conclusive several mechanisms have been proposed to explain the link between endometriosis and infertility:[4-6]

- *Distorted pelvic anatomy*: Adhesion, which could be ranging from minimal to the frozen pelvic state, can definitely impair oocyte release from the ovary and inhibit the transportation of ovum.
- *Altered uterotubal transport*: A reduction in physiologic uterotubal transportation is seen in women with endometriosis as compared to control subjects.
- *Altered peritoneal function*: An increase volume of peritoneal fluid with increased concentrations of prostaglandins, cytokines including interleukin-8 (IL-8), IL-6 and tumor necrosis factor α (TNFα), protease, and vascular endothelial growth factor (VEGF) produced by macrophages.[7,8] An increase level of inflammatory cytokines has been reported in serum of women affected with endometriosis. These alterations may have adverse effects on oocyte, sperm, embryos, and fallopian tube function.
- *Endocrine and ovulatory abnormalities*: Women with endometriosis are known to have luteinized unruptured follicle syndrome, abnormal follicular growth, and luteal phase defects. Women with endometriosis are also known to have abnormal and premature LH surges leading to deranged estradiol and progesterone secretions.[9]
- *Impaired implantation*: Immunoglobulin G (IgG) and IgA antibodies and lymphocytes may be increased in the endometrium of women with endometriosis. Similarly, reduced endometrial expression of integrins and proteins required for implantation is seen in women with endometriosis.[10] These abnormalities may alter endometrial receptivity and embryo implantation.
- *Oocyte and embryo quality*: Altered progesterone and cytokine concentration in follicular fluid of women with endometriosis supports the findings of poor oocyte quality and subsequent poor embryogenesis in patients affected with endometriosis.[11] Embryos derived from women with endometriosis have been reported to grow slowly compared to embryos derived from women with tubal disease.[12] In oocyte donation cycles, women with severe endometriosis who receive oocytes from disease free women appear to have normal endometrial receptivity and PRs.

DIAGNOSIS

Good history and physical examination can yield significant findings suggestive of endometriosis, which could range but not limited to chronic or cyclic pain, dysmenorrhea, dyspareunia, retroverted fixed uterus, adnexal mass, thickening and nodularity of uterosacral ligament, and tenderness. Though ultrasound can pick up an endometrioma and severe pelvic adhesions but cannot really image peritoneal implants.

Laparoscopy remains the gold standard in the definitive diagnosis of endometriosis within the peritoneal cavity from the diaphragm to the pelvis, but performing laparoscopy for asymptomatic women with infertility simply to rule out or confirm endometriosis is unwarranted as the therapeutic benefit of laparoscopy to increase fecundity in a women with mild disease is minimal.[13] On laparoscopy, many typical and atypical peritoneal lesions ranging from a single 1 mm peritoneal implant to more than or equal to 10 cm endometriomas and cul-de-sac obliteration have been described.[14] Histologic evaluation is warranted whenever the diagnosis is not apparent on visual inspection at surgery. Many staging systems have been proposed to allow clinicians to quantify the extent of disease and to permit standardization and comparison of outcomes. The American Society for Reproductive Medicine Classification System for Endometriosis (ASRM 1996) is the most widely accepted. Unfortunately, no staging system correlates well with the chance of pregnancy following therapy.

CLASSIFICATION

Revised American Society of Reproduction Medicine Classification

The Revised American Society of Reproduction Medicine Classification is given in **Figure 2**.

Koninckx and Martin (1992) Classification:

It is based on laparoscopic findings:

- *Type 1*: Large pelvic area of typical or subtle lesions surrounded by wide sclerotic tissue
- *Type 2*: Formed by retraction of bowel and recognized clinically as a small classical lesion associated with retraction
- *Type 3*: Nodular endometriosis of rectovaginal septum. It is the most severe and often spreads laterally to involve the ureter.

We classified the disease on the basis of our first overview on laparoscopy:

- *Minimal disease:* Characterized by isolated implants and no significant adhesions.
- *Mild endometriosis:* Consist of superficial implants less than 5 cm in aggregate, scattered on peritoneum, and ovaries, no significant adhesions are present.
- *Moderate endometriosis:* It exhibits multiple implants both superficial and invasive, peritubal, and periovarian adhesions may be evident.
- *Severe disease*: multiple superficial and deep implants including large ovarian endometriomas, Flimsy and dense adhesion are usually present.
- *Advanced*: Severe disease including rectovaginal endometriosis.
- *Extensive*: Frozen pelvis represents most complex and severe pattern.

MANAGEMENT OF ENDOMETRIOSIS WITH INFERTILITY

Medical Therapy

Though medical therapy is effective in relieving pain associated with endometriosis, there is little evidence that medical treatment improves fertility. Most of the medical treatments inhibit ovulation, thereby eliminating fertility chance. The options for medical management of endometriosis include:

- Progestins and combined estrogen-progestin therapy
- Gonadotropin-releasing hormone agonists (GnRhs)
- Danazol
- Aromatase inhibitors
- Dienogest.

In a meta-analysis that included seven studies comparing medical treatment to no treatment or placebo, the common odds ratio (OR) for pregnancy was 0.85 [95% confidence interval (CI), 1.22].[15] A review of 13 randomized clinical trials (RCTs) that included nearly 800 infertile women with endometriosis reported no evidence that ovulation suppression was superior to placebo in women who wished to conceive.[16] Thus hormonal treatment does not improve the fertility of women with stage I or II disease. At present, there is insufficient data to evaluate the efficacy of aromatase inhibitors, selective estrogen receptor modulators (SERMs), and progesterone antagonists in the medical management of endometriosis for fertility.

Surgical Treatment

The advent of laparoscopy has revolutionized surgical treatment of endometriosis. Laparoscopy provides magnification and better illumination, and various techniques have been developed to destroy endometriotic deposits. These include excising the lesions using sharp scissors, diathermy or ablating them using monopolar or bipolar coagulation, or using laser or argon beam.

Stage I/II

Laparoscopic ablation of endometrial implants has been associated with a small but significant improvement in live birth rates. In literature, two studies, viz (1) Italian and (2) Canadian are commonly quoted with only one study demonstrating benefit.[13,17] Both studies permitted surgical discretion in the intervention regarding excision or ablation.

REVISED AMERICAN SOCIETY FOR REPRODUCTIVE MEDICINE CLASSIFICATION OF ENDOMETRIOSIS 1985

Patient's Name ____________________ Date: ____________________

Stage I (Minimal) 1–5 Laparoscopy________Laparotomy________Photography__________
Stage II (Mild) 6–15 Recommended Treatment ____________________
Stage III (Moderate) 16–40 ____________________
Stage IV (Severe) > 40
Total ______________ Prognosis ____________________

	ENDOMETRIOSIS	< 1 cm	< 1–3 cm	> 3 cm
Peritoneum	Superficial	1	2	4
	Deep	2	4	6
Ovary	R Superficial	1	2	4
	Deep	4	16	20
	L Superficial	1	2	4
	Deep	4	16	20
	POSTERIOR CUL-DE-SAC OBLITERATION	Partial		Complete
		4		40
	ADHESIONS	<1/3 Enclosure	1/3–2/3 Enclosure	>2/3 Enclosure
Ovary	R Filmy	1	2	4
	Dense	4	8	16
	L Filmy	1	2	4
	Dense	4	8	16
Tube	R Filmy	1	2	4
	Dense	4	8	16
	L Filmy	1	2	4
	Dense	4*	8*	16

*If the fimbriated end of the fallopian tube is completely enclosed, change the point assignment to 16

Additional Endometriosis:____________________

Associated Pathology:____________________

To be used with normal Tubes and Ovaries

L R

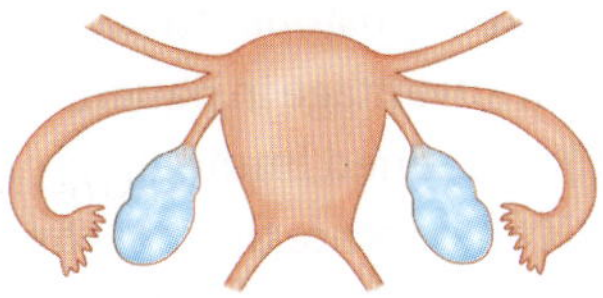

To be used with abnormal Tubes and/or Ovaries

L R

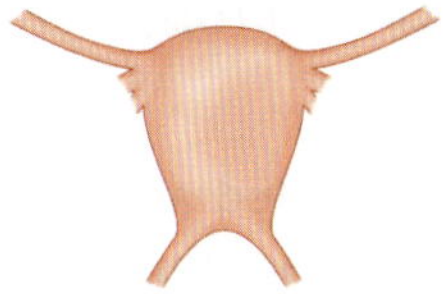

Fig. 2: Revised American Society for Reproductive Medicine Classification.

The Canadian study showed a marginal benefit (29% vs 17%) in the treated and untreated groups. The study concluded that for every 12 patient having stage I/II endometriosis diagnosed at laparoscopy, there will be one additional successful pregnancy if ablation or excision of visible endometriosis is performed compared to no treatment. It also concluded that the outcome is not affected by the method of ablation, either electro surgery or laser delivery systems.

Stage III/IV

In a nonrandomized study of 216 patient's laparoscopic cystectomy for ovarian endometrioma greater than 4 cm improved fertility compared to cyst drainage and coagulation, which is associated with increased risk of cyst recurrence. This and many other observational studies suggest that for stage III/IV endometriosis with no other identifiable infertility factors, conservative surgical treatment with laparoscopy and possible laparotomy may increase fertility. But one must emphasize, a possible adverse consequence is the loss of ovarian cortex and there by ovarian reserve.[18] There is insufficient evidence to indicate that resection of endometriomas prior to in vitro fertilization (IVF) improves outcomes. After an initial surgery, additional surgery has only rarely increased fecundability, and these patients may be better served by using assisted reproductive technology (ART).[19]

Surgical Treatment for Other Conditions in Endometriosis: Rectovaginal Lesions and Recurrent endometriosis

Rectovaginal endometriosis usually results in severe pain that is a consequence of deep, infiltrating endometriosis. The primary objective of surgical treatment of rectovaginal endometriosis is pain relief. The resection of the rectovaginal lesion has been reported to significantly relieve the pain, but is ineffective for fertility enhancement. Few studies have been performed that examine options for second-line surgery for patients with recurrent endometriosis. Repeated surgery has only rarely increased fecundity and ASRM has recommended ART for patients who have a history of at least one surgical treatment. The results of another meta-analysis suggested that expectant management followed by ART may result in a better prognosis for pregnancy compared with repeated surgery in women with recurrent endometriosis. However, if the patients suffer from severe pain or from endometrioma more than 4 cm, the Royal College of Obstetricians and Gynecologists (RCOG) has recommended that repeated surgery could be considered.

Basic Guidelines for Surgical Therapy in Endometriosis

- Endometrial implants if detected accidentally in laparoscopy being performed for other indications, should be tackled taking care of vital structures like ureter, colon, etc.
- If pain is to be relieved, good clearance should be attempted. The basic goal of surgical treatment for endometriosis should be to restore normal tubo-ovarian anatomy, in the presence of adhesions associated with endometriosis.
- If endometrioma is present, one must rule out false chocolate cyst. The endometrioma should be separated from its adhesions with pouch of Douglas, colon, and tubes.
- Excision of the cyst wall is superior to ablation only as recurrence chances are less. If bilateral endometriotic cyst is present, cystectomy of both side will lead to greater loss of ovarian reserve, and should be avoided. In endometriomas of less than 2 cm, excision should be avoided as it can lead greater loss of ovarian tissue. During cystectomy, correct plane should be achieved to prevent loss of ovarian tissue and one must be careful near hilum. In difficult situations, diluted vasopressin has been used to good effect to achieve a correct plane and reduce bleeding.
- As endometriosis is as such a recurring disease all possible attempts should be made to clear all possible visible lesions or else the recurrence will be faster and every repeat surgery will lead to more decrease of ovarian reserve.
- Surgery should be performed by a well-versed endoscopic surgeon, with due respects to all fertility aspects.

Medical and Surgical Therapy Combination

There is no evidence in literature that combination medical-surgical treatment significantly enhances fertility, and one must also bear that the combination may in fact delay further fertility therapy. Preoperative therapy may help reduce vascularity and the size of implants, thus minimizing blood loss and reduced surgical time. Also because of reduced vascularity, postsurgery adhesions could be reduced. Postsurgical medical therapy has been advocated as a means of eradicating residual implants in the presence of extensive disease in whom resection of all implants is not possible. Use of postoperative GnRh agonists depot has been used with advantage in patients in whom IVF-embryo transfer (ET) is planned immediately following surgery.

The GnRH analogs are the most frequently used medical therapy in endometriosis and these are used in following conditions:

- Inflamed endometriosis or endometrioma
- Frozen pelvis or previous abdominal surgery for endometrioma
- Recurrent endometrioma treated by surgery
- Rectovaginal endometriosis or adenomyosis
- Postoperatively as a follow-up treatment to improve the PRs.

In stimulation protocols for ART in patients with endometriosis of all grades

Guidelines

European Society of Human (ESHRE), ASRM, and RCOG commissions have suggested guidelines for infertility management in women with endometriosis that have mostly coincided **(Table 1)**. Surgical treatment has demonstrated benefit in stage I/II endometriosis in ESHRE and RCOG guidelines, but insufficient benefit to be recommended solely to increase the likelihood of pregnancy in ASRM guideline. Surgical treatment is a possible treatment modality for stage III/IV endometriosis in all three guidelines. Postoperative adjuvant management is not currently recommended; because there is little evidence that the postoperative ovarian suppression effects may improve future fertility. Although controversial, all three committees recommended that surgical treatment can be performed before ART for patients with endometrioma more than 3–4 cm especially to improve endometriosis-associated pain or accessibility of follicles or to detect occult malignancy. The ASRM committee opinion was that ART rather than repeated surgical procedures should be used for women with recurrent endometriosis.[20]

Intrauterine Insemination

Several studies have reported success with intrauterine insemination (IUI) when it is combined with ovarian stimulation in the treatment of endometriosis-associated infertility. The ASRM guideline level II evidence suggests that superovulation (SO) or IUI may be a viable option for women who have had a surgical diagnosis and treatment of stage I or II endometriosis as an alternative to IVF-ET or further surgical therapy, as this is a progressive disease and a delay may alter the tubo-ovarian anatomy. But there is insufficient evidence to determine if SO/IUI is more successful after endometriosis is diagnosed and treated compared to minimal or mild endometriosis left undiagnosed or untreated.

ART in Endometriosis

The IVF may represent a viable option that overcomes the influence of distorted pelvic anatomy in infertile women with endometriosis. However, because few studies have been performed that evaluate whether IVF is superior to expectant management for patients with endometriosis, it is not a treatment of choice for infertile women with endometriosis. Although most of the results from recent studies have suggested that endometriosis does not affect the IVF outcome after adjusting for age, some discrepancies have been reported. Some of the studies have reported lower fertilization or implantation rates altered oocyte quality and PRs in endometriosis patients, compared with the controls. In the early 2000s, a meta-analysis that included 27 trials compared the outcome of IVF for patients with endometriosis with that of women undergoing IVF for other indications.[20] The chance of achieving pregnancy was significantly lower in endometriosis patients (OR 0.56, 95% CI 0.44–0.70), compared with the tubal controls. Fertilization and implantation rates were also significantly lower. Fewer oocytes were retrieved from the endometriosis patients after adjusting for age, stimulation protocol.

The effect of existing endometrioma on ART outcome has been debated. There have been no randomized studies comparing IVF or ICSI outcomes between expectant management and surgical treated groups. Moreover, the effect of endometrioma on IVF outcome is difficult to evaluate because endometrioma rarely occurs without peritoneal lesions or adhesions. Surgical removal of endometrioma can have possible benefits, particularly for larger endometriomas, and can prevent incidental or iatrogenic rupture of the endometrioma during oocyte retrieval, early detection of ovarian malignancy, and easier oocyte retrieval. The disadvantages of surgical removal include potential surgical complications, decreased ovarian reserve after surgery, economic costs, and lack of definitive evidence for a positive effect on ART outcome. There are no studies evaluating impact of size of the endometrioma on outcome. The study by Basheer AlKudmani et al. concludes that presence of endometriomas did not have an impact on IVF outcome when comparing patients with severe (stage 3 and 4) endometriosis.[21] The same study also concludes that the interval from endometriosis surgery to IVF had a significant effect on the PR. The highest ongoing PR was achieved in patients who underwent their IVF cycle 6–25 months after their endometriosis surgery. The exact mechanism of for impaired fertility during first 6 months needs to be investigated, the reduced PRs after 2 years may be explained by either recurrence and/or age factors. The results of a case control study indicated that there is no effect on ART outcome when endometrioma is removed laparoscopically before IVF. The authors of a recent Cochrane review concluded that neither aspiration nor cystectomy before ART in asymptomatic women further improves PR.

The systematic review that summarized three RCTs concluded that administrating GnRH agonists for 3–6 months prior to ART in women with endometriosis increases the odds of clinical pregnancy (OR 4.28, 95% CI 2.00–9.15).

The study by Basheer AlKudmani showed that clinical and ongoing PRs per cycle to be lower than the control group by 1.8% and 2.2% in patients with mild endometriosis and 17 % and 22% in patients with severe endometriosis. Another recent study by Kemal Ozgur et al. concludes that in patients with endometriosis, segmental IVF that is freezing of embryos after IVF and transferring frozen embryos in subsequent cycle have shown better PRs (i.e. 58% vs 31% reported in the reviews).[22]

PREGNANCY OUTCOMES

Women with endometriosis have been shown to have adverse obstetrical outcomes compared to those without endometriosis, like:

- Increased risk of preterm birth
- Higher risk of preeclampsia
- Higher risk of antepartum bleeding or placental complications
- Higher C-section rates.

RECOMMENDATIONS[1]

- Before formulating management plan for infertility patients with endometriosis, complete counseling of the couple should be done considering the age, duration of infertility, presence of pelvic pain, and stage of endometriosis and ovarian reserve.
- Current evidence of laparoscopy in minimal or mild endometriosis shows no benefit and should not be recommended solely to increase the likelihood of pregnancy, in the absence of pain.
- During laparoscopy for other indications and if endometriosis is detected, one must consider excising or ablating all visible lesions.
- In stage I/II endometriosis in younger women with normal ovarian reserve, expectant management or ovulation induction (OI)/IUI can be considered as first-line therapy. For older women or with decrease ovarian reserve, aggressive treatment such as OI/IUI or IVF may be considered.
- In young women with stage III/IV endometriosis conservative surgical therapy with laparoscopy may be beneficial.
- Surgical management of endometrioma should include cystectomy or ablation rather than drainage, with cystectomy preferred with proper vigilance on ovarian reserve
- For women with stage IV endometriosis who fail to conceive following conservative surgery or because of advancing reproductive age, IVF ET is an effective alternative.

CONCLUSION

Though endometriosis is such a debilitating disease, if managed by a competent gynecologist who has scientific knowledge of endoscopic surgery as well as ART and TVS, it has the most promising results. Laparoscopy is a common approach for the diagnosis and treatment of endometriosis, especially with regard to pelvic pain, and infertility. Last but not the least, active fertility management and resorting to ART earlier gives higher PRs.

REFERENCES

1. Practice Committee of the American Society for Reproductive Medicine. Endometriosis and Infertility: a committee opinion. Fertil Steril. 2012;98:591-8.
2. Verkauf BS. Incidence, symptoms, and signs of endometriosis in fertile and infertile women. J Fla Med Ass. 1987:74:671-5.
3. Missmer SA, Hankinson SE, Spiegelman D, et al. Incidence of laparoscopically confirmed endometriosis by demographic, anthropometric, and lifestyle factors. Am J Epidemiol. 2004;160:784-96.
4. Schenken RS, Treatment of human infertility: the special case of endometriosis. In: Adashi EY, Rock JA (Eds). Reproductive endocrinology. Philadelphia, PA: Lippincot-Raven; 1996. pp. 2122-39.
5. Bulun SE. Endometriosis. N Engl J Med. 2009;360:268-79.
6. Giudice LC. Clinical practice. Endometriosis. N Engl J Med. 2010;362:2389-98.
7. Bedaiwy MA, Falcone T, Sharma RK, et al. Prediction of endometriosis with serum and peritoneal fluid markers: a prospective controlled trial. Human Reprod. 2002;17:426-31.
8. Pizzo A, Salmeri FM, Ardita FV, et al. Behaviour of cytokine levels in serum and peritoneal fluid in women with endometriosis. Gynecol Obstet Invest. 2002;54(2):82-7.
9. Schenken RS, Asch RH, Williams RF, et al. Etiology of Infertility in monkeys with endometriosis: luteinized unruptured follicles, luteal phase defects, pelvic adhesions, and spontaneous abortions. Fertil Steril. 1984;41:122-30.
10. Lessey BA, Castlebaum AJ, Sawin SW, et al. Aberrant integrin expression in the endometrium of women with endometriosis. J Clin Endocrinol Metab. 1994;79:643-9.
11. Garrido N, Navarro J, Remohi J, et al. Follicular hormonal environment and embryo quality in women with endometriosis. Hum Reprod Update. 200;6:67-74.
12. Pellicer A, Oliveira N, Ruiz A, et al. Exploring the mechanisms of endometriosis-related infertility: an analysis of embryo development and implantation in assisted reproduction. Hum Reprod. 1995;10(Suppl 2):91-7.
13. Marcoux S, Maheux R, Berube S. Laparoscopic surgery in infertile women with minimal or mild .endometriosis.

Canadian Collaborative Group on Endometriosis. N Engl J Med. 1997;337:217-22.
14. American Society for Reproductive Medicine. Revised American Society for Reproductive Medicine classification of Endometriosis: 1996. Fertil Steril. 1997;67:817-21.
15. Hughes EG, Fedorkow DM, Collins JA. A quantitative overview of controlled trials in endometriosis-associated infertility. Fertil Steril. 1993;59:963-70.
16. Hughes E, Brown J, Collins JJ, et al. Ovulation suppression for endometriosis. Cochrane Databas Syst Rev. 2007: CD000115.
17. Parazzini F. Ablation of lesions or no treatment in minimal-mild endometriosis in infertile women. A randomized trial. Hum Reprod. 1999;14:1332-4.
18. Crosignani C, Vercillini P, Biffignandi F, et al. Laparoscopy versus laparotomy in conservative surgical treatment for severe endometriosis. Fertil Steril. 1996;66:706-11.
19. Donnez J, Nisolle M, Gillet N, et al. Large Ovarian endometriomas. Human Reprod. 1996;11:641-6.
20. Yun BH, Choi YS, Lee BS. Management of Endometriosis-Associated Infertility. J Androl Gynaecol. 2014;2(2):7
21. AlKudmani B, Gat I, Buell D, et al. In Vitro Fertilization Success Rates after surgically treated Endometriosis and effect of Time Interval Between Surgery and In Vitro Fertilization. J Minim Invasive Gynecol. 2018;25:99-104.
22. Kemal Ozgur, Hasan Bulut, Murat Berkkanoglu et al. Reproductive outcomes of Segmented In Vitro fertilization in Patients Diagnosed with Endometriomas. J Minim Invasive Gynecol. 2018;25:105-10.

Adenomyosis: Newer Trends in Assisted Reproductive Technology

11

KD Nayar, Kuldeep Jain, Amiti Agrawal, Nupur Agarwal

INTRODUCTION

Since the very inception of adenomyosis, it has been the most perplexing disorder for the treating gynecologist. Lack of substantial evidence in literature and standard treatment guidelines makes it a crucial topic of discussion.[1]

DEFINITION

Adenomyosis is the occurrence of heterotopic endometrial glands and stroma in the myometrium of uterus. It is usually accompanied by a myometrial hyperplasia and inflammatory cells infiltration in the surrounding myometrium.

HISTORICAL BACKGROUND

The first description of the current day adenomyosis was by Thomas Stephan Cullen in the year 1896.

Frankl, in the year 1925, used the term "Adenomyosis uteri" to clearly distinguish adenomyoma, an adenomyosis. In adenomyoma, there is autochthonous growth of the glands within the myoma, whereas in adenomyosis, endometrium is directly connected with islands of mucosa of musculature. It was in the year 1972, that Bird stated that: "Adenomyosis can be defined as invasion of endometrium into myometrium, leading to a diffusely enlarged uterus which is seen microscopically as ectopic non-neoplastic, endometrial glands and stroma bordered by hypertrophic and hyperplastic myometrium".

PREVALENCE AND INCIDENCE

Due to the lack of standard criteria for diagnosis of adenomyosis, the true incidence is not known. In one of the largest cross-sectional study done at Spain, the prevalence of adenomyosis was 24.4% among the patients undergoing assisted reproductive technology (ART).[2]

PATHOGENESIS

Invagination of the Endometrial Basalis

- Invagination due to myometrial weakness
- Invagination due to altered immunological activity
- Embryologic misplaced pleuripotent Mullerian remnants.
- More number of estradiol receptors are expressed in adenomyotic tissue which leads to increased estrogen enhancing the endometriotic tissue invagination into the myometrium.
- Basalis endometrium invagination in the myometrium can be due to altered immunological activity at the endometrial-myometrial.
- Junction zone of the endomyometrium is altered due to cytokines stimulation by antibiotic produced by T and B cells.
- Basalis can invaginate beside the intramyometrial lymphatic system.

MORPHOLOGICAL FEATURES

Gross: Pinpoint/small cystic areas of hemorrhage seen within the myometrium with hyperplastic myometrium.

Microscopic: The main diagnostic features are ectopic endometrial stroma and glands in the myometrium. The diagnosis can be made either by the distance between the lower border of endometrium and the affected myometrial area should be more than half of a low power field, or when

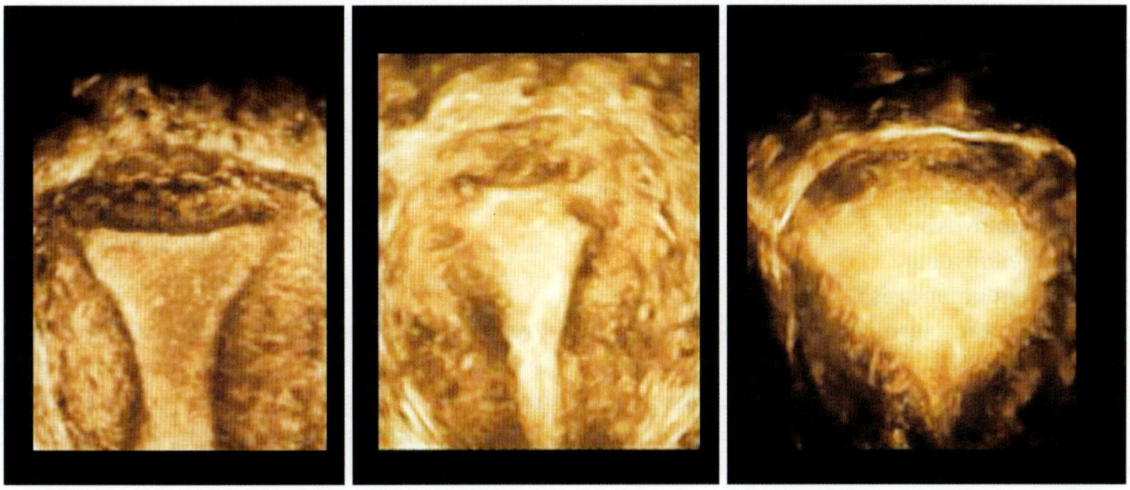

Fig. 1

endometrial glands and stroma are deeper than 2.5 mm below the endometrial surface on a low power field.

CLASSIFICATION

Various authors have designed different classifications.

Levgur et al. devised a grading system to describe the depth of adenomyotic foci—deep (>80%), intermediate (40–80%), and superficial (<40%).[3]

Surgical/Histological Classification of Adenomyosis

Diffuse Adenomyosis

- Smooth muscle hyperplasia with ectopic endometrium (junctional zone)
- Micro-dilated ectopic endometrial glands throughout hyperplastic myometrium.

Focal Adenomyosis

- Adenomyomas
- Cystic adult adenomyosis
- Juvenile cystic adenomyosis.

Polypoid Adenomyosis

- Typical polypoid adenomyomas
- Atypical polypoid adenomyomas.

Special Categories

- Adenomyomas of endocervical type
- Retroperitoneal adenomyosis or rectovaginal endometriosis

Ken Tamai from Japan classified adenomyosis in three categories, based on the magnetic resonance imaging (MRI) features.[4]

Adenomyoma: Common presentations of this pathological process is a well-circumscribed and localized form, known as adenomyoma. The presentation of this condition is most similar to that of a leiomyoma.

The clinical as well as the imaging pattern is usually similar. The main advantage of this form is that it is amenable to surgical resection.

Adenomyomatous polyp (polypoid adenomyoma): This form usually appear as sessile or pedunculated polypoid mass in the endocervix or lower uterine endometrium. It usually occurs in the premenopausal women, with presentation as abnormal genital bleeding.

Adenomyotic cyst (cystic adenomyosis): This presents as hemorrhagic cyst due to severe menstrual bleeding in ectopic endometrial gland. It can be completely within the myometrial, submucosal or subserosal tissue.

RISK FACTORS

- Age
- Increasing parity—multiparous patients. This may be due to the elevated levels of estrogen as described above or secondary to trophoblast invasion into the myometrium at implantation
- Premature menarche (≤10 years of age)
- Short menstrual cycles (≤24 days)
- Elevated BMI (>24.9)

- *Smoking*: A history of smoking was associated with a decreased risk (OR: 0.7). The postulated mechanism was that cigarette smoking alters hormonal metabolism, leading to a reduced incidence of endometrial abnormalities.
- Previous uterine surgery leading to endometrial trauma can cause adenomyosis
- Concomitant leiomyoma
- Concomitant endometriosis
- Previous pregnancy termination (>1)—leading to endometrial trauma
- Previous cesarean section was more often associated with adenomyosis as compared to a history of previous normal vaginal delivery.
- *Tamoxifen therapy*: Tamoxifen binds to selective estrogen receptors and can stimulate both normal and ectopic endometrial tissue fostering the development of adenomyosis.

CLINICAL MANIFESTATIONS

Symptoms

- *Age group*: 40 years and 50 years
- Abnormal uterine bleeding (65% of patients)
- Heavy menstrual bleeding (40–60%)
- Intermenstrual bleeding in cases of an adenomyotic polyp.

Dysmenorrhea and Dyspareunia

It occurs in 15–30% of patients presenting with adenomyosis. The extent of pain is usually related to the size of adenomyotic foci and depth of invasion.

Infertility

The incidence of adenomyosis in the infertile population has reported to be around 20.9–24.4%.[5]

Vercellini et al. did a meta-analysis and found that women with adenomyosis undergoing in vitro fertilization (IVF)/ICSI with autologous oocytes had 28% lower likelihood of clinical pregnancy.[6]

There are multiple factors responsible for the decreased pregnancy amongst these patients.

Histologically, it has been observed that increased estrogen by aromatase P450 and endometrial glands inflammation causes inflammation. Few authors have hypothesized a detrimental effect due to altered uterine peristalsis and decreased endometrial receptivity.

Some authors have also reported that there is no statistically significant difference in pregnancy and implantation rates in women having adenomyosis or no adenomyosis diagnosed at TVS.[6-8]

Early Pregnancy Losses

Adenomyosis was associated with almost a doubled risk of miscarriage, indicating a causal relation.

Pressure symptoms: Enlarging uterus causes a pressure on the surrounding structures. The most common symptom due to the enlarging uterus is increased frequency of urination. Others symptoms of constipation and pedal edema are also seen in cases of big uteri.

Signs

There is a diffuse uterine enlargement presenting as a globular uterus. The probable mechanism is proliferation of the ectopic endometrial tissue, which causes smooth muscle cell hyperplasia and hypertrophy. Some women may have a tender uterus on physical examination.

Adenomyosis can also be present in the endometrial cavity as a polypoidal mass or it can form adenomyomas which are focal areas of circumscribed nodular aggregates of smooth muscle.

Diagnostic Modalities

The two primary modalities of diagnosis are the imaging and histopathological analysis. Imaging

Ultrasound

This is the primary modality used for diagnosing adenomyosis in cases of clinical suspicion.

Two-dimensional transvaginal ultrasound (2D-TVUS): USG parameters used to define adenomyosis are:

- The most common heterogeneous myometrial echotexture.
- Globular asymmetrically enlarged uterus, usually with a uterine length of not more than 12 cm.
- In the myometrium, there are presence of irregular cystic spaces, myometrial linear striations and poor definition of endometrial myometrial junction which also gives the appearance of pseudowidening of the endometrium.
- There is asymmetry of anterior-posterior myometrium, which is observed as thickening of anterior and

posterior myometrial wall and increased or decreased echogenicity.

- Furthermore, a diffuse spread of small vessels within the myometrium has also been described as a diagnostic feature of adenomyosis.
- An adenomyoma is a focal confined nodular collection of ectopic endometrium commonly identified on the posterior uterine wall.
- Two-dimensional transvaginal ultrasound volume measurement (cm^3) is calculated by the ellipsoid formula (uterine longitudinal diameter × transverse diameter × anteroposterior diameter × 0.532).[9]
- Myometrial cysts will be observed in 50% of patients. Cysts are dilated glands or hemorrhagic foci in the heterotopic endometrium. These are usually less than 5 mm in diameter.
- Cystic adenomyosis, these can be larger (>5 mm in diameter). These can appear as echogenic nodules on ultrasound due to the hemorrhagic content.

Three-dimensional transvaginal ultrasound (3D-TVUS): 3D-TVUS helps us to see the junctional zone clearly compared to 2D-TVUS.

On the coronal view the junctional zone can be identified as a hypoechoic area surrounding the endometrium, an ill-defined junctional zone, and a distortion or infiltration of the inner myometrium.[9]

Color Doppler Studies

Usage of color Doppler studies helps us to improve the diagnostic accuracy of ultrasound findings. Presence of anechoic areas of myometrial thickness of more than or equal to 1 mm, intramyometrial cysts and negative color Doppler were diagnostic of adenomyosis. Overall there is an increased vascularity in the stroma of the myometrium.

Magnetic Resonance Imaging

Features are:

- Enlarged uterus with presence of a distinct or an ill-defined myometrial mass of low intensity.
- Diffuse or local widening of junctional zones on T2-weighted image.
- Junctional zone thickness is increased to more than equal to 0.15 mm, this could be localized or diffuse.
- Champaneria et al. did a systematic review to compare the diagnostic precision of MRI and ultrasound. 2,312 women and 23 articles were included and found that TVUS had pooled sensitivity of 72%, specificity of 81%, positive likelihood ratio of 3.7 and negative likelihood ratio of 0.3. Pooled sensitivity of MRI was 77%, specificity of 89%, positive likelihood ratio of 6.5, and negative likelihood ratio of 0.2. They found that both MRI and TVUS had high precision in diagnosing adenomyosis.[10]

Histological Features

This forms the final reference standard for the diagnosis of adenomyosis. The features on gross and microscopic examination have been discussed above.

TREATMENT MODALITIES

The main treatment can be divided into:

- *Medical management*:
  - Non-hormonal therapy
  - Analgesics and anti-inflammatory agents
  - Anti-angiogenic drugs
  - Hormonal therapy
  - Oral contraceptives
  - Danazol—oral and intrauterine system
  - Levonorgestrel intrauterine system
  - Gonadotropin-releasing hormone agonists (GnRH agonists)
  - Estrogen receptor inhibitors
  - Selective estrogen receptor modulators (SERMs)
  - Selective progesterone receptor modulators (SPRMs)
  - Progestins and progestational agents
  - Antiprogestins
  - Aromatase inhibitors
- *Surgical management*:
  - Minimal surgical intervention
  - Radical procedures
  - Hysterectomy.

Medical Management

Nonsteroidal Anti-inflammatory Drugs

Women may experience symptom improvement by taking non-steroidal anti-inflammatory drugs, which inhibit the production of prostaglandins by inhibiting cyclo-oxygenase enzyme. Although not devoid of potential adverse effects nonsteroidal anti-inflammatory drugs (NSAIDs) form the first line of management dysmenorrhea.

Anti-angiogenic Agents

Neovascularization forms an integral part in the pathogenesis of adenomyosis. Although an emerging concept various drugs like growth factor inhibitors, endogenous angiogenesis inhibitors, fumagillin analogs, endogenous angiogenesis inhibitors, statins, cyclo-oxygenase-2 inhibitors, statins, phytochemical compounds, immunomodulators, dopamine agonists, immunomodulators, peroxisome proliferator-activated receptor agonists have been used in adenomyosis and endometriosis patients. These drugs have still been used in experimental settings and are a great potential for further research.

Hormonal Therapy

Oral Contraceptive Pills

Patients may show symptomatic improvement of dysmenorrhea and heavy menstrual bleeding when taking oral contraception continuously or cyclically.

The main mechanism is prevention of ovulation and thereby the hormonal action. However, these medications help improve symptoms by inducing amenorrhea and may induce regression of adenomyosis for a short period, however randomized control trials are lacking.

Danazol

Danazol can be given by routes—oral and danazol-loaded intracervical injections and intrauterine devices. Danazol acts by suppressing pituitary release of FSH and LH, therefore causes atrophy of both normal and ectopic endometrial tissue. Systemic treatment with danazol may decrease aromatase cytochrome P450 expression in eutopic endometrium; this may contribute to improvement of symptoms and reduced uterine size.

Oral: However, it is not well tolerated by many patients because of its side effect profile which can include acne, depression, deepening of the voice, hirsutism, hot flushes, increased liver enzyme concentrations, decreased high-density lipoprotein levels, oily skin, muscle cramps, reduced breast size, and weight gain.

Selective Estrogen Receptor Modulators

Selective estrogen receptor modulators, e.g. tamoxifen, raloxifene, etc. have differential estrogen receptor (ER) expression in tissues so may be preferred agents in management of Adenomyosis due to binding to the ER co-regulator proteins. Ideal SERM should have an antagonist estrogenic activity on endometrium with an agonist activity in the bone and serum.[11,12]

Selective Progesterone Receptor Modulators

It has been observed that progesterone is produced by adenomyotic lesions, although levels of progesterone receptor (PR) with endometrium are significantly lower. It has been observed that SPRMs interact with the PR, leading to the binding of antiprogestins with both agonist and antagonist properties, thereby decreasing the pain associated with adenomyosis.

In 2016, retrospective analysis of a prospectively collected database conducted in Italy on patients with adenomyosis and fibroids, who took three months of ulipristal acetate observed an improvement in bleeding but pain was worsened, following administration for a period of 3 months.[13]

Progestins

The main mechanism by which progestational agents act is causing atrophy and decidualization of the endometrium. The most commonly used progestational agents are medroxyprogesterone acetate and norethisterone are more commonly used in cases of adenomyosis. Studies have shown significant symptomatic benefit in terms of pain and bleeding, with the use of these agents.

Dienogest

Dienogest is a synthetic oral progestin and progestational 19-norsteroid derivative which binds selectively to PRs. It has an antiovulatory, antiproliferative activity on endometrial cells with mild hypoestrogenic effects as well.

Dienogest helps in decreasing pain in endometriosis and adenomyosis.

A randomized, multicenter, double-blind, placebo-controlled phase III study of dienogest in patients of adenomyosis was conducted at Japan. The efficacy and safety profile of the drug in symptomatic adenomyosis patients was analyzed. They concluded that this drug is helpful in pain associated with adenomyosis not having severe uterine enlargement or severe anemia.[14]

Antiprogestins (Gestrinone)

Anti-progestational drugs, like gestrinone (ethylnorgestrienone) have been used for treatment of adenomyosis.

It causes ovarian steroidogenesis inhibition and progestational withdrawal effect at the endometrial cellular level.

Gonadotropin-releasing Hormone Agonists

Gonadotropin-releasing hormone agonists cause a suppression of pituitary gonadotropins and thus induce ovarian quiescence, resulting in a medical menopausal, hypoestrogenic state thereby reducing the manifestations of adenomyosis.

Mode of action: Subcutaneous injections or intranasal spray.

Effect: Studies have shown that patient's symptoms of heavy menstrual bleeding and dysmenorrhea completely resolved and her uterine volume decreased.

Side effects: Hot flushes, vaginal atrophy, and accelerated bone demineralization. However, after discontinuation of therapy, symptoms may return and uterine volumes may increase to pretreatment size. Further research is required to determine the duration of GnRH analog treatment that will result in symptomatic improvement while minimizing risk of long-term side effects and delay in patients wanting to conceive.[15]

Aromatase Inhibitors

Aromatase cytochrome P-450 converts androgens to estrogens and its expression has been observed in both eutopic and ectopic endometrium in patients with endometriosis. Improved lesion size, mean pain scores, and quality of life scores in patients with adenomyosis treated with aromatase inhibitors have been shown by studies.

Also various studies depicted that aromatase inhibitors along with progestins or oral contraceptives decreased the intensity of pain due to endometriosis and improved quality of life.[16]

Estrogen Receptor Inhibitor

Fulvestrant, an anti-estrogen has high affinity for ER, got approval for hormonal receptor positive metastatic breast cancer treatment by the US Food and Drug Administration in 2002.

It attenuates ER ability to inhibit or activate transcription leading to estrogen action blockade. We still need further trials to prove its efficacy in adenomyosis.

Surgical Management

Hysteroscopic procedures form the main stay of conservative uterine surgeries, in case of adenomyosis.

They can be divided in ablative or excisional procedures.

Endometrial Ablation and Hysteroscopic Resection

These procedures can be used as a treatment option in patients who have completed childbearing.

It has been divided in two categories:

1. Nonresectoscopic, e.g. bipolar radiofrequency, cryotherapy, circulating hot water, microwave, and thermal balloon
2. Resectoscopic, e.g. wire loop resection, laser or roller ball ablation and radiofrequency ablation.

Disadvantages

Levgur, in the year 2007, reviewed over 2,000 patients with abnormal bleeding treated by YAG laser.

He concluded that there was a higher failure rates in adenomyotic patients if foci was more than 2.5 mm and where hysterectomy was unavoidable.

- Depth of the adenomyotic lesions limits the success of the treatment.
- Deep ectopic endometrium can become trapped behind the ablated edge resulting in pain and bleeding.
- Resection is often limited to superficial lesions as there is risk of causing significant bleeding from arteries present around 5 mm below the myometrial surface.
- Predictors of amenorrhea were uterine length less than 9 cm, endometrial thickness less than 4 mm, age more than 45 years of age and the use of radiofrequency ablation instead of thermal balloon ablation.
- Predictors of treatment failure included parity of 5 or more, prior tubal ligation, age less than 45 years, and dysmenorrhea.

In 2009, Mayo Clinic, Rochester, MN, USA, did a retrospective cohort study which was done in menorrhagia patients undergoing global endometrial ablation either thermal balloon ablation or radiofrequency ablation. They concluded that global endometrial ablation for adenomyotic women had higher failure rates and required repeat procedure or hysterectomy finally.[17]

Adenomyoma Excision

Complete excision of the ectopic endometrium of adenomyotic foci is a moderately good therapeutic modality.

However the lesions often are not clearly defined and the adenomyosis is present diffusely throughout the myometrium. This can be performed by various routes as in vaginal, laparoscopic or by hysteroscopic means.

One of the largest study on 165 women undergoing adenomyomectomy or combined surgical-medical treatment (surgery followed by 6 months administration of a GnRH agonist) was conducted.

The adenomyomectomy was done by laparoscopy, mini-laparotomy or ultramini-laparotomy. There was a statistically significant symptomatic relief and all symptom scores at the end of the 2-year follow-up period. 77.5% had clinical pregnancy rate and 69.0 had a successful delivery.

Disadvantages: The success following excisional treatment is on an average 50% and the risk of relapse is always there.

Advantage: Good reproductive outcomes following treatment.[18]

Uterine Artery Embolization

Patients report improvement in symptoms following uterine artery embolization with significant improvement in menorrhagia and dysmenorrhea at follow-up. Kim et al. in 2005 observed the effectiveness and pregnancy outcome after uterine artery embolization in adenomyotic patients. 83.3% live birth rate was seen after a 35 months follow up.[19]

Side effects: Pelvic pain, fever and due to ischemic necrosis. 5% of patients suffer a major complication such as infection, hemorrhage, or unplanned surgical procedure. Few cases of decreased ovarian function following uterine artery embolization have also been documented.

Myometrial Reduction

Myometrial reduction is an approach to treating patients with diffuse adenomyosis by removing the abnormal tissue and then completing metroplasty during laparoscopy or laparotomy.

Approaches

Classical reduction method where the uterus is dissected in the midline longitudinally and the anterior and posterior portions of the myometrium are resected. They found this method was not very successful as women developed adenomyosis and required hysterectomy within 1 year.

Modified method a transverse H incision: Adenomyoma is removed by one vertical and two crossing horizontal incisions to allow easy removal of adenomyotic tissue. The operative time, blood loss, and volume of specimen removed was almost the same but the symptomatic improvement was more obvious in the transverse H technique.

The modified group had a greater improvement in pain, return of the reproductive function and lower risk of perforation.[20]

Triple flap method—Osada et al. described this method of adenomyomectomy where the adenomyotic tissues were excised and by a triple-flap repair the uterine wall reconstruction was done.[21] All 104 women had adenomyosis of more than 80% of anterior and posterior uterine walls with wall thickness of more than 6 cm as diagnosed by ultrasound and MRI.

The uterus was delivered intraoperatively and a tourniquet was applied supracervically. Then uterus was bisected in the sagittal plane in the midline and opened the uterine cavity. A 1 cm of myometrial thickness was left from the serosa and the endometrium above and below respectively after excision of adenomyotic tissue from surrounding myometrium. Myometrium was repaired with the triple-flap after the approximation of endometrial lining.

The results showed a definitive improvement in the degree of dysmenorrhea, menstrual blood loss, and anemia. On following up the patients there was a reduced recurrence rate. The main advantage was that utilizing this method was the reduced risk of rupture during pregnancy.

Disadvantage: Post-procedure there is a reduction in the uterine volume, which may hamper the future pregnancy outcome. Patients may be predisposed to spontaneous abortion or premature labor. Uterine scaring caused due to the procedure can lead to decreased uterine wall strength and increased risk of uterine rupture.[22,23]

As compared to classical method of adenomyomectomy which involved uterine incision and stepwise resection and closure of adenomyotic tissue, the new modified reduction surgery uses H-shape incision and adenomyomatous tissue excision and had 50% pregnancy rate, as compared to older classical method with no pregnancy. The old classical method in comparison to newer technique had 0.14 (95% CI, 0.00 and 4.47) odd of having a live birth.[20]

Laparoscopic transient occlusion of bilateral uterine arteries: A prospective study in 2017 described the laparoscopic transient occlusion of bilateral uterine arteries as therapeutic in cases of focal adenomyosis cases. In a 7-month follow-up of the 105 patients he operated there was a marked improvement in the clinical symptoms of the patient with reduced intraoperative blood loss.[24]

Robotic assisted adenomyoma excision: First case report in 2010 of robot-assisted cystic adenoma excision was reported in an adolescent girl.[25]

Magnetic resonance imaging-guided focused ultrasound surgery for adenomyosis: This procedure uses MRI-guided ultrasound energy to remove the areas of adenomyosis in patients who are willing for reproductive function preservation.

Mode of action: The treatment causes cell death and necrosis of the targeted adenomyotic tissue, preserving the surrounding myometrium and uterine walls. The ultrasound beams, with high thermal imaging sensitivity and good anatomic resolution, are focused on the target and cause thermal coagulation and consequent necrosis.

Side effects: Risk of skin burn, nausea and vomiting, and sciatic nerve palsy. It is also found that posttreatment the patients has significantly smaller mean uterine volume and lower scores related to heavy menstrual bleeding and bulk during a period of 3–6 months.[26-28]

EFFECT OF ADENOMYOSIS AFTER ENDOMETRIOSIS SURGERY ON REPRODUCTIVE OUTCOME

Pregnancy rate was good in women with endometriosis, but without adenomyosis, compared with those with concurrent endometriosis and adenomyosis after laparoscopic excision of deep, infiltrated endometriosis. Presurgical hormone treatment (GnRH agonists for 3 months) was used in two studies. Surgery was performed in three studies with laparoscopy and with laparotomy or laparoscopy in 2 studies.[29]

ADENOMYOSIS AND ASSISTED REPRODUCTIVE TECHNOLOGY

There are different conclusions of various studies pertaining to the results of ART in adenomyosis relating to the type of protocol used. Thalluri and Tremellen conducted a retrospective study in women with adenomyosis undergoing IVF cycle with an antagonist stimulation protocol. Their results concluded that in the adenomyosis group clinical pregnancy rates were reduced as compared to the group without adenomyosis. A study used a long agonist stimulation protocol in ART cycles found live-birth rate per cycle to be same between controls and women with adenomyosis. GnRH downregulation may have had affected endometrium, correcting endometrial alterations related to the presence of adenomyosis and thus increasing live-birth rates.[30]

Oocyte Donation

In a retrospective cohort study, in oocyte recipients with adenomyosis, implantation rates were comparable to those of women with endometriomas or controls without endometriosis and adenomyosis. In women with adenomyosis early miscarriage rates were higher as compared to women with endometriosis or controls. Reason postulated is the disruption of the junctional zone in adenomyosis which could alter early stages of embryo invasion and later on placentation.[8]

Pretreatment in Frozen-thawed Embryo Transfer Cycles

Long-term pituitary downregulation prior to frozen-thawed embryo transfer (FET) cycles may improve pregnancy outcomes in women with adenomyosis. The implantation, pregnancy and ongoing pregnancy rates were significantly higher compared to the non-leuprolide acetate group.

KEY POINTS

- Adenomyosis is a common condition, not only found in the multiparous population, but also has an increasing incidence amongst the infertile patients.
- Adenomyosis is a majorly under discussed and researched topic.
- There are no formal guidelines given by any apical body in this regards.
- Unlike endometriosis, surgical modality is not the preferred modality in patients with infertility.
- Although, MRI has a better diagnostic value as compared to other modalities, still on a cost benefit analysis, a good 3D ultrasound also is equally effective in diagnosing adenomyosis.
- Newer drugs like dienogest, others like ulipristal have shown a symptomatic improvement in this condition.

REFERENCES

1. Owolabi TO, Strickler RC. Adenomyosis: a neglected diagnosis. Obstet Gynecol. 1977; 50(4):424-7.
2. Puente JM, Fabris A, Patel J, et al. Adenomyosis in infertile women: prevalence and the role of 3D ultrasound as a marker of severity of the disease. Reprod Biol Endocrinol. 2016:14:60.
3. Levgur M, Abadi MA, Tucker A. Adenomyosis: symptoms, histology, and pregnancy terminations. Obstet Gynecol. 2000;95(5):688-91.
4. Tamai K, Koyama T, Umeoka S. Spectrum of MR features in adenomyosis. Best Pract Res Clin Obstet Gynaecol. 2006;20:583-602.
5. Naftalin J, Hoo WL, Pateman K, et al. How common is adenomyosis? A prospective study of prevalence using transvaginal ultrasound in a gynaecology clinic. Hum Reprod. 2012:27(12): 3432-9.
6. Vercellini P, Consonni D, Dridi D, et al. Uterine adenomyosis and in vitro fertilization outcome: a systematic review and meta-analysis. Hum Reprod. 2014;29(5):964-77.
7. Tremellen KP, Russell P. The distribution of immune cells and macrophages in the endometrium of women with recurrent reproductive failure. II: adenomyosis and macrophages. J Reprod Immunol. 2012;93:58-63.
8. Martı´nez-Conejero JA, Morgan M, Montesinos M, et al. Adenomyosis does not affect implantation, but is associated with miscarriage in patients undergoing oocyte donation. Fertil Steril. 2011;96:943-50.
9. Exacoustos C, Brienza L, Di Giovanni A, et al. Adenomyosis: three-dimensional sonographic findings of the junctional zone and correlation with histology. Ultrasound Obstet Gynecol. 2011;37(4):471-9.
10. Champaneria R, Abedin P, Daniels J, et al. Ultrasound scan and magnetic resonance imaging for the diagnosis of adenomyosis: systematic review comparing test accuracy. Acta Obstet Gynecol Scand. 2010;89(11):1374-84.
11. Pinkerton JV, Thomas S. Use of SERMs for treatment in postmenopausal women. J Steroid Biochem Mol Biol. 2014;142:142-54.
12. Chen YJ, Li HY, Huang CH, et al. Oestrogen-induced epithelial-mesenchymal transition of endometrial epithelial cells contributes to the development of adenomyosis. J Pathol. 2001;222:261-70.
13. Ferrero S, Scala C, Racca A, et al. Leone Roberti Maggiore changes in adenomyosis after treatment with ulipristal acetate. Fertil Steril. 2016;106:e281-e282.
14. Osuga Y, Fujimoto-Okabe, Haginob A. Evaluation of the efficacy and safety of dienogest in the treatment of painful symptoms in patients with adenomyosis: a randomized, double-blind, multicenter, placebo-controlled study. Fertil Steril. 2017;108(4):673-7.
15. Huang FJ, Kung FT, Chang SY, et al. Effects of short-course Buserelin therapy on adenomyosis: A report of two cases. J Reprod Med Obstet Gynecol. 1999;44(8):741-4.
16. Patwardhan S, Nawathe A, Yates D, et al. Systematic review of the effects of aromatase inhibitors on pain associated with endometriosis. BJOG. 2008;115(7):818-22.
17. El-Nashar SA, Hopkins MR, Creedon DJ. et al. Prediction of treatment outcomes after global endometrial ablation. Obstet Gynecol. 2009;113:97-106.
18. Wang PH, Liu WM, Fuh JL, et al. Comparison of surgery alone and combined surgical medical treatment in the management of symptomatic uterine adenomyoma. Fertil Steril. 2009;92(3):876-85.
19. Kim MD, Kim NK, Kim HJ, et al. Pregnancy Following Uterine Artery Embolization with Polyvinyl Alcohol Particles for Patients with Uterine Fibroid or Adenomyosis. Cardiovasc Interven Radiol. 2005:28:611-5.
20. Fujishita A, Masuzaki H, Khan KN, et al. Modified reduction surgery for adenomyosis. Gynecol Obstet Invest. 2004;57: 132-8.
21. Osada H, Silber S, Kakinuma T, et al. Surgical procedure to conserve the uterus for future pregnancy in patients suffering from massive adenomyosis. Reprod Biomed Online. 2011;22:94-9.
22. Pepas L, Deguara C, Davis C. Update on the surgical management of adenomyosis. Curr Opin Obstet Gynecol. 2012;24:259-64.
23. Nishida M, Takano K, Arai Y, et al. Conservative surgical management for diffuse uterine adenomyosis. Fertil Steril. 2010;94(2):715-9.
24. Kwack YJ, Kwon YS. Laparoscopic Surgery for Focal Adenomyosis. J Soc Laparoendosc Surg. 2017;21(2):e2017. 00014.
25. Akar ME, Leezer KH, Yalcinkaya TM. Robot-assisted laparoscopic management of a case with juvenile cystic adenomyoma. Fertil Steril. 2010;94:e55-e56.
26. Rabinovici J, Inbar Y, Eylon SC, et al. Pregnancy and live birth after focused ultrasound surgery for symptomatic focal adenomyosis: a case report. Hum Reprod. 2006;21(5):1255-9.
27. Fukunishi H, Funaki K, Sawada K, et al. Early results of magnetic resonance guided focused ultrasound surgery of adenomyosis: analysis of 20 cases. J Minim Invasive Gynecol. 2008;15(5):571-9.
28. Zhou M, Chen JY, Tang LD, et al. Ultrasound-guided high-intensity focused ultrasound ablation for adenomyosis: the clinical experience of a single center. Fertil Steril. 2011;95(3):900-5.
29. Landi S, Mereu L, Pontrelli G, et al. The influence of adenomyosis in patients laparoscopically treated for deep endometriosis. J Minim Invasive Gynecol. 2008;15:566-70.
30. Costello MF, Lindsay K, McNally G. The effect of adenomyosis on in vitro fertilisation and intracytoplasmic? Sperm injection treatment outcome. Eur J Obstet Gynecol Reprod Biol. 2011;158:229-34.

New Trends in Fibroids and Infertility

12

Parul Kotdawala, Mala Raj, Ishwaran, Parzan Mistry

INTRODUCTION

Fibroids or leiomyomas are one of the most common issues with which a childbearing woman presents in her reproductive age. Fibroids are smooth muscle tumors of benign etiology.[1] They are the most common tumors of the female genital tract and are perhaps one of the most common tumors in women. Most of these tumors go unnoticed, it is only when they present with symptoms like menorrhagia or dysmenorrhea that they are generally diagnosed. With ultrasound being one of the mainstay diagnosis in a workup of infertility, these tumors are picked up early, which may result sometimes to unnecessary interventions and overenthusiastic management. In the yesteryears, the treatment options for management of fibroids were very limited and were mostly surgical removal of the tumors or the removal of uterus (hysterectomy) in the cases where the patient's family was complete. The routes of retrieval of these tumors have also undergone a lot of changes from abdominal to vaginal to laparoscopy to the present-day use of robotics. Nowadays, the development of several noninvasive surgical techniques and the recent clinical introduction of newer pharmacological agents have implicated that some of these patients, who initially had surgical indication, may have an alternative and conservative treatment due to which the patients are spared from the surgeries and are being able to preserve the fertility.

CLASSIFICATION

It is essential for us to know the classification of these tumors as the management and the pathogenesis through which they cause infertility depends on them. Fibroids are generally classified on the basis of their position in the uterus. The fibroid projecting inside the endometrial cavity is known as a submucous myoma. The ones inside the myometrium are called intramural myomas and the ones projecting on the peritoneal surfaces are called subserous variety. If the bulk of myoma is outside the myometrium and attached to the uterus with only a stalk, they are called pedunculated fibroids.

Fibroids were also classified by Wamstekar et al. (1993) based on their penetration in the myometrium. This was later adopted by European Society for Gynecological Endoscopy (ESGE).

- G0—fibroid is completely within the cavity and attached to the cavity with a pedicle
- G1—more than 50% of the fibroid is within the cavity
- G2—more than 50% of the fibroid is within the myometrium.

Lasmer et al. (2005) proposed a classification for surgical management of fibroid. This preoperative classification of fibroid is based on the degree of penetration, and other parameters like the extension of the base of the fibroid with respect to the uterus, the size of the fibroid and the topography of uterine cavity. A total score of 0–2 is counted for each parameter and the patient is allocated into one of the three groups of classification based on the score. The surgical plan is suggested based on the score **(Fig. 1)**:

- *Score 0–4:* Low complex hysteroscopic myomectomy
- *Score 5–6:* High complexity myomectomy, can consider gonadotropin-releasing hormone (GnRH) agonists, or can consider two step hysteroscopic myomectomy.
- *Score 7–9:* Consider alternatives to hysteroscopic techniques.

Leiomyoma subclassification system

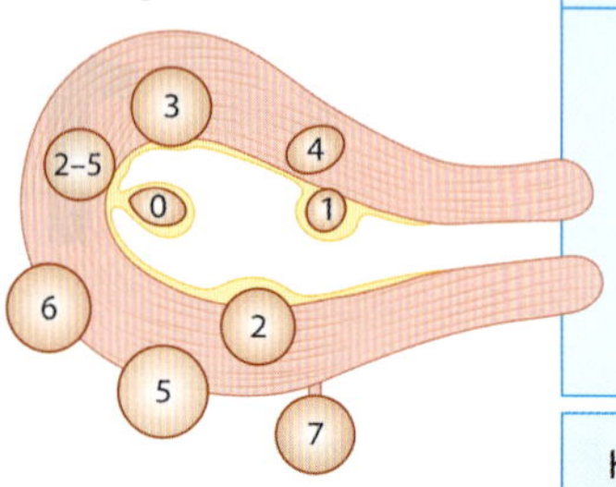

SM–submucosal	0	Pedunculated intracavitary
	1	<50% intramural
	2	≥50% intramural
O–other	3	Contacts endometrium: 100% intramural
	4	Intramural
	5	Subserosal ≥50% intramural
	6	Subserosal <50% intramural
	7	Subserosal pedunculated
	8	Other (specify e.g., cervical, parasitic)
Hybrid leiomyomas (impact both endometrium and serosal)	Two numbers are listed separated by a hypen. By convetion, the first refers to the relationship with the endometrium, while the second refers to the relationship to the serosa. One example given below	
	2–5	Submucosal and subserosal, each with less than half the diameter in the endometerial and peritoneal cavities, respectively

Fig. 1: FIGO leiomyoma subclassification system.
(FIGO: International Federation of Gynaecology and Obstetrics)
Source: Munro MG, Critchley HO, Broder MS, et al. FIGO classification system (PALM-COEIN) for causes of abnormal uterine bleeding in nongravid women of reproductive age. Int J Gynaecol Obstet. 2011;113(1):3-13.

MECHANISM OF INFERTILITY WITH FIBROIDS

Various factors are attributed to infertility in case of fibroids:

- *Physical factors:* By impeding the transport of sperm, eggs, and embryo.
- *Alteration of uterine contractions*: Fibroids increase the myometrial peristalsis and induce a chronic inflammatory reaction and impair implantations. Many anti-inflammatory factors like the cytokines, growth factors, neurotensin, neuropeptides, encephalin, and oxytocin modulators are found in the fibroid capsule, which would increase the myometrial contractility and interfere with the fertility.[2]
- *Cytokine factors:* Cytokines like interleukin-10 (IL-10) and glycodein are mainly responsible for implantation and early embryonic development. These are reduced in women with submucosal fibroids.
- *Genetic factors:* Endometrial receptivity is modulated by endometrial HOXA 10, HOXA II, and BT EB1 gene expression. There is reduction or absence of HOXA 10 in the endometrium in women with fibroids, which may lead to infertility due to implantation failure. This reduction is noticed throughout the entire endometrium and not over the endometrium overlying the fibroid.[3]
- *Alteration in endomyometrial functional (EMJ) zone:* The EMJ zone is the inner one-third of the myometrium adjoining the endometrium. It has the macrophages and the uterine natural killer (NK) cells, which are responsible for endometrial decidualization in the mid luteal window of implantation. There is reduction in the concentration of both macrophages as well as uterine NK cells in EMJ zone in women with fibroids, and this would impair the implantation.[4]

MANAGEMENT

It is essential for us to differentiate the patients who would desire fertility to those who have completed their families. Approximately, half of the fibroids will not cause problems in the gestation, but on the other hand, a third could induce abortions and premature births.[5]

In both cases, it is not easy to correctly assess these patients, although compromise of the endometrial cavity and the location of fibroids are essential to define. As a general rule, submucous fibroids (0, 1, and 2) should be operated on by hysteroscopy. However, type 4 intramural fibroids larger than 5 cm and types 5 and 6 larger than 6–7 cm should be treated

We obviously reject hysterectomy as an option for treatment, but it should be noted and included in the informed consent as an unexpected consequence, if a myomectomy is to be performed. However, the risk is low and should never exceed 2%–3% of myomectomies. However, the treatment with one or two ulipristal acetate cycles could be tried in patients with type 3 myomas or those where a slight decrease in size may improve cavity condition. In these cases, the volume reduction of the fibroids may achieve a regular endometrial cavity free of fibroids. Patients could then safely gestate after the second, and probably the first menstruation. The effects in gestation seem to be beneficial because gestation appears to inhibit fibroids' growth through apoptosis that occurred during the treatment period. No adverse teratogenic effect has been reported.[6,7] Ulipristal acetate treatment should be a valid alternative also in polymyomatous uterus and those presenting myometrial scars, with uncertain surgical outcome. In any case, the situation could be reassessed after treatment, evaluating the effect on the fibroids and the influence on the endometrial cavity. When the desire of pregnancy is deferred over time, it is recommended to delay the intervention until the moment when the patient is desirous of pregnancy. Recurrence of fibroids is frequent and surgery becomes more difficult each time, worsening the prognosis and increasing the risks of hysterectomy. Therefore, we should follow-up and assess the growth of these fibroids.

For some women with myomas who are mildly or moderately symptomatic, watchful waiting may allow surgery to be deferred, perhaps indefinitely. Studies are needed to determine whether this strategy works for a longer period of time.

MEDICAL MANAGEMENT

- *Nonsteroidal anti-inflammatory drugs (NSAIDs):* NSAIDs have not been shown to be effective in women with myomas. In various observational studies, it has been seen that the use of NSAIDs decreases the mean blood loss by 36% in the idiopathic cases of menorrhagia as compared to those with fibroids.[8]
- *Gonadotropin-releasing hormone agonists:* The effects of this group of drugs on the uterus and myoma volume appear to be the result of decreased levels of estrogen and progesterone, but other mechanisms, including induction of myoma degeneration and hyaline necrosis, a decrease in the size or number of leiomyoma cells, decreased levels of growth factors [vascular endothelial growth factor, fibroblast growth factor, and *EDGF* (VEGF, FGF, *and EDGF)]* a reduction in extracellular matrix, or a decrease in blood flow to the uterus, may be important.
- *Gonadotropin-releasing hormone antagonist*: The GnRH antagonist ganirelix was given [daily by subcutaneous (SC) injection] for the treatment of these tumors. The immediate suppression of endogenous GnRH, without an initial flare, resulted in a rapid decrease in myoma and uterine volumes.[9]
- *RU 486 (mifepristone):* The reduction in uterine size after treatment with the progesterone-blocking drug RU-486 is similar to that found with GnRH antagonist. A prospective randomized controlled trial using either 5 or 10 mg of RU-486 for 1 year found that both doses induced a 48% decrease in mean uterine volume after 6 months.[10]
- *Asoprisnil:* A selective progesterone receptor modulator binds to progesterone receptors, which are increased in myoma tissues. Doses of 10 and 25 mg are effective in shrinking myomas and suppress both abnormal and normal uterine bleeding, with no effects on circulating estrogen levels, no clinical symptoms of estrogen deprivation, and no breakthrough bleeding have been reported.
- *Levonorgestrel-releasing intrauterine system (LNG-IUS)*: In women with myomas, uterine size of less than 12 weeks, and a normal uterine cavity, LNG-IUSs have been shown to substantially reduce menstrual bleeding.[11]
- *Newer treatments:* Forthcoming medical treatments for myomas will include compounds that block the action of growth factors that regulate cellular proliferation and/or collagen production.[12] Myoma cells, however, express aromatase in situ, perhaps in amounts sufficient to support their own growth, and large myomas have higher aromatase expression than do small myomas. One hopes that new aromatase inhibitors can be found that avoid systemic hypoestrogenic symptoms by inhibiting myoma, but not ovarian, estrogen production.
  - Myomas have increased production of collagen. Pirfenidone, an antifibrotic compound (Marnac, Inc., Dallas, TX) decreases expression of collagen type I and III messenger RNA in cultured myometrial cells. Results of these studies, however, suggest that pirfenidone may inhibit new myoma growth but not affect myomas already present

SURGICAL TREATMENT

Myomectomy has been stated to relieve symptoms in 80% of women.[13] In cases of fibroids with anemia erythropoietin alfa and epoetin, recombinant forms of erythropoietin, commonly are used to increase preoperative hemoglobin concentrations. A prospective, nonrandomized study of preoperative epoetin found a significant increase in hemoglobin concentrations before and after gynecologic surgery.[14] GnRH agonist may be used preoperatively to stop abnormal bleeding, with a resultant increase of hemoglobin concentration.

Experience and expertise of the operating surgeon: The various surgical options are:

- Laparoscopic myomectomy
- Hysteroscopic myomectomy
- Abdominal myomectomy
- Uterine artery embolization (UAE)
- Magnetic resonance imaging (MRI)-guided focused ultrasound surgery.

Laparoscopic Myomectomy

Laparoscopic myomectomy is the procedure of choice in the subserosal and intramural fibroids. It is also preferred in certain submucosal fibroids as it provides improved vision, magnification, decreased blood loss, quicker recuperation, and reduced post-operative pain. With increase in the expertise of suturing skills, the incidence of rupture during pregnancy following laparoscopic myomectomy is almost same as abdominal myomectomy. It is almost mandatory to perform multilayer suturing of the myoma bed, occluding the potential dead space, to avoid scar dehiscence during pregnancy. The overall incidence of uterine rupture during pregnancy following laparoscopic myomectomy appears to be low.

As laparoscopic myomectomy would involve morcellation, it is mandatory to counsel women regarding the complications of the morcellation, including the fact that in rare cases it may upstage the disease if leiomyosarcoma is morcellated inadvertently.

Hysteroscopic Myomectomy

Hysteroscopic myomectomy (myoma resection) is the first-line conservative surgical option for managing symptomatic intracavity fibroids. The resection of a submucous fibroid can be performed in single or double sitting based on the size and depth of the myoma. The resection is performed using either a monopolar or a bipolar energy source. The monopolar energy requires the use of a nonelectrolyte solution (glycine, etc.) as distension medium, whereas the bipolar energy would require an electrolyte solution (normal saline or lactated ringer) as the distension medium. In case of fluid overload as a result of opening of vascular channels, the severity of the consequences would be more when a hypotonic solution is used (in monopolar resection) compared to an isotonic solution (in bipolar resection), as hypotonic solution may exaggerate the overload and lead to electrolyte disturbances, by reducing the osmotic pressure in the blood stream. A well-experiences person only should attempt to resect a large type 1 and type 2 fibroids (>3 cm). A laparoscopic myomectomy is a better option, if the submucosal fibroid is very large (>5 cm) and there is very little myometrium (<5 mm) surrounding it.

A new technique of mechanical hysteroscopic morcellation of the submucous myoma has now been introduced. It is a quicker surgery than the traditional electrocautery resection, with reduction in operating time as simultaneous clearing of resected pieces saves time. The limitation of this technique is that it cannot reach deeper part of myomas, necessitating second procedure in such situation.

Laser ablation can be employed in fibroids of less than 2 cm size. The disadvantage of laser is a longer operative time, high costs of the equipment, and reduced opportunity to evaluate tissue specimen.

Abdominal Myomectomy

Abdominal myomectomy can be performed by traditional myomectomy principles. The introduction of vasopressin has reduced the blood loss at the surgery, and is a safe option, when a myoma is very big (7–10 cm +, according to surgeon's choice), or when the medical condition of the patient does not allow general anesthesia.

Uterine Artery Embolization

Uterine artery embolization is performed by introducing a retrograde catheter through the femoral artery to the internal iliac artery and to the branches of the uterine artery supplying the fibroids (Ravina et al. 1995). Embolization agents are injected into the catheter, which will block the blood flow to the fibroid/s. This anoxia would cause the fibroids to shrink, reducing the bulk of the myoma, and thereby reducing the menstrual bleeding. This is not suitable for an infertile patient, or for a woman desirous of future childbearing. Nevertheless, pregnancies have been reported after UAE. Of 34 pregnancies subsequent to UAE, 32% of women had a spontaneous abortion.[15]

MRI-guided Focused Ultrasound Surgery

High intensity ultrasound energy is used to deliver focused heat to the target tissues and cause the destruction of the tissue. This is used to reduce the size of the fibroid and its associated symptoms (Hindley et al. 2004). It is a non-invasive procedure, but again is not suitable for infertile patients.

REFERENCES

1. Walker CL, Stewart EA. Uterine fibroids: the elephant in the room. Science. 2005;308(5728):1589-92.
2. Mahfoudh AL. Role of angiogensis on uterine fibroids. Gynecol Endocrinology; 2013.
3. Cakmak H, Taylor HS. Implantation failure: molecular mechanisms and clinical treatment. Hum Reprod Update. 2011;17(2):242-53.
4. Kitaya K, Yasuo Y. Leukocyte density and composition in human cycling endometrium with uterine fibroids. J Hum Immunol. 2010;17(2):158-63.
5. Yamada T, Ikeda A, Okamoto Y, et al. Intraoperative blood salvage in abdominal simple total hysterectomy for uterine myoma. Int J Gynaecol Obstet. 1997;59:233-6.
6. Mais V, Ajossa S, Guerriero S, et al. Laparoscopic versus abdominal myomectomy: a prospective, randomized trial to evaluate benefits in early outcome. Am J Obstet Gynecol. 1996;174:654-8.
7. Seracchioli R, Rossi S, Govoni F, et al. Fertility and obstetric outcome after laparoscopic myomectomy of large myomata: a randomized comparison with abdominal myomectomy. Hum Reprod. 2000;15:2663-8.
8. Ylikorkala O, Pekonen F. Naproxen reduces idiopathic but not fibromyoma-induced menorrhagia. Obstet Gynecol. 1986;68:10-2.
9. Flierman PA, Oberye JJ, van der Hulst VP, et al. Rapid reduction of leiomyoma volume during treatment with the GnRH antagonist ganirelix. BJOG. 2005;112:638-42.
10. Murphy AA, Morales AJ, Kettel LM, et al. Regression of uterine leiomyomata to the antiprogesterone RU486: dose-response effect. Fertil Steril. 1995;64:187-90.
11. Grigorieva V, Chen-Mok M, Tarasova M, et al. Use of a levonorgestrel-releasing intrauterine system to treat bleeding related to uterine leiomyomas. Fertil Steril. 2003;79:1194-8.
12. Nowak RA. Novel therapeutic strategies for leiomyomas: targeting growth factors and their receptors. Environ Health Perspect. 2000;108(Suppl 5):849-53.
13. Buttram VC Jr, Reiter RC. Uterine leiomyomata: etiology, symptomatology, and management. Fertil Steril. 1981;36:433-45.
14. Sesti F, Ticconi C, Bonifacio S, et al. Preoperative administration of recombinant human erythropoietin in patients undergoing gynecologic surgery. Gynecol Obstet Invest. 2002;54:1-5.
15. Goldberg J, Pereira L, Berghella V, et al. Pregnancy outcomes after treatment for fibromyomata: uterine artery embolization versus laparoscopic myomectomy. Am J Obstet Gynecol. 2004;191:18-21.

Polycystic Ovary Syndrome

13

Shivanand Sukhare, Manisha Bhagat, Kundan Ingale

INTRODUCTION

Polycystic ovary syndrome (PCOS) is a common, multifactorial endocrine disorder of uncertain etiology. There are three criteria used to make the diagnosis of PCOS and prevalence varies according to the criteria used. According to Rotterdam criteria the prevalence is 6–8%.[1] The syndrome complex consisting of amenorrhea, hirsutism and enlarged ovaries was described by Stein and Leventhal in 1935 **(Fig. 1)**.

There are many theories which explain the origin of PCOS. The most recent being genetic[2] theory which states that the gene alteration found in PCOS is a result of adverse condition like famine causing changes at the genetic level, which will manifest in the adulthood only if the person has associated obesity, sedentary lifestyle and unhealthy eating habits. Not everyone with abnormal gene for PCOS will manifest the disease, but they will be at a higher incidence for metabolic diseases like diabetes mellitus and coronary artery disease.

According to Frank and Berga, the origin of PCOS is due to excessive in-utero hyperandrogenism.[3]

ETIOPATHOGENESIS OF PCOS

It is a multifactorial disorder of unexplained etiology. Various etiologies have been proposed for its origin.[4] The diagram chart **(Fig. 2)** explains the etiology.

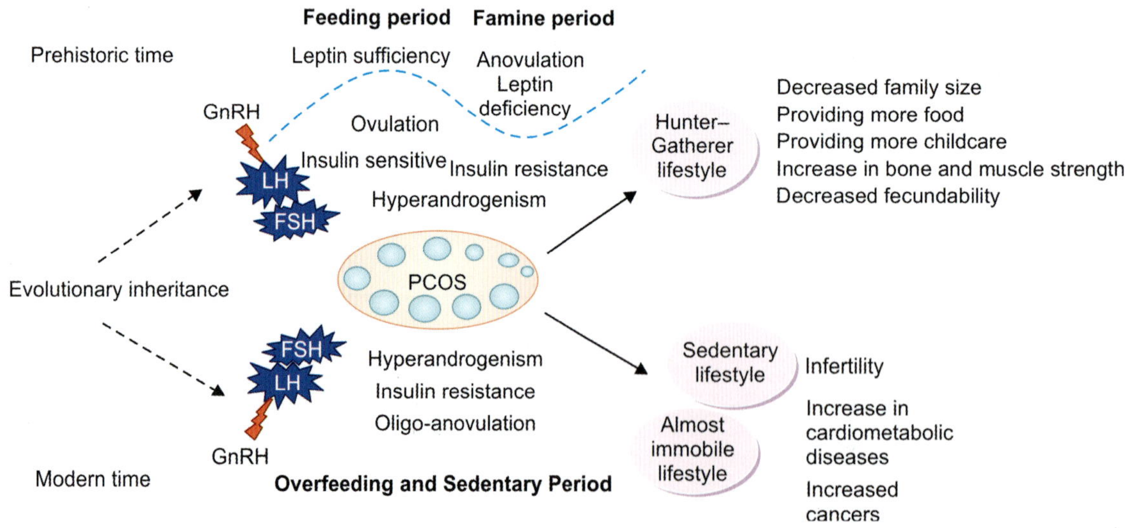

Fig. 1: Evolutionary advantages and disadvantages of polycystic ovary syndrome (PCOS). From an evolutionary perspective, although susceptibility genes for PCOS may have constituted protective factors for human beings during prehistoric times, these inheritances would have turned into genetic triggers for complex metabolic diseases through changing lifestyle conditions.

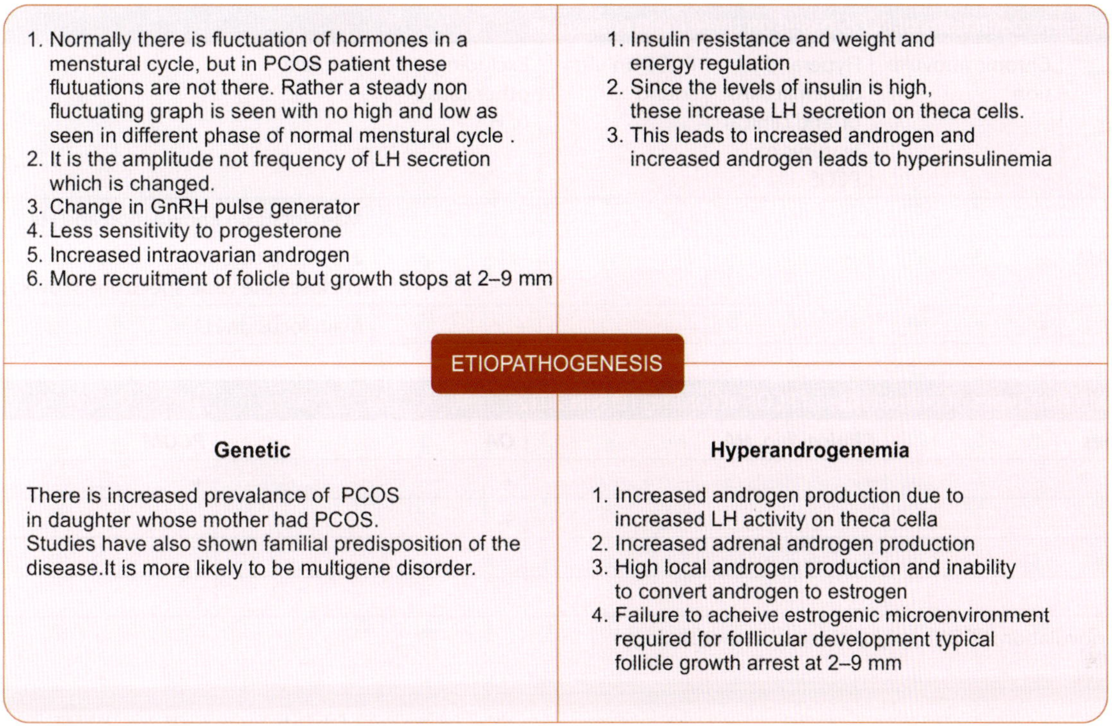

Fig. 2: Etiology of PCOS.

SEQUEL OF PCOS

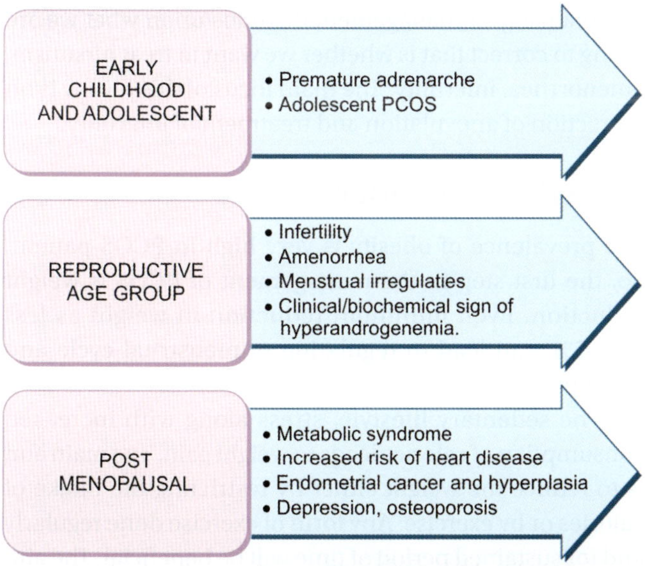

HOW TO DEFINE PCOS?

There are many different definitions of PCOS. Three major definition based on three main consensus is given below **(Table 1)**:

1. NIH criteria (National Institute of Health)[5]
2. ASRM/ESHRE Rotterdam criteria[6]
3. AEPCOS (Androgen Excess Society) criteria[7]

Regarding ultrasound criteria: there should be 12 or more follicles of 2–9mm, ovarian volume of more than 10 cc, taken in one ovary. A longitudinal scan is done, ovary is measured from inner margin to outer with a 7 MHZ probe. (Some people use the criteria 25 or more follicles per ovary on 3D USG). Scan can be done in any day for amenorrhoeic female or day 2/3 after withdrawal bleed.[8]

CLINICAL PRESENTATION OF PCOS

PCOS patient presents with a wide variety of symptoms. Menstrual abnormalities like anovulation, oligomenorrhoea and in some amenorrhea. Clinical sign of hyperandrogenism like hirsutism, acne, and male pattern of baldness.

DIFFERENT PHENOTYPES OF PCOS (TABLE 2)

The phenotypes help us in management as what type of patient will require monitoring having high risk for coronary artery disease, diabetes mellitus, etc. For example, phenotype A more prone for these ailments then phenotype D.

Anti-Mullerian Hormone (AMH): It has come up with as a very important tool in the armamentarium of the gynecologist. AMH is the principal regulator of early follicular recruitment from the primordial pool.[4] It also help to predict the response to ovarian stimulation. In case

Table 1: Different definitions of PCOS based on three main consensus.

	Chronic anovulation	Hyperandrogenemia (HA) or/and clinical features of PCOS	PCOS on ultrasound	Excluding other cause of HA	Remarks
NIH	+	+	–	–	Main focus on anovulation and HA
ROTTERDAM	+	+	+	–/+	2/3 of the criteria Encloses the wide spectrum of disease
AEPCOS	+	+	–	+	Main focus on HA

Table 2: Different types of phenotypes of PCOS according TO NIH 2012[9]

Phenotypes	***Clinical/bio. HA***	***OA***	***PCOM***
A	+	+	+
B	+	+	–
C	+	–	+
D	_	+	+

(OA: oligoanovulation; PCOM: polycystic ovarian morphology)

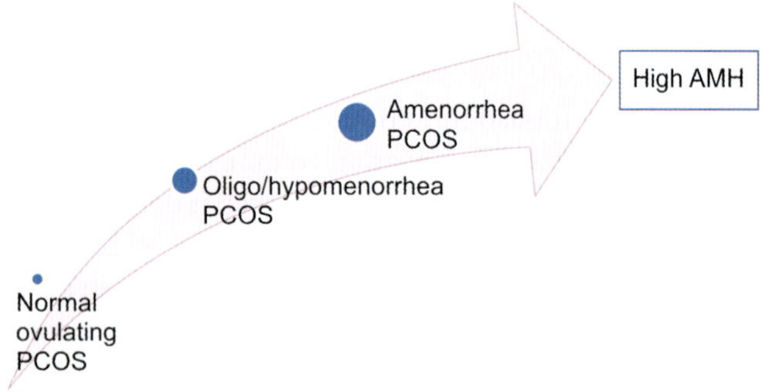

Fig. 3: Women with amenorrhea will have more anti-Mullerian hormone than that of oligo/normal PCOS patient.

of PCOS patients more severe the menstrual abnormality higher the level of AMH. It means women with amenorrhea will have more AMH than that of oligo/normal PCOS patient **(Fig. 3)**.

Patient with low body mass index (BMI), previous history of ovarian hyperstimulation syndrome (OHSS) and those with high AMH (>3.4ng/mL) and antral follicle count (AFC) (>24) and retrieval of more than 24 oocytes have high chance in going into OHSS.[10] In case of high responders AMH helps to identify females who will have high chances of hyper responding to the stimulation and going into OHSS. Patient can be started with low dose of gonadotropin 150 IU, with antagonist protocol which per se decreases the incidence of OHSS. Also with antagonist protocol we can use of agonist trigger in case of there is excessive stimulation.

So in case of high responders AMH can predict treatment outcome and prognosis

MANAGEMENT (FIG. 4)

The mainstay of management depends upon what we are trying to correct that is whether we want to treat hirsutism, amenorrhea, infertility. The main focus of this review is on correction of anovulation and treatment of infertility.

Lifestyle Modification

The prevalence of obesity is very high in PCOS patient. So, the first step in the management of PCOS is weight reduction. Even minimum reduction in weight as less as 2–5%[4] can lead to regulation of menstrual cycle and conception.

The sedentary lifestyle, stress along with increased consumption of calories leads to weight gain. The main aim is to reduce the weight either by restricting the intake of calories or by exercise. Any form of exercise done regularly and for sustained period of time will be beneficial. The aim is at least 5% weight reduction.[11]

There are many types of diets available, however no one is preferred over the other. The goal should be calories restriction with avoidance of junk food. The weight loss by both diet and exercise will lead to decrease in free testosterone levels by increasing the production of sex hormone binding globulin (SHBG) by liver.

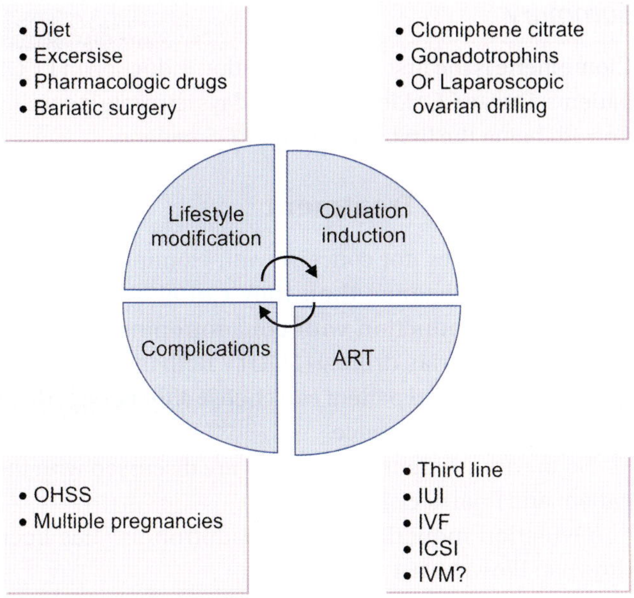

Fig. 4: Management plan of PCOS.

Advice the patient to stop smoking, take folate 5mg/day supplementation preconceptionally.

Pharmacologic

Drugs used either to suppress appetite or increasing the peripheral utilization of glucose.

1. *Insulin sensitizing agents:*
   a. Metformin
   b. Thiazolidinediones: Rosiglitazone, pioglitazone
   c. D-chiro inositol
2. *Appetite suppressant:* Sibutramine
3. *Anti-obesity:* Orlistat

Metformin

When patient is unable to control weight with lifestyle modifications and is having impaired glucose tolerance, metformin can be used. It acts by increasing the uptake of glucose in intestine and by increasing insulin sensitivity. Though it causes weight loss in some patients it should not be used solely for the purpose of weight reduction. It is started as a minimum dose of 500 mg per day and advised slowly over 4–6 weeks to increase the dose to 1500–2000mg/day[11] (which is the desired dose). The main side effect is nausea which can be overcome by taking tablet along with meals.

Other side effects are vomiting, bloating, flatulence, indigestion. Lactic acidosis is very rare.

Indication for metformin usage: Patient having impaired glucose tolerance, diabetes mellitus type 2, severe insulin resistance and women having metabolic syndrome. Practice committee(2017)[12] has found that increases clinical birth rates along with CC undergoing ovulation induction but it does not increase the chance of having a live birth.[13] Also in patient undergoing IVF it does decrease the chance of OHSS in PCOS patient.

Thiazolidinediones, orlistat, sibutramine, statins are other drugs which are purposed for management but are not used routinely.

OVULATION INDUCTION

PCOS is one of the main causes of chronic anovulation leading to infertility. In PCOS patients not only there is anovulation, the oocyte quality, endometrium and implantation is impaired. Ovulation induction is done with the goal of forming good quality single oocyte without overstimulation. The problem with PCOS patients is that they have lots of small follicles which when stimulated in slightly higher doses can lead to OHSS. We start with oral drugs such as clomiphene citrate (first line in the management of PCOS) and then if required gonadotropins **(Fig. 5)**.

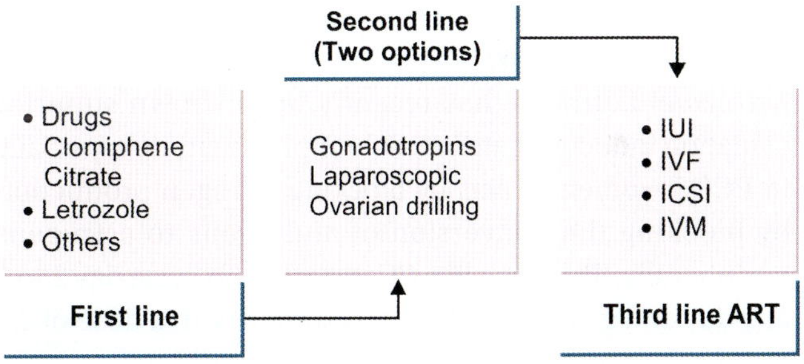

Fig. 5

Clomiphene Citrate

Clomiphene citrate is an antiestrogen, with both weak agonist and strong antagonist activity. It is a selective estrogen receptor modulator.[13] It is the preferred drug for treatment of PCOS because it is safe, inexpensive ,well tolerated with less side effects. CC binds to the nuclear central estrogen receptor ,there is receptor depletion which leads to decreased E2 levels .So less negative feedback to hypothalamus, increase in GnRH levels which leads to increase in FSH levels and increased follicular recruitment.[4] It is started typically between cycle day 2–5 and given for 5 days starting with a initial dose of 50 mg /day and increasing up to 150 mg/day.[13] Maximum 250 mg/day can be given but maximum response that is ovulation is observed at 150 mg /day and increasing the dose further will not be beneficial. Clomiphene is typically given for 6 cycles if no response till then, then think of second line therapy of add metformin or other alternatives discussed below. The efficacy of inducing ovulation with clomiphene is reported to be 75% but the live birth rate is just 22%.[13]

Normally no need for monitoring but we usually monitor the first cycle to see whether the drug is effective in causing ovulation .This can also be checked by using LH kit usually started day 11 of the cycle to detect ovulation.

Combined Therapy

- *Clomiphene citrate with metformin:* Metformin can be added especially in CC resistant cases and also patient having high[14] BMI> 35kg/m^2.
- *Clomiphene citrate along with corticosteroids[4]:* Especially in patients with raised dehydroepiandrosterone sulfate (DHEAS) use prednisolone 5 mg /day starting day 5 to day 14 of the menstrual cycle along with CC.
- Give preliminary suppression with oral contraceptive pills in previous two cycle .It suppress LH and androgen levels.[4]

Alternative Therapy

Aromatase inhibitor:

Letrozole: Letrozole has recently been shown superior ovulation induction rates over clomiphene citrate especially in PCOS women. It acts by blocking estrogen production by blocking the conversion of androgens to estrogens peripherally. This drug like CC is started on cycle day 2 to 5 any day and given for 5 days .It is started with a dose of 2.5 mg/day and increased to maximum 7.5 mg/day.

Another protocol similar to CC stair step has also been proposed for letrozole. In this protocol, start with 2.5 mg of letrozole for 5 days, sonography is done after 7 days, immediately increase the dose to 5 mg and repeat sonography after 1 week. If no response still increase it to 7.5 mg.[15]

	Clomiphene citrate	***Aromatase inhibitor***
MOA	At central level	At peripheral level
Multiple pregnancy	more	less
endometrium	Affected can be thin	No adverse effect on endometrium
Cervical mucus	Affected decreases	No adverse effect

Summary

Clomiphene is the first line for ovulation induction in PCOS patients. Due to CC side effects now days letrozole is coming up with being the first choice[16] in PCOS patients.

Second Line of Treatment

If the patient does not conceive with clomiphene citrate, there is CC resistance then they can either continue the ovulation induction with gonadotropins or can get laparoscopic ovarian drilling (LOD).[11] Both the options are equally effective and patient can choose either one of them according to his preference.

So the above-mentioned points are discussed with the patient and final decision is made.

Ovulation induction with gonadotropins[17] has been shown in **Flowchart 1**.

There are two ways of performing ovulation induction with gonadotropins the above mentioned that is step up and step down .Usually step up is preferred in PCOS patients since there is less chances of OHSS with this protocol and more chance of unifollicular development.

Table 4

	GONADOTROPINS[11]	***LOD[11]***
Risk of OHSS	Increased	No
Risk of multiple pregnancy	Increased	Decreased
Risk of surgery and anesthesia	No	Yes
Advantage	If patient still not pregnant after LOD she has to undergo OI with gonadotropins	Patients tubal status is checked ,other pathologies are checked
Monitoring required	Yes	No
Cost of therapy	Probably more	Comparatively less since one time procedure
Adhesions	No	Chances of adhesions increases, decreases ovarian reserve
Ovulation rate Pregnancy rate	70% 20%	40–50% 20%

Give progesterone one to induce withdrawal bleed. Start on day 2 of menses. Do an ultrasound check for cyst (<10 mm), endometrial thickness (<5 mm)

↓

- Start with gonadotropins (usually recombinant is preferred) 37.5 /75 IU per day (depending on patient's weight, previous response to stimulation) for 7 days.
- Do a scan after 7 days (no follicle of >10 mm) continue for another 7 days. still no response increase the dose 50% of the previous dose.

↓

Maximum you can give upto 225 IU/day. if no response after three weeks cancel the cycle and start with increased dose in the next cycle. If the response is fine continue till the follicle size is 18 mm to give trigger

↓

- TRIGGER: Ideally one but not more than two follicles of 16–18 mm is present give trigger. S. estradiol150–300 pg/mL per dominant follicle
- Inj HCG 5000 IU stat/recombinant 250 μg is given
- Luteal support is given with vaginal progesterone twice a day for 14 days

↓

When to cancel the cycle?
>3 follicle of >18 mm
Large intermediate follicle (10–15 mm)
E2 levels>1500 pg/mL

Flowchart 1: Ovulation induction with gonadotropins.

NOTE: Before starting gonadotropins, you have to check tubal status by either doing a HSG or saline infusion sonography.

In some cases we can also give clomiphene citrate 100mg/day for 5 days of menses and add gonadotropins on day 5. This will decrease the cost of the therapy and decreases the chance of OHSS and multiple pregnancies.

Laparoscopic Ovarian Drilling

Surgical intervention for PCOS dated back in 1935 when Stein and Leventhal did ovarian wedge resection to restore the ovulation for PCOS patient but due to open laparotomy the procedure was abandoned in favor of drugs and gonadotropins. With the advent of laparoscopy the interest was again revived since ovarian drilling is equally effective than gonadotropins and other pelvic pathology can be visualized .Also in patients where intensive monitoring is not possible this can be done as one time procedure. By destroying the ovarian stroma there is a decrease in both intraovarian and systemic androgens which restores ovulation. Hence leading to conception. A live birth rate of 37% is achieved with LOD.[18]

There is rule of 4 followed. 4 punctures in each ovary, 4 second current is applied, 4 mm depth stroma is cauterized and 40 W current is used.

Complications: increased risk of adnexal adhesions, decrease in ovarian reserve in some patients.

Third Line (ART)

Even after ovulation induction with gonadotropins there will be a subset of patients that will not be pregnant. Also, along with PCOS there is another factor of infertility like male factor, tubal factor, in these patients IVF/ICSI is indicated.

For mild male factor infertility IUI can be tried initially.

Treatment Regimen

Patient can be offered multiple regimens ranging from classical long protocol to antagonist to mild stimulation protocol.

Long protocol: Not preferred now due to increased risk of OHSS

GnRH ANTAGONIST PROTOCOL

This is the protocol commonly used in PCOS since the chances of OHSS decreased by 50% and trigger can be modified this the protocol preferred in PCOS.

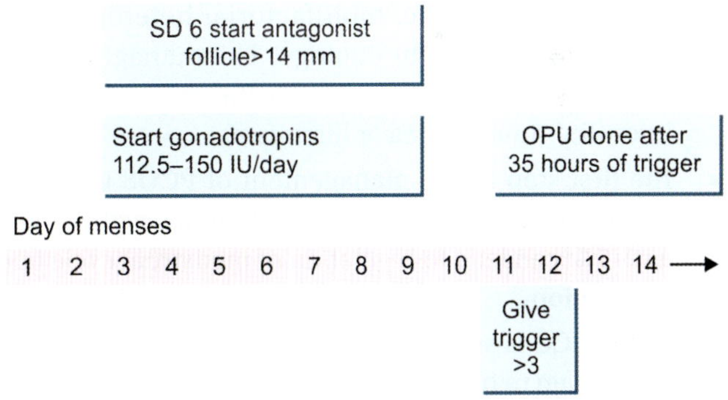

Antagonist

Antagonist either cetrorelix/ganirelix 0.25mg/day starting on stimulation day 5/6(fixed protocol) or when the dominant follicle is more than 14 mm (flexible protocol). *Trigger* is given when >3 follicle of 18 mm. HCG can be given either 10000 IU or recombinant HCG 250 μg.

With antagonist protocol, there is a possibility of triggering follicle with agonist trigger which can lead to decrease in incidence of OHSS. According to Cochrane

2016[19] antagonist protocol decreases the risk from 11% (in agonist) to 6–9% in antagonist protocol without decreasing the live birth rate.

When the follicle count is more than 14, serum estradiol is more than 3500 ng/mL agonist trigger is used in antagonist protocol to decrease the chances of OHSS.

The only problem is short luteal phase with agonist trigger which can be overcome by either doing frozen embryo transfer, giving dual or double trigger. If we want a fresh transfer either give supplemented luteal support or HCG 1500 IU on the day of ovum pickup.

IN-VITRO MATURATION

The main challenge while inducing a PCOS patient is risk of having OHSS. To overcome this many strategy has been adopted and tried, one of them is in-vitro maturation In this procedure immature oocytes are retrieved transvaginally from antral follicles and kept in culture. ICSI is done and fertilization is assessed. The transfer is done either in same cycle or next cycle. Since we do not stimulate the ovary there is no chance of early OHSS. Especially useful in patients who are prone for PCOS. The disadvantage is that the technique is still experimental, done at some centers and has low success rates.

SUMMARY

- PCOS is a polygenic, multifactorial heterogeneous disorder of uncertain etiology. The management of PCOS is dependent on whether the main concern is infertility, amenorrhea or hirsutism.
- The first step in the management of PCOS is weight reduction. Even minimum reduction in weight as less as 2–5%[4] can lead to regulation of menstrual cycle and conception.
- Though CC is still the first choice for OI, but letrozole has proven to be more efficacious then clomiphene.
- If CC fails then patient can opt from either gonadotropins or LOD.
- With gonadotropins start with lowest possible dose preferably 37.5 IU/day.
- LOD if preferred in cases where there is associated tubal factor, patient's choice.
- For IVF the preferred protocol is antagonist because it lowers the risk of OHSS and agonist trigger can be used.

REFERENCES

1. Azziz R, Woods KS, Reyna R, et al. The prevalence and features of the polycystic ovary syndrome in an unselected population. J Clin Endocrino Metab. 2004; 89(6):2745-9.
2. Ugar U, Sezgin E. Evolutionary determinants of polycystic ovary syndrome: part 1. Fertil Steril. 2016;106:33-41.
3. Franks S, Berga SL. Does PCOS have development origin. Fertil Steril. 2012;97:2-6.
4. Speroff L, Fritz MA. Clinical gynaecologic endocrinology and infertility, 8th ed. Philadelphia: Lippincott Williams and Wilkins; 2011. Chapter 12, Chronic Anovulation and the Polycystic Ovary Syndrome; p.495-532.
5. Zawadski JK, Dunaif A. Diagnostic criteria for polycystic ovary syndrome: towards a rational approach. In: Dunaif A, Givens JR, Haseltine FP, Merriam GR (Eds). Polycystic ovary syndrome. Boston, MA: Blackwell Scientific Publications, 1992:377-84.
6. The Rotterdam ESHRE/ASRM-sponsored PCOS consensus workshop group. Revised 2003 consensus on diagnostic criteria and long-term health risks related to polycystic ovary syndrome (PCOS). Hum Reprod. 2004; 19:41-7.
7. Azziz R, Dewailly D, Kandarakis DE, et al.Task Force on the the Androgen Excess and PCOS Society criteria for the polycystic ovary syndrome: the complete task force report. Fertil Steril. 2009;91:456-88.
8. Botrosrizk, AbhoulgharM. Ultrasound in Reproductive medicine and infertility published Cambridge university press. 2010. pp. 75-81.
9. National Institutes Of Health Evidence-based Methodology Workshop on Polycystic Ovary Syndrome. December 3-5, 2012.
10. Prevention and treatment of moderate and severe ovarian hyperstimulation syndrome. Practice Committee of the American Society for Reproductive Medicine, and other DOI. Fertil Steril. 2016;106(7):1634-16.
11. Consensus on infertility treatment related to polycystic ovary syndrome. The Thessaloniki ESHRE/ASRM-Sponsored PCOS consensus Workshop. Fertil Steril. 2008;89:505-22.
12. Role of metformin in ovarian induction in infertile patients with polycystic ovary syndrome(PCOS): a guideline. Practice committee of ASRM. Fertil Steril. 2017;108:426-41.
13. Use of clomiphene citrate in infertile women: a committee opinion. The Practice Committee of the American Society for Reproductive Medicine. Fertil Steril. 2013;100:341-8.
14. Legro RS, Barnhart HX, Schlaff WD, et al. Clomiphene, metformin, or both for infertility in the polycystic ovary syndrome. N Engl J Med. 2007;356:551-66.
15. Rhoda J. Karl R, Latasha Craig. Letroz stairstep protocol in polycystic ovary patient. Fertil Steril. 2016;107(3).
16. Effect of Letrozole versus Clomiphene on live birth in women with anovulatory infertility due to polycystic ovary syndrome (PCOS): a randomized double-blind multi-center trial. Fertil Steril. 2013;100(3):51.

17. Gardner DK, Weissman A, Howles CM, et al. Textbook of Assisted Reproductive Techniques. London.Informa healthcare. 2012. Chapter 38. The role of FSH and LH in ovulation induction: Current concepts; pg 75-98.
18. Farquhar C, Lilford RJ, Marjoribanks J, et al. Laparoscopic "drilling" by diathermy or laser for ovulation induction in anovulatory polycystic ovary syndrome. Cochrane Database Syst Rev 2012.CD 001122.DOI: 10.1002/14651858.CD001122.pub4.
19. Al-Inany HG, Youssef MAFM, Brockmans FJ, et al. Gonadotrophin - Releasing hormone antagonists for assisted reproductive technology. Cochrane Database of Systematic Reviews 2016, DOI: 10.1002/14651858.CD001750.

Tubal Factor in Infertility

14

Muralidhar V Pai

INTRODUCTION

Fallopian tubes play a pivotal role in fertilization and hence fertility. The fimbrial ends pick up the ovum, remaining parts of the tubes form the bridge for ova and sperms to travel and meet in the ampullary region for fertilization. Tubes should not only be anatomically patent but functionally viable also.

Tubal factor accounts for 25–35% of female factor infertility, with more than half the cases due to salpingitis.[1] In the past, tubal diseases were corrected surgically, but now tubal factor infertility is mostly overcome through in vitro fertilization (IVF). In fact, tubal factor was the indication for first IVF and it remained so for some time. It accounts for 9–18% of all the indications for IVF.[2]

ANATOMY

Fallopian tubes are derived from paramesonephric ducts and are situated at both cornual ends of the uterus. They are lined by ciliated columnar epithelium. They are around 10 centimeters in length consisting of interstitial, isthmic, ampullary, infundibular, and fimbrial parts. Fimbrial end contains a specialized fimbria named fimbria ovarica, which captures the ovum after ovulation. Ampulla is where the fertilization occurs.

PHYSIOLOGY

The fallopian tube transports the ovum from the ovary to the ampulla where it is fertilized by the sperm during ovulatory period and then the fertilized zygote is transported to the uterus. The cilia and tubal fluid assist in the transport. Impedance to this either in the form of an anatomical blockade, either extrinsic or intrinsic, or a functional disruption results in tubal factor infertility.

PATHOPHYSIOLOGY/PATHOLOGY

The tubal pathologies are broadly divided into proximal and distal, latter being more severe and irreparable in most instances. Genital tuberculosis is the major cause of tubal obstruction and ciliary damage, as it most commonly affects the fallopian tubes (95–100%), leading to infertility, especially in developing countries.[3] Mycobacterium tuberculosis is responsible for disease in approximately 90–95% of cases and produces granulomatous salpingitis.[3] Salpingitis due to other sexually transmitted diseases also may end up in hydro/pyosalpinx and cause blocks and damage of the cilia. Though the blocks can be surgically corrected, if cilia are damaged, one has to resort the IVF to bypass the tubal factor.

ASSESSMENT OF FALLOPIAN TUBE PATENCY

Hysterosalpingography

Despite recent advances in imaging tools, such as computerized tomography (CT) scan, magnetic resonance imaging (MRI), and ultrasonography, hysterosalpingography (HSG) is still the standard first-line screening test for evaluation of tubal infertility, especially in short-term infertile patients with no apparent pelvic pathology.[4] It is less invasive compared to laparoscopic chromopertubation. It is performed between day 7 and day 10 of the cycle using water or lipid-soluble contrast. It has the advantage of knowing the site of block and luminal changes, especially in cases of tubal damage due to tuberculosis (beaded tubes, golf club tubes, pipe-stem tubes, cobblestone tubes, and leopard skin tubes).[3] It also provides additional information on uterine anomalies, intrauterine adhesions (Asherman's syndrome), T-shaped tuberculosis uterus, pseudounicornuate uterus (also seen in tuberculosis), submucous fibroids, and polyps. HSG also has therapeutic benefits. There is evidence of effectiveness of tubal flushing with oil-soluble contrast media in increasing the odds of pregnancy and live birth versus no intervention.[5] However, HSG is not useful for detecting peritubal adhesions or endometriosis.

The HSG appears to have very high specificity and sensitivity for diagnosing distal tubal occlusion or major distal tubal adhesions, but much lower specificity for diagnosing proximal tubal occlusion.[6] Proximal occlusion could be due to tubal spasm at cornual ends (referred to as "Pseudo blocks") as the procedure is done without general anesthesia.

Fluoroscopic/Hysteroscopic-guided Tubal Evaluation

The corneal blocks could be confirmed using fluoroscopic or hysteroscopic selective tubal perfusion. Fluoroscopic/hysteroscopic-guided tubal evaluation not only helps in diagnosing the block, in selected cases of cornual block ("Beak" type of blocks) but it also helps in cannulation of the tubes through ostia and overcomes flimsy/mild blocks.

Hysterosalpingo-contrast Sonography

In this procedure, saline is injected through cervix while performing transvaginal sonography for evaluation of uterus and adnexa. If the tubes are patent, one can see saline escaping from fimbrial ends—"waterfall sign". It is quick, a safe, and well tolerated.[7]

Laparoscopic Chromopertubation

In long-term infertility, in women with suspected pelvic pathology and when the diagnosis is in doubt (as in cases of "pseudo blocks"), laparoscopic chromopertubation is preferred. In addition to diagnosing tubal block, it also throws light on pelvic pathologies such as endometriosis, tuberculosis, and adhesions due to previous pelvic inflammatory disease, and helps in providing concurrent therapeutic intervention.

Falloposcopy

This procedure is performed either through hysteroscopy or laparoscopy. However it is not routinely performed to evaluate the functional patency of the tubes.

The choice of test is determined by the indication and availability of different testing modalities.

MANAGEMENT

The tubal factor infertility may be managed either by surgical correction of blocks or by IVF. The choice and success of surgical correction depend upon the cause of block (tubes damaged due to tuberculosis have poor prognosis), site (fimbrial blocks are difficult to correct and success rates are also poor so also shoulder type of cornual blocks due to fibrosis), nature/extent of the block (if good length of the tubes are blocked/damaged, the postcorrection length of tubes will be insufficient for proper transport and fertilization), and the surgical skill. Tuboplasty may be performed either laparoscopically or through laparotomy. One must observe microsurgical techniques while performing the recanalization surgeries. The advantage of surgical correction of tubes is the lower cost of procedure compared to IVF. Moreover, it is one time procedure and patients may attempt conception cycle after cycle without further intervention or cost and they may conceive more than once.

However, in the era of Assisted Reproductive Techniques, IVF is preferred method of management for tubal factor infertility, as it can address other factors of infertility also. There is good evidence to consider surgical removal or plugging of hydrosalpinx prior to IVF as that fluid can be toxic to the embryo and prevent implantation by washing out the embryo.[2]

It goes without saying that whether surgical correction or IVF one must also look into the other factors such as ovarian reserve, uterine, and male factors for overall success.

The IVF has higher per cycle pregnancy rate.[2] However, end-to-end anastomosis, especially for reversal of tubal sterilization, has higher cumulative pregnancy rate and is cost effective.

REFERENCES

1. Honore GM, Holden AE, Schenken RS. Pathophysiology and management of proximal tubal blockage. Fertil Steril. 1999;5:785-95.

2. ASRM Committee Opinion. Role of Tubal surgery in the era of assisted reproductive technology: a committee opinion. Fertil Steil. 2015;103:e37-43.
3. Ahmadi F, Zafarani F, Shahrzad G. Hysterosalpingographic appearances of female genital tract tuberculosis: Part I. Fallopian Tube. Int J Fertil Steril. 2014;7:245-52.
4. Papaioannou S, Bourdrez P, Varma R, et al. Tubal evaluation in the investigation of subfertility: a structured comparison of tests. BJOG. 2004;111:1313.
5. Luttjeboer F, Harada T, Hughes E, et al. Tubal flushing for subfertility. Cochrane Database Syst Rev. 2007;(5):CD003718.
6. Swart P, Mol BW, van der Veen F, et al. The accuracy of hysterosalpingography in the diagnosis of tubal pathology: a meta-analysis. Fertil Steril. 1995;64:486.
7. Saunders RD, Shwayder JM, Nakajima ST. Current methods of tubal patency assessment. Fertil Steril. 2011;95:2171-9.

ART in Seropositive Couples

15

Nandita Palshetkar, Hrishikesh D Pai, Deepa Talreja, Nikita Lad, Shammim Khandaker

INTRODUCTION

Along with the increase in number of couples seeking fertility services, there is increase in medical issues as well that needs to be addressed. Sexually-transmitted infections are one of these major problems. Infections such as human immunodeficiency virus (HIV), hepatitis C, and hepatitis B are heading the lists, as these infections can be transmitted to an uninfected partner during the process of conception.

Since last two decades, intensive research in sexually transmitted viruses has provided information on mechanisms and risk factors underlying these infections, thus suggested the strategies for risk reduction. The introduction and widespread use of HAART and prophylaxis against opportunistic infections have decreased morbidity and mortality in this group of patients.[1] Due to increase in life expectancy, perception of HIV has been changed from a lethal disease to a chronic illness. The management of HIV infection during pregnancy has also been changed over the last decade.[2] Decrease in the perinatal transmission rates to 2–4% with the use of aggressive antiretroviral therapy has allowed a number of couples to have their own children.

Development of assisted reproductive technologies and newer approaches to decrease viral load in genital secretions have resulted in negligible rates of horizontal transmission. It helps in the prevention of HIV transmission for fertile and infertile HIV-infection discordant couples by decreasing the number of exposures (unprotected intercourse) necessary to conceive.

The ethical guidelines provided by the *American College of Obstetricians and Gynecologists* and by the *American Society for Reproductive Medicine (ASRM)* also concurred that "assisted reproductive technologies should not be denied to individuals with chronic viral infections, including HIV, solely on the basis of their positive serostatus".[3,4]

MANAGEMENT PROTOCOLS IN ART

Management of these patients should be done according to the recommendations provided by *ASRM* based on scientific principles and clinical experience. These recommendations are aimed at following:[5]

- Reducing the viral load in infected partner(s)
- Reducing exposure and susceptibility of a noninfected partner
- Frank and detailed discussion of available scientific evidence and risk-reduction strategies to provide a basis for informed consent.

Management approach includes the following:

1. *Multidisciplinary approach*: Management of these patients needs multidisciplinary approach, ideally including maternal–fetal medicine specialists, HIV/AIDS specialists, neonatologists, pediatricians, psychiatrists, social workers, and reproductive endocrinologists. Availability of an efficient maternal and child care institution that can care for pregnant patients with HIV and the child delivered under these circumstances is also a prerequisite to beginning fertility treatment. In addition, the program's staff should be properly trained in processing specimens and separate freezing facilities for gametes/embryos from infected patients.
2. *Proper explanation of procedure and informed consent*: Before starting the fertility treatment, couple should be properly informed about the diagnosis, purpose of

treatment, risks, and benefits related with the treatment. Common risks involved are risk of transmission to partners and offspring, side effects related to procedure, and complications related to pregnancy.

3. *Initial evaluation*: Similar to the any other patient undergoing assisted reproductive therapy (ART), patient or the couple with infections should undergo evaluation of factors that could affect fertility out-comes. This assessment includes:
   - Assessment of ovulatory function and ovarian reserve.
   - Assessment of tubal patency. However, if in vitro fertilization (IVF) is indicated, tubal patency evaluation is not necessary.
   - Assessment of the uterine cavity is important before IVF to rule out any abnormality that might interfere with pregnancy, such as submucous fibroid or uterine septum. Common methods used are hysterosalpingography, sonohysterography, or hysteroscopy.
   - Semen analysis is an important initial evaluation as semen parameters affect the choice of treatment. Presence of leukocytospermia may increase the risk for transmission of HIV.
4. *Assessment of medical problems*: Both partners should be evaluated medically by their primary care provider and/or infection specialist before initiating fertility therapy and appropriate preventive measures should be taken.

Virus-specific Management in ART

HIV and ART

The HIV I and II belong to retrovirus family, which primarily affects the immune cells especially T lymphocytes. Infection with HIV leads to AIDS and death in most of the untreated cases. High-risk groups for HIV include intravenous drug users, users of infected blood products, sex workers, etc. It is found in blood, vaginal secretions, and semen of infected persons. In case of seminal fluid, leukocytes are the main mode of HIV infection. It is important to recognize that serum viral load does not always correlate with the seminal viral load and semen from males with undetectable peripheral viral loads can still test positive for HIV.

Before starting the treatment, following strategies should be followed to reduce the risk of transmission in couple:

- Disease should be stable with undetectable viral load in serum.
- Ideally, these patients should be under the specialist's care and treatment with HAART should be started to aim the viral load and CD4 count within acceptable limit, generally taken as viral load less than 200 copies/mL and CD4 count more than 250 cells/mm^3 for the preceding 6 months.
- In case of discordant couple, uninfected partner should be tested for HIV serology and viral load at 3-month interval during treatment and pregnancy.

Management options depend on seropositive status of patient and the partner.

Virus-positive males: When the male partner is infected, goal of the treatment is to prevent infection transmission to female partner and offspring. According to *Centers for Disease Control and Preventions Guidelines, 2014*,[6] couple with a virus-positive male may be given options of intrauterine insemination (IUI), IVF or intracytoplasmic sperm injection (ICSI), if the virus-positive semen undergoes procedures removing seminal fluid containing HIV.

- *IUI with processed sperms*: When the husband is HIV positive and the wife is a good candidate for IUI then it is a cost-effective treatment. However, the main concern is the risk of transmission. Although studies have confirmed cases of zero post-wash contamination, it is not guaranteed that final sample for IUI is free from HIV viral particles.[7]

  During IUI, precaution should be taken to minimize trauma to the cervix and uterus.
- *IVF with ICSI*: Despite being simple treatment, with IUI, still there is a chance of seminal fluid containing possible remnants of HIV to come into contact with the female partner. The use of IVF with ICSI is a reasonable option. It is the first-line treatment with low-sperm count insufficient for IUI and theoretically to decrease the viral exposure.

  Beside the higher pregnancy rate with ICSI in comparison to IUI, major advantage of ICSI is that it provides the least exposure of seminal or prostatic secretions.
  - *Sperm wash technique*: For processing of semen sample, no other expertise is needed except for the properly taken universal precautions. Recommended technique of sperm preparation is density gradient method followed by an additional swim-up step of sperm from the pellet resulting from density gradient. If available, testing of washed sample for HIV RNA by polymerase chain reaction (PCR) method may further reduce

the risk. Using this method, chance of getting positive sperm samples is reduced to less than 1%.[8] However, a recent *Cochrane review*[9] has noted that no randomized controlled trial has assessed the benefit or risk of sperm washing to prevent HIV transmission from HIV-infected men and identified the need for a multicenter randomized controlled trial assessing the benefits and possible risks of sperm washing in preventing HIV transmission from HIV-infected men.

- *Donor insemination*: If the couple is not willing to take least possible risk of transmission, donor insemination is the safest option. However, donor sample should also be properly screened. *Food and Drug Administration (FDA)* recommends that all semen donors should be screened for high-risk factors and be tested serologically for chronic viral infections including HIV, HBV, HCV, HTLV-I and II, and *Cytomegalovirus (CMV)*. It states that individuals diagnosed positive for HIV by ELISA are ineligible for donation, even if they test negative by subsequent Western blot.[10]

Virus-positive females: In these cases, fertility options include IUI or IVF/ICSI without any risk of infection to male partner. In case of IUI, processing of female gamete in laboratory is not required. However in IVF/ICSI, precautions should be taken for handling of virus-positive oocytes. For these patients, ICSI is a better option than IVF, in order to reduce the number of cumulus and granulose cells in culture and to minimize handling of these cells by embryologists.

The main concern with the virus-positive females is the risk of vertical transmission to the child. However with appropriate medical management, especially with HAART during pregnancy or labor, use of cesarean section, and avoidance of breastfeeding, this risk has been reduced to less than 2%.[11]

Another concern in these patients related with ART is risk of multiple pregnancies. Problems such as prematurity due to multiple gestations along with obstetrical complications increase the risk of maternal-to-fetal HIV transmission. Due to these reasons, single embryo transfer is preferable in these patients (especially in women <40 years old).[12]

Hepatitis B and ART

Hepatitis B virus (HBV) is a double-stranded DNA virus and is one of the major causes of liver disease worldwide. According to WHO report, about 5% population is a chronic carrier of HBV (defined as hepatitis B surface antigen positive for 6 months).[13] It can be transmitted sexually, parenterally, and vertically.

Virus-positive male: Donor insemination is the safest option to be given but couples willing for autologous methods can be counseled to agree reasonable interventions to reduce the risk of transmission. In case of serodiscordant couple for HBV infection, female partner who is seronegative should be vaccinated against HBV and once the anti-hepatitis B surface antibody titer (HBsAB) is positive, fertility treatment can be initiated. Modified sperm-washing technique is not needed when the female partner is immunized for HBV.[14]

Virus-positive female: When female partner is HBsAG positive, main concern is the risk of vertical transmission and couple should be properly counseled before starting ART. Newborn should receive immunoprophylaxis within 12 hours after birth, which includes HBV vaccination and immunoglobulin. A review by *Dunkelberg et al.*[15] has shown that mother-to-child transmission (MTCT) has reduced to about 5% in countries that have instituted postpartum neonatal immunoprophylaxis for HBV.

Hepatitis C and ART

Hepatitis C virus (HCV) is a RNA virus, which affects 1% of world's population. It is transmitted mainly through the parenteral route such as blood products, needle injuries, and shared needles. HCV is a highly pathogenic virus and since unlike HBV there is no vaccine for HCV, risk reduction is important during ART. Management involves following approaches:

- When the male partner is HCV positive, sperm washing is recommended, similar to HIV in order to reduce the viral load in semen.
- Chronically infected partner with HCV should be treated with *peginterferon-alpha* and *ribavirin* before starting fertility treatment to decrease the viral load. Duration of treatment is 48 weeks, during which two forms of contraception be used and pregnancy should be avoided for an additional 6 months after completion of therapy in either partner to reduce teratogenic risk of ribavirin.
- Risk of vertical transmission is related with the maternal viral load and there is no vaccine available to treat newborn with HCV-positive mother.

Other Sexually Transmitted Viruses

Other sexually transmissible viruses include T-cell lymphotropic viruses (HTLV) I and II hepatitis A virus (HAV), human papilloma viruses (HPV), and several members of the herpes virus family such as Epstein–Barr virus (EBV), cytomegalovirus (CMV), herpes simplex virus 2 (HSV-2), and human herpes viruses (HHV)-types 6 and 8. Recently, two new viruses, i.e. Ebola and Zika, have attracted attention due to their catastrophic outcomes in infected mothers and fetuses.

In case of *Ebola virus*, it is recommended that there should be a waiting period of 21 days after returning from an Ebola-infected country before starting fertility treatment.

Infection with *Zika virus* may be asymptomatic or with mild symptoms, but effects on fetus are catastrophic. So, *Centers for Disease Control* recommends a waiting period of at least 8 weeks for women and at least 6 months for men who have Zika virus disease after symptom onset to attempt conception.[16]

RISK REDUCTION STRATEGIES IN ASSISTED REPRODUCTION

Following precautions should be taken during ART:[16]

1. *General precautions*:
    - Universal precautions and proper decontamination of work area
    - Use of personal protection and equipment such as laboratory coat, gloves, shoe cover, hair cover, mask, face shield, or goggles
    - Proper labeling of containers and samples
    - Avoid sharp and splash injuries and needle punctures
    - Proper waste management
    - Avoid mouth pipetting.
2. *Precautions to be taken while handling of gametes*:
    - Schedule such procedures at the end of daily work flow to isolate the patient
    - Use of disposable materials such as counting chambers for sperm
    - If possible, processing should be done in a biosafety cabinet. Otherwise, turn off the fan in laminar flow hood and hood should be used to process the semen.
    - Aerosol formation should be avoided during procedures such as pipetting, centrifugation, and mixing.
    - For processing of sperms, centrifugation should be done with gradient method to first separate leukocytes and other seminal constituents followed by separation of motile sperms from the resulting pellet by swim-up.
    - During oocyte retrieval, follicular fluid may contain viral particles, so granulose and cumulus cells should be removed and oocyte wash should be done thoroughly in sterile medium to dilute the viral titer.
    - Gametes and embryos should be cultured in separate incubator.
    - At the end of procedure, surface should be wiped out with 6% hydrogen peroxide followed by distilled water.
3. *Precautions to be taken during cryopreservation*: Viruses such as HIV, HCV, and HBV can survive in liquid nitrogen, so there is a possibility of cross-contamination of samples in liquid nitrogen. *Practice Committee of American Society of Reproductive Medicine* has provided the following guidelines to reduce the risk of cross-contamination in liquid nitrogen:
    - Use of specimen containers guaranteed by the manufacturer to withstand freezing temperatures and thawing cycles
    - Use of "double bagging" or sealing techniques to prevent the direct contact of cryo-containers with liquid nitrogen
    - Storage of samples in liquid nitrogen vapor instead of in liquid nitrogen itself
    - Use of "sperm-washing" techniques to decrease the viral load before freezing semen samples.

Freezing in heat-sealed and leak-proof *"High Security Straws"*, i.e. closed system of cryopreservation, is a safe option of storage.

ETHICAL ISSUES

As recommended by American College of Obstetricians and Gynecologists (ACOG) and ASRM, individuals with infected disease should not be refused to access fertility treatments. Physicians have right of assisting these patients to achieve their reproductive goals. Providing fertility services is supported by the facts that with the use of medical interventions including antiretroviral therapy prognosis of these patients has improved and perinatal transmission has also decreased significantly. ART helps in decreasing the risk of viral transmission to the unaffected partner.

On the contrary, points in disfavor to offer infertility treatment to these individuals such as, due to the uncertain prognosis of parents—it is not in the best interest of the child, when parent may not be available to provide long-term care for that child. Other point is the risk of the child acquiring infections from the parent.

So considering above facts, it has been advised that whatever decision is taken about the treatment, it is the responsibility of medical team to explain the decision and its rationale thoroughly to the couple.

KEY POINTS

- Individuals with chronic viral infections, including HIV, should not be denied from fertility services, if the center has the appropriate resources to provide care.
- There should be a case-by-case basis management of serodiscordant couples and the choice of treatment should depend on the available resources.
- Whenever possible, HIV viremia should be reduced with the use of antiretroviral therapy before starting fertility treatment.
- In case of infected male partner with HIV and HCV, sperm-washing technique to reduce the viral load should be used.
- In case of HBV, uninfected partner should be vaccinated against HBV.
- Once the female partner is immunized for HBV, sperm washing solely to decrease HBV viral load is not needed.
- HCV-infected partners are advised to take treatment with peginterferon-alpha and ribavirin before starting fertility treatment.
- For the recent Ebola and Zika viruses, no recommendations are available for semen processing. However, counseling, precautions, and procedures should be followed similar to other viruses.
- Standard universal precautions and laboratory safety measures should be taken during handling of infected gametes.

REFERENCES

1. Panel on Clinical Practices for Treatment of HIV Infection. (2002). Guidelines for the use of antiretroviral agents in HIV-infected adults and adolescents. HIV/AIDS Treatment Information Service. February 4, 2002. [online] Available from https://aidsinfo.nih.gov/ContentFiles/AdultandAdolescentGL04232001006.pdf. [Last accessed February, 2019].
2. HIV/AIDS Treatment Information Service. (2001). Public Health Service Task Force recommendations for the use of antiretroviral drugs in pregnant HIV-1-infected women for maternal health and interventions to reduce perinatal HIV-1 transmission in the United States. May 4, 2001.
3. Committee on Ethics of the American College of Obstetricians and Gynecologists (ACOG). Human immunodeficiency virus: ethical guidelines for obstetricians and gynecologists. Ethics in Obstetrics and Gynecology. Washington, DC: ACOG; 2002. pp. 42-7.
4. Ethics Committee of the Society for Reproductive Medicine. Human immunodeficiency virus and infertility treatment. Fertil Steril. 2002;77:218-22.
5. Practice Committee of American Society for Reproductive Medicine. Guidelines for reducing the risk of viral transmission during fertility treatment. Fertil Steril. 2008;90:S156.
6. Centers for Disease Control and Prevention, National Institutes of Health, American Academy of HIV Medicine, International Association of Providers of AIDS Care, National Minority AIDS Council. (2014). Recommendations for HIV Prevention with Adults and Adolescents with HIV in the United States, 2014. [online] Available from https://aidsetc.org/resource/recommendations-hiv-prevention-adults-and-adolescents-hiv-united-states-2014.
7. Barnes A, Riche D, Mena L. Efficacy and safety of intrauterine insemination and assisted reproductive technology in populations serodiscordant for human immunodeficiency virus: a systematic review and meta-analysis. Fertil Steril. 2014;102:424-34.
8. Politch JA, Xu C, Tucker L, et al. Separation of human immunodeficiency virus type 1 from motile sperm by the double tube gradient method vs other methods. Fertil Steril. 2004;81:440-7.
9. Eke AC, Oragwu C. Sperm washing to prevent HIV transmission from HIV-infected men but allowing conception in serodiscordant couples. Cochrane Database Syst Rev. 2011;CD008498.
10. Food and Drug Administration. (2005). Part 1271—Human Cells, Tissues and Cellular and Tissue Based Products; Donor Screening and Testing, and Related Labeling; Interim Final Rule 5/24/05. [online] Available from https://www.federalregister.gov/documents/2005/05/25/05-10583/human-cells-tissues-and-cellular-and-tissue-based-products-donor-screening-and-testing-and-related. [Last accessed February, 2019].
11. Practice Committee of the American Society for Reproductive Medicine. Recommendations for reducing the risk of viral transmission during fertility treatment with the use of autologous gametes: a committee opinion. Fertil Steril. 2013;99:340-6.
12. Ohl J, Partisani M, Wittemer C, et al. Encouraging results despite complexity of multidisciplinary care of HIV-infected women using assisted reproduction techniques. Hum Reprod. 2005;20:31-6.
13. WHO Hepatitis B Fact sheet N 204 Updated July 2015.
14. Molina I, Del Carmen Gonzalvo M, Clavero A, et al. Assisted Reproductive Technology and Obstetric Outcome in Couples when The Male Partner Has A Chronic Viral Disease. Int J Fertil Steril. 2014;7:291-300.
15. Dunkelberg JC, Berkley EM, Thiel KW, et al. Hepatitis B and C in pregnancy: a review and recommendations for care. J Perinatol. 2014;34:882-91.
16. Jindal SK, Rawlins RG, Muller CH, et al. Guidelines for risk reduction when handling gametes from infectious patients seeking assisted reproductive technologies. Reprod Biomed Online. 2016;33:121-30.

Isthmocele: An Under Diagnosed Cause of Infertility

16

Singh VP, Walker P

INTRODUCTION

Cesarean section is one of the most commonly performed surgeries and rates are continuing to increase all over the world. Well known complications of a cesarean section scar include placenta accreta, placenta previa, scar ectopic, and scar dehiscence (either antenatally or intrapartum). However, we are less familiar with the implications from a cesarean scar defect such as dysfunction uterine bleeding, pelvic pain and secondary infertility.

HISTORY

Isthmocele also known as cesarean scar defect, uterine scar deficiency, uterine niche or pouch was first described by the Obstetrician Gynecologist Morris in 1995.[1] This entity is only just being identified and described in the literature, and is becoming a subject of attention, especially in those who present with secondary infertility. The reported incidence of isthmocele ranges from 24–84%.[2,3] With the incidence of cesarean section increasing, it is important that we are aware that isthmocele could be a cause of these symptoms.

PRESENTATION

Isthmocele may present with secondary infertility, menstrual disturbance (typically postmenstrual spotting), continuous brown discharge, dysmenorrhea, pelvic pain, and/or dyspareunia.[1,2,4] Isthmocele can also be asymptomatic. The intensity of symptoms is thought to be related to the size of the isthmocele.[1] As other pathology may present with these symptoms, there is often a delay in diagnosis.[5]

DEFINITION AND DIAGNOSIS

There is no international standardized definition or diagnosis for isthmocele. It can be identified on imaging with transvaginal ultrasound scan (TVUS), magnetic resonance imaging (MRI), or at the time of hysteroscopy. Isthmocele or cesarean scar defect has been defined as "any visible filling defects in the anterior isthmus of the uterus on transvaginal ultrasound scan".[6] A "larger" isthmocele is thought to be when the remaining myometrial thickness is less than 2.5–3.0 mm.[7]

PREVALENCE

Studies have found wide prevalence ranges. Bij de Vaate Aj et al. estimated the incidence to between 24–84%, CB Wang et al. reported 6.6–69%.[8] While Florio, Tower and Frishman reported and incidence or 30–52% and 19.4–88% respectively.[8]

Although isthmocele is quite prevalent, it is not always associated with secondary infertility.

One of the largest systematic reviews on cesarean section scar associated with secondary infertility showed an association between cesarean delivery and increased odds of subfertility when compared to vaginal delivery of 1.6 (95% CI 1.45-1.76, p <0.00001).[9]

There is growing evidence that IVF success rates are lower in patients who deliver via cesarean section when using embryos from the same cohort,[10] suggesting a possible impact of embryo implantation.

RISK FACTORS

A number of risk factors are thought to be implicated in the development of isthmocele. The list includes more than one cesarean section, retroflexed uterus, preeclampsia, maternal age less than or equal to 30 years, duration of labor more than 5 hours, cervical dilation more than or equal to 5 cm at time of delivery, lower station at delivery (below pelvic inlet), incision in the cervical area, use of oxytocin, exclusion of endometrial layer during repair, one layer closure of myometrium, delayed absorbable sutures, and more ischemic closure.[1, 6]

INVESTIGATIONS

Transvaginal ultrasound scan (TVUS) and MRI are considered to be the gold standard when investigating for isthmocele,[7] although ultrasound is usually considered as the first diagnostic tool.[1] The depth and length of the defect are measured along with the remaining myometrial wall thickness. Other key sonographic findings to consider are inward and outward protruding of the scar, scar retraction and hematoma.[6] On TVUS the defect is seen as a triangular hypoechogenic zone in the uterine scar area, the term for this is known as "niche".[1] Saline infusion sonohysterography and hysterosalpingography have also been used to detect isthmocele **(Fig. 1)**.

PATHOPHYSIOLOGY

The exact mechanism of how isthmocele or cesarean scar defect occurs is not completely understood.[8] It is possible that two mechanisms are at play; inadequate healing of the cesarean section scar and the resulting thickness of the myometrium.[11] Reduced scar contractility and abnormal myocontraction, along with the presence of functional endometrium leads to the accumulation and impaired drainage of menstrual blood in the cavity.[2,12] This results in intermenstrual bleeding and pelvic pain.[11]

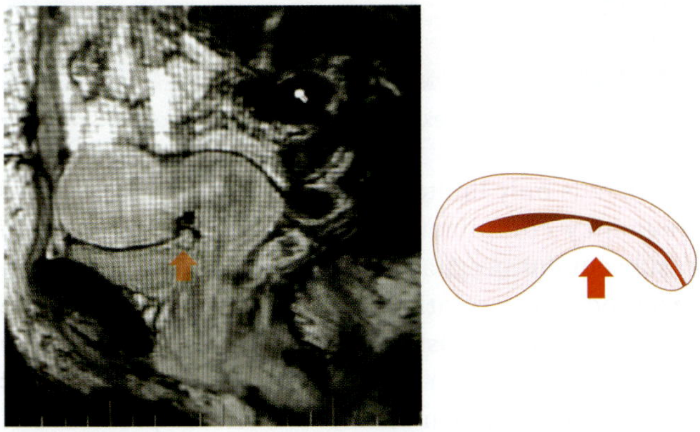

Fig. 1: MRI showing isthmocele and pictorial diagram.

The retained menstrual fluid is likely to impair the quality of cervical mucous, sperm viability, and disrupt sperm swim-up. Bleeding may cause the blastocyst to be washed out of the uterus interfering with embryo implantation.[1,2]

In addition, endometrial abnormalities around the scar defect such as overhanging endometrium and/or inclusion of endometrium within the scar could lead to abnormal bleeding.[2] Careful re-approximation of the endometrial layer during uterine closure could reduce endometrial abnormalities and dysfunctional bleeding.[2]

TREATMENT

Treatment should be offered to symptomatic women.[7] There is no "gold standard" or treatment protocol for isthmocele repair, and no technique that has shown a statistically superior outcome.[7]

Although some report medical therapy can help to improve symptoms by suppressing menstruation,[11] others would argue that medical treatment with the combined oral contraceptive or Mirena shows no benefit.[13] Hormonal treatment is also not suitable for patients who are planning a pregnancy.

Both hysteroscopic resection and laparoscopic resection and repair of isthmocele have high success rates of treating both infertility and bleeding disturbance, and a variety of different surgical approaches have been described.[1]

Isthmocele repair was first performed laparoscopically by Jacobson in 2003.[7] The laparoscopic method has the advantage of increasing the thickness of the myometrial layer after repair.[14] It is the preferred surgical approach particularly if the residual myometrium is less than 3 mm thick.[7,9] Restoring normal myometrial thickness is important in those patients planning a pregnancy to help reduce the risk of scar rupture.[7] Furthermore, the laparoscopic approach has a reduced risk of incomplete removal of scar tissue, uterine perforation and bladder injury which is associated with hysteroscopic resection.[1,7]

The crucial step of laparoscopic repair is to correctly identify the uterine scar defect.[7] A popular technique described in the literature is the "Rendezvous technique".[1] This is a combined technique where the isthmocele is identified at laparoscopy with the simultaneous use of hysteroscopy to outline the defect with its light source.

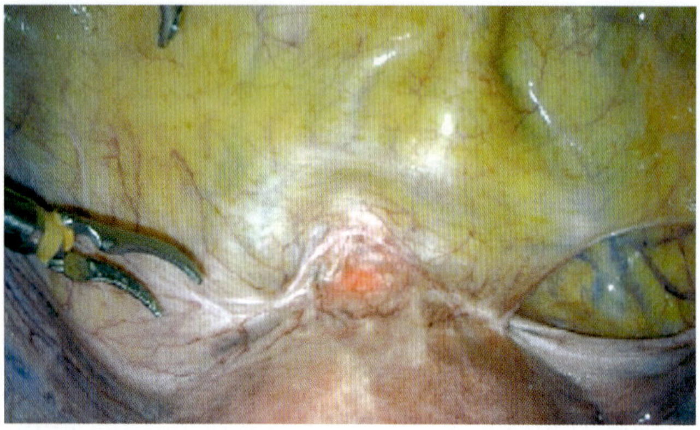

Fig. 2: Isthmocele seen at laparoscopy.

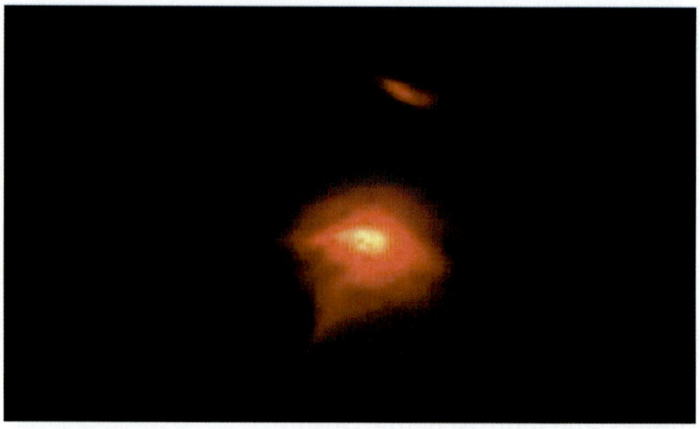

Fig. 3: The defect can be seen under the light of the hysteroscope "Halloween sign".

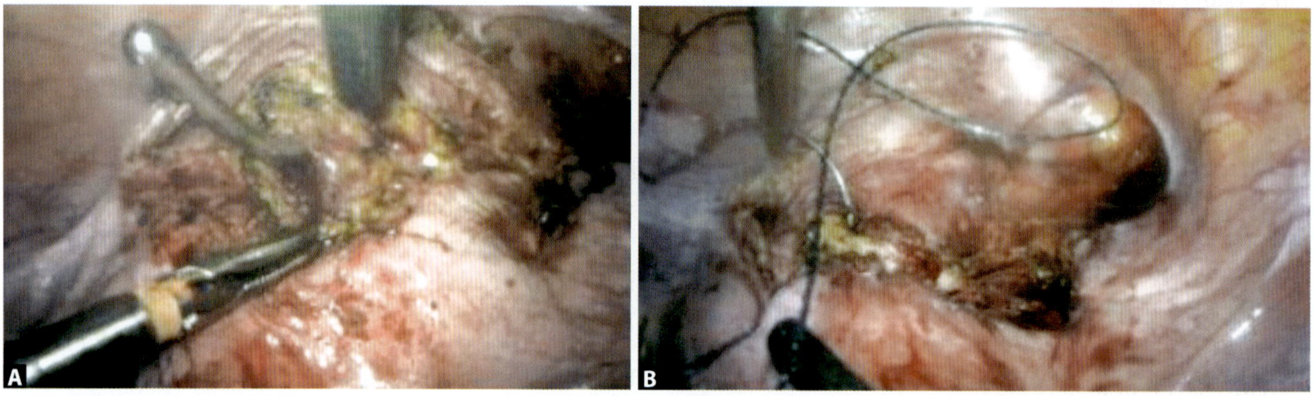

Figs. 4A and B: Intraoperative laparoscopic excision and repair of isthmocele.

The defect can be seen under the light of the hysteroscope and is known as the "Halloween sign"[1] **(Figs. 2 and 3)**. A Foley catheter or TVUS can also be used during laparoscopy to help identify the location of the isthmocele.[11,15] It is unclear which type of energy source or suture material is best to repair the scar defect with.[1]

Symptoms are generally improved after repair of isthmocele, with one study reporting a 97% improvement in pain **(Figs. 4 and 5)**.[5]

FUTURE PREGNANCY

Secondary infertility is an indication for treatment, and the reported pregnancy rates after endoscopic repair of isthmocele are 44–92%.[1,16] As with cesarean section, the risk following treatment of isthmocele is scar dehiscence in subsequent pregnancies. The current recommendation is to wait at least 3 months after repair to get pregnant.[1] It is also recommended that delivery is by cesarean section at term,[1] although successful vaginal deliveries after surgical repair of isthmocele have been reported in the literature.

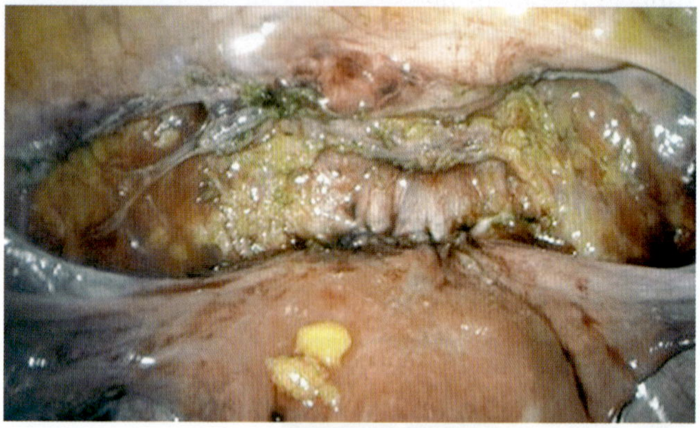

Fig. 5: After laparoscopic excision and repair of isthmocele.

There is only limited data regarding isthmocele and pregnancy complications including uterine rupture in subsequent pregnancies.[17] However, what has been observed is the relationship between the size of the isthmocele and the risk of scar rupture, where the larger the defect the greater the risk of scar rupture.[17] Lower uterine thickness near term could also be predictive of uterine rupture.[17]

FUTURE TRENDS

Isthmocele is common following cesarean section and is associated with infertility. We need a prospective multicenter database to develop an understanding of this condition with regards to diagnosis, surgical techniques, and outcomes of surgery so that we can give robust information to our patients.

CONCLUSION

Isthmocele must be considered in patients with a history of cesarean section who presents with secondary infertility, abnormal bleeding or pelvic pain. With cesarean section rates' rising globally it is predicted that we will encounter this issue with increasing frequency. By increasing awareness of this common complication, we can help to prevent a delay in diagnosis.

There are few modifiable risk factors in preventing the development of isthmocele following cesarean section. Attention to surgical technique, in particular avoiding incision into the cervical area, not performing a one layer closure, and not using delayed absorbable sutures could all be taken into consideration at the time of cesarean section.

One of the first steps in diagnostic workup is TVUS, however often other imaging modalities are employed. Surgical treatment needs to be considered for symptomatic patients, including those who present with secondary infertility. The laparoscopic approach appears to be gaining popularity as the preferred method for treatment primarily because it aims to restore normal myometrial thickness. However, no technique has actually shown a statically superior outcome.

Patients need to be counseled to wait at least 3 months after treatment before they try for pregnancy, that it does not eliminate the risk of uterine rupture, and that the recommended mode of delivery is cesarean section at term.

SUMMARY

- Isthmocele also known as cesarean scar defect is only just being identified and described in the literature, and is becoming a subject of attention especially in those who present with secondary infertility.
- Cesarean section is one of the most commonly performed surgeries, and rates are continuing to increase all over the world.
- Isthmocele is an underdiagnosed cause of infertility.
- Isthmocele may present with secondary infertility, menstrual disturbance, dysmenorrhea, pelvic pain or dyspareunia. Isthmocele must be considered in patients with a history of cesarean section whom present with these symptoms.
- One of the first steps in diagnostic workup is TVUS, although other imaging modalities such as MRI are often employed.
- Surgical treatment should be offered to patients who present with secondary infertility.
- Reported pregnancy rates after endoscopic repair of isthmocele are high.
- The laparoscopic approach appears to be gaining popularity as the preferred method for treatment, primarily because it aims to restore normal myometrial thickness. However, no technique has actually shown a statically superior outcome.
- With cesarean section rates raising globally it is predicted that we will encounter this issue with increasing frequency. Raising awareness of this common complication can help to prevent a delay in diagnosis.

REFERENCES

1. Bakavičiūtė G, Špiliauskaitė S, Meškauskienė A, et al. Laparoscopic repair of the uterine scar defect-successful treatment of secondary infertility: a case report and literature review. Acta Med Litu. 2016;23:227-231.
2. Masuda H, Uchida H, Maruyama T, et al. Successful treatment of atypical cesarean scar defect using endoscopic surgery. BMC Pregnancy Childbirth. 2015;15:342.
3. Bij de Vaate AJ, Brolmann HA, van der Voet LF, et al. Ultrasound evaluation of the cesarean scar: relation between a niche and postmenstrual spotting. Ultrasound Obstet Gynecol. 2011;37:93-9.
4. Urman B, Arslan T, Aksu S, et al. Laparoscopic Repair of Cesarean Scar Defect "Isthmocele". J Minim Invasive Gynecol. 2016;23:857-8.
5. Bij de Vaate AJ, van der Voet LF, Naji O, et al. Prevalence, potential risk factors for development and symptoms related to the presence of uterine niches following Cesarean section: systematic review. Ultrasound Obstet Gynecol. 2014;43:372-82.
6. Tower AM, Frishman GN. Cesarean scar defects: an underrecognized cause of abnormal uterine bleeding and other gynecologic complications. J Minim Invasive Gynecol. 2013;20:562-72.
7. Setubal A, Alves J, Osorio F, et al. Treatment for Uterine Isthmocele, A Pouchlike Defect at the Site of a Cesarean Section Scar. J Minim Invasive Gynecol. 2018;25:38-46.

8. Istvan F, Ekine AA, Istvan T, et al. Isthmocele: Successful Surgical Management of an Under-Recognized Iatrogenic Cause of Secondary Infertility. Womens Health Gynecol. 2017;3:1-5
9. Keag OE, Norman JE, Stock SJ. Long-term risks and benefits associated with cesarean delivery for mother, baby, and subsequent pregnancies: Systematic review and meta-analysis. PLoS Med. 2018;15:e1002494.
10. Hayes MK, Bergh PA, Bergh CM, et al. Repeat in vitro fertilization success rates are lower in patients who deliver via caesarean section when using embryos from the same cohort. Fertil Steril. 2016;106:e48.
11. Nazik H, Nazik E. A new problem arising after the cesarean, cesarean scar defect (isthmocele) a Case Report. Obstet Gyncol Int J. 2017;7:00264.
12. Murji A, Glass K, Leyland N. Isthmocele. J Obstet Gynaecol Can. 2013;35:779.
13. Zhang X et al. Prospective evaluation of five methods used to treat cesarean scar defects. Int J Gynaecol. Obstet. 2016;134:336-9.
14. Aimi G, Buggio L, Berlanda N, et al. Laparoscopic repair of a symptomatic post-cesarean section isthmocele: a video case report. Fertil Steril 2017;107:e17-e18.
15. Akdemir A, Sahin C, Ari SA, et al. Determination of Isthmocele Using a Foley Catheter During Laparoscopic Repair of Cesarean Scar Defect. J Minim Invasive Gynecol. 2018;25:21-22.
16. Donnez O, Jadoul P, Squifflet J, et al. Laparoscopic repair of wide and deep uterine scar dehiscence after cesarean section. Fertil Steril. 2008;89:974-80.
17. Bolla D, Raio L, Favre D, et al. Laparoscopic Ultrasound-Guided Repair of Uterine Scar Isthmocele Connected With the Extra-Amniotic Space in Early Pregnancy. J Minim Invasive Gynecol. 2016;23:261-4.

SECTION 4: Fertility Enhancing Endoscopic Surgeries

Hysteroscopy: Instrumentation 17

S Krishnakumar, Aditi Joshi, Rachana Kaveri

INTRODUCTION

Though Pantaleoni reported the first successful hysteroscopy in the year 1869, major advancements and improvements in this field of has happened only in the last two decades. Diagnostic and operative hysteroscopy are now considered the "gold standard" for evaluation and treatment of any intrauterine pathology such as intrauterine fibroids, polyps, uterine septae, and intrauterine adhesions. As with any other procedure, appropriate instrumentation and good visualization together with distension media like electrolyte and nonelectrolyte solutions is the key to a correct diagnosis and a precise treatment. The essential elements for any optimal endoscopic surgery include:

- High-definition medical grade monitor
- High-definition endocamera
- Light source (Xenon/LED) and light cable
- Recording device

The layout of the operating room is as shown in **Figures 1 and 2**.

Modern hysteroscopy can be classified as:

- Operative hysteroscopy—done with smaller diameter sheaths with 5 Fr operative channel requiring no dilation of cervix
- Resectoscopic surgery: Require dilatation of cervix.

DISTENSION MEDIA

Both diagnostic and operative procedures can be performed using normal saline making it the distension media of choice. It is easily available and economical. Also in modern hysteroscopy, if energy is required it can be safely used with bipolar energy. The features and safety of various distension media is shown in **Tables 1 and 2**.

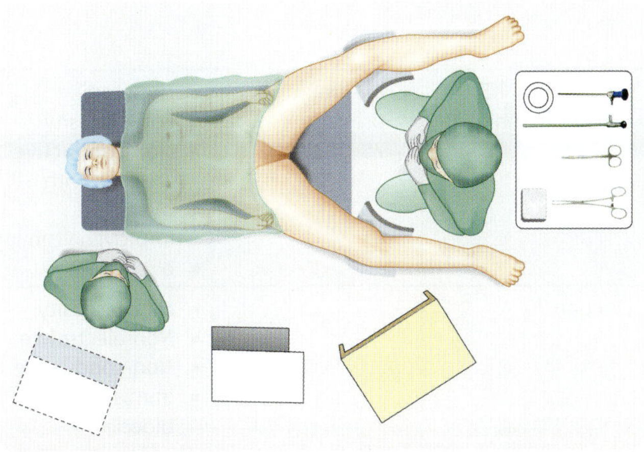

Fig. 1: Position of patient, surgeon, anesthetist and instruments in operating room (OR).

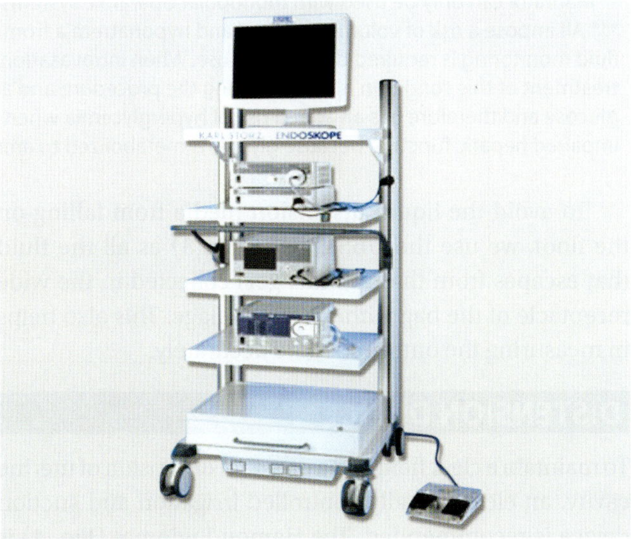

Fig. 2: Fully equipped mobile cart.

Table 1: Features of distension media.

Media type	*Maximum flow rate*	*Pros*	*Cons*	*Volume discrepancy*	*Complications*
CO_2 gas	▪ Cannot use laparoscopic insufflators ▪ Flow rate of 40–60 mL/min ▪ Maximum pressure 100 mm Hg	▪ Rapidly absorbed gas easily flows through narrow channels in office	▪ Cannot clear blood from the scope		▪ Higher pressures and rates can cause cardiac arrhythmias embolism and arrest
0.9% Saline and lactated ringers	▪ Maximum pressure 75–100 mm Hg	▪ Isotonic ▪ Conductive ▪ Low viscosity ▪ Safe with mechanical	▪ Miscible with blood (increased pressures to clear field) ▪ Excellent conductivity (precludes standard monopolar*)		
3% Sorbitol, 1.5% glycine, mannitol**	▪ Maximum pressure 75–100 mm Hg	▪ Hypotonic ▪ Low viscosity ▪ Non-conductive ▪ Miscible with blood but improved visibility ▪ over saline		Stop at 2 L***	▪ Risk of volume overload and hyponatremia with intravascular absorption
Dextran 70		▪ High viscosity ▪ Non-electrolyte ▪ Non-conductive ▪ Immiscible with blood		Stop at 500 mL	▪ Allergic reactions and anaphylaxis ▪ Fluid overload ▪ Disseminated intravascular coagulopathy ▪ Destruction of instruments

* Monopolar systems with the ERA sleeve or Opera Star systems may be used with these solutions

** Mannitol can only be used with monopolar operative systems

*** All impose a risk of volume overload and hyponatremia from intravascular absorption (particularly > 2 L). Therefore, careful fluid monitoring is required during their use. When intravasation of 5% mannitol occurs, It stays in the extracellular compartment; treatment of this condition is discontinuing the procedure and administering diuretics. 3% sorbitol is broken down into fructose and glucose and therefore has an added risk of hyperglycemia when absorbed in excess. Use 1.5% glycine with caution in patients with impaired hepatic function because glycine is metabolized to ammonia.

To avoid the liquid distension media from falling on the floor, we use the OBSTI bag **(Fig. 3)** as all the fluid that escapes from the introitus gets collected in the wide receptacle of the bag without any spillage. This also helps in measuring the outflow of fluid accurately.

DISTENSION DEVICE

To maintain a clear field and a constant distension of uterine cavity, an electronically controlled irrigation and suction device is recommended. The Hamou Endomat **(Fig. 4)** is

Table 2: Electrolyte properties of distension media.

Solution	*Na mEq/L*	*Cl mEq/L*	*mOsm/L*
0.9% Sodium chloride	154	154	308
Lactated ringers	130	110	275
0.45% Sodium chloride	77	77	155
3% Sorbitol	–	–	178
1.5% Glycine	–	–	200
5% Mannitol	–	–	275
5% Dextrose in water	–	–	250

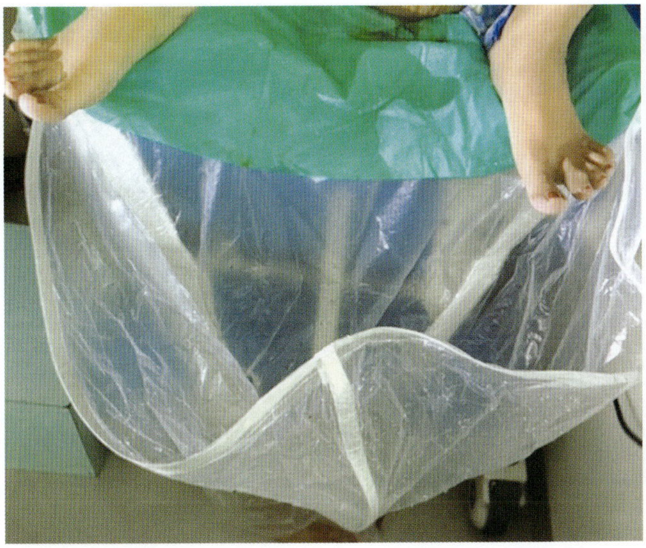

Fig. 3: OBSTI bag.

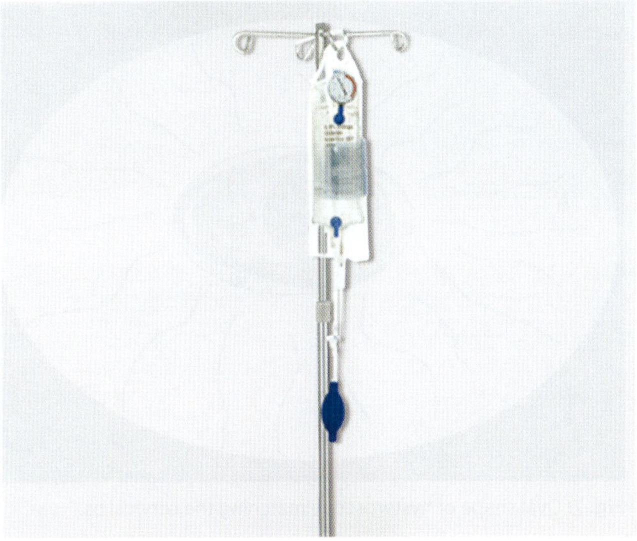

Fig. 5: Medex pressure with TUR set.

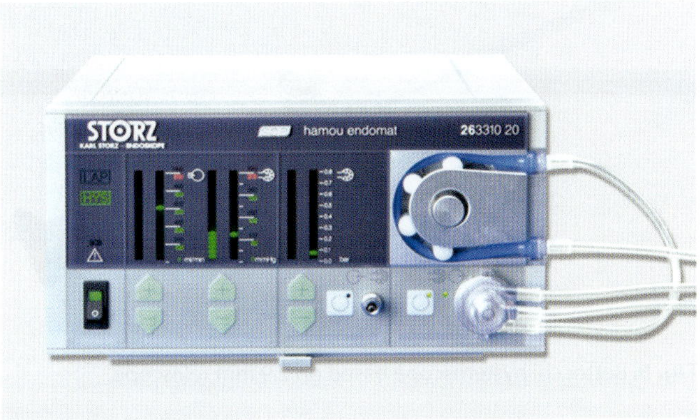

Fig. 4: Hamou Endomat.

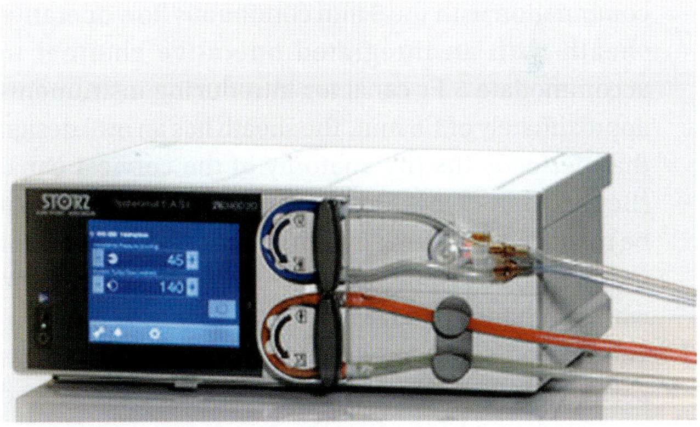

Fig. 6: EASI Endomat.

particularly suitable for office operative hysteroscopy. The various parameters like flow, pressure, and aspiration are set so as to obtain a constant distension of 30–40 mm Hg.

The saline solution may be insufflated at atmospheric pressure by means of 2, 3 or 5 L bags connected by a urologic "Y" outflow and located 1.5 m above the patient or at a pressure generated by a pressure bag **(Fig. 5)**.

EASI Endomat

This new device has specific setting for various types of sheaths and procedures. It also has different settings for resectoscopic surgery. The intrauterine pressure and fluid flow rate is fixed in this device and gives alarm if the pressure goes above the set limit. It also has a blood and mucous mode which when activated, the flow of fluid automatically increases to clear the field rapidly. Apart from the initial learning curve, this pump seems to have all the safety features desired of a Hysteromat **(Fig. 6)**.

Telescopes and Sheaths

Bettocchi et al. created the awareness that the internal cervical os is oval horizontally and introduction of conventional 4 mm telescopes with 5 mm rounded diagnostic sheath necessitates dilatation of cervix and anesthesia. They also modified the hysteroscopes **(Fig. 7)** so that it negotiates the internal os without dilatation.

With the introduction of small diameter telescopes, ranging from 1.9 mm to 2.9 mm, very thin diagnostic sheaths and operative sheaths (including the working channel and continuous flow features) with a diameter equal or less than 5 mm, have been manufactured. The possibility of making a visual examination of the uterine cavity and at the same time exploiting the contextual operative facilities represents the so-called "see and treat" philosophy, even called "Office Operative Hysteroscopy". Various operative hysteroscope sets are available as follows:

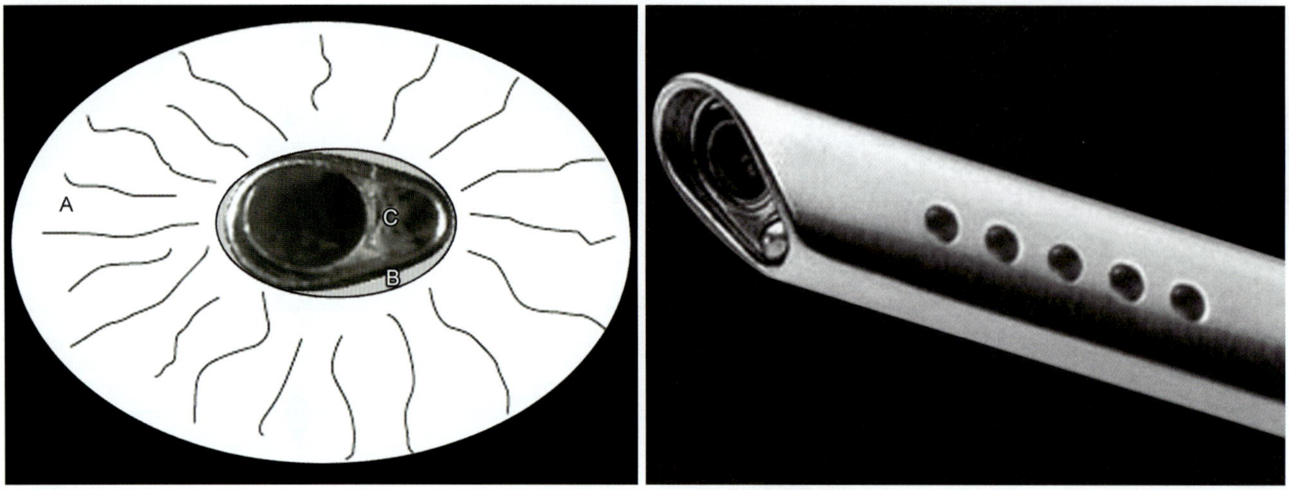

Fig. 7: Oval shape of hysteroscope matching the cervical os.

1. 2.9-mm 30° fore-oblique view telescopes can be used with single-flow operating sheath of 4.3 mm in combination with the 5 mm continuous flow operative sheath with an integrated operative channel to accommodate 5 Fr canal for introducing instruments approximately of 1.6 mm. The sheath has an oval design that perfectly fits the anatomy of the cervical canal (Bettocchi system). Most anatomical difficulties can be managed with such hysteroscopes as they allow for introduction grasping forceps or scissors through the working channel **(Fig. 8)**.
2. The true office hysteroscope, also called "size 4" has 2.0 mm telescope (30°) with an outer diameter reduced to 4 mm, ideal for office hysteroscopy, but is very delicate to handle and has an increased risk of damage **(Fig. 9)**.

   Both instruments adhere more strictly to the anatomy of the cervical canal and create continuous flow system as they feature two sheaths (one for irrigation and other for suction).
3. Bettocchi integrated office hysteroscope (BIOH) **(Fig. 10)**, which is fitted with a handle compatible for use with the Bettocchi system includes operating sheath, fiber-optic light connector and connections for irrigation and suction tubes. It is available with short or long handle.
4. The TROPHY scope or CAMPO compact hysteroscope **(Fig. 11)** has a thin outer diameter of 2.9 mm that can be loaded with either a diagnostic sheath or a 4.4 mm operating sheath. It may be used without a sheath for diagnostic hysteroscopy in single-flow mode. If needed, the continuous flow diagnostic sheath or continuous-flow operating sheath is used in conjunction with the compact hysteroscope.

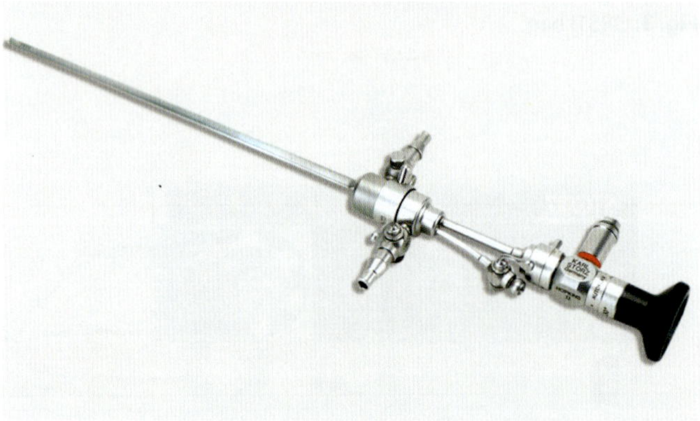

Fig. 8: Bettocchi hysteroscope based on 2.9 mm telescope.

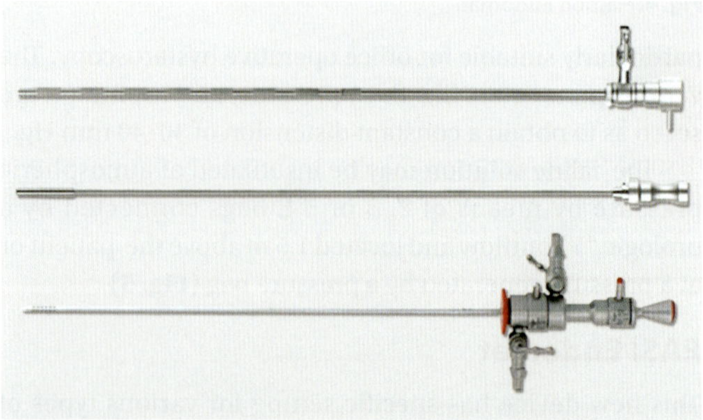

Fig. 9: Betocchi hysteroscope based on 2 mm telescope.

MECHANICAL INSTRUMENTS

The commonly used mechanical instruments used through the operative channel of operative sheath **(Fig. 12)** are available either in 5Fr or 7Fr. Among the most commonly used are alligator forceps (grasping forceps with teeth), the spoon or biopsy forceps, the pointed scissors (used for

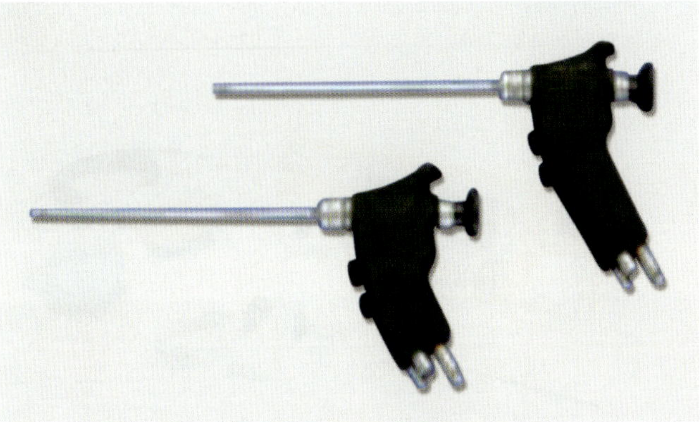

Fig. 10: Bettocchi integrated office hysteroscope (BIOH).

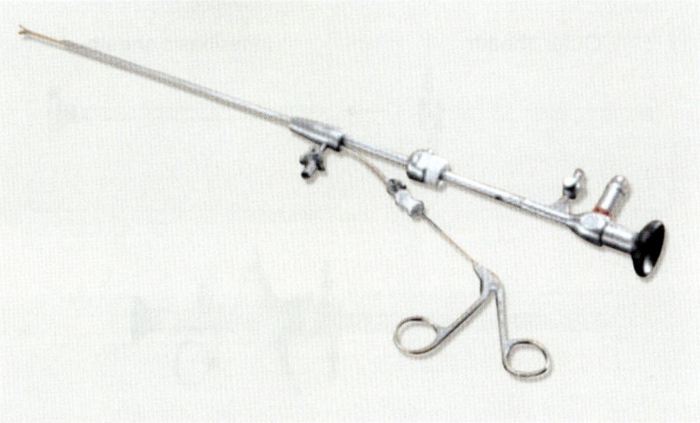

Fig. 11: TROPHY scope-CAMPO compact hysteroscope.

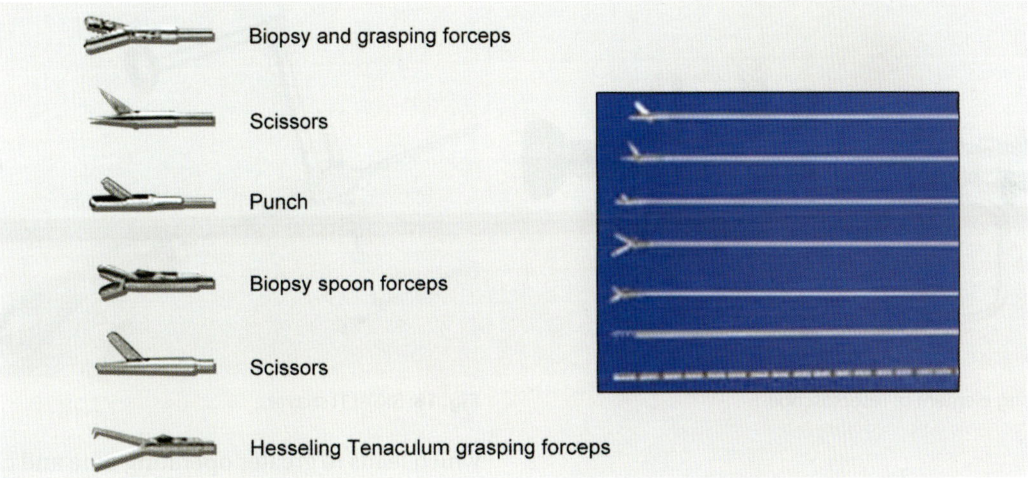

Fig. 12: Basic set of instruments.

metroplasty or small septum), and the tenaculum grasping forceps (used for removal of myoma fragments and polyps). The 7 Fr instrument allows removal of a larger chunk of tissues. The myoma spiral can be used to extract submucous fibroids to make it project more into the cavity.

Bipolar Needle (Fig. 13)

These 5 Fr instruments use energy for slicing of large polyps, cutting of septum, and coagulating small bleeders.

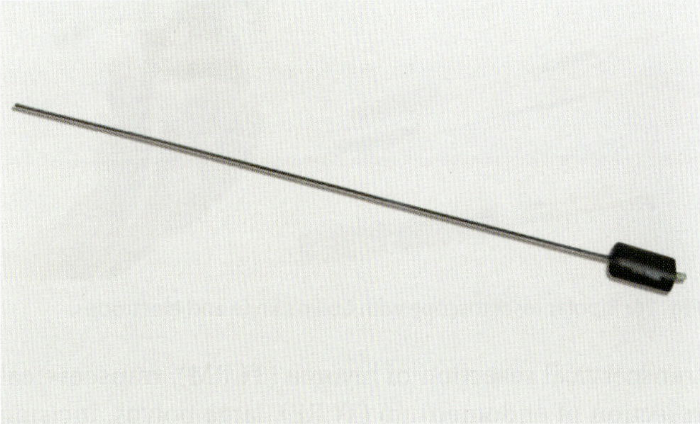

Fig. 13: Bipolar needle.

Resectoscope

Typically, a resectoscope includes inflow and outflow channels **(Fig. 14)** with the working element, which is passive **(Fig. 15)**.

They are available either to be used with bipolar or monopolar current. Traditionally, resectoscope was available only in 26 Fr size, which was used with 4 mm 30° telescopes. Presently resectoscopes are available in 22 Fr and 18 Fr also. The telescopes used are narrower with 12° angle. The various electrodes to be used with resectoscope include—Collins knife, loop electrode, roller ball, and cylinder **(Fig. 16)**. Resectoscopic surgery is restricted to

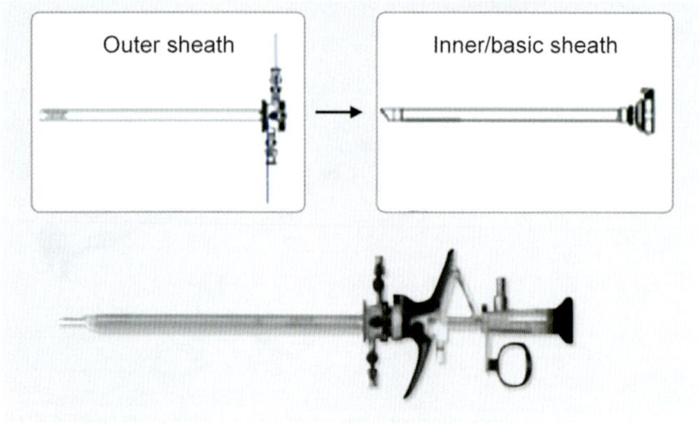

Fig. 14: Resectoscope with outer and inner sheath.

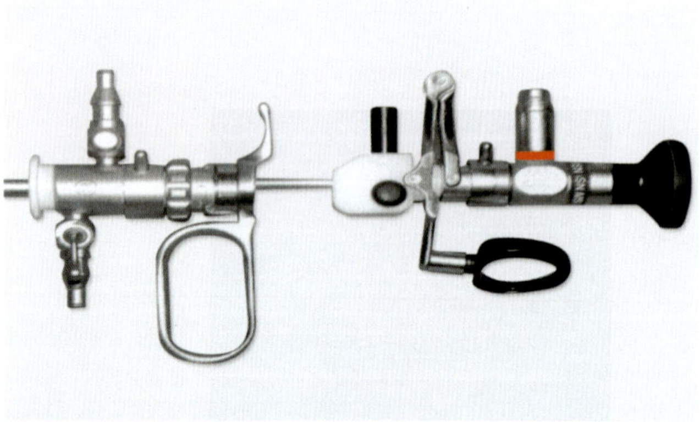

Fig. 15: Working element of resectoscope.

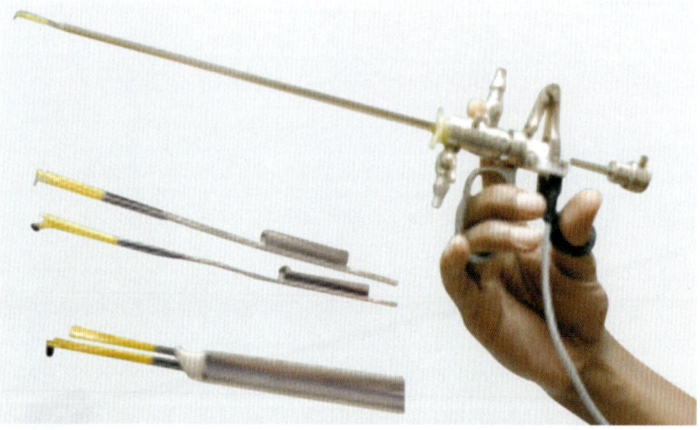

Fig. 16: Bipolar resectoscope with Collin's knife and electrodes.

transcervical resection of myoma (TCRM), transcervical resection of endometrium (TCRE), large polyps, incising of broad and fleshy septum. With the advancement of underwater bipolar generators **(Fig. 17)**, monopolar surgery should be avoided during resectoscopic surgery.

Hysteroscopic Morcellators

During resectoscopic surgeries, the resected tissue remains floating within the cavity, thereby reducing the visibility,

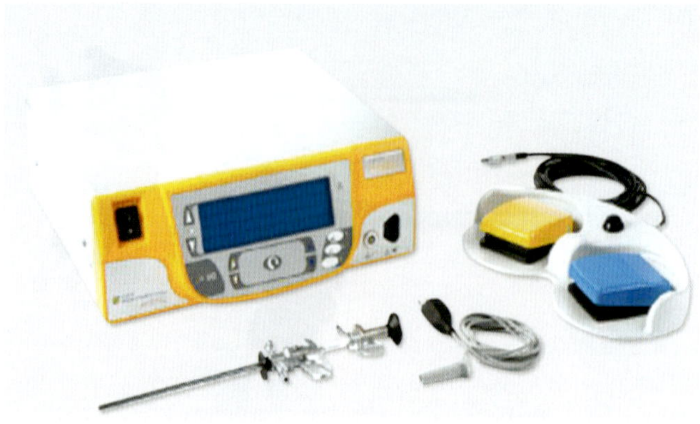

Fig. 17: Bipolar generator.

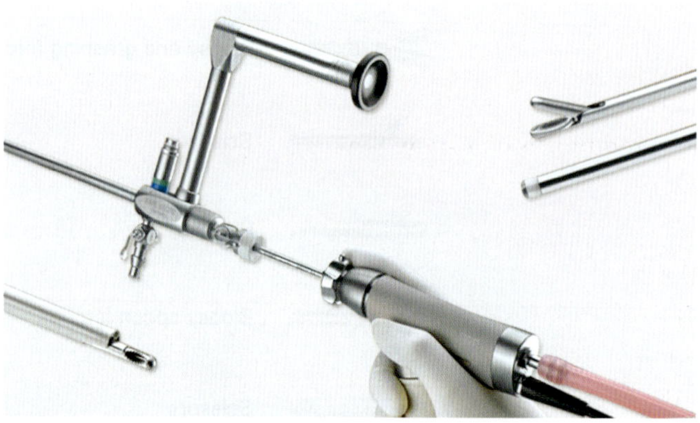

Fig. 18: BIGATTI shaver.

which leads to greater operating time and chances of fluid overload. Hence need for intrauterine morcellators was always desired, this led to the development of the following commonly used devices:

Intrauterine Bigatti Shaver

It is introduced into a straight operative channel of a 90° angulated and 6° panoramic optic. The outer sheath diameter of the optic is 24 Fr (8.5 mm). The Intrauterine BIGATTI Shaver (IBS®) system consists of two hollow metal tubes which fit into each other. The inner tube oscillates within the outer tube and is connected to a handpiece (Drill cut-X), a motor unit (Unidrive SIII) and to a roller pump (Endomat EASI) and controlled by foot pedal. The movements of the shaver tip and the roller pump's aspiration are controlled simultaneously by the foot pedal. This maintains a continuous suction power of solution and tissue through the hollow blade during procedure. The IBS helps in effectively enucleating the myoma from their fovea and the intramural site of insertion without causing thermal injury to the surrounding healthy endometrium as compared to the less precise behavior of conventional resectoscope **(Fig. 18)**.

TruClear Hysteroscopic Morcellator (Smith and Nephew)

This is the first mechanical morcellator for intrauterine pathology, approved by US Food and Drug Administration (FDA). It comprises of a rigid single-use metallic inner tube consisting of cutting edges that rotate within a 4 mm rigid outer tube. The outer tube, at its distal end incorporates a side-facing cutting window. This assembly is secured to a reusable handpiece to which a suction tube is attached. The handpiece is in turn connected to a motor control unit. Following this suction pressure is applied to the inner tube and the tissue is then pulled into the cutting window as the inner tube rotates at 1,100 rpm. All of the resected material is then aspirated into a collecting bag. The entire device is introduced into the uterine cavity with a 9-mm outer diameter, rigid, continuous-flow, 0°; hysteroscope that requires a high-flow Smith and Nephew fluid pump for proper functioning **(Figs. 19A to C)**.

MyoSure Morcellator

This was the second hysteroscopic morcellation device approved by FDA in 2009—the "MyoSure Tissue Removal System". Similar to TruClear device, this also is suction-based, uses mechanical energy and has a rotating tubular cutter system to remove tissue. However, this has the advantage of having a smaller (2.5 mm) inner blade that rotates within a 3 mm outer tube at speeds of 6,000 rpm and presents an outer bevel on the rotating blade edge. The blade and handpiece are combined into a single-use device that is then attached to suction and a motor control unit. The device is introduced into the uterus through a 6.25 mm 0° lens; custom-designed continuous flow hysteroscope that is compatible with all currently available fluid management systems **(Figs. 20A and B)**.

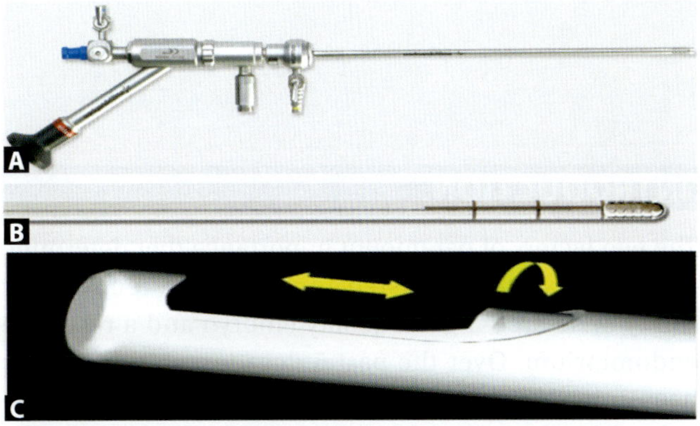

Figs. 19A to C: TruClear hysteroscopic morcellator: (A) TruClear hysteroscope with cutting blade; (B) TruClear rotating cutting blade; and (C) TruClear reciprocating blade.

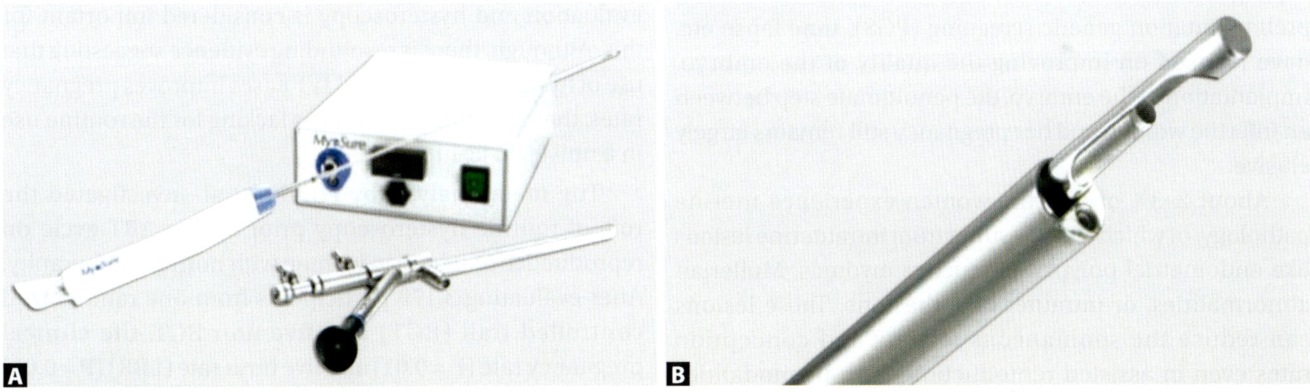

Figs. 20A and B: MyoSureTissue removal system: (A) MyoSure system hysteroscope, handpiece, and motor drive and (B) MyoSure system blade inserted through hysteroscope.

SUGGESTED READING

1. Bigatti G. IBS® Integrated Bigatti Shaver, an Alternative Approach to Operative Hysteroscopy. Gynecol Surg. 2011; 8:187-91.
2. Instructions for use: disposable hysteroscopic morcellators. Andover, MA: Smith & Nephew, Inc.; 2007.
3. Interlace Medical Inc. (2009). MyoSURE™ Hysteroscopic Tissue Removal System 501(k) summary. Framingham, MA: Interlace Medical. [online] Available from http://www.accessdata.fda.gov/cdrh_docs/pdf9/K091100.pdf [Last accessed February, 2019].
4. Mencaglia L, De albuquerque Neto LC, Alfonso Arias Alvarez R. Manual of Hysteroscopy—Diagnostic, Operative and Office Hysteroscopy. Tuttlingen: Endo: Press; 2014.
5. Silander T. Hysteroscopy through a transparent rubber balloon in patients with carcinoma of the uterine endometrium. Acta Obstet Gynecol Scand. 1963;42:284-99.
6. Vilos GA, Abu-Rafea B. New developments in ambulatory hysteroscopic surgery. Best Pract Res Clin Obstet Gynaecol. 2005;19:727-42.

Fertility Enhancing Hysteroscopic Surgery

18

Asha Baxi, Apoorva Pallam Reddy

INTRODUCTION

The two factors of paramount importance that determine the success of an assisted reproductive technology (ART) cycle are—a good quality embryo and a receptive endometrium. Over the past 5 decades, since ART has been introduced, various advances in technology have helped fertility specialist improve the pregnancy rates in a systematic manner. Much of these expansions, like embryo grading, blastocyst development, single step media, triple gas environment, assisted hatching, metabolomics, preimplantation genetic screening (PGS), time lapse etc. have focused on improving the quality of the embryo. Implantation of the embryo, the penultimate step between an infertile woman and her pregnancy still remains largely elusive.

About 2–3% of infertile women experience uterine pathology, of which 40–50% suffer from intrauterine lesions like endometrial polyps, submucous myomas, Mullerian abnormalities, or intrauterine adhesions. These lesions can reduce the spontaneous fertility and conception rates even in assisted reproduction. Various modalities like transvaginal sonography (TVS), 3D sonography, hysterosalpingography (HSG), sonohysterography, hystero-contrast sonography (HyCoSy), and hysteroscopy are used to assess the intrauterine milieu. The advent of hysteroscopy in fertility assessment has transformed the diagnosis and management of intrauterine pathology. Safety, efficacy, and cost efficiency have been improved over time in both diagnostic and operative fields with the introduction of newer technology like smaller scopes, bipolar energy devices, hysteroscopic morcellators, etc. There has been lot of debate on the technical feasibility, patient compliance and effect of hysteroscopy can increase the pregnancy rates in subfertile woman. This chapter aims at summarizing the available data.

ROLE OF HYSTEROSCOPY

Routine Hysteroscopy

Assessment of the uterine cavity in in vitro fertilization (IVF) patients is of paramount importance in female fertility evaluation and hysteroscopy is considered important for this. Although, there is resounding evidence suggesting that use of hysteroscopy in failed IVF cases improves pregnancy rates, the substantial research is lacking for the routine use in a universal fashion.

The meta-analysis by Pundir et al. investigated the role of routine hysteroscopy prior to first ART cycle on reproductive outcome in women with normal sonography. After evaluating 3,179 participants from one randomized controlled trail (RCT) and five non-RCT, the clinical pregnancy rate ($P = 0.01$) and live birth rate (LBR) ($P = 0.05$) were significantly higher in the routine pre-IVF hysteroscopy group. However, for every additional clinical pregnancy and additional live birth 10 and 11 hysteroscopies should be done, respectively. The authors however concluded that more RCTs were required to authenticate this finding.

In view of its cost and invasive nature, the American Society for Reproductive Medicine (ASRM) and NICE guidelines recommend the use of hysteroscopy only to evaluate abnormalities suspected noninvasive modalities like HSG and sonohysterography.

FIBROIDS

The interference of fibroids on fertility, submucous fibroids should be removed in infertile patients, regardless of the size or the presence of symptoms.[1]

Diagnosis

Fibroids can be diagnosed efficiently by using a HSG, showing a filling defect in uterine cavity or a saline infusion sonohysterography (SIS) with the added benefit of defining their location and attachment more precisely. Only type 0 and type 1 submucosal fibroids are amenable to hysteroscopic myomectomy **(Fig. 1)**.

In a systematic review, Cynthia et al. have compared the efficacy of HSG, hysteroscopy, and SIS for evaluation of submucosal fibroids and concluded that SIS is comparable with hysteroscopy in the sensitivity and specificity for diagnosis and superior to that of HSG. However, the American Association of Gynecological Laparoscopists (AAGL) says that magnetic resonance imaging (MRI) is the gold standard and endoscopic techniques in illustrating the relationship of submucous leiomyomas with the myometrium and uterine serosa.[2]

Myomectomy in these cases improves fertility in various ways:[3]

- Removes the physical impedance to sperm, egg movement, or embryo attachment.
- Decrease the contractility of the myometrium
- Improvement in progesterone-regulated glycoprotein mainly IL 10 and glycodelin that promotes angiogenesis and suppresses natural killer (NK) cells.
- Enhanced endometrial HOXA1 gene expression.

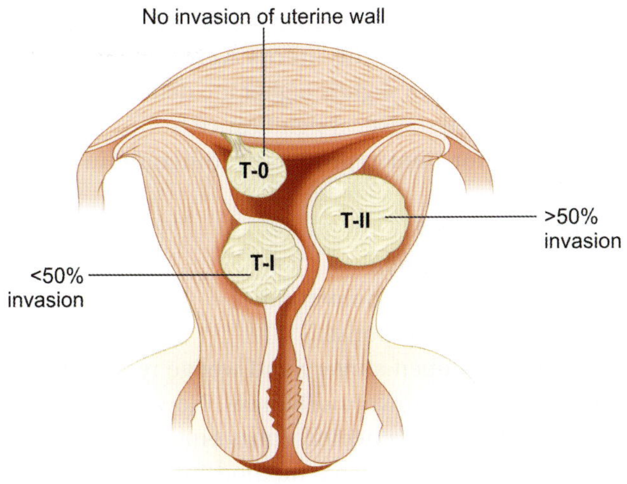

Fig. 1

These benefits postmyomectomies have translated into improved reproductive outcome. In the meta-analysis of Pritts et al., there were significantly higher spontaneous abortion rates in women with submucous myomas (two studies, RR 1.68, 95% CI 1.37-2.05, p 5.022), a difference that seemed to vanish after resectoscopic myomectomy.[4]

Shokeir et al. randomized 215 women with submucous myomas to group 1—transcervical resectoscopic myomectomy (TCRM) and group 2 no treatment. The spontaneous conception rate was significantly higher in the TCRM group as compared to no intervention group (63% vs 28%).[5]

Tips to Consider during Myomectomy

- Type 1 fibroids and larger fibroids (> 3 cm) may be resected in multiple sitting in order to reduce complications.
- Morcellation decreases the time of operation and reduces the amount of damage to surrounding tissue.
- The use of bipolar resectoscope for hysteroscopic myomectomy is associated with lesser risk of hyponatremia compared to unipolar resectoscope.[6]

Conclusion

All woman with type 0 and type 1 submucosal fibroids should be offered hysteroscopic myomectomy **(Fig. 2)**.

POLYPS

Endometrial polyps are more often than not diagnosed during the process of infertility work up or during the course of treatment and are known to negatively impact endometrial receptivity through various mechanisms.

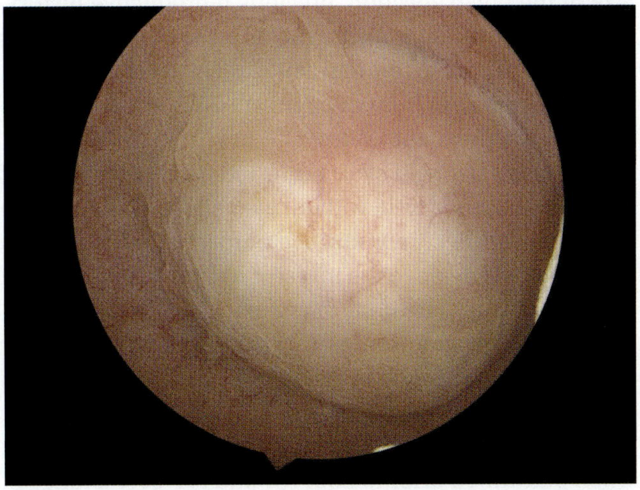

Fig. 2

The prevalence of polyps varies from 32% to 41% amongst infertile population. Although the mechanism of this effect is poorly understood, studies have suggested that endometrial polyps lead to mechanical meddling with sperm transport, embryo implantation, through intrauterine inflammation or even abnormalities in expression of NF-κB1 and NF-κB p65, which may contribute to endometrial receptivity and thus leading to polyp-related subfertility.[7]

Overall, most studies point to a favorable effect of hysteroscopic polypectomy on subsequent fertility. Some studies have reported spontaneous regression in as many as 27% cases. Hysteroscopic polypectomies under vision using an operative office hysteroscope or resectoscope (using scissors, a loop electrode, electric probe. or a morcellator) have lower recurrence rates as opposed to a blind curettage. Performing it under vision minimizes the damage to the surrounding endometrium and ensures the polyp has been removed completely.

Hysteroscopic polypectomy seems to improve fertility potential not only in intrauterine insemination (IUI) and ARTs but also in natural conceptions.

Spiewankiewicz et al. reported spontaneous pregnancy rate of 76% within 12 months after hysteroscopic polypectomy.[8]

In a prospective comparative study by Shohayeb et al. 120 women with endometrial polyp were divided into an intervention group with polypectomy and a nonintervention group prior to IUI. The woman in the intervention group showed a significantly higher cumulative pregnancy rate over the period of next 4 IUIs (38.3 vs 18.3%; p = 0.015).[9]

Polyps, which were found incidentally during the stimulation for IVF, or frozen embryo transfer is controversial. Size of the polyp, location, previous reproductive history, number of available embryos, and time to pregnancy (TTP) are various factors that could affect decision making. Removal of polyps 1.5 cm prior to ART did not seem to enhance the pregnancy rates.[10]

Although Batioglu et al. suggested we could remove of polyp in the same cycle without cancellation using a wire loop and not affect reproductive outcome (before Day 9), the practice is deemed too invasive by most clinicians.[11]

Youssef et al. have done a systematic review on the cost-effectiveness of performing either an office hysteroscopy or operative hysteroscopy in patients diagnosed with polyps prior to fertility treatment. They concluded that office or operative hysteroscopic polypectomy was cost-effective when performed prior to both IUI and IVF over a range of plausible pregnancy rates and procedural costs.[12]

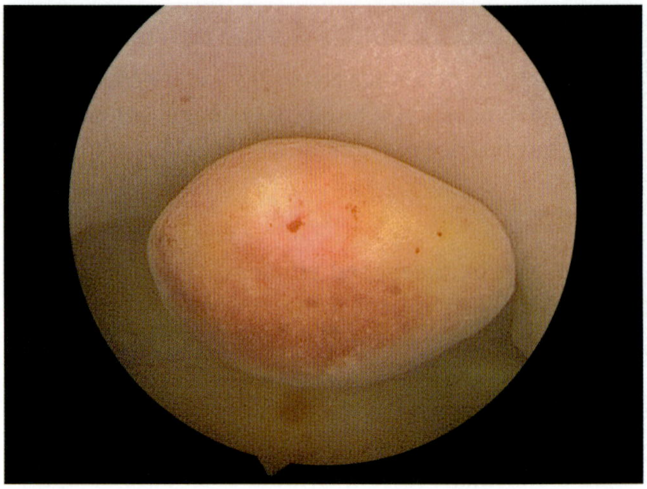

Fig. 3

Conclusion

Hysteroscopic polypectomy of polyps larger than 1.5 cm improves the pregnancy rates **(Fig. 3)**.

MULLERIAN ANOMALIES

Uterine septa arise from impaired fusion of the bilateral paramesonephric ducts. 5–12% of women with infertility experience Mullerian malformation of which 80–90% are uterine septum. Despite HSG being a useful tool for screening of uterine malformations, a 3D ultrasonography (USG) or hysterolaparoscopy is required to differentiate between different Mullerian anomalies. Whether uterine septum causes infertility or not has been a matter of debate. A meta-analysis of 25 studies where the ASRM classification was used to categorize the canalization defects, an increase in TTP was seen in patients with a uterine septum.[13] In another study, 153 women with various anomalies of the uterus were compared with controls, there was a slightly higher incidence of infertility but did not reach statistical significance.[14]

Reasons for poor reproductive outcome in septate uterus are:

- Poor vascularity
- Higher fiber content
- Poorly receptive endometrium
- Low hormonal response.

In the past, open surgery and wedge resection were associated with its own morbidities. Now hysteroscopic septum resection or rather incision is a much more simpler surgery and is the decisive method for both diagnosis and management of uterine septum.

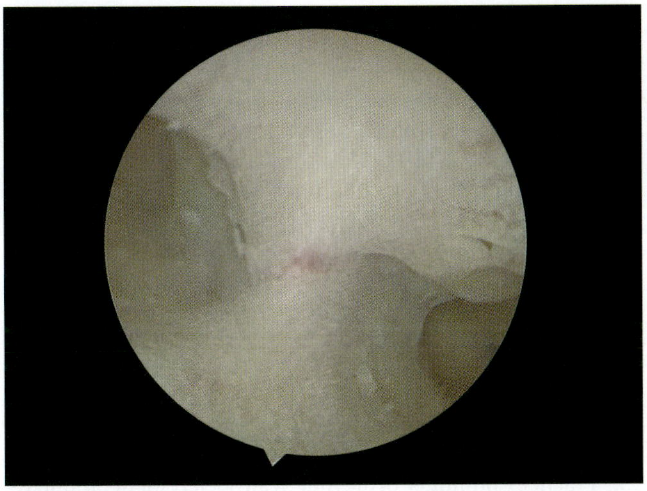

Fig. 4

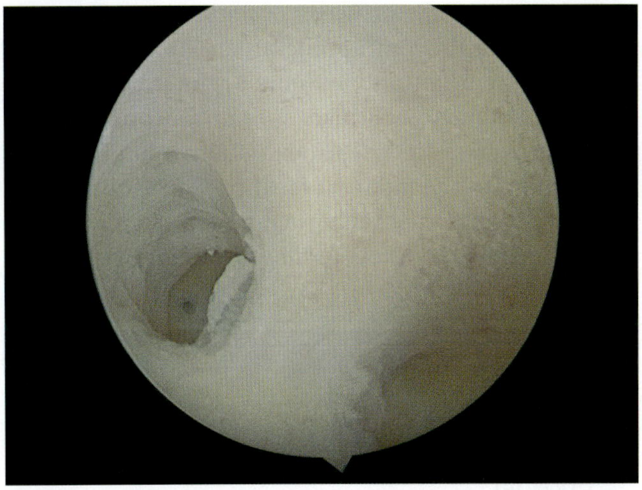

Fig. 5

As per practice committee report of ASRM in 2016, there is less evidence to conclude that uterine septum is associated with infertility.[15] However, many observational studies have shown that septum resection is shown to improve the pregnancy rates.

In a retrospective analysis of 64 patients with septate uterus with infertility, hysteroscopic septoplasty was shown to be safe and effective with pregnancy in 60% patients.[16]

Other conditions associated with uterine septum are miscarriage, premature birth, abnormal fetal position, and other poor reproductive outcome.

Resection or incision of the septum can be done with hysteroscopic scissors, as it is avascular and fibrous. If a resectoscope is to be used, a bipolar resectoscope is in vogue these days owing to its greater safety profile when compared with the monopolar resectoscope. Hysteroscopic morcellator has been used to remove the septum.[17]

Postoperative second look hysteroscopy has shown complete healing of the cavity in 8 weeks,[18] however, there are no randomized trials to find out the optimum time to conceive after the septoplasty. In a retrospective study of 193 women who underwent septum resection, 10% conceived in the first 6 months, 18.1% in 6–12 months and 23.3% after 18 months **(Fig. 4)**.[19]

INTRAUTERINE ADHESIONS

Intrauterine adhesions are seen in about 2.5–13% of infertile patients. Miscarriage, endometritis, and history of operative hysteroscopy are various risk factors for development of intrauterine adhesions, which result in poor reproductive outcome.[20]

In a prospective cohort study by Sameer et al., 61 patients presenting with infertility (primary or secondary) or recurrent pregnancy losses caused by IUAs were managed with adhesiolysis. Conception rate escalated from 18% to 65.5%, while LBR increased from 14.7 to 36% in the study group with a mean TTP of 10.2 months posthysteroscopic adhesiolysis. There was significant negative correlation between the grade of IUAs and the improvement in reproductive performance.[21]

In a retrospective cross-sectional study, Chen et al. evaluated 357 patients with intrauterine adhesions (135 with mild IUAs, 116 with moderate IUAs, and 106 with severe IUAs). In the follow-up period over 2 years, the overall conception rate posthysteroscopic adhesiolysis was 48.2%, which dropped significantly with increased IUA severity with a mean TTP was 9.7 ± 3.7 months. The incidence of complication was less with 11 patients (7.9%) having postpartum hemorrhage, of which six (4.3%) had adherent placenta and three (2.1%) had placenta accreta.[22]

Conclusion

Intrauterine hysteroscopic adhesiolysis significantly improves the reproductive outcome **(Fig. 5)**.

CERVICAL STENOSIS

In patients with tight cervical stenosis and history of difficult embryo transfers, partial excision of the canal with hysteroscopic scissors, resectoscope or morcellator can be used to ease the subsequent transfers.

ISTHMOCELE

Isthmocele is a defect on the anterior uterine wall at the level of the isthmus located at the site of a previous cesarean delivery scar. The menstrual blood may accumulate in the niche because of the presence of fibrotic tissue, causing pelvic pain in the suprapubic area. The accumulated menstrual pool not only influences the mucus quality negatively but also obstructs sperm transport through the cervical canal, interferes with embryo implantation, and leading to secondary infertility. Correction of this defect can be performed either laparoscopically or hysteroscopically to either restore fertility or improve symptoms, respectively.[23]

REFERENCES

1. Bosteels J, Kasius J, Weyers S, et al. Hysteroscopy for treating subfertility associated with suspected major uterine cavity abnormalities. Cochrane Database Syst Rev. 2013;(1): CD009461.
2. American Association of Gynecologic Laparoscopists (AAGL): Advancing Minimally Invasive Gynecology Worldwide. AAGL practice report: practice guidelines for the diagnosis and management of submucous leiomyomas. J Minim Invasive Gynecol. 2012;19(2):152-7.1
3. Purohit P, Vugbeswaran K. Fibroids and Infertility. Curr Obstet Gynecol Rep. 2016;5:81-88.
4. Pritts EA, Parker WH, Olive DL. Fibroids and infertility: an updated systematic review of the evidence. Fertil Steril. 2009;91:1215-23.
5. Shokeir T, El-Shafei M, Yousef H, et al. Submucous myomas and their implications in the pregnancy rates of patients with otherwise unexplained primary infertility undergoing hysteroscopic myomectomy: a randomized matched control study. Fertil Steril. 2010;94:724-9.
6. Roy KK, Metta S, Kansal Y, et al. A Prospective Randomized Study Comparing Unipolar Versus Bipolar Hysteroscopic Myomectomy in Infertile Women. J Hum Reprod Sci. 2017;10(3):185-93.
7. Bozkurt M, Şahin L, Ulaş M. Hysteroscopic polypectomy decreases NF-κB1 expression in the mid-secretory endometrium of women with endometrial polyp. Eur J Obstet Gynecol Reprod Biol. 2015;189:96-100.
8. Spiewankiewicz B, Stelmachow J, Sawicki W, et al. The effectiveness of hysteroscopic polypectomy in cases of female infertility. Clin Exp Obstet Gynecol. 2003;30:23-5.
9. Shohayeb A, Shaltout A. Persistent endometrial polyps may affect the pregnancy rate in patients undergoing intrauterine insemination. Middle East Fertil Soc J. 2011;16: 259-64.
10. Tiras B, Korucuoglu U, Polat M, et al. Management of endometrial polyps diagnosed before or during ICSI cycles. Reprod Biomed Online. 2012;24:123-8.
11. Al Chami A, Saridogan E. Endometrial Polyps and Subfertility. J Obstet Gynecol India. 2017;67(1):9-14.
12. Mouhayar Y, Yin O, Mumford SL, et al. Hysteroscopic polypectomy prior to infertility treatment: A cost analysis and systematic review. Eur J Obstet Gynecol Reprod Biol. 2017;213:107-15.
13. Venetis CA, Papadopoulos SP, Campo R, et al. Clinical implications of congenital uterine anomalies: a meta-analysis of comparative studies. Reprod Biomed Online. 2014;29(6):665-83.
14. Shuiqing M, Xuming B, Jinghe L. Pregnancy and its outcome in women with malformed uterus. Chin Med Sci J. 2002;17: 242-5.
15. Practice Committee of the American Society for Reproductive Medicine. Uterine septum: a guideline. Fertil Steril. 2016; 106(3):530-40.
16. Nouri K, Ott J, Huber JC, et al. Reproductive outcome after hysteroscopic septoplasty in patients with septate uterus—a retrospective cohort study and systematic review of the literature. Reprod Biol Endocrinol. 2010;8:52.
17. Simons M, Hamerlynck TW, Abdulkadir L, et al. Hysteroscopic morcellator system can be used for removal of a uterine septum. Fertil Steril. 2011;96(2):e118-21.
18. Yang JH, Chen MJ, Chen CD, et al. Optimal waiting period for subsequent fertility treatment after various hysteroscopic surgeries. Fertil Steril. 2013;99(7):2092-6.
19. Saygili-Yilmaz E, Yildiz S, Erman-Akar M, et al. Reproductive outcome of septate uterus after hysteroscopic metroplasty. Arch Gynecol Obstet. 2003;268(4):289-92.
20. Hooker A, Fraenk D, Brölmann H, et al. Prevalence of intrauterine adhesions after termination of pregnancy: a systematic review. Eur J Contracept Reprod Health Care. 2016;21(4):329-35.
21. Sanad AS, Aboulfotouh ME. Hysteroscopic adhesiolysis: efficacy and safety. Arch Gynecol Obstet. 2016;294(2): 411-6.
22. Chen L, Zhang H, Wang Q, et al. Reproductive Outcomes in Patients With Intrauterine Adhesions Following Hysteroscopic Adhesiolysis: Experience From the Largest Women's Hospital in China. J Minim Invasive Gynecol. 2017;24(2): 299-304.
23. Florio P, Filippeschi M, Moncini I, et al. Hysteroscopic treatment of the cesarean-induced isthmocele in restoring infertility. Curr Opin Obstet Gynecol. 2012;24(3):180-6.

Fertility Enhancing Laparoscopic Surgeries

19

Alka Kriplani, Bharti Dhorepatil, Reeta Mahey

INTRODUCTION

In last 3–4 decades with advancement in assisted reproduction techniques (ART), the need of laparoscopy has decreased and is considered controversial and debatable in infertile women. But its role still stands beneficial in some infertility problems.

In patients with decreased or compromised ovarian reserve and moderate to severe male factor infertility, ART is the only option so laparoscopy is not indicated. The main controversy regarding role and indications of laparoscopy is in polycystic ovarian syndrome (PCOS), endometriosis, adenomyosis, pelvic inflammatory disease (PID), leiomyoma distorting endometrial cavity, and unexplained infertility.

Before making any plan for the infertile couple, complete infertility work up is necessary; and individualization and case-based approach is must to select when there is need of fertility enhancing laparoscopic surgeries. The indications and procedural steps of commonly done fertility enhancing laparoscopic surgeries are discussed in this chapter.

LEIOMYOMA

Leiomyoma with infertility is a unique combination. When significant myoma-related symptoms occur, myomectomy is indicated irrespective of fertility issues. In asymptomatic myomas, first other causes of infertility should be ruled out. The prevalence of myoma among infertile population is around 5–10%. But after ruling out other causes, fibroids are found in only 1–2% of infertile women.[1]

Which myomas to be removed?[2]

- All symptomatic myomas presenting with heavy menstrual bleeding or pressure symptoms should be removed. Medical management may be tried before myomectomy depending upon size, location and number of myoma, and severity of symptoms.
- All submucous myomas have negative impact on fertility and these should be removed before planning conception or ART.
- Subserous myomas usually do not affect the fertility and myomectomy is not advised for fertility reasons.
- Effect of intramural myomas on fertility is unclear. Those indenting endometrial cavity should be removed. The exact effect of fibroid size on fertility is unclear. If there is no distortion of endometrial cavity confirmed on hysteroscopy, intramural myoma may not be removed regardless of size of myoma.
- Myomectomy may be considered in women with previous implantation failures or recurrent abortions even if myoma is not distorting the endometrial cavity. With advent of minimally invasive surgery, most of the myomectomies are done laparoscopically when surgical expertise is not the issue. All intramural myomas and submucous myomas more than 5 cm are managed laparoscopically.

PREOPERATIVE EVALUATION BEFORE LAPAROSCOPIC MYOMECTOMY

- Proper fibroid mapping with ultrasonography (USG) or magnetic resonance imaging (MRI)
- Build up hemoglobin to at least 11 g/dL before planning myomectomy

- Other causes of infertility should be ruled out before proceeding for myomectomy
- In patients with large myomas (>18 weeks gravid uterus size) or vascular myomas, preoperative injections of GnRH analog can be given. There is clear evidence that GnRH analog injections reduce fibroid volume and vascularity thus decreasing blood loss during surgery.[3]

Laparoscopic Myomectomy (Figs. 1A to F)

After giving general anesthesia, port placement is done according to surgeon's discretion and pneumoperitoneum is created.

- After initial inspection of abdomen, fibroid mapping is done. After informing the anesthetist, 20 units vasopressin diluted in 200 mL normal saline is injected in subcapsular space to decrease the blood supply to the myoma. Other agents, which have been used to reduce blood loss during myomectomy are unilateral or bilateral uterine artery ligation, hypotensive anesthesia, and preprocedure rectal misoprostol (400–800 μg).[4] Combination of these can also be used depending upon size and vascularity of myoma and surgeon's expertise.
- A transverse incision is given on the myoma bulge with harmonic scalpel or unipolar scissors or unipolar hook. Care is taken to avoid going too near to the cornual ends. Incision is continued till cleavage plan is found and myoma is delineated from the surrounding myometrium.
- *Enucleation*: Once myoma is exposed, either with toothed grasping forceps or myoma screw; myoma is held and enucleated with traction and counter traction.
- *Suturing*: The myoma bed is closed with delayed absorbable polyglactin (1 or 0 vicryl) or with barbed sutures (V-Loc™180; 03.5 Metric; M/s Covidien, United States Surgical, Middletown Avenue North haven, CT, 06473, USA). The advantages of barbed sutures are tight myoma bed closure and less chances of hematoma formation.
- *Specimen retrieval*: The traditional technique of power morcellation was questioned and warning has been issued due to risk of peritoneal dissemination of myoma fragments. With availability of specimen retrieval bags, the specimen can be retrieved safely without any fear of dissemination and its potential complications.
- Tubal patency should always be checked before or after myomectomy especially if patient is not going for ART. Myomas near cornu can cause tubal stretching and

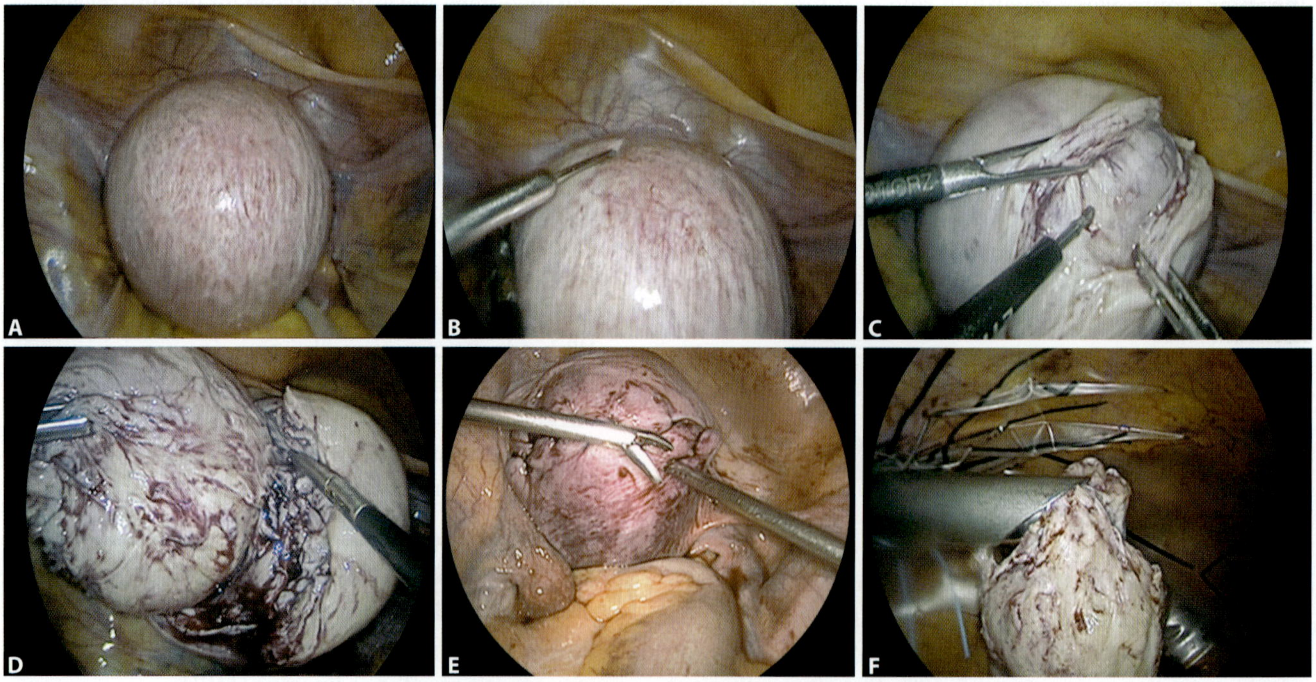

Figs. 1A to F: Steps of laparoscopic myomectomy: (A) laparoscopic view showing fundal myoma; (B) vasopressin injection in subcapsular space; (C) incision on the myoma bulge; (D) enucleation with traction and counter traction; (E) suturing the myoma bed; and (F) specimen retrieval with in-bag morcellation.

tubal block. If patency not confirmed preprocedure, it may be repeated after myomectomy and should be documented so that plan can be made for fertility after myomectomy.

ADENOMYOSIS AND ADENOMYOMA

Main symptoms of adenomyosis are pain abdomen, heavy menstrual bleeding, dysmenorrhea, dyspareunia, and infertility. It can be diffuse and scattered throughout the myometrium (diffuse adenomyosis) or focal circumscribed nodule of hypertrophic and distorted endometrium within the myometrium (focal adenomyoma).

Transvaginal ultrasound (TVUS) and MRI are used to confirm the diagnosis of adenomyosis and its extent and spread. First-line management for infertility and pain in adenomyosis is medical management. Those who do not respond to medical management or have focal adenomyoma on imaging, surgical intervention is indicated as second-line option.

In view of debatable benefits of surgery and potential adverse pregnancy outcomes in diffuse adenomyosis, clinicians should take crucial case-by-case decision for surgery. It should be reserved for:

- Symptomatic women presenting with chronic pelvic pain, dysmenorrhea, and heavy menstrual bleeding
- Young infertile women who have failed medical management
- Older women with infertility despite ART
- Those with a history of recurrent pregnancy loss or implantation failure.

The basic steps are same as described in myomectomy **(Figs. 2A to F)**.

Main difficulty is encountered in separating the lesion from the surrounding myometrium, as there are no planes and no capsule. Various techniques and modifications have been devised and documented in literature to improve the quality of surgery and better reproductive outcome in adenomyosis.[5]

- Incision is given over the bulge of the lesion either vertical, horizontal, or H-shaped.
- Suturing is done through U-shaped technique, overlapping flap technique, or triple flap method (Osada's technique).[6] These modifications have been devised for tight and strong closure of myometrium after debulking surgery especially in women willing for future fertility.

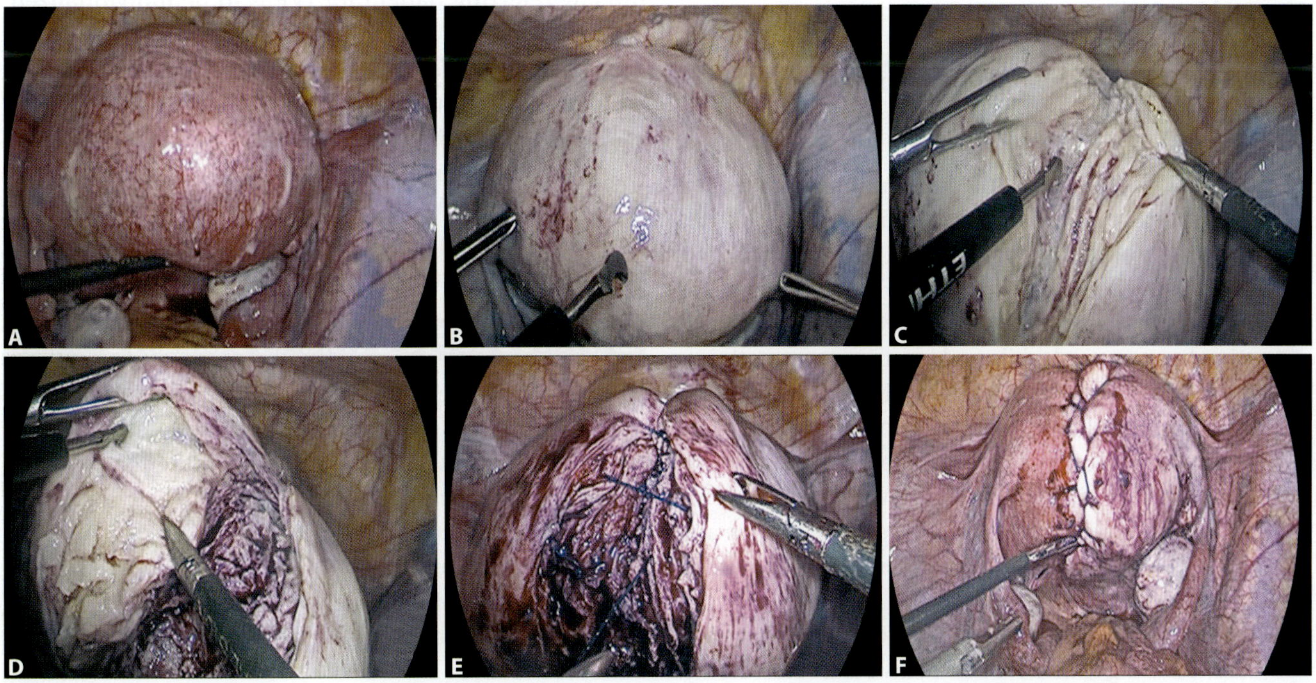

Figs. 2A to F: Steps of laparoscopic adenomyomectomy: (A) laparoscopic view of large fundal adenomyoma; (B) vasopressin injection to reduce vascularity; (C) incision with Harmonic hook and separating the lesion from serosa; (D) dissecting the lesion with traction and counter traction; (E) suturing the bed with barbed sutures; and (F) final picture after adenomyoma resection.

ENDOMETRIOSIS

The causes of infertility in endometriosis are due to decreased ovarian reserve, altered tubo-ovarian relationship, chronic inflammation, pelvic adhesions and defective oocyte, and embryo transport.

Surgery is recommended in women with endometriosis if:
- Symptomatic endometriosis (dysmenorrhea, dyspareunia, etc.)
- Infertility if there is no previous surgery for endometrioma
- Diagnosis not clear on USG
- According to European Society of Human Reproduction and Embryology (ESHRE) 2013:[7]
- In infertile women with American Society for Reproductive Medicine (ASRM) stage I/II, endometriosis operative laparoscopy (excision preferred to drainage in cases of endometrioma) should be performed instead of diagnostic laparoscopy alone to increase ongoing pregnancy rates.
- In patients undergoing in-vitro fertilization (IVF), laparoscopic cystectomy of endometriomas more than 3 cm should only be performed to improve endometriosis associated pain or accessibility of follicles.

Endometriotic Cystectomy

After making the laparoscopic ports and creating pneumoperitoneum, assessment is done and size of ovaries, tubo-ovarian relationship, adhesions, endometriotic implants in peritoneum, and pouch of Douglas are inspected for severity of disease.
- Adhesiolysis is done with sharp and blunt dissection and hydrodissection. Ovary is freed from the uterosacral ligaments and pouch of Douglas. Most of the cysts drain spontaneously while doing adhesiolysis. This occurs at the weakest point where ovarian cortex invagination has occurred while endometrioma formation.
- The cyst lining is identified, held with toothed grasper, and is stripped off from the normal ovarian tissue using traction and counter traction. The method of endometrioma stripping is preferred over endometrioma drainage and fulguration as chances of recurrence and damage to normal ovarian tissue is less and spontaneous conceptions rate is better.[8]
- There has been debate regarding use of bipolar cautery versus suturing to achieve hemostasis after cystectomy. Use of bipolar cautery is negatively associated with ovarian reserve and should be avoided.[9,10] Approximation with sutures (2-0 vicryl) should be used for hemostasis especially when future fertility is required.
- Specimen is removed either through one of the ports or in cystectomy bag. A modified bag made from surgical glove or plastic bag can be used, if cystectomy bag not available.
- Tubal patency is checked and documented before the procedure or after the procedure, if no patency documented before cystectomy.

Effect of Endometriotic Cystectomy on Ovarian Reserve

There is concern about effect of endometriotic cystectomy on ovarian reserve. Studies have shown decrease in anti-Mullerian hormone (AMH) levels after endometriotic cystectomy though it has been studied up to 9–12 months only. The declines in AMH levels are more especially, if age is more than 38 years and in severe endometriosis.[11]

Laparoscopic Surgery for Recurrent Endometriosis

After first surgery, if there is no conception either spontaneous or with ovulation induction and there is recurrence of endometriosis, further plan for repeat surgery or directly referring patient for IVF is to be individualized. There is concern for decrease in ovarian reserve after repeated surgery for endometriosis. Surgery for recurrent endometriosis should be planned only if symptomatic relief is desired. For fertility purpose only, surgery does not give any added advantage especially if patient is going for IVF.[12] Studies have not been able to demonstrate a difference between pregnancy rates of women with and without surgical management of endometriomas undergoing IVF.[13]

LAPAROSCOPIC OVARIAN DRILLING

In patients with clomiphene resistance or failure or no conception with 3–4 cycles of letrozole, second-line option is either ovulation induction with gonadotropins or laparoscopic ovarian drilling (LOD). The advantages of LOD over gonadotropins are:
- One time procedure
- Less chances of multiple pregnancy
- More chances of spontaneous conception
- Cost effective
- Less chances of ovarian hyperstimulation syndrome (OHSS)

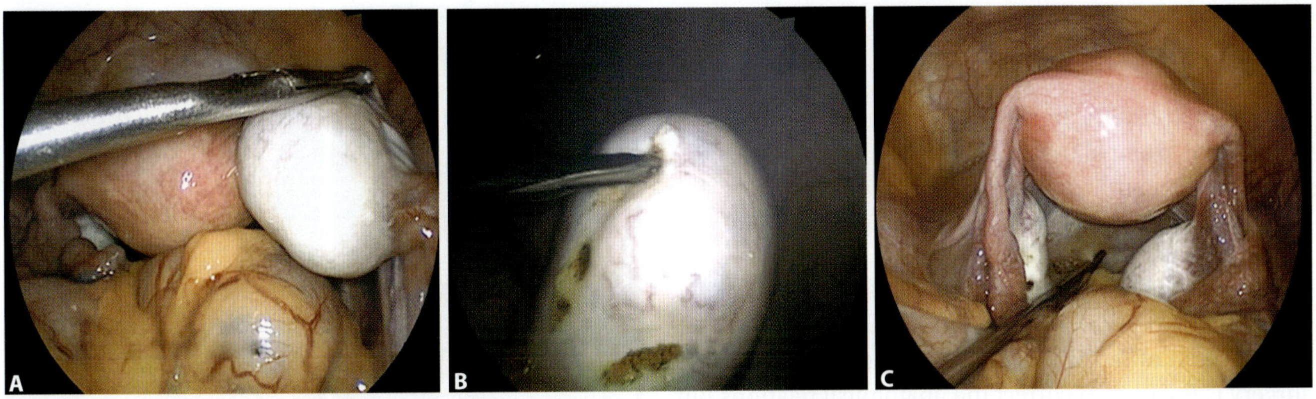

Figs. 3A to C: Laparoscopic ovarian drilling: (A) Fixing the ovary against uterus; (B) Making punctures with unipolar drilling needle; and (C) hydroflotation at end of procedure.

- Less frequent monitoring
- Simultaneous assessment of other pelvic structures.

The LOD works by converting the androgen dominant intrafollicular environment to estrogen dominant one and restores the normal physiology of ovarian pituitary feedback system. Both local and systemic effects are thought to promote follicular recruitment, maturation, and ovulation.

Procedure of LOD (Figs. 3A to C)

- After making laparoscopy ports and creating pneumoperitoneum, pelvis and abdomen inspection is done.
- Tubal patency is documented.
- With help of 5 mm atraumatic grasper, the ovary is lifted and rested against the uterine body. This provides a firm and stable platform to the ovary while drilling. Stabilization of ovary is must because if ovary slips, the charged monopolar cautery may hit the adjacent vital structures causing serious complications **(Fig. 3A)**.
- Unipolar drilling needle is inserted through the contralateral lower port.
- Visible bluish follicles are punctured. About 4–5 punctures are made with 40 W current up to a depth of 4 mm for 4 second duration **(Fig. 3B)**.
- Care is taken to make all the punctures away from the tubal side of the ovary, as there is risk of peritubal adhesions.
- The number of punctures made depends on ovarian volume, hormonal levels, ovarian reserve, and previous treatment history. This discretion is must as there is growing concern of declining ovarian reserve after overzealous drilling of ovaries.
- Thorough irrigation of the ovaries is done after the procedure to cool down the temperature of the ovaries. Hydroflotation also helps to check any bleeding, which may cause postoperative adhesions **(Fig. 3C)**.

LOD and AMH Levels

There is growing concern regarding negative affect of ovarian drilling on ovarian reserve in terms of AMH levels. In a recent meta-analysis by Amar SA et al. authors concluded that though LOD seems to markedly reduce circulating AMH, it remains uncertain whether this reflects a real damage to ovarian reserve or normalization of the high preoperative serum AMH levels. Further long-term studies on ovarian reserve after LOD are required to address this uncertainty and also effect of LOD on serum follicle stimulating hormone (FSH) levels.[14]

LOD before ART

In PCOS women going for IVF, antagonist protocol is the gold standard along with prophylactic cabergoline from the day of trigger to reduce the risk of OHSS. If there is previous history of OHSS, LOD can also be considered as an option to decrease chances of OHSS in subsequent IVF cycles.[15]

TUBAL FACTOR INFERTILITY

Tubal pathology is one of the most common causes of infertility. It accounts for 25–35% of the cases of all infertile couples.[16] With advent of ART, though role of reconstructive tubal surgery has decreased but it still stands beneficial in some patients. The following points should be considered when planning reconstructive tubal surgery in infertile patient.

- Age of the patient
- Previous obstetric history
- Site and extent of tubal disease
- History of antitubercular treatment (ATT) intake
- Presence of other factors contributing to infertility
- Semen analysis
- Patient willingness for donor intrauterine insemination (IUI) if semen abnormalities present

The goal of fertility enhancing reconstructive tubal surgery is not only to correct the anatomical relations but also to establish the functional integrity. The success of reconstructive surgery depends upon the site of block, extent of mucosal damage, associated ovarian, and peritoneal factors. Tubal pathologies can either affect the proximal or distal part of the tube or, at times, the entire tube may be affected (bipolar tubal disease).

Proximal Tubal Block

Blockage of the tube at the proximal end is a common finding in hysterosalpingogram (HSG). Its incidence is around 10–30% of all infertile women going for HSG. Common causes include obstruction due to mucus plugs, occlusion due to adhesive disease like endometriosis, PID, or uterotubal ostium spasm.[17] Very often patients with bilateral cornual block show free spill on hysterolaparoscopy.

Hysteroscopic Tubal Cannulation under Laparoscopic Guidance (Figs. 4A to B)

The procedure is done in postmenstrual phase under general anesthesia and under lap guidance:

- Cervix is dilated and operative hysteroscope with operating channel is inserted
- 5Fr catheter with obturator is inserted through operating channel **(Fig. 4A)**
- The obturator is removed and catheter is curved and directed into the tubal ostium
- Diluted methylene blue dye is injected through the catheter. If free spill is seen from the fimbrial end, the tubal patency is confirmed and procedure is repeated on opposite site.
- If no dye is seen filling the tube, inner system of cannulation set (inner catheter with guidewire) is introduced through the catheter.
- The guidewire is advanced slowly through the cornual end and under lap vision, it is advanced into the isthmic portion of tube **(Fig. 4B)**.

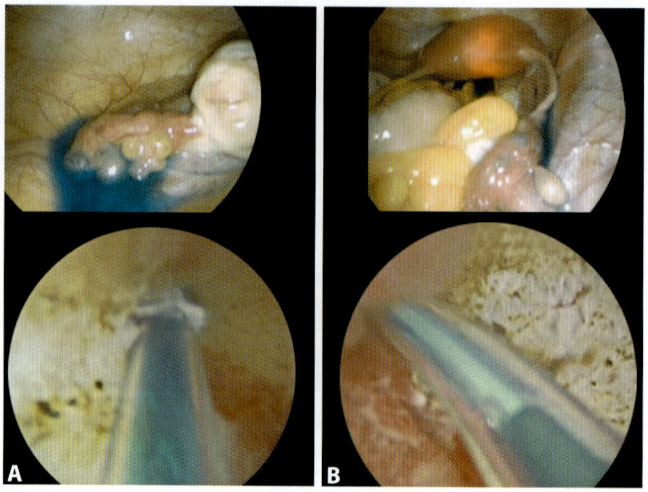

Figs. 4A and B: Laparoscopic tubal recanalization (previous lap ligation).

- If resistance is felt to passage of guidewire or catheter, lap assistant is asked to straighten the tube.
- Inner guidewire is removed and diluted dye is injected under lap guidance.
- If dye is seen through fimbrial end, the procedure is considered successful and complete.
- Failure to cannulate tube may be due to fibrosis or associated mid segment block.

Distal Tubal Disease

Fimbrial Block

Distal tubal block of varying degrees can be treated laparoscopically by either fimbriolysis or fimbrioplasty. Fimbriolysis is separation of adherent fimbria. Fimbrioplasty refers to correction of phimotic but patent fimbrial end. The success of a favorable outcome depends inversely on the degree of disease. Most pregnancies occur within first two years of treatment. Milder forms of disease after correction can achieve a pregnancy rate of almost 60%, compared to 20–30% with severe disease.[18]

There is almost no role of treatment in presence of both proximal and distal tubal block as even after treatment live birth rates are rarely more than 10%.[19]

Hydrosalpinx

Hydrosalpinx is a chronic pathological condition of the fallopian tube. Most often it occurs following occluded fimbrial end, resulting in distended distal half of the tube. Common causes include PID, endometriosis, previous ectopic pregnancy, previous abdominal or tubal surgery, and tuberculosis. Hydrosalpinx is known to be associated with lower implantation rate per embryo and lower clinical pregnancy rate.[20]

Treatment options for hydrosalpinx include salpingectomy, tubal occlusion, and aspiration. Salpingectomy is largely useful in treatment of hydrosalpinx prior to IVF although there is no consensus on its role in absence of hydrosalpinx. A systematic review suggested absence of variation in ovarian reserve markers after unilateral salpingectomy, while contradictory results were observed following bilateral salpingectomy. Their data suggested significant improvement in ongoing pregnancy rate and live birth rate following IVF without significant reduction in ovarian response to gonadotropin stimulation.[21] Effect of hydrosalpinx aspiration is doubtful and needs to be assessed.

Sterilization Reversal or Tubal Recanalization

Women wishing to conceive after tubal sterilization have availability of two options—either IVF or anastomosis (tubal recanalization).

Advantages of tubal reanastomosis include:

- Chance of natural conception
- Lower rates of multiple gestation
- Cost of IVF is omitted.

Disadvantages mainly include:

- Higher uncertainty of conception
- Risk of ectopic pregnancy
- Future need of contraception.

Procedural steps ***(Figs. 5A to E)****:*

- Removing the mid tubal segment where ligation has been done and freshening the ends of proximal and distal tubal segments.
- Distention of proximal segment of tube with transcervical instillation of dye to identify exact position of tubal lumen.
- Confirmation of patency of distal segment by pushing dye through the fimbrial end.
- Once tubal patency is confirmed at both ends, mesosalpinx of both sides is sutured with 6-0 polypropylene or 6-0 vicryl.

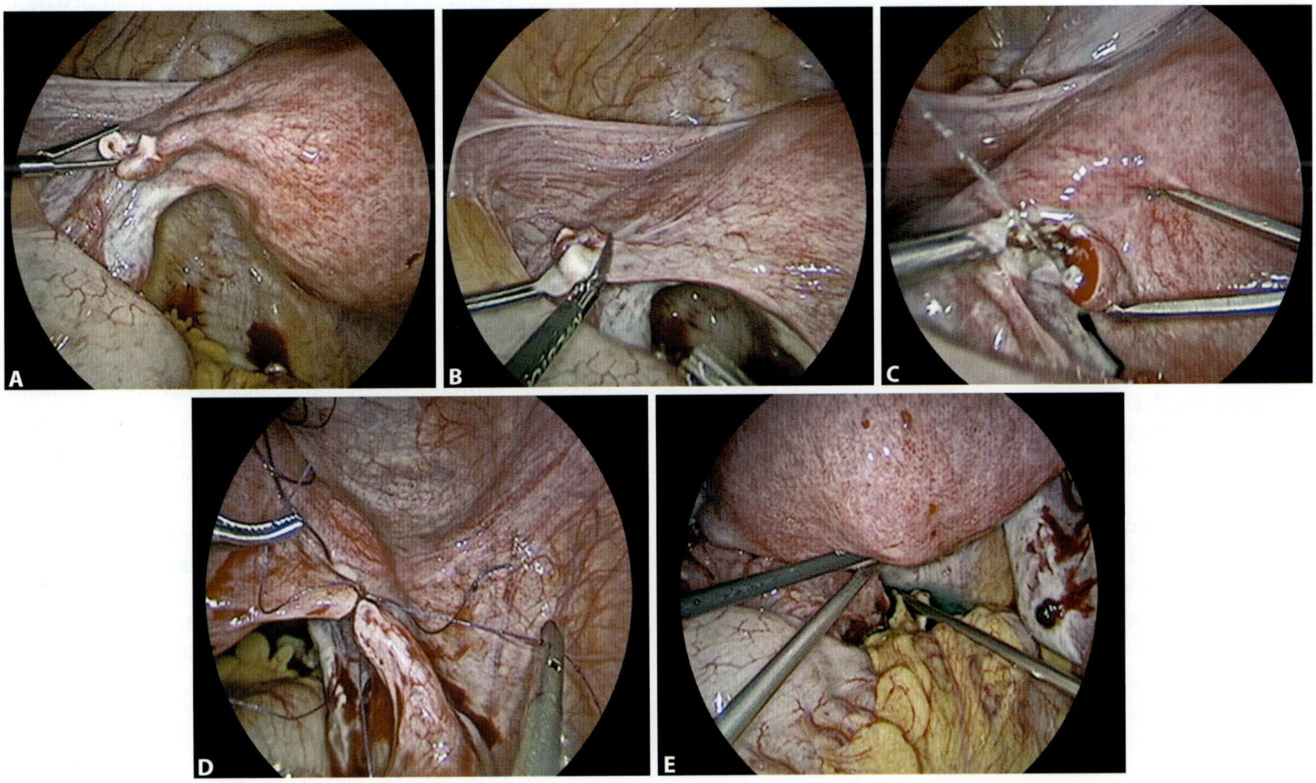

Figs. 5A to E: Procedural steps for tubal recanalization

- With 5-0 vicryl or 5-0 polypropylene, sutures are taken at 12, 3, and 9 o' clock positions taking mucosa—muscularis layer.
- Second layer of sutures is taken with same suture taking muscularis—serosal layer.
- Tubal patency is checked at the end of procedure.

Laparoscopically sterilized tubes had higher conception rate after reanastamosis (50%) as compared to Pomeroy's technique (30%).[22]

CONCLUSION

- Laparoscopy and ART are complementary to each other rather than competitors.
- The clinician should decide and individualize the plan according to woman age, cause of infertility, options available, previous treatment history, and patient's choice.

REFERENCES

1. Cook H, Ezzati M, Segars JH, et al. The impact of uterine leiomyomas on reproductive outcomes. Minerva Ginecol. 2010;62:225-36.
2. Carranza-Mamane B, Havelock J, Hemmings R. The management of uterine fibroids in women with otherwise unexplained infertility. J Obstet Gynaecol Can. 2015;37(3): 277-85.
3. Lethaby A, Puscasiu L, Vollenhoven B. Preoperative medical therapy before surgery for uterine fibroids. Cochrane Database Syst Rev. 2017;11:CD000547.
4. Frederick S, Frederick J, Fletcher H, et al. A trial comparing the use of rectal misoprostol plus perivascular vasopressin with perivascular vasopressin alone to decrease myometrial bleeding at the time of abdominal myomectomy. Fertil Steril. 2013;100(4):1044-9.
5. Younes G, Tulandi T. Conservative surgery for adenomyosis and results: A systematic review. J Minim Invasive Gynecol. 2018;25(2):265-76.
6. Osada H, Silber S, Kakinuma T, et al. Surgical procedure to conserve the uterus for future pregnancy in patients suffering from massive adenomyosis. Reprod Biomed Online. 2011;22(1):94-9.
7. Dunselman GA, Vermeulen N, Becker C, et al. ESHRE guideline: management of women with endometriosis. Hum Reprod. 2014;29(3):400-12.
8. Hart RJ, Hickey M, Maouris P, et al. Excisional surgery versus ablative surgery for ovarian endometrioma. Cochrane Database Syst Rev. 2008(2):CD004992.
9. Deckers P, Ribeiro SC, Simões RDS, et al. Systematic review and meta-analysis of the effect of bipolar electrocoagulation during laparoscopic ovarian endometrioma stripping on ovarian reserve. Int J Gynaecol Obstet. 2018;140(1):11-17.
10. Ata B, Turkgeldi E, Seyhan A, et al. Effect of hemostatic method on ovarian reserve following laparoscopic endometrioma excision; comparison of suture, hemostatic sealant, and bipolar dessication. A systematic review and meta-analysis. J Minim Invasive Gynecol. 2015;22(3):363-72.
11. Saito N, Yamashita Y, Okuda K, et al. Comparison of the impact of laparoscopic endometriotic cystectomy and vaporization on postoperative serum anti-Mullerian hormone levels. Asian J Endosc Surg. 2018;11(1):23-9.
12. Cranney R, Condous G, Reid S. An update on the diagnosis, surgical management, and fertility outcomes for women with endometrioma. Acta Obstet Gynecol Scand. 2017;96(6): 633-43.
13. Tsoumpou I, Kyrgiou M, Gelbaya TA, et al. The effect of surgical treatment for endometrioma on in vitro fertilization outcomes: a systematic review and meta-analysis. Fertil Steril. 2009;92(1):75-87.
14. Amer SA, Shamy TT, James C, et al. The impact of laparoscopic ovarian drilling on AMH and ovarian reserve: a meta-analysis. Reproduction. 2017;154:R13-21.
15. Seyam E, Hefzy E. Laparoscopic ovarian drilling versus GnRH antagonist combined with cabergoline as a prophylaxis against the re-development of ovarian hyperstimulation syndrome. Gynecol Endocrinol. 2018;15:1-7.
16. Jose Miller AB, Boyden JW, Frey KA. Infertility. Am Fam Physician. 2007;75:849-56.
17. Neerja, Jain K. Role of laparoscopy hysteroscopy in cases of infertility with pregnancy outcome. J Indian Med Assoc. 2014;112(2):85-6, 88.
18. Canis M, Mage G, Pouly JL, et al. Laparoscopic distal tuboplasty: report of 87 cases and a 4-year experience. Fertil Steril. 1991;56:616-21.
19. The role of tubal reconstructive surgery in the era of assisted reproductive technologies. Fertil Steril. 2008;90: S250-3.
20. Liu S, Shi L, Shi J. Impact of endometrial cavity fluid on assisted reproductive technology outcomes. Int J Gynaecol Obstet. 2016;132(3):278-83.
21. Noventa M, Gizzo S, Saccardi C, et al. Salpingectomy before assisted reproductive technologies: a systematic literature review. J Ovar Res. 2016;9:74.
22. Ramalingappa A, Yashoda. A Study on Tubal Recanalization. J Obstet Gynaecol India. 2012;62(2):179-83.

Medicolegal Aspects of Endoscopy 20

Nikhil Datar

INTRODUCTION

Endoscopy has revolutionized the medical care. The field of gynecology has not stayed away from the effect of this advancement of science and technology. Use of telescope to examine the endometrial cavity namely, hysteroscopy and peritoneal cavity namely, laparoscopy have created numerous opportunities to create newer treatment options. The treatment of intrauterine adhesions or removal of intrauterine septum by hysteroscopy are the examples of new surgeries. Whereas replacing conventional route of surgeries such as hysterectomy or myomectomy have helped patients to recover quicker and faster.

Innovative terms such as "keyhole surgery" or "minimally invasive" surgery have created massive interest amongst patients. One does not realize that the operation inside the abdomen is of the same magnitude. Surgeons and patients must stay aware of the fact that endoscopy poses different challenges and can sometimes be more challenging than open surgery.

HOW IS ENDOSCOPY DIFFERENT?

On comparing endoscopy with the open surgery one can notice some unique features in endoscopic surgery.

- Distention of the cavity (by carbon dioxide in laparoscopy and normal saline or glycine in hysteroscopy) is a unique to endoscopy. Problems related to distention media, their prevention and early detection need a special mention.
- Entry to the abdominal cavity by Veress needle or trocar has specific complications such as vascular injury associated with it.
- Tunnel vision is produced by the use of optics, making surgeon aware of the surrounding structures.
- The three-dimensional open field gets converted to two-dimensional surgical field posing challenges in depth perception.
- Use of energy sources leading to passage of current to nearby structures may lead to thermal injury.
- The surgeon needs to learn newer skills such as hand-eye coordination and different types of instruments. The surgeon cannot use the touch sensation while operating.

Thus the surgery and anesthesia both need to be planned in a different manner as compared to open surgery. These surgeries have different types of complications.

PREVENTION IS THE BEST SOLUTION

Prevention of a disease can be explained on the concept of primary, secondary and tertiary prevention. The same theme can be used to describe prevention of medicolegal litigation. Primary prevention is to avoid adverse events or complications by making the surgery safer. Secondary prevention means preventing a litigation when a complication or adverse event has already occurred. Tertiary prevention is to strategize medicolegal defense and mitigate the damage.

Primary Prevention: Avoiding Adverse Events or Complications to the Level Best

The man, machine and technique all are important in this regards. Studies have shown that human factors, system factors, and circumstantial factors contribute to adverse events. As the complexity of the system increases the chances of adverse events increase.[1] Simple techniques such as measuring input, output and deficit in distention medium can significantly prevent complications in hysteroscopy. Use of capnography can prevent anesthesia related complications in laparoscopy.

Training

There is no doubt that endoscopic surgery needs special or additional surgical skill set. A doctor who completes his/her specialist training in India may have a limited exposure to endoscopy.[1] He/she may acquire the skills during working in this field. However, there is no process of validation of these skills by the national or state medical council. The only exception to this is laparoscopic tubal ligation. Under the quality assurance scheme of the Government of India, specific criteria regarding training have been laid down. Upon fulfilling the criteria, doctors are certified and authorized to perform laparoscopic sterilization surgery. Similar system needs to evolve in India so that newly acquired skills are validated formally by licensing body. This shall lead to medicolegal safety.

Machine

Endoscopy is significantly dependent on high take equipment. These machines require a regular maintenance. India has just begun its journey toward safety regulation of medical devices. In 2018, the Drug Controller of India has issued draft guidelines on the subject under medical devices rules. At this point in time, most of the equipment manufacturers do not provide maintaninance or calibration services for the equipment. If a certain machine is not required to be calibrated, the manufacturer should expressly provide such a statement in writing. Accreditation and regular audit are helpful in ensuring good quality of maintenance of equipment.

The sterilization of equipment such as endoscopes is another major area of concern. In India, mobile endoscopy units are not uncommon. Thus when the mobile unit moves along with all equipment from place to place; malfunction, lack of back up, sterilization of the used instruments pose definite safety concern.

Technique

The interplay between the man and the machine is termed as technique. Most of the complications related to laparoscopy are related to one of the following:

- Selection of patient for the surgery and fitness for anesthesia.
- Positioning of the patient.
- Entry to the abdominal cavity. Many international organizations have created evidence based guidelines to improve the safety.[2]
- Safe use of energy devices to avoid inadvertent thermal injuries.
- Prevention of venous thromboembolism.

It is important that guidance from professional organizations such as RCOG, BSGE be adhered to.

Secondary Prevention

Complications can be minimized but cannot be eliminated. It is indeed difficult to differentiate a complication from an error. There is a possibility that every complication is classified as error by hindsight bias. Interestingly, magnitude of the damage, not the error decides whether it is negligence or error. A report published in 1999 by the Institute of Medicine titled " To err is human: Building a safer health system" has vividly discussed the etiology of medical errors.[3]

If the complication or error occurs, one must prevent it from turning into a medicolegal case. Appropriate documentation, counseling (before and after the procedure) and communication are important.

The author finds following common flaws in documentation in general:

1. Absence or insufficient documentation: Many a times the events are not recorded on case sheet. It is also found that the events are not recorded in chronological order. Date and time are not mentioned. The author of the entry cannot be traced.
2. It is a common practice to simply record the patient parameters in the case sheet. The case notes should showcase the thought process behind decision making. It is important that provisional diagnosis, final diagnosis, and the plan of action are documented. If the plan is changed the same must be documented.
3. Use of unauthorized abbreviations should be avoided.

Communication

Communication failure is a major problem in the healthcare industry. Communication failure amongst caregivers can lead to an adverse event. Improper communication with the patients is highly associated with the medicolegal liability. Bismark et al. have reiterated that actual negligence is much lesser than perceived negligence in health care.[4]

In India, it is a common practice that the primary doctor does not communicate to his/her patient that another surgeon would be preforming the surgery. This practice is risky and may attract medicolegal liability.

Consent

Consent is the cornerstone of defense in negligence cases. It has been found that consent and the process of taking consent are challenged in close to 85% cases of medico-legal negligence. Consent means permission given by the patient. Surgery without such express permission amounts to battery and assault. The Supreme Court of India has dealt with practical issues related to consent and has laid down following principles:

- In India, the principle of real consent shall prevail.
- The consent should cover:
  - The nature and procedure of the treatment and its purpose, benefits and effect
  - Alternatives if any available
  - Adverse consequences of refusing treatment
  - An outline of the substantial risks.
- A surgeon should not go beyond the scope of the consent except in life-saving situations.
- A surgeon can do the diagnostic and therapeutic procedure if a patient is well informed beforehand.

Indian surgeons who see many more patients face following genuine challenges in this regard.

- How much information is "legally" sufficient?
- How to provide the information related to risks without frightening the patient?
- How to manage the language barrier?
- How to give sufficient time?
- How to improve patient recall?

The author has been working on developing an audio-visual standard format consent that shall significantly improve the patient experience and also provide medicolegal safety to the doctors.

Tertiary Prevention

Tertiary prevention is to mitigate the damage when the matter has reached the court. It is obvious that legal professional plays an important role at this point in time. Careful selection of lawyer or medicolegal expert is vital at this time.

Interaction with the lawyer:

- Giving inputs to the lawyer while preparing a reply or written statement
- Providing necessary medical evidence to defend.

It is important to understand the legal definition of the word "negligence ". The doctor has to prove that

- The practice adopted by him/her is the standard or common norm.
- Any professional man with ordinary skills would have adopted the same practice.[5]

Laws, government rules, textbooks and guidelines from medical organizations play a vital role in this regard. The standards laid down by foreign textbooks may not be feasible to adhere to in India. Hence Indian textbooks play a more important role.

Role of Medical Organizations

It may be stated that the local or regional medical organizations have vital role in setting up minimum standards. These standards can be a reference point to adjudge whether the care given by a particular provider was as per standards or not. The author is of the opinion that such move can go a long way in defending the litigation matters.

Role of Indemnity Insurance

It is important to ensure that one has sufficient professional indemnity insurance. The quantum of compensation awarded by Indian courts has been exponentially rising.

SPECIAL SITUATIONS

Pregnancy and Endoscopy

Doing laparoscopy in pregnancy poses a different dimension to the problem. Risk of general anesthesia to the mother and the fetus is one such important attribute. Pelvic surgery may become more difficult due to the presence of soft vascular mass which cannot be maneuvered. Preterm labor and fetal demise may be higher after laparoscopy. Diagnostic laparoscopy should be judiciously used only when other safer modalities such as USG or MRI are not able to conclude on the diagnosis. The salient guidelines from Society of American Gastrointestinal and Endoscopists in this regards are as follows:

- Traditional viewpoint of avoiding laparoscopy in first and third trimester, respectively to avoid spontaneous abortion and preterm labor are not supported by good quality evidence.
- A patient should be put into left lateral decubitus, entry to the abdomen should be done with the help of open technique or Hasson's technique.

- Tocolysis should not be used routinely but should be started when signs of preterm labor are seen.
- Adnexal masses which are not expected to be malignant should only be observed. Laparoscopy is acceptable method even in case of adnexal torsion.

CONCLUSION

- Although endoscopy has a significant role in modern medicine it poses different challenges.
- Prevention of medicolegal problem is the best strategy.
- Healthcare organizations providing endoscopy services must take active interest in maintaining the quality of equipment used.
- Consent taking must be practiced seriously and should not be left to junior staff.
- National medical organizations must come up with minimum standards or practice management guidelines that can help practitioners.
- A doctor must take indemnity insurance before starting the practice.
- The medical council must lay down criteria for doctors who can perform endoscopy.

REFERENCES

1. World Health Organization. Patient Safety Curriculum Guide for Medical Schools. Geneva: WHO; 2009.
2. National Board of Examinations. (2006). Revised curriculum for competency based training of dnb candidates.[online] Available from https://www.natboard.edu.in/notice_for_dnb_candidates/obg.pdf. [Last Accessed on February, 2019].
3. Royal College of Obstetricians and Gynaecologists. (2008). Laparoscopic Injuries (Green-top Guideline No. 49). [Online] Available from https://www.rcog.org.uk/en/guidelines-research-services/guidelines/gtg49/. [Last Accessed on February, 2019].
4. PSNET: Agency for Healthcare Research and Quality. (2000). To Err Is Human: Building a Safer Health System. [Online] Available from https://psnet.ahrq.gov/resources/resource/1579/to-err-is-human-building-a-safer-health-system#. [Last Accessed on February, 2019]
5. Bismark M, Dauer E, Paterson R, et al. Accountability sought by patients following adverse events from medical care: the New Zealand experience. CMAJ. 2006;175(8):889-94.

Genetic, Lifestyle, and Environmental Factors in Male Infertility

21

Skand Shekhar, Anne Martini, Alan DeCherney

INTRODUCTION

Male infertility (MI) affects 50% of infertile couples. The evaluation of the male factor is an essential aspect of the diagnostic evaluation and encompasses various elements. The purpose of this chapter is to review the genetics, lifestyle factors, and environmental exposures in the causation and evaluation of MI.

GENETICS OF MALE INFERTILITY

Although approaches to diagnosis vary, commonly the first step in the diagnosis of MI after a thorough history and physical is a semen analysis. The results of the semen analysis influence the genetic approach to the diagnosis of MI.

Spermatozoa Defects

Broadly, the genetic approach is based on whether the semen defects are quantitative or qualitative. The summary of spermatozoa and genetics is provided in **Tables 1 and 2**.

Defects in the Hypothalamic Pituitary Testicular Axis—Congenital Hypogonadotropic Hypogonadism

Congenital hypogonadotropic hypogonadism (CHH) is characterized by delayed puberty, reduced or absent pubic or axillary hair and eunuchoid habitus. Two main forms of CHH include (1) normosmic hypogonadotropic hypogonadism and (2) Kallmann syndrome (hyposmic hypogonadotropic hypogonadism). More than 30 genes have been implicated in its causation including the KAL1 gene, and the list continues to grow. CHH is reversible with androgen replacement but a period of treatment is recommended, since spontaneous reversal of CHH has been reported after a period of treatment.

Mitochondrial Genetic Defects

Spermatozoa have high-energy requirements postejaculation in order to have normal motility. Conceivably to meet

Table 1: Quantitative defects (spermatogenesis).

Etiology	*Defect*	*Test*
Azoospermia (<10 million sperm/mL)	Chromosomal anomalies	Karyotyping, deletion screening
	Y-chromosome deletions	
	Partial androgen insensitivity	Androgen receptor testing
Severe azoospermia (<5 million sperm/mL)	Y chromosome deletions	Deletion screening, PCR testing
	Congenital bilateral absence of vas deferens	CFTR testing—mutation panel followed by whole genome sequencing
Oligozoospermia (10–20 million sperm/mL)	GR deletion (AZFc region)	Deletion screening, PCR

(AZF: azoospermia factor; CFTR: cystic fibrosis transmembrane conductance regulator; PCR: polymerase chain reaction)

this requirement, multiple mitochondria are present in each sperm. With increasing oxidative stress including advancing paternal age and other environmental factors, the mitochondrial deoxyribonucleic acid (DNA) is susceptible to damage, which in turn can reduce motility and fertility. The most commonly implicated mutations include 4977bp and A3243G, as the list continues to grow.[1]

Table 2: Qualitative defects (spermatogenesis).		
Etiology	***Defect***	***Test***
Globozoospermia	DPY19L2	Targeted mutation testing with PCR, consider whole genome sequencing
Sperm macrocephaly	AURKC	Mutation panel for AURKC testing, consider whole genome sequencing
Multiple morphological Abnormalities of the Sperm Flagella	DNAH1	Targeted mutation testing
Primary ciliary dyskinesia	DNAH1 + 26 other genes	Gene panel testing
Oligozoospermia (10–20 million sperm/mL)	GR deletion (AZFc region)	Deletion screening, PCR

(AZF: azoospermia factor; PCR: polymerase chain reaction)

Implications in Assisted Reproductive Technology

The objectives of genetics in MI are threefold. Firstly, it allays anxiety in couples by providing a diagnosis for the infertility. Secondly, it can assist the treating team in choosing the optimal assisted reproductive technology (ART) strategy and deliver a cost-effective treatment method. Lastly, it also provides the couple crucial genetic information which may also affect the offspring and hence facilitate early diagnosis and management in their offspring.

LIFESTYLE FACTORS IN MALE INFERTILITY (TABLE 3)

Stress

Animal models have, for long, demonstrated the negative impact of both acute and chronic stress on Sertoli, Leydig, and germ cells mediated by the glucocorticoid receptor (GR). In humans too, the polymorphism of GR leads to variable yet detrimental response to stress. Social factors such as major life events, work related, or other psychosocial stressors have significant negative impacts on sperm quality.[2] Stress can further worsen after a diagnosis of infertility and in turn lead to failed IVF treatments. Some studies have also demonstrated a negative linear association between perceived stress and semen

Table 3: Summary of lifestyle factors in male infertility.		
Etiology	***Effects***	***Actions recommended***
Stress	Oligozoospermia, hypothalamic pituitary gonadal effects	Professional counseling, stress reducing measures, *Yoga*, *Taiichi*, etc.
Advanced age	Increase reactive oxygen species (ROS), hypogonadism	Preconception counseling
Caffeine consumption	Unclear effects in adult males but some data suggests a negative effect	Avoidance of excessive caffeine intake
High ambient temperature	Heat reduced spermatogenesis	Avoidance of prolonged heat, tight clothes, etc.
Metabolic syndrome (MS): ▪ Physical exercise ▪ Obesity ▪ Poor diet-saturated fats, low vegetable or fiber intake	*Multifactorial:* ▪ Balanced exercise helps in reducing obesity ▪ Oligozoospermia ▪ Possible increase in ROS, DNA damage to sperm	▪ Combination of aerobic and anaerobic exercise ▪ Combination of exercise and a healthy diet. ▪ Diet rich in antioxidants, avoidance of high caloric diets
Recreational agents: ▪ Tobacco ▪ Heavy alcohol use ▪ Chronic marijuana use	▪ Oligozoospermia ▪ HPG suppression ▪ Hypogonadism	▪ Discourage consumption in all forms ▪ Avoidance of heavy use ▪ Avoidance

quality.[3] Since psychosocial stress is a modifiable risk factor for MI, clinicians should pay special focus to both its diagnosis and management in couples seeking infertility treatment.

Diet

Multiple observational studies have demonstrated a positive relationship between healthy dietary choices and male fertility. A recent systematic review concluded that diets rich in antioxidants such as vitamins A, C and E, and omega 3 fatty acids and poor in unhealthy fats were associated with better semen quality.[4] Other studies indicate that a diet rich in vegetables, fruits, legumes, and fish and low in whole fat milk, processed meats, and foods improved sperm quality.[5] Thus, the positive impact of a healthy diet and regular physical activity cannot be overstated in the management of MI.

Age

Strong evidence exists suggesting the negative impacts of advanced paternal age on a variety of male factors including a declining male endocrine milieu, increased seminal oxidative stress, and a higher prevalence of certain congenital disorders in offspring. Use of caution is advisable in counseling men of advanced age seeking fertility treatments.

Exercise

The role of physical exercise and maintenance of a healthy body habitus has been demonstrated in multiple studies, to have improved male fertility. Although a rigorous continuous exercise regimen can be detrimental to male fertility, a healthy exercise regimen including a balanced combination of aerobic and anaerobic exercise is advisable in the treatment of MI.[6]

Caffeine Consumption

Caffeine is the most widely used central nervous system stimulant used across the world. Prenatally, caffeine can impair gonadal development, but the data is less clear in adult gonadal function.[7] Since current data does not prove a causal relationship between caffeine and infertility, it is best to only encourage patients to limit excess consumption rather than advocate complete abstinence.

Ambient Temperature

Human testes are very temperature sensitive and respond to even minor rises in ambient temperature. Activities such as bicycling, using laptops, exposure to cellphone electromagnetic radiation, prolonged sitting in vehicles, tight clothing, and others that raise scrotal temperature can impair semen quality. Active avoidance of all such factors is highly advisable.

Metabolic Syndrome

Metabolic syndrome (MS) is a cluster of multiple disorders including central adiposity, dyslipidemia, hypertension, and type 2 diabetes. While each of these disorders is independently associated with infertility, their compounded effects tend to be much larger. Each of these conditions increases the prevalence of erectile dysfunction(ED), low testosterone (T) levels and reduced semen quality. Given the epidemic of MS globally, infertility treatments should play special emphasis on the encouraging healthy lifestyles in order to improve both overall health as well as fertility.

Obesity

While obesity is a major component of MS, it deserves special mention due to its continuously rising prevalence globally. In a J-shaped curve fashion, rising body mass index (BMI) seems to be associated with MI. Morbidly obese men were found to have a twofold risk of oligozoospermia, compared to healthy controls, according to a recent study. Additionally, obesity adversely impacts sperm morphology, circulating T levels and estradiol to T ratio compounding MI treatment in obese men.[8]

Alcohol, Tobacco, and Illicit Drug Use

Alcohol has been shown to suppress the hypothalamic pituitary testis axis in both animal and human male studies. It has also been linked to defective spermatogenesis and direct testicular cell damage. Tobacco use has been linked to decreased sperm concentration across many studies and reviews, and is presumed to be related to exposure to the various chemicals contained in tobacco smoke. Illicit drug use, particularly chronic marijuana use, has also been associated with decreased serum testosterone levels and oligospermia.[9]

ENVIRONMENTAL FACTORS IN MALE INFERTILITY (TABLE 4)

Male spermatogenesis is more vulnerable to environmental hazards when compared to oogenesis in females.[10] Various chemicals, pesticides, heavy metals, and pollution have been implicated in impacting male reproductive fitness through either direct effects on gonadal tissues, genetic alterations or through disrupting critical endocrine pathways. Some studies suggest that these effectors may impact men across multiple generations.[11] Despite clear associations in animal studies, human studies are less able to control for confounding variables. Understanding these limitations is critical when drawing conclusions on the impacts of environmental exposures on MI.[9]

Endocrine Disrupting Chemicals

Endocrine disrupting chemicals arise from both natural and synthetic sources and can act directly or indirectly to impair the actions of male reproductive hormones. The clinical impact on MI is inconsistent across studies.

Polychlorinated biphenyls (PCBs) have chemical stability and resistance to degradation that is responsible for their continued presence in many areas of the world. Animal studies have demonstrated associations between PCB exposure and poorer semen analysis parameters, alterations in testis architecture, change in Sertoli cell estrogen and androgen-related gene expression, and impaired testicular steroidogenesis.[10,11] Few studies have demonstrated these same effects in humans.[9]

Bisphenol A (BPA), found in many consumer products, is widely detectable in human serum samples from varying populations. BPA has been demonstrated in animal studies to alter serum gonadotropin and sex steroid levels, damage the sperm acrosome and mitochondria, and downregulate androgen receptor expression and genes involved spermatogenesis. Research on the effects of BPA on human males has yielded conflicting results, but one review suggested that BPA exposure in utero can lead to feminization of male fetuses as well as gonadal, hormonal, and genitourinary abnormalities.[10,11]

Phthalate, a nearly ubiquitous compound, has been linked to MI in both human and animal studies. The most commonly used phthalate compounds, diethyl phthalate (DEHP) and di-N-butyl phthalate (DBP), have been discovered to act in an antiandrogenic fashion and have been implicated in decreased sperm motility, increased sperm DNA damage and abnormal levels of sex steroids.[10,11]

Pesticides and Herbicides

Pesticides are potent endocrine disruptors that possess the ability to mimic reproductive hormones. These compounds are most commonly encountered through dietary consumption or occupational exposure. Organophosphates are a widely used group of pesticides that have been associated with impaired sperm motility, decreased sperm counts, lower testosterone levels and reduced testicular weight, particularly notable after long exposure durations.

Table 4: Environmental exposures and proposed mechanisms leading to male infertility.

Environmental exposure	*Source*	*Theorized mechanisms of action*
Endocrine disrupting chemicals: ▪ Polychlorinated biphenyls (PCBs) ▪ Bisphenol A (BPA) ▪ Phthalate	Various foods and industrial solvents	▪ Interference with the action (stimulation and inhibition) or elimination of sex steroid and gonadotropin hormones ▪ Competitive binding to sex steroid receptors ▪ Direct damage to sperm acrosome and mitochondria ▪ Interference with spermatogenesis-related gene expression
Pesticides and herbicides: ▪ Organophosphates ▪ Dichlorodiphenyldichloro-ethylene (DDT)	Dietary consumption, occupational exposures	▪ Mimicry of sex steroids
Heavy metals: ▪ Lead ▪ Cadmium ▪ Mercury	▪ Old house paint, brass water fixtures, ceramics, and smoking ▪ Smoking, fertilizers, plastics, and ceramics ▪ Soil, fish, and shellfish	▪ Competitive binding to sex steroid receptors ▪ Increased formation of reactive oxygen species (ROS) in the testes leading to apoptosis of spermatozoa
Pollution	Air and water	▪ Unclear, possibly through epigenetic modification or direct sperm DNA damage

Dichlorodiphenyldichloroethylene (DDT), used in developing countries in attempts to control the spread of malaria, has the ability block androgen receptors and interferes with the metabolism of estrogen. Studies evaluating male fertility after occupational exposure demonstrated inhibition of spermatogenesis, abnormal semen analysis parameters and reduced testicular weights.[10,11]

Heavy Metals

Heavy metals including lead, cadmium, and mercury impair male fertility through direct and indirect mechanisms. They can exert direct gonadotoxic effects through increasing production of reactive oxygen species in the testes that induces DNA damage and ultimately leads to destruction of spermatozoa. Indirectly, they have the potential to competitively binding of sex steroid receptors. Though distinct associations between these exposures and decreased sperm counts have been demonstrated in animal studies, these results have not been consistently replicated in human studies.[10,11]

Pollution

Associations have been described between outdoor air pollution and altered semen quality, with most studies describing at least one affected semen parameter.[10] Sperm counts, however, have not been consistently impacted.[9] A recent review evaluating semen from men exposed to air pollution demonstrated higher rates of epigenetic changes and sperm DNA damage.[10] The effect of water pollution on semen parameters is currently unknown.[9]

CONCLUSION

When evaluating an infertile male, it is essential that providers consider the impact of genetic, lifestyle, and environmental factors. Though a detailed history and physical exam can provide clues to lifestyle and environmental causes, karyotyping, Y-chromosome microdeletion testing, and screening for targeted mutations are the primary methods to evaluate for genetic etiologies. Elimination of modifiable factors and offering assisted reproductive technology should be primary considerations in the treatment of such patients. Future directions should focus on designing studies with proper control of confounders to more fully understand the gravity of various exposures on male reproduction.

KEY POINTS

- Genetic, lifestyle, and environmental factors should be primary considerations in the evaluation of the infertile male
- Genetic anomalies can manifest as both quantitative and qualitative aberrations in spermatogenesis
- Modifiable and nonmodifiable lifestyle factors including stress, diet, age, obesity, substance use, and activities that lead to be elevated ambient scrotal temperatures have been linked to abnormalities in male reproduction
- Environmental exposures including endocrine disrupting chemicals, pesticides, heavy metals, and pollution have strong associations between abnormal reproductive function in male animal studies which have been demonstrated to a lesser degree in human studies.

REFERENCES

1. Kao SH, Chao HT, Wei YH. Multiple deletions of mitochondrial DNA are associated with the decline of motility and fertility of human spermatozoa. Mol Hum Reprod. 1998;4(7):657-66.
2. Anderson K, Nisenblat V, Norman R. Lifestyle factors in people seeking infertility treatment—A review. Aust NZ J Obstet Gynaecol. 2010;50(1):8-20.
3. Janevic T, Kahn LG, Landsbergis P, et al. Effects of work and life stress on semen quality. Fertil steril. 2014;102(2):530-8.
4. Salas-Huetos A, Bullo M, Salas-Salvado J. Dietary patterns, foods and nutrients in male fertility parameters and fecundability: a systematic review of observational studies. Hum Reprod Update. 2017;23(4):371-89.
5. Braga DP, Halpern G, Figueira Rde C, et al. Food intake and social habits in male patients and its relationship to intracytoplasmic sperm injection outcomes. Fertil Steril. 2012;97(1):53-9.
6. Hajizadeh Maleki B, Tartibian B. Combined aerobic and resistance exercise training for improving reproductive function in infertile men: a randomized controlled trial. Appl Physiol Nutr Metab. 2017;42(12):1293-306.
7. Dorostghoal M, Erfani Majd N, Nooraei P. Maternal caffeine consumption has irreversible effects on reproductive parameters and fertility in male offspring rats. Clin Exp Reprod Med. 2012;39(4):144-52.
8. Martins AD, Majzoub A, Agawal A. Metabolic Syndrome and Male Fertility. World J Mens Health. 2018;36.
9. Gabrielsen JS, Tanrikut C. Chronic exposures and male fertility: the impacts of environment, diet, and drug use on spermatogenesis. Andrology. 2016;4(4):648-61.
10. Mima M, Greenwald D, Ohlander S. Environmental Toxins and Male Fertility. Curr Urol Rep. 2018;19(7):50.
11. Jenardhanan P, Panneerselvam M, Mathur PP. (2016). Effect of environmental contaminants on spermatogenesis. Semin Cell Dev Biol. 2016;59:126-40.

Medical Management of Male Infertility

22

Kedar Ganla, Rana Choudhary

INTRODUCTION

Male factor infertility is responsible for up to 50% of the cause of infertility in couples. Generally these men have abnormal semen parameters or the male partner is having ejaculatory or erectile problems leading to coital difficulties in the couple. This alteration in the semen parameters could be due to low sperm count and/or motility and/or morphology. These semen analysis findings must be consistently reported in at least two different semen analyses, which comply with the World Health Organization (WHO) 2011 guidelines. Identifying the cause of this semen abnormality and treating it may allow couple to improve their fertility potential and conceive naturally. However, despite technological advances, the cause of male infertility remains unknown in almost 25–30%. This is known as idiopathic male infertility or unexplained male infertility according to semen quality **(Table 1)**.

Oligoasthenoteratozoospermia (OATS) is a condition that includes oligozoospermia (low number of sperm), asthenozoospermia (poor sperm movement), and teratozoospermia (abnormal sperm shape). OATS is the most common cause of male subfertility **(Box 1)**.

Table 1: WHO (2010 Guidelines)—Lower limit of normal reference values for different sperm parameters.

Parameter	***Lower reference limits (WHO 2010)***
Semen volume	1.5 mL
Sperm concentration	15 million sperm/mL
Progressive motility	32%
Total motility	40%
Vitality	58% live
Morphology (Strict criteria)	4% normal form

The aims of medical management of male therapy are listed below in **Box 2**.

Male factor infertility can be managed by medical treatment as discussed below: Specific and nonspecific. Specific treatments are used for certain etiologies such as hypogonadotropic hypogonadism, male accessory gland infection and retrograde ejaculation. When the cause of abnormal semen is not known empirical nonspecific therapy may be tried in selected cases.

SPECIFIC MEDICAL THERAPY

1. *Chronic scrotal fungal dermatitis*:
   - Can cause thickening of scrotal skin and ↑ local temperature.
   - *Treatment*: Topical antifungal and steroids.

Box 1: Factors affecting choice of therapy.

- Age of couple and duration of infertility
- Severity of OATS
- Past illness (mumps-related orchitis)
- Reversible, correctable gonadotoxic factors such as exposure to hot environmental conditions (furnaces, etc.)
- Antioxidants trial already given
- Socioeconomic status
- Psychosocial pressure

Box 2: Aims of medical therapy.

- To improve count, motility and morphology of sperms
- Increase rates of spontaneous conception
- Lower rates of miscarriages due to DNA abnormalities in sperm.

2. *Genital tract infections*: Leukocytospermia (WBC count in semen > 1 × 10^6/mL). Prevalence 10–20%.
   - Semen culture
   - *Common organisms*: *Streptococcus fecalis, E. coli, Chlamydia trachomatis, Ureaplasma urealyticum.*
   - Because of the difficulty of culturing, doxycycline 200 mg/day is given for 15 days on empirical basis
   - Antibiotics may be added later as per culture reports, e.g. fluoroquinolones 0.5–1 g/day, cotrimoxazole or erythromycin 1.5–2 g/day for 2–3 weeks.
   - *Culture negative patients*: Anti-inflammatory therapy and frequent ejaculations.
   - *Refractory leukocytospermia*: Sperm washing and intrauterine insemination (IUI).
3. *Immunological infertility*:
   - *Oral steroids*: To suppress antibody production, but efficacy not confirmed by double blind randomized trial.
   - Pregnancy rates are 0–44%, with maximum pregnancy seen after treatment for more than 3 months.
   - *Treatment*: Tablet predinisolone 5 mg, thrice a day for 10 days with tapering of dose.
4. *Chronic epididymo-orchitis*:
   - Clinical evidence of chronic filarial epididymo-orchitis such as enlarged adherent epididymis, thickened cord, etc.
   - *Treatment*: Diethylcarbamazine (DEC) 100 mg thrice a day for 20 days + doxycycline 100 mg twice a day for 10 days, followed by low dose steroids.

NONSPECIFIC OR EMPERICAL THERAPY

1. *Hormonal agents*:
   - *Androgens*: The effect of androgens on semen parameters in male infertility is explained by the following theories:
     - *Direct stimulatory theory*: According to this theory, the androgens have a direct stimulatory effect on spermatogenesis. They also help in sperm transport and maturation without affecting the pituitary gonadotropin hormones.
     - *Rebound theory*: According to this theory, androgens initially suppress gonadotropin secretion and spermatogenesis. However, once they are suddenly withdrawn, it causes a transient increase in gonadotropin hormones and also in spermatogenesis.

     Literature review shows that there is only one randomized double blind control trial in which treatment with androgens lead to marginally significant improvement in sperm morphology and improved pregnancy rates. Contradictory to these findings there are several meta-analyses which showed that androgens may not be effective. Further it is important to note that any supplementation of testosterone from outside will suppress the hypothalamic-pituitary axis. This will cause further reduction in intratesticular testosterone and adversely affect spermatogenesis. However many clinicians, especially urologist, still prescribe this therapy. For example,
     - Mesterolone 25 mg thrice a day.
     - Testosterone undecanoate 80–160 mg/day
   - *Antiestrogen*: Inhibit the negative feedback effect of estrogen by blocking estrogen receptors in hypothalamus and thus ↑ gonadotrophins. ↑ Follicle-stimulating hormone (FSH) and luteinzing hormone (LH) stimulate sertoli Leydig cells and improve spermatogenesis.
     - *Aromatase inhibitors increase FSH*: This may be helpful against the traditional testosterone supplementation to improve testosterone levels especially in older men who have late-onset of hypogonadism.
     - Who will benefit? Idiopathic male infertility
     - Who will not be benefited? High baseline fluorescence in situ hybridization (FISH), severe OATS, and azoospermia.
     - A Cochrane Database review showed that both clomiphene and tamoxifen cause increase in serum testosterone levels. However evidence is insufficient regarding their effect on pregnancy outcomes. Moreover, a recent meta-analysis with 11 randomized controlled trials found that anti-estrogen therapy was associated with a statistically significant increase in the pregnancy rate, sperm concentration, and sperm motility. The authors concluded that these drugs had a statistically significant beneficial effect on the pregnancy rate. For example,
       - Clomiphene citrate 25 mg/day
       - Tamoxifen citrate 10–20 mg/day
   - *Aromatase inhibitors*: Inhibit peripheral conversion of testosterone to estrogen and enhance spermatogenesis.

- Normal testosterone (T)/Esterogen (E2) is 1:16
- Low T/E ratio indicates high aromatase activity
- Useful in a subpopulation of patients with low T/E2 ratio (e.g. obese men)
- There are very few studies related to pregnancy outcome and use of aromatase inhibitors for male factor infertility. Literature review shows only a single double-blinded crossover randomized trial. During this study high-dose testolactone was used for 15–16 months. However, there was no improvement in semen parameters or conception rate. However, there was decrease in sex hormone-binding globulin (SHBG) binding capacity and increase in free testosterone in the study participants. Further there are many small nonrandomized studies where letrozole or anastrozole has been used. These have shown a significant increase in sperm count as well as motility along with improvement in serum testosterone levels.
- Aromatase inhibitors are effective when used for men who have obesity and high estrogen or low testosterone-to-estrogen (T/E) ratios (<10). Unfortunately the normal T/E ratio is not well defined for Indian population. For example,
  - Letrozole 2.5 mg daily orally.

- *Gonadotrophins*: Helpful in men with idiopathic infertility (subclinical endocrinopathy) with normal hormonal levels.

  According to published literature, this is the only therapy which is effective for improving the semen count and motility in men with abnormal semen. Certain studies have also demonstrated its positive effect on ultrastructural features of sperm. A recent systematic review which included six RCTs (456 subjects) further showed that gonadotrophins improve the live birth and pregnancy rate in idiopathic male infertility. However, the pregnancy rate did not improve significantly after IUI and intracytoplasmic sperm injection (ICSI) cycles within the gonadotropin treatment period. For example,
  - hCG 1,500 IU or hMG 37.5–75 IU thrice a week
  - Injection r-FSH 300 IU daily followed by 3–6 cycles of IUI followed by ICSI.

2. *Antioxidants*: In spite of doing IVF/ICSI, there is high incidence of implantation failure and early pregnancy loss. If the DNA of sperm is damaged, it will result in a poor pregnancy outcome. Oxidative stress on the sperm may be the cause of almost 30–80% of idiopathic male subfertility.

   Men with normal semen parameters have a balance between ROS (reactive oxygen species) production and total antioxidant capacity. Various conditions may adversely affect this balance and damage the sperms. These include infections like mumps, autoimmune conditions, increasing age, chronic disease, and lifestyle factors like excessive alcohol consumption or smoking. There are studies demonstrating the role of stress and obesity leading to increase in oxidative stress and damage to the sperms. The defense mechanism of the antioxidants against ROS can be either by an enzymatic or nonenzymatic process. The cellular cytoplasm having the scavenging enzymes along with the antioxidants from seminal fluid are important defense mechanisms. If there is a decrease in these enzymes or increase in the polyunsaturated fatty acids in membranes, spermatozoa become susceptible to ROS arsing by lipid peroxidation. Antioxidants may help in preventing this damage. For example, glutathione 250 mg/day, lycopene 4–8 g/day, vitamin E 400–800 mg/day, and vitamin C.
3. *Sperm vitalizers*: Energizes the sperms (improves motility) and increases fertilization. May assist in sperm maturation and some have antioxidant properties. For example,

   L- and acetyl carnitine 1 g thrice a day

   Coenzyme Q10 100–300 mg/day

   Carnitines are used by spermatozoa for mitochondrial membrane stabilization and energize the sperm.
4. *Nutritional supplements*: May be of some benefit in nutritionally depleted patients.

A recent Cochrane Database review highlighted the benefit of vitamin E supplementation in increasing live births compared to placebo. However, there was no fixed dosage of vitamin E in these studies, e.g. multivitamins with zinc, selenium, folic acid, and vitamin B_{12} **(Flowcharts 1 to 3)**.

TAKE HOME MESSAGES

- Give patients a very clear roadmap of therapy.
- Individualized treatment with timeline and endpoints established beforehand.
- Treatment should be of at least 3 months to incorporate full 74-day spermatogenesis cycle, followed by semen analysis.
- Patient should be counseled about realistic expectations.

Flowchart 1: Management of male infertility by optimization of sperms.

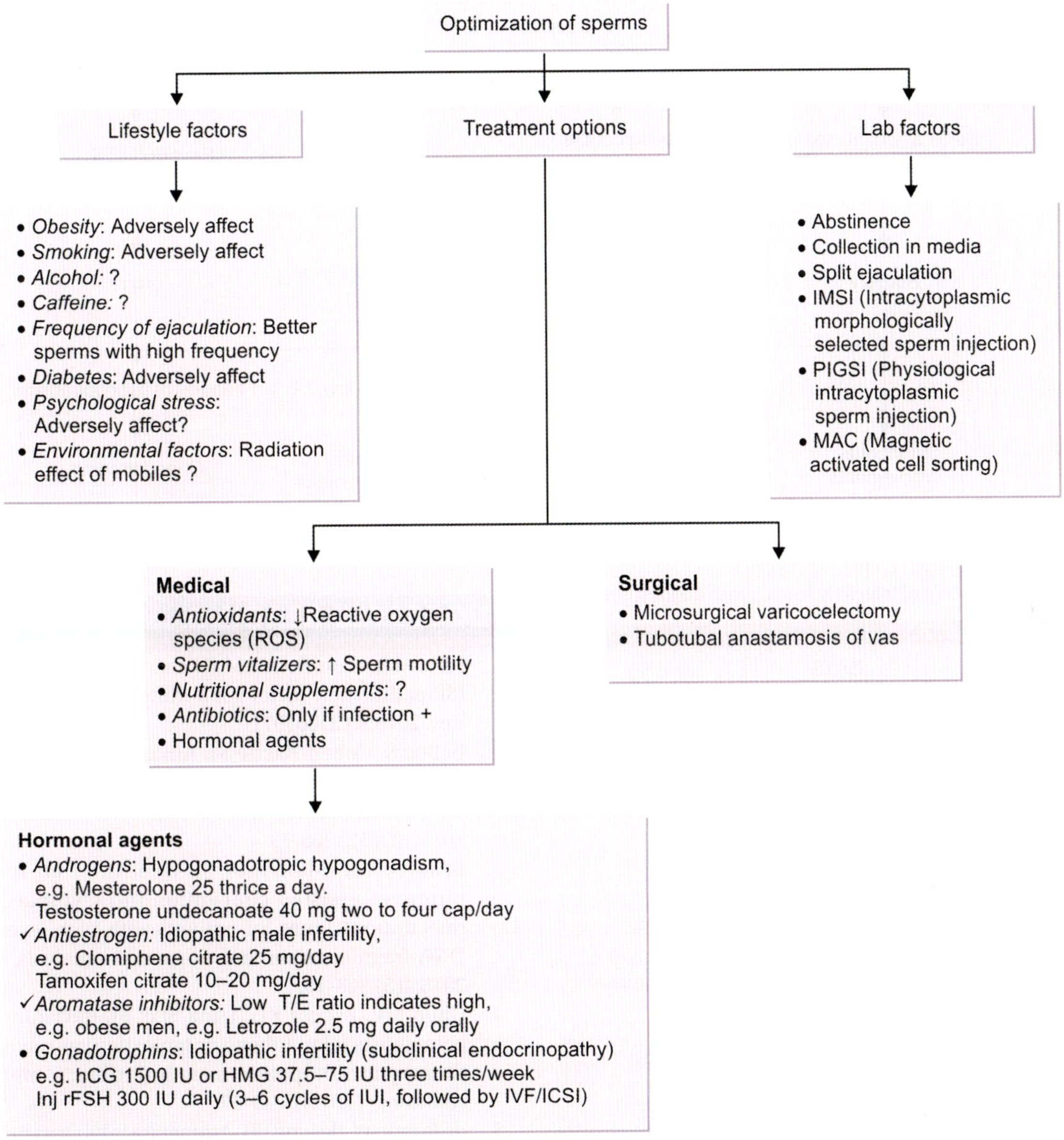

(FSH: follicle-stimulating hormone; hCG: human chorionic gonadotropin; hMG: human menopausal gonadotropin; ICSI: intracytoplasmic sperm injection; IUI: intrauterine insemination; IVF: in vitro fertilization)

- Do not waste time and money over medical therapy if the circumstances call for assisted reproductive therapy.

CONCLUSION

- Various types of empiric medical therapy (EMT) have been used over the years for idiopathic male infertility.
- Hormonal agents and modulators are the most commonly used agents. Selective estrogen-receptor response modulators (SERMs) and aromatase inhibitors are the mainstay of hormonal therapy.
- Exogenous testosterone should never be used for the treatment of male infertility as it inhibits spermatogenesis.
- There are not many large randomized control trials which have evaluated gonadotropin (hCG, FSH, and GnRH) use in idiopathic male infertility. However, there are a few smaller studies which show some improvement in pregnancy rates.
- Due to unavailability of data and studies other treatments such as clomiphene citrate and letrozole

Flowchart 2: Medical management of male infertility.

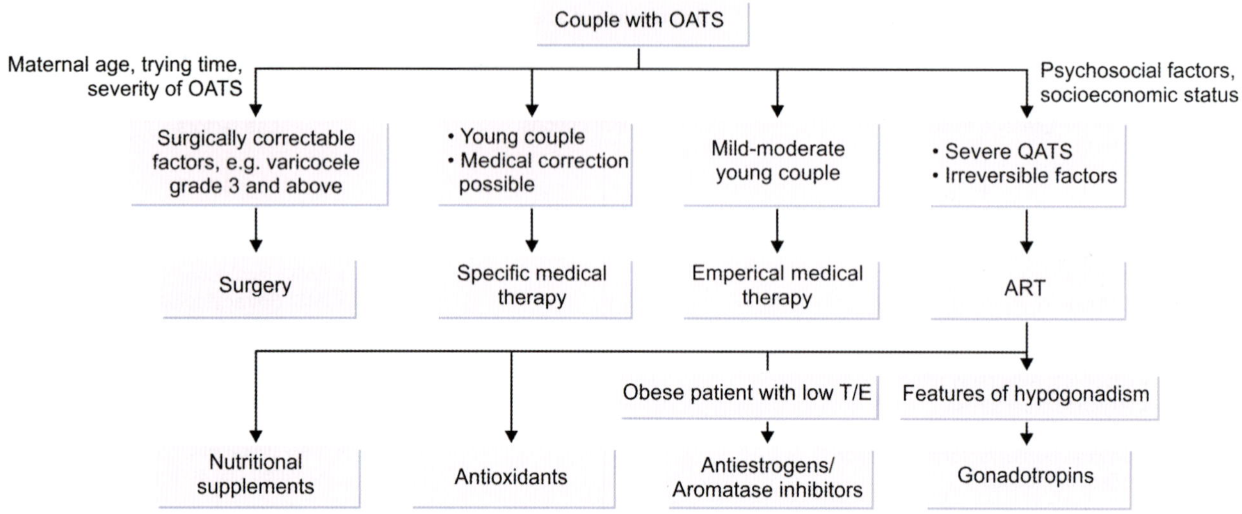

(ART: assisted reproductive techniques; OATS: oligoasthenoteratozoospermia)

Flowchart 3: Management of infertility in men with oligoasthenoteratozoospermia (OATS).

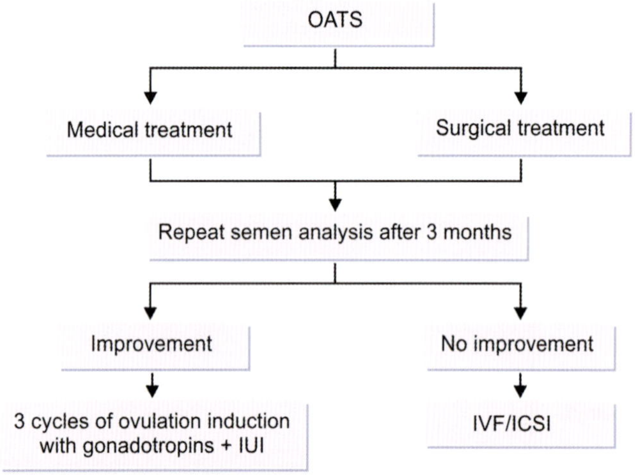

(ICSI: intracytoplasmic sperm injection; IUI: intrauterine insemination; IVF: in vitro fertilization)

which are cheaper, easily available, easier to administer and monitor are used instead of gonadotropins.

- Aromatase inhibitors (letrozole) are useful in men with low serum testosterone and elevated estradiol levels and obese men. Their use in men with normal testosterone and estradiol remains controversial.
- Clomiphene citrate (CC) has been used for decades to improve male fertility. However there is no clear data or trials to prove efficacy. However, CC is still the safest and most effective empiric treatment for idiopathic male infertility.

SUGGESTED READING

1. Attia AM, Abou-Setta AM, Al-Inany HG. Gonadotrophins for idiopathic male factor subfertility. Cochrane Database Syst Rev. 2013;8:CD005071.
2. Belloc S, Cohen-Bacrie M, Amar E, et al. High body mass index has a deleterious effect on semen parameters except morphology: results from a large cohort study. Fertil Steril. 2014;102(5):1268-73.
3. Bradley CK, McArthur SJ, Gee AJ, et al. Intervention improves assisted conception intracytoplasmic sperm injectionoutcomes for patients with high levels of sperm DNA fragmentation: a retrospective analysis. Andrology. 2016;4(5):903-10.
4. Chua ME, Escusa KG, Luna S, et al. Revisiting oestrogen antagonists (clomiphene or tamoxifen) as medical empiric therapy for idiopathic male infertility: a meta-analysis. Andrology. 2013;1:749-57.
5. de Ronde W, de Jong FH. Aromatase inhibitors in men: effects and therapeutic options. Reprod Biol Endocrinol. 2011;9:93.
6. Fariello RM, Pariz JR, Spaine DM, et al. Association between obesity and alteration of sperm DNA integrity and mitochondrial activity. BJU Int. 2012;110(6):863-7.
7. Fronczak CM. The insults of illicit drug use on male fertility. J Androl. 2012;33:515-28.
8. Gil M, Sar-Shalom V, Melendez Sivira Y, et al. Sperm selection using magnetic activated cell sorting (MACS) in assisted reproduction: a systematic review and meta-analysis. J Assist Reprod Genet. 2013;30(4):479-85.
9. Gnoth C. Definition and prevalence of subfertility and infertility. Hum Reprod. 2005;20:1144-7.
10. Gosálvez J, González-Martínez M, López-Fernández C, et al. Shorter abstinence decreases sperm deoxyribonucleic acid fragmentation in ejaculate. Fertil Steril. 2011;96(5):1083-6.

11. Ho CC, Tan HM. Treatment of the Hypogonadal Infertile Male—A Review. Sex Med Rev. 2013;1(1):42-9.
12. Hussein TM, Elariny AF, Elabd MM, et al. Effect of repeated sequential ejaculation on sperm DNA integrity in subfertile males with asthenozoospermia. Andrologia. 2008.
13. Jensen TK. Antioxidants and male subfertility: a survey of a Cochrane review. Ugeskr Laeger. 2011;173:3253-5.
14. Jeve YB, Potdar N, Blower JA, et al. Strategies to improve fertilisation rates with assisted conception: a systematic review. Hum Fertil (Camb). 2018;21(4):229-47.
15. Juárez Bengoa A, Díaz Pérez Mde L, Sánchez Martínez M, et al. Sperm capacitation with double ejaculate of short interval. A choice in assisted reproduction. Ginecol Obstet Mex. 2009;77(12):550-5.
16. Ko EY. Empirical medical therapy for idiopathic male infertility: a survey of the American Urological Association. J Urol. 2012;187:973-8.
17. Marshburn PB, Giddings A, Causby S, et al. Influence of ejaculatory abstinence on seminal total antioxidant capacity and sperm membrane lipid peroxidation. Fertil Steril. 2014;102(3):705-10.
18. Mayorga-Torres BJ, Camargo M, Agarwal A, et al. Influence of ejaculation frequency on seminal parameters. Reprod Biol Endocrinol. 2015;13:47.
19. Owen RC, Elkelany OO, Kim ED. Testosterone supplementation in men: a practical guide for the gynecologist and obstetrician. Curr Opin Obstet Gynecol. 2015;27(4):258-64.
20. Palmieri A, Imbimbo C, Longo N, et al. Ejaculatory abstinence influences intravaginal ejaculatory latency time: results from a prospective randomized trial. Urol Int. 2012;88(4): 459-62.
21. Patel DP, Chandrapal JC, Hotaling JM, et al. Hormone-based treatments in subfertile males. Curr Urol Rep. 2016;17(8): 56.
22. Sánchez-Martín P, Sánchez-Martín F, González-Martínez M, et al. Increased pregnancy after reduced male abstinence. Syst Biol Reprod Med. 2013;59(5):256-60.
23. Separation efficiency of a microfluidic sperm sorter to minimize sperm DNA damage. Fertil Steril. 2016;105(2):315-21.e1.
24. Showell MG. Antioxidants for male subfertility. Cochrane Database Syst Rev. 2011:CD007411.
25. Tadros NN, Sabanegh ES. Emperic medical therapy with hormonal agents for idiopathic male infertility. Indian J Urol. 2017;33(3):194-8.
26. Uppangala S, Mathai SE, Salian SR, et al. Sperm Chromatin Immaturity Observed in Short Abstinence Ejaculates Affects DNA. Integrity and Longevity In Vitro. PLoS One. 2016;11(4):e0152942.
27. Valenti D, La Vignera S, Condorelli RA, et al. Follicle-stimulating hormone treatment in normogonadotropic infertile men. Nat Rev Urol. 2013;10:55-62.
28. Valko M. Free radicals and antioxidants in normal physiological functions and human disease. Int J Biochem Cell Biol. 2007;39:44-84.
29. Vandekerckhove P. Clomiphene or tamoxifen for idiopathic oligo/asthenospermia. Cochrane Database Syst Rev. 1996;4: CD000151.

Azoospermia

23

Mohit Saraogi, HD Pai

INTRODUCTION

About 10–15% of all couples in the world suffer from infertility. In about 50% of these cases, the cause of the infertility can be attributed to a male factor.

Azoospermia, which is defined as the complete absence of sperm in the ejaculate is identified in approximately 1% of all men and in approximately 10–15% of all infertile men.[1.]

Azoospermia is often associated with underlying genetic conditions or predisposing medical conditions and hence requires detailed evaluation prior to further management. However, with the onset of assisted reproductive technology (ART) techniques such as intracytoplasmic sperm injection (ICSI), a number of azoospermic men are now able to produce their own biological children.

DIAGNOSIS AND DEFINITION OF AZOOSPERMIA

Azoospermia is defined as complete absence of sperm in the ejaculate sample. If no sperms are seen in the wet preparation of the semen sample, The World Health Organization (WHO) recommends centrifugation of the semen sample at 3,000 g for 15 minutes at room temperature followed by a high-powered microscopic examination of the pellet formed. If still no sperms are seen, a second semen analysis with similar centrifugation is repeated at least 2 weeks apart. If no sperms are seen in two successive samples, the man is labeled as azoospermic. If even a few sperms are seen in the pellet, the condition is described as cryptozoospermia.[2]

ETIOLOGY AND CLASSIFICATION OF AZOOSPERMIA

Azoospermia can be broadly classified into:

- Obstructive azoospermia (post-testicular azoospermia)
- Nonobstructive azoospermia (pretesticular and testicular azoospermia).

Obstructive azoospermia is less common than nonobstructive azoospermia and accounts for about 15–20% of all azoospermia cases.

Nonobstructive azoospermia can further be classified as:

- *Pretesticular azoospermia:*
    - This is caused by endocrine abnormalities due to disease or injury affecting the hypothalamo-pituitary axis. It is characterized by low levels of gonadotropins and sex steroids. It can be congenital or acquired.
    - Congenital causes of pretesticular azoospermia include conditions like Kallmann syndrome. Acquired causes of pretesticular azoospermia include conditions affecting the hypothalamus or the pituitary such as tumors, trauma, infection of the hypothalamus or pituitary or as a consequence of secondary adverse effects of medicines.
- *Testicular azoospermia:*
    - Testicular azoospermia is characterized by a failure of production of sperms at the level of the testis due to either congenital or acquired causes.
    - Congenital causes include cryptorchidism, Sertoli cell only syndrome (germ cell aplasia), Y chromosome microdeletion (YCMD), and other genetic

mutations such as Klinefelters syndrome (47 XXY), 47 XXY syndrome, mixed gonadal dysgenesis, pure testicular dysgenesis, and spermatogenesis arrest.
  - Acquired causes of testicular azoospermia include tumors, trauma, infection of the testis, torsion of testis, exposure to radiation or chemotherapy or as a consequence of adverse effects to medication.
- *Obstructive or post-testicular causes of azoospermia:*
  - These include congenital or acquired conditions, which have caused obstruction in the vas deferens, the ejaculatory ducts, or the epididymis.
  - Congenital conditions include congenital bilateral absence of vas deferens, Young's syndrome (triad of sinusitis, bronchiectasis, and obstructive azoospermia at the level of the epididymis), and congenital obstruction of ejaculatory ducts by Müllerian or Wolffian duct cysts.
  - Acquired causes of ductal obstruction would include vasectomy, accidental damage to vas deferens in hernia repair, and secondary to infections such as tuberculosis, which can cause blockage at different levels in the vas, epididymis, and the ejaculatory ducts.

EVALUATION OF AN AZOOSPERMIC MALE

History Taking

A good history taking is of paramount importance in evaluation of azoospermic males. Specific points to be evaluated during the history should any history of trauma to the genital organs in childhood, any history of childhood surgeries, cryptorchidism, or recent vasectomy. History of chronic substance abuse should also be elicited. Patients with testicular azoospermia have low testosterone levels leading to low sex drive causing dysfunctional coital life.

Systemic disease such as diabetes mellitus, cirrhosis of the liver, or chronic kidney disease can be associated with azoospermia, and specific history related to these should be taken. Previous malignancies need to be identified especially if treated with chemotherapy or radiotherapy.

Physical Examination

General Examination

A general examination of the height, stature, distribution of body hair, and development of secondary sexual characteristics is of utmost importance. Absence of body hair and failure of well-developed secondary sexual characteristics suggest testosterone deficiency, which suggests pretesticular or testicular causes of azoospermia. Gynecomastia, eunuchoid stature in the male, and previous surgery scars point toward specific causes of azoospermia.

Genital Examination

A systematic genital examination must be performed in a patient of azoospermia.

- *Testicular examination*: Presence of both the testis in the scrotal sac rules out persistent missed cryptorchidism.
- Bilateral testis must be examined for the size and consistency. The normal testicular dimensions are about 4 x 3 cm and the normal testicular volume is about 18–20 cc. In cases of defective spermatogenesis, the testis is smaller and soft in consistency. In such cases, the testicular volume will be less than 15 cc. This is because 85% of the testicular volume is accounted for by spermatogenesis at the level of the Sertoli cells. An exception to this rule are cases of Klinefelters syndrome, where the testicular volume is less than 5 cc but the testis is hard and stone like.
- Varicocele should be ruled out by examining the patient in both supine and standing up position. Grade 3 or 4 varicoceles can be associated with azoospermia in rare cases. However, azoospermia is not usually found in low-grade varicoceles.
- Examination of the penis may reveal other subtle abnormalities such as hypospadias. Conditions like micropenis may be found in Klinefelters Syndrome.
- Scrotal palpation can help to rule out conditions like congenital bilateral absence of vas deferens. Digital rectal examination helps in evaluating the size and consistency of prostate. The seminal vesicles may be palpable in cases of ejaculatory duct obstruction.

Semen Examination

A good semen examination can give us insight into the cause of azoospermia.

- *Semen volume:* A low semen volume less than 1.5 mL is usually found in the following conditions:
  - Ejaculatory duct dysfunction
  - Ejaculatory duct obstruction
  - Cases of retrograde ejaculation in which sperms can be isolated from the postcoital urine sample on centrifugation.

- *Semen PH:* A low semen PH goes in favor of obstruction at the level of the ejaculatory ducts.
- *Fructose in semen:* Absence or low levels of fructose in semen again suggest obstruction at the level of the ejaculatory ducts.

Radiological Examination

Scrotal USG to rule out varicocele, transrectal ultrasonography (TRUS), TRUS-guided seminal vesiculography, endorectal magnetic resonance imaging, abdominal USG, and cranial imaging are the various methods, which can be used to evaluate males with azoospermia.

Endocrinological Examination

The endocrinological examination primarily involves measurement of serum follicle-stimulating hormone (FSH), luteinizing hormone (LH), testosterone, prolactin, and a thyroid profile.

- Elevated prolactin levels can suppress gonadotropin-releasing hormone (GnRH) pulsatile release from the hypothalamus, occasionally causing azoospermia.
- Elevated FSH and LH levels with decreased testosterone levels suggest primary testicular failure.
- Low FSH, LH, and testosterone levels suggest hypogonadotropic hypogonadism
- A normal FSH, LH, and testosterone level in an azoospermic patient suggest an obstructive cause of azoospermia.

Testicular Biopsy

A testicular biopsy [testicular sperm extraction (TESE or micro TESE)] can be performed as a confirmation tool in cases of azoospermia. In cases, where the cause of azoospermia is obstruction at any level in the ejaculatory system, TESE or micro TESE should be able to yield adequate number of sperms to perform ICSI for the couple.

In conditions, where the FSH levels are normal, a testicular biopsy may help differentiate between a normally functioning testis and disorders of spermatogenesis such as maturation arrest, Sertoli cell only syndrome, etc.

Genetic Examination

A genetic examination and karyotyping should be performed in men with testicular causes of azoospermia. Cytogenetic tests such as YCMD test, and CFTR (cystic fibrosis transmembrane conductance regulator gene) mutation should be ruled out.

MANAGEMENT OF CASES OF AZOOSPERMIA

Obstructive Azoospermia

- *Reversal of obstruction:*
  - *Vasovasostomy*: This is the most commonly done procedure and is the gold standard for vassal reconstructive procedures. Following microsurgical vasovasostomy, the success rates have been reported at 86% patency rates and 52% pregnancy outcomes.
  - *Vasoepididymostomy*: This is done in cases of proximal vas blockage. About 20–40% couples achieve pregnancy through timed intercourse following vasoepididymostomy.
  - *Trans-urethral resection of ejaculatory ducts (TURED):* It is the treatment of choice in cases of ejaculatory duct obstruction. After TURED sperms return to the ejaculate in approximately 50–75% men and almost 20% men achieve pregnancy. Complications can include hematuria, hematospermia, urinary tract infection (UTI), and a watery ejaculate due to reflux of urine.
- Microsurgical sperm extraction from the testis by percutaneous epididymal sperm aspiration (PESA), testicular sperm aspiration (TESA), or micro TESE. The different methods of surgical sperm extraction include:
  - Percutaneous methods such as PESA and TESA.
  - In these methods, a wide bore needle is introduced into either the epididymis or the testis and testicular tissue including seminiferous tubules are aspirated out and examined under a microscope for viable sperms.
  - Incisional methods such as conventional testicular sperm extraction and microdissection testicular sperm extraction. Microdissectional TESE is known to have the highest sperm retrieval rate as compared to conventional TESE or TESA or PESA.
  - The sperms retrieved by such techniques can be utilized for performing ICSI.

Nonobstructive Azoospermia

This could be due to either a testicular failure or a failure of the hypothalamo hypophyseal pituitary axis to secrete adequate hormones to stimulate the testis to perform proper spermatogenesis. Intrinsic testicular impairment rarely responds to medication. Options of management include:

- *Human chorionic gonadotropin (hCG) supplementation:* Biweekly or thrice a week administration of hCG 2,500 units subcutaneously for 3–6 months can induce spermatogenesis. This is especially useful in cases of hypogonadotropic hypogonadism.
- *Follicle-stimulating hormone and gonadotropin administration*: FSH in doses of 37.5 IU–150 IU thrice a week for 3–6 months especially in conjunction with hCG administration can significantly improve spermatogenesis. FSH is known to help in the completion of spermiogenesis.
- *Antioxidant administration*: The role of antioxidants in management of cases of spermatogenesis arrest is highly debatable with a number of papers both supporting and opposing the outcomes. The proponents suggest that increased oxidative stress can cause spermatogenesis arrest and this can be reversed by prolonged use of antioxidants.
- *Aromatase inhibitors*: In men with nonobstructive azoospermia having low testosterone levels and high estradiol levels, administration of aromatase inhibitors such as letrozole or anastrozole can help to correct this imbalance by preventing the peripheral conversion of testosterone to estradiol. This correction is knows to facilitate spermatogenesis by increasing intratesticular levels of testosterone.
- *Management of varicocele associated nonobstructive azoospermia:* In rare cases, grade 3 and 4 varicocele may be associated with nonobstructive azoospermia with raised FSH levels. Surgical correction of the varicocele is known to restore sperm in the ejaculate in up to 44% patients according to a recent review.[3,4] As the restoration of sperm to the ejaculate is often transient, it is often advisable to freeze the semen sample containing the sperm for future use.
- *Genetic evaluation of patients with nonobstructive azoospermia:* This may reveal a variety of conditions such as Klinefelters syndrome, YCMD, etc. This diagnosis requires concurrent management with a genetic counselor who can advise on the impact of the genetic condition on the health of the patients as well as the possibility of successful surgical sperm retrieval through microdissection techniques. In conditions such as YCMDs, where the patient harbors complete AZFa or AZF b deletion the patient should be advised to opt for donor sperm. Patients having AZF c YCMD should be forewarned that any male child that they may conceive will also likely suffer from nonobstructive azoospermia.
- *Pulsatile administration of GnRH agonist:* GnRH can be administered subcutaneously or intravenously or intranasally. It is used as a second-line treatment when treatment with gonadotropins fails. It will only be effective, if the man has an intact pituitary gland. The dose administered is 5–20 μ subcutaneously every 2 hours for 12–24 months. Spermatogenesis results in 77% of azoospermic men. However, it is an expensive treatment and the frequency of doses makes compliance an issue. It is again useful in cases of hypogonadotropic hypogonadism.

Men with nonobstructive azoospermia with high serum FSH levels and low testosterone levels are likely to have a lower chance of sperm retrieval by any other surgical sperm retrieval techniques. They will benefit from donor sperm treatment or adoption.

REFERENCES

1. Cocuzza M, Alvarenga C, Pagani R. Epidemiology and etiology of azoospermia. Clinics Sao Paulo. 2013;68 (suppl 1): 15-26.
2. Gudeloglu A, Parekattil S. Update in the evaluation of the azoospermic male. Clinics Sao Paulo. 2013;68(suppl 1): 27-34.
3. Esteves SC, Miyaoka R, Roque M, et al. Outcome of varicocele repair in men with nonobstructive azoospermia: systematic review and meta-analysis. Asian J Androl. 2016;18(2): 246-253.
4. Practice Committee of the American Society for Reproductive Medicine. Management of nonobstructive azoospermia: a committee opinion. Ferti Steril. 2018;110:1239-45.

Oligozoospermia

24

Vineet Mishra, Pawan Dhir

INTRODUCTION

Infertility is a major issue faced by the married couples globally. According to World Health Organization (WHO), 60–80 million of married couple worldwide live under the stress of infertility. The burden of infertility affecting the Indian couples ranges between 3.9% and 16.8%.[1] Male factor infertility accounts for 40–50% of the cases with about 2% of the men having suboptimal semen parameters. On an average male infertility affects 1 in 20 men.[2]

Male factor infertility accounts to altered semen parameters in terms of low sperm concentration and/or decreased motility and/or altered morphology in at least one sample of two semen, analyzed at 1 week and 4 weeks apart. The most common presentation in males is a suboptimal sperm count, which is termed as oligozoospermia. The term oligospermia is defined as sperm density below the fifth centile in fertile men that is a sperm count below 15 million spermatozoa/mL.[1] Male infertility in 90% of cases is centered around sperm count. The abnormal semen parameters are positively associated with sperm count.[1]

NORMAL SEMEN ANALYSIS (WHO REVISED LOWER REFERENCE LIMITS)

- *Volume*: 1.5 mL [95% confidence interval (CI): 1.4–1.7]
- *Sperm concentration*: 15 million spermatozoa/mL (95% CI: 12–16)
- *Total sperm number*: 39 million spermatozoa per ejaculate (95% CI: 33–46)
- *Morphology*: 4% normal forms (95% CI: 3–4), using "strict" Tygerberg method
- *Vitality*: 58% live (95% CI: 55–63)
- *Progressive motility*: 32% (95% CI: 31–34)
- *Total (progressive + nonprogressive motility):* 40% (95% CI: 38–42).

OLIGOZOOSPERMIA RISK FACTORS

Semen quality may be affected by varied factors, it may be environmental, occupational, or a genetic cause. Thus pining down one particular risk factor or a causative factor for oligozoospermia is difficult.[3] Semen quality can be affected by occupational hazard like working in hot environment or causing mechanical trauma on the pelvic contents. Environmental factors like psychological stress, toxins, etc. affect the sperm count.

Health issues like weight gain or febrile illness can have a significant impact on the semen quality, decreasing the count. Stress is another cardinal factor, which can affect sperm parameters and it reduces sperm morphology.[3] Stress causes hormonal imbalance resulting in reducing levels of testosterone, progesterone, cortisol, and prolactin. Varicocele causes deterioration of semen quality by decreasing the sperm count and morphology. Repair of varicocele shows improvement in semen quality.

The severity of oligospermia is graded as follow:

- *Mild oligospermia*: 14–5 million sperm/mL
- *Moderate oligospermia*: 5–1 million sperm/mL
- *Severe oligospermia*: Less than 1 million sperm/mL.

Pretesticular causes:

- Central cause causing hormonal imbalance
- Health issues like febrile illness
- Food habits, smoking, and drinking.
- Microdeletions in the Y chromosome.

Testicular causes:
- Cryptorchidism
- Hydrocele
- Genital injuries
- Varicocele.

Post-testicular causes:
- Obstruction in vas deferens
- Absent vas deferens
- Inflammation in the urethra.

It is seen that oligozoospermia related to hormonal imbalances due to stress and high fevers with inflammation of the testicular zone is reversible. However, those due to genetic cause or testicular atrophy is irreversible.

CONDITIONS ASSOCIATED WITH OLIGOZOOSPERMIA

Androgen Deficiency

Androgen deficiency can affect spermatogenesis. A morning sample for serum testosterone should be evaluated. In case of subnormal levels, serum LH is done. It is imperative to evaluate the patient for secondary testicular failure in case of low undetectable serum gonadotropin and testosterone levels with or without persistent hyperprolactinemia.

Asymptomatic cases of mildly elevated LH levels do not warrant treatment with testosterone. However, follow-up is essential. In case of overt symptoms of androgen deficiency, testosterone therapy may be given only after the infertility issue is addressed. If not sperm, cryopreservation should be done followed by testosterone replacement. Testosterone replacement will suppress the gonadotropin levels by negative feedback and thus suppressing spermatogenesis.

Genetic Defect

Oligozoospermia may often be associated with chromosomal aberration. Most common associated chromosomal anomaly is autosomal translocation and inversions accounting for 3% of the cases, whereas sex chromosome anomalies are associated with 1.6% cases. The prevalence of chromosomal anomalies is 8- to 10-fold higher in infertile men as compared to fertile men even in the absence of any phenotypic features.[2]

Fertility is often normal in these men expect for a lower sperm count while some may be azoospermic. The risk of chromosomal anomalies like trisomy 21 or 13, or of uniparental disomy is significantly increased in the offsprings born to these patients. 0.7% of severely oligo- or azoospermic men may have reciprocal translocation between an autosome and sex chromosome or autosome. Genes responsible for spermatogenesis may be interrupted by breakpoints causing meiotic arrest or sperm that are chromosomally unbalanced.[2] In oligozoospermic men with sperm densities of 0.1–5 million/mL, the prevalence of Yq microdeletion is approximately 4%, however, in case of azoospermia, the prevalence is still higher. 60% of Y microdeletions are formed by the AZFc deletion where one-third have severe oligozoospermia, while another third the sperm is surgically recoverable for ART.

Secondary Testicular Failure

Hypothalamo-pituitary disorders can lead to secondary testicular failure. It can lead to hypogonadotropic hypogonadism (HH) leading to androgen deficiency may be attributed to certain adult-onset disease like surgery, radiotherapy, pituitary adenoma, hemochromatosis, and trauma.

Hypogonadotropic Hypogonadism

Low undetectable gonadotropin and testosterone, with or without persistent elevated prolactin may warrant the diagnosis of HH.

The HH may result from Hyperprolactinemia of any cause (adenoma drug-related, idiopathic) thus affecting fertility. Macroprolactinoma is the most common of functional lesion leading to androgen deficiency and pressure symptoms (headache and visual field defects) but less frequently, these patients may present with infertility due to sexual dysfunction and/or oligozoospermia.

Systemic Illness and Drug Effects

A number of drugs can affect the release of gonadotropin-releasing hormone (GnRH) causing HH. Chronic use of opioids or glucocorticosteroids can suppress GnRH release. Antipsychotic drugs are known to cause HH by inducing hyperprolactinemia. Severe systemic illness and malnutrition are also known to affect GnRH release leading to androgen deficiency and oligozoospermia.

Sex Steroid Suppression of Hypothalamic-pituitary-testis Axis

Prolong exposure to exogenous androgens may lead to an undetectable level of serum LH and low sex hormone-binding globulin (SHBG). Serum testosterone may be high.

However, synthetic androgens (e.g. nandrolone) do not cross-react in the testosterone immunoassay thus giving a false negative result of low or undetectable testosterone levels. With cessation of exposure, sperm output return back to normal by 3–12 months.

Endogenous Sex Steroid Production

Oligozoospermia and infertility secondary to HH may result in patients with sex steroid-secreting adrenal or testicular neoplasms.

Environmental Insults causing Oligozoospermia

The germ cell lineage can be readily damaged in patients undergoing Chemo- and radiotherapy for malignant or other diseases. Salazopyrin is the classic drug causing reversible oligozoospermia.

Evaluation of a Case of Oligozoospermia

The evaluation of male infertility is centered around the semen analysis report, which forms the decisive factor for further investigations. A normal semen report virtually rules out any, endocrine abnormalities, and further hormonal evaluation is not needed. However, in case of abnormal semen, thorough historical, physical, and laboratory evaluations need to be performed, in order to pinup a specific diagnosis.[4]

SEMEN ANALYSIS

Semen is collected after 3-4 days of sexual abstinence in the aseptic condition in the clean, dry, sterile, and leak-proof container. The sample is taken to the laboratory for further analysis without any delay. Temperature should be maintained to 37°C **(Fig. 1, Flowchart 1, and Table 1)**.

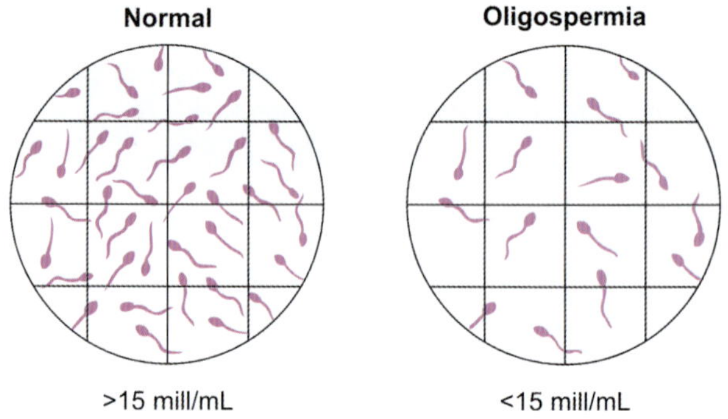

Fig. 1: Semen analysis.

Flowchart 1: Semen analysis algorithm.

Abnormal semen analysis
↓
FSH, LH, T, PRL

- **Hypergonadotropic hypogonadism** ↑FSH, ↑LH, ↓T
  → R_x:
  - T replacement
  - Donor insemination
  - IVF
  - Micromanipulation
- **Testicular injury** ↑FSH, nl LH, nl T
  → R_x:
  - Donor insemination
  - IVF
  - Micromanipulation
- **Eugonadotropic oligoazoospermia** nl FSH, nl LH, nl T
  → **Rule out:**
  - Infection
  - Autoimmunity
  - Varicocele
  - Obstruction
  - Retrograde ejaculation
  → **Idiopathic oligospermia**
  → R_x:
  - Empiric
  - IUI
  - Donor insemination
  - IVF
  - Micromanipulation
- **Partial androgen insensitivity** nl FSH, ↑LH, ↑T
  → R_x:
  - Donor insemination
  - IVF
  - Micromanipulation
- **Hypogonadotropic hypogonadism** ↓FSH, ↓LH, ↓T
  → **Rule out:**
  - Hyperprolactinemia
  - Mass lesion
  - Adrenogenital syndrome
  → R_x:
  - Gonadotropins
  - GnRH

(FSH: follicle stimulating hormone; IVF: in vitro fertilization; LH: luteinizing hormone; PRL: prolactin; nl: normal; ↑: high; ↓: low)

Table 1: Semen classification based on an average between two samples.

	Potential for natural coception		
Variables	***High***	***Moderate***	***Low***
Volume (mL)	>2	1–2	<1
Concentration (x 10^6/mL)	>20	10–20	<10
Motility (% motile)	>50	40–50	<40
Morphology (% normal)	>14* >30**	4–14* 20–30**	<4* <20**

*Classified according to Kruger strict criteria, 1986.
**Classified according to World Health Organization, 1999.

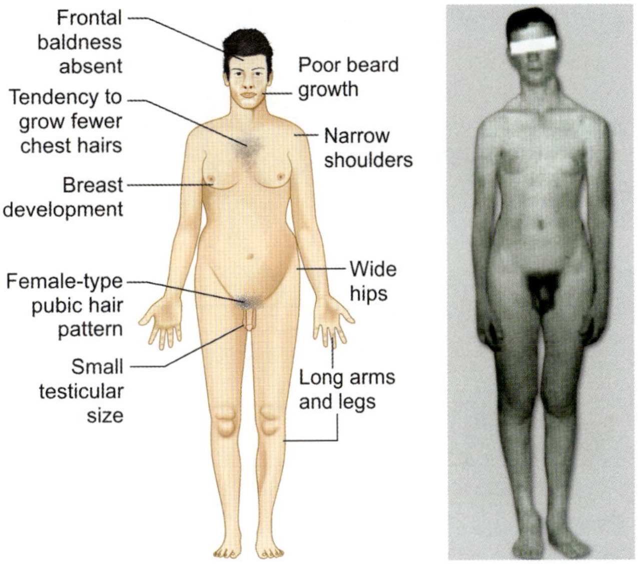

Fig. 2: Klinefelter's syndrome.

Semen Analysis Algorithm

The semen analysis algorithm has been given in **Flowchart 1.**

HISTORY

History forms a pivotal part in evaluating a couple with male factor infertility. It is essential to differentiate between primary and secondary infertility. A complete medical and sexual history should be obtained. It is imperative that we identify those few patients who have a treatable specific etiology.

Starting with the onset of puberty it is important to determine, if pubertal development and virilization was normal or not. Patient's sexual history including changes in libido, potency, etc. should be evaluated. History of any endocrine or anatomic abnormality like hypospadias, microphallus is asked for. Any voiding difficulty or changes in voiding pattern including and medical history of diabetes mellitus or neuropathology should be obtained.

Any insult at the testicular level like testicular torsion, infection, mumps, and genitourinary surgery should be ruled out. Any history of exposure to excessive heat should be asked for, especially at work place. Environmental exposure to toxins plus and history addiction should be asked for. Alcohol smoking, etc. can have severe impact on decreasing sperm count. Any history of abuse of anabolic steroids common in athletes must be ruled out. Any malignant condition treated with chemotherapy or irradiation can permanently damage the germ cells. There are commonly used medications (e.g. allopurinol, spironolactone, valproic acid, ketoconazole, cimetidine, sulfasalazine, cyclosporine, diethylstilbestrol, colchicine, nitrofurantoin, minocycline, and calcium-channel blockers) that can adversely affect semen parameters.

PHYSICAL EXAMINATION

A complete physical examination of external genitalia including secondary sexual characteristics should be examined. Attention should be paid to virilization of external genitalia. Any systemic disease including evaluation of genitourinary system to rule out hypospadias should be done. Testicular size should be measured and extracorporeal location of testis should be confirmed. The epididymis and prostate palpated to detect tenderness or swelling, indicative of possible infection, or obstruction. Look for gynecomastia. Rule out Klinefelter's and Kallmann's syndromes **(Fig. 2)**.

Examination of bilateral vasa deferentia and spermatic cord is done. Congenital absence of vas is ruled out. Spermatic cord examination in standing and supine position is done to rule out varicocele. Rule out retrograde ejaculation **(Fig. 3)**.

LABORATORY TESTING IN OLIGOZOOSPERMIA

Hormonal profile including serum testosterone, luteinizing hormone (LH), and follicle stimulating hormone (FSH) are performed on a morning sample. Sperm density and serum FSH are inversely related, in patients with primary

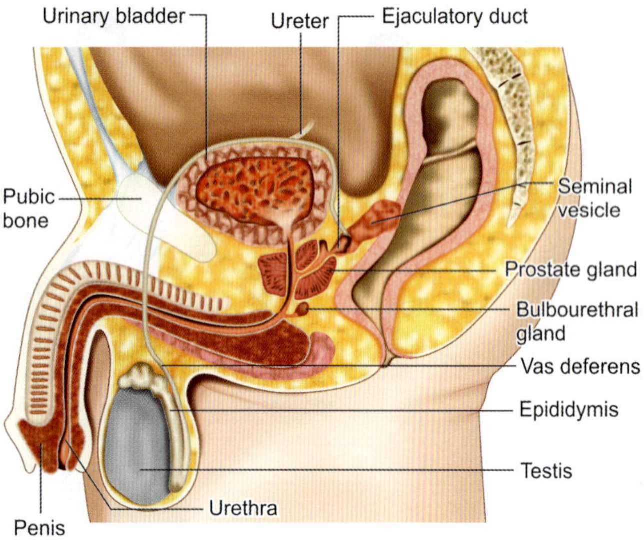

Fig. 3: Male reproductive tract.

spermatogenic failure, reflecting reduced feedback by Sertoli cell inhibin B secretion. Elevated FSH levels are seen in case of nonobstructive azoospermia thus differentiating it from obstructive azoospermia, which has normal FSH levels. A consensus value for the upper limit in reproductively normal young men across 7 immunoassays was 8.4 IU/L; similarly, 7.6 IU/L was found most discriminatory in testicular biopsy-determined obstructive versus nonobstructive azoospermia.

Patients with primary spermatogenic failure have a serum FSH of about 8 IU/L, which is suggestive of the diagnosis, while a value of 12 IU/L makes it certain as the cause for oligozoospermia.

TREATMENT

Lifestyle Modification and Age

Obesity has found to have a positive correlation between oligozoospermia and subfertility (but not always), many potential explanations are offered, however, beneficial effect of weight loss on fertility outcome is unclear. Smoking has shown to have detrimental effect on the semen parameters causing oligozoospermia, poorer sperm DNA integrity, and health of offspring.

IDIOPATHIC OLIGOZOOSPERMIA

About 30% of couples with sperm densities of 1–5 million/mL conceive spontaneously over a 2–3 years period. Indeed well-powered placebo-controlled, randomized clinical trials (RCTs) have shown many proposed therapies to be ineffective in improving live birth rates.

Clomiphene or Aromatase Inhibitors

These agents cause a rise in the gonadotropins levels by the relief of estrogenic feedback, and/or by a reduction in intratesticular estrogen exposure. Evidence is limited, and no agents are approved for this indication.

Clomiphene citrate in the dose of 25 mg daily for 25 days with 5 days rest is given for 3 months.[5]

HYPOGONADOTROPIC HYPOGONADISM

Sperm production is obtained in 50–80% of patients, treated with gonadotropins for HH with high (40–80%) pregnancy rates.

In couples with HH, attempting to have children the usual dose of hCG is 1,000–2,500 IU, two to three times per week, intramuscularly (IM) or subcutaneously (SC). Human menopausal gonadotropin (hMG), IM or SC, or highly purified or recombinant FSH, at the dose of 75, 100, or 150 IU, SC, three times per week, is used. If the HH has not been treated for a long period with gonadotropins or the patient has received only testosterone before, initial monotherapy with hCG for stimulation of their own testosterone production is recommended for 4–6 weeks, adding hMG thereafter. The onset of spermatogenesis can be observed in more than 90% of patients. The average time taken for the spermatozoa to appear in the ejaculate is 6–9 months; however, in individual patients this period can be much longer

REFERENCES

1. Kumar N, Singh AK. Trends of male factor infertility, an important cause of infertility: A review of literature. J Hum Reprod Sci. 2015;8(4):191-6.
2. McLachlan RI. Approach to the patient with oligozoospermia. J Clin Endocrinol Metab. 2013;98(3):873-80.
3. Hadi P, Ahmadi HR, Yasemi M, et al. Prevalence and Risk Factors of Oligospermia in Infertile Men. J Clin Diagnost Res. 20148(9):FC11-3.
4. Damani M, Shaban S, Glob libr women's med. (2008). Medical Treatment of Male Infertility. [online] Available from: https://www.glowm.com/section_view/heading/Medical%20Treatment%20of%20Male%20Infertility/item/333 [Last Accessed February, 2019].
5. Patankar SS, Kaore SB, Sawane MV, et al. Effect of clomiphene citrate on sperm density in male partners of infertile couples. Indian J Physiol Pharmacol. 2007;51(2):195-8.

Sperm DNA Fragmentation: Methods to Determine, Clinical Implications and Approaches of its Reduction

25

Himanshu Patel, Vidisha Bhatt, Madhuri Patel

INTRODUCTION

The term *infertility* described by World Health Organization (WHO) and the American Society for Reproductive Medicine (ASRM) is that when within a 1-year of time if the woman is not able to conceive without use of any contraceptive method.[1] In infertile couple, the male part contributes to 20% the prime cause of infertility while rest 30–40% because of both male and the female partners.[2]

The chromatin structure and the DNA integrity of sperm, both are important for effective fertilization and transmission of the genome to the future generation.[1] The sperm DNA fragmentation (SDF) test is the substantial tool to determine the integrity of DNA that is ultimately the predictive marker for the fertility in men. Though there are some disagreements regarding performing the assay but the fact resides in that there is a higher level of DNA fragmentation in semen from infertile men as compared to fertile ones. The increased level of DNA fragmentation not only causes the fertilization failure but also is the reason for spontaneous pregnancy loss. Higher level of DNA fragmentation index (DFI) also obstructs assisted reproductive techniques (ART) outcomes in terms of fertilization of oocyte, quality of embryo, clinical pregnancy and live birth rate.[3]

There are various methods to determine DNA fragmentation in sperm.[4] The most routinely used laboratory methods are sperm chromatin structure assay (SCSA), terminal deoxynucleotidyl transferase dUTP nick end labeling (TUNEL) and sperm chromatin dispersion assay (SCD or Halo test).[3]

STANDARD SEMEN ANALYSIS

Since long the fertility tests for men has been depend mostly on a basic semen analysis criteria, which evaluates semen volume, sperm concentration, sperm morphology, vitality and motility. Though many couples are facing difficulties related to infertility and the reasons are not clear. This can be interpreted as a basic semen analysis is insufficient when it comes to assessing male fertility potential. Though it beneficial to check for the number of motile sperm that are morphologically normal in shape, it does not provide the amount of DNA fragmentation that ultimately contributes to a successful pregnancy.

Under the routine semen analysis procedure, followed by liquefaction, semen samples are evaluated for volume, pH, viscosity and appearance. The semen analysis is performed as per the WHO guidelines to determine the concentration and motility of the sperm. Vitality can be determined by eosin-nigrosin stain and the morphology by preparing smear and staining with papanicolaou stain.[5]

SPERM DNA FRAGMENTATION

The chromatin structure of the sperm is highly compact and stable, and is organized in a specific manner to achieve the unique condense state. These condense state of DNA organization provides more secure transfer of genetic information to the next generation from the paternal side to the oocyte.[6] Mammalian sperm DNA is structurally different in organization from that of somatic cell **(Fig. 1)**.[7] During the compaction of chromatin structure, the transition of histone protein takes place. The histone proteins are replaced by

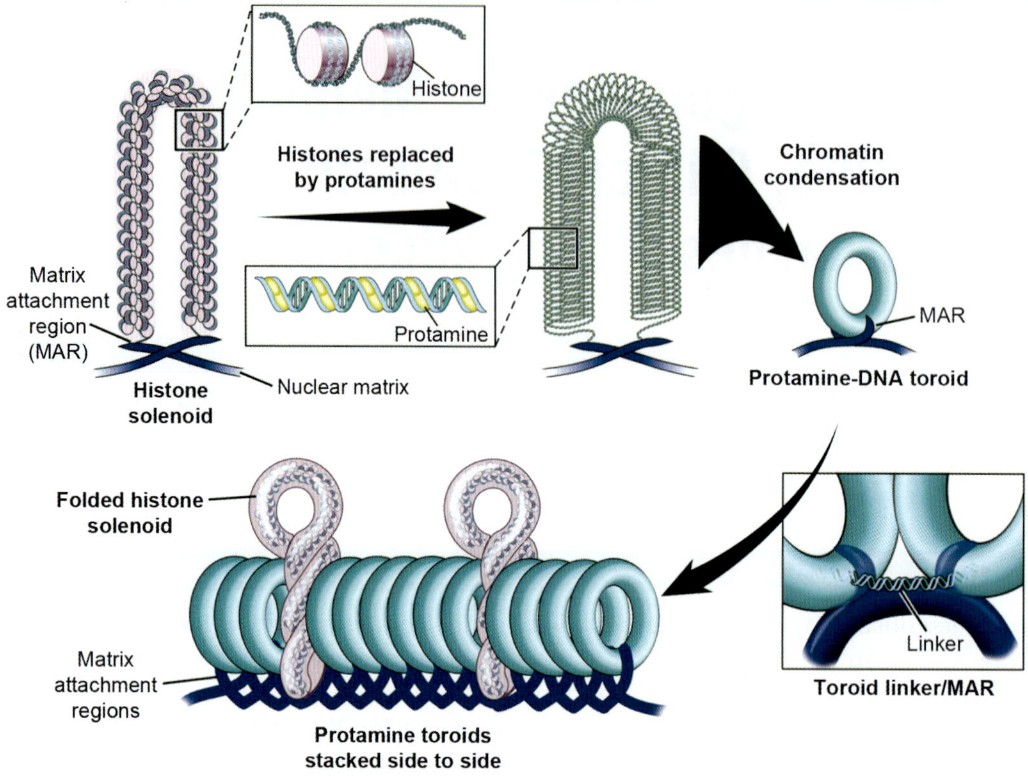

Fig. 1: Sperm DNA organization.
Source: Agrawal A, Singh A. Sperm DNA damage and antioxidant use: roles in male fertility. In: Parekattil S, Agarwal A (Eds). Male Infertility. New York: Springer; 2012. pp. 307-15.

the protamines (P1, P2) that are mainly responsible for the final condensation and stabilization of DNA of the sperm. The DNA of the sperm then interacts with the protamines and converts the coiled DNA into toroidal subunits called "Doughnut loops".[6]

The abnormal development of DNA loop domain and histone-protamine replacement enhances the defects and that can arise at any stage of the process. The endogenous nicks assist to form DNA loop and is consider as reducing the torsional stress. During the transition of elongated spermatids from round and before complete protamination the nicks are thought to form. Topoisomerase II helps to create the loop domain and the defect in packaging of the DNA in sperm causes the infertility in male. The increase in the internal DNA break is enhanced by the enzyme inhibitors that prevents the repair and increases the susceptibility of DNA toward the damage.[6]

Causes of Sperm DNA Fragmentation

The main cause for DNA fragmentation and DNA base oxidation is oxidative stress that is caused after release of sperm from the testis.[8] The concentration of reactive oxygen species (ROS) increases when the excess production is not being neutralized by the cellular antioxidants.[6]

External factors have thought to be the main cause for the DNA damage like change in lifestyle, exposure to radiation, heat and medications. Lifestyle as cigarettes, recreational drugs, and caffeine all have an impact on the amount of DNA damage found in spermatozoa. These factors are either directly linked with rises in strand breaks or indirectly via secondary oxidative methods **(Fig. 2)**.[6]

CLINICAL CONSEQUENCES OF SPERM DNA FRAGMENTATION

The chromatin integrity of sperm is directly correlated with the fertility of men, as it has been found that in the unexplained conditions the routine semen analysis parameters appears normal while the percentage of DFI appears higher. The quality of embryo, development of the embryonic stage and the ongoing pregnancy is related to the concentration of DNA fragmentation in the sperm.[6] The semen with a lesser amount of DNA fragmentation is

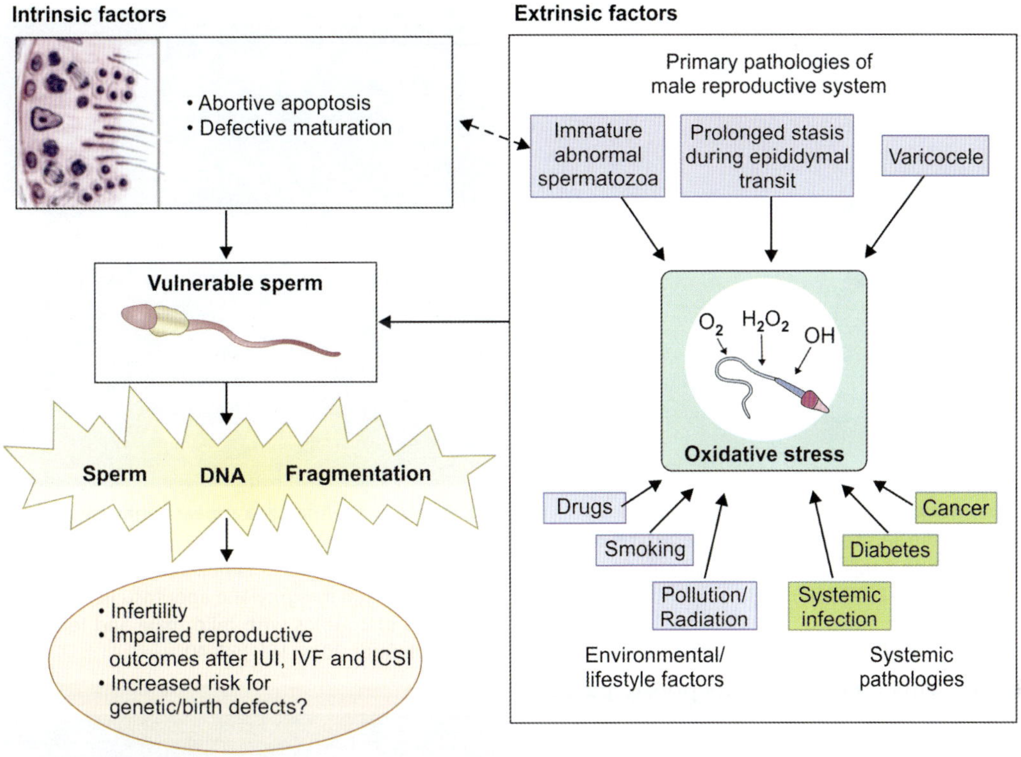

Fig. 2: Factors affecting DNA fragmentation.
Source: Cho CL, Agarwal A. Role of sperm DNA fragmentation in male factor infertility: a systematic review. Arab J Urol. 2018;16(1):21-34.

associated with the less time to achieve natural pregnancy as compared to the semen with higher level of DNA fragmentation.[9]

Methods to Determine Sperm DNA Fragmentation

For clinical use of a sperm, DNA test must have strong predictive capacity for pregnancy with slight overlap among fertile and infertile samples. The tests to determine DNA fragmentation includes acidic aniline blue (AAB) and toluidine blue (TB) stains, SCD test, chromomycin A3 (CMA3), DNA breakage detection–fluorescence in situ hybridization assay (DBD–FISH), in situ nick translation (NT), and flow cytometric-based sperm chromatin structure assay (SCSA). The regularly less used method is high-performance liquid chromatography (HPLC).[10]

Acidic Aniline Blue Stain

In this procedure the core or the processed samples can be used to prepare the slides. Prepare smear by placing 5 µL of the sample on the slide and allow it to get air dry. Fix the slide with 3% glutaraldehyde in phosphate buffer saline (PBS) for 30 minutes. Drain the excess solution and cover the slide with 5% aqueous aniline blue solution (pH 3.5) for 5 minutes is taken on the slide. Slides are prepared by smearing 5 µL of either raw or washed semen sample. The slides are air-dried and fixed for 30 minutes in 3% glutaraldehyde in phosphate-buffered saline (PBS). The smear is dried and stained for 5 minutes in 5% aqueous aniline blue solution (pH 3.5). The sperm with immature nuclear chromatin is stained blue, while those with mature nuclei do not take up the stain.[10] This is a simple and inexpensive technique requiring a simple bright field microscope for analysis **(Fig. 3)**.

Chromomycin A3 Assay

Prepare the smear and fix with 3:1 of methanol-glacial acetic acid solution at 4°C for 20 minutes. Drain the excess solution and allow the slides to get air dry at room temperature for 20 minutes. Overlay 100 µL CMA3 solution over the slide and treat for 20 minutes. Rinse the slide with buffer and mount with 1:1 v/v PBS-glycerol. Keep the slide at 4°C overnight and evaluate next day using fluorescence microscope for emission of fluorescence. The spermatozoa with bright yellow fluorescence are CMA3 positive while

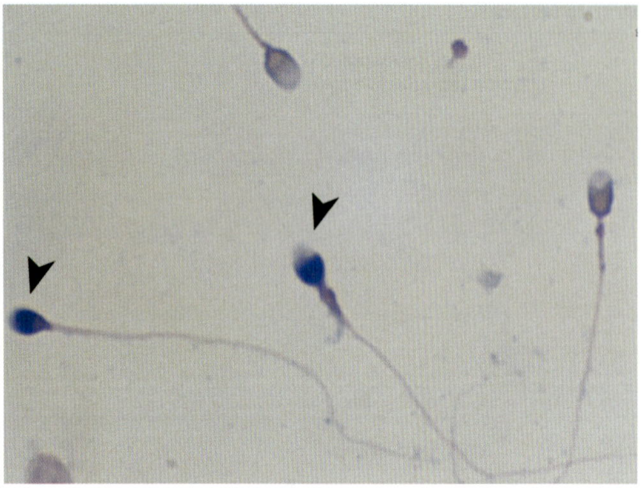

Fig. 3: Immature sperm stained dark blue by eosin stain.
Source: Kim HS, Kang MJ, Kim SA, et al. The utility of sperm DNA damage assay using toluidine blue and aniline blue staining in routine semen analysis. Clin Exp Reprod Med. 2013;40(1):23-8.

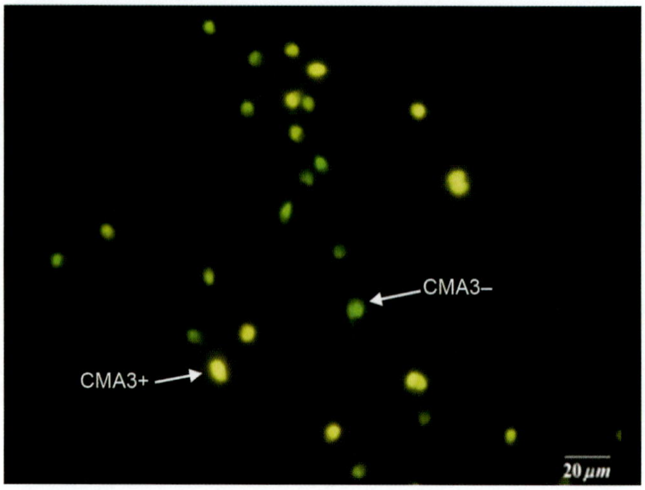

Fig. 4: CMA3+ spermatozoa appear bright yellow; CMA3- spermatozoa appear yellowish green.
Source: Khalili MA, Nazari S, Firouzabadi RD, et al. Comparing the roles of sperm chromatin integrity and apoptosis in intrauterine insemination outcomes of couples with mild male and female factor infertility. J Reprod Infertil. 2014; 15(1):35-40.

the spermatozoa with dull yellow fluorescence are CMA3 negative **(Fig. 4)**.[10] This method reveals poorly packed chromatin.

Acridine Orange Assay

Prepare the smear and fix the slide in Carnoy's fixative (methanol:acetic acid, 1:3) for at least 2 hours. Stain the slide with AO buffer solution for 5 minutes and rinse gently with deionized water. The spermatozoa emitting green color indicated intact DNA while spermatozoa emitting spectrum of yellow-orange to red color indicated fragmented DNA. This is a fast, simple and inexpensive method to perform.[10] Lack of test reproducibility makes AO a less reliable test of SDF.

The Comet Assay

The comet assay is a second generation SDF analysis test. The sperms are embedded in an agarose matrix and are treated with hypertonic lysis solution containing non-ionic detergents that eliminates the cytoplasm, nucleoplasm and the cell membrane. Then the sperms are treated with high alkali solution that unwinds super coiled DNA and enhances the labile sites which appears as break. When the charge is applied via electrophoretic system the fragmented part travels toward anode and forms comet like structure.[11] Hence it is termed as comet assay. This method is sensitive, have reproducible results, estimate both single and double stranded break. DNA damage can be assessed from even low concentration of sperm, quantifies actual amount of DNA damage per sperm **(Fig. 5)**.

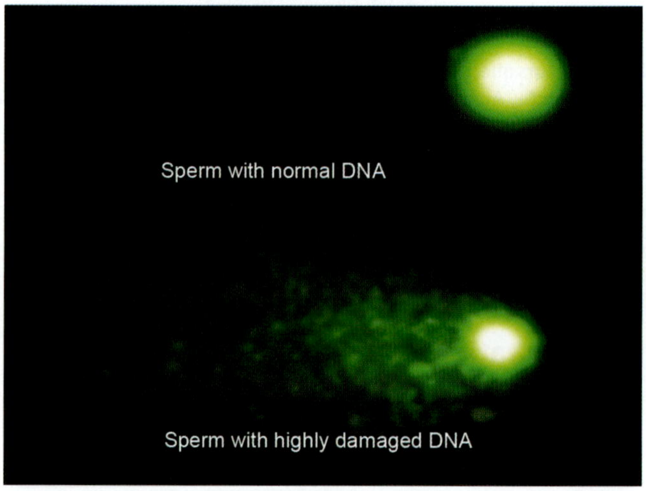

Fig. 5: Visual scoring of DNA damage.
Source: Chi HJ, Chung DY, Choi SY, et al. Integrity of human sperm DNA assessed by the neutral comet assay and its relationship to semen parameters and clinical outcomes for the IVF-ET program. Clin Exp Reprod Med. 2011;38(1):10-7.

TUNEL Assay

To determine the DNA fragmentation by TUNEL assay, initially fix the sperm with 1% formaldehyde for 10 minutes at room temperature. Wash the sample with PBS by centrifuging the sample at 10,000 *g* for 4 minutes. Resuspend the pellet in 100 μL prewash buffer containing single-strength One-Phor-All® buffer for 10 minutes at room temperature. The sample is then centrifuged again

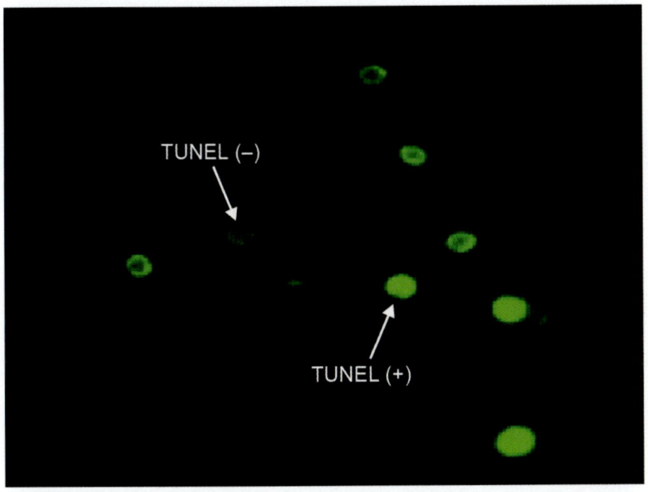

Fig. 6: Under fluorescence microscopy normal DNA (non-apoptotic sperm) was is seen light green and damaged DNA (apoptotic sperm) was is seen bright green.

Source: Ghasemzadeh J, Talebi AR, Khalili MA, et al. Sperm parameters, protamine deficiency, and apoptosis in total globozoospermia. Iran J Reprod Med. 2015;13(8):495-502.

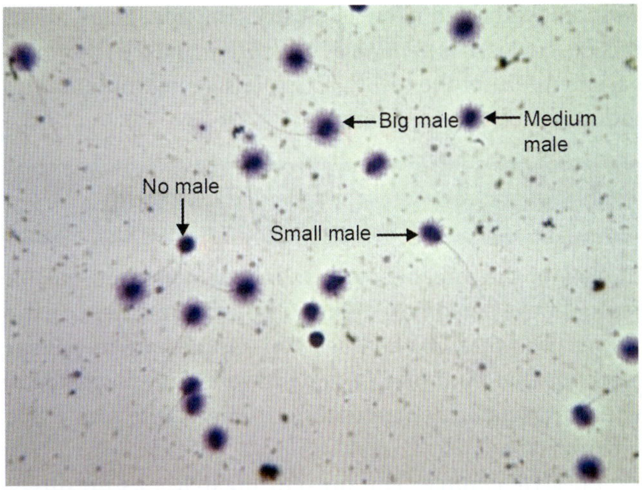

Fig. 7: Under bright field microscopy, sperm with normal DNA shows big halo.

resuspended in 50 µL of TdT buffer (3 µmol/L biotin-16-dUTP, 12 µmol/L deoxyadenosine triphosphate (dATP), 0.1% Triton X-100, and 10 U of TdT enzyme) and incubated at 37°C for 60 minutes. Then wash the sample twice with PBS and then fix the sperms in 100 µL of staining buffer (0.1% Triton X-100 and 1% streptavidin/Texas red antibiotin) and incubated for 30 minutes in dark at 4°C **(Fig. 6)**. Interpret the result by flow cytometer.[10,12] This is an extremely sensitive and reliable assay, samples can be stored for longer time after fixing but costly and time consuming.

The Sperm Chromatin Structure Assay

The SCSA method provides high reproducibility of result, rapid and accurate estimation of the percentage of DNA damage. All the steps are performed at 4°C, the sample is diluted with TNE buffer (0.15 mol/L NaCl, 0.01 mol/L Tris, 0.001 mol/L EDTA, pH 7.4) for the final concentration of sperm less than or equal to 2×10^6 sperm/mL. A 200-µL of the suspended sperm solution is mixed with 400 µL of a low-pH detergent solution (0.15 mol/L NaCl, 0.08N HCl, 0.01% Triton X-100, pH 1.4). Add 1.2 mL staining solution (6 µg/mL AO, chromatographically purified in 0.2 mol/L Na_2HPO_4, 1 mmol/L disodium EDTA, 0.15 mol/L NaCl, 0.1 mol/L citric acid monohydrate, pH 6.0) after 30 seconds in the above mentioned mix, and place the sample into the flow cytometer sample chamber.[10] The results are analyzed with the help of the software where a scatter plot is created, displaying the ratio of green and red sperm. The sperm with the fragmented DNA gives red emission and sperm with intact DNA gives green emission.

Sperm Chromatin Dispersion Assay

The principle of the SCD test is based on interpreting the difference between the fragmented and the non-fragmented DNA in the spermatozoa depending on the formation of halos. When the embedded sperms are exposed to the buffer solution, the membrane and the proteins are removed resulting in the formation of nucleoids with a central core and a peripheral halo of dispersed DNA loops. The dispersion of halos depends on the amount of DNA fragmentation in the sperm. The spermatozoa with the intact DNA shows big halos while spermatozoa with the fragmented DNA shows minimal or no halos. The halos are visualized either by fluorescent stain or by bright field microscopy stain.[13]

The SCD assay is a kit based method and in that the semen sample is diluted with flushing media/PBS to get the concentration of 15–20 million/mL. Mix the diluted semen sample with melted agarose and pipette onto the precoated slides. Cover the mix of semen and melted agarose with coverslip and place the slide at 4°C to solidify the gel. Remove the coverslip gently and process rest of the steps on horizontal position. The sperms are then treated with acid solution for 7 minutes followed by lysis solution for 20 minutes. Wash the slide with 20 mL of distilled water and dehydrate sequentially with 70%, 90%, and 100% ethanol. Allow the slide to get air dry and then stain with mix of Giemsa staining solution and PBS (1:1) for 10–15 min with continuous airflow **(Fig. 7)**. Briefly wash the slides with tap water and allow to air dry. The advantage about this method is, *it is available in kit format*, easy to perform, easy to interpret the result, no expensive instrumentation require, cheap and convenient.[14]

APPROACH TO REDUCE SPERM DNA DAMAGE

In view of the impact sperm DNA fragmentation has on reproductive outcomes, it is important to implement on the preventive measures and develop appropriate treatment methods that minimize DNA damage in the spermatozoa used in assisted reproduction. Some of the strategies include:

- *Lifestyle change:* The present lifestyle has no direct impact on spermatogenesis via fragmentation of sperm DNA. The prevalence of overweight young couples in the reproductive age of life is steadily increasing. Obesity is also associated with male fertility because of lifestyle changes, internal hormonal environment alterations, and sperm genetic factors. Avoid consumption of alcohol, smoking tobacco, physical stress, radiations, hot bath, ingestion of acrylamide and glycidamide containing foods. It ultimately reduces sperm count, motility and morphology.[15]
- *Short abstinence:* The short abstinence and repeated ejaculation has been a potential means in reducing SDF in raw semen. The reduction of 22–25% in DNA fragmentation is observed when the ejaculatory abstinence is 1–2 days without any change in the conventional semen parameters. Antibiotics are effective in reducing the DFI when it caused because of an infection.[16-18]
- *Role of antioxidants:* Certain amounts of free radicals are required for the normal sperm function but the excess amount affects the sperm function, fertilization potential and offspring health. Free radicals are engrossed from the food or environment. The use of oral antioxidants and daily ingestion of vitamin C and E decreases SDF.[16]
- *Varicocelectomy:* Varicocele repair is an efficient method to increase sperm with the normal DNA than the level of DNA fragmentation in the patient with the varicocele.[16]
- Laboratory methods
    - *Sperm preparation method:* Sperm preparation should be aimed at minimizing damage to the spermatozoa and can be accomplished by performing density gradient wash.[19-22]
    - Sperm selection method
        - *Morphologically selected sperm injection (IMSI):* It is designed with advances in microscope optics and computer enhancement of digital images. Newly designed lenses and microscope condensers allow 600X magnification. IMSI allows to see the sperm head in a lot more detail, and in particular features inside the sperm head which are thought to be associated with incorrect packing of DNA.[23]
        - *Hyaluronic acid:* Sperm binding to hyaluronic acid is one of the methods of sperm selection for intracytoplasmic sperm injection (ICSI), commercial products of hyaluronic acid coated slides and/or petri dishes are available for clinical use.[24] The ability of sperm bindings to hyaluronic acid is documented as being related to normal sperm morphology, maturity and DNA integrity.[25,26] Remolding of the sperm plasma membrane occurs, leading to the formation of hyaluronic acid binding sites during late spermatogenesis. Therefore, the presence of hyaluronic acid binding sites on the sperm plasma membrane can be considered as a sign of sperm maturity.[27] However, the ability of hyaluronic binding for identifying functional better quality sperm is limited as compare to routine techniques.[28] There is some evidence that using these sperms may increase the pregnancy rate and reduce the miscarriage rate.[29]
        - *Microfluidics:* Microfluidics is a pump-less hydrostatic pressure device in which the sperm swim through laminar flows to reach a collecting area for motile sperm **(Fig. 8)**. This device differentiates motile sperm from immotile sperm,

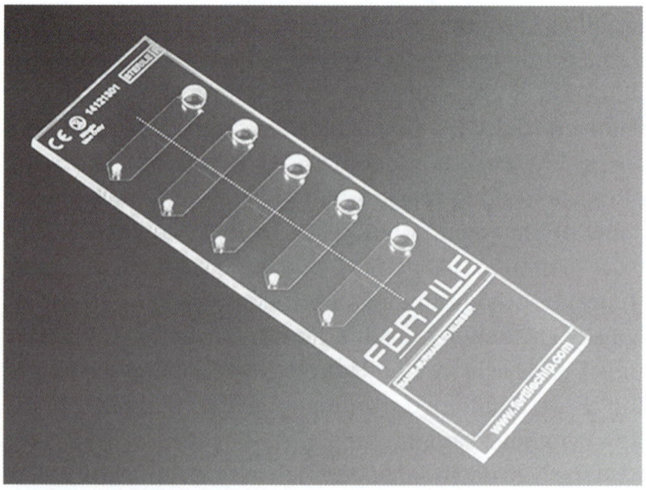

Fig. 8: Microfluidics chamber.

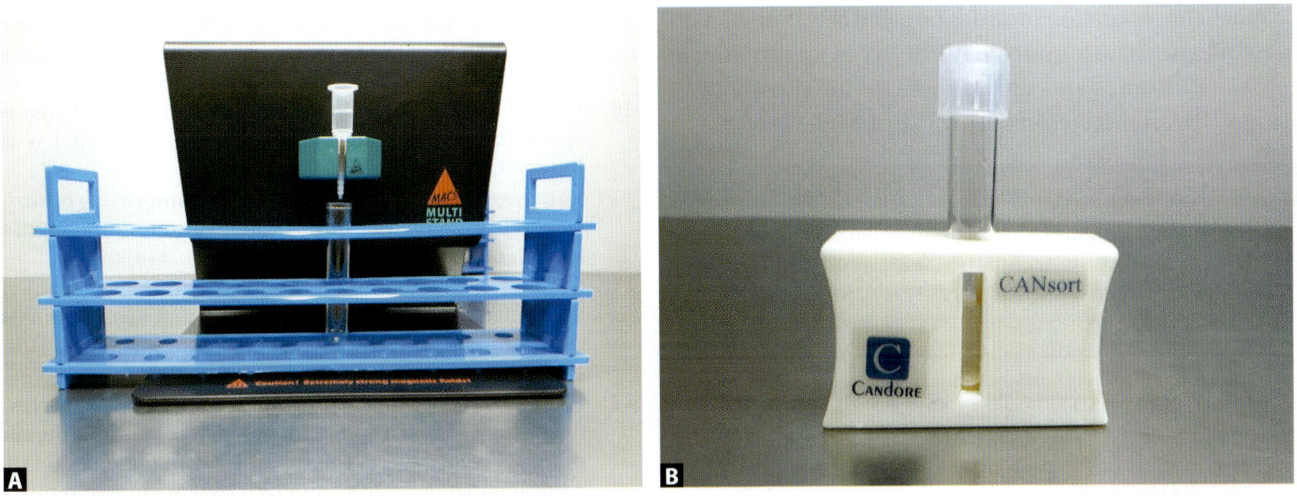

Figs. 9A and B: Sperm separation via (A) MACS or (B) CANsort method.

dead sperm or dead cells, and debris in raw semen, and thus opened a new era of applications in ART.[30-33] As the number of sperms retrieved by this method is very less this methodology is only suitable to perform ICSI.

- *Sperm sorting using magnetic separator:* Magnetic cell separation is an efficient method to select non-apoptotic sperm. Apoptosis (programmed cell death) is a physiological phenomenon that involves a series of morphological and biochemical changes that eventually result in cellular death.[34] Apoptosis-related features have been reported in human spermatozoa. It has been suggested that damage to the plasma cellular membrane occurs at an early stage of apoptosis that precedes extensive nuclear damage and irreversible apoptosis. The extrusion of phosphatidylserine (PS), which is normally present in the inner leaflet of the plasma membrane, to the outer surface has been identified as one of the early apoptotic changes in human spermatozoa. Externalization of PS (EPS), mitochondrial dysfunction, and nuclear DNA damage are all markers of sperm apoptosis that were detected at significantly higher levels in infertile men and those with varicoceles.[35,36] This is a non-invasive method and effectively reduces the sperm with the fragmented DNA and the non-apoptotic sperm from the apoptotic one.[37] The technique employs paramagnetic microbeads (~50 nm) conjugated with annexin V, a 35–36 kDa phospholipid binding protein, which has a selective affinity to bind with PS.[38] As one of the early manifestations of apoptosis, EPS allows for binding with annexin V microbeads and separation of spermatozoa using a CANsort System (Candore Bioscience, India) or MACS system (MiltenyiBiotec, Germany) **(Figs. 9A and B)**. The magnet included in the system retains the apoptotic sperm labeled with microbeads. The unlabeled spermatozoa can be considered as non-apoptotic and collected for use in IUI/IVF/ICSI.

CONCLUSION

Semen analysis is a primary test to evaluate male fertility in spite of its limitations of its prediction for reproductive outcome. Sperm DNA fragmentation assessment is a useful tool to predict IVF and ICSI outcomes. Various literatures show correlation between Sperm DNA fragmentation and outcome in IVF and ICSI though there are certain limitations to draw any conclusion due to the heterogeneity of the study material. Though the etiology and implication of sperm DNA fragmentation is incomplete, it still provides an additional information regarding its role in development and maintenance of pregnancy. SCSA, TUNEL and SCD are the widely used method to determine sperm DNA fragmentation. As the advantage of SCD method over other is its availability as a kit format, easy to perform and interpret the result is the reason it is widely accepted. Routine sperm preparation techniques such as swim up or DGC can isolate motile, morphologically normal sperm but they lack the ability to specifically target sperm based on apoptosis manifestations. Separation of good quality sperm via magnetic separation provides targeted selection of non-apoptotic spermatozoa prior to IVF/ICSI can prevent similar negative outcomes and should increase the possibility of using a DNA-intact sperm during IVF/ICSI.

REFERENCES

1. Durmaz A, Dikmen N, Gundus C, et al. Fluctuation of "sperm DNA integrity" in accordance with semen parameters, and it's relationship with infertility. J Assist Reprod Genet. 2014;31:1665-71.
2. Schulte R, Ohl D, Sigman M, et al. Sperm DNA damage in male infertility: etiologies, assays, and outcomes. J Assist Reprod Genet. 2010;27:3-12.
3. Mohamed A, Bardisi H. Clinical implication of DNA fragmentation in male infertility. Transl Androl Urol. 2017;6(4):S656-S657.
4. Evenson DP, Wixon R. Clinical aspects of sperm DNA fragmentation detection and male infertility. Theriogenology. 2006;65(5):979-91.
5. WHO. WHO Laboratory Manual for the examination and processing of human semen, 5th edition. Geneva: WHO; 2010.
6. Hekmatdoost A, Lakpour N, Sadeghi MR. Sperm chromatin integrity: etiologies and mechanisms of abnormality, assays, clinical importance, preventing and repairing damage. Avicenna J Med Biotech. 2009;1(3):5-9
7. Singh A, Agarwal A. The Role of Sperm Chromatin Integrity and DNA Damage on Male Infertility. Open Reproduct Sci J. 2011;3:65-71.
8. Tamburrino L, Marchiani S, Montoya M, et al. Mechanisms and clinical correlates of sperm DNA damage. Asian J Androl. 2012;14:24-31.
9. Cho CL, Agarwal A. Role of sperm DNA fragmentation in male factor infertility: a systematic review. Arab J Urol. 2018;16(1):21-34.
10. Agarwal A, Said TM. Sperm chromatin assessment. In: Gardner DK, Weissman A, Howles CM (Eds). Textbook of Assisted Reproductive Techniques. New York: CRC Press; 2012. pp. 93-106.
11. Nandhakumar S, Parasuraman S, Shanmugam MM, et al. Evaluation of DNA damage using single-cell gel electrophoresis (Comet Assay). J Pharmacol Pharmacother. 2011;2(2):107-11.
12. Sharma R, Masaki J, Agarwal A. Sperm DNA fragmentation analysis using the TUNEL assay. Methods Mol Biol. 2013;927:121-36.
13. Amar E, Cornet D, Cohen M, et al. Treatment for high levels of sperm dna fragmentation and nuclear decondensation: sequential treatment with a potent antioxidant followed by stimulation of the OneCarbon Cycle vs One-Carbon Cycle Back-up Alone. Austin J Reprod Med Infertil. 2015;2(1):1006.
14. Fernández JL, Muriel L, Rivero MT, et al. The Sperm Chromatin Dispersion Test: A Simple Method for the Determination of Sperm DNA Fragmentation. J Androl. 2003;24(1):59-66.
15. Esteves SC, Agarwal A, Majzoub A. Comparison of strategies to reduce sperm DNA fragmentation in couples undergoing ICSI. Transl Androl Urol. 2017;6(Suppl 4):S570-S573.
16. Pons I, Cercas R, Villas C, et al. One abstinence day decreases sperm DNA fragmentation in 90% of selected patients. J Assist Reprod Genet. 2013;30:1211-8.
17. Campagne D. Can male infertility be improved prior to assisted reproduction through the control of uncommon considered factors? Int J Fertil Steril. 2013;6(4):214-23.
18. Larson KL, Brannian JD, Timm BK, et al. Density gradient centrifugation and glass wool filtration of semen remove spermatozoa with damaged chromatin structure. Hum Reprod. 1999;14(8):2015-9.
19. Hammadeh ME, Kuhnen A, Amer AS, et al. Comparison of sperm preparation methods: Effect on chromatin and morphology recovery rates and their consequences on the clinical outcome after in vitro fertilization embryo transfer. Int J Androl. 2001;24(6):360-8.
20. Tomlinson MJ, Moffatt O, Manicardi GC, et al. Interrelationships between seminal parameters and sperm nuclear DNA damage before and after density gradient centrifugation: implications for assisted conception. Hum Reprod. 2001;16(10):2160-5.
21. Marchetti C, Obert G, Deffosez A, et al. Study of mitochondrial membrane potential, reactive oxygen species, DNA fragmentation and cell viability by flow cytometry in human sperm. Hum Reprod. 2002;17(5):1257-65.
22. O'Connell M, McClure N, Powell LA, et al. Differences in mitochondrial and nuclear DNA status of high-density and low-density sperm fractions after density centrifugation preparation. Fertil Steril. 2003;79(Suppl 1):754-62.
23. Schuster TG, Cho B, Keller LM, et al. Isolation of motile spermatozoa from semen samples using microfluidics. Reprod Biomed Online. 2003;7:75-81.
24. Huszar G, Ozkavukcu S, Jakab A, et al. Hyaluronic acid binding ability of human sperm reflects cellular maturity and fertilizing potential: Selection of sperm for intracytoplasmic sperm injection. Curr Opin Obstet Gynecol. 2006;18:260-7.
25. Huszar G, Jakab A, Sakkas D, et al. Fertility testing and ICSI sperm selection by hyaluronic acid binding: Clinical and genetic aspects. Reprod Biomed Online. 2007;14(5):650-63.
26. Nasr-Esfahani MH, Razavi S, Vahdati AA, et al. Evaluation of sperm selection procedure based on hyaluronic acid binding ability on ICSI outcome. J Assist Reprod Genet. 2008;25(5):197-203.
27. Said T, Mahfouz R, Del Valle A. Advanced sperm selection techniques for intracytoplasmic sperm injection. In: Gardner DK, Weissman A, Howles CM (Eds). Textbook of Assisted Reproductive Techniques. New York: CRC Press; 2012. pp. 117-27.
28. Worrilow KC, Eid S, Woodhouse D, et al. Use of hyaluronan in the selection of sperm for intracytoplasmic sperm injection (ICSI): significant improvement in clinical

outcomes—multicenter, double-blinded and randomized controlled trial. Hum Reprod. 2013;28(2):306-14.
29. Erberelli RE, Salgado RM, Mendes Pereira DH, et al. Hyaluronan-binding system for sperm selection enhances pregnancy rates in ICSI cycles associated with male factor infertility. JBRA Assist Reprod. 2017;21(1):2-6.
30. Tsai VFS, Chang HC, Hsieh JT, et al. M. Application of microfluidic technologies to the quantification and manipulation of sperm. Urological Sci. 2016;27(2):56-9.
31. Schuster TG, Cho B, Keller LM, et al. Isolation of motile spermatozoa from semen samples using microfluidics. Reprod Biomed Online.2003;7:75-81.
32. Park JY, Kricka LJ. Male infertility and microchips. Clin Chem. 2013;59:457-8.
33. Kjelland ME, Stroud T, Ayliffe HE, et al. Portable automated microfluidic device for rapid determination of sperm counts. Reprod Fertil Dev. 2013;26:203-4.
34. Vaux D, Korsmeyer S. Cell death in development. Cell. 1999;96:245-54.
35. Bucar S, Ana Gonçalves A, Rocha E, et al. DNA fragmentation in human sperm after magnetic-activated cell sorting. J Assist Reprod Genet. 2015;32:147-54.
36. Nandhakumar S, Parasuraman S, Shanmugam MM, et al. Evaluation of DNA damage using single-cell gel electrophoresis (Comet Assay). J Pharmacol Pharmacother. 2011; 2(2):107-11.
37. Said TM, Grunewald S, Paasch U, et al. Advantage of combining magnetic cell separation with sperm preparation techniques. Reprod Biomed Online. 2005;10:740-6.
38. Grunewald S, Paasch U, Glander HJ. Enrichment of non-apoptotic human spermatozoa after cryopreservation by immunomagnetic cell sorting. Cell Tissue Bank. 2001; 2(3):127-33.

Ultrasound and Color Doppler in Infertility

26

Narendra Malhotra, Diksha Goswami, Jaideep Malhotra

INTRODUCTION

Ultrasound is one of the most indispensable investigation as far as an infertile couple is concerned. A comprehensive ultrasound examination can replace multiple diagnostic tests needed in an infertile female often at different sites and over multiple visits. Two-dimensional (2D) ultrasound is a primary tool to evaluate the pelvis and can be combined with a three-dimensional (3D) scan to enable volume reconstruction. Color Doppler adds valuable information for the diagnosis and treatment of infertile female. Dynamic changes of the menstrual cycle in a reproductively active female are picked up very well by transvaginal color Doppler and definite conclusions can be drawn regarding the diagnosis, prognosis, and treatment of infertile patients.

ROLE OF ULTRASOUND AND DOPPLER IN INFERTILE COUPLE

- Help in understanding the anatomy and physiology and rule out major pelvic pathologies
- To predict fertility potential before starting infertility treatment by means of antral follicle count (AFC) to determine the ovarian reserve
- To monitor intrauterine insemination (IUI) and in vitro fertilization (IVF) cycles, decide dose and type of drugs.
- Prediction of the response to ovarian stimulation in assisted conception, assessment of oocyte quality based on perifollicular flow and parameters influencing implantation following embryo transfer using Doppler.
- To prevent complications in assisted reproduction technology (ART) like hyperstimulation or poor response to stimulation.

BASELINE SCAN IN INFERTILITY

Baseline scan is a performed between day 3 and day 7 of the cycle. It is known as a baseline scan because at this time of the cycle, endometrium is thin like a single line as it has shed off during menstruation and this is an absolute baseline status of the ovaries. It should comprise of a systematic approach in which first transabdominal scanning should be done, following which after emptying the bladder transvaginal scanning for cervix, uterus, and bilateral ovaries. All the findings should be documented and saved electronically. The proposed sequence of examination is to evaluate the uterus first using both 2D and 3D ultrasound to determine the appearance and symmetry of the endometrium, myometrium, and junctional zone, and to rule out the presence of congenital or acquired anatomic abnormalities. The adnexa should be evaluated next for any tubal or ovarian pathology and for evidence of polycystic ovaries. The sonohysterogram performed at this juncture allows detailed evaluation of the endometrial cavity combining with hystero-contrast sonography (HyCoSy) to test for tubal patency.

Technical Aspects of Transvaginal Sonography

Transvaginal sonography (TVS) probe consists of a head, shaft, and handle (grip). It may be straight or bend type. Straight probes one better for examination, bent probes may be better for TVS-guided interventional procedures. An ideal set up should have privacy, a female attendant should be present and a comfortable gynecological chair.

Cervix

Cervix is evaluated for echotexture cervicitis, nabothian cysts, and cervical mucus **(Fig. 1)**.

Uterus

Transvaginal ultrasound is done to rule out any myometrial, endometrial abnormalities, or uterine anomalies. The uterus should be scanned completely in transverse and sagittal planes. Imaging of the uterus helps in identifying pathologies like fibroids, adenomyosis, polyps, and congenital malformations. Fibroids appear as hypoechoic, well defined, and discrete masses with distal acoustic shadowing on 2D scan with peripheral blood flow **(Fig. 2)**.[1] Different sonographic features of adenomyosis include globular uterus, poor definition of the endometrial–myometrial junction, asymmetrical thickening of the anterior or posterior wall **(Fig. 3)**, anechoic lacunae or cysts of poorly circumscribed areas within the myometrium 1–7 mm diameter, subendometrial echogenic linear striations, and heterogeneous myometrium.[2] Polyps usually appear as echogenic structures within the endometrium, often containing a feeder vessel easily demonstrated with color Doppler imaging **(Table 1)**.

Endometrium: The endometrial cavity should be visualizable as a separate entity within the uterus in virtually all menstruating patients. It is generally centrally located in the uterus. Endometrium might be difficult to visualize in axially positioned uteri or in case of uterine rotation due to endometriosis or previous surgery-related adhesions. Endometrial thickness is measured in sagittal plane at maximum thickness including both endometrial layers placing the callipers at two opposite endometrial-myometrial interface. In case of fluid, thickness of both single layers is measured and is added **(Fig. 4)**. Assessment of the endometrial morphology should include endometrial echogenicity **(Figs. 5A to D)**, endometrial midline **(Figs. 6A to D)**, and endometrial-myometrial interface.[3]

The cyclic histologic changes and changes in the thickening of the endometrium with hormonal stimulation can be imaged using transvaginal ultrasound during the different phases of the menstrual cycle. Sakamoto described the characteristic sonographic image noted during the menstrual cycle in 1985.[4,5] The proliferative endometrium is characterized by:

- The presence of a well-defined three line sign
- A hypoechogenic functional layer
- A minimal or absent posterior acoustic enhancement.

The three line sign is formed by the central hyperechoic reflection representing the endometrial cavity and the additional hyperechoic reflection representing the thin developing layer of endometrium. There is also a surrounding hypoechoic halo.

Luteal phase endometrium is (1) hyperechoic; (2) posterior enhancement is present; and (3) three line sign and halo are absent.

Various studies have compared endometrial thickness in predicting pregnancy outcome in ART cycles with varied results. Although an appropriate conclusion has not been made, it is accepted that a very thin endometrium below 7 mm negatively impacts implantation rates.

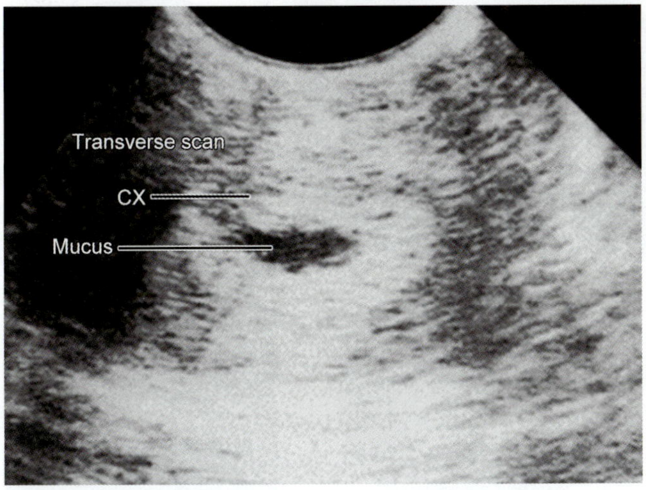

Fig. 1: Cervical mucus.

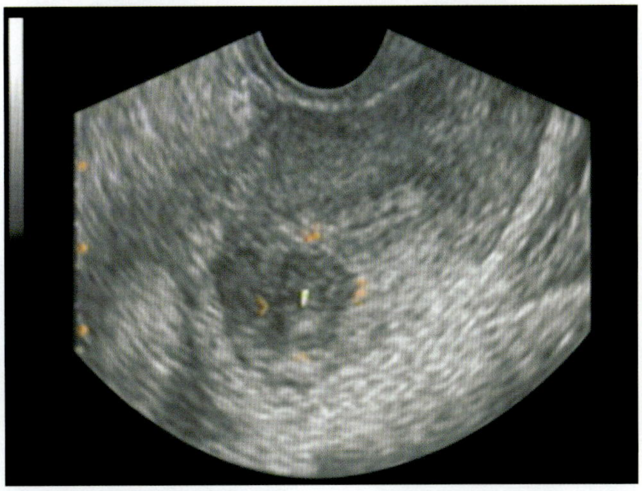

Fig. 2: Fibroid.

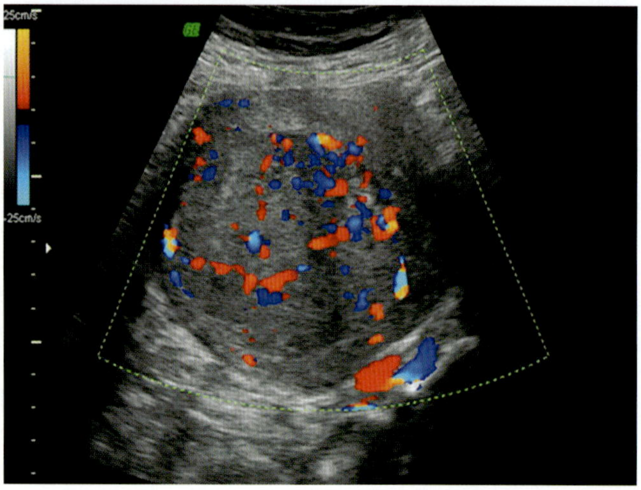

Fig. 3: Penetrating vessels in adenomyosis.

Tubes

Fallopian tubes are isoechoic and cannot be normally seen on ultrasound unless pathological or fluid surrounds the tubes. 3D ultrasound is the key to differentiating a tubal from an ovarian mass because the entire tube can be

Table 1: Distinguishing features between fibroid and adenomyoma.

Fibroid	*Adenomyoma*
▪ Iso-hypoechoic ▪ Cavity distorting ▪ Distal acoustic shadowing ▪ Doppler-peripheral draping vessel	▪ Hyperechoic ▪ Cavity displacing ▪ Pencil line/streaky shadows ▪ Doppler-penetrating vessel

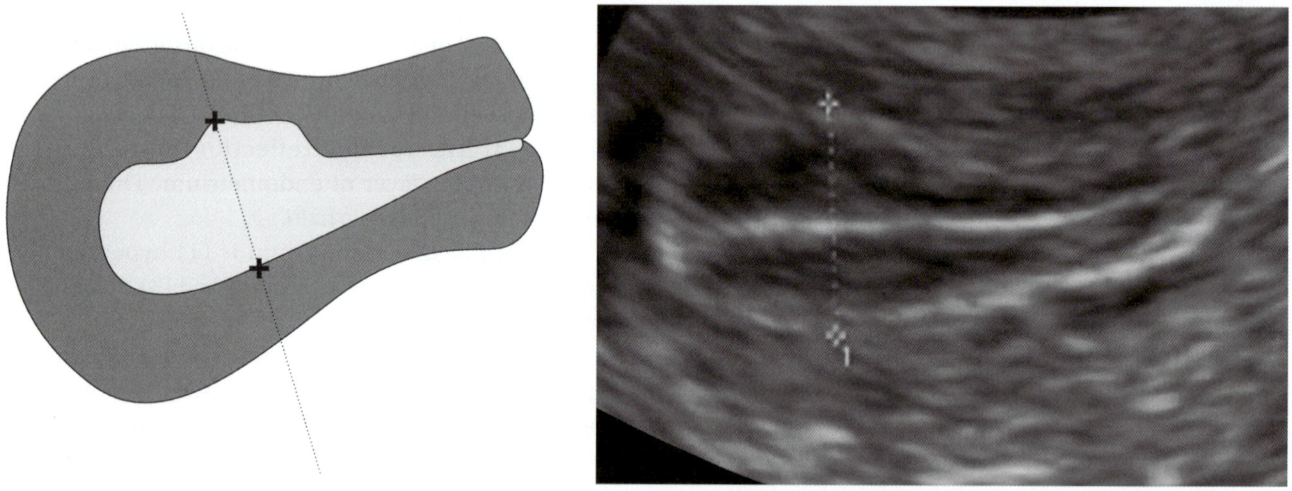
Fig. 4: Measurement of endometrial thickness.

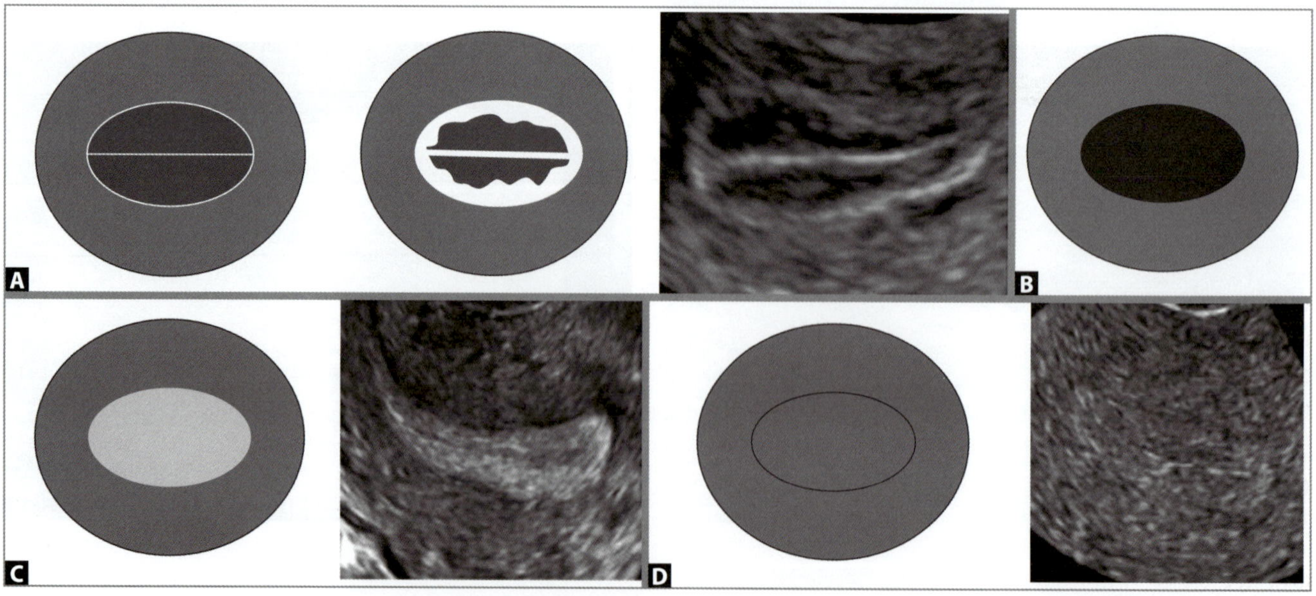

Figs. 5A to D: Endometrial echogenicity (A) Hypoechoic; (B) Iso; and (C and D) Hyperechoic.

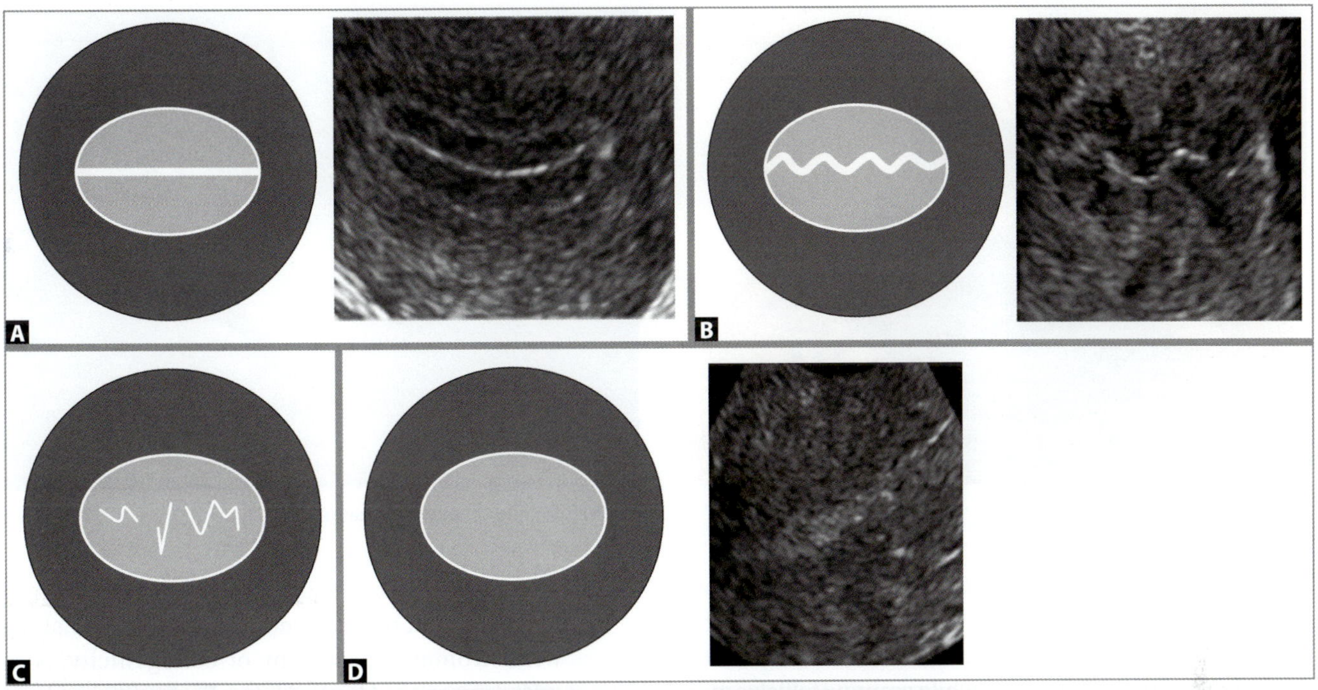

Figs. 6A to D: Endometrial midline—(A) Linear; (B) Nonlinear; (C) Irregular; and (D) Not defined.

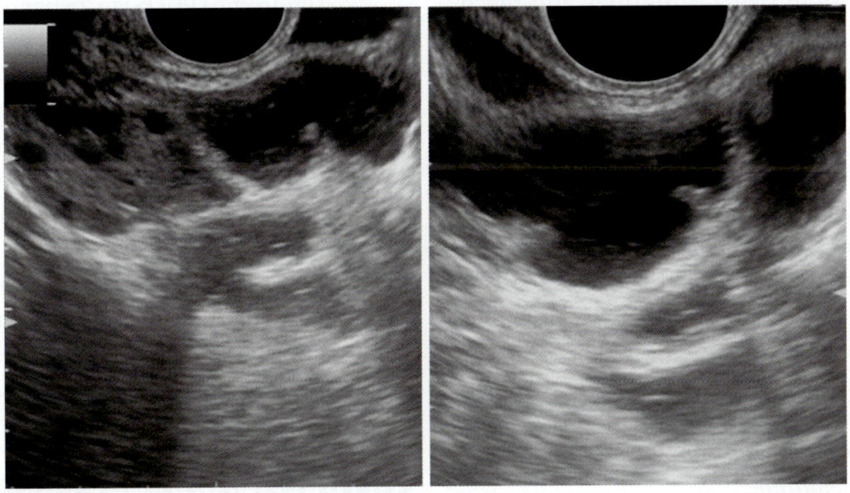

Fig. 7: Hydrosalpinx.

displayed within the volume. On 2D scan, hydrosalpinx usually appears as a fusiform cystic lesion, cogwheel sign, and adnexal cyst with incomplete septae and has a thickened cyst wall in all acute inflammations **(Fig. 7)**.

Ovary

The TVS is the modality of choice for imaging of the ovaries and detects common pathologies. The ovaries are placed medial to the internal iliac vessels on either side of the uterus. TVS can accurately track follicular development, predict, and confirm ovulation.

- *Antral follicle count*: Healthy antral follicles more than 2 mm usually respond to follicle stimulating hormone (FSH) stimulation and reflect the primordial follicle pool, being described as "selectable". A scan to determine the AFC should be performed in the early follicular phase of the menstrual cycle when there are less chances of including coexisting ovarian cysts or the corpus luteum in the AFC. It is recommended that all

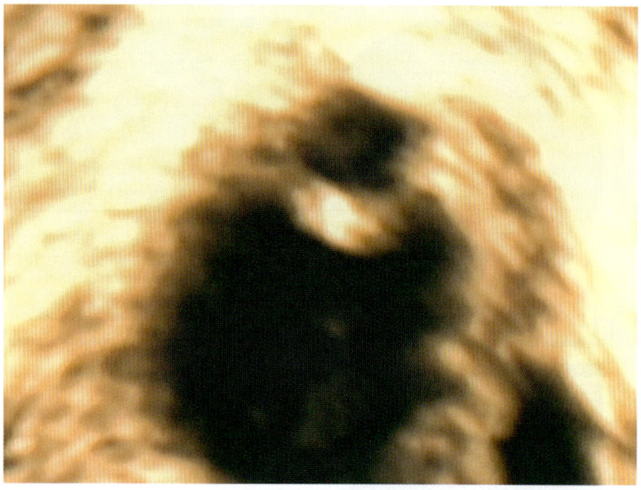

Fig. 8: Cumulus oophorus.

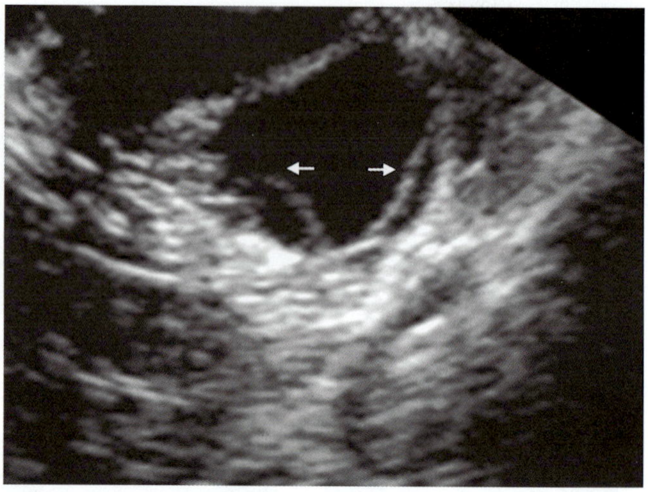

Fig. 9: Infolding of inner cell mass.

antral follicles 2–10 mm in diameter, appearing as round or oval transonic structures should be counted within the entire ovary. AFC is obtained as a sum of all antral follicles in both the ovaries, while omitting follicles more than 10 mm.

- *Follicular development:* Developing follicles destined to ovulate increase in size 2–3 mm/day and reach a maximum diameter of 16–33 mm before ovulation. Selection of the dominant follicle is thought to occur by cycle days 5–7 but is not apparent sonographically until cycle days 8–12. Other antral follicles of the developing cohort will generally undergo atresia and will not exceed 14 mm in diameter.
- *Potential signs seen in a preovulatory follicle are:*[6]
  - Presence of a dominant follicle (usually > 16–18 mm)
  - Anechoic area, double contour, around the follicle (possible ovulation within 24 hours)
  - Separation and folding of the follicle lining (ovulation within 6–10 hours) **(Figs. 8 and 9)**
  - Thickened proliferative endometrium.
- *Confirmation of ovulation:*[7]
  - Disappearance of the follicle (91% cases)
  - Decrease in follicle size (9% cases)
  - Fluid in cull de sac when not present in a previous scan
  - Development of intrafollicular echoes suggesting the formation of a hemorrhagic corpus luteum.
- *Common ovarian pathologies:*
  - Ultrasound diagnosis of polycystic ovarian morphology according to Rotterdams criteria is presence of more than or equal to 12 follicles in each ovary of 2–9 mm in size or ovarian volume more than 10 mL in at least one of the ovaries. Distribution may be peripheral or scattered in dense stroma along with stromal hypertrophy or echogenicity. New criteria proposed by Androgen Excess Society have proposed to increase the follicle number per ovary (FNPO) for establishing diagnosis of polycystic ovary syndrome (PCOS) to 25 per ovary.
  - A good 2D ultrasound can help differentiate between common pathologies of the ovary. Dermoid cysts are usually unilocular cysts with mixed echogenicity due to varying composition of fat, bone, and fluid. Rokitansky nodule, which appears as a distinct hyperechoic mural nodule is pathognomonic of dermoid cyst and represents areas of floating hair. Endometriotic cysts are commonly unilocular with diffuse low-level echoes—ground glass appearance in 82–95 and low-level blood flow in the wall. Atypical endometriomas can have papillary projections and malignancy should be ruled out.

ULTRASONOGRAPHY EVALUATION OF TUBAL PATENCY

Sonosalpingography (SSG) also known as "Sion test" is a test to assess the tubal patency using ultrasound and Doppler. Sion test is a noninvasive, cheap outdoor screening procedure for tubal testing but cannot replace hysterosalpingography (HSG) or laparoscopy as it cannot determine the site of block or intratubal pathology.

Method—No. 8 Foley's catheter is put inside the uterus. The bulb is inflated with 2 mL of distilled water. Prior to procedure, the patient is asked to evacuate the bladder and

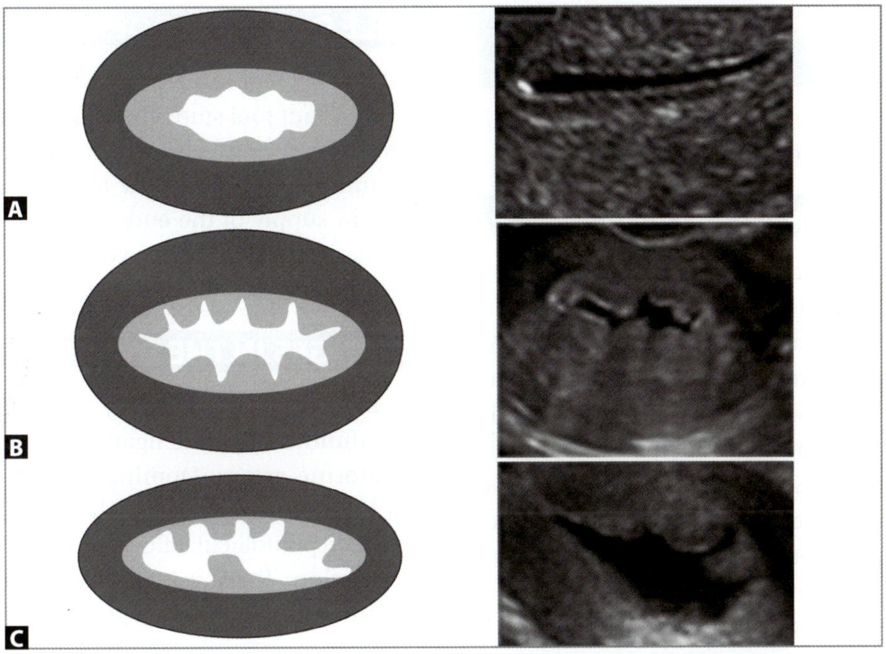

Figs. 10A to C: Sonohysterography nomenclature. (A) Smooth cavity; (B) Endometrial folds; (C) Polypoidal, irregular.

baseline vaginal scan is performed. 20–60 mL of solution containing dipoles, hyalase, and dexamethasone is taken in 50 mL catheter tip syringe and pushed via Foley's catheter; spill is confirmed as turbulence from the fimbrial end or presence of periovarian or fluid in pouch of Douglas.

UTERINE CAVITY EVALUATION (FIGS. 10A TO C)

The SSG can be combined with sonohysterography (SHG) for a complete infertility workup. It can very accurately delineate the cavity and pick up pathologies like irregular endometrium, polyps, Asherman syndrome, submucous fibroids, septum, unicornuate, and T-shaped uterus. Saline infusion SHG can establish the location of the fibroid with respect to the endometrial lining **(Table 2)**.

Sonohysterography is done in the proliferative phase by introducing a No. 8 Foley's catheter or an infant feeding tube into the uterine cavity and injecting a sterile fluid media under ultrasound visualization (normal saline, hydrotubation fluid, or commercially available echo-contrast media—ECHOVIST).

Table 2: Distinguishing features between polyps and fibroid on SHG (Fig. 8).

Intracavitary lesion	
Polyp	***Fibroid***
▪ Echogenicity-similar to endometrium ▪ Epicenter-endometrial based ▪ Vascularity-feeder vessel at pedicle	▪ Echogenicity-similar to myometrium ▪ Epicenter-myometrial based ▪ Vascularity-peripheral draping vessel

ROLE OF ULTRASONOGRAPHY MONITORING IN STIMULATED CYCLES

Follicular monitoring is important to assess the follicular response to stimulation in IUI or IVF cycles. This scan should be done on the day 5/6 of stimulation for an assessment of both number and size of follicles and helps to adjust the dosage of gonadotropins along with estradiol estimation. Hackelor et al. (1979) reported a good correlation between follicular diameter and plasma estradiol levels in women in spontaneous menstrual cycles. The follicular diameters must be measured in the transverse and longitudinal planes to get the average diameter.

Follicular sizes also help to decide timing of human chorionic gonadotropin (hCG) trigger, which is usually 20 mm in clomiphene cycle and 17–18 mm in gonadotropin cycles. In IVF cycles, trigger is given when at least 2–3 lead follicles more than 18 mm and majority more than 14 mm. Total number of follicles on day of trigger also helps to assess the risk of ovarian hyperstimulation syndrome (OHSS) so that preventive measures can be initiated.

ULTRASONOGRAPHY-GUIDED PROCEDURES

Ultrasound is an integral part of key IVF procedures like oocyte retrieval and embryo transfer.

ROLE OF 3D SCAN IN INFERTILITY

Müllerian duct anomalies are estimated to occur in 3–4% of all women, 7% of infertile women, 5–10% of patients with recurrent early miscarriages and more than 25% of women who present with recurrent late miscarriages and preterm deliveries.[8] 3D sonography has a sensitivity and specificity of 100% for diagnosing Müllerian abnormalities. In comparison, HSG has a sensitivity of 78% and accuracy of 86% as there is nonvisualization of the fundal contour and cannot distinguish between bicornuate and septate uterus on HSG.[9] 3D ultrasound provides an accurate picture of the uterine cavity, serosal surface, and the myometrium in-between **(Fig. 11)**. 3D ultrasound is also paramount for detecting polyps and pinpointing the location of fibroids. Scoring systems like STEPW (size, topography, extension, penetration, wall) or Lasmar score have been devised which help to decide feasibility of hysteroscopic surgery for submucous fibroids **(Table 3)**.[10]

Sonography-based automated volume count (SonoAVC) ***(Fig. 12)*** is a software that automatically calculates the volume and mean diameter of all hypoechoic regions, and depicts them pictorially in different colors to help study follicular development in the ovary. It is found to be highly accurate and reproducible in assessing individual antral follicles and exact follicular size saving time but needs postprocessing and was not found to improve the clinical outcomes.[11]

ROLE OF COLOR DOPPLER IN INFERTILITY

Addition of color to a 2D TVS while evaluating infertility is an important tool study the whole of the menstrual cycle. Color Doppler provides vital information about follicular dynamics like blood flow to the growing follicle, the vascular supply of the endometrium, and corpus luteum vascularization, which are very important for a successful outcome in terms of pregnancy.

CHANGES IN THE OVARY

The blood supply is to ovary is by the ovarian artery via the infundibulopelvic ligament and ovarian branch of the uterine artery. Dominant follicle within the ovary can be identified by Doppler usually day 8–10 by its increased perifollicular flow appearance due to the neovascularization. These vessels become more abundant and prominent as the follicle grows in size. In general, the

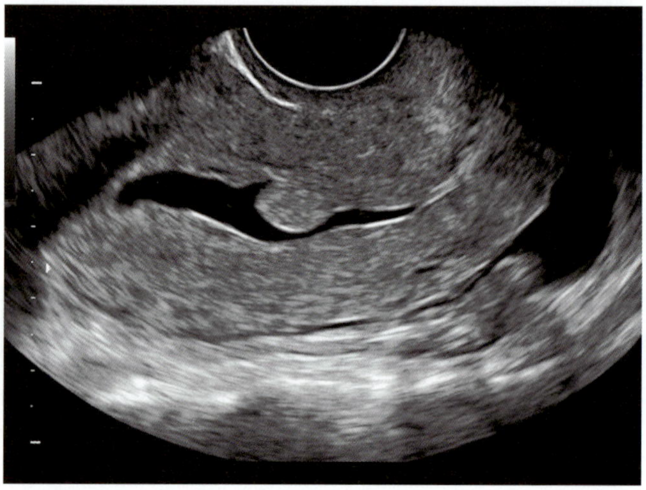

Fig. 11: Cavity lesion on sonohysterography.

Table 3: STEPW score.

	Size (cm)	*Topography*	*Extension of the base*	*Penetration*	*Lateral wall*	*Total*
0	<2	Low	< 1/3	0	+1	
1	>2–5	Middle	>1/3–2/3	<50%		
2	>5	Upper	>2/3	>50%		
Score	+	+	+	+	+	

Score	*Group*	*Complexity and therapeutic options*
0 to 4	I	Low complexity hysteroscopic myomectomy
5 to 6	II	High complexity hysteroscopic myomectomy. Consider GnRH use? Consider two-step hysteroscopic myomectomy
7 to 9	III	Consider alternatives to the hysteroscopic technique

(GnRH: gonadotropin-releasing hormone; STEPW: size, topography, extension, penetration, and wall)

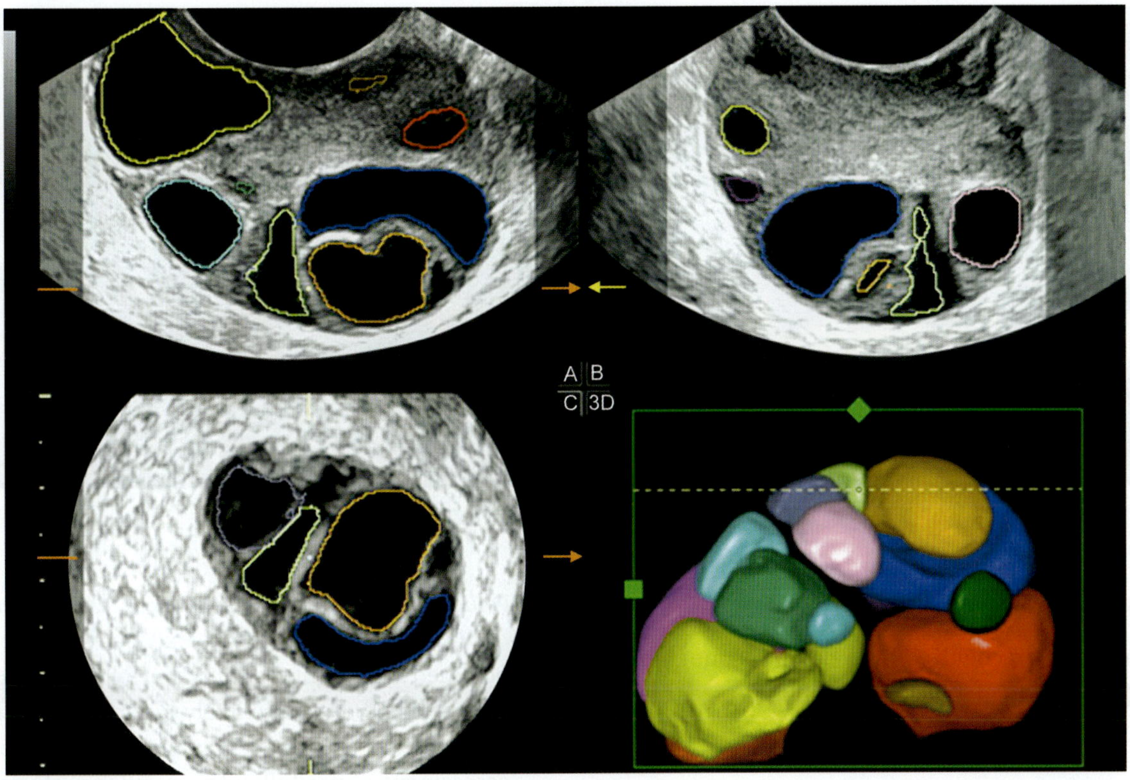

Fig. 12: Sono-based automated volume calculation (AVC).

Doppler index values are high in the early part of menstrual cycle and fall as ovulation approaches. According to Kurjak et al., the perifollicular resistance index (RI) in the early proliferative phase is 0.54 +/– 0.04 and falls the day before ovulation [luteinizing hormone (LH) peak] when it is about 0.44 +/– 0.04.[12]

This is the best time for administration of surrogate hCG. Impending ovulation is heralded by an increase in peak systolic velocity (PSV) with a relatively constant RI. The lowest RI values were obtained during the mid luteal phase (RI 0.42 ± 0.06) with a return to higher vascular resistance (0.50 ± 0.04) during the late luteal phase. If the ovary having corpus luteum shows high RI (>0.50), it is associated with nonviable outcome.

Uterine Perfusion (Fig. 13)

Uterus receives its blood supply by the uterine artery via the arcuate arteries located in the outer one-third of the myometrium. These arcuate vessels branch into radial arteries at the endomyometrial border and further into basal arteries and the spiral arteries.

Usually, uterine artery RI remains around 0.88+– 0.04 in the follicular phase, with an increase in uterine artery impedance 3 days after the LH peak (day 16). This is due to the compression of vessels traversing the uterine wall, which decreases their diameter and consequently causes higher resistance to flow. The uterine artery impedance again declines to its lowest in the mid luteal phase (RI = 0.84 ± 0.04) favoring implantation.

Similarly, blood flow changes in the spiral arteries can be used to predict implantation more precisely than uterine artery waveforms. Blood flow velocity waveform changes in the spiral arteries during normal ovulatory cycles are characteristics of by lower velocity and lower impedance to blood flow than in the uterine arteries.

Changes in the Endometrium

Michael Applebaum in his study with transvaginal color Doppler divided the endometrium and periendometrial areas into four zones. In the study conducted by him, no pregnancy was reported in IVF patients unless vascularity was demonstrated in zone III or with in zone III or IV prior to transfer.

1. *Zone 1:* 2 mm thick area surrounding the hyperechoic outer layer of the endometrium
2. *Zone 2:* The hyperechoic outer layer of the endometrium
3. *Zone 3:* The hypoechoic inner layer of the endometrium
4. *Zone 4*: The endometrial cavity.

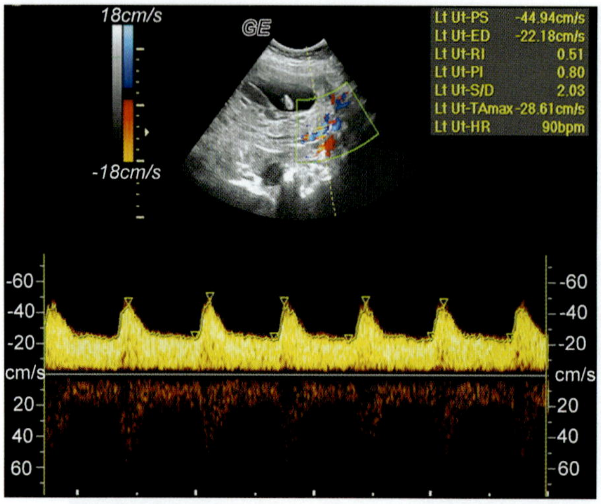

Fig. 13: Uterine artery waveform.

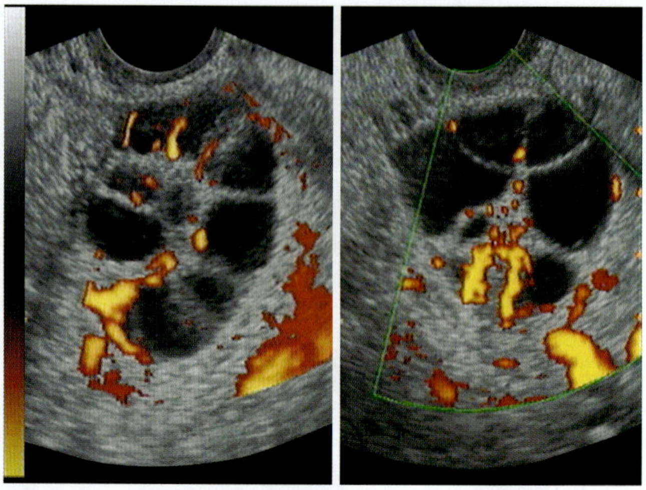

Fig. 14: Perifollicular blood flow.

Luteinized Unruptured Follicle

This condition is recognized by serial ultrasonography to monitor the growth of follicle, with failure to see expected changes at the time of ovulation. Luteinized unruptured follicle (LUF) can be identified by means of color Doppler. Rising PSV with steady low RI suggests that follicle is close to rupture while steady or declining PSV with rising RI is indicative of follicle proceeding to LUF.

Luteal Phase Defect

This is due to decreased vascularization of corpus luteum. In the LPD group, no difference was obtained in terms of intraovarian RI during the follicular phase. The mean RI throughout the luteal phase (0.56 ± 0.04) was significantly higher compared to that in the normal women. Furthermore, it did not show any difference between the early, middle, and late luteal phase. In the LPD group, no difference occurred in terms of intraovarian RI between the sides.

Color Doppler in In vitro Fertilization

Color Doppler could prove valuable in the prediction of the response of patients to ovarian stimulation in assisted conception, assessment of oocyte quality based on perifollicular flow and parameters influencing implantation following embryo transfer.

- *Prediction of patient response to ovulation stimulation:* It is seen that women with greater ovarian stromal peak systolic blood flow velocity have increased intraovarian perfusion and need less amount of gonadotropins.
- *Follicular characteristics assessment in predicting oocyte quality* ***(Fig. 14)****:* Nargund et al.[13] showed that oocytes obtained from highly vascularized follicle were of higher quality and were more likely to fertilize and result in pregnancy. From the available data, it appears that assessment of perifollicular vascular perfusion could lead to a better selection of oocytes and ultimately a higher pregnancy rate.
- *Implantation:* Friedler et al. showed that the uterine artery impedance was different in the mid luteal phase in women with subinfertility compared with those with normal fertility. They grouped the patients according to whether the pulsatility index (PI) was low (1–1.99), medium (2–2.99), or high (> 3.0). There were no pregnancies in high PI group and the PI was significantly lower in women who become pregnant as compared with those who did not.[14,15]

The ability to predict implantation before the administration of hCG allows the clinician the option to delay giving hCG until the uterine artery PI improves.

CONCLUSION

Ultrasonography offers a reproducible method of comprehensive complete infertility evaluation of the female patient, which can replace a multitude of other diagnostic tests and give information about the entire pelvis. Addition of color gives us more information about organ perfusion and addition of 3D has opened a new dimension to diagnosis of pelvic pathologies.

REFERENCES

1. Fedele L, Bianchi S, Dorta M, et al. Transvaginal ultrasonography in the differential diagnosis of adenomyoma versus leiomyoma. Am J Obstet Gynecol. 1992;167:603-6.
2. Caoili EM, Hertzberg BS, Kliewer MA, et al, Refractory Shadowing from Leiomyoma. Am J Radiology. 2000:174:97-101.
3. Botsis D, Kassanos D, Antoniou G, et al. Adenomyoma and leiomyoma: differential diagnosis with transvaginal sonography. J Clin Ultrasound. 1998;26:21-5.
4. Leone FP, Timmerman D, Bourne T, et al. Terms, definitions and measurements to describe the sonographic features of the endometrium and intrauterine lesions: a consensus opinion from the International Endometrial Tumor Analysis (IETA) group. Ultrasound Obstet Gynecol. 2010;35(1):103-12.
5. Sakamoto C. Sonographic criteria of phasic changes in human endometrial tissue. Int J Gynaecol Obstet. 1985;23(1):7-12.
6. Broekmans FJ, de Ziegler D, Howles CM, et al. The antral follicle count: practical recommendations for better standardization. Fertil Steril. 2010;94(3):1044-51.
7. Picker RH, Smith DH, Tucker-MH, et al. Ultrasonic signs of imminent ovulation J. Clin Ultrasound. 1983;11:1-2.
8. Jaffe R. Ben Aderet N. Ultrasonic screening in predicting the time of ovulation. Gynecol Obstet Invest. 1984;18:303-5.
9. Chan YY, Jayaprakasan K, Zamora J, et al. The prevalence of congenital uterine anomalies in unselected and high-risk populations: a systematic review. Hum Reprod Update. 2011;17(6):761-71.
10. Saravelos SH, Cocksedge KA, Li TC. Prevalence and diagnosis of congenital uterine anomalies in women with reproductive failure: a critical appraisal. Hum Reprod Update. 2008;14(5)415-29.
11. Lasmar RB, Xinmei Z, Indman PD, et al. Feasibility of a new system of classification of submucous myomas: a multicenter study. Fertil Steril. 2011;95:2073-7.
12. Raine-Fenning N, Jayaprakasan K, Deb S, et al. Automated follicle tracking improves measurement reliability in patients undergoing ovarian stimulation. Reprod Biomed Online. 2009;18(5):658-63.
13. Kujak A, Kupesic S. (1995) Transvaginal Color Doppler and Pelvic tumor vascularity: Lessons learned and future challenges. Ultrasound Obstet Gynaecol. 1995;6:145-9.
14. Nargund G, Doyle PE, bourne TH, et al. Ultrasound derived indices of follicular blood flow before HCG administration and prediction of oocyte recovery and preimplantation embryo quality. Hum Reprod. 1996;11:2512-17.
15. Freidler S, Schenker JG, Herman A, et al. (1996) The hole of ultrasonography in the evaluation of endometrial receptivity following assisted reproductive treatments: a critical review. Hum Reprod Update. 1996;2:323-35.

Ultrasound Mapping of Fibroids

27

Mamata Deenadayal, Aarti Deenadayal Tolani, Anupama Deenadayal Mettler

INTRODUCTION

"The uterus is an organ that should bear something, if not a child then a fibroid"—is an age-old saying. Fibroids, also called leiomyomas, are benign and the most common tumors of the uterus. They are benign neoplasms of smooth muscle origin with various degrees of fibrous connective tissue. These tumors can develop in any part of the female genital track diagnosed with a fibroid/s. Fibroids mostly remain asymptomatic but sometimes are the causes of menorrhagia, pelvic pain, infertility, dysmenorrhea, and pressure symptoms. Submucous fibroids lower the pregnancy rates by 70% and surgical removal appeared to improve pregnancy rates [relative risk (RR 2.03)]. The surgical removal of intramural fibroids should be a well-calculated decision weighing all the pros and cons and after considering if the fibroid is really the cause of the symptoms or not. Women with no fibroids and subserous fibroids appear to have similar pregnancy outcomes.

Ultrasound has been proven to be a cost-effective and adequate means to identify, map, and evaluate single to multiple fibroids as less as 4–5 mm in diameter. Accurate fibroid mapping not only works as a diagnostic tool but also can help guide the doctor toward the appropriate management (medical therapy, surgery, uterine artery embolization, or conservative management).

SETTING UP AND ADJUSTING THE MACHINE

Before beginning an ultrasound examination especially for mapping of fibroids (where our main aim is to understand the position of the fibroid in the uterus and its relationship to the endometrium and serosa), the following settings have to be adjusted according to the sonologist's comfort and habit whether using an abdominal or transvaginal probe.

Listed below are salient points related to technique and knobs of the ultrasound machine

- *Probe:* A high frequency probe always gives better images and can make mapping of fibroids an easy task. A transvaginal scan is superior to an abdominal scan when possible. But, when necessary, an abdominal probe needs to be used. The latest electrical abdominal probes give superior imaging.
- *Orientation of the image:* The image needs to be oriented to the comfort of the sonologist in order to prevent confusion of anterior-posterior and right-left. The probe marker (dot on the probe) should be orientated toward the patient's right side. In case of doubt, the anatomical landmark of the bladder can be used to confirm the anterior position of the fibroid. It is important for the sonologist to be confident about which side of the screen image is right and which side is left.
- *Preset:* On some machines, the optimum settings for a vaginal and abdominal scan can be preset and chosen just before performing the scan to improve the quality of the scan and decrease the time taken to optimize the image.
- *Depth:* The examination is started at a high depth for better orientation and to bring the uterus to the center of the screen before decreasing the depth to concentrate on the uterus.
- *Frequency:* Frequency improves the quality of the image at the expense of depth. Use the highest frequency that gives a reasonable image. The "penetration mode"

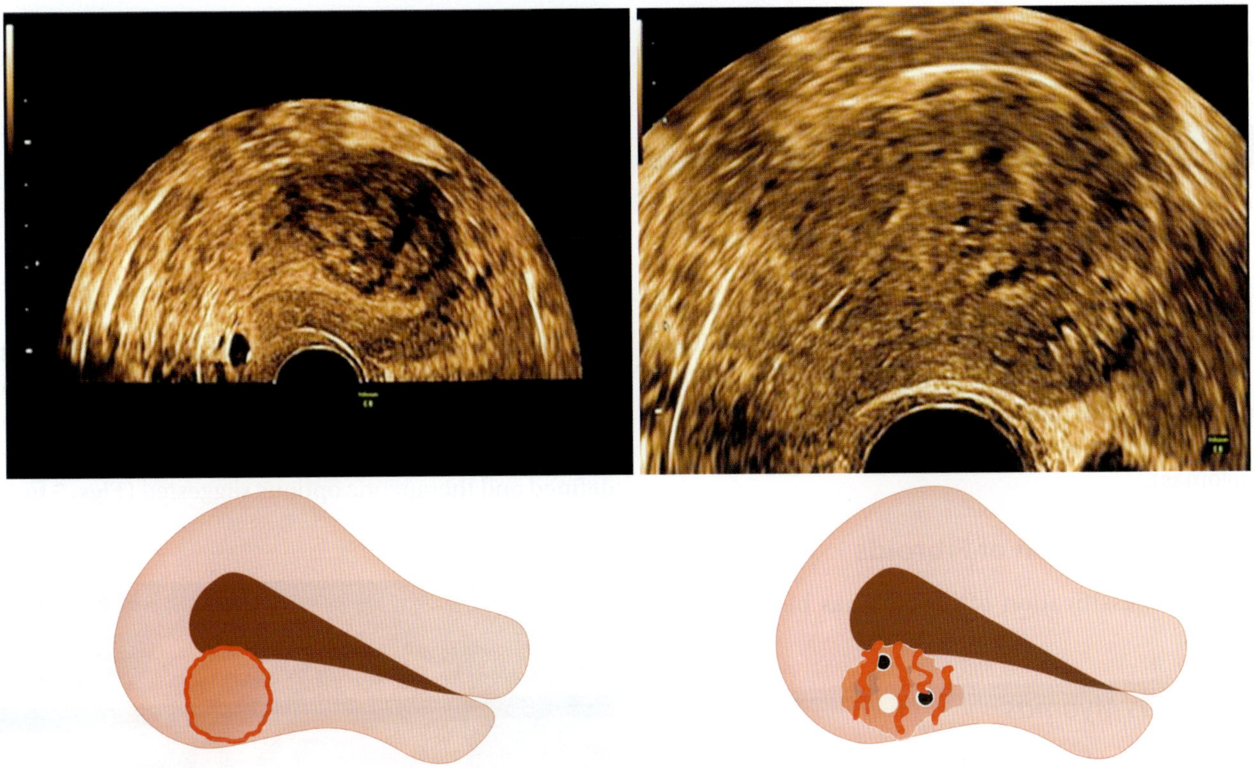

Fig. 1: Fibroid and adenomyosis on ultrasound—ultrasound image on the left of the uterus in sagittal section with a posterior wall fibroid. Ultrasound image on the right showing sagittal section with a posterior adenomyosis.

can be used for viewing a large uterus by transvaginal sonography (TVS).

- *Gain:* It should be adjusted so that fluid is black, tissues are mild gray and some bits of the image are white. Using the gain knobs, the brightness of the near, middle and far parts of the image can be changed for a clear image.
- *Practical tip regarding technique:* For best images use lots of gel, press hard, and use a darkened room. Myometrial contractions can be mistaken for uterine fibroids.[1] However, the contractions are transient, and therefore the masses will disappear on subsequent scans. Sapir mode assesses fibroids better.

TYPICAL ULTRASONOGRAPHY FEATURES OF FIBROID

- Hypo, iso, hyperechoic, or complex[2] (cystic degeneration, hyalinization, and myxoid change) **(Fig. 1)**
- Edema within these tumors is also another type of degenerative process which, when less severe, is often referred to as hydropic change[3] or hydropic degeneration.[4] Cyst formation can be an exaggeration of this process, and is associated with increasing amounts of edematous fluid in some tumors. Cystic change itself is a recognized degenerative phenomenon.[5]
- Linear stripy fan-shaped internal shadowing edge shadows-significant shadowing from its edges **(Fig. 2)**

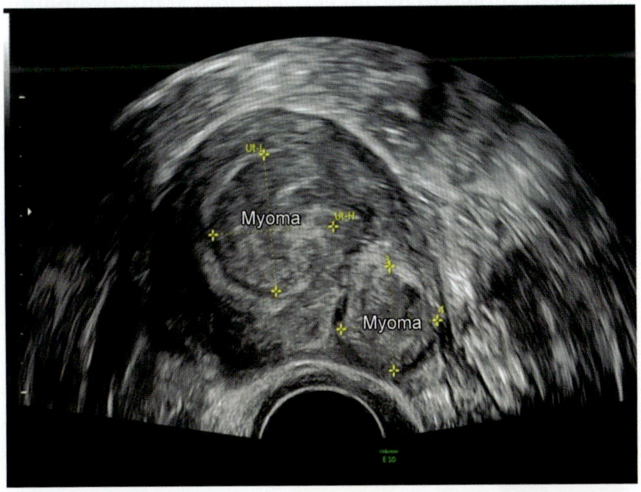

Fig. 2: 2D sagittal section of the uterus on TVS shows two well-defined myomas, which are isoechoic with typical edge shadow appearance on gray scale.

- Calcification—posterior acoustic shadowing
- Peripheral calcification—egg shell appearance, and cavitations.

CLASSIFICATION OF FIBROIDS

Numerous classifications of myomas can be found in the literature. All of them take into account the degree of intramural extension and uterine cavity distortion. There is the European Society for Gynaecological Endoscopy (ESGE) fibroid classification. More recently, International Federation of Gynaecology and Obstetrics (FIGO) classification was published, describing the types of fibroids as well as a hybrid class (association of two types of myomas).

FIGO Classification of Fibroids

The FIGO classification of fibroids has been given in **Figure 3**.

Submucous Myomas

The importance of a separate presurgical classification is to evaluate the viability of hysteroscopic surgical treatment.

The classification of ESGE/FIGO considers only the level of penetration of the myoma in to the myometrium and it was shown to be not very efficient at discriminating the complexity of hysteroscopic myomectomy.

Hysteroscopic myomectomy is the therapeutic option for patients with abnormal uterine bleeding and/or infertility where there is a need to cause as little myometrial damage as possible.

The objective of having separate classification like Lasmars STEPW (size, topography, extension, penetration, and wall) classification was to analyze specific parameters that make surgery more difficult, as that the hysteroscopic myomectomies can be planned based on the expected degree of technical difficulty in carrying out the procedure and to recommend the most suitable course of action in each situation **(Fig. 4)**.

STEPW Classification of Submucous Myomas

The STEPW classification of submucous myomas has been given in **Table 1**.

A score is given to the submucous myoma based on the size, topography, extension of the base penetration into the myometrium, and presence of the myoma in the lateral wall. Based on the total score, complexity of the surgery was defined and therapeutic options suggested **(Figs. 5 to 7)**.

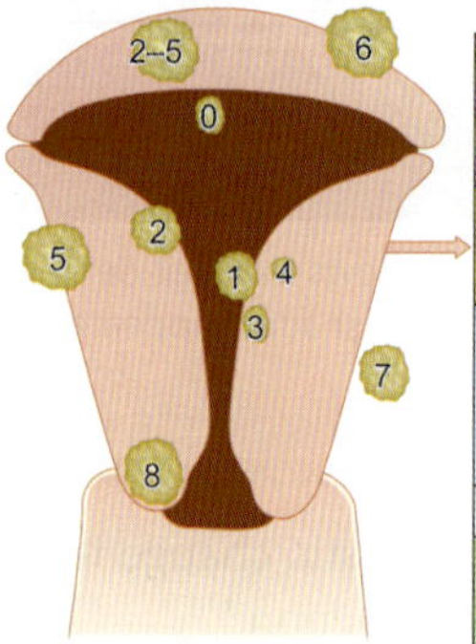

Submucosal	0	Pedunculated intracavity
	1	< 50% intramural
	2	> 50% intramural
Intramural	3	Contracts endometrium; 100% intramural
	4	Intramural
Subserosal	5	Subserosal, >50% intramural
	6	Subserosal, <50% intramural
	7	Subserosal pedunculated
	8	Other type (e.g. Cervical parasitic)
Transmural	2–5	Submucosal and subserosal, each with less than half the diameter in the endometrial and peritoneal cavities respectively

Fig. 3: FIGO classification of fibroids.

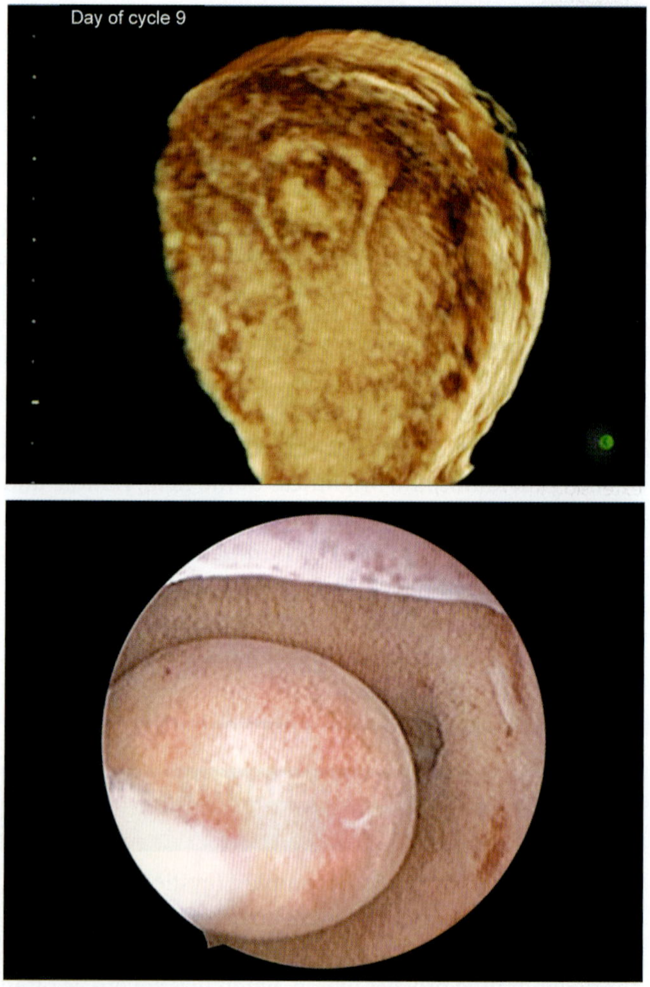

Fig. 4: 3D reconstruction of a uterine cavity—a virtual hysteroscopy. Picture on the left showing submucous myoma. A 3D reconstructed image of a submucous myoma in the uterus. Image on the right is the hysteroscopy of the same patient.

Table 1: STEP-W classification of submucous myomas.

<table>
<tr><th>Number</th><th>Size in cm</th><th>Topography</th><th>Extension of the base</th><th>Penetration</th><th>Lateral wall</th></tr>
<tr><td>0</td><td><2</td><td>Low</td><td><1/3</td><td>0</td><td rowspan="3">+1</td></tr>
<tr><td>1</td><td>>2–5</td><td>Middle</td><td>>1/3–2/3</td><td><50%</td></tr>
<tr><td>2</td><td>>5</td><td>Upper</td><td>>2/3</td><td>>50%</td></tr>
<tr><td>Score</td><td>+</td><td>+</td><td>+</td><td>+</td><td>+</td></tr>
<tr><td>Score</td><td>Group</td><td colspan="4">Complexity and Therapeutic option</td></tr>
<tr><td>0–4</td><td>I</td><td colspan="4">Low complexity hysteroscopic myomectomy</td></tr>
<tr><td>5–6</td><td>II</td><td colspan="4">High complexity hysteroscopic myomectomy. Consider Gn RH use? Consider Two-step hysteroscopic myomectomy.</td></tr>
<tr><td>7–9</td><td>III</td><td colspan="4">Consider alternative to the hysteroscopic technique</td></tr>
</table>

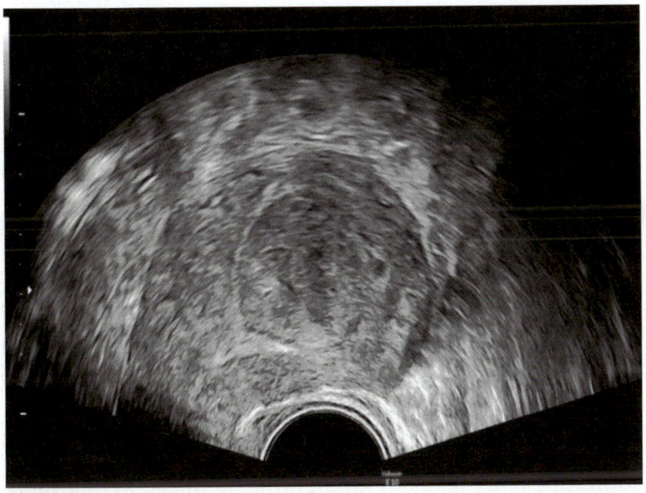

Fig. 5: A 3D coronal section of a rendered image of the uterus on a TVS—showing a FIGO stage 1 submucous fibroid with a less than 50% extension in to the myometrium and a LASMARS score—4 indicating need for low complexity hysteroscopic myomectomy.

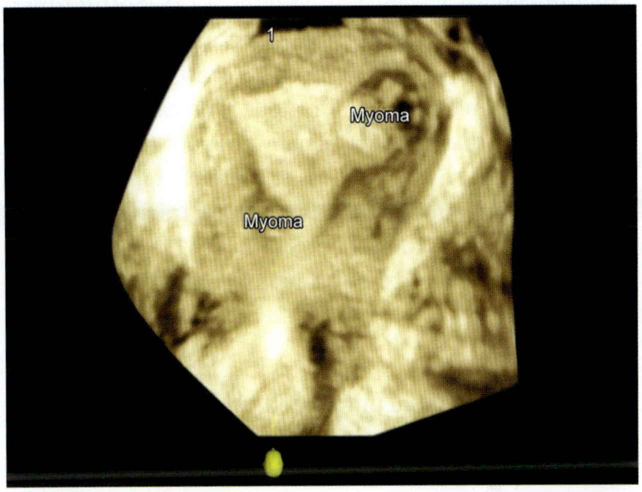

Fig. 6: 2D sagittal section of the uterus on TVS showing a well-defined myometrial mass in the upper part of the uterus distorting the endometrial cavity and the endomyometrial junction. The 3D coronal image can further clarify the location and allow precise grading of the submucous myoma as per LASMARS classification.

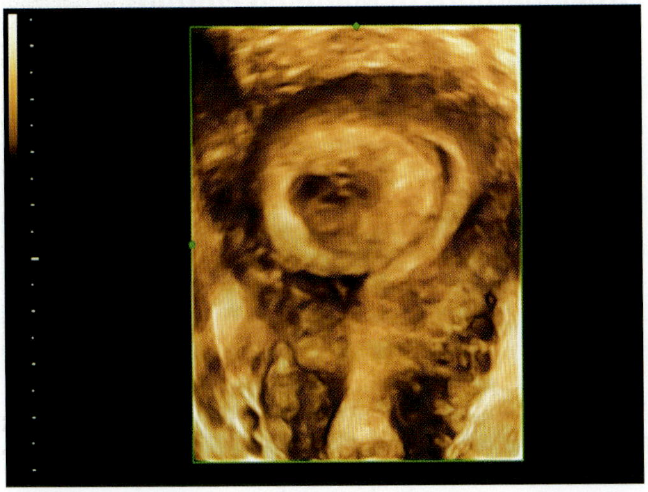

Fig. 7: This shows a 3D coronal section of a rendered image of the uterus on TVS, showing a large submucous fibroid more than 5 cm in size with a large bone in the lateral wall and extending across the upper, middle and lower corpus of the uterus with less than 50% myometrial extension. As per the FIGO classification, it is a stage-1 submucous myoma, but as per LASMARS classification, its score is 8 which mean it is a complicated mass to operate on hysteroscopy.

MODALITIES COMMONLY USED TO MAP FIBROIDS

2D Transvaginal and Transabdominal Ultrasound

Both transabdominal scan TAS and TVS should be done as they complement one another. Though TVS is more sensitive in diagnosis of small leiomyomas especially in retroflexed and retroverted uteri, TAS is essential in a large uterus as the TVS is suboptimal in such situations. Sometimes, the uterus fills the pelvis and a full bladder is not necessary for the TAS. In the TVS of a patient with a large cervical fibroid, shadowing prevents the assessment of structures above it. Hence, an additional TAS is of uttermost importance. As TAS is difficult in obese patients and gives less information, an additional TVS or in certain cases, a transrectal scan might be indicated (Sabrina Q et al. 2015). Large leiomyomas can occasionally obstruct the ureters and cause secondary hydronephrosis. Therefore, an ultrasound examination should include the urinary tract whenever a large pelvic mass is identified (Sabrina Q 2015) **(Fig. 8)**.

The kidneys need to be evaluated for hydronephrosis.

3D Ultrasound

- Three-dimensional ultrasound is very good for volume measurement of uterine leiomyomas and vascularity assessment by using vascularity index or vascularity volume display.[6]

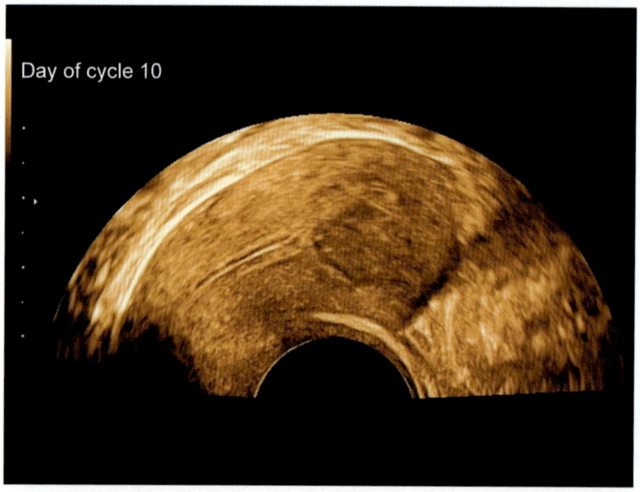

Fig. 8: This sagittal session of the uterus on TVS shows a well-defined mass in the myometrium distorting the endometrial cavity and endo-myometrial junction. The need for 3D will further map the location of the fibroid in the uterus clearly.

- A 3D reconstruction gives a clear picture regarding the outer contour of the uterus, shape of uterine cavity, junctional zone (JZ), and relation of myometrial pathologies to the endometrium and serosa.
- In addition to the multiplanar mode, the volume data may be also utilized for a multislice mode, rendered display mode, thick slice mode, or other modes (e.g. invert mode). In patients with a distorted endometrium on 2D ultrasound, 3D hysterosonography may readily demonstrate submucosal leiomyomas, help distinguish a pseudopolyp or an endometrial polyp, and allow for accurate assessment of intrauterine abnormalities.[6,7]
- In a 3D rendered coronal image, a walk through the image will show how anterior or posterior the fibroid is.

Role of MRI in Fibroid Mapping

Magnetic resonance imaging (MRI) is the preferred method for accurately characterizing pelvic masses.[8] It does not involve the use of ionizing radiation and it can demonstrate the zones of the uterus very well. Submucosal, intramural, and subserosal fibroids are well demonstrated and very small fibroids and cervical fibroids can be detected by MRI. MRI should be considered when there are more than 5 fibroids or the uterus is larger than 375 cc. The diagnosis of uterine leiomyomas on ultrasound is usually reasonably straightforward, although focal adenomyosis can mimic a leiomyoma and a pedunculated uterine leiomyoma can sometimes be mistaken for an adnexal mass.[8] When there is doubt about the origin of a pelvic mass at ultrasound, further evaluation with MRI should be performed. MRI sequences should include axial and sagittal T1 weighted (T1W) and T2 weighted (T2W) images.[9]

Other Methods of Mapping Fibroids

Elastography

Elastography is an ultrasound-based imaging modality that is based to assess tissue stiffness. Considering the fact that endometrial polyps desire from soft endometrial tissue, and submucosal fibroids are made of hard muscle, and fibrous tissue elastography seems a perfect tool for differentiating such intramural masses.

Sonohysterography

Another modalities, which can add informative value and complement the traditional sonographic evaluation is 2D and 3D sonohysterography. In patients with a distorted endometrium on 2D ultrasound, 3D hysterosonography may readily demonstrate submucosal leiomyomas, help distinguish a pseudopolyp or an endometrial polyp, and allow for accurate assessment of intrauterine abnormalities.[10] A 3D TVS can be combined with saline instillation into the uterine cavity to complement diagnostic hysteroscopy for the assessment of a submucosal leiomyoma. Three-dimensional saline contrast sonohysterography may provide even more information than conventional 3D TVS in this aspect.[6,7]

STEPS FOR FIBROID MAPPING

Vaginal Entry

- During entry, evaluate the vaginal wall and the bladder mucosa and its relationship to the uterus.
- Observe the cervix for any abnormality and document it. If there is an abnormality that needs further in detail evaluation (e.g. fibroid, large cyst, and multiple cysts), it is preferable to finish the general assessment of the pelvis before concentrating on one part.

Evaluating the Uterus

- Observe the uterus while rotating the probe to achieve true axial, coronal, and sagittal views. Use the depth setting to fill at least three-fourths of the screen with the uterus to avoid missing any pathology. Increase or decrease the gain to have a clear and sharp image **(Fig. 9)**.
- While observing the uterus in various planes, if any pathology (e.g. fibroids) is identified, a mental picture is made of the following.
- Observe if the fibroid is fundal, below the fundus or cervical in the axial (transverse) plane while moving the probe to assess the uterus from the fundus of the uterus through both the cornue to the cervix (external os). Observe the relation of the fibroids in the coronal plane while moving the probe from the front of uterus to the back.
- Observe if the fibroid is the anterior or posterior walls while in the sagittal plane and moving one side of the uterus to the other including the uterine cornue. Measure the distance from the serosa and the endometrium of each fibroid.
- A 3D coronal view further enhances the visualization of the position of the fibroid.
- If asymmetry is noticed between the anterior and posterior walls, then the thickness of each wall is noted (including JZ) for follow-up in the future to assess the advancement of the pathology. If the walls are symmetrical, no measurement is made.
- The total number of fibroids observed is documented.

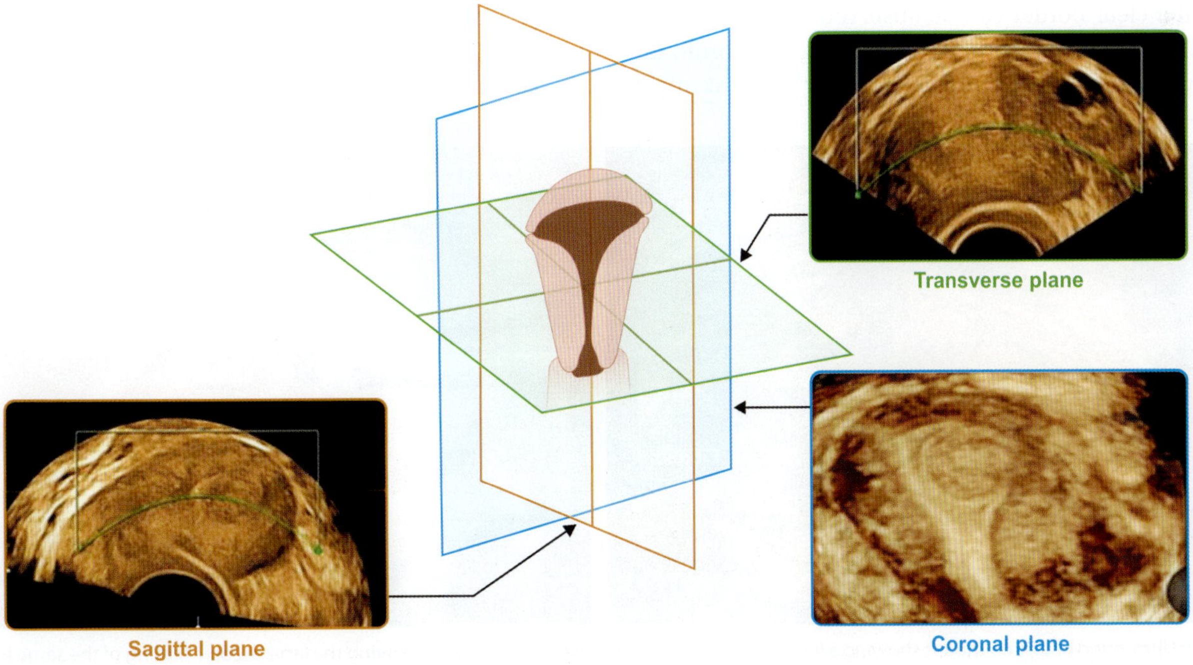

Fig. 9: A pictorial explanation of the different planes in which the uterus is observed during ultrasound.

Location of Each Fibroid in the Uterus

- To identify the location of a fibroid in the uterus, it is important to first delineate the endometrial cavity to identify the center of the uterus. It is advisable to find the cervical canal and trace it upwards in to the endometrial cavity especially in challenging cases of multiple fibroids. It is easier to give the location of fibroid once the endometrium stripe is marked out **(Fig. 10)**.
- Position of the fibroid can be:
  - Anterior, posterior, lateral wall (more posterior or anterior). Anterior wall to be documented if there is a significant relationship to the bladder and if there is infiltration of the bladder wall
  - Fundal, upper corpus, mid-corpus, lower-corpus, cervix, cornual fundal—to be documented if there is additional cornual distortion due to the presence of the fibroid. Cornual if right or the left cornu is involved.
  - Right, left, and middle
  - Cervical—to be documented if it is a pure cervical fibroid.

Measurements of the Fibroids

- Fibroid should be measured in three orthogonal dimensions.
- Ill-defined lesions are difficult to measure. In such cases, the probe should be twisted in different planes till a clear border can be observed for measurement. If this does not work, try measuring the fibroid after switching on the power Doppler and taking the circumferential flow as the border (mention this in the report).
- Volume of each fibroid is calculated and mentioned.

Echogenicity

- To define the echogenicity of a lesion, the myometrium is used as standard for comparison. Isoechoic lesions are difficult to define.
- Fibroids can be hyperechoic (white on the screen), hypoechoic (gray on the screen), anechoic (black on the screen), or a mixture.
- The reason for heterogeneity of a fibroid could be myometrial cysts or shadowing.
- When it is localized, it is usually a fibroid or adenomyoma and, if it is diffused, it may be adenomyosis.
- Fibroid usually shows edge shadows because of its well-defined margins.

Relationship of the Fibroid to the Endometrium

- Fibroid mapping is the term used to understand where the fibroid lies in the uterus in relation to the endometrium and noting the exact distance of the fibroid from the mucosa or serosa, which in turn is useful for surgical management of the cases. It is best done in the secretory phase of the cycle.
- Use the FIGO classification of fibroids to explain the position of each fibroid. This will help the surgeon to decide on the need for the myomectomy, whether it should be hysteroscopic or laparoscopic.

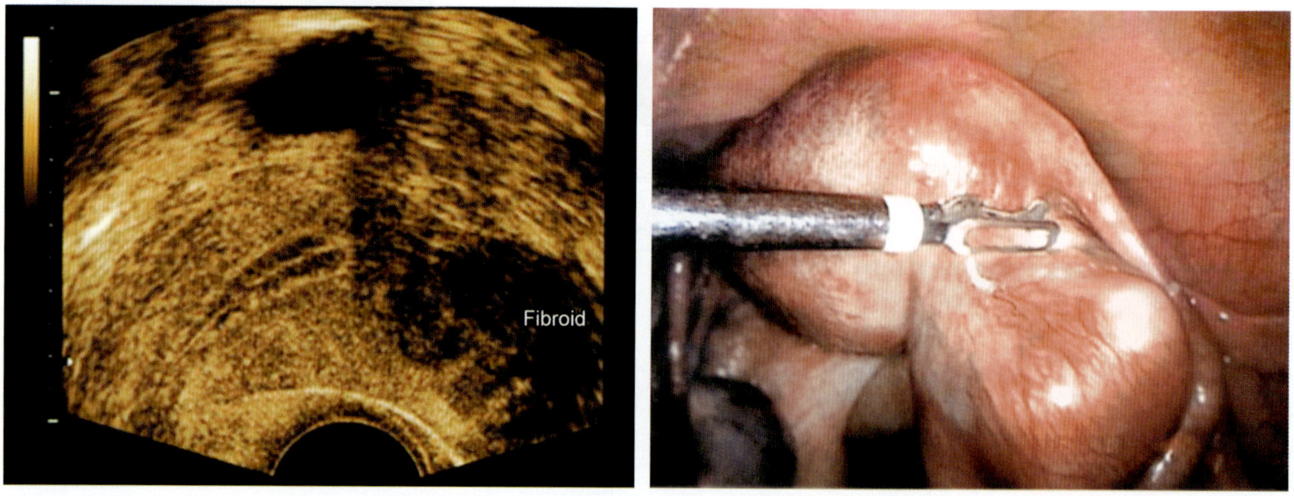

Fig. 10: Ultrasound image on the left showing a fundal subserosal fibroid. Image on the right showing the laparoscopic finding of the same patient.

Endomyometrial Junction

- *Junctional zone:* Innermost layer of the myometrium. Hypoechoic or dark halo just beyond eno. Best viewed by 3D-rendered images and 3D sectional planes using the volume contrast imaging (VCI).
- Presence of distortion of the endomyometrial junction may occur due to a submucous myoma or an intramural myoma close to the endometrial cavity.

Vascularity

- Power Doppler is more sensitive in detecting flow in small vessels and low velocity flows. Color Doppler ultrasound typically shows circumferential vascularity. However, leiomyomas that are necrotic or have undergone torsion will show a lack of blood flow. Adenomyosis has intralesional flow.
- Vascular morphology is best seen with 3D power Doppler using glass body display.
- Subjective color scoring is used [from 1 (absent flow) to 4(abundant flow)], spectral flow analysis to assess flow resistance, which is estimated by the flow indices—resistive index (RI) or pulsatility index (PI). Flow velocity, which is estimated by the PSV.
- Put the Doppler on and look for the site of origin of the fibroid and also look for the pedicle sign.
- Combined gray scale and color Doppler ultrasound may help in distinguish a uterine leiomyosarcoma from a leiomyoma.
- When the diameter of the myoma is more than or equal to 8 cm with mark central vascularity with RI less than 0.42 and peak systolic velocity (PSV) more than 42 with presence of cystic degeneration, all these together are considered high suspicion for leiomyosarcoma.

REPORTING

Report mentions all the above findings in a systematic and detailed method, which makes the report valuable and understandable to the treating physician or the surgeon.

- *Location and number:*
  - Wall (anterior/posterior/lateral) + position (fundal/upper corpus/lower corpus/cervix) + type (subserous/intramural/submucous/transmural) fibroid.
- *Distance of fibroid from the endometrium and serosa:*
  - X cm from the endo or serosa. Relevant 2D and 3D images should be provided.
- Diagrammatic representation of the fibroids sketched in one or more planes
- Measurement of the fibroids
- If the uterus is riddled with fibroids or mapping is suboptimal, it should be mentioned and the relevant fibroids, if possible should be numbered as F1, F2...so on, measured, and mapped.
- Vascularity of the fibroid to be mentioned.

CONCLUSION

Ultrasound has been shown to be an adequate and cost-effective means of evaluating size, number, and location of fibroids. Both TAS and a TVS should ideally be performed for precise detection and 3D ultrasound is very good for volume measurement vascularity assessment and spatial orientation of the fibroids.

The MRI can be preferred when there are five or more fibroids, and when origin of large pelvic masses needs to be known. A 3D saline contrast sonohysterography provides more information and is complementary in the assessment of intrauterine abnormalities. Knowledge of the various appearances of fibroids enables an accurate diagnosis and prefers the treatment. Fibroids need to be differentiated from the adenomyosis and endometrial polyps. Although most myomas are benign, 0.23–0.7% of apparently benign uterine leiomyomas are actually leiomyosarcomas based on the pathological examination. So, it is important to always look at a myoma with suspicion and be more careful when a patient presents with a pelvic mass that has had a recent or rapid increase in size and use Doppler (2D and 3D) to further assess clinically such suspicious masses.

Variants of leiomyomas occur when they undergo cystic degeneration, hyalinization, or calcification. In such situation, determining a diagnosis is sometimes difficult. MRI can be used in this situation for an accurate diagnosis.

Understanding various methodologies available to assess simple straightforward and atypical fibroids is important. Mapping these fibroids in detail in the above mentioned systematic methods give the treating physician or surgeon, the necessary information to decide on modality of treatment and prepare him to counsel the patient about the pathology and prognosticate his treatment plans.

ACKNOWLEDGMENT

Authors thank Dr Suhasini Donthi for her assistance in draft preparation.

REFERENCES

1. Rashid SQ, Chou Y, Tiu C. Ultrasonography of Uterine Leiomyomas. J Med Ultrasound. 2016;24(1):3-12.
2. Zaloudek C, Hendrickson MR. Mesenchymal tumors of the uterus. In: Kurman RJ (Ed). Blaustein's pathology of the female genital tract, 5th edition. New York (NY): Springer; 2002. pp. 561-615.
3. Hendrickson MR, Kemson RL. Surgical pathology of the uterine corpus. In: Bennington J (Ed). Major problems in pathology. Philadelphia (PA): WB Saunders; 1980. pp. 473-84.
4. Clement PB, Young RH, Scully RE. Diffuse perinodular, and other patterns of hydropic degeneration within and adjacent to uterine leiomyomas. Problems in differential diagnosis. Am J Surg Pathol. 1992;16:26-32.
5. Coard K, Plummer J. Massive multilocular cystic leiomyoma of the uterus: an extreme example of hydropic degeneration. South Med J. 2007;100:309-12.
6. Makris N, Kalmantis K, Skartados N, et al. Three-dimensional hysterosonography versus hysteroscopy for the detection of intracavitary uterine abnormalities. Int J Gynaecol Obstet. 2007;97:6-9.
7. Muniz CJ, Fleischer AC, Donnelly EF, et al. Three-dimensional color Doppler sonography and uterine artery arteriography of fibroids. J Ultrasound Med. 2002;21:129-33.
8. Weinreb JC, Barkoff ND, Megibow A, et al. The value of MR imaging in distinguishing leiomyomas from other solid pelvic masses when sonography is indeterminate. AJR Am J Roentgenol. 1990;154:295-9.
9. Rha SE, Byun JY, Jung SE, et al. CT and MRI of uterine sarcomas and their mimickers. AJR Am J Roentgenol. 2003;81:1369-74.
10. Yang T, Pandya A, Marcal L, et al. Sonohysterography: principles, technique and role in diagnosis of endometrial pathology. World J Radiol. 2013;5:81-7.

Ovulation Induction and Superovulation

28

Rishma Dhillon Pai, Madhoo Loomba, Rutvij Dalal

This section attempts to summarize the latest evidence regarding various agents currently used for ovulation induction. A brief review about the origin of ovulation induction and the relevant physiology is mentioned.

INTRODUCTION

Normal menstrual cycle is under the control of various paracrine and endocrine mechanisms through neuro-endocrine system via hypothalamic-pituitary-ovarian axis (HPO axis). Changes occur both in ovary and uterus, which result in egg production and preparation of endometrium, which is utmost important for reproduction.[1] Induction of ovulation in anovulatory women is a landmark achievement in the history of reproductive endocrinology. The last century has seen major advancement in the field of infertility and the discovery of various medical and surgical methods of ovulation induction has changed the face of treatment worldwide. Women, in yesteryears who had little hope of normal menstruation, can now successfully ovulate and bear children. Ovulation induction is the treatment of choice in anovulatory infertility. Anovulation and oligo-ovulation are the etiological factors for almost 21% of infertile couples. Aim is to combat any subtle fault in ovulatory function and luteal phase defect (LPD) that are not detected with recent investigations. Superovulation has been useful in conditions such as mild-to-moderate male factor infertility, transient anovulation, minimal-to-mild endometriosis, cervical factor, and unexplained infertility. It is done in women already ovulating with subtle defects.

CATEGORY OF PATIENTS BENEFITING FROM OVULATION INDUCTION

Patients belonging to WHO (World Health Organization) class 1 and 2 benefit the most. WHO classification of ovulatory disorders is enlisted in **Box 1**.

The WHO type I ovulatory dysfunctions (hypothalamic pituitary failure or hypothalamic amenorrhea or

Box 1: WHO classification of anovulation.[2]

Class 1—hypogonadotropic hypogonadal anovulation:
- FSH low/normal
- Estradiol low
- Pituitary is less or unresponsive to GnRH

Class 2—normogonadotropic normoestrogenic anovulation:
- Pituitary-ovarian dysfunction
- FSH normal
- Estradiol normal
- 70–80% are PCOS, rest are other hyperandrogenic disorders

Class 3—hypergonadotropic hypoestrogenic anovulation:
- FSH high
- Estradiol low
- Suggestive of ovarian failure/insufficiency

Class 4—hyperprolactinemic anovulation:
- High-prolactin levels
- Normal FSH
- Low estradiol

(FSH: follicle-stimulating hormone; GnRH: gonadotropin-releasing hormone; PCOS: polycystic ovary syndrome; WHO: World Health Organization)

hypogonadotropic hypogonadism) are characterized by low-gonadotropin levels, low-estrogen levels, and normal prolactin levels and account for 10% of all ovulatory disorders. They typically have amenorrhea and do not have withdrawal in response to a progestin challenge test. They require pulsatile gonadotropin-releasing hormone (GnRH) infusions or injectable gonadotropins to ovulate.

The WHO type II ovulatory dysfunction (hypothalamo-pituitary dysfunction) comprises of women with gonadotropin disorder and normal estrogen levels accounting for 85% of patients with ovulatory dysfunction. Other causes of anovulation include hyperprolactinemia, hypothyroidism, pituitary tumors, etc. In these conditions, it is always prudent to treat the cause first.

BRIEF REVIEW OF EVOLUTION OF OVULATION INDUCTION

Before 1960s, treatment of anovulatory infertility was restricted to psychological support and proper timing and frequency of intercourse. In 1961, Greenblatt and colleagues published their first experience of successful induction of ovulation and results with clomiphene. 60 years have passed and clomiphene still remains the first-line treatment for polycystic ovary syndrome (PCOS) and this simple and inexpensive treatment has resulted in innumerable pregnancies. Gemzell, in 1958, and Bettendorf, in 1961, achieved a major leap forward with successful induction of ovulation using human pituitary gonadotropins. They were independently able to achieve successful pregnancies in hypophysectomized individuals. In 1963, Lunenfeld and co-workers isolated the gonadotropins from urine of postmenopausal women and reached another landmark since this inexpensive source helped in isolating large quantities of the hormone for widespread use. Insler and Lunenfeld were able to achieve pregnancies in large number of amenorrheic women. GnRH was isolated and synthesized in the laboratory in 1978 but it was Knobil in 1980 who demonstrated its clinical efficacy by pulsatile administration of the drug. Though these were the foremost milestones in the history of ovulation induction, management has indeed come a long way today with advent of controlled ovarian stimulation (COS) and GnRH agonists (GnRHa) and antagonist protocols used in assisted reproduction.

PHYSIOLOGY OF OVULATION

Folliculogenesis and ovulation occur because of a complex interplay between cellular, endocrine, and paracrine factors.[3] Germ cells or oogonia that migrate from the genital ridge to the fetal ovary undergo mitosis and reach their maximum number of 6–7 million at mid-gestation. Onset of meiosis and follicular atresia result in decline in their number after birth and at puberty only about 300,000 oocytes are left. The final development of ovarian follicles begins about 3–6 months before ovulation. In response to unknown signals independent of gonadotropins, a cohort of primordial follicles is recruited to grow. During early follicular development, the oocyte enlarges and granulosa cells around it proliferate to form preantral follicles. Over a period of 3–6 months, these follicles acquire follicle-stimulating hormone (FSH) and luteinizing hormone (LH) receptors and the follicle forms a fluid-filled space within it, called the antrum.[4] From this stage onward, the antral follicles are dependent on gonadotropins for further growth as depicted in **Figure 1**. Oogonia are transformed into primary oocytes after the first meiotic division and are arrested at prophase of the first meiotic division until just before ovulation.

As the levels of estradiol, inhibin A, and progesterone decrease with regression of the corpus luteum in the latter part of the cycle, the concentrations of FSH and LH rise. When this intercycle rise of FSH exceeds the critical level, it activates the largest antral follicles (2–5 mm) present at this time. This activation involves induction of key enzymes like aromatase and appearance of LH receptors. LH stimulates the production of androstenedione from the thecal cells. Androstenedione diffuses into the granulosa cells and is here converted to estradiol by the action of aromatase, the production of which is stimulated by FSH. The emerging dominant follicle produces increasing amounts of estrogen and inhibin A and this induces a negative feedback of FSH. The fall in FSH prevents further recruitment of follicles. As the follicle further acquires LH receptors, it matures and at LH surge, the first meiotic division is completed and it transforms into a secondary oocyte. The two-cell-two gonadotropin theory states that FSH concentration must exceed a certain threshold before follicular development will proceed. The duration for which the FSH level exceeds the threshold is called the "FSH window" and it is the short duration of this window in normal ovulation that permits monofollicular selection.

The physiological principles of ovulation induction include either increasing the number of antral follicles available in the ovary at the time of selection, releasing the ovary from inhibitory influences, or by maintaining the level of FSH above the threshold level for longer either by enhancing endogenous gonadotropins or administration of exogenous gonadotropins. This effect is illustrated in **Figure 2**.

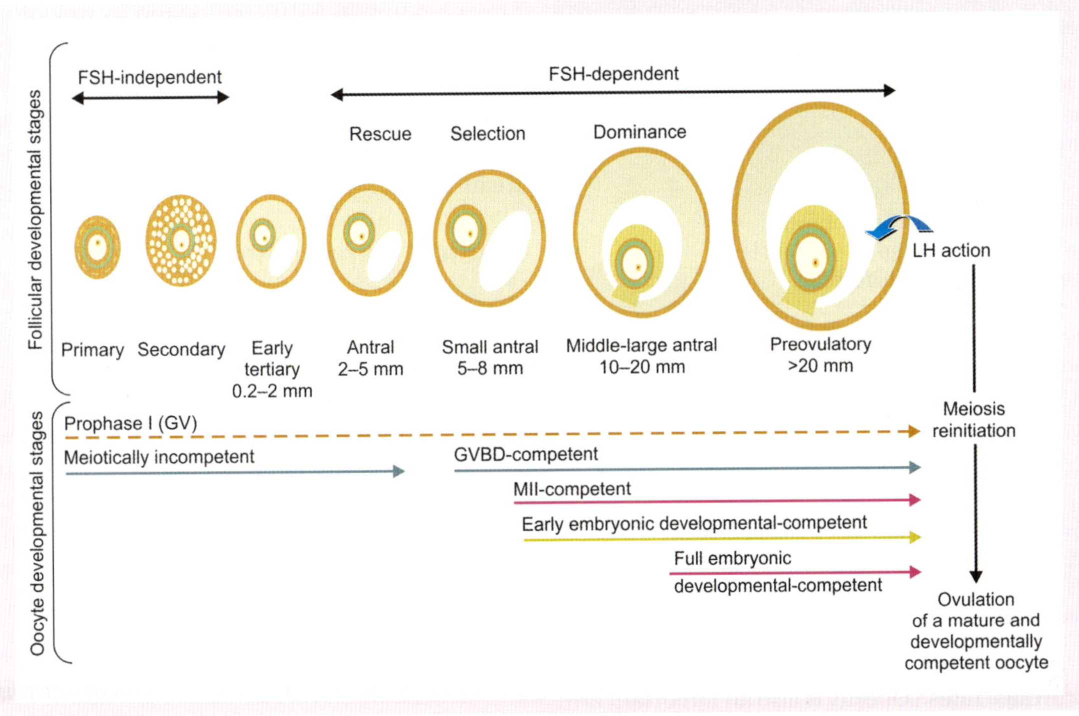

Fig. 1: Folliculogenesis and oogenesis. (FSH: follicle-stimulating hormone; LH: luteinizing hormone; GV: germinal vesicle; GVBD: germinal vesicle breakdown; MII: metaphase II)

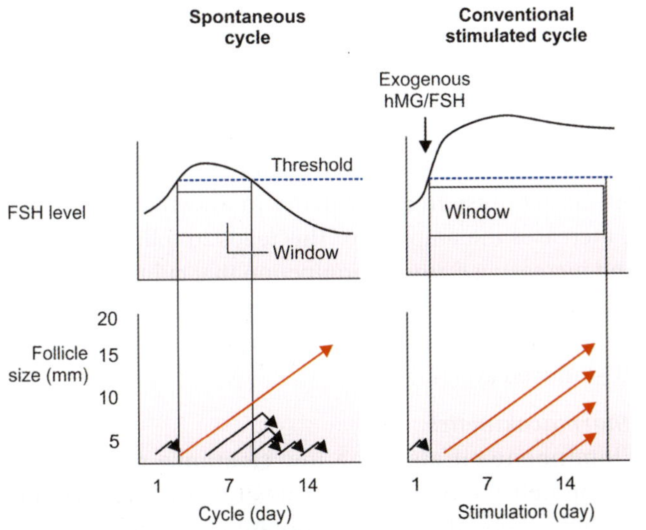

Fig. 2: Follicle-stimulating hormone threshold and window in spontaneous and stimulated cycle. (FSH: follicle-stimulating hormone; hMG: human menopausal gonadotropin)

Dominant follicle should have LH exposure for particular period of time and concentration for final follicular maturation. LH threshold and ceiling concept has been described in **Box 2**.

MANAGEMENT OPTIONS FOR OVULATION INDUCTION[6]

Management options for ovulation induction are:

- Lifestyle modifications in form of diet and exercise
- Medical management with:
  - Antiestrogens
  - Aromatase inhibitors (AIs)
  - Insulin sensitizers
  - Gonadotropins
  - Dopamine agonists
  - Gonadotropin-releasing hormone
  - Gonadotropin-releasing hormone agonists and antagonists
- Surgical methods.

Lifestyle Modification for Obesity-related Infertility

Obesity has been known to have an adverse effect on ovarian function and fertility.[7] It is defined as a body mass index (BMI) of over 25 kg/m^2, obesity is associated with lower fertility rates—both at natural conception and ovulation induction, higher doses of ovulation-inducing drugs, and

Box 2: Concept of luteinizing hormone (LH) threshold and ceiling.[5]

- Suppression of granulosa cell proliferation
- Oocyte development compromised
- Follicular atresia
- Premature luteinization

LH ceiling

Normal follicular growth and development
- Paracrine signaling activated by FSH and LH
- Adequate granulosa cell proliferation
- Functional maturation
- Androgen and estrogen biosynthesis
- Oocyte maturation

LH window

LH threshold

- No paracrine signaling between granulosa cells and theca cells
- Androgen and estrogen biosynthesis hampered
- Impaired oocyte maturation
- Improper granulosa cell proliferation
- Decreased activation of aromatase activity by LH

higher miscarriage rates.[8] Obesity is also an important arm of the PCOS triad and is seen in 50% of women with PCOS. 80% of obese patients are insulin resistant as well. These women have a higher tendency to multifollicular response even on low-dose FSH and greater tendency for cycle cancellation and ovarian hyperstimulation.

Obesity evidently expresses and exaggerates the signs and symptoms of insulin resistance. Weight loss can be achieved either by exercise, diet, or both. Studies have shown that a weight loss of just 5–10% through diet or exercise restores reproductive function in 55–100% of individuals within a period of 6 months. Reduction in weight results in a 30% fall in visceral fat restoring ovulation and reducing the markers for metabolic disease. Weight loss in patients with PCOS has been observed to decrease elevated androgen and LH levels, enhance insulin sensitivity, and reestablish mono-ovulation and improve response to ovulation-inducing agents.[9]

Exercise helps in weight loss, improving insulin resistance, and restoration of reproductive function. Exercise burns visceral fat more than subcutaneous fat. Aerobic exercise should last for at least 20–30 minutes thrice a week sufficient to cause sweating to be effective. A diet that is low in calorie, fat, and carbohydrate with a low-glycemic index is recommended.[10] Thus, weight loss is an intervention that is effective, inexpensive, and without adverse effects. It has an added advantage in decreasing the long-term complications of diabetes and cardiovascular disease. Since a minimal 5–10% reduction in weight is sufficient to reinstate ovarian function, it should be advised as the first line of treatment in obese subjects. In patients with a BMI more than 28–30 kg/m^2 who would respond poorly to ovulation induction, it is wise to advise weight loss prior to treatment.[11]

Medical Management

Antiestrogens

In normogonadotropic anovulation, administration of small amounts of FSH will induce ovulation. This can be achieved by antiestrogens, pulsatile GnRH, or low-dose gonadotropins. Clomiphene citrate (CC) and tamoxifen are the two antiestrogens [SERM (selective estrogen receptor modulator)] used. It is the best treatment for ovulatory dysfunction and normal estrogen levels (WHO type II). Combined with intrauterine insemination (IUI), CC enhances fecundity in unexplained infertility.[12]

Chemical structure and mechanism of action: Clomiphene citrate is a nonsteroidal triphenylethylene derivative and a competitive nonselective estrogen receptor (ER) modulator. It has both agonistic and antagonistic actions at the level of ERs.[13] It binds to the nuclear ER in the hypothalamus for extended periods (weeks rather than hours) and depletes ER concentrations by interfering with the normal process of ER replenishment. It thus blocks the negative feedback effect of estrogen, alters the pulsatile release of GnRH, and stimulates gonadotropin secretion from the pituitary gland. In ovulatory women, it increases the GnRH pulse frequency; and in anovulatory women, it increases the amplitude. This leads to follicle selection and increasing estrogen production that culminates in LH surge.[14] Hence, there is normally no need to administer exogenous human chorionic gonadotropin (hCG) in CC-induced cycles.[15]

Pharmacokinetics: Clomiphene citrate has a low clearance rate and has a long half-life of 5 days.[16] It has two distinct isomers: enclomiphene that is more potent and responsible for the ovulation-inducing action of CC and zuclomiphene (Zu) that is less active, longer lasting, and cleared more slowly from the body. The enclomiphene levels rise rapidly and fall to insignificant levels after a few days. Significant levels of the Zu isomer can be detected up to 4 weeks after administration of the drug **(Table 1)**. The starting dose of CC is 50–100 mg and CC can be begun from day 2–5 of a

Table 1: Differences between two isomers of clomiphene.[17]

Enclomiphene	*Zuclomiphene*
62% concentration	38% concentration
Antiestrogenic action is more	Less antiestrogenic and more estrogenic
Potency is more than zuclomiphene	Less potent
T1/2 of 2.5–11.8 hours	T1/2 of 14.2–33.4 hours

normal period or a withdrawal bleed without any impact on outcome. If there is no response in three cycles, the dose is increased as women who do not respond to 50 mg, two-thirds will not do so in the first cycle. The maximum dose should not be more than 150 mg as higher doses do not enhance ovulation and pregnancy rates and only add to side effects. CC treatment generally should be limited to the minimum effective dose and to no more than six ovulatory cycles per attempt and not more than 12 total cycles. Failure to conceive after successful CC-induced ovulation is indication for further evaluation to exclude other contributing causes of infertility. CC is excreted through stools and cleared mainly by the liver.

Caution has to be exerted as CC treatment is futile in women with elevated FSH values, hypogonadotropic hypogonadism, severe male factor infertility, and uterine or tubal factor infertility. It is also prudent to confirm tubal patency before embarking on any ovulation-induction regime.

Monitoring response:

Response to treatment should be monitored by measurement of basal body temperature, serum progesterone levels (day 21 and 28), urinary LH levels, or ultrasound.[18] No studies have evaluated the advantage of using more intensive monitoring methods like ultrasound to assess treatment response. But ultrasound, when available, should be used to monitor IUI cycles and preferably the first cycle to determine the minimum effective dose.[19]

About 20–25% of women fail to ovulate despite maximum doses of clomiphene and this is called "clomiphene resistance". This commonly occurs in obese, hyperandrogenic, and insulin-resistant women with high LH levels. Failure to conceive despite successful ovulation is called "clomiphene failure".[20]

Results with treatment:

Ovulation rates following treatment with clomiphene in properly selected patients are usually 70–85% and conception rates are 40–50%.[21] The cycle fecundity in patients who respond to clomiphene is approximately 15%. Three-fourths of the pregnancies reportedly occur in the first three cycles. Cumulative pregnancy rates can be as high as 60% after six cycles and may reach almost 97% after 12 cycles. 20% of pregnancies that occur due to clomiphene may end in a spontaneous abortion and the estimated risk of multiple pregnancies is about 8–13%; majority being twins. The discrepancy between ovulation and pregnancy rates is commonly due to lack of persistence of therapy or other associated causes of infertility. The reasons for the relatively low-pregnancy rate are unclear, but may be related to high-LH levels, to antiestrogenic effects of clomiphene, and to adverse effects on the oocytes. Because of the long half-life of clomiphene isomers, they may exert an antiestrogenic effect on the quality and quantity of cervical mucus and growth and maturation of the endometrium. These effects are thought to occur with prolonged therapy and at larger doses. Traditionally, the antiestrogenic effect of CC on the endometrium has been implicated to be responsible for the discrepancy in ovulation and pregnancy rates. Successful implantation depends on an adequate endometrial thickness and a receptive endometrium. A reduction in endometrial thickness below the minimum, thought to be necessary for pregnancy to occur, was seen in 30% of patients on clomiphene. Another study found the endometrium deleterious to implantation in clomiphene-induced cycles in having a reduction in glandular density and presence of vacuolated cells.[22] Due to the inability to define a minimum endometrial thickness necessary for pregnancy to occur and tremendous individual variability in the antiestrogenic effect of CC, the significance of these effects is difficult to quantify.[23] The antiestrogenic effect of CC on the cervix has been reported to occur in about 15% of cases and, if demonstrated, the adverse effect can be circumvented by IUI.[24]

A systematic review of four cross-over randomized controlled trials (RCTs), that compared CC with placebo in patients with PCOS, found that all doses of CC were associated with increased pregnancy rates per treatment cycle [odds ratio (OR) 3.41, 95% confidence interval (CI) 4.23–9.48] and with increased ovulation (OR 4.6, 95% CI 2.84–7.45). Life-table analysis of the largest and most reliable studies indicates a conception rate of up to 22% per cycle in those ovulating on CC (Hammond et al., 1983; Kousta et al., 1997; Eijkemans et al., 2003).

Routine administration of hCG adds little to improving conception rates. It is indicated only when there is an absent or delayed LH surge or for timing IUI or intercourse. Both recombinant and urinary hCG are equally effective though urinary hCG is reported to have more local reactions. Steroids have been tried as adjunctive agents with CC in women with elevated dehydroepiandrosterone (DHEAs) levels (>200 μg/dL). Dexamethasone helps to decrease the adrenal production of androgens and increases ovulation rates by reducing the inhibitory effect of local androgens. It suppresses the action of estradiol on the pituitary gland and increases serum growth hormone and insulin-like growth factor-1 (IGF-1) levels. It is usually administered at a dose of 0.5 mg at bedtime for 1 month (low dose), or prednisolone that is administered at a dose of 5 mg. Long-standing use of oral steroids caution in view of their adverse effects. An increased appetite and weight gain would further deteriorate the metabolic profile of any patient with PCOS. Two recent studies have proposed a high-dose and short-course regimen that is more convenient to the patient with higher ovulation (75–88%) and pregnancy rates (40–40.5%). It has also lately been tried in clomiphene-resistant women but with normal DHEAS levels with successful outcome.[25]

Clomiphene resistance:

Failure to ovulate after three cycles of CC treatment with maximum dose of 150 mg is called clomiphene resistance. Resistance to CC treatment occurs in obese, hyperandrogenic, and insulin-resistant individuals with elevated LH levels. Alternatives to management include higher doses of CC, weight reduction, extended CC therapy for 8 days, pretreatment with oral contraceptive pills (OCPs) (to lower LH levels), concomitant use of GnRH agonist to suppress LH, and adjunctive therapy with dexamethasone or insulin-sensitizing agents. Alternative drugs such as AIs and gonadotropins can be tried.[26]

Clomiphene failure:

Failure to conceive despite successful ovulation for six cycles calls for seeking other causes for infertility. Combination and alternative strategies can be attempted. Lack of pregnancy despite 12 successful ovulatory cycles in the absence of other causes is usually an indication for assisted reproduction.

Indications of antiestrogens:[27]

- Anovulation
- Luteal phase deficiency
- Unexplained infertility
- Hypothalamic or pituitary dysfunction
- IUI or in vitro fertilization (IVF)—mild stimulation
- Endometriosis—stage 1 and 2. Prerequisites for CC are:
    - Male partner evaluation
    - History and physical examination
    - Age, duration, and cause of infertility
    - Normal thyroid and prolactin function
- Normal functioning of pituitary. Adverse effects:
    - Vasomotor flushes are temporary and seen in about 10% of patients. They cease once treatment ends
    - Mood swings and nausea
    - Blurred vision, double vision, scotoma, light sensitivity, and optic neuropathy (severe and persistent). Visual disturbances (<2%) are mostly uncommon and reversible. In the eventuality of persistent or severe complications, treatment needs to be stopped and alternative methods should be considered.[12] Breast tenderness (2–5%).
    - Pelvic discomfort
- Effect on endometrium and cervical mucus:[28]
  Multiple pregnancy is lowest with CC. The incidence of multiple pregnancy can be further reduced by ultrasound monitoring and withholding hCG and IUI when there are more than two follicles more than 18 mm. The earlier notion that CC-induced successful pregnancies have higher incidence of spontaneous abortions has not been proved in any study. Recent reports have shown that abortion rates are not increased compared to normal (20%).[15]
    - *Ovarian cancer*: Some case reports and epidemiological studies have suggested an association between epithelial ovarian cancer and fertility drugs. But there is little evidence for an increased risk of invasive epithelial ovarian cancer in women exposed to fertility treatment. Those studies that have found higher rates of the disease report a twofold increased risk at the most, although this has rarely been statistically significant. These facts must be viewed in the context of the considerable methodological difficulties that frustrate these studies. There is a clear need for larger studies employing longer periods of follow-up, detailing precisely the types, doses, and duration of treatments patients have received, and controlling for potential confounding reproductive factors.
    - *Ovarian hyperstimulation syndrome (OHSS)*: Mild OHSS is relatively common but severe OHSS rarely occurs.

Contraindications:

- Suspected pregnancy
- Hypersensitivity to drug
- Liver failure and dysfunction
- Functional ovarian cysts

- Visual disorders. Other selective ER modulators:
    - *Tamoxifen*: Tamoxifen has been useful in patients with anovulation even in failed CC treatment cycles. One recent study has shown comparable results of ovulation and pregnancy rates when efficacy of tamoxifen with that of CC was tested. Some studies suggest superiority of tamoxifen, as it has no effect on endometrium.[29] Raloxifene has recently been tried in trials but not in use presently.

Aromatase Inhibitors

The two compounds currently being used for ovulation induction are the selective nonsteroidal AIs namely—letrozole and anastrozole.[30] Aromatase is a microsomal cytochrome P450 hemoprotein-containing enzyme that catalyzes the rate-limiting step in estrogen biosynthesis, i.e., conversion of androstenedione and testosterone to estrone and estradiol. Aromatase activity is present in the ovary, adipose tissue, brain, muscle, liver, and breast tissue.

Three generations of AIs have been developed over the past three decades but the first two generation drugs were clinically not found useful owing to significant adverse effects and low potency. Generations of AIs are given in **Table 2**. Till recently, they were approved for use in treatment of postmenopausal breast cancer; but letrozole has been lately approved for use as an ovulation-inducing agent.

Classification:

- *Steroidal*: It competes with endogenous androstenedione and testosterone for P450 causing irreversible enzymatic inhibition.
- *Nonsteroidal*: It competes with endogenous substrates for cytochrome P450 forming a reversible bond.

Aromatase inhibitors are also classified as:

- *First generation of AI*: It induces hepatic enzymes and inhibits cortisol, aldosterone, thyroxine, and aromatase.
- *Second generation of AI*: Its potency is twice than first generation.

Table 2: Classification of aromatase inhibitors.

Generation	*Nonsteroidal/reversible*	*Steroidal/irreversible*
First	Aminoglutethimide	None
Second	Fadrozole	Formestane
Third	Anastrozole/letrozole/ exemestane	Exemestane

- *Third generation of AI*: It inhibits aromatase enzyme only. Potency is three to four times more than that of second-generation AI.

Mechanism of action:

- Aromatase inhibitors block conversion of androgens to estrogens and thus increase testosterone levels.
- Aromatase inhibitors block inhibitory feedback of testosterone on hypothalamo-pituitary-gonadal (HPG) axis and convert into more potent estrogen without any increase in circulating estrogens and estradiol (E2) receptor modulators.[31]

Letrozole and anastrozole are competitive, potent, and reversible AIs and reduce estrogen levels by 97–99%. They inhibit release of estrogen from various sources, namely ovarian, adipose tissue, and locally produced estrogen in the brain and thus release the hypothalamopituitary axis from the negative feedback effect of estrogen.[32] The consequent increase in the release of gonadotropins stimulates follicular growth. Unlike CC, which has a prolonged duration of action and causes depletion of ERs, letrozole does not deplete ERs and central feedback mechanisms remain intact. As the dominant follicle grows, it produces estrogen that exerts a negative feedback at the center and decreases FSH release. Suppression of FSH secretion results in atresia of smaller follicles and monofollicular growth. Studies have also proposed peripheral mechanisms of action. Inhibition of aromatase in the ovary would result in the temporary accumulation of androgens. It has been postulated that this increased androgen level stimulates follicular growth by increasing its sensitivity to FSH. By decreasing follicular estrogen levels, the ER levels in the endometrium are upregulated leading onto a rapid endometrial growth once the drug is stopped and estrogen secretion resumes. This results in thicker and more receptive endometrium in patients receiving AIs. In patients with PCOS, FSH production in the early follicular phase may be blunted because of high androgen levels being aromatized to estrogen in the brain and exerting a negative feedback. Thus, AIs may be particularly useful in PCOS patients. A recent study has evaluated expression of HOXA10 and integrin $\alpha(v)\beta(3)$ in rat endometrium exposed to either letrozole or clomiphene. This study found that letrozole affects HOXA10 expression but not integrin in uterine endometrium and concluded that clomiphene suppresses endometrial receptivity more than letrozole.[33]

Pharmacokinetics:

Letrozole is used in a dose of 2.5–5 mg orally from day 2 to day 3 of the cycle for 5 days. These compounds are completely absorbed after oral administration with a mean terminal half-life of about 30–60 hours. Because of this short half-life of 45 hours, they are ideal ovulation-inducing agents, as they are eliminated from the circulation rapidly and do not continue to exert their action after cessation of the drug.

Evidence from controlled studies (Table 3):[34-36]
Theoretically and by earlier studies, evidence emerged that letrozole use is associated with monofollicular response, lower multiple pregnancy rates, thicker and more receptive endometrium, and consequently better pregnancy rates.

Though earlier studies did show a thicker endometrium and a trend toward higher pregnancy rates, evidence accumulating from recently published randomized studies is conflicting. Studies have shown greater follicular number and estradiol levels with CC on the day of hCG and no significant difference in pregnancy rates, endometrial thickness, and ovulation rates.

Aromatase inhibitors have been tried in patients with clomiphene failures either alone or in conjunction with gonadotropins. In patients with CC failures, letrozole alone has shown 75% ovulation rates and 20–25% pregnancy rates. In comparative studies with gonadotropins and letrozole in patients with CC failure or advanced age, gonadotropins have been found to have better pregnancy rates. When used in a sequential regime with gonadotropins, women who received letrozole and FSH had fewer follicles and E2 levels on the day of hCG, similar or higher endometrial thickness, equivalent pregnancy rates, and lower multiple pregnancy. In comparison with gonadotropins alone, similar pregnancy rates could be achieved with 40–50% lower gonadotropin usage and lower multiple pregnancy rates. Recently, one double-blinded randomized trial by Amer et al.[37] had shown higher pregnancy rates with letrozole as compared to CC, but live birth rates were not statistically significant among them.

Indications for use:
- Clomiphene failure cases[38]
- Persistent thin endometrium with clomiphene cases
- Ovarian stimulation in women having breast cancer, as it does not cause high estrogen levels but give good oocyte yield.[39]

Advantages over CC:
- No antiestrogenic effect on endometrium and cervical mucus
- Absence of ER depletion
- Better uterine blood flow
- Rapidly eliminated from body due to short half-life of 45 hours
- Limited follicles[40]
- Reduced multiple pregnancy rates[41]
- Decreased chances of OHSS.[42]

Adverse effects:
- Vasomotor symptoms such as hot flushes
- Nausea and fatigue
- Alopecia
- Vaginal bleeding after long-term use in cases of breast cancer.

Contraindications:
- Women at risk of endometrial hyperplasia and endometrial neoplasia
- Osteoporosis.

Insulin Sensitizers

Insulin sensitizers are discussed in chapter on "Role of Adjuvants in Ovarian Stimulation".

Evidence:
Metformin has been better than placebo for ovulation rate and pregnancy rate in PCOS women but there is significant statistical heterogeneity in that.[43] Combined analyses of

Table 3: Evidence from controlled studies to show various evidences on clomiphene and letrozole.

Author	*Year*	*Study*	*Patient group*	*Follicles*	*Endometrial thickness*	*Ovulation rates*	*E2 level*	*Pregnancy rate*
Casper[34]	2007	CC vs letrozole	PCOS	Similar				Similar
Badawy[35]	2007	CC vs letrozole*	PCOS	CC > L	CC > L	Not significant	CC > L	Similar
Bayar	2006	CC vs letrozole*	PCOS	Similar	Similar	Not significant	CC > L	Similar
Atay[36]	2006	CC vs letrozole*	PCOS	CC > L	L > CC	L > CC	L > CC	L > CC
Bayar	2006	CC vs letrozole*	Ovulatory		Similar	Similar	CC > L	Similar

(*; randomized trials; CC: clomiphene citrate; PCOS: polycystic ovary syndrome; L: letrozole) all women demonstrated a benefit of metformin over placebo without statistical heterogeneity for pregnancy rate. Limited data shows no difference between metformin and placebo for live birth rate or miscarriage rate. Metformin induced more minor gastrointestinal-related adverse events compared to placebo. Metformin, therefore, improves ovulation and pregnancy rate, but there is currently inadequate data for an effect on live birth rates. It is generally recommended, if using metformin, that doses are initiated at 500 mg daily and increased by 500 mg daily every 2 weeks. There is considerable controversy over when metformin should be ceased, if pregnancy occurs. In general, there is inadequate evidence to support continuing metformin following conception with more research needed. There was no benefit of metformin over CC for live birth rate, and CC was better than metformin for live birth rate in those with a BMI more than or equal to 30 kg/m^2. Metformin, therefore, did not result in improved reproductive outcomes compared to CC.

Current evidence-based guidelines recommend intensive lifestyle modification, particularly in those with a BMI more than or equal to 30 kg/m^2, including frequent multidisciplinary engagement for 3–6 months as first-line therapy—level of evidence 1B. This recommendation was underpinned by RCTs, which found that there was no benefit of metformin over lifestyle.

Gonadotropins

Exogenous gonadotropins are used in the treatment of WHO type I infertility and WHO type II infertility who have failed to conceive with antiestrogens despite ovulation (clomiphene failure) or have failed to ovulate with CC (clomiphene resistance). Gonadotropins are more effective than CC but are expensive, require parenteral administration, and have higher risk for ovarian hyperstimulation and multiple pregnancy. The principle of gonadotropin induction of ovulation is to mimic the normal physiological cycle of follicular selection, maturation, and ovulation. To use gonadotropins successfully for ovulation induction requires a sound knowledge of the normal endocrinologic processes that govern ovulation. Ovarian hyperstimulation, multiple follicular development, and multiple pregnancy are serious complications that can occur with uncontrolled stimulation.

As mentioned earlier, it is the duration of the "FSH window" during which the FSH levels are above the threshold required to stimulate the growing follicles that determines the number of follicles that will be recruited. The essence of monofollicular achievement in gonadotropin induction of ovulation is to identify the FSH threshold dose that results in the selection of a single follicle. Administration of an FSH dose higher than the threshold for a period of time inevitably results in multifollicular recruitment. Earlier, higher dose conventional gonadotropin stimulation was in vogue but had associated with it a higher incidence of hyperstimulation and multiple pregnancy. It involved starting with a dose of 2 ampoules (150 IU) of gonadotropins and increasing the dose every 3–5 days by 75 IU. Though ovulation rates were high, this regime was associated with high-complication rates. Currently used protocols are—low-dose step-up regime, step-down regimen, or sequential regimen.

These aim to increase the FSH concentrations gradually to reach the threshold level and, at the same time, avoid an explosive ovarian response that is typical of patients with PCOS.

Low-dose step-up protocol: This has been the preferred method of gonadotropin induction in PCOS patients. This is based on a threshold concept that initiation of follicular growth requires only a 10–30% increase in dose of exogenous FSH. This small dose increase is done at weekly intervals. This protocol is begun with a low starting dose of 75 IU daily for 7 days.[44] An ultrasound is done at the end of 1 week and, if the dominant follicle is more than 10 mm in diameter, the same dose is continued and, if it is less than 10 mm, the same dose is maintained for another week. At the end of the 2nd week, if the follicular size is still less than 10 mm, the dose of gonadotropin is increased by half ampoule weekly up to a maximum of 225 IU/day **(Flowchart 1).** This regime has the disadvantage that it is prolonged and requires multiple injections. But studies have shown that it maintains fair pregnancy rates (20%) and incidence of complications like multiple pregnancy (6%) and OHSS (0.14%) is low.

Step-down protocol: This protocol aims to mimic the normal physiological rise of FSH in the early follicular phase and subsequent decreasing dependence of the dominant growing follicle toward FSH. The starting dose is higher than the step-up protocol and once a follicular response is seen on ultrasound, the dose is reduced to a baseline level that is persisted with till it reaches 18 mm. This protocol warrants experience and judgment to determine the effective starting dose that should neither be administered high nor long enough to stimulate multifollicular growth. It thus calls for more stringent monitoring. The duration of treatment is smaller. It is depicted in **Flowchart 2.**

Flowchart 1: Chronic low-dose step-up protocol.

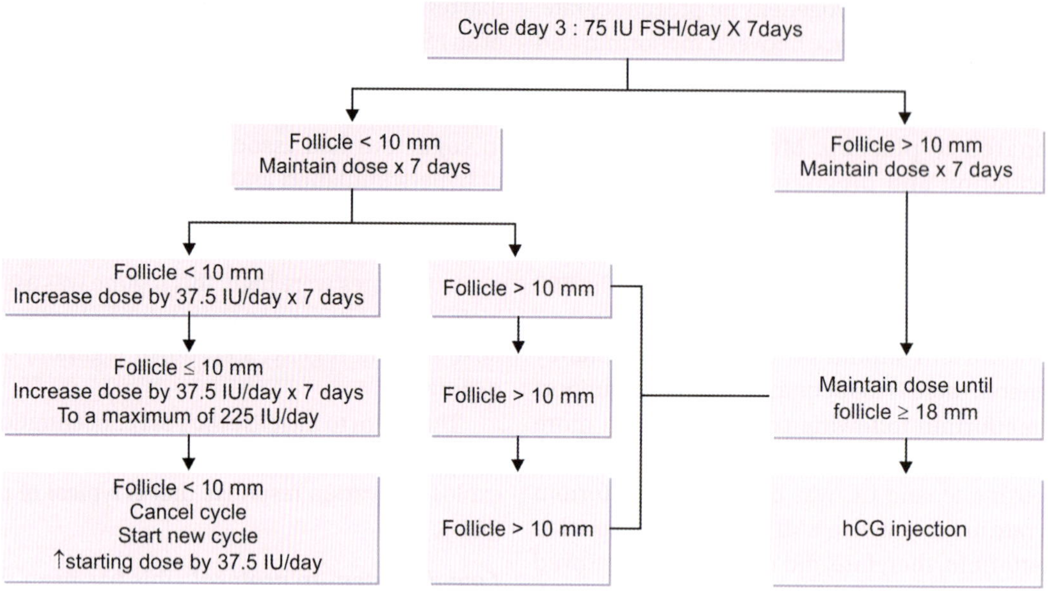

(FSH: follicle-stimulating hormone; hCG: human chorionic gonadotropin)

Flowchart 2: Chronic step-down protocol.

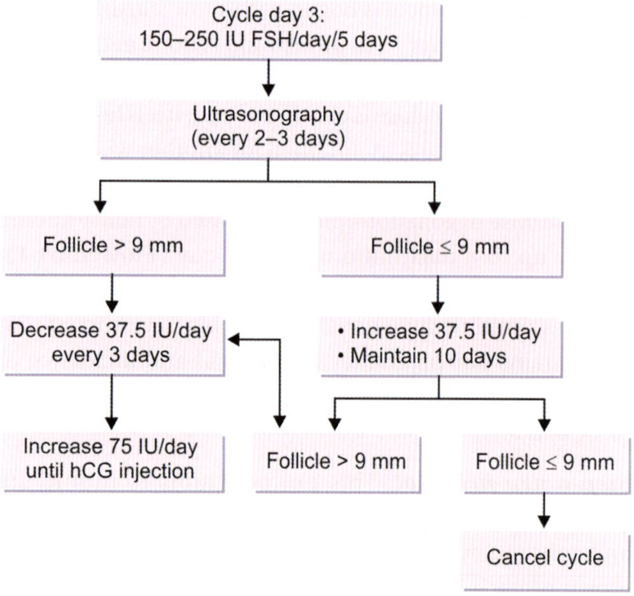

(FSH: follicle-stimulating hormone; hCG: human chorionic gonadotropin)

Oral ovulogens when used with gonadotropins, they result in almost equivalent pregnancy rates as gonadotropins alone and have the advantage of reducing gonadotropin use by 45–55%, lower cost per cycle, and no antiestrogenic side effects.[45]

Dopamine Agonists

Study and understanding of pathophysiology of OHSS has explained the use of cabergoline as dopamine agonist. It reduces vascular permeability, hemoconcentration, and ascites. With proper informed consent, it can be used in high-risk situations.[46]

Mechanism of action: Dopamine agonists decrease receptor expression for vascular endothelial growth factor (VEGF), which is responsible for causing OHSS.[47]

Dosage and risks: It should start on day of trigger at a dose of 0.5 mg daily for 8 days. No significant risk is seen with administration for 8 days at low dose. Most common side effects are headache, nausea, and dizziness. With long-term treatment, valvular heart disease was rarely observed with doses higher than 0.5 mg with incidence of 3/1,000 cases.

Gonadotropin-releasing Hormone

Pulsatile GnRH therapy can be given in women with intact pituitary gland, idiopathic hypogonadotropic hypogonadism, and weight loss-related amenorrhea. It can be given with the help of computerized mini-pump at pulse intervals of 60–180 minutes. More than 90% ovulation rates can be achieved with cumulative pregnancy rates up to 96% after six cycles. Incidence of multiple pregnancy rates is about 17.4%.

Disadvantages:

- Pump needs to be connected to the body at all times
- Development of antibodies
- Allergic skin reactions.

Gonadotropin-releasing Hormone Analogs

They are seldom used for ovulation induction treatment.

Surgical Methods

Stein and Leventhal in 1935 first performed ovarian wedge resection in infertile patients with PCOS. Though it was followed by promising results, the procedure was soon abandoned in view of extensive postoperative adhesions, tissue loss, and emergence of easier medical methods for ovulation induction. The introduction of minimally invasive surgery or laparoscopy created resurgence of interest in surgical methods. The process of laparoscopic ovarian drilling has been controversial and evolving, and its current status must be evaluated in the context of newer theories of pathogenesis of PCOS, newer definition of the disease, and the growing popularity of insulin sensitizers.

The first-line of treatment in PCOS still remains CC or letrozole. Options to treat women who are clomiphene resistant are insulin sensitizers, ovarian drilling, and gonadotropic induction. Ovulation induction with gonadotropins is expensive, requires experience since response can be explosive in later stages, and is associated with higher rates of multiple pregnancies. Ovarian drilling relatively is a more invasive procedure and is associated with irreversible complications like adhesion formation and poor ovarian reserve.

Laparoscopic ovarian drilling was first introduced by Gjonnaess in 1984. This procedure is less invasive when compared to wedge resection and involves producing multiple holes on the ovarian surface using either electrocautery or laser. Electrosurgical reduction in the volume of ovarian stroma decreases ovarian androgen production and provides a better follicular environment. Reduction in androgen production causes lesser peripheral aromatization and elevated FSH levels and reestablishment of HPO axis. Controversies continue to persist as to whether electrocautery is better than laser; the type of laser preferred, the number of holes per ovary, duration, strength, and nature of current to be used. In a review by Saleh et al. in 2004 involving 18 articles, the authors concluded that there was no difference in rates of ovulation between electrocoagulation and laser.

REFERENCES

1. Baerwald AR, Adams GP, Pierson RA. Ovarian antral folliculogenesis during the human menstrual cycle: a review. Hum Reprod Update. 2012;18(1):73-91.
2. Santbrink EJV, Eijkemans MJ, Laven JSE, et al. Patient-tailored conventional ovulation induction algorithms in anovulatory infertility. Trends Endocrin Metab. 2005;16(8):381-9.
3. Oktem O, Urman B. Understanding follicle growth in vivo. Hum Reprod. 2010;25(12):2944-54.
4. Vegetti W, Alagna F. FSH and folliculogenesis: from physiology to ovarian stimulation. Reprod Biomed Online. 2006;12(6):684-94.
5. Balasch J, Fabregues F. LH in the follicular phase: neither too high nor too low. Reprod Biomed Online. 2006;12(4):406-15.
6. Ludwig M, Felberbaum RE, Diedrich K, et al. Ovarian stimulation: from basic science to clinical application. Reprod Biomed Online. 2002;5(Suppl. 1):73-86.
7. Derosa G, Maffioli P. Anti-obesity drugs: a review about their effects and their safety. Expert Opin Drug Saf. 2012;11(3):459-71.
8. Homburg R, Insler V. Ovulation induction in perspective. Hum Reprod Update. 2002;8(5):449-62.
9. Macklon NS, Stouffer RL, Giudice LC, et al. The science behind 25 years of ovarian stimulation for in vitro fertilization. Endocr Rev. 2006;27:170-207.
10. ESHRE Capri Workshop Group. Mono-ovulatory cycles: a key goal in profertility programmes. Hum Reprod Update. 2003;9(3):263-74.
11. van Santbrink EJ, Fauser BC. Ovulation induction in normogonadotropic anovulation (PCOS). Best Pract Res Clin Endocrinol Metab. 2006;20(2):261-70.
12. ESHRE Capri Workshop Group. Health and fertility in World Health Organization group 2 anovulatory women. Hum Reprod Update. 2012;18(5):586-99.
13. Brown J, Farquhar C, Beck J, et al. Clomiphene and anti-estrogens for ovulation induction in PCOS. Cochrane Database Syst Rev. 2009;4:CD002249.
14. Kosmas IP, Tatsioni A, Fatemi HM, et al. Human chorionic gonadotropin administration vs. luteinizing monitoring for intrauterine insemination timing, after administration of clomiphene citrate: a meta-analysis. Fertil Steril. 2007;87(3):607-12.
15. George K, George S, Chandy A, et al. hCG administration offers no outcome benefit over spontaneous ovulation in anovulatory women treated with clomiphene citrate. Fertil Steril. 2007;87(4):985-7.
16. Goldstein SR, Siddhanti S, Ciaccia AV, et al. A pharmacological review of selective oestrogen receptor modulators. Hum Reprod Update. 2000;6(3):212-24.
17. Young SL, Opsahl MS, Fritz MA. Serum concentrations of enclomiphene and zuclomiphene across consecutive cycles of clomiphene citrate therapy in anovulatory infertile women. Fertil Steril. 1999;71(4):639-44.
18. Randall JM, Templeton A. Transvaginal sonographic assessment of follicular and endometrial growth in

spontaneous and clomiphene citrate cycles. Fertil Steril. 1991;56(2):208-12.
19. Jirge PR, Patil RS. Comparison of endocrine and ultrasound profiles during ovulation induction with clomiphene citrate and letrozole in ovulatory volunteer women. Fertil Steril. 2010;93(1):174-83.
20. Eden JA, Place J, Carter GD, et al. The effect of clomiphene citrate on follicular phase increase in endometrial thickness and uterine volume. Obstet Gynecol. 1989;73:187-90.
21. Hughes E, Collins J, Vandekerckhove P. Clomiphene citrate for ovulation induction in women with oligo-amenorrhoea. Cochrane Database Syst Rev. 2000;(2):CD000056.
22. Sammour A, Biljan MM, Tan SL, et al. Prospective randomized trial comparing the effects of letrozole (LE) and clomiphene citrate (clomiphene citrate) on follicular development, endometrial thickness and pregnancy rate in patients undergoing super-ovulation prior to intrauterine insemination (IUI). Fertil Steril. 2001;76(Suppl 1):S110.
23. Badawy A, Elnashar A, Totongy M. Clomiphene citrate or aromatase inhibitors for superovulation in women with unexplained infertility undergoing intrauterine insemination: A prospective randomized trial. Fertil Steril. 2009;92(4):1355-9.
24. Mahani IM, Afnan M. The pregnancy rates with intrauterine insemination (IUI) in superovulated cycles employing different protocols (clomiphen citrate (CC), human menopausal gonadotropin (HMG) and HMG+CC) and in natural ovulatory cycle. J Pak Med Assoc. 2004;54(10):503-5.
25. Elnashar A, Abdelmageed E, Fayed M, et al. Clomiphene citrate and dexamethasone in treatment of clomiphene citrate resistant polycystic ovary syndrome: a prospective placebo-controlled study. Hum Reprod. 2006;21(7):1805-8.
26. Holzer H, Casper R, Tulandi T. A new era in ovulation induction. Fertil Steril. 2006;85(2);277-84.
27. Homburg R, Insler V. Ovulation induction in perspective. Hum Reprod Update. 2002;8(5):449-62.
28. Annapurna V, Dhaliwal LK, Gopalan S. Effect of two anti-estrogens, clomiphene citrate and tamoxifen, on cervical mucus and sperm-cervical mucus interaction. Int J Fertil Womens Med. 1997;42(3):215-8.
29. Boostanfar R, Jain JK, Mishell DR Jr, et al. A prospective randomized trial comparing clomiphene citrate with tamoxifen citrate for ovulation induction. Fertil Steril. 2001;75(5):1024-6.
30. Franik S, Kremer JA, Nelen WL, et al. Aromatase inhibitors for subfertile women with polycystic ovary syndrome. Cochrane Database Syst Rev. 2014;(2):CD010287.
31. Yasser E, Ibrahim F. Aromatase inhibitors in the treatment of male infertility. Human Andrology. 2011;1(2):35-8.
32. Mitwally MF, Casper RF. Aromatase inhibition: a novel method of ovulation induction in women with polycystic ovary syndrome. Reprod Technol. 2000;10:244-7.
33. Bao SH, Sheng SL, Peng YF, et al. Effects of letrozole and clomiphene citrate on the expression of HOXA10 and integrin alpha v beta 3 in uterine epithelium of rats. Fertil Steril. 2009;91(1):244-8.
34. Fisher SA, Reid RL, Dean A, et al. A randomized double-blind comparison of the effects of clomiphene citrate and the aromatase inhibitor letrozole on ovulatory function in normal women. Fertil Steril. 2002;78(2):280-5.
35. Badawy A, Abdel Aal I, Abulatta M. Anastrozole or letrozole for ovulation induction in clomiphene resistant women with polycystic ovarian syndrome: A prospective randomized trial. Fertil Steril. 2008;89(5):1209-12.
36. Atay V, Cam C, Muchu M, et al. Comparison of letrozole and clomiphene citrate in women with polycystic ovaries undergoing ovarian stimulation. J Int Med Res. 2006;34(1):73-6.
37. Amer SA, Smith J, Mahran A, et al. Double-blind randomized controlled trial of letrozole versus clomiphene citrate in subfertile women with polycystic ovarian syndrome. Hum Reprod. 2017;32(8):1631-8.
38. Legro RS, Brzyski RG, Diamond MP, et al. Letrozole versus clomiphene for infertility in the polycystic ovary syndrome. N Engl J Med. 2014;371(2):119-29.
39. Geisler J, Haynes B, Anker G, et al. Influence of letrozole and anastrozole on total body aromatization and plasma estrogen levels in postmenopausal breast cancer patients evaluated in a randomized, cross-over study. J Clin Oncol. 2002;20(3):751-7.
40. Mitwally MF, Casper RF. Aromatase inhibition reduces gonadotrophin dose required for controlled ovarian stimulation in women with unexplained infertility. Hum Reprod. 2003;18(8):1588-97.
41. Palomba S, Orio F Jr, Zullo F. What is the best first-step therapeutic approach in treating anovulatory infertility in patients with polycystic ovary syndrome? Questions that are still unanswered. Gynecol Endocrinol. 2007;23(5):245-7.
42. Mitwally MF, Biljan MM, Casper RF. Pregnancy outcome after the use of an aromatase inhibitor for ovarian stimulation. Am J Obstet Gynecol. 2005;192(2):381-6.
43. Sohrabvand F, Ansari Sh, Bagheri M. Efficacy of combined metformin-letrozole in comparison with metformin-clomiphene citrate in clomiphene-resistant infertile women with polycystic ovarian disease. Hum Reprod. 2006;21(6):1432-5.
44. Thessaloniki ESHRE/ASRM-Sponsored PCOS Consensus Workshop Group. Consensus on infertility treatment related to polycystic ovary syndrome. Hum Reprod. 2008;23(3):462-77.
45. Fields E, Chard J, James D, et al.; Guideline Development Group. Fertility (update): summary of NICE guidance. BMJ. 2013;346:f650.
46. Alverez C, Marti-Bonmati L, Novella-Maestre E, et al. Dopamine agonist cabergoline reduces hemoconcentration and ascites in hyperstimulated women undergoing assisted reproduction. J Clin Endocrinol Metab. 2007;92(8):2931-7.
47. Soares SR, Gomez R, Simon C, et al. Targeting the vascular endothelial growth factor sys-tem to prevent ovarian hyper-stimulation syndrome. Hum Reprod Update. 2008;14(4):321-33.

Ultrasonography in Follicular Monitoring

29

Sonal Panchal, CB Nagori

INTRODUCTION

Follicular monitoring is an absolute essential for any fertility therapy in which ovulation induction is done. The aim is to assess the follicle maturity and endometrial receptivity to determine the time of ovulation trigger. This can be done by hormonal assessments and/or ultrasound. The follicular maturity can be assessed by estradiol levels, but frequent assessment of blood estradiol level is a cumbersome procedure as it might demand multiple fresh blood samples at times. With the advent of high end ultrasound machines the diagnosis and monitoring of ovulation induction has become very precise.[1] Transvaginal ultrasound supplemented with Doppler today is the most accepted modality for follicular monitoring and endometrial scoring. Follicular maturation, endometrium growth, ovulation, and luteinization are the complex biochemical, morphological and vascular phenomenon. The color Doppler denotes the vascular changes which in turn are indicative of biochemical changes in the endometrium. The 3D ultrasound in comparison to the 2D ultrasound assesses the endometrial as well as the follicular size more superiorly. The 3D power Doppler is useful in diagnosing qualitative and quantitative idea of vascularity which is a marker of physiological/functional maturity. Another advantage of the ultrasound is that even when there are multiple follicles, every individual follicle can be studied from the time it has been recruited as antral follicle to the stage when it matures, ruptures, gets converted into corpus luteum. This discussion can be divided into monitoring follicular changes and monitoring endometrial changes.

FOLLICULAR MONITORING

Secondary antral follicles are the first follicular structures that become evident on ultrasound. These grow till the size of 6–7 mm under the effect of androgen alone, but beyond that these develop follicle-stimulating hormone (FSH) receptors. The dominant follicle is selected very early during the menstrual cycle and becomes apparent as early as 5th day on ultrasound. A follicle that is of more than 10 mm in diameter, is FSH dependent dominant follicle has a growth rate of 2–3 mm per day and has no internal echogenicity and has thin (pencil line like) walls, and is not only more likely to become the leading follicle but will also give mature healthy ovum.

The growing follicle can be assessed by transvaginal sonography. The shape changes from round to polygonal when there are multiple follicles due to pressure effect from adjacent follicles. In such follicles the follicular volume would has to be considered instead of a single diameter and is calculated as $(D1 \times D2 \times D3) \times 0.523$, where D1, D2 and D3 are three diameters of follicles in perpendicular planes using B-mode ultrasound. The reason why optimum pressure must be applied during a transvaginal ultrasonography over the probe is that the follicle shape may become ellipsoid under excess pressure.

B-mode Features of a Mature Follicle

A mature follicle, is 16–18 mm **(Fig. 1A)**, has thin walls and regular round shape. It shows a thin hypoechoic rim surrounding the follicle and sometimes (about 35–40%) cumulus like shadow may be seen. This thin hypoechoic

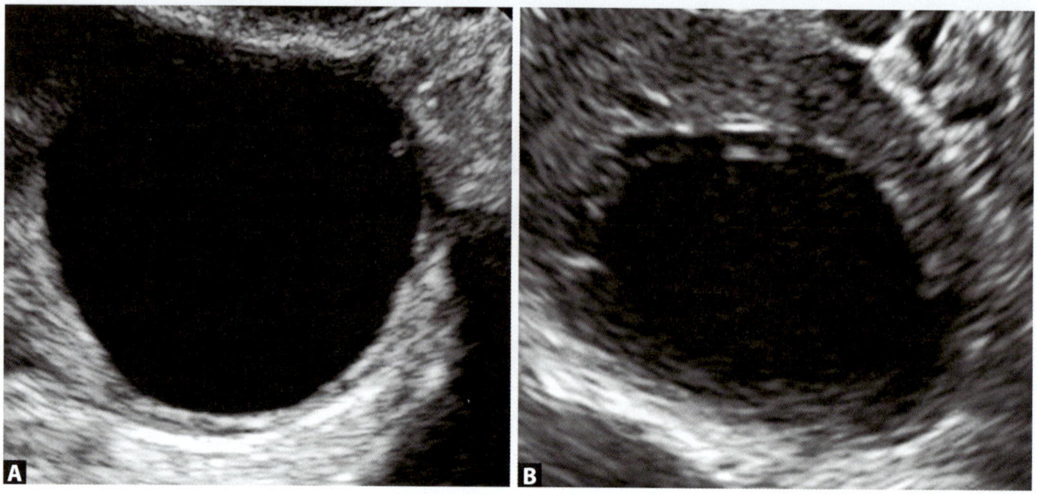

Figs. 1A and B: (A) Preovulatory follicle on B-mode; (B) 6–8 hours before rupture.

rim and cumulus like shadow develop approximately 24–36 hours before rupture. About 6–10 hours before rupture of follicle an irregular flimsy line is visualized within the follicle parallel to the wall **(Fig. 1B)**.

Doppler Features of a Good Pre-hCG Follicle

As early as 8th day of the cycle the perifollicular vascularity increases in the theca layer of the dominant follicle. Decrease in perifollicular resistance index (RI) starts 2 days before ovulation, reaches baseline at ovulation, remains low for 4 days and then with gradual rise reaches 0.5 in mid-luteal phase.[2] When the follicle matures functionally the Doppler demonstrates blood vessels covering at least three-fourths of the follicular circumference **(Fig. 2)**. Perifollicular vessels are only those that obliterate the follicular margins and overlap those margins. When in a single cross area slice, the flow covered less than 25%, 25–50%, 50–75% and more than 75% of follicular circumference, the grade of follicular flow was graded as 1 to 4 by Chui et al. The conception was related to grade 3–4 vascularity.[3] On pulse Doppler perifollicular blood vessels should show RI of 0.4–0.48[4] and PSV of more than 10 cm/ sec **(Fig. 3)**. The PRF settings for color Doppler are set at 0.3 and wall filter at the lowest.

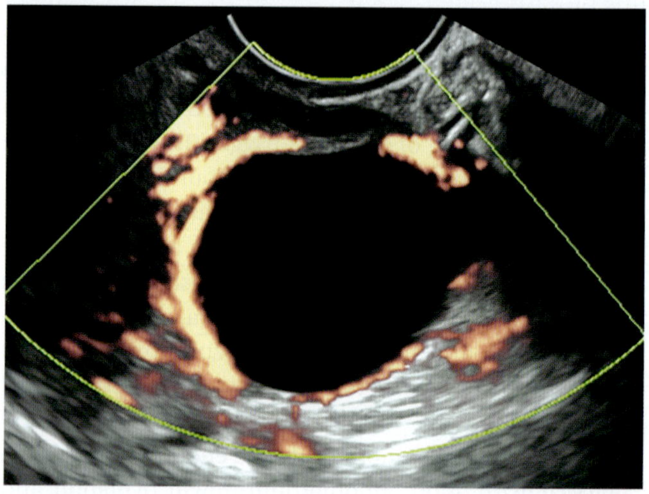

Fig. 2: Preovulatory follicle with vascular ring surrounding the follicle.

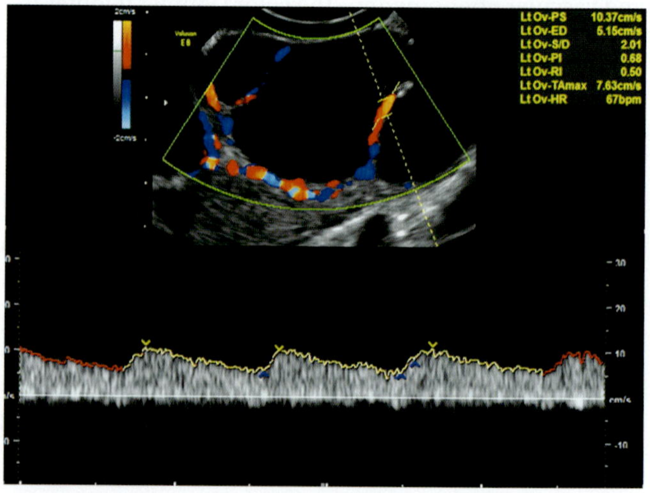

Fig. 3: Preovulatory follicle with pulse Doppler showing low resistance flow.

IMPLICATIONS OF FLOW PARAMETERS ON OVUM QUALITY

The appropriate time to administer hCG to optimize the recovery rate is determined by the ovarian flow. Higher RI indicates higher resistance flow to the follicle meaning lower flow during diastolic phase and so reduced phasic oxygen supply to the ovum and hence lack of maturity. A study by

Nargund et al.[5,6] stated that the chances of having grade 1 embryos are reduced and the risk of having chromosomal malformations was higher in the ova from follicles which had a perifollicular PSV of less than 10 cm/sec. In the same study it has been shown that the probability of developing a grade 1 or 2 embryo is 75% if PSV was more than 10 cm/sec, 40% if PSV was less than 10 cm/sec, 24% if there was no perifollicular flow. There is yet another study that supports this finding. High frequency of abnormalities of organization of chromosomes on metaphase spindle and which may lead to segregation disorders and catastrophic mosaics in embryo are seen in oocytes from severely hypoxic follicles.[7]

Our Data

Our unpublished data of more than 1,000 intrauterine insemination (IUI) cycles has shown that when the perifollicular RI more than 0.53 and PSV less than 9 cm/sec, 12 hours before hCG injection, the conception rates were only 8.3% and 10% respectively as compared to 32.8% and 28.2 % respectively and individually when perifollicular RI less than 0.50 and PSV more than 11 cm/sec.

Follicular RI (1,025 cases)

Follicular RI	***0.56–0.53***	***0.53–0.50***	***< 0.50***
Conc.	05	71	170
Nonconc.	58	373	348
Total	63	444	518

Follicular PSV (1,025 cases)

Follicular PSV	***<9***	***9–10***	***10–11***	***> 11***
Conc.	04	14	38	190
Nonconc.	36	92	168	483
Total	40	106	206	673

(Conc.: conceived cases, Nonconc.: nonconceived cases)

So, it would be best to wait with no extra medication when patient is on clomiphene citrate (CC) stimulation or continue with the same dose of gonadotropin till we get proper perifollicular RI and PSV, though sometimes the follicular size may reach up to 22 mm. Almost 90% of the times the desired RI and PSV are reached by the time follicular size is 20 mm maximum.

VOLUME ULTRASOUND FOR FOLLICULAR ASSESSMENT

Assessment of these follicles can be done efficiently with 3D US and 3D power Doppler. We studied 500 IUI cycles that were all monitored for ovulation by 2D and color Doppler. When the follicles appeared mature as per the abovementioned features, 3D and 3D power Doppler was done for all and the values of 3D and 3D power Doppler indices were studied and plotted on the graphs for conception and nonconception cycles. We used Voluson 730 Expert (GE) for our studies. Once the follicles of more than or equal to 16 mm for gonadotropin stimulation or more than or equal to 18 mm for CC stimulated cycle is seen and assessed by color Doppler, the volume box is switched on. The size of the volume box should be enough to include the whole follicle and at least a surrounding 5–7 mm margin. The angle of the volume should be large enough to cover the whole follicle from edge to edge. The acquired volume is seen as follicle in three perpendicular planes on the screen. Using the VOCAL (Virtual organ computer aided analysis), software with 15° angle the follicle is traced at its circumference at every 15° rotation **(Fig. 4)** and at the end the command "done" is given, the volume is ultimately accepted, or any corrections required may be made and the machine then calculates the volume of the follicle.

Volume Ultrasound Parameters of Good Pre-HCG Follicle

Follicular Volume

A study by Witmack et al.[8] shows that—in IVF-ET cycles, optimal rates of oocyte recovery, fertilization and cleavage are associated with follicles with mean follicular diameter of 12–24 mm. This corresponds to the follicular volumes of between 3 mL and 7 mL. The accuracy of 3D US measurement of follicular volume compared to the standard

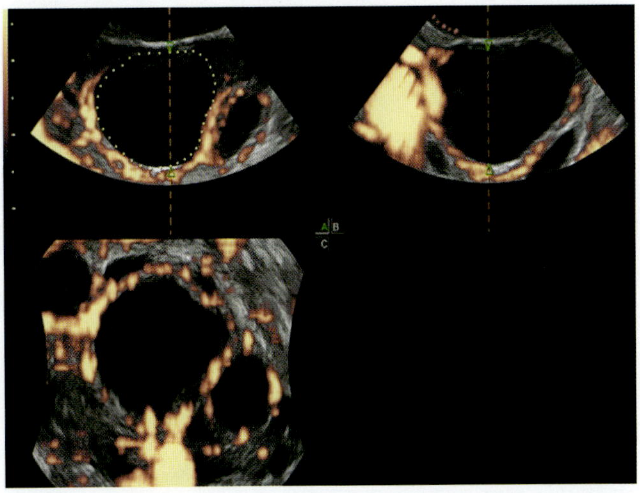

Fig. 4: Calculation of follicular volume by Virtual Organ Computer-aided AnaLysis (VOCAL).

2D techniques by comparing the volume of individual follicles estimated by both methods with the corresponding follicular aspirates: using the formula of ellipse the limits of agreement between aspirates and calculated volume was +3.47 to –2.42 as compared to +0.96 to –0.43 when calculated by 3D US using VOCAL.[9] This is because 3D US measurement is not affected by the follicular shape as the changing contours are outlined serially to obtain the specific volume measurement.

Cumulus

After the volume calculation the follicle is seen plane by plane in the acquired volume by translation and rotation that is walking through the volume and rotating the volume. If it is seen on one plane it is confirmed on the other two planes and also on the rendered image. Using a combination of surface smooth and light gradient mode for rendering with high threshold can show cumulus **(Fig. 5)**. We in our study of 500 IUI cycles have been able to locate the cumulus in 94.6% of cases in conception cycles and in 53% of nonconception cycles by surface rendering. In IVF cycles also, we have been able to predict the number of ova that we would obtain on retrieval by the number of cumulus containing follicles. Presence of cumulus in follicles more than 15 mm by 3D US have been shown in a study by Feichtinger et al.[10] Follicles in which cumulus is not visualized in all three planes are not likely to contain mature oocytes. Appearance of the intrafollicular cumulus structures by 3D US was correlated with the recovery rate of the mature oocytes was shown in a study by Poehl et al.[11] They also found a significant correlation between the number of detected cumuli and the number of retrieved oocytes ($P < 0.0001$), mature oocytes ($P < 0.0001$) and number of fertilized oocytes ($P < 0.0001$). Therefore visualization of the cumulus by 3D US is a good indicator of mature oocytes in IUI and in vitro fertilization (IVF) procedures and has been found to be a marker of successful fertilization in IVF cycles.

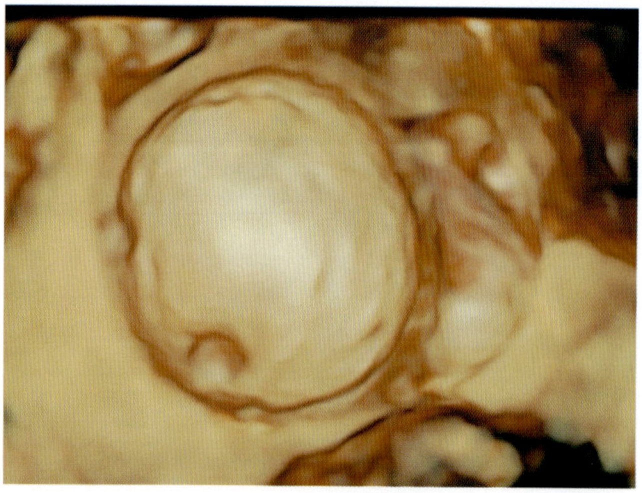

Fig. 5: Cumulus oophorus in preovulatory follicle.

3D PD for Follicular Assessment

Follicular fluid concentrations of leptine, a follicular angiogenesis related factors are inversely related to the stromal blood flow index.[12] It has also been suggested that the follicles containing oocytes capable to produce a pregnancy have a perifollicular vascular network more uniform and distinctive.[13]

After having measured the volume of the follicle and looking for the presence of the cumulus, we switch over to power Doppler. The PRF settings are fixed at 0.3, and wall filter at the lowest. A 3D volume with power Doppler is taken, with the volume angle to include the entire follicle is selected. Again on the screen, the follicle is seen in three perpendicular planes but this time with blood vessels as seen on power Doppler. Again switch on the VOCAL and calculate the follicular volume. At the end of the last trace around the follicle, click the "done" switch and the options are open to accept the ROI or to select one of the options for the shell volume. We select an option for the outside shell with the wall thickness of 2 mm, which has been found to be the most appropriate to include the perifollicular vessels **(Fig. 6A)**. Then accept this and switch on the volume histogram. When this volume is accepted it gives you the follicular volume as the reference volume, the shell volume as the volume of the wall and the whole combined volume. Then switch over to volume histogram, to get a graph that shows the calculation of the gray voxels and the color voxels in the given volume and these values are displayed on the screen as VI, FI and VFI values. VI indicates the abundance of the color voxels in the given volume, FI indicates the intensity of the color in the given volume and VFI is the ratio of the abundance and intensity, meaning it gives idea about the general perfusion status of the given volume **(Fig. 6B)**. This means volume histogram or the 3D power Doppler indices gives the quantitative assessment of global vascularization and perfusion of the given volume.

3D PD Indices and Follicular Quality

In our study[14] we have found perifollicular VI of between 6 and 20 and perifollicular FI less than 35 as most optimum.

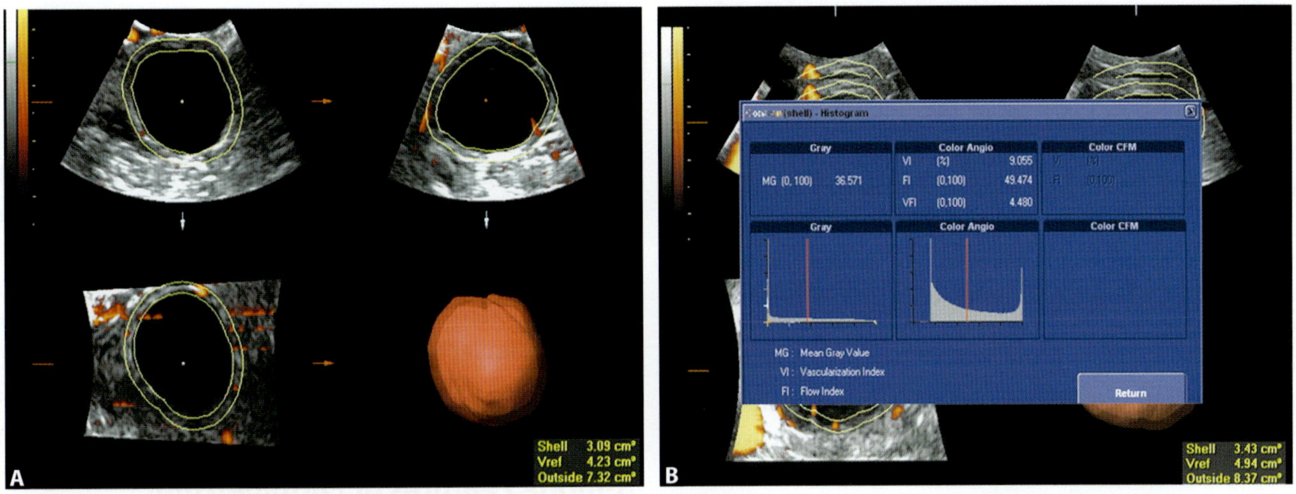

Figs. 6A and B: (A) Calculating the shell volume of the follicle for perifollicular 3D-PD assessment; (B) Histogram for perifollicular flow giving vascularity index (VI), flow index (FI), and vascularity flow index (VFI) values.

68.4% of patients conceived when the VI was between 6 and 18 and 50% when it was between 18 and 20. However, the pregnancy rates were less than 25% when VI was less than 6 and only 7.4% when VI was more than 20. It was only 7.4% of patients with FI less than 27 who conceived whereas beyond 27, the conception rates rose consistently. It was 50% with FI between 27 and 35, 70% when FI was between 35 and 43 and almost all patients had conceived when FI was more than 43.

Follicular Volume (500 cases)

Follicular Volume	***< 3***	***3–5***	***5.1–7***	***> 7***
Conc.	15	94	85	20
Nonconc.	46	89	66	95
Total	61	173	151	115

Follicular VI (500 cases)

Follicular VI	***<6***	***6–18***	***18.1–20***	***> 20***
Conc.	6	115	83	10
Nonconc.	20	55	83	128
Total	26	170	166	138

Follicular FI (500 cases)

Follicular FI	***< 27***	***27–35***	***35.1–43***	***> 43***
Conc.	12	100	76	26
Nonconc.	153	100	32	1
Total	165	200	108	27

(Conc.: conceived cases, Nonconc.: nonconceived cases)

Meaning that even when the follicle appeared mature according to the 2D US and color and pulse Doppler parameters, the pregnancy rates were significantly better only when the follicular volume was between 3 and 7.5 cc, cumulus was present and the perifollicular VI and FI values were as mention earlier.

A study, by Kupesic and Kurjak, shows that when the ratio of follicular volume to blood flow index (FV/FI) is between 0.4–0.6 the pregnancy rates are 39%, if more than 0.6, it is 52% and when less than 0.4 is only 21%.[15] Although it is possible to assess the follicular flow as expressed by the peak systolic velocity and perifollicular color map,[16] it is the 3D power Doppler which proves the most precise information about the vascularization and follicular blood flow.[17] The 3D and the 3D power Doppler assessment may explore the hidden causes of failure of conception in treatment cycles.

DOPPLER PARAMETERS OF FOLLICLE AND TIME OF INTRAUTERINE INSEMINATION

Going a little further from this stage, hCG plays a major role in inducing influx of blood within follicles. Vascular changes at the time of impending ovulation include increased vascularity of the inner wall of the follicle and a coincident surge in blood velocity just prior to eruption.[18] A marked increase in the peak systolic velocity around the follicle, in the presence of a relatively constant pulsatility index (PI), could be a sign of follicle maturity and impending ovulation.[19] At the LH surge the perifollicular PSV is 10 cm/sec. The follicular PSV goes as high as 45 cm/sec before an hour of ovulation under the effect of rising LH. This means that if the follicle is said to be functionally mature when PSV is 10 cm/sec that is the time when the LH surge starts and under the effect of that LH, the perifollicular PSV keeps on rising constantly. This derives that a rising PSV with steady low RI suggests that the follicle is close to rupture.

Based on these facts, we did a study to find out if double IUI can increase the pregnancy rate in patients who have a pre-hCG perifollicular PSV more than 15 cm/sec. 300 IUI cycles were studied, with three different stimulation protocols. The protocols were only CC 100 mg from day 5 to day 9, aromatase inhibitor tablet Letrozole 100 mg from day 3 to 7, followed by recombinant FSH (rFSH) 75 IU till the follicle size of 16–18 mm was achieved, and only rFSH from 3 of the cycle till the desired follicular size was achieved. All the patients had unexplained infertility, were between 23 years and 29 years of age, and had a body mass index (BMI) of between 23 and 27. Color and pulse Doppler was done for all patients. Stimulation was continued till optimum flows were also seen apart from the size of the follicle. hCG 10,000 was given to all patients for follicular rupture. Every alternate patient was taken for double IUI, irrespective of color Doppler findings. Single IUI was done between 36 hours and 38 hours and double IUI were done at 12–14 hours and 36–38 hours postwash sperm count between 7 million/mL and 10 million/mL. The results clearly showed that no matter what protocol was used, the conception rates were significantly high in patients in whom double IUI was done when perifollicular PSV was more than or equal to 20 cm/sec on the day of hCG, as compared to when single IUI was done. When perifollicular PSV on the day of hCG was between 15 cm/sec and 20 cm/sec the conception rates were only minimally increased with double IUI. Though the conception rates were similar for single or double IUI when perifollicular PSV on the day of IUI was less than 15cm/sec.

Endometrial Evaluation

Weakest link in the success of infertility treatment is implantation. Endometrium plays a major role in the success of the infertility treatment as it is the receptor organ for all the major hormones involved hence a detailed study of the endometrium is of utmost importance. Therefore, like follicle, a similar transvaginal 2D US and color Doppler of the endometrium is done before planning for hCG during any assisted reproductive technologies.

B-mode Features of Endometrium with Good Receptivity

On transvaginal sonography, an endometrial thickness of minimum 6 mm is required on the day of hCG, but 8–10 mm is optimum. Endometrial thickness has more negative predictive value for implantation. In all the healthy endometria, the endometrial-myometrial interface is always seen as a clear hypoechoic halo surrounding the whole endometrium **(Fig. 7)**. Breach or irregularity of endometrial-myometrial junction is an indication of unhealthy endometrium and therefore poor receptivity.

Morphology of the endometrium is as important as thickness of the endometrium. Grade A is considered to be morphologically suitable grade for the implantation, when it is a triple line endometrium with the intervening area showing echogenicity not more than the anterior

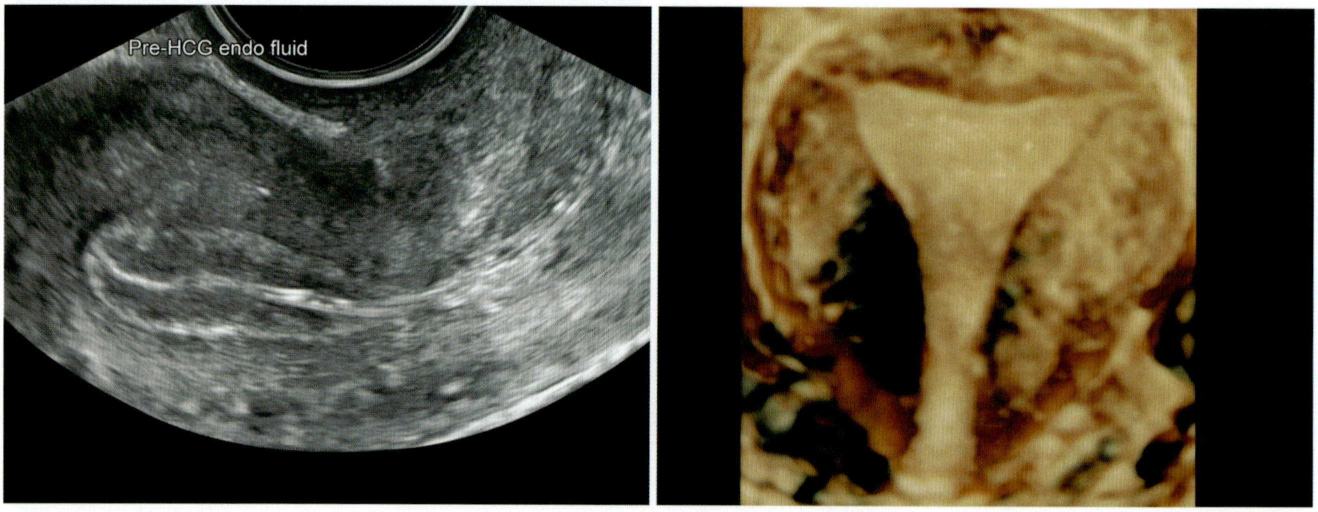

Fig. 7: Endometrial–myometrial junction (EMJ).

myometrium. The echogenicity is attributed to stromal edema, development of multiple vessels penetrating in the endometrium producing multiple tissue interfaces and therefore causing the echogenicity and due to glycogen storage in the endometrial columnar epithelium **(Fig. 8)**. Grade B or intermediate grade is when it **(Fig. 9)** is multilayered or triple line with hypo to anechoic intervening area, mildly suitable for implantation. The Grade C is considered the most unfavorable endometrium as it is a homogenous isoechoic endometrium **(Fig. 10)**.[20] This endometrium is typically hyperestrogenic endometrium. Though some studies have shown no significant difference in pregnancy rates amongst different morphological patterns.

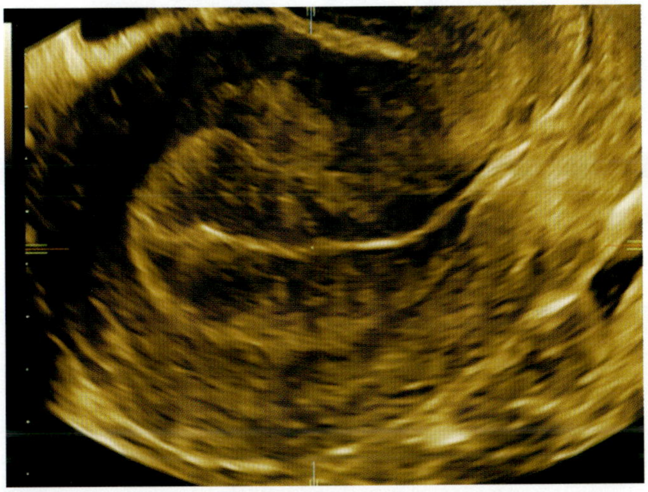

Fig. 8: Most receptive endometrium grade A—multilayered.

Doppler Features of Endometrium with Good Receptivity

There are several reports by different groups[21] that agree on the fact that implantation rates can be more correlated to the vascularity of the endometrium rather than the thickness and morphology of the endometrium. The presence of endometrial blood flow significantly improves cycle outcome in hormone replacement therapy-FET cycles.[22]

Segmental uterine artery perfusion demonstrates significant correlation with hormonal and histological markers of uterine receptivity, reaching the highest sensitivity for subendometrial blood flow.[15] On color Doppler the endometrium that is mature shows vascularity in zone 3 and 4 or may be called subendometrial and endometrial layers **(Fig. 11)**. The zones of vascularity are defined according to Applebaum[23] as: zone 1 when the vascularity on power Doppler is seen only at endometrial-myometrial junction, zone 2 when vessels penetrate through the hyperechogenic endometrial edge, zone 3 when it reaches intervening hypoechogenic zone and zone 4 when they reach the endometrial cavity.

One more comparison of two studies have also shown markedly better conception rates with vascularity in zone 3 and 4:[24]

▪ Zone 1	3.5– 7.5%	5.2%
▪ Zone 2	15.8–29.7%	28.7%
▪ Zone 3	24.2–47.8%	52%
▪ Zone 4	67.3%	74%

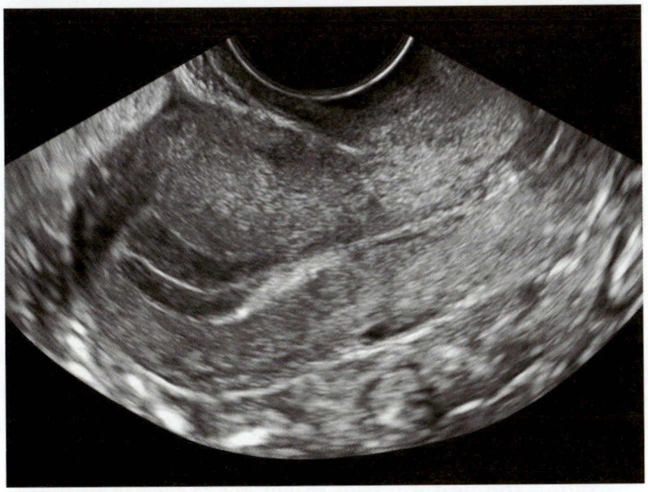

Fig. 9: Multilayered endometrium grade B—intermediate.

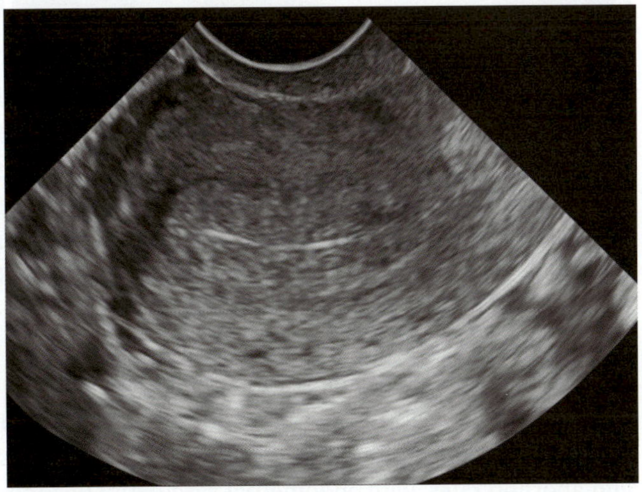

Fig. 10: Isoechoic homogeneous grade C endometrium.

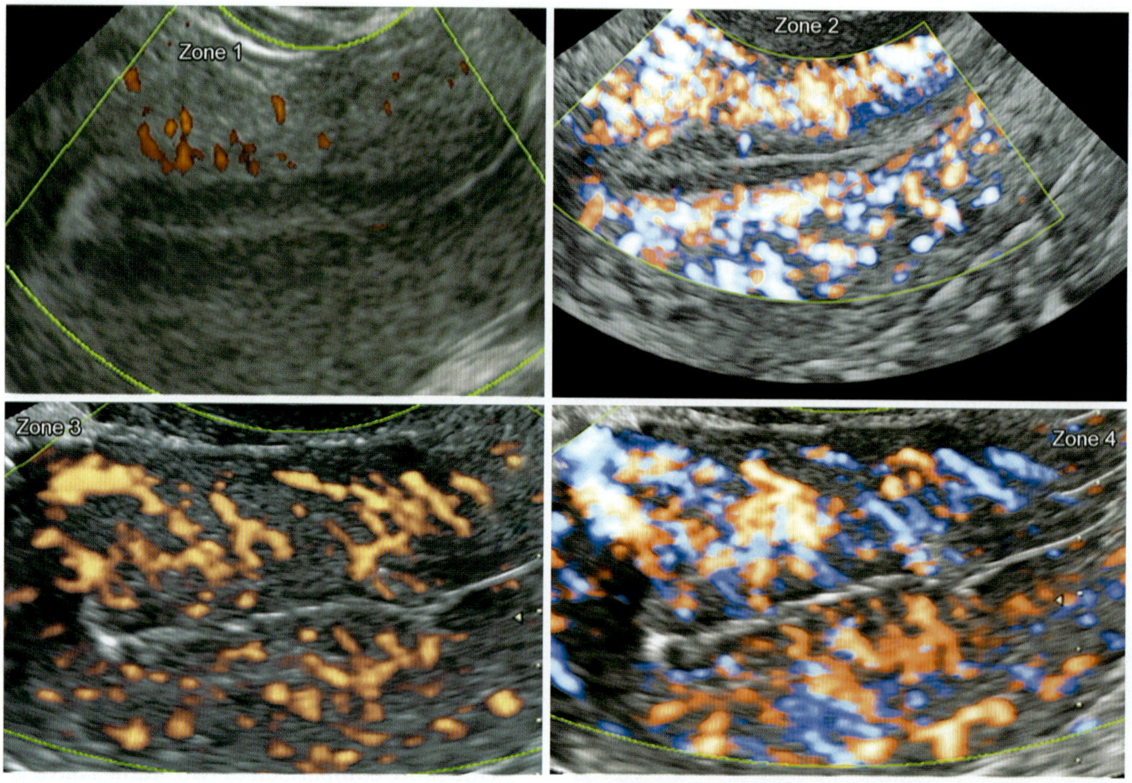

Fig. 11: Endometrial vascularity zones (1, 2, 3 and 4).

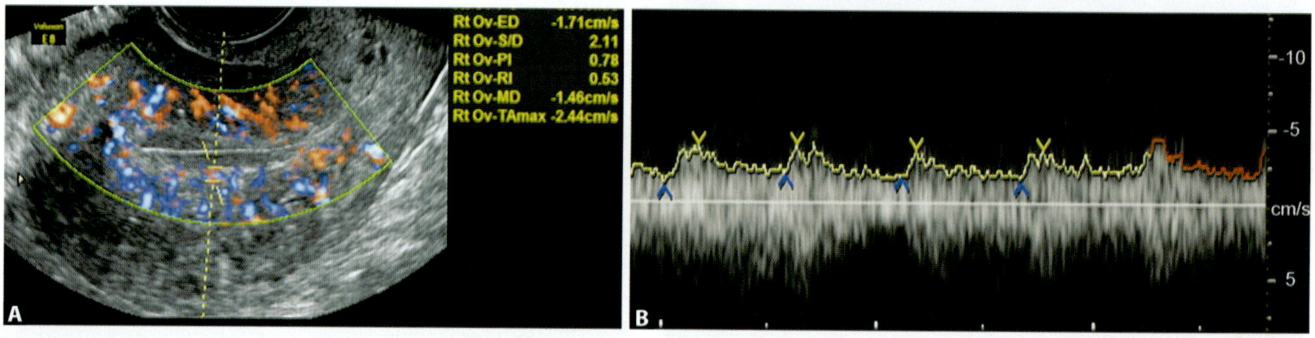

Figs. 12A and B: Pulse Doppler of endometrial vascularity.

Zaidi et al. found that absence of flow in the endometrial and subendometrial zones on day of hCG indicate total failure of implantation.[22] The vessels that reach the endometrium are the spiral arteries. The pulse Doppler of these arteries should have an RI of between 0.6 and 0.8 and PI of between 1.1 and 2.3 for the endometrium to be called mature for implantation **(Figs. 12A and B)**. This vascularity should cover at least 5 mm^2 area of the endometrium. Below this cutoff, the pregnancy rates are extremely low.[25]

In one of our studies we have found a significant difference in conception rates, ongoing pregnancy rates and abortion rates, with endometrial vascularity in zones 1, 2, 3, and 4 **(Table 1)**.[26]

Table 1: Zones of vascularity.

Vascularity zone	*1*	*2*	*3*	*4*
% of patients	6.69%	20.73%	58%	14.47%
B-hCG	19%	21.87%	39.77%	70.14%
Gestational sac	9.6%	14.58%	36.8%	68.65%
Abortion rate	50%	23.8%	5.6%	1.5%

When pregnancy is achieved in absence of endometrial and subendometrial flow on the day of embryo transfer, more than half of these pregnancies will finish as spontaneous miscarriage.[24]

When the endometrial thickness is less than 8 mm, and if there are non-triple endometrial line and non-favorable blood flow zone on day of hCG in IVF/ICSI cycles, pregnancy is unlikely and embryo transfer should be canceled with freezing of all embryos for future transfer to increase the success rate.[27]

Uterine Artery Doppler

Moreover the pulse Doppler analysis of the uterine artery waveform is done and its PI should be less than 3.2 **(Fig. 13)**. Several authors have shown that the optimum uterine receptivity was obtained when average pulsatility index (PI) of the uterine artery was between 2 and 3 on the day of transfer or on the day of hCG.[24,28] Coulam et al. have also shown that no pregnancy was achieved after embryo transfer when uterine artery PI was above 3.3 in an IVF program.[29] Tsai and colleagues[30] evaluated the prognostic value of uterine perfusion on day of hCG for IUI cycles and showed that no pregnancy occurred when the PI of ascending branch of uterine artery was less than 3. Fecundity rate was 18% when PI less than 2 and 19.8% when between 2 and 3. This probably can be explained on the basis that the uteri having fibroids or adenomyosis show fairly high uterine artery blood flow velocities but lower resistance indices. A study by Cacciatore et al. suggest that implantation is unlikely when PI is more than 3.3 and RI more than 0.95 or when no velocities are seen at the end of the diastole.[31] Though uterine artery impedance is usually low in superovulated cycles. In our unpublished data of more than 1,000 IUI cycles, when color Doppler studies were done 12 hours before hCG injection, we have found no conceptions when uterine artery PI is more than 3.5.

VOLUME ULTRASOUND ASSESSMENT OF ENDOMETRIUM

When endometrial and the uterine artery parameters are optimum as described earlier, the volume of the endometrium with power Doppler is acquired and then the endometrial volume is calculated by VOCAL, tracing the outer edge of the hyperechoic outer rim of the endometrium and accept the volume **(Fig. 14)**. The endometrium up to the internal os is taken into calculation. For accurate measurements, a good contrast in the image is necessary. Select smaller angles of rotation for VOCAL. Fluid in the endometrial cavity can be a source of error.

3D and 3D-PD Features of Good Endometrial Receptivity

Our study[14] showed that at endometrial volume of less than 2 cc no pregnancies occurred. With endometrial volume of 2–3 cc only 16.66% of patients conceived, between 3 and 5 cc 47% of patients conceived and when the endometrial volume was between 5 and 7 cc 61.5% patients conceived.

Endometrial volume (500 cases)					
Endometrial volume	***< 2***	***2–3***	***3.1–5***	***5.1–7***	***> 7***
Conc.	0	26	70	67	41
Nonconc.	20	132	78	42	24
Total	20	158	148	109	65

Decline in conception rates at endometrial volumes of more than 7 cc is seen. This can be explained by

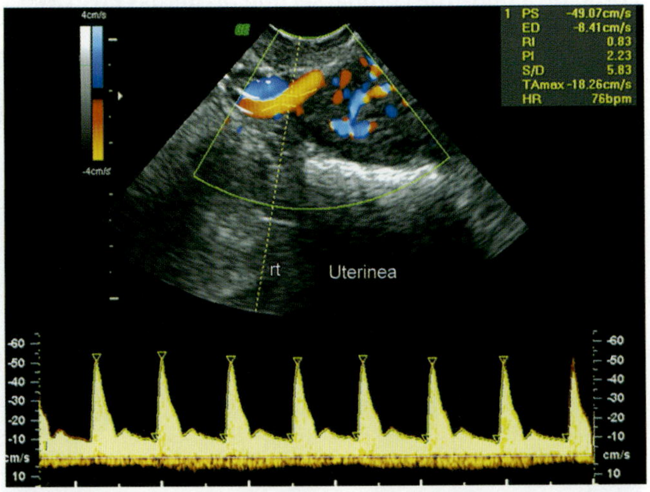

Fig. 13: Preovulatory uterine artery waveform.

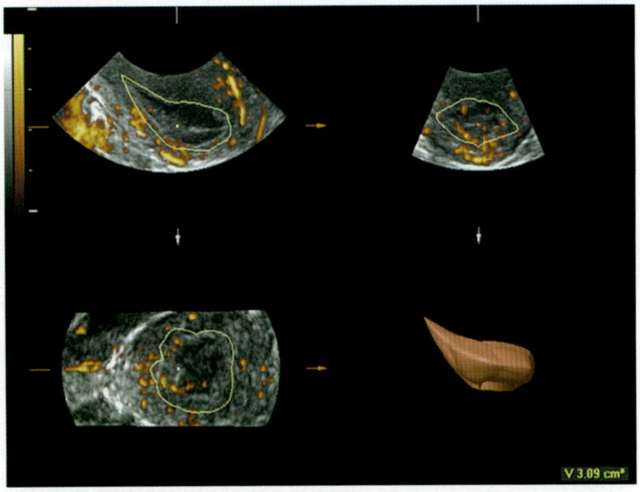

Fig. 14: Calculating endometrial volume by Virtual Organ Computer-aided AnaLysis (VOCAL).

pathological increase in endometrial thickness and volume like hyperplasia or large polyps that significantly decrease the implantation rates. For endometrial volume the inter CC definition of internal os and (interobserver variation) was 0.82 and intra CC (intraobserver variation) was 0.90, the chief source of error being definition of endometrial margins.[34] Endometrial volume by 3D US volume calculation of the endometrium may help to correlate the cycle outcome with quantitative parameter rather than endometrial thickness.[8] A study by Raga et al.[32] shows pregnancy and implantation rates were significantly lower when endometrial volume less than 2 mL, while no pregnancy was achieved when endometrial volume was less than 1 mL. Study by Kupesic et al. also shows no pregnancy when endometrial volume was less than 2 mL, or when exceeded 8 mL.[33] For the same calculated volume, volume histogram is switched on and it calculates the endometrial VI, FI and VFI. In our series[14] the endometrial VI values were not very conclusive. Endometrial FI when was less than 20, only 23% of patients showed conception, between 20 and 40 it was almost 50% but when FI was more than 40, 68% of patients showed conception.

Endometrial FI (500 cases)				
Endometrial FI	***< 20***	***20–30***	***30.1–40***	***> 40***
Conc.	37	68	75	34
Nonconc.	125	76	68	17
Total	162	144	143	51

Endometrial VFI when was more than 20 the conception occurred in 71.2% of patients and when VFI was less than 1.0 no conception was seen. Though between VFI 5 and 20 the percentage of conception was 49–56%.

Endometrial VFI (500 cases)					
Endometrial VFI	***< 2***	***2–5***	***5.1–12***	***12.1–20***	***> 20***
Conc.	00	96	64	45	09
Nonconc.	44	136	66	36	04
Total	44	232	130	81	13

A scoring system reported by Kupesic et al.,[34] for uterine receptivity, done on the day of embryo transfer shows that subendometrial FI less than 11 was a cutoff limit. (Subendometrial indices are calculated in the same way from the endometrial volume as we calculate the perifollicular indices from the follicular volume, i.e. by shell volume of 2 mm thickness.) No pregnancies occurred when it was less than 11 and the conception group showed its values of 13.2 ± 2.2. These values differ from our values probably because we have done calculations on whole endometrium as compared to the calculations made for the subendometrial layers here, but is common in both that higher FI values are associated with higher pregnancy rates.

Whereas Ng et al.[35] documented a low endometrial VI and VFI in pregnant group on the day of oocyte retrieval and also a non-significant trend of higher implantation and pregnancy rates in patients with absent subendometrial and endometrial flow. This probably can be explained on the basis that hCG administration/LH peak causes increased uterine artery resistance and hence decrease in endometrial perfusion also on the day of oocyte retrieval. This also correlates with the observation made by Ng et al.,[36] which says that subendometrial vascularization flow indices are significantly lower in patients with uterine artery RI more than or equal to 0.95. They concluded that number of embryos replaced and endometrial VFI were the only two predictive factors for pregnancy. Wu et al.[37] reported that endometrial VFI was more reliable than VI and FI, and best prediction rate was achieved by VFI cutoff value of more than 0.24.

Uterine Contractions and Maximum Implantation Point

Apart from these criteria, there are another few that have been worked upon in some studies. It has been shown that uterine motility on the day of embryo transfer has an impact on implantation rates. Number of uterine peristaltic contractions is counted per minute in longitudinal scan of the uterus. More than 5 contractions per minute, has considered as unfavorable sign and less than 3 has been considered as a favorable sign for implantation.[38] Point of maximum implantation also has been worked out. This point is an intersection of two lines that are drawn parallel to both cornu on a mid-true coronal section of uterus **(Fig. 15)**.[39]

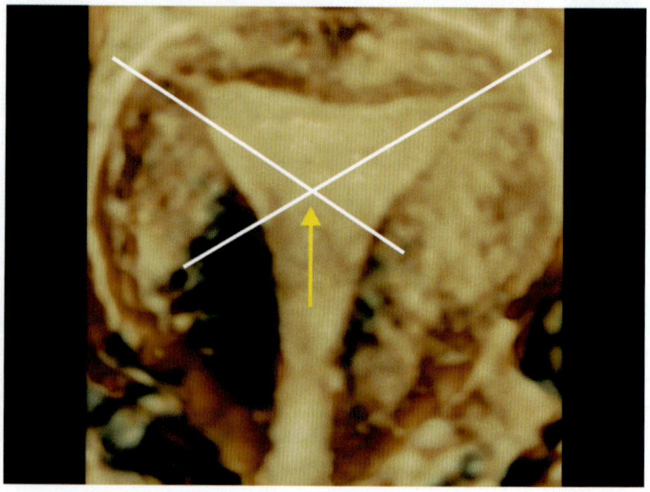

Fig. 15: Maximum implantation point.

SUMMARY

	Follicle	*Endometrium*
Size/thickness	16–18 mm	8–10 mm
Morphology	Thin wall, no internal echoes, halo	Grade A/B
Vascularity	3/4th circumference	Zone 3–4
RI	0.4–0.48	<0.5
PSV	>10 cm/sec	-
Uterine artery PI	-	<3.2
volume	3–7 cc	3–7 cc
3D morphology	Cumulus	Intact endo-myo junction
3D Power Doppler	More symmetrical the better	Higher the better

3D ultrasound is much accurate for volume assessment both for follicle and the endometrium, and is much more reliable parameter than follicular diameter or endometrial thickness. The presence of cumulus can be confirmed by 3D ultrasound increases the surety of the presence of a mature ovum in the follicle. The 3D power Doppler gives idea about the global vascularity of follicle and endometrium. Though still larger studies and standardization of ultrasound parameters and settings are required to establish more precise values for follicular and endometrial VI, FI and VFI, the results are fairly promising. We can hope to understand the follicular and endometrial physiological status better with these parameters and achieve better pregnancy rates with ART procedures and reduce the span of unexplained infertility.

REFERENCES

1. Kyei-Mensah A, Zaidi J, Pittrof R, et al. Transvaginal three dimensional ultrasound: accuracy of follicular volume measurements. Fertil Steril. 1996;65:371-6.
2. Jokubkeine L, Sladkevicius P, Rovas L, et al. Assessment of changes in volume and vascularity of ovaries during the normal menstrual cycle using three-dimensional power Doppler ultrasound. Hum Reprod. 2006;21(10):2661-8.
3. Chui D, Pugh N, Walker S, et al. Follicular vascularity—the predictive value of transvaginal power Doppler ultrasonography in an in vitro fertilization program: a preliminary study. Hum Reprod. 1997;12(1):191-6.
4. Kupesic S, Kurjak A. Uterine and ovarian perfusion during the periovulatory period assessed by transvaginal colour Doppler. Fertil Steril. 1993;3:439-43.
5. Nargund G, Doyle PE, Bourne TH, et al. Ultrasound-derived indices of follicular blood flow before HCG administration and prediction of oocyte recovery and preimplantation embryo quality. Hum Reprod. 1996;11:2512-17.
6. Nargund G, Bourne TH, Doyle PE, et al. Association between ultrasound indices of follicular blood flow, oocyte recovery and preimplantation embryo quality. Hum Reprod. 1996;11:109-13.
7. Blerkom V, Davis P, Alexander S. Inner mitochondrial membrane potential (DeltaPsim), cytoplasmic ATP content and free Ca^{2+} levels in metaphase II mouse oocytes. Hum Reprod. 2003;18(11):2429-40
8. Wittmack FM, Kreger DO, Blasco L, et al. Effect of follicular size on oocyte retrieval, fertilization, cleavage and embryo quality in in vitro fertilization cycles: a 6 year data collection. Fertil Steril. 1994;62:1205-10.
9. Kyei-Mensah A, Zaidi J, Pittrof R, et al. Transvaginal three-dimensional ultrasound reproducibility of ovarian and endometrial volume measurements. Fertil Steril. 1996;66:718-22.
10. Feichtinger W. Transvaginal three dimensional imaging for evaluation and treatment of infertility. In: Merz E (Ed). 3D Ultrasound in Obstetrics and Gynecology. Philadelphia: Lippincott Williams & Wilkins; 1998. pp. 37-43.
11. Poehl M, Hohlagschwandtner M, Doerner V, et al. Cumulus assessment by three-dimensional ultrasound for in vitro fertilization. Ultrasound Obstet Gynecol. 2000;16:251-3.
12. Wu MH, Tsai SJ, Pan HA, et al. Three dimensional power Doppler imaging of ovarian stromal blood flow in women with endometriosis undergoing in vitro fertilization. Ultrasound Obstet Gynecol. 2003;21:480-5.
13. Vlaisavljevic V, Reljic M, Gavric Lovrec V, et al. Measurement of perifollicular blood flow of the dominant preovulatory follicle using three-dimensional power Doppler. Ultrasound Obstet Gynecol. 2003;22:520-6.
14. Panchal SY, Nagori CB. Can 3D PD be a better tool for assessing the pre HCG follicle and endometrium? A randomized study of 500 cases. Presented at 16th World Congress on Ultrasound in Obstetrics and Gynecology, 2006, London. J Ultrasound Obstet Gynecol. 2006;28(4):504.
15. Kupesic S, Kurjak A. Prediction of IVF outcome by three dimensional ultrasound. Hum Reprod. 2002;17:950-5.
16. Merce LT. Ultrasound markers of implantation. Ultrasound Rev Obstet Gynecol. 2002;2:110-23.
17. Merce LT, Barco MJ, Kupesic S, et al. 2D and 3D power Doppler ultrasound from ovulation to implantation. In: Kurjak A, Chervenak F (Eds). Textbook of Perinatal Medicine. London: Parthenon Publishing; 2005.
18. Bourne TH. Transvaginal colour Doppler in gynecology. Ultrasound Obstet Gynecol. 1991;1:53.
19. Tan SL, Zaidi J, Campbell S, et al. Blood flow changes in the ovarian and uterine arteries during the normal menstrual cycle. Am J Obstet Gynecol. 1996;175:625-31.
20. Porter R, Ahuja K, Craft I. (1984) Ultrasonic assessment of endometrial changes in stimulated cycles in an in vitro fertilization and embryo transfer program. J In Vitro Fertil. Embryo Transf. 1984;1:233-8.
21. Zaidi J, Campbell S, Pittrof R, et al. Endometrial thickness, morphology, vascular penetration and velocimetry in

predicting implantation in an in vitro fertilization program. Ultrasound Obstet Gynecol. 1995;6:191-8.
22. Sardana D, Upadhyay AJ, Deepika K, et al. Correlation of subendometrial-endometrial blood flow assessment by two-dimensional power Doppler with pregnancy outcome in frozen-thawed embryo transfer cycles J Hum Reprod Sci. 2014;7(2):130-5.
23. Applebaum M. The 'steel' or 'Teflon' endometrium–ultrasound visualization of endometrial vascularity in IVF patients and outcome. Presented at The third World Congress of Ultrasound in Obstetrics and Gynaecolgy. Ultrasound Obstet Gynecol. 1993;3(Suppl 2):10
24. Chien LW, Au HK, Chen PL, et al. Assessment of uterine receptivity by the endometrial-subendometrial blood flow distribution pattern in women undergoing IVF-ET. Fertil Steril. 2002;78:245-51.
25. Yang JH, Wu MY, Chenet CD, et al. Association of endometrial blood flow as determined by a modified colour Doppler technique with subsequent outcome of IVF. Hum Reprod. 1999;14:1606-10.
26. Nagori C, Panchal S. Endometrial Vascularity: its Relation to Implantation Rates. Int J Infertil Fetal Med. 20102;3(2):1-13.
27. Kader MA, Abdelmeged A, Mahran A, et al. The usefulness of endometrial thickness, morphology and vasculature by 2D Doppler ultrasound in prediction of pregnancy in IVF/ICSI cycles. Egyptian J Radiol Nuc Med. 2016;47(1):341-6.
28. Zaidi J, Pittrof R, Shaker A, et al. Assessment of uterine artery blood flow on the day of human chorionic gonadotrophin administration by transvaginal colour Doppler ultrasound in an in vitro fertilization program. Fertil Steril. 1996;65:377-81.
29. Coulam CB, Stern JJ, Soenksen DM, et al. Comparison of pulsatility indexes on the day of oocyte retrieval and embryo transfer. Hum Reprod. 1995;10:82-4.
30. Tsai YC, Chang JC, Tai MJ, et al. Relationship of uterine perfusion to outcome of intrauterine insemination. J Ultrasound Med. 1996;15:633-6.
31. Cacciatore B, Simberg N, Fusaro P, et al. Transvaginal Doppler study of uterine artery blood flow in in vitro fertilization embryo transfer cycles. Fertil Steril. 1996;66:130-4.
32. Kyei-Mensah A, Zaidi J, Pittrof R, et al. Transvaginal three dimensional ultrasound: accuracy of follicular volume measurements. Fertil Steril. 1996;65:371-6.
33. Raga F, Bonilla-Musoles F, Casan EM, et al. Assessment of endometrial volume by three-dimensional ultrasound prior to embryo transfer: clues to endometrial receptivity. Hum Reprod. 1999;14:2851-4.
34. Kupesic S, Bekavac I, Bjelos D, et al. Assessment of endometrial receptivity by transvaginal colour Doppler and three dimensional power Doppler ultrasonography in patients undergoing in vitro fertilization procedures. J Ultrasound Med. 2001;20:125-34.
35. Ng EH, Chan CC, Tang OS, et al. The role of endometrial and subendometrial blood flows measured by three dimensional power Doppler ultrasound in prediction of pregnancy during IVF treatment. Hum Reprod. 2006;21(1): 164-70.
36. Ng EH, Chan CC, Tang OS, et al. Relationship between uterine blood flow and endometrial and subendometrial blood flows during stimulated and natural cycles. Fertil Steril. 2006;85(3):721-7.
37. Wu HM, Chiang CH, Huang HY, et al. Detection of subendometrial vascularization flow index by three-dimensional ultrasound may be useful for predicting pregnancy rate for patients undergoing in vitro fertilization-embryo transfer. Fertil Steril. 2003;79(3):507-11.
38. Fanchin R, Righini C, Olivennes F, et al. Uterine contractions at the time of embryo transfer alter pregnancy rates after in-vitro fertilization, Hum Reprod. 1998;13(7):1968-74.
39. Gergely RZ, DeUgarte CM, Danzer H, et al. Three dimensional/ four dimensional ultrasound-guided embryo transfer using the maximal implantation potential point. Fertil Steril. 2005;84(2):500-3.

Intrauterine Insemination

30

Ameet Patki, Kedar Ganla, Rana Choudhary

INTRODUCTION

The history of intrauterine insemination (IUI) goes back to the 18th century when Scottish surgeon John Hunter performed an effective procedure with the use of the husband's sperm. In 1884, after William Pankhurst from Philadelphia in the United States applied the donor's sperm, live birth was reported.[1,2] There are still ongoing discussions about the role of IUI in this era of assisted reproductive technology, i.e. in vitro fertilization (IVF)/intracytoplasmic sperm injection (ICSI).

The popularity of the IUI results from the fact that it is a relatively simple procedure and the cost of treatment is lower compared with IVF. In countries where the access to IVF/ICSI is significantly limited by, e.g. the lack of even partial coverage of costs, insemination treatment remains an important therapeutic step that can be offered to a couple who is unsuccessfully trying to have a child. The European Society of Human Reproduction and Embryology (ESHRE) data indicate that the pregnancy rate (PR) per cycle after IUI-H is 12.4% compared with 28.9% after IVF and the results have not changed over the last few years.[3]

WHAT IS IUI?

Procedure to treat infertility in which washed and prepared sperms are introduced into the woman's uterus, with timed ovulation, with the aim of getting the sperms nearer to the ovum and achieving pregnancy.[4]

INDICATIONS

- Mild male infertility
- Unexplained infertility
- Ovulatory dysfunction, polycystic ovarian syndrome (PCOS)
- Mild endometriosis (Grade 1 and 2)
- Cervical factors
- Coital issues
- Immunological factors
- Human immunodeficiency virus (HIV), surface antigen of the hepatitis B virus (HBsAg) infection
- Donor Sperm.

Prerequisite: At least one fallopian tube must be normal and patent.

CASES IN WHICH IUI IS INEFFECTIVE

- Blocked or damaged fallopian tube
- Ovarian failure
- Severe seminal fluid abnormality
- Severe endometriosis
- Long standing unexplained infertility.

POSITIVE PREDICTIVE FACTORS FOR IUI SUCCESS

- Age of female partner <35 years
- Duration of infertility <5 years
- At least one functional normal fallopian tube and no uterine factor leading to infertility
- Adequate ovarian reserve [based on serum anti-Müllerian hormone (Sr. AMH), Antral follicular count, Day 2 follicle stimulating hormone (FSH)]
- Mild male factor infertility with good semen parameters.[5]

VARIABLES AFFECTING IUI SUCCESS

Treatment with ovulation induction and IUI is more successful in anovulatory women. Various factors that affect the success rate of IUI include:[6-8]

- Age of female—As age advances, the chances of pregnancy after ovulation induction and assisted reproductive procedures (ART) procedures like IUI, decreases[2]
- Unexplained Infertility—Addition of IUI to super ovulation produces better results (20.47%) than super ovulation and timed intercourse (11.37%) especially in cases of unexplained infertility[3]
- Endometriosis—Mild or minimal endometriosis may benefit from IUI (pregnancy rates 7% to 18%), however in severe cases it is not advisable (4.5%)
- Cervical Factor—Conception rate in natural cycle is 14% and in IUI plus Gonadotropins is 17%[4]
- Male factor infertility—Total motile sperm count (TMSC) >5 million/mL and sperm morphology are most valuable sperm parameters to predict IUI outcome.

EVALUATION PRIOR TO IUI

Female Partner

- Routine—Thyroid stimulating hormone (TSH), prolactin, viral markers [HIV, HBsAg, hepatitis C virus (HCV)], detailed transvaginal ultrasound for Antral follicular count (AFC) on D2 or D3.
- Specific— Sr. AMH
- Specific—Day 2 FSH, luteinizing hormone (LH), blood sugar/insulin; in suspected case of polycystic ovarian syndrome
- Tubal patency—Hysterosalpingogram (HSG) or diagnostic laparoscopy [depending on the specific history/duration of infertility /presence of abnormal ultrasonography (USG) findings].

Male Partner

- Semen analysis—In clinical practice, male factor infertility is identified by *Abnormal Semen Parameters* from authenticated laboratory within the last 3 months
- Any abnormality—Do sperm function tests (SFT) and genetic evaluation (depending on the history and other clinical findings)
- Sperm Count <5 million/mL—Do Sr. FSH. High FSH suggests testicular failure. Semen sample freezing must be offered in these cases
- Varicocele—Grade 1 and 2: No surgery is required
- Varicocele—Grade 3: Surgery is required
- A trail of medical therapy can be given for at least 3 months followed by IUI.

Success of IUI depends on Total Motile Sperm Count (TMC) and Morphology

- TMSC = Count x Volume x % Motility {e.g.:10 million x 4 mL x 5 % = (10 x 4 x 50) × 100 = 20 million TMSC}
- Optimal cut-off level = 5 million (1-5 million IVF, <1 million ICSI)
- Success in IUI is highest with ≥14% sperms with normal morphology, intermediate with 4-14% and poor with <4%.

OVULATION INDUCTION DRUGS

Oral—Clomiphene Citrate (CC) and Letrozole (Aromatase Inhibitor) (Table 1)

Clomiphene citrate (CC) contains unequal mixture of two isomers, enclomiphene and zuclomiphene. Enclomiphene is more potent antiestrogenic isomer and primarily responsible for ovulation induction. While letrozole is an aromatase inhibitor.[5,9,10]

Advantages

- Oral tablets
- Ovulation and pregnancy rates are 73% and 36% respectively
- Less risk of hyperstimulation and multiple pregnancy.

Practical Problems

- CC Resistance—Inability to induce ovulation
- CC failure—Ovulation restored, but no pregnancy
- Maybe due to peripheral antiestrogenic effects of CC on endometrium, cervical mucus or hypersecretion of LH[5,11]
- Should be used for a maximum of 12 months in patient's lifetime and for a maximum of 6 months continuously [Royal College of Obstetricians and Gynecologists (RCOG) and American College of Obstetricians and Gynecologists (ACOG)].

Injectables—Gonadotropins

Preparations

- HMG
- FSH
- LH
- rFSH + rLH (2:1)
- Long-acting gonadotropins.

Table 1: Effects of clomiphene and letrozole.

	Clomiphene	*Letrozole*	*Effect*
↓ E2 receptors in Endometrium	Yes	No	CC—Poor endometrium
Endometrial thickness	Thin < 0.5 cm	Adequate (0.7–0.9 cm)	↓ Pregnancy Rate
Mechanism of action	Estrogen receptor blocking	Competitive inhibition	
Half-life	Long	Short (2 days)	Letrozole does not affect ovulation and implantation
Uterine blood flow	Decreased	Increased	Letrozole—Better implantation rates
Pregnancy rate	Low	High	

Indications

- Failure to respond to antiestrogen therapy
  - At least 3 cycles of oral induction and no ovulation
  - At least 6 ovulatory cycles and not conceived.
- Side effects to antiestrogen therapy irrespective of ovulation
- Two or more miscarriages after CC therapy.

Disadvantages

- High cost
- Intense and close monitoring of IUI cycle
- Increased ovarian hyperstimulation syndrome (OHSS), Risk of ovarian torsion, increased multiple pregnancies (5%)
- Premature LH surge can cause failure of follicles to rupture—(Serum LH >10 mIU/mL, Progesterone >2 ng/mL before dominant follicle is 18 mm in diameter). Leads to abandoning the cycle or cycle failure
- Review of current literature indicates use of Gonadotropin-releasing hormone (GnRH) antagonist along with gonadotropin in selected cases to prevent premature luteinization of follicle and may increase pregnancy rates.

Advantages of use of Letrozole in combination with gonadotropins

- Increases follicular sensitivity of FSH
- It increases the number of preovulatory follicles
- Optimal endometrial thickness
- It decreases gonadotropin requirements without a negative effect on pregnancy rates
- Induces moderate, safe and effective ovarian hyperstimulation.

Disadvantages of use of Clomiphene citrate/Letrozole in combination with gonadotrophins[12-14]

- Adding gonadotrophins does not reduce antiestrogenic actions of clomiphene
- Difficult to titrate the dose
- Many a times, excessive response is seen.

Adjuvants

- Insulin Sensitizing Drugs—Metformin (Oral biguanide), Inositols—Myoinositol and D-chiro-inositol. These may benefit in obese PCOS and anovulatory women
- Dexamethasone
- Oral contraceptive pills (OCPs)
- Estrogen
- Sildenafil
- N-acetylcysteine

Gonadotropins

- HMG preparations
  - Equal amounts of FSH/LH
  - Urinary/highly purified (HP).
- FSH preparations
  - Only FSH with varying degree of purity
  - Urinary/HP/recombinant.
- No difference in live birth and OHSS rates (Cochrane Database Syst Rev 2015 Sep.)

Dose of Gonadotropins

Dose of gonadotropins have been discussed in **Table 2**.

Points to Remember

- Be careful in increasing the dose
- Step up by 30-50 % [37.5 IU]
- Multi dose vials helpful
- Response may be sudden and explosive once the threshold is crossed

- Give the higher dose for 3 days and monitor again
- Use gonadotropins only if proper monitoring facilities are available
- Start with softer stimulations and become bolder as experience increases
- Do not use multiple protocols at the same time. Get familiar with one
- No matter how careful you are, OHSS is likely to occur and you should be ready to tackle it
- Remember that response varies from patient to patient and in the same patient from cycle to cycle.

Success Rate with Different Agents

The pregnancy rates discussed in **Table 3** are seen when infertility is due to unexplained cause. The pregnancy rates will be lower, if there is an added contributory factor like male factor infertility or endometriosis etc.[14-16]

Incidences of multiple pregnancies with:

- Clomiphene citrate: 5–10% almost exclusively due to twins
- Letrozole: 5–10% equivalent or less than CC.
- Conventional step up protocol: 15–36%
- Step down protocol: 10%
- Low dose step up protocols: 6% (twins: 88%)

Table 2: Doses of gonadotrophins.

Age	*PCOS/ Hyperresponder*	*Normal responder*	*Poor responder*
<30 years	37.5–75 IU	75 IU	150 IU
30–35 years	75 IU	150 IU	225 IU
35 years	150 IU	225 IU	300 IU

- IVF Programmes: 20–30%
- Spontaneous conception: 1%.

IDEAL PROTOCOL FOR OVULATION INDUCTION

There is no ideal protocol for ovulation induction as each patient is different, however recent studies have shown that the following protocol may give better pregnancy rates.

IUI TIMING

- 24 hr after LH surge
- 34-46 hr (average 38 hr) after ovulation trigger
- Double insemination at 12 and 36 hr
- Pregnancy rates are same if IUI is done after short 32–34 hr interval or long (38-40 hr interval after HCG).[7]

SEMEN PREPARATION TECHNIQUES

- Direct overlay method—Swim up without centrifugation
- Swim up—Based on self-migration of spermatozoa
- Density gradient centrifugation (DGC) —Using different density gradient preparations.

IUI—ESHRE GUIDELINES

- Success rates are better after mild stimulation and maturation of a 2/3 follicles
- Cycle must be monitored by USG and hormonal analysis and if there are too many mature follicles, the attempt maybe cancelled
- Majority of pregnancies occur during the first six cycles

Table 3: Success rate with different agents.

Drug	*Ovulation Rate*	*Clinical Pregnancy Rate*	*Important*
Natural cycle	------	8%	
Clomiphene citrate (CC)	74–76%	8–9 %	▪ May have thin endometrium due to antiestrogenic effect
Letrozole	80–82%	12–14%	▪ Better endometrial thickness ▪ More dominant follicles, as compared to CC
Letrozole + Gonadotropins	80–90%	20–22%	▪ Expensive ▪ Difficult for beginners ▪ Increase in multiple pregnancy
Gonadotropins	80–90%	25%	▪ Expensive ▪ Increase in multiple pregnancy
Gonadotropins + Antagonist	80–90%	38%	▪ Can be used only in selected patients ▪ Increase in multiple pregnancy

- No difference in outcome between gradient techniques and swim-up for semen preparation
- No difference in outcome after single or double IUI. (Double IUI is beneficial only in mild male factor infertility).

PROCEDURE FOR IUI

- IUI should be around the time of ovulation (34-36 hr after trigger)
- Consent of both the husband and wife
- Should be done in a separate IUI room [as recommended by Indian Council of Medical Research (ICMR) guidelines]
- Take care to label samples properly
- Use nontoxic, non-powdered gloves
- Expose cervix, do not hold
- Excessive mucus, if any can be removed by a small cotton swab
- Inseminate prepared sample just 1-2 cm above internal OS (i.e. *2 cm from the fundus)*
- Inseminate with infused semen *volume of 0.3–0.5 mL,* can significantly improve pregnancy rate in patients undergoing IUI with the husband's semen[7]
- Inseminate slowly over 3–5 min
- Wait for few seconds, prevent reflux
- Lay patient supine for 10 min
- No need of prolonged bed rest, head low, pain killers, or antibiotics.

Softer vs. hard catheters: A softer catheter:

- Allows tip to follow the path
- Minimize trauma to endometrium
- Less bleeding, mucus plugging and uterine contraction
- However, they are difficult to negotiate.

DIFFICULT IUI AND THEIR MANAGEMENT

- Acutely anteverted/retroverted uterus—Filling the bladder can straighten the acute anteversion—
- Stenosed cervix/intracervical crepts—Consider using the Maklers or metal catheter (standard). Double lumen catheters may be used in difficult IUI
- Hold the cervix with tenaculum/Allis forceps and give traction to manipulate the Utero-Cervix angle (straighten the utero-cervical angle) and also to stabilize the cervix
- If there was difficultly in the previous IUI, one can do cervical dilatation on D2/3 of the next cycle and perform IUI with a partially full bladder under USG guidance
- Regurgitation during IUI in documented patent tubes could be due to:
  - Semen injected too fast
  - Anxiety or fear of the procedure leading to spasm
  - Endometrial contractions
  - Large semen sample volume in the catheter.

Sometimes there may be problem in visualizing the cervix and doing IUI due to the different angulation of the uterus and cervix. In these cases, one should use a tenaculum or Allis forceps and give traction to manipulate the utero-cervix angle and also to stabilize the cervix. Maklers or metal catheter (standard) also help in these cases.

Various Positions of the Uterus During Difficult IUI

- *Empty bladder and acutely anteverted uterus:* In these cases, it is better to have a full Bladder and or use Allis (instrument) traction in the opposite direction.
- *Full bladder and acutely retroverted uterus:* In these cases, patient should empty her bladder and traction should be applied using Allis forceps or tenaculum in the opposite direction.

In cases of difficult IUI, one must consider cervical dilatation with smallest dilator (helps to identify the direction and also to negotiate the stenosis). Also, it is very important to make a note on the paper and consider for cervical dilatation on the 1st or 2nd day of next menses.

IS ULTRASOUND-GUIDED IUI BETTER?

Studies have shown that ultrasound-guided IUI does not produce better results than blind insemination, because the pregnancy rate per cycle is similar.[11]

COMPLICATIONS

- Accidental wrong/mismatch samples—Can be prevented by proper labelling of semen sample containers with husband and wife's full name and reconfirm the same when doing the insemination
- Preferably process one semen sample at a time, to avoid mixing incidents
- Infections—If plenty of pus cells in the semen sample
- Trauma and bleeding
- Pain—Traumatic/unsatisfactory sample preparation leading to release of prostaglandins and hence the pain
- Vasovagal syncope (rare).

POST IUI SUPPLEMENTATION

Supplementation of luteal phase with progesterone significantly increases live birth among women undergoing IUI when receiving gonadotropins for ovulation induction.[9] Some patients may require exogenous estrogen to maintain the estrogen progesterone ratio important for implantation. Adjuvants such as Sildenafil, L-arginine and Ecosprin may be used to overcome thin endometrium and poor vascularity in selected cases. Recently, a few studies have reported good results with GnRH analogue single dose on the 5–7th day post ovulation. This causes flare up response and increase in LH, which may increase intrinsic progesterone and help in the implantation process.

Methods of Semen Preparation

- Simple wash
- Overlay technique
- Swim up technique
- Density gradient technique

The effectiveness of specific semen preparation techniques for increasing pregnancy rates in subfertile couples undergoing IUI is unknown. It is known that white blood cells, bacteria and dead sperm in semen can impair fertilization of the egg. However, the Cochrane review found that there is insufficient evidence to recommend any specific semen preparation technique for subfertile couples undergoing intrauterine insemination as there was no differences in pregnancy rates using the different techniques and more research is needed in this area.

SETTING UP OF IUI LAB

- Basic laboratory requirements—essential equipment
  - Microscope (Phase contrast preferred)
  - Counting chamber (Makler, Neubauer)
  - Centrifuge
  - Refrigerator
  - CO_2 Incubator (optional)
  - Laminar air flow (optional)
  - Heating block
  - Autoclave
  - pH meter (optional)
  - LN2 and cryopreservation unit (optional).
- Disposables
  - Semen collection containers
  - Tissue paper/mediwipes
  - Microscope
  - Slides, coverslips
  - Pasteur pipettes or micro pipettes and tips
  - Falcon tubes 6 mL and 13 mL.
- Culture media (sperm washing and density gradient).

CONCLUSION[17]

Success rate depends on a couple's fertility problem and age. Studies have found that for couples with unexplained infertility, the pregnancy rate for each natural IUI cycle is about 4-5%, and when fertility drugs are used, the pregnancy rate is about 5-16%, with lowest being for oral ovulogens (5-10%) and maximum when only gonadotrophins (14-16%) are used. Pregnancy rates for patients aged 38-40 years remained stable even after more than 3 cycles, up until 6 cycles. However, no more than 3 insemination cycles should be attempted in these women. Patients seeking to become pregnant should be given detailed information about this point. It could play an important role in the choice of method by older couples.

The success rate of IUI varies and depends upon the age of female partner, extent of male factor, cause of infertility, ovulation induction and laboratory. The disadvantages of ovulation induction are risk of hyperstimulation and multiple pregnancies. But overall, IUI is a reasonable initial treatment and should be utilized for its simple, inexpensive and effective.

REFERENCES

1. Dickey RP, Brinsden PR, Pyrzak R. Manual of intrauterine insemination and ovulation induction. Cambridge: Cambridge University Press;2010.
2. Jędrzejczak P, Talarczyk J. Inseminacjadomaciczna. In: Putowski L (Ed.) Leczenienieplodności. Med Pharm Polska; 2011.
3. Ferraretti AP, Goossens V, de Mouzon J. et al. Assisted reproductive technology in Europe, 2008: results generated from European registers by ESHRE. Hum Reprod. 2012; 27;2571-84.
4. Wang R, Kim BV, van Wely M, et al. Treatment strategies for women with WHO group II anovulation: systematic review and network meta-analysis. BMJ. 2017;356:138.
5. Hendin BN, Falcone T, Hallak J, et al. The effect of patient and semen characteristics on live birth rates following intrauterine insemination: A Retrospective study. J Assist Rep Gen. 2000;17(5):245-52.
6. Bou NL, Weitzman VN, Arheart KL, et al. In Vitro Fertilization Versus Mild Stimulation Intrauterine Insemination in Women Aged 40 and Older. Reprod Sci. 2017;24(4):609-12.
7. Liu WJ, Li WT, Zhang RL, et al. Factors influencing the clinical pregnancy rate following intrauterine insemination. Zhonghua Nan KeXue. 2015;21(11):992-6.

8. Zhu WJ, Li XM, Chen XM, et al. Effects of catheter depth and infused semen volume on the pregnancy of intrauterine insemination. Zhonghua Nan KeXue. 2003;9(8):572-4.
9. Imani B, Eijkemans MJ, te Velde ER, et al. A nomogram to predict the probability of live birth after clomiphene citrate induction of ovulation in normogonadotropic oligoamenorrheic infertility. Fertil Steril. 2002;77(1):91-7.
10. Bae SA, Joo JK2, Choi JR, et al. Clinical outcomes of three- or five-day treatment with clomiphene citrate combined with gonadotropins and a timed intercourse cycle in polycystic ovary syndrome patients. Clin Exp Reprod Med. 2015;42(3):106-10.
11. Bates GW, Hickman JM, Matthews ML, et al. Novel clomiphene protocol in polycystic ovarian syndrome. Am J Obstet Gynecol. 2009;200(5):e1-3.
12. Samia ME, Shakweer MM. Effect of Late Luteal Phase Clomiphene Citrate on Ovulation Induction and Endometrial Blood Flow in Patients with Polycystic Ovary Syndrome. Clin Med Diag. 2014;4(4):65-70.
13. Erdem A, Erdem M, Atmaca S, et al. Impact of luteal phase support on pregnancy rates in intrauterine insemination cycles: a prospective randomized study. Fertil Steril. 2009;91(6):2508-13.
14. Erdem M, Abay S, Erdem A, et al. Recombinant FSH increase live birth rates as compared to clomiphene citrate in intrauterine insemination cycles in couples with subfertility: a prospective randomized study. Eur J Obstet Gynecol Reprod Biol. 2015;189:33-7.
15. Peeraer K, Debrock S, De Loecker P, et al. Low dose human menopausal gonadotrophin versus clomiphene citrate in subfertile couples treated with intrauterine insemination: a randomized controlled trial. Hum Reprod. 2015;30(5):1079-88.
16. Azmoodeh A, Pejman MM, Akbari AF, et al. Effects of Letrozole-HMG and Clomiphene-HMG on Incidence of Luteinized Unruptured Follicle Syndrome in Infertile Women Undergoing Induction Ovulation and Intrauterine Insemination: A Randomised Trial. Glob J Health Sci. 2015;8(4):244-52.
17. Kyrou D, Kolibianakis EM, Fatemi HM, et al. Increased live birth rates with GnRH agonist addition for luteal support in ICSI/IVF cycles: a systematic review and meta-analysis. Hum Reprod Update. 2011;17(6):734-40.

Individualization of Controlled Ovarian Stimulation

31

Damodar R Rao, Abarajda V, Asha R Rao

INTRODUCTION

Over the years, there has been a constant evolution in controlled ovarian stimulation in IVF (in vitro fertilization). The availability of gonadotropin preparations, like recombinant follicle-stimulating hormone (rFSH) and recombinant luteinizing hormone (rLH), option of small dosage adjustments in gonadotropins, gonadotropin-releasing hormone (GnRH) antagonists, and better freezing techniques of embryos and oocytes have enriched the armamentarium of an infertility specialist. Good-quality oocytes and sperms can also be selected. These advancements allow a physician to tailor the treatment according to the patient's variable requirements.

The ultimate goal of an individualistic approach in IVF is to design a management protocol specific to each patient, which suits best to her clinical profile, so as to improve treatment outcomes. In addition, every treating gynecologist must make every effort to achieve reduction in drug induced and preventable risks due to ovarian stimulation by reducing the possibility of either hypo-response or hyper-response. This will reduce the costs of IVF treatment and case dropouts.

PREDICTION OF OVARIAN RESPONSE

The endocrine and follicular reactions of ovaries to exogenous hormones have been described as ovarian response.[1] Ovarian reserve refers to the quantification of residual pool of primordial follicles in the ovary and represents the reproductive age of the women.

Treatment individualization in IVF should be based on predicting the ovarian response for each individual. The primary task is to classify the patient based on expected outcome: normal, poor, or a hyper-responder and then choose the ideal treatment protocol.[2]

Based on this, we can give them more precise information regarding the possible outcomes during their IVF cycle including prolonged treatment, cycle cancellation, ovarian hyperstimulation syndrome (OHSS), treatment burden, and reduced success. Predicting the ovarian response should be based on the most sensitive markers of ovarian reserve.[2]

The approach toward induction of ovulation depends on many parameters such as demographics, biomarkers (hormonal, functional, and genetic), and dynamic tests. However, the most common parameters frequently used have been enlisted in **Box 1**.

Oliveira et al. calculated ovarian reserve prediction index (ORPI) = Anti-Müllerian hormone (AMH) × antral follicle count (AFC) / Age. ORPI helps to predict low and excessive ovarian response and prediction of pregnancy in infertile women. ORPI helps to decide the protocol and dosage thereby reducing treatment cost according to the actual needs of the patient.[3]

Box 1: Predictors of ovarian response.

- Age
- Body mass Index (BMI)
- Menstrual cycle characteristics
- Previous IVF response
- Anti-Müllerian hormone (AMH)
- Antral follicle count (AFC)

(IVF: in vitro fertilization)

Based on AFC and AMH, it is possible to classify women as: (1) poor responders, (2) normal responders, and (3) hyper-responders **(Fig. 1)**.

Poor Responders

The response is considered to be poor, either in case of cancellation of a cycle (due to the development of less than three growing follicles) or if the collection of oocytes is less than or equal to 4, following a conventional IVF protocol.[4] The incidence of poor responders is 10–20% and the prevalence increases with increasing age.

Poor ovarian responders are identified based on characteristics (age, short menstrual cycle, outcomes of previous IVF cycles, and previous surgery on ovaries) and the clinical profile. The disadvantage of using ovarian reserve markers is that there is no accurate cut-off level for predicting poor response. The studies show varying values for AMH and AFC in the predicting of the poor response. This variation is due to the small study population and differences in the laboratory quantification of biomarkers.

Nelson et al.[5] in his study of 340 women showed that the cut-off value for AMH was 5 pmol/L (0.7 ng/mL) (DSL assay), which was associated with a sensitivity and specificity of 75% and 91%. Al-Azemi et al.[6] in 2011 found an AMH value of 1.36 ng/mL (9.7 pmol/L) (IBC assay) to be associated with sensitivity and specificity of 75.5% and 74.8% respectively among 356 women. A cut-off value of AMH ranging between 0.7 ng/mL and 1.3 ng/mL is considered acceptable for predicting poor response in IVF.[5-7] An AFC of less than 5–7 has been reported ideal for predicting poor response.[8-10] These markers are not very accurate to predict pregnancy.[11] Despite the poor chance, pregnancy rates are still considered reasonable particularly in the younger population.

Predicting poor response may not result in significant improvement in treatment outcome.[12,13]

Treatment Strategy for Poor Responders

- *Choice of protocol*:
  - Use of GnRH antagonist protocol
  - Microdose flare protocol
  - Minimal stimulation protocols
  - Modified natural cycle.
- *Gonadotropins*:
  - Type of gonadotropin—FSH and LH
  - Dose of gonadotropin.
- Adjuvant treatment.

Choice of protocol:

- *Antagonist protocol*: The stimulation protocols are simple, cheap, and associated with lower total gonadotropin dosage and fewer days of treatment. A meta-analysis comparing GnRH agonist and antagonist in poor responders showed an increased number of oocytes with the GnRH antagonist regimen.[14,15] Natural selection of chromosomally competent oocytes and

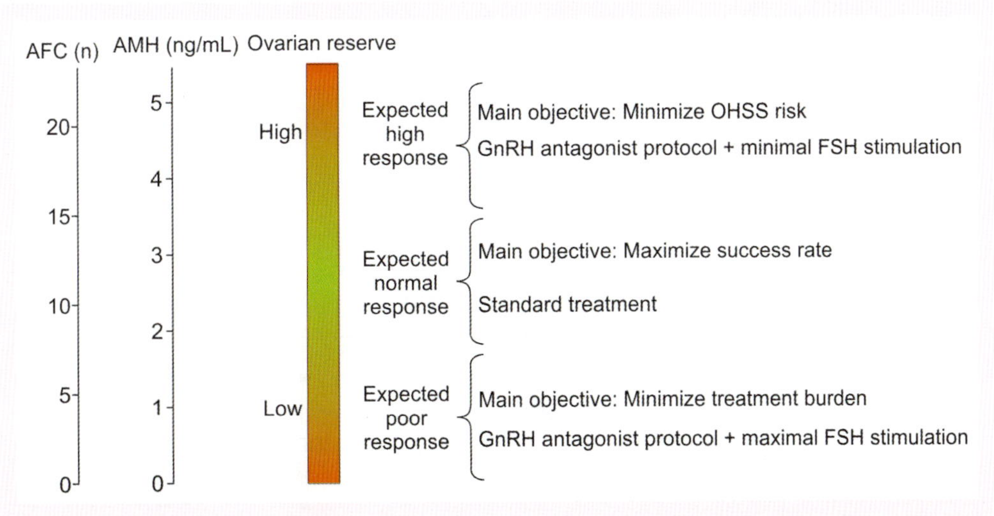

Fig. 1: Categorize patients according to ORT (La Marca and Sunkara, 2013). (AFC: antral follicle count; AMH: anti-Müllerian hormone; FSH: follicle-stimulating hormone; GnRH: gonadotropin-releasing hormone; OHSS: ovarian hyperstimulation syndrome)

hence good-quality euploid embryo yield is better with antagonist protocol **(Fig. 2)**.

- *Microdose flare protocol*: Small doses of GnRH agonist are used during the follicular phase. The initial stimulatory effect on pituitary hormones improves the ovarian response **(Fig. 3)**.
- *Minimal stimulation protocols*: It is an easy practice with a minimal dose of gonadotropins, fewer days of monitoring, and a lower cost. A recent multicenter randomized trial demonstrated the non-inferiority of a mild ovarian stimulation strategy with a GnRH antagonist compared with conventional GnRH agonist regime. The ongoing pregnancy rate for mild ovarian stimulation versus for conventional ovarian stimulation was 12.8% and 13.6%, respectively. The duration of ovarian stimulation and amount of gonadotropins used were significantly lower in the mild stimulation strategy.[16]
- *Modified natural cycle (mnIVF)*: mnIVF is a viable alternative option in poor responders, with patients below 35 years having a good prognosis.[17] The outcome of modified natural IVF was comparable to conventional COS protocols in terms of reducing the need for gonadotropins and stimulation length.[18]

Gonadotropins:

- *Deciding the initial dose of gonadotropins*:

The dose of gonadotropin is based on age, classification of response, ovarian reserve tests, and the decision to use an

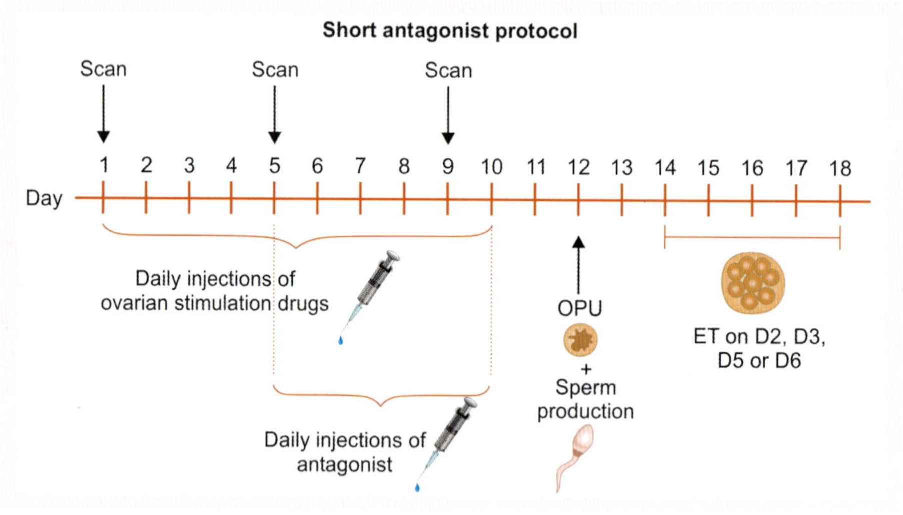

Fig. 2: Antagonist protocol. (OPU: ovum pick-up)

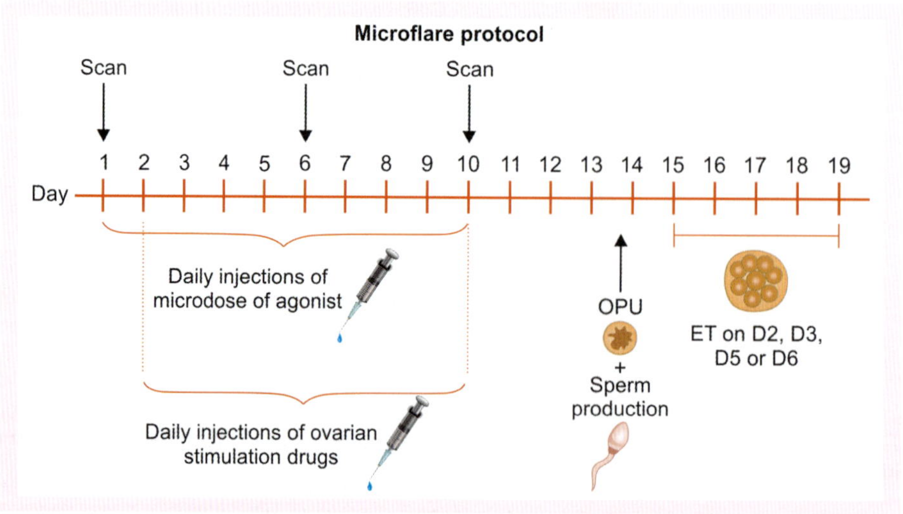

Fig. 3: Microflare protocol. (OPU: ovum pick-up)

antagonist or agonist protocol. For poor responders, a dose of 300–450 IU may be started. Unfortunately, there has been no study so far which has documented better outcomes with very high doses. Many models have been tried by combining different markers of ovarian reserve using either clinical, hormonal, or ultrasound based markers for FSH dosing **(Table 1)**.[19,20]

Naether et al. in his study observed that the physician-recommended starting dose of rhFSH for COS was generally higher than the CONSORT-calculated dose. This suggested a lack of certainty by the physicians in the CONSORT-calculated dose.

Nelson et al., in 2009, and Yates et al., in 2011, published simple models for gonadotropin dose selection according to AMH profile[21,22] **(Fig. 4)**.

Table 1: Predictive model incorporating more than one ovarian reserve test for follicle-stimulating hormone (FSH) dosing.

Name of model	***Parameters combined in model***
Popovic–Todorovic	AFC, ovarian stromal blood flow, age, and smoking status
Howles (CONSORT study)	Basal FSH, BMI, age, AFC
La Marca	Age, AMH, FSH
PIVET	Age, day-2 FSH, AFC, AMH, BMI, and smoking status

(AFC: antral follicle count; AMH: anti-Müllerian hormone; FSH: follicle-stimulating hormone; GnRH: gonadotropin-releasing hormone; BMI: body mass index)

High dose of FSH more than 300 did not correlate with the number of oocytes retrieved. The utmost number of oocytes that can be obtained in women was strongly limited by number of recruitable follicles and a higher gonadotropin dose was not able to compensate for lack of substrate.[23] High dosage of gonadotropin is useful when FSH threshold is not reached or because of FSH receptor polymorphism.

- *Addition of LH*:

The addition of LH is shown to benefit a subset of older patients, decreased ovarian reserve, and carriers of LH mutation.[24] There is a concept according to which recombinant FSH is started and LH is added on day 5 or 6, but it is better to start LH from day 2 of the cycle.

The LH supplementation during the latter half of the follicular phase has no effect on reproductive outcome or on ovarian response in women above 35 years undergoing GnRH antagonist IVF/ICSI cycles (Konig et al., 2013).

Adjuvant treatment:

- *Growth hormone supplementation (GH)*: Combined treatment with GH improves assisted reproduction outcome in poor responders. Although generally GH supplements did not increase controlled ovarian stimulation response or number of oocytes, the supplements improved pregnancy and live-birth rates, thus speaking for an effect on oocyte quality.[25]
- *Androgens or androgen-modulating agents*: Androgens [dehydroepiandrosterone (DHEA) and testosterone]

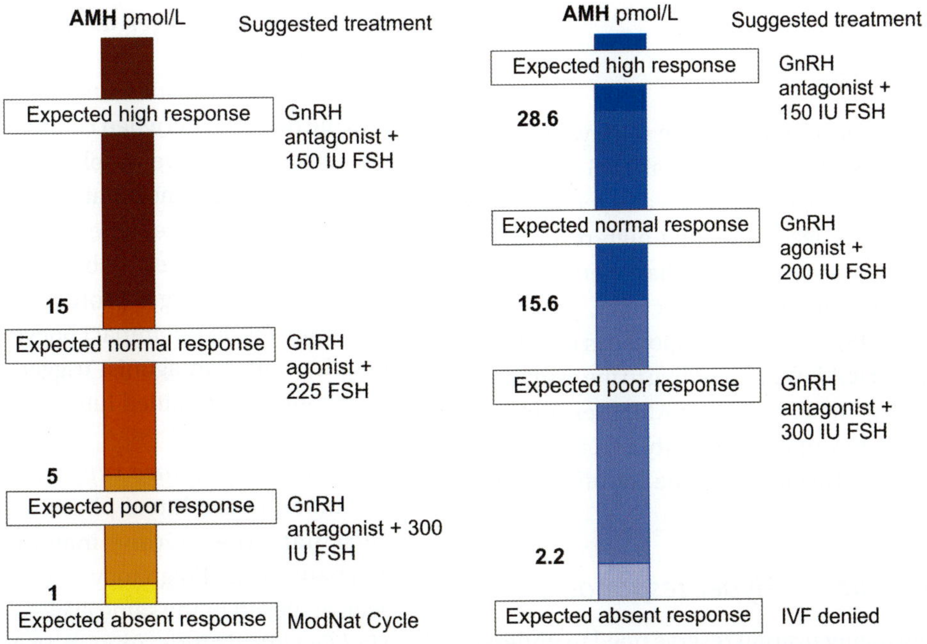

Fig. 4: Individualizing ovarian stimulation as per predicted response. (AFC: antral follicle count; AMH: anti-Müllerian hormone; FSH: follicle-stimulating hormone; GnRH: gonadotropin-releasing hormone; OHSS: ovarian hyperstimulation syndrome)

have the ability to regulate follicular recruitment and improve ovarian environment. In a randomized controlled trial (RCT) by Moawad et al.,[26] higher number of oocytes was retrieved and significantly higher pregnancy rates per cycle (20.9% vs 15.2%, respectively; P = 0.048) were observed in the DHEA group compared to the control group.

- *Letrozole*: It improves intra-ovarian micro-environment and endometrial receptivity. CPR is significantly lower and duration of gonadotropin stimulation is lower with antagonist/letrozole group compared with microflare protocol.[27]
- *Pyridostigmine*: Acetylcholine esterase inhibitor increases growth hormone secretion. But the number of studies and study population is limited.
- *Aspirin*: Meta-analysis concluded that there is no difference in CPR by adding aspirin.
- *L-arginine*: Addition of L-arginine increases number of retrieved oocytes but has no benefit in terms of pregnancy outcome.

Normal Responders

These patients have an *AMH* values between 1.3 ng/mL and 3.4 ng/mL and AFC between 8 and 14. These patients respond well to the standard agonist downregulation as well as antagonist protocol. Associated male factor should be considered to decide stimulation protocol. FSH dose of 225 U is ideal for normal responders in either agonist or antagonist protocol.

Hyper-responders

The term "hyper-response" refers to the retrieval of more than 15 oocytes following a conventional COS protocol.[28] The incidence of hyper-responders is 7% and reduces with the increasing patient's age. Predicting high response is based on clinical criteria and patient characteristics such as younger age, prolonged menstrual cycles, polycystic ovary syndrome (PCOS), and hyper-response in a previous cycle.[29,30] AMH cut-off levels vary according to the assay used (DSL, IBC, or AMH generation II), but AMH serum levels more than 3.5 ng/mL have good sensitivity and specificity.[2] AFC of more than 16 was defined to be the cut-off for hyper-response.

Treatment Strategies for Hyper-responders

Individuals having higher ovarian reserve need to undergo tailored COS protocol so as to avoid OHSS and therefore improve treatment outcomes. The following options are to be considered in such scenarios:

- GnRH antagonist protocols
- Reducing the doses of gonadotropins (100–150 IU/day)
- Coasting
- Ovulation trigger—GnRH agonist and low-dose human chorionic gonadotropin (hCG)
- Role of metformin.

GnRH antagonist protocols:

- GnRH antagonist protocols are associated with a reduction in ovarian hyperstimulation syndrome, reduction in cycle cancellation, and patient hospitalization.[31]
- Slightly reduced number of retrieved oocytes compared with GnRH agonist protocols.
- Duration of stimulation is lesser than the GnRH agonist protocol—9 days versus 13 days.
- Similar reproductive outcome compared with a GnRH agonist protocol.[31]
- GnRH analog can be used as a trigger rather than hCG hence decreasing the risk of OHSS.

Reducing the doses of gonadotropins:

The FSH dose should be tailored on the basis of ovarian reserve tests (the higher the ovarian reserve, the lower the dose).

Addition of LH in late follicular stages leads to differentiation of dominant follicles and atresia of smaller follicles thus reducing chance of OHSS.

- *GnRH agonist trigger as a substitute for hCG in antagonist cycles*:

  The GnRH agonist, due to its short half life, significantly reduces the risk of OHSS when compared to hCG protocols. It is associated with lower implantation rates in fresh IVF cycles, because of an undesirable effect on endometrium receptivity due to irreversible luteolysis.[32] Reproductive outcome of frozen-thawed embryos is similar in both hCG and GnRH agonist trigger protocols. Henceforth, GnRH agonist protocols do not impact oocyte quality.[33] There are three options after an agonist trigger: (1) intensive luteal phase support, (2) modified luteal phase support, and (3) freeze all and FET.

1. *Intensive luteal phase support*: Aggressive supplementation of the luteal phase with high-dose intramuscular progesterone may help to improve the pregnancy rate. Pregnancy rates as high as 27% have been achieved in the same cycle.
2. *Modified luteal phase support*: An approach to improve reproductive outcomes in GnRH agonist-triggered

cycles is the addition of a low dose (1,500 IU) of hCG, administered 35 hours per 5 days after the triggering bolus of GnRH agonist; however, this approach does not eliminate severe OHSS.[34]

3. *Freeze all and FET*: Owing to the improvement in vitrification methods, in GnRH agonist-triggered cycles, frozen embryo transfer in the following cycles may be the best strategy to eliminate the risk of OHSS.[32,35]

Coasting: In GnRH agonist protocol, omission of gonadotropins and continued administration of GnRH agonist can be used to prevent or decrease the severity of OHSS. Withdrawal of FSH causes the larger follicles to continue growth while the intermediate and smaller follicles undergo atresia. This alters the ability of granulosa cells to produce vascular endothelial growth factor (VEGF).[36] Significant reduction in OHSS with coasting was reported when it was continued until serum estradiol levels fell below 3,000 pg/mL.[37] However, some studies have found no benefit in coasting.[38]

Role of metformin: Even though the outcome of pregnancy has not improved with metformin in PCOS patients, a decrease in the incidence of hyperstimulation has been observed. Metformin may be given to PCOS and high-AMH patients.

Type of response	***Stimulation protocol***	***Gonadotropin dose***	***Gonadotropin type***
Poor	Antagonist/flare/minimal/modified natural/GH supplementation	300–450 IU	HP-hMG/rFSH+rLH
Normal	Agonist/antagonist	225 IU	HP-hMG/FSH
High	Antagonist with hCG/agonist trigger	100–150 IU	rFSH

(rFSH: recombinant follicle-stimulating hormone; hCG: human chorionic gonadotropin)

CONCLUSION

In spite of the long history beyond IVF, clinicians have always found it difficult to negate the adverse effects of ineffective induction protocols leading to either maximal or suboptimal ovarian response. However, the accessibility of new markers of ovarian reserve, the methodological advances made in these measurements, and the recent clinical studies using these markers have enabled us to appropriately characterize and predict the outcomes of stimulation. It is vital to use these markers especially AFC and AMH to strategize and design a therapeutic protocol, which is unique for each individual. This individualization in IVF is the way forward and would reduce morbidity and treatment burden of IVF.

REFERENCES

1. Fauser BC, Diedrich K, Devroey P. Predictors of ovarian response: progress towards individualized treatment in ovulation induction and ovarian stimulation. Hum Reprod Update. 2008;14:1-14.
2. La Marca A, Sunkara SK. Individualization of controlled ovarian stimulation in IVF using ovarian reserve markers: from theory to practice. Hum Reprod Update. 2014;20:124-40.
3. Oliveira JB, Baruffi RL, Petersen CG, et al. A new ovarian response prediction index (ORPI): Implications for individualised controlled ovarian stimulation. Reprod Biol Endocrinol. 2012:10:94.
4. Ferraretti AP, La Marca A, Fauser BC, et al. ESHRE consensus on the definition of 'poor response' to ovarian stimulation for in vitro fertilization: the Bologna criteria. Hum Reprod. 2011;26:1616-24.
5. Nelson SM, Yates RW, Fleming R. Serum anti-Mullerian hormone and FSH: prediction of live birth and extremes of response in stimulated cycles—implications for individualization of therapy. Hum Reprod. 2007;22:2414-21.
6. Al-Azemi M, Killick SR, Duffy S, et al. Multi-marker assessment of ovarian reserve predicts oocyte yield after ovulation induction. Hum Reprod. 2011;26:414-22.
7. Nelson SM. Biomarkers of ovarian response: current and future applications. Fertil Steril. 2013;99:963-9.
8. Frattarelli JL, Levi AJ, Miller BT, et al. A prospective assessment of the predictive value of basal antral follicles in in vitro fertilization cycles. Fertil Steril. 2003;80:350-5.
9. Jayaprakasan K, Campbell B, Hopkisson J, et al. A prospective, comparative analysis of anti-Müllerian hormone, inhibin-B, and three-dimensional ultrasound determinants of ovarian reserve in the prediction of poor response to controlled ovarian stimulation. Fertil Steril. 2010;93:855-64.
10. Jayaprakasan K, Deb S, Batcha M, et al. The cohort of antral follicles measuring 2–6 mm reflects the quantitative status of ovarian reserve as assessed by serum levels of anti-Müllerian hormone and response to controlled ovarian stimulation. Fertil Steril 2010;94:1775-81.
11. Kwee J, Elting ME, Schats R, et al. Ovarian volume and antral follicle count for the prediction of low and hyper responders with in vitro fertilization. Reprod Biol Endocrinol. 2007;5:9.
12. Popovic-Todorovic B, Loft A, Lindhard A, et al. A prospective study of predictive factors of ovarian response in 'standard' IVF/ICSI patients treated with recombinant FSH. A suggestion for a recombinant FSH dosage nomogram. Hum Reprod. 2003;18:781-7.
13. Howles CM, Saunders H, Alam V, et al. FSH Treatment Guidelines Clinical Panel. Predictive factors and a

corresponding treatment algorithm for controlled ovarian stimulation in patients treated with recombinant human follicle stimulating hormone (follitropin alfa) during assisted reproduction technology (ART) procedures. An analysis of 1378 patients. Curr Med Res Opin. 2006;22:907-18.
14. Oudendijk JF, Yarde F, Eijkemans MJ, et al. The poor responder in IVF: is the prognosis always poor? a systematic review. Hum Reprod Update. 2012;18:1-11.
15. Griesinger G, Diedrich K, Tarlatzis BC, et al. GnRH-antagonists in ovarian stimulation for IVF in patients with poor response to gonadotrophins, polycystic ovary syndrome, and risk of ovarian hyperstimulation: a meta-analysis. Reprod Biomed Online. 2006;13:628-38.
16. Youssef MA, van Wely M, Al-Inany H, et al. A mild ovarian stimulation strategy in women with poor ovarian reserve undergoing IVF: a multicenter randomized non-inferiority trial. Hum Reprod. 2017;32:112-8.
17. Morgia F, Sbracia M, Schimberni M, et al. A controlled trial of natural cycle versus microdose gonadotropin releasing hormone analog flare cycles in poor responders undergoing in vitro fertilization. Fertil Steril. 2004;81:1542-7.
18. Kim CH, Kim SR, Cheon YP, et al. Minimal stimulation using gonadotropin-releasing hormone (GnRH) antagonist and recombinant human follicle-stimulating hormone versus GnRH antagonist multiple-dose protocol in low responders undergoing in vitro fertilization/intracytoplasmic sperm injection. Fertil Steril. 2009;92:2082-4.
19. La Marca A, Papaleo E, Grisendi V, et al. Development of a nomogram based on markers of ovarian reserve for the individualisation of the follicle-stimulating hormone starting dose in in vitro fertilisation cycles. BJOG. 2012;119:1171-9.
20. La Marca A, Grisendi V, Giulini S, et al. Individualization of the FSH starting dose in IVF/ICSI cycles using the antral follicle count. J Ovarian Res. 2013;6:11.
21. Nelson SM, Yates RW, Lyall H, et al. Anti-Müllerian hormone-based approach to controlled ovarian stimulation for assisted conception. Hum Reprod. 2009;24:867-75.
22. Yates AP, Rustamov O, Roberts SA, et al. Anti-Mullerian hormone-tailored stimulation protocols improve outcomes whilst reducing adverse effects and costs of IVF. Hum Reprod. 2011;26:2353-62.
23. Berkkanoglu M, Ozgurk. What is the optimum maximal gonadotopin dosage used in microdose flare up cycles in poor responders? Fertil Steril. 2010;94:662-5.
24. Esteves S. (2015). The Role of LH in Controlled Ovarian Stimulation, January 2015. [online] Available from https://www.researchgate.net/publication/303728109. [Last accessed February, 2019].
25. de Ziegler D, Streuli I, Meldrum DR, et al. The value of growth hormone supplements in ART for poor ovarian responders. Fertil Steril. 2011;96:1069-76.
26. Moawad A, Shaeer M. Long-term androgen priming by use of dehydroepiandrosterone (DHEA) improves IVF outcome in poor-responder patients. A randomized controlled study. Middle East Fertil Soc J. 2012;17:268-74.
27. Song Y, Li Z, Wu X. Effectiveness of the antagonist/letrazole protocol for treating poor responder undergoing IVF/ICSI. A systematic review and meta-analysis. Gynaecol Endocrinol. 2014;30:330-4.
28. La Marca A, Sighinolfi G, Radi D, et al. Anti-Mullerian hormone (AMH) as a predictive marker in assisted reproductive technology (ART). Hum Reprod Update. 2010;16:113-30.
29. Papanikolaou EG, Humaidan P, Polyzos N, et al. New algorithm for OHSS prevention. Reprod Biol Endocrinol. 2011;9:147.
30. Aflatoonian A, Oskouian H, Ahmadi S, et al. Prediction of high ovarian response to controlled ovarian hyperstimulation: anti-Müllerian hormone versus small antral follicle count (2-6 mm). J Assist Reprod Genet. 2009;26:319-25.
31. Toftager M, Bogstad J, Bryndorf T, et al. Risk of severe ovarian hyperstimulation syndrome in GnRH antagonist versus GnRH agonist protocol: RCT including 1050 first IVF/ICSI cycles. Hum Reprod. 2016;31:1253-64.
32. Griesinger G, Schultz L, Bauer T, et al. Ovarian hyperstimulation syndrome prevention by gonadotropin-releasing hormone agonist triggering of final oocyte maturation in a gonadotropin-releasing hormone antagonist protocol in combination with a "freeze-all" strategy: a prospective multicentric study. Fertil Steril. 2011;95:2029-33.
33. Eldar-Geva T, Zylber-Haran E, Babayof R, et al. Similar outcome for cryopreserved embryo transfer following GnRH-antagonist/GnRH-agonist, GnRH-antagonist/HCG or long protocol ovarian stimulation. Reprod Biomed Online. 2007;14:148-54.
34. Olivennes F, Howles CM, Borini A, et al. Individualizing FSH dose for assisted reproduction using a novel algorithm: the CONSORT study. Reprod Biomed Online. 2009;18:195-204.
35. Casper RF. Introduction: Gonadotropin-releasing hormone agonist triggering of final follicular maturation for in vitro fertilization. Fertil Steril. 2015;103:865-6.
36. Tozer AJ, Iles RK, Iammarrone E. The effects of 'coasting' on follicular fluid concentrations of vascular endothelial growth factor in women at risk for developing ovarian hyperstimulation syndrome. Hum Reprod. 2004;19:522-8.
37. Levinson-Tavor O, Friedler S, Schachter M, et al. Coasting—what is the best formula? Hum Reprod. 2003;18:937-40.
38. D'Angelo A, Brown J, Amso NN. Coasting (withholding gonadotrophins) for preventing ovarian hyperstimulation syndrome. Cochrane Database Syst Rev. 2011;6:CD002811.

Mild Ovarian Stimulation Protocol

32

Korula George, Abha Khurana

INTRODUCTION

Infertility is a worldwide health issue. The first in vitro fertilization (IVF) baby was born in 1978. Currently, IVF is expensive and the cost is increasing with every passing year. Funding from the government or through insurance differs all over the world. Cost factor is a major constraint for couples, which often results in abandonment for further treatment options in the developing countries. Whereas in the developed world, most patients will go ahead with the treatment since financial problems may not be a major issue. In the developing world, if there is a high population then the government is likely to disregard the infertility issues. In the developing world, the proportion of population getting married is significantly high and at an early age. The moment fertility becomes a problem, stress and emotional burden arise, often with annoyance from the family members. Since infertility is not a life-threatening issue, it is not a priority for the policy makers in the health sector and hence the dearth of inexpensive IVF in the government sector. Mild stimulation is a step toward providing these people affordable treatment.

Initially when Robert Edwards started IVF, ovarian stimulation was not practiced. Oocyte retrieval was done in natural cycles. The practice of using ovarian stimulation in IVF with human menopausal gonadotropin (hMG) was started by the US group in 1981. hMG 150 IU was initiated on day 2–3 and continued for about 7–10 days, which would usually result in retrieval of around 10 oocytes. Gonadotropin-releasing hormone (GnRH) agonist was introduced to ensure that pituitary hormones were suppressed (downregulation) and continued to prevent the LH surge. High dose of gonadotropins was initiated, once the downregulation was confirmed in the early follicular phase to maximize the follicular recruitment and optimize the pregnancy rates. Larger doses were also considered essential for low responders.

Due to the increasing concerns regarding patient safety, increased discomfort with high hormonal dosages, and high costs of conventional stimulation protocols, there was rekindled interest in novel treatment protocols. Mild/soft stimulations promise reduced risk of ovarian hyperstimulation, multiple pregnancy, emotional stress, and financial burden to the patient.

THEORETICAL CONCEPT: BASIS OF MILD STIMULATION

It is a well-known fact that follicle-stimulating hormone (FSH) is an absolute requirement for development of large antral follicles. Once the most mature follicle, i.e. the one with maximum FSH receptors in the granulosa cells, gains dominance, there is release of estrogen and inhibin B. These exert a negative feedback on the hypothalamic–pituitary axis, which causes a decline in the FSH levels during the mid-late follicular phase, causing atresia of the smaller follicles.

The physiological basis of mild IVF is to allow initial recruitment of follicles by endogenous FSH. A lower dose of gonadotropins is delayed in mild IVF until the mid-follicular phase (around day 5). This extends the FSH window, which leads to growth of several follicles. In women with normal ovarian reserve, multiple follicle development can be achieved even when FSH is initiated up to 7th day of cycle. It is, however, initiated usually on day 5 to avoid risk of a monofollicular response **(Fig. 1)**.

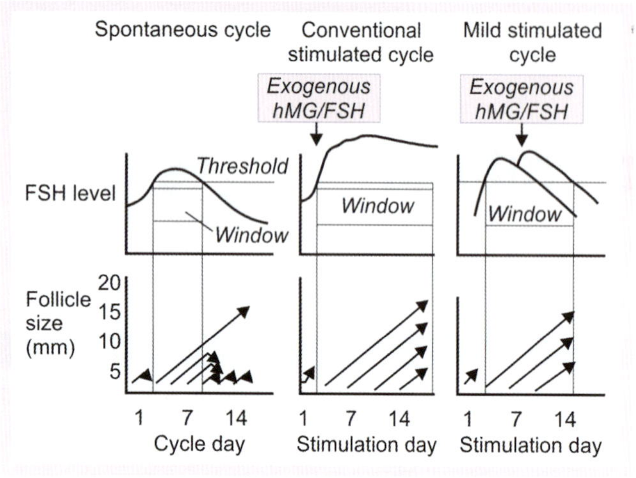

Fig. 1: Schematic representation of the follicle-stimulating hormone (FSH) threshold/window concept in relation to single dominant follicle selection during the follicular phase of the normal menstrual cycle, multiple follicle development, and high FSH levels in conventional ovarian hyperstimulation when compared with more subtle mild in vitro fertilization (IVF). (hMG: human menopausal gonadotropin)

DEFINITION

With an aim to limit the number of oocytes retrieved to be less than 8, mild stimulation is considered the option by giving either low dose/fewer days of either gonadotropins/anti-estrogens/aromatase inhibitors or even a combination of these. Following the ISMAAR (International Society for Mild Approaches in Assisted Reproduction) meeting, revised definition of mild IVF was recommended.[1]

Mild IVF is defined as the method when FSH or hMG is administered at lower doses and/or shorter duration in a GnRH antagonist cotreated cycle, or when oral compounds (antiestrogens or aromatase inhibitors) are used alone or in combination with gonadotropins. Human chorionic gonadotropin (hCG) injection and luteal phase support are also administered. The aim was to collect between 2 and 7 oocytes. It was also recommended that term "mild IVF" be used instead of soft, minimal stimulation, or "friendly" IVF.

Mild IVF, protocols usually used are:

- *Low dose of gonadotropins*: 100–150 IU started on day 2–3 of the period. GnRH antagonist is added after 5–7 days to prevent LH surge, usually once the leading follicle reaches 12–13 mm in size and continued till the day of hCG trigger.
- Clomiphene citrate (CC)/letrozole can also be started on day 2–3 of period for 5 days and then gonadotropins at a lower dose (100–150 IU) to be started around day 5–6 of period. The GnRH antagonist is added within next 2–3 days when the leading follicle reaches 12–13 mm in size.

The remaining steps of triggering oocyte maturation with hCG trigger, oocyte retrieval, embryo transfer, and luteal phase support are followed in the same fashion as conventional IVF protocols.

Significantly reduced pregnancy rates as compared to conventional IVF limit its widespread use in spite of the reduced cost. A large randomized trial compared the live birth rates in mild simulation protocol with conventional protocol.[2] The pregnancy rate per treatment cycle was significantly lower following mild stimulation (17.6% vs 28.6%). However, the cumulative pregnancy rates at the end of 1 year were similar in both groups (43.4% vs 44.7%). The multiple pregnancy rates were significantly lower with mild stimulation (0.5%) as compared to the conventional protocol (13.5%).

ADDITIONAL MEASURES TO BRING DOWN THE COST

- Continuation of use of CC, till the day of hCG trigger, helps in preventing the premature LH surge. CC blocks the estrogen receptors in the hypothalamus and pituitary. Estrogen rise by the growing follicles is not perceived by the pituitary and thus LH surge does not occur.[3] Antagonists is not required.
- Use of indomethacin prior to oocyte retrieval also prevents follicle rupture. Indomethacin is an NSAID (non-steroidal anti-inflammatory drug), which inhibits the production of prostaglandins, a necessary agent for follicle rupture and ovulation. However, when evaluated in a randomized controlled trial by TM Rijken-Zijlstra et al., in modified natural cycle IVF, it was found that indomethacin is effective in preventing premature ovulation only in a subgroup of patients without LH surge prior to oocyte retrieval.[4] Indomethacin is given in a doses of 50 mg thrice daily from the day of hCG triggering until the morning of oocyte retrieval, especially when CC is given for prevention of LH surge.

BENEFITS OF MILD STIMULATION

- Lower cost of medication
- Less intense monitoring
- Fewer injections with lower dose—lesser patient discomfort
- *Lower risk of ovarian hyper-stimulation syndrome (OHSS)*: Mild stimulation may be particularly beneficial

for patients at risk of developing OHSS. These are the patients with high anti-Mullerian hormone (AMH) levels, antral follicles, and those with polycystic ovaries. These women when given higher gonadotropin doses may hyper-respond and display risk factors for development of OHSS in the form of high estrogen values (>3,000 pg/mL), and a higher number of oocytes retrieved (>20). If these patients are properly identified and counseled for mild IVF, the risk of OHSS will be substantially reduced.

In the study by Heijnen et al.,[2] the incidence of OHSS was 1.4% with mild IVF protocol compared with 3.7% in the long protocol. Aleyamma TK et al. reported no cases of OHSS in a study of 143 normal responder women undergoing mild IVF with CC with hMG.[3] However, these studies were in a group of normal responders.

- Decreased rates of multiple pregnancies.
- *Better endometrial receptivity in patients given mild IVF*:
- Haouzi et al. found altered endometrial receptivity with negative effect on embryo implantation in gonadotropin-stimulated cycles.[5] This was due to altered gene expression in normal stimulated cycles. Mild IVF may reduce this negative effect on endometrial receptivity, which may translate into improved implantation rates.
- Lower rates of aneuploid embryos were evaluated by preimplantation genetic screening (PGS): Transfer of these embryos was also shown to have a higher pregnancy outcome. In a randomized controlled trial by Baart et al., the embryo aneuploidy rates following conventional and mild IVF stimulation protocols were evaluated using PGS.[6] Even though retrieved oocytes were less following milder stimulation, the average normal euploid embryos were similar in both groups, making the proportion of euploid embryos significantly higher in the milder stimulation group.

  The benefits of mild IVF need to be explored in patients with recurrent implantation failure in view of above two anticipated benefits.
- *Benefits in poor responders*: When mild IVF stimulation is used for poor responders, the number of oocytes retrieved is found similar to conventional or stimulation methods using higher doses. The additional advantage of mild stimulation is that the oocyte quality is often better. Better embryo quality and implantation due to improved endometrial receptivity may translate into acceptable pregnancy rates.

  Mohsen et al. compared minimal IVF stimulation protocol using letrozole versus microdose flare-up GnRH agonist protocol in women with poor ovarian response and obtained similar pregnancy rates (18.3% in mild simulation vs 16.6% in microdose flare protocol).[7] Youssef et al., in a multicenter randomized trial, evaluated a mild ovarian stimulation strategy in women with poor ovarian reserve undergoing IVF.[8] 394 couples were randomized to mild ovarian stimulation strategy or conventional stimulation. Ongoing pregnancy was 12.8% for women who received mild stimulation and 13.6% who received conventional stimulation. They concluded that a mild ovarian stimulation strategy is noninferior to conventional ovarian stimulation in terms of the ongoing pregnancy rates and is associated with shorter duration of stimulation, lower amount of gonadotropins, and less costs required for ovarian stimulation. Thus, mild ovarian stimulation should be the treatment of choice in women with poor reserve undergoing IVF.
- *Role in normal responders*: Mild ovarian stimulation is usually not advised to patients who are expected to be normal responders undergoing their first IVF cycles for the concern of retrieving a lower number of oocytes. A meta-analysis studied the clinical significance of retrieval of a low number of oocytes following mild ovarian stimulation in first treatment IVF cycles.[9] Data showed that mild stimulation yielded significantly less number of oocytes as compared to conventional stimulation. Optimal embryo implantation rates were observed with 5 oocytes retrieved following mild stimulation (31%) versus 10 oocytes following conventional stimulation (29%).

  Letrozole use with gonadotropins has been mentioned in an article by Haas et al. to increase endometrial receptivity by increasing integrin expression in the endometrium and by lowering the estrogen concentration.[10]
- *Reduced emotional stress*: Patients undergoing standard IVF protocols are often emotionally stressed due to multiple injections and intense biochemical and radiological monitoring. Cost factor and family pressure also adds on to the stress. Minor symptoms like abdominal pain and nausea although not very common may also deter patients from undergoing a repeat IVF cycle after a failed attempt.

  Some studies suggest that women who underwent mild IVF were less likely to drop-out from treatment than women undergoing conventional IVF. This is the reason why cumulative pregnancy rates were found to be equivalent to pregnancy rates achieved by conventional IVF.

One cannot, however, overlook the fact that lower pregnancy rates associated with mild IVF can itself lead to emotional stress. De Klerk et al.[11] conducted a randomized controlled trial (RCT) to evaluate the psychological impact of mild stimulation with single embryo transfer compared with conventional IVF and concluded that, during first IVF cycle, mild ovarian stimulation with single embryo transfer (SET) does not lead to more psychological complaints than conventional IVF.

LIMITATIONS OF MILD STIMULATION PROTOCOLS

1. Lower pregnancy rates as compared to conventional IVF in case of normal responders.
2. Lack/less numbers of vitrified embryos bring down cumulative pregnancy rates following single completed cycle.
3. Higher rates of cycle cancellation.
4. Lower margin for suboptimal laboratory performance.

During mild IVF, lesser oocytes are available, any compromise on the laboratory performance will cause unacceptable decline in the pregnancy rates.[12] Hence, fertilization rates, embryo development rates, and implantation rates, which are the quality control parameters of an IVF setup should be optimum. This was also mentioned by Aleyamma et al. in their study of couples offered affordable ART.[3] They specified that the equipment used and procedures followed during low-cost ART were similar to those used during conventional ART. The "laboratory air quality" also was not compromised at any stage.

PERSONAL EXPERIENCE

In 2008, at Christian Medical College (CMC) Vellore, I had many patients who required IVF due to major infertility issues. However, out of 10, only three to four would actually agree for IVF treatment. The reason was mainly financial problems. Since CMC is a mission hospital we wanted to ensure that patients with financial problems can be provided the facility at a reasonable cost. An uncommonly used, but proven to be of benefit, combination of CC with low dose of gonadotropins was offered to such patients at a much lower cost. It was, however, offered only to women who were less than 35 years of age and had a BMI of less than 26 with a normal ovarian reserve as evaluated by TVS (antral follicle count > 10). The couples were counseled and explained the cost factor and the possible pregnancy outcomes.

Clomiphene citrate, 50 mg per day, was started on day 2 of the menstrual cycle and continued till the day of hCG trigger. Injection hMG 150 IU was started from day 5 and given on alternate days. Follicular monitoring was started on day 8. Oocyte pick-up was planned after 35 hours of hCG trigger, when at least two follicles greater than 18 mm in size were seen on ultrasound. Oocyte pick-up was planned as a day-care procedure, under conscious sedation, and patient discharged the same day after luteal support, 400 mg vaginal progesterone given twice daily.

The IVF was done for all indications other than male factor. Intracystoplasmic sperm injection (ICSI) was done only for male factor. Embryo transfer was done on day two or three depending upon numbers and quality. Not more than three embryos were transferred. Since it was a mild stimulation protocol, vitrification was not required for majority of patients. However, it was done in case surplus embryos were remaining. Clinical pregnancy rates were around 25%. The overall cost was approximately rupee 40,000–45,000, which was definitely beneficial to patients with financial problems.

CONCLUSION

Reproductive medicine clinicians are facing ever increasing challenges of having to deal with special subcategories of patients such as poor responders, patients at high risk of OHSS, older age group, and recurrent implantation failure. This has led to rekindled interest in the benefits of mild IVF. However, there is still a lot of resistance among clinicians to use mild IVF because of concerns regarding lower pregnancy rates. Larger RCTs are hence required in all these subsets of patients to give clinicians a clear picture of the success rates and to lay guidelines for using such protocols.

REFERENCES

1. Nargund G, Fauser BC, Macklon NS, et al.; Rotterdam ISMAAR Consensus Group on Terminology for Ovarian Stimulation for IVF. The ISMAAR proposal on terminology for ovarian stimulation for IVF. Hum Reprod. 2007;22(11): 2801-4.
2. Hejinen EMEW, Eijkemans MJC, De Klerk C, et al. A mild treatment strategy for in vitro fertilisation: a randomised non-inferiority trial. The Lancet. 2007;369(9563):743-9.

3. Aleyamma TK, Kamath MS, Muthukumar K, et al. Affordable ART: a different perspective. Hum Reprod. 2011;26(12):3312-8.
4. Rijken-Zijlstra TM, Haadsma ML, Hammer C, et al. Effectiveness of indomethacin to prevent ovulation in modified natural cycle IVF: a randomised controlled trial. Reprod Biomed Online. 2013;27(3):297-304.
5. Haouzi D, Assou S, Mahmoud K, et al. Gene expression profile of human endometrial receptivity: comparison between natural and stimulated cycles for the same patients. Hum Reprod. 2009;24(6):1436-45.
6. Baart EB, Martini E, Eijkemans MJ, et al. Milder ovarian stimulation for in vitro fertilisation reduces aneuploidy in human preimplantation embryo: a randomized controlled trial. Hum Reprod. 2007;22(4):980-8.
7. Mohsen IA, El Din RE. Minimal stimulation protocol using letrozole vs. microdose flare up GnRH agonist protocol in women with poor ovarian responds undergoing ICSI. Gynecol Endocrinol. 2013;29(2):105-8.
8. Youssef MA, van Wely M, Al-Inanry H, et al. A mild ovarian stimulation strategy in women with poor ovarian reserve undergoing IVF: a multicenter randomized non-inferiority trial. Hum Reprod. 2017;32(1):112-8.
9. Verberg MF, Eijkemans MJ, Macklon NS, et al. The clinical significance of retrieval of a low number of oocytes following mild ovarian stimulation for IVF: A meta analysis. Hum Reprod Update. 2009;15(1):5-12.
10. Jigal Haas, Bassil R, Meriano J, et al. Does daily co-administration of letrozole and gonadotropins during ovarian stimulation improve IVF outcome? Reprod Biol Endocrinol. 2017;15(1):70.
11. De Klerk C, Macklon NS, Hejinen EM, et al. The psychological impact of IVF failure after two or more cycles of IVF with a mild vs. standard treatment strategy. Hum Reprod. 2007;22(9):2554-8.
12. Fauser BC, Nargund G, Andersen AN, et al. Mild ovarian stimulation for IVF: 10 years later. Hum Reprod. 2010;25(11):2678-84.

Stimulation Protocols in Cancer Patients

33

N Sanjeeva Reddy, Kamala Selvaraj, Erika Desai

INTRODUCTION

Cancer is no more considered an incurable disease due to the immense advances in medical care especially in reproductive-aged women. Since the long-term survival rates have increased in these women in recent times, issues concerning to fertility and fertility preservation are now of paramount importance. Eighty-three percent of women under the age group of 45 years with cancer have survived during the impending period 2002–2012 in the United States.[1]

Cancer treatment in these reproductive age women usually includes chemotherapy, radiotherapy or surgical removal of reproductive organs.[2] All of these lead to reduced fertility and menopause-related complications in young age.[3]

When a young patient is diagnosed with a cancer, it is the responsibility on the part of the surgeon or oncologist to educate the patient about the options of fertility preservation. Controlled ovarian stimulation (COS) followed by oocyte or embryo cryopreservation is the most preferred method for fertility preservation in cancer patients and is also the only technique endorsed by American Society of Reproductive Medicine (ASRM).[4]

OVARIAN RESERVE TESTS

Before starting any stimulation, it is important to assess the ovarian reserve tests.

The frequently used tests are:

- *Follicle-stimulating hormone (FSH)*: It is not very reliable since it is cycle day-specific and sometimes the stimulation needs to be started in luteal phase.
- *Antral follicle count (AFC)*: It is an accurate test but can be measured only till day 5 of the cycle.
- *Anti-Müllerian hormone (AMH)*: More reliable as compared to other test since it can be done on any day of the cycle prior to starting stimulation. AMH is also used as a prognostic tool for ovarian reserve post chemotherapy.[5]

Effects of Cancer on Ovarian Response

In cancer patients, the hypothalamic-gonadal axis is affected due to various factors like increased stress hormone levels, increased catabolic state and malnutrition.[6] Hence, it becomes difficult to predict the ovarian response to various stimulation protocols.

TIMING OF STIMULATION

In order to obtain maximum oocyte yield and prevent delay in cancer treatment, early referral to a fertility specialist and random-start protocols are very important. The decision to start ovarian stimulation depends on the type of tumor as well as time left for chemotherapy or radiotherapy. In hematological cancers, the tumor burden is very high at the outset of diagnosis and hence random-start protocol is recommended to start immediate stimulation. In other cancers where surgery is the first line of management, the patient either has a time frame of 4–6 weeks before surgery or in between surgery and adjuvant therapy. Hence random-start protocol can be started during this period.

GONADOTROPIN DOSE DURING OVARIAN STIMULATION

Since there is only one chance at ovarian stimulation in cancer patients, the aim is to get maximum oocyte/embryo yield. One of the strategies used for this is using higher doses of gonadotropins. However, there are theories that suggest that use of higher doses of gonadotropins may cause recruitment of chromosomally abnormal or incompetent oocytes.[7] Although, higher doses of gonadotropins may be required in patients with poor ovarian response.

OVARIAN STIMULATION PROTOCOLS

1. Conventional COS (early follicular)
2. Luteal halt:
   - Anderson's protocol
   - Michael Wolff's protocol
3. Random-start protocol:
   - Late follicular start
   - Luteal start
4. DuoStim protocol (Shanghai protocol).

Conventional Controlled Ovarian Stimulation (Early Follicular)

Amongst the various COS protocols used, the majority of patients are treated with a gonadotropin-releasing hormone (GnRH) antagonist-based protocol. The advantage of antagonist protocol is that they decrease the interval from patient presentation to oocyte cryopreservation.[8]

In conventional protocol, gonadotropins are started from second day of menstrual cycle and GnRH antagonists are started when the lead follicle reaches 12–14 mm **(Fig. 1)**.

Luteal Halt

If the patient is in luteal phase, initiating menses by breaking down the corpus luteum to stop progesterone production was proposed. By doing so ovarian stimulation can be initiated more quickly.

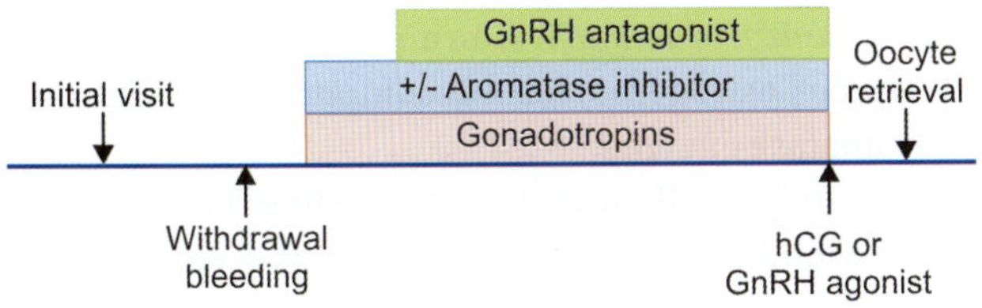

Fig. 1: Conventional controlled ovarian stimulation.

Anderson's Protocol[9]

After giving GnRH antagonist (e.g. single dose of 3 mg cetrorelix subcutaneously) during the midluteal phase, menses ensues a few days later. Gonadotropin stimulation started from day 2 of menses and GnRH antagonist is restarted when the lead follicle is at 12–14 mm to prevent premature luteinizing hormone (LH) surge **(Fig. 2)**.

Michael Wolff's Protocol[10]

In this protocol, both gonadotropins and GnRH antagonist are started simultaneously without waiting for menses to ensue. However, only FSH is used since use of exogenous LH may prevent luteolysis.

Random-Start Controlled Ovarian Hyperstimulation

Sometime in cancer patients there is an urgency for cancer treatment and hence it is undesirable to wait for next menstrual period. Random-start protocols were proposed for such patients.[11,12] In this protocol, stimulation is initiated at the time of patient presentation instead of waiting for spontaneous menses.[12]

Late Follicular Start

The late follicular phase was defined as after menstrual cycle day 7 with emergence of a dominant follicle (>13 mm) and/or progesterone level less than 2 ng/mL.[11]

When the patient presents in late follicular phase, one of the following may be done:

- If the follicles are less than 12 mm and remain less than 12 mm before a spontaneous LH surge, stimulation is started without GnRH antagonist. After the LH surge, GnRH antagonist is initiated when the secondary follicle cohort reached 12 mm in order to prevent premature secondary LH surge **(Fig. 3)**.
- If the follicular cohort reaches 12 mm before spontaneous LH surge, GnRH antagonist is started and continued till trigger is given for final oocyte maturation **(Fig. 4)**.

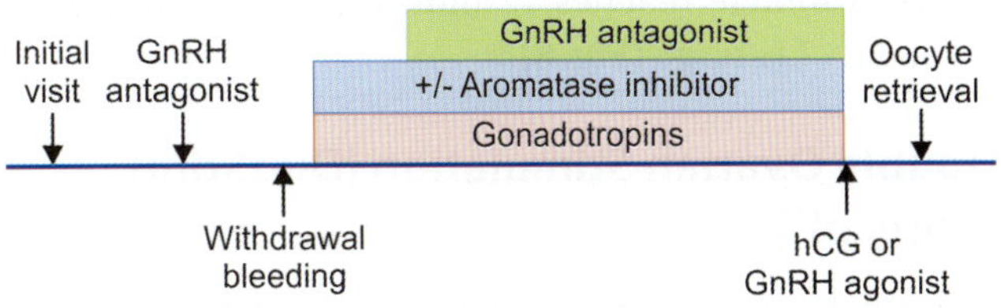

Fig. 2: Luteal halt—Anderson's protocol.

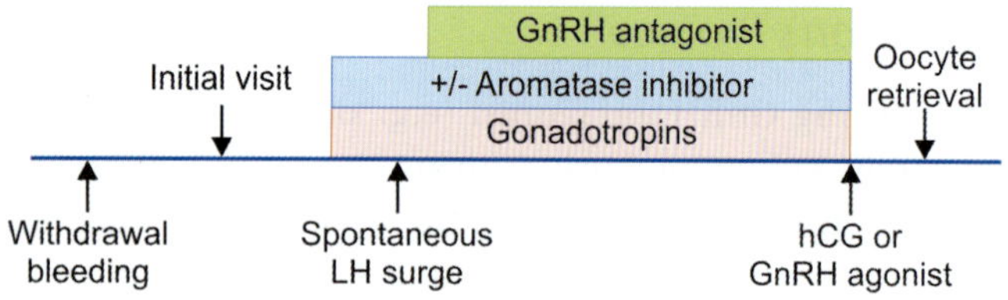

Fig. 3: Late follicular phase start.

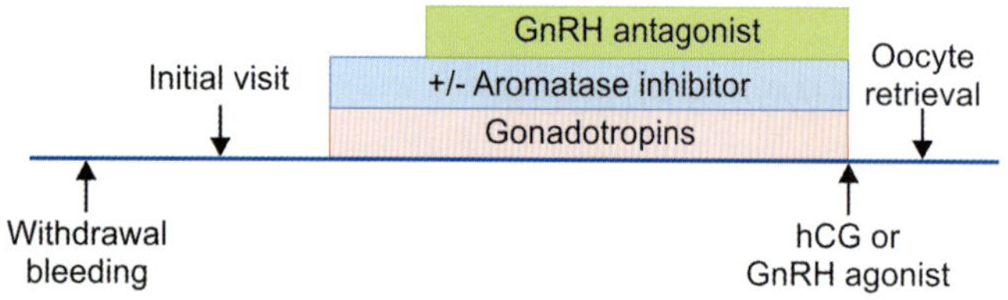

Fig. 4: Luteal phase following spontaneous luteinizing hormone (LH) surge.

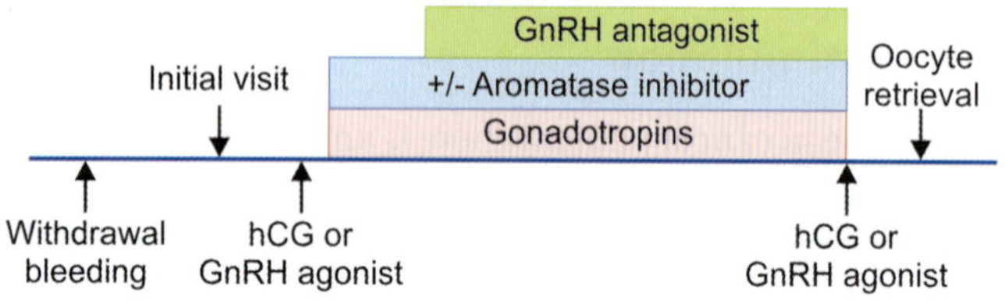

Fig. 5: After ovulation induction with human chorionic gonadotropin (hCG) or GnRH agonist.

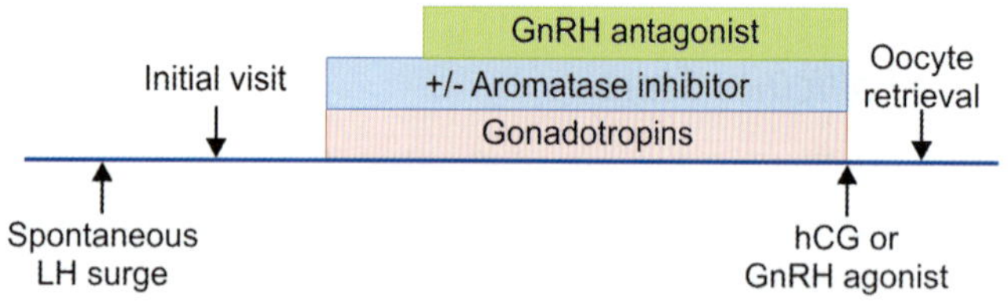

Fig. 6: Luteal phase start.

- If the dominant follicle has reached 18 mm in diameter then human chorionic gonadotropin (hCG) or GnRH agonist was given to trigger ovulation and stimulation started in luteal phase after 2–3 days **(Fig. 5)**.

Luteal Start

When the cancer patient presents in the luteal phase after ovulation was induced, COS is started with only gonadotropins and GNRH antagonist is added later when the lead follicle reaches 12 mm to prevent premature secondary LH surge **(Fig. 6)**.[10]

Double Ovarian Stimulation (DuoStim) Protocol[13]

Recently Kuang et al. suggested dual stimulation for these patients (Shanghai protocol). It is based on the belief that there are more than one follicle recruitment waves during menstrual cycle. It is beneficial to do multiple cycles of stimulation prior to cancer treatment to obtain maximum oocyte/embryo yield especially in patients with poor ovarian reserve.

In this protocol, patients were started with random-start antagonist protocol. Ovulation trigger was given with 5,000 IU of hCG when more than three follicle were greater than 17 mm in diameter and oocyte retrieval was performed 35 hours later. A second consecutive stimulation was started with gonadotropins either on day of oocyte retrieval or a few days later. Second trigger was given when more than three follicles were greater than 17 mm. The oocytes retrieved from both stimulation cycles were cryopreserved for future use.

CONTROLLED OVARIAN STIMULATION IN PATIENTS WITH ESTROGEN-SENSITIVE CANCERS

It is essential to keep a check on COS-induced rise in estrogen levels while ovarian stimulation in estrogen-sensitive cancers. These high levels of estrogen may promote the growth of tumors like breast (estrogen receptor-positive) and endometrial cancers.[14]

Safer protocols in estrogen-sensitive tumors are:

1. Natural cycle: It is not considered practical to do a natural cycle since there is a high rate of cycle cancellation and these patients may not have time for a second cycle of in vitro fertilization (IVF) before their chemotherapy.
2. Tamoxifen-based protocol:
   Mechanism of action:
   - Antiestrogenic effect on breast tissue[15]
   - Antagonist action on estrogen receptors in the brain.

   Tamoxifen 20–60 mg/day is started on day 2–5 of the menstrual cycle, either alone or in combination with gonadotropins.[16] Tamoxifen when used in combination with gonadotropins further increases the number of oocytes and embryos obtained.[17]
3. Letrozole:
   Mechanism of action: It is an aromatase inhibitor which reduces estrogen levels by competitive inhibition of aromatase enzyme.
   In a study by Oktay et al.,[18] it was shown that letrozole in combination with gonadotropins yielded similar number of oocytes as compared to standard protocol while keeping the peak estrogen levels lower. In this

study, they also restarted letrozole after oocyte retrieval till the estrogen levels were less than 50 pg/mL **(Fig. 7)**.

Controlled ovarian stimulation with letrozole plus gonadotropins in estrogen-sensitive cancer patients is safe and yields similar number of oocytes and embryos compared to standard protocols while minimizing the risk of increased estrogen levels and cancer recurrence.[19] Hence the routine use of letrozole is recommended for ovarian stimulation in patients with estrogen-sensitive cancers.

PREVENTION OF COMPLICATIONS AND OTHER MEDICAL CONSIDERATIONS

Ovarian Hyperstimulation Syndrome

Ovarian hyperstimulation syndrome (OHSS) in cancer patients may lead to delay in lifesaving cancer treatment.[20] Hence it is very important to prevent OHSS in these patients. GnRH agonist trigger in GnRH antagonist-based protocols reduces the risk of OHSS.[21] It is also convenient in these patients since they do not require luteal support. When GnRH agonist trigger is given, its effects must be confirmed the next morning by doing serum LH levels which should be greater than 12 mIU/mL. If less than that then hCG trigger can be given on the same day.

Thromboembolic Events

In cancer patients, there is a hypercoagulable state due to both their malignancy as well as high estrogen levels due to COS.[22] In order to prevent any thromboembolic events, low-molecular weight heparin may be started in high-risk patients. It is stopped 24 hours prior to oocyte retrieval and restarted 12 hours post retrieval.[19] Secondly, letrozole helps in these high-risk groups by keeping the estrogen levels low.

Bleeding

There is a tendency of bleeding during oocyte retrieval in patients with liver involvement or hematological malignancies. Hence platelet or fresh frozen plasma transfusion should be given prior to oocyte retrieval in these patients.[19]

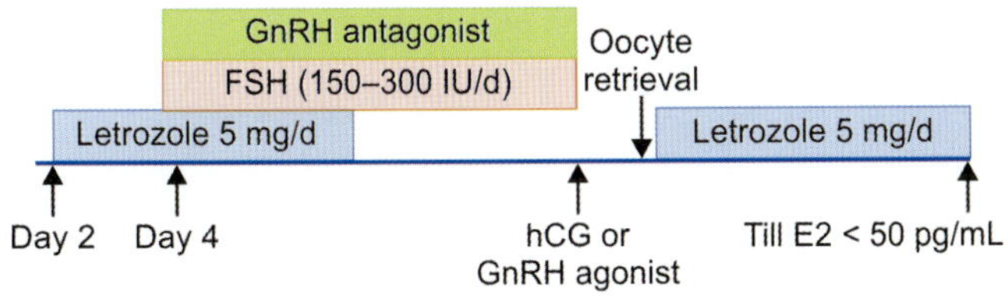

Fig. 7: Controlled ovarian stimulation with letrozole.

Infection

Patients with neutropenia are at high risk of infection and hence should be considered for prophylactic antibiotics. Alternatively, after consultation with the oncologist, granulocyte colony-stimulating factor may be administered to increase the neutrophil count.

Cancer-related Medical Conditions

Anesthesia consultation should be obtained in advance for the patients with conditions involving the respiratory system. Antiepileptic drugs must be continued during stimulation. If the patient is on imatinib, it must be stopped as it has adverse effects on ovarian hormone production.[23]

CONCLUSION

It is very important that patients undergoing cancer treatment are given proper counseling regarding fertility preservation prior to starting their therapy. Although there is no proper data regarding clinical pregnancy rates and live birth rates of these new protocols, they are efficient in obtaining appropriate number of oocytes and embryos. In cases of emergency, random-start protocols are considered to be the most appropriate. The dose and type of gonadotropins can be individualized based on patient's ovarian reserve. The main aim in cancer patients is to obtain maximum number of oocytes/embryos for cryopreservation while minimizing the risk for OHSS and other complications. Letrozole along with gonadotropins is an effective method of ovarian stimulation in estrogen-sensitive cancers. Although more clinical studies are required to determine the live birth rates from using these cryopreserved oocytes and embryos in cancer patients.

REFERENCES

1. Howlader N, Noone AM, Krapcho M, et al. SEER cancer statistics review, 1975-2009 (Vintage 2009 populations). Bethesda, MD: National Cancer Institute; 2012. [online] Available from http://seer.cancer.gov/csr/1975_2009_pops09/. [Last accessed February, 2019].
2. Rodriguez-Wallberg KA, Oktay K. Options on fertility preservation in female cancer patients. Cancer Treat Rev. 2012;38:354-61.
3. Letourneau JM, Ebbel EE, Katz PP, et al. Acute ovarian failure underestimates age-specific reproductive impairment for young women undergoing chemotherapy for cancer. Cancer. 2012;118:1933-9.

4. Ethics Committee of the American Society for Reproductive Medicine. Fertility preservation and reproduction in cancer patients. Fertil Steril. 2005;83:1622-8.
5. Rama Raju GA, Chakraborty B. Individualized Controlled Ovarian Stimulation. Philadelphia: Elsevier; 2016. pp. 175-6.
6. Pal L, Leykin L, Schifren JL, et al. Malignancy may adversely influence the quality and behaviour of oocytes. Hum Reprod. 1998;13:1837-40.
7. Baart EB, Martini E, Eijkemans MJ, et al. Milder ovarian stimulation for in-vitro fertilization reduces aneuploidy in the human preimplantation embryo: a randomized controlled trial. Hum Reprod. 2007;22:980-8.
8. McLaren JF, Bates GW. Fertility preservation in women of reproductive age with cancer. Am J Obstet Gynecol. 2012;207:455-62.
9. Anderson RA, Kinniburgh D, Baird DT. Preliminary experience of the use of a gonadotrophin-releasing hormone antagonist in ovulation induction/in vitro fertilization prior to cancer treatment. Hum Reprod. 1999;14:2665-8.
10. von Wolff M, Thaler CJ, Frambach T, et al. Ovarian stimulation to cryopreserve fertilized oocytes in cancer patients can be started in the luteal phase. Fertil Steril. 2009;92:1360-5.
11. Cakmak H, Katz A, Cedars MI, et al. Effective method for emergency fertility preservation: random-start controlled ovarian hyperstimulation. Fertil Steril. 2012;98:S170.
12. Sonmezer M, Turkcuoglu I, Coskun U, et al. Random-start controlled ovarian hyperstimulation for emergency fertility preservation in letrozole cycles. Fertil Steril. 2011;95:2125. e9-11.
13. Kuang Y, Chen Q, Hong Q, et al. Double stimulations during the follicular and luteal phases of poor responders in IVF/ICSI programmes (Shanghai protocol). Reprod Biomed Online. 2014;29:684-91.
14. Reddy J, Oktay K. Ovarian stimulation and fertility preservation with the use of aromatase inhibitors in women with breast cancer. Fertil Steril. 2012;98:1363-9.
15. Early Breast Cancer Trialists' Collaborative Group. Systemic treatment of early breast cancer by hormonal, cytotoxic, or immune therapy. 133 randomised trials involving 31,000 recurrences and 24,000 deaths among 75,000 women. Lancet. 1992;339:71-85.
16. Rodriguez-Wallberg KA, Oktay K. Fertility preservation in women with breast cancer. Clin Obstet Gynecol. 2010;53: 753-62.
17. Oktay K, Buyuk E, Libertella N, et al. Fertility preservation in breast cancer patients: a prospective controlled comparison of ovarian stimulation with tamoxifen and letrozole for embryo cryopreservation. J Clin Oncol. 2005;23: 4347-53.
18. Oktay K, Hourvitz A, Sahin G, et al. Letrozole reduces estrogen and gonadotropin exposure in women with breast cancer undergoing ovarian stimulation before chemotherapy. J Clin Endocrinol Metab. 2006;91:3885-90.
19. Cakmak H, Rosen MP. Ovarian stimulation in cancer patients. Fertil Steril. 2013;99(6):1476-84.
20. Delvigne A, Rozenberg S. Epidemiology and prevention of ovarian hyperstimulation syndrome (OHSS): a review. Hum Reprod Update. 2002;8:559-77.
21. Engmann L, DiLuigi A, Schmidt D, et al. The use of gonadotropin-releasing hormone (GnRH) agonist to induce oocyte maturation after cotreatment with GnRH antagonist in high-risk patients undergoing in vitro fertilization prevents the risk of ovarian hyperstimulation syndrome: a prospective randomized controlled study. Fertil Steril. 2008;89: 84-91.
22. Aurousseau MH, Samama MM, Belhassen A, et al. Risk of thromboembolism in relation to an in-vitro fertilization programme: three case reports. Hum Reprod. 1995; 10:94-7.
23. Zamah AM, Mauro MJ, Druker BJ, et al. Will imatinib compromise reproductive capacity? Oncologist. 2011;16: 1422-7.

Management of Poor Responders in ART

34

Nimish R Shelat

It may not be possible to have superior outcome from ovaries in terms of oocytes, by finding efficacious management in this class of patients. There are about 9–24% of infertile patients who exhibit poor response to oocyte development, but seem to have increased even more in day-to-day practice.

Recent criteria on low-ovarian oocyte maturation outcome by the Bologna ESHRE working group on poor ovarian responders show new risk factors that lead to reduced ovarian reserve besides genetic factors.[1]

"Bologna Criteria" have lead to higher results of ovarian induction strategies with long-acting gonadotropins.[2]

INTRODUCTION

With gonadotropin-releasing hormone (GnRH) analogs added to gonadotropins induction cycle, results are still related to number of oocytes.[3]

There are less embryos to choose with less eggs obtained and transfer them, resulting in diminished conception rate per transfer and degraded cumulative pregnancy rates per initiated cycle, when seen in light with normal outcome of patients.

Varying definitions of poor responders cause confusion, but, as per ESHRE guidelines, poor responders are defined as the one in which out of three, minimum two criteria are evident:[4-7]

1. Higher mother's age or other issues with overall health
2. Former reduced ovarian outcome in terms of oocytes
3. Ovarian reserve test abnormality.

Mildly raised in last 10 years, the incidence is over 24%.

From 37 years to 38 years,[8] the follicular disappearance in ovaries is markedly increased. Thereafter, 10–13 years later, menopause sets in. Ovarian surgery for endometriosis,[9-12] treatment of cancer, by radiation, chemotactic drugs, immunological diseases, single ovary, causes related to genetic abnormalities and infertility related to unknown causes.[13,14] New risk factors include:

1. Diabetes mellitus type-1[15]
2. Beta thalassemia, which is due to transfusion[16]
3. Embolization of uterine artery for the myoma ablation[17,18]
4. Why the follicle depletion occurs is not known.[13] The term "aging process" is casual term because Caucasian women despite longer age do not deplete their follicles, in comparison to Asian women by at least 5 years.

The mechanism leads to reduction of quality with reduced implantation rates and increased pregnancy loss.[19] Poor responders by themselves not necessarily be stamped with low-success rates because it is known that, even with a few follicles and lesser eggs, pregnancies and live births are on record. It is the age related to genetic racial factors, which predict live birth rate.[20-25] Here, with difficult cases, one should tailor and plant the best stimulation protocol to obtain maximum yield of ovarian reserve so as to optimize retrieval of oocytes in larger numbers. This is possible with new biomarkers of ovarian reserve that are a tool for superior strategies for managing poor responders in ART.[15]

PREDICTION OF OVARIAN RESPONSE

- *Age*: *Much reduced after 35 years in Asia.*
- *Basal serum follicle-stimulating hormone (FSH)* is, in deciding ovarian output of quality oocytes in IVF (in vitro fertilization), the most crucial indicator. This rise is seen almost 10 years before onset of menopause,[26,27] reduce the negative feedback the inhibin B and inhibin

A from ovary are proteins that control FSH to reduce negative effects.[28,29] FSH modulating, proteins from the ovary. This is secondary to early antral follicle diminution. With higher degrees of FSH threshold, more than 12 mIU/mL is the quantum required to qualify as a good predictor that shows very low-depleted ovarian reserve.[30] The preantral follicles producing anti-Mullerian hormone (AMH) provide the qualitative estimate of developing oocytes that are not measured by ultrasonic antral follicle count (AFC), aromatase activity, and follicular growth.[31-33] AMH inhibits FSH-mediated granulosa cell modification. During menstrual cycle, the inter- and intracycle variability are very low with AMH, which is stable, making it a very reliable marker. AMH is an indicator to find poor expression of ovaries in terms of egg development. This characteristic of AMH[34] is not changed by the lag of time period between AMH in serum and the start of follicular stimulation up to 1 year.

Again, age remains most important factor related to live birth rates[35] when compared to AMH and AFC alone or in combination by a meta-analysis that did not show better prediction on going pregnancy rate.

The nonobese poor responders have better pregnancy rates than obese poor responders by estimated body mass index (BMI).[36,37]

THE BOLOGNA CRITERIA FOR POOR OVARIAN RESPONSE

These criteria are used in management of poor responders in ART.

By definition, the number of matured follicles on the day of injecting human chorionic gonadotropin (hCG) is:

1. Less than 2 to less than 5[38-40]
2. Less than 4 to less than 6 oocyte number obtained[41,42]
3. On day 5 of stimulation, serum estradiol level—100 pg/mL, or less than 300 to less than 600 pg/mL on hCG administration,[39,41,43] Or
4. Overall dose of gonadotropin use and/or daily stimulation dose,[43-45] and/or
5. Longer time of gonadotropin stimulation.[46,47]

MANAGEMENT BY GONADOTROPINS

- There is a need to increase the dose, if the standard dose of 225–300 IU does not produce proper follicular growth.
- Some[38,48,49] have not substantiated superior ovarian performance with oocyte production or higher pregnancy rates upon initiating the above doses, in prospective and retrospective studies, except[50] by raising the initial dose of FSH, better conception rates are not achieved irrespective of the dosage and there is no difference between 300 IU, 450 IU, or 600 IU of gonadotropins with respect to rate of successful pregnancy, embryo numbers, or eggs recovered as shown by Berkkanoglu and Ozgur.[51] No de-novo follicles can be manufactured in spite of stimulations, except only dose administered supports the cohort of follicles.

Management by GnRH Analogs

Combination of GnRH agonists with gonadotropins, with long protocol, will have lower cancellation rates raising number of preovulatory follicles and numbers of oocytes retrieved and will produce good-qualities embryos for transfer in normal responders with better pregnancy rates.[52] However, in poor responders, this will act adversely by excessive ovarian suppression leading to reduced or absent follicular response.[53,54]

Therefore, for poor responders:

- Decrease duration of GnRh agonist protocol thereby decreasing duration of suppression to lower short, ultra-short, mini, and micro dose flare-up regimen[39,55-57]
- Lower or stopped GnRH agonists started from luteal phase[41,58,3]
- GnRH antagonist use in combination to control aberrant early luteinizing hormone (LH) peak wave during any time after early follicular phase.[59]

For more than 20 years, flare-up of short or ultra-short regimens, though widely used, has not demonstrated significant beneficial effect.[39,50,56,57,60,61]

Clinical pregnancy rates did not show significant difference between flare-up short regimen and antagonist, agonist GnRH protocols.[62]

Duration or in the management with GnRH, there was no difference between stimulation by GnRH agonists stopped regime and standard agonist regime stimulation when assessing the number of gonadotropin ampoules on the number of oocytes retrieved. GnRH agonist stopped protocol and standard agonist protocol.[62,63]

Management with GnRH Antagonist

For poor responders, the appropriate right regime is gonadotropins continued with GnRH antagonist, wherein immature LH surge is prevented without suppression in early follicular phase obtaining more natural follicles recruited without any inhibitory effect induced by GnRH agonist.[63-67]

This does not disturb the normal follicular development in early period of the cycle that can be included as well. The use of GnRH antagonist can have reduction of live birth rates compared to GnRH agonist protocol due to difference in patients' population selections, which is not statistically significant.[68]

Less time is needed to produce desired stimulation with GnRH antagonist regimes than those with GnRH agonist without significantly different number of cancellations of egg retrieval and positive conception rate on clinical scenario.[69,70]

There is not a stimulation protocol as a yardstick of ideal reproductive medical treatment to make better, significantly, improve the clinical outcome in poor responders.

On ultrasound, patients with mean follicular number of less than 5 have considerable variation from one cycle to another in count of antral follicles from –2 to + 5[71] and 2–3 to +7.[72]

NEW TOOLS OF STRATEGY IN POOR RESPONDERS TO ART

A high-breed gonadotropin corifollitropin, the protein from anterior pituitary, quoted by many, a molecule with prolonged half life corifollitropin alpha supports follicle cohort receptive to stimulate with GnRH antagonist for preventing premature LH rise. This long-acting gonadotropin helps to rapidly increase serum FSH concentration exposing small antral follicle in a higher way with follicular phase bolus of FSH, thereafter, boosting the reduced ovarian reserve.[73,74]

Better pregnancy rates have been reported in patient age of 40 years who subjected to GnRH antagonist protocol-controlled administration of highly purified human menotropin (HP-HMG) with corifollitropin alpha in poor responders.[75]

The reduced ovarian reserve is fully exploited by peculiar pharmacokinetics of corifollitropin alpha reducing the number of daily injections thereby less physical and psychological stress to patients.[76]

OTHER APPROACHES TO MANAGEMENT OF POOR RESPONDERS

Addition of estradiol, in the former luteal period of the previous menstrual cycle:

- This addition decreases the risk of cycle cancellation and increases the probability of achieving a viable pregnancy in poor responders.[77]
- The luteal estradiol priming in previous cycle improves pools of follicles in the next cycle, which synchronize in one batch to be available for stimulation.[78,79]

Recombinant LH

In poor responders, larger cohort of eggs is collected with superior clinical pregnancies achieved with combining both recombinant hFSH and recombinant hLH compared to only single recombinant hFSH by 30%, beneficial to such poor responders.[80-83]

Growth Hormone

It modulates actions by promoting focused production of IGF-1, insulin-like growth promoting factor, to act on FSH that modulates granulosa cells of FSH[84-86] that amplifies FSH effect on theca cells and granulosa cells.[87,88]

This positively improves the chances of healthy delivery at term.[6,62]

Routinely, it is not advisable to subject poor ovarian responding patients to the addition of growth hormone (GH).[89,90]

Androgens

Androgens produced by theca cells play crucial role in control of steroid production in ovarian follicles[91] and proper follicular and granulosa cell development in early stage.[92] Androgen may increase FSH receptor expression and, therefore, low level results in decreased sensitivity of ovaries to FSH and low-pregnancy rates.[93-95]

Addition of dehydroepiandrosterone (DHEA) in poor responders shows significant pregnancy rate in androgen supplementation group.[96] Though multicenter randomized control trials are required.[97-99]

Aspirin

Improving delivery of gonadotropins or other growth factors requires increased intraovarian vascularity and impaired blood flow leads to lower ovarian response.[100,101]

Aspirin being vasoactive enhances ovarian vascularization to improve ovarian response.[102-107]

Another study[108] of prospective randomized control trials shows no such improvement and the evidence is conflicting.[109]

Natural Cycle IVF

- Eight percent is the highest birth rate per patient on cumulative basis.[110]

- Natural cycle IVF is better option with same chance of pregnancy and implantation.[111,112]
- In a younger woman less than 35 years, a study by Schimberni et al.[113] with 500 patients reported very good results of IVF outcome in poor responders that showed 31% pregnancy rate per patient, 29% per transfer, and 18% per cycle started.
- How poor responder patients characterize with natural cycle IVF in terms of effect of natural cycles IVF in terms of the "Bologna criteria"?

Oocyte Cryopreservation

Egg vitrification (a technique of freezing or cryopreservation) has opened new doors to success in ART, as the most important milestone of success in last 10 years. Highly efficient procedure that helps streamline support for day-to-day fertility care management.[114]

European Society of Human Reproduction and Embryology (ESHRE), American Society for Reproductive Medicine (ASRM), and American Society of Clinical Oncologists (ASCO).[115]

Various methods are found useful for low responders by the technique of egg freezing. A high number of eggs can be collected by storing vitrified frozen eggs over multiple induction cycles, mimicking the same scenario as in otherwise those patients who show a standard response.[116]

For those women, who over time are likely to, passively by aging process, give away their reserved eggs to apoptosis and atrophy, the technique of fertility preservation is best enhanced by early age healthy egg cryopreservation, which will hold the aging in a static phase, till wanted to be reactivated at a convenient time, when pregnancy is desired.

CONCLUSION

Inadequate evidence is prevailed by evidence-based medicine of meta-analyses and comprehensive reviews to support most of the regimes for improving fertility in poor ovarian responders.

It is a challenging task to discover the most efficacious induction regime in treatment of low-ovarian output of good-quality eggs, despite the huge numbers of indexed scientific content at our disposal from journals and publications.

Any other modality of adjuvant molecules proposed for this group of poor responders meets with poor success.

The long-acting gonadotropin corifollitropin alpha combination has GnRH antagonist protein combined with highly pure HMG; is the only possible route in the current scenario to achieve a viable response in poor responders, however, more randomized controlled trials will further validate the advantages of this modality of treatment.

It is prudent to give the alternative of egg freezing for future conception before the downhill road to egg storage, as there are no deleterious effects of vitrification of eggs as per evidence on record.[117,118]

REFERENCES

1. Polyzos NP, Devroey P. A systematic review of randomized trials for the treatment of poor ovarian responders: is there any light at the end of the tunnel? Fertil Steril. 2011;96: 1058-61.
2. Keay SD, Liversedge NH, Mathur RS, et al. Assisted conception following poor ovarian response to gonadotrophin stimulation. Br J Obstet Gynaecol. 1997;104:521-7.
3. Ben-Rafael Z, Bider D, Dan U, et al. Combined gonadotropin releasing hormone agonist/human menopausal gonadotropin therapy (GnRH-a/hMG) in normal, high, and poor responders to HMG. J In Vitro Fert Embryo Transf. 1991;8: 33-36.
4. Jenkins JM, Davies DW, Devonport H, et al. Comparison of "proof" responders with "good" responders using a standard buserelin/human menopausal gonadotrophin regime for in-vitro fertilization. Hum Reprod. 1991;6:918-21.
5. Surrey ES, Schoolcraft WB. Evaluating strategies for improving ovarian response of the poor responder undergoing assisted reproductive techniques. Fertil Steril. 2000;73:667-76.
6. Kolibianakis EM, Venetis CA, Diedrich, Tarlatzis BC, et al. Addition of growth hormone to gonadotrophins in ovarian stimulation of poor responders treated by in-vitro fertilization: a systematic review and meta-analysis. Hum Reprod Update. 2009;6:613-22.
7. Ferraetti AP, La Marca A, Fauser BC, et al. ESHRE consensus on the definition of "poor response" to ovarian stimulation for in vitro fertilization: the Bologna criteria". Hum Reprod. 2011;26:1616-24.
8. Faddy MJ, Gosden RG, Gougeon A, et al. Accelerated disappearance of ovarian follicles in mid-life: implications for forecasting menopause. Hum Reprod. 1992;7:1342-6.
9. de Ziegler D1, Borghese B, Chapron C. Endometriosis and infertility: pathophysiology and management. Lancet. 2010;376:730-8.
10. Bengalia L, Somigliana E, Vighi V, et al. Rate of severe ovarian damage following surgery for endometriomas. Hum Reprod. 2010;25:678-82.
11. Streuli I, de Ziegler D, Gayet V, et al. In women with endometriosis anti-Mullerian hormone levels are decreased only in those with previous endometrioma surgery. Hum Reprod. 2012;27:3294-303.
12. Raffi F, Metwally M, Amer S. The impact of excision of ovarian endometrioma on ovarian reserve: a systematic review and meta-analysis. J Clin Endocrinol Metab. 2012;97:3146-54.

13. De Vos M, Devroey P, Fauser BC. Fauser, Primary ovarian insufficiency. Lancet. 2010;376:911-21.
14. Fritz MA, Speroff L. Clinical Gynecologic Endocrinology and Infertility. Philadelphia, PA, USA: Wolters Kluwer Health/ Lippincott Williams & Wilkins; 2011.
15. Soto N, Iñiguez G, López P, et al. Anti-Mullerian hormone and inhibin B levels as markers of premature ovarian aging and transition to menopause in type 1 diabetes mellitus. Hum Reprod. 2009;24:2838-44.
16. Chang HH, Chen MJ, Lu MY, et al. Iron overload is associated with low anti-mullerian hormone in women with transfusion dependent -B-thalassaemia. Br J Obstet Gynaecol. 2011;118:825-31.
17. Hehenkamp WJK, Volkers NA, Broekmans FJM, et al. Loss of ovarian after uterine artery embolization: a randomized comparison with hysterectomy. Hum Reprod. 2007;22:1996-2005.
18. Tropeano G, Di Stasi D, Amoroso S, et al. Long term effects of uterine fibroid embolization on ovarian reserve: a prospective cohort study. Fertil Steril. 2010;94:2296-300.
19. Reproductive Endocrinology and Infertility Committee, Family Physicians Advisory Committee, Maternal-Fetal Medicine Committee, Executive and Council of the Society of Obstetricians, Liu K, Case A. Advanced reproductive age and fertility. JOGC. 2011;33;1165-75.
20. Ulug U, Ben-Shlomo I, Turan E, et al. Conception rates following assisted reproduction in poor responder patients; a retrospective study in 300 consecutive cycles. Reprod Biomed Online. 2003;6:439-43.
21. Zhen XM, Qiao J, Li R, et al. The clinical analysis of poor ovarian response in-vitro-fertilization embryo—transfer among Chinese couples. J Assist Reprod Genet. 2008;25;17-22.
22. Sunkara SK, Tuthill J, Khairy M, et al. Pituitary suppression regimens in poor responders undergoing IVF treatment: a systematic review and meta-analysis. Reprod Biomed Online. 2007;15:539-46.
23. El-Toukhjy T, Khalaf Y, Hart R, et al. Young age does not protect against the adverse effects of reduced ovarian reserve—an eight year study. Hum Reprod. 2002;17:1519-24.
24. Polyzos NP, Nwoye M, Corona R, et al. Live birth rates in Bologna poor responders treated with ovarian stimulation for IVF/ICSI. Reprod Biomed Online. 2014;28:469-74.
25. Al-Azemi M, Kilick SR, Duffy S, et al. Multi-marker assessment of ovarian reserve predicts oocyte yield after ovulation induction. Hum Reprod. 2011;26:414-22.
26. Ebbiary NA, Lenton EA, Cooke ID. Hypothalamic-pituitary ageing: progressive increase in FSH and LH concentrations throughout the reproductive life in regularly menstruating women. Clin Endocrinol. 1994;41:199-206.
27. Groome NP, Illingworth PJ, O'Brien M, et al. Measurement of diametric inhibin B throughout the human menstrual cycle. J Clin Endocrinol Metabol. 1996;81:1401-5.
28. Burger HG, Cahir N, Robertson DM, et al. Serum inhibins A and B fall differentially as FSH rises in perimenopausal women. Clin Endocrinol. 1998;48:809-13.
29. Welt CK, McNicholl DJ, Taylor AE, et al. Female reproductive aging is marked by decreased secretion of dimeric inhibin. J Clin Endocrinol Metab. 1999;84:105-11.
30. Broekmans FJ, Kwee J, Hendriks DJ, et al. A systematic review of tests predicting ovarian reserve and IFV outcome. Hum Reprod Update. 2006;12:685-718.
31. La Marca A, Stabile G, Artenisio AC, et al. Serum anti-Mullerian hormone throughout the human menstrual cycle. Hum Reprod. 2006;21:3103-7.
32. La Marca A, Giulini, A. Tireli et al. Anti-Mullerian hormone measurement on any day of the menstrual cycle strongly predicts ovarian response in assisted reproductive technology. Hum Reprod. 2007;22:766-71.
33. Dolleman M, Faddy MJ, van Disseldorp J, et al. The relationship between anti-Mullerian hormone in women receiving fertility assessments and age at menopause in subfertile women: evidence from large production studies. J Clin Edocrinol Metab. 2013;98:5:1946-53.
34. Polyzos NP, Nelson SM, Stoop D, et al. Does the time interval between anti-Mullerian hormone serum sampling and initiation of ovarian stimulation affect its predictive ability in in-vitro fertilization-intracytoplasmic sperm injection cycles with a gonadotropin-releasing hormone antagonist. A retrospective single-center study. Fertil Steril. 2013;100;438-44.
35. Broer SL, Dolleman M, van Disseldorp J, et al. Prediction of an excessive response in in-vitro fertilization from patient characteristics and ovarian reserve tests and comparison in subgroups: an individual patient data meta-analysis. Fertil Steril. 2013;100:420.e7-429.e7.
36. Oudendijk JF, Yarde F, Eijkemans MJ, et al. The poor responder in IVF: Is the prognosis always poor? A systematic review. Hum Reprod Update. 2012;18:1-11.
37. Koning AMH, Kuchenbecker WKH, Groen H, et al. Economic consequences of overweight obesity in infertility: a framework for evaluating the costs and outcomes of fertility care. Hum Reprod Update. 2010;16:246-54.
38. Land JA, Yarmolinskaya MI, Dumoulin JCM, et al. High-dose human menopausal gonadotropin stimulation in poor responders does not improve in-vitro fertilization outcome. Fertil Steril. 1996;65:961-5.
39. Surrey ES, Bower J, Hill DM, et al. Clinical and endocrine effects of a microdose GnRH agonist flare regimen administered to poor responders who are undergoing in-vitro fertilization. Fertil Steril. 1992;69:419-24.
40. Lashen H, Ledger W, Lopez-Bernal A, et al. Poor responders to ovulation induction: is proceeding to in-vitro fertilization worthwhile?" Hum Reprod. 1999;14:964-9.
41. Faber BM, Mayer J, Cox B, et al. Cessation of gonadotropin-releasing hormone agonist therapy combined with high-dose gonadotropin stimulation yields favourable pregnancy results in low responders. Fertil Steril. 1998;69:826-30.
42. Rombauts L, Suikkari A, MacLachlan V, et al. Recruitment of follicles by recombinant human follicle-stimulating hormone commencing in the luteal phase of the ovarian cycle. Fertil Steril. 1998;69:665-9.
43. Ibrahim ZHZ, Matson PL, Buck P, et al. The use of biosynthetic human growth hormone to augment ovulation induction with buserelin acetate/human menopausal gonadotrophin in women with a poor ovarian response. Fertil Steril. 1991;55:202-4.

44. Hughes SM, Hung ZH, Morris ID, et al. A double-blind cross-over controlled study to evaluate the effect of human biosynthetic growth hormone on ovarian stimulation in previous responders to in-vitro fertilization. Hum Reprod. 1994;9:13-8.
45. Vishvanath K, Morris R, Rinehart J, et al. Limited success using the "flare" protocol in poor responders in cycles with low basal follicle stimulating hormone levels during in-vitro fertilization. Fertil Steril. 1997;67:900-3.
46. Toth TL, Awwad JT, Veeck LL, et al. Suppression and flare regimens of gonadotropin-releasing hormone agonist: use in women with different basal gonadotropin values in an in-vitro fertilization program. J Reprod Med Obstet Gynaecol. 1996;41:321-6.
47. Younis JS. The Bologna criteria for poor ovarian response; has the job been accomplished. Hum Reprod. 2012;27:1874-5.
48. Karnade VC, Jones GS, Muasher SJ, et al. High dose follicle stimulating hormone stimulation at the onset of the menstrual cycle does not improve the in-vitro fertilization outcome in low-responder patients. Fertil Steril. 1990;53:486-9.
49. Van Hoof MHA, Alberda AT, Huisman GJ, et al. Doubling the human menopausal gonadotrophin dose in the course of an in-vitro fertilization treatment cycle in low responders, a randomized study. Hum Reprod. 1993;8:369-73.
50. Hofmann GE, Toner JP, Muasher SJ, et al. High dose follicle-stimulating hormone (FSH) ovarian stimulation in low responder patients for in-vitro fertilization. J In Vitro Fertil Embryo Trans. 1989;6:285-9.
51. Berkkanoglu M, Ozgur K. What is the optimum maximal gonadotropin dosage used in microdose flare-up cycles in poor responders? Fertil Steril. 2010;94:662-5.
52. Hughes EG, Fedorkow DM, Daya S, et al. The routine use of gonadotropin-releasing hormone agonists prior to in-vitro fertilization and gamete intrafallopian transfer: a meta-analysis of randomized controlled trials. Fertil Steril. 1992;58:888-96.
53. Yoshimura Y, Nakamura Y, Ando M, et al. Direct effect of gonadotropin-releasing hormone agonists on the rabbit ovarian follicle. Fertil Steril. 1992;57:1091-7.
54. Kowalik A, Barmat L, Ando M, et al. Ovarian estradiol production in vivo. Inhibitory effect of leuprolide acetate. J Reprod Med. 1998;43:413-17.
55. Lindheim SR, Barad DH, Witt B, et al. Short-term gonadotropin suppression with oral contraceptives benefits poor responders prior to controlled ovarian hyperstimulation. J Assist Reprod Genet. 1996;13:745-7.
56. Schoolcraft W, Schlenker T, Gee M, et al. Improved controlled ovarian hyperstimulation in poor responder in-vitro fertilization patients with a microdose follicle stimulating hormone flare, growth hormone protocol. Fertil Steril. 1997;67:93-7.
57. Padilla SL, Dugan K, Maruschak V, et al. Use of the flare-up protocol with high does human follicle stimulating hormone and human menopausal gonadotropins for in-vitro fertilization in poor responders. Fertil Steril. 1996;65:796-9.
58. Karande V, Gleicher N. A rational approach to the management of low responders in in-vitro fertilization. Hum Reprod. 1999;14:1744-8.
59. Craft I, Gorgy A, Hill J, et al. Will GnRH antagonists provide new hope for patients considered "difficult responders" to GnRH agonist protocols. Hum Reprod. 1999;14:2959-62.
60. Akman MA, Erden HF, Tosun SB, et al. Addition of GnRH antagonist in cycles of poor responders undergoing IVF. Hum Reprod. 2000;15:2145-7.
61. Leondires MP, Escalpes M, Segars JH, et al. Microdose follicular phase gonadotropin-releasing hormone agonists (GnRH-a) compared with luteal phase GnRH-a for ovarian stimulation at in-vitro fertilization. Fertil Steril. 1999;72:1018-23.
62. Kyrou D, Kolibianakis EM, Venetis CA, et al. How to improve the probability of pregnancy in poor responders undergoing in-vitro fertilization: a systematic review and meta-analysis. Fertil Steril. 2009;91:749-66.
63. Pinkas H, Orvieto R, Avrech OM, et al. Gonadotropin stimulation GnRH-a priming for poor responders in in-vitro fertilization—embryo transfer programs. Gynaecol Endocrinol. 2000;14:11-4.
64. Schachter M, Friedler S, Raziel A, et al. Improvement of IVF outcome in poor responders by discontinuation of GnRH analogue during the gonadotropin stimulation phase-a function of improved embryo quality. J Assist Reprod Genet. 2001;18:197-204.
65. Dirnfeld M, Fruchter O, Yshai D, et al. Cessation of gonadotropin-releasing hormone analogue (GnRH-a) upon down-regulation versus conventional long GnRH-a protocol in poor responders undergoing in-vitro fertilization. Fertil Steril. 1999;72:406-11.
66. Garcia-Velasco JA, Isaza V, Requena A, et al. High does of gonadotrophins combined with stop versus non-stop protocol of GnRH analogue administration in low responder IVF patients: a prospective, randomized, controlled trial. Hum Reprod. 2000;15:2292-6.
67. Kenigsberg D, Littman BA, Hodgen GD. Medical hypophysectomy: I. Dose—response using a gonadotropin-releasing hormone antagonist. Fertil Steril. 1984;42:112-5.
68. Al-Inany HG, Youssef MA, Aboulghar M, et al. Gonadotrophin-releasing hormone antagonists for assisted reproductive technology. Cochrane Database Syst Rev. 2011;(5):CD001750.
69. Griesinger G, Diedrich K, Tarlatzis BC, et al. GnRH-antagonists in ovarian stimulation for IFV in patients with poor response to gonadotrophins, polycystic ovary syndrome, and risk of ovarian hyperstimulation: a meta-analysis. Reprod Biomed Online. 2006;13:628-38.
70. Pu D, Wu J, Liu J. Comparisons of GnRH antagonist versus GnRH agonist protocol in poor ovarian responders undergoing IVF. Hum Reprod. 2011;26:2742-9.
71. Scheffer GJ, Broekmans FJM, Dorland M, et al. Antral follicle counts by transvaginal ultrasonography are related to age in women with proven natural fertility. Fertil Steril. 1999;72: 845-51.
72. Bancsi LF1, Broekmans FJ, Looman CW, et al. Predicting poor ovarian response in IFV :use of repeat basal FSH measurement. J Reprod Med Obstet Gynaecol. 2004;49:187-94.
73. van Schanke A1, van de Wetering-Krebbers SF, Bos E, et al. Absorption, distribution, metabolism and excretion of corifollitropin alfa, a recombinant hormone with a sustained follicle stimulating activity. Pharmacology. 2010;85:77-87.

74. Polyzos NP, Devos M, Humaidan P, et al. Corifollitropin alfa followed by rFSH in a GnRH antagonist protocol for poor ovarian responder patients: an observational pilot study. Fertil Steril. 2013;99:422-6.
75. Polyzos NP, DeVos M, Corona R, et al. Addition of highly purified HMG after corifollitropin alfa in antagonist-treated poor ovarian responders, a pilot study. Hum Reprod. 2013;28:1254-60.
76. Mahmoud Youssef MA, Van Wely M, Aboulfoutouh I, et al. Is there a place for corifollitropin alfa in IVF/ICSI cycles? A systematic review and meta-analysis. Fertil Steril. 2012;97:876-85.
77. Reynolds KA, Omurtag KR, Jimenez PT, et al. Cycle cancellation and pregnancy after luteal estradiol priming in women and defined as poor responders: a systematic review and meta-analysis. Hum Reprod. 2013;28:2981-8.
78. Fanchin R, Salomon L, Castelo-Branco A, et al. Luteal estradiol pre-treatment coordinates follicular growth during controlled ovarian hyperstimulation with GnRH antagonists. Hum Reprod. 2003;18:2698-703.
79. Polyzos NP, Tournaye H. Poor Ovarian responders: to meta-analyse or not, that is the question. Hum Reprod. 2014;29:634-5.
80. Hill MJ, Levens ED, Levy G, et al. The use of recombinant luteinizing hormone in patients undergoing assisted reproductive techniques with advanced reproductive age: a systematic review and meta-analysis. Fertil Steril. 2012;97:1108,e1-1114,e1.
81. Bosdou JK, Venetis CA, Kolibinanakis EM, et al. The use of androgens or androgen-modulating agents in poor responders undergoing in-vitro fertilization: a systematic review and meta-analysis. Hum Reprod Update. 2012;18:127-45.
82. Fan W, Li S, Chen Q, et al. Recombinant Luteinizing Hormone supplementation in poor responders undergoing IVF: a systematic review and meta-analysis. Hum Reprod Update. 2013;29:278-84.
83. Lehert P, Kolibianakis EM, Venetis CA, et al. Recombinant human follicle-stimulating hormone (r-hFSH) plus recombinant luteinizing hormone versus r-hFSH alone for ovarian stimulation during assisted reproductive technology: Systematic review and meta-analysis. Reprod Biol Endocrinol. 2014;12:17.
84. Davoren JB, Kasson BG, Li CH, et al. Specific insulin-like growth factor (IGF) I- and II binding sites on rat granulose cells; relation to IGF action. Endocrinology. 1986;119:2155-62.
85. Hsu CJ, Hammond JM. Concomitant effects of growth hormone on secretion of insulin-like growth factor I and progesterone by cultured porcine granulose cells. Endocrinology. 1987;121:1343-8.
86. Barreca A, Artini PG, Del Monte P, et al. In vivo and in vitro effect of growth hormone on estradiol secretion by human granulose cells. J Clin Endocrinol Metab. 1993;77:61-7.
87. Adashi EY, Resnick CE, D'Ercole AJ, et al. Insulin-like growth factors as intra-ovarian regulators of granulose cell growth and function. Endocrine Rev. 1985;6:400-20.
88. Jia XC, Kalmijn J, Hsueh AJW. Growth hormone enhances follicle-stimulating hormone-induced differentiation of cultured rat granulosa cells. Endocrinology. 1986;118:1401-9.
89. Dor J1, Seidman DS, Amudai E, et al. Adjuvant growth hormone therapy in poor responders to in-vitro fertilization: a prospective randomized placebo-controlled double-blind study. Hum Reprod. 1995;10:40-3.
90. Eftekhar M, Aflatoonian A, Mohammadian F, et al. Adjuvant growth hormone therapy in antagonist protocol in poor responders undergoing assisted reproductive technology. Arch Gyanecol Obstet. 2013;287:1017-21.
91. Ryan KJ, Petro Z, Kaiser J. Steroid formation by isolated and recombined ovarian granulose and thecal cells. J Clin Endocrinol Metab. 1968;82:355-8.
92. Weil SJ, Vendola K, Zhou J, et al. Androgen receptor gene expression in the primate ovary: cellular localization, regulation, and functional correlations. J Clin Endocrinol Metab. 1998;83:2479-85.
93. Vendola KA, Zhou J, Adesanya SJ. et al. Androgens stimulate early stages of follicular growth in the primate ovary. J Clin Invest. 1998;101:2622-9.
94. Frattarelli JL, Peterson EH. Effect of androgen levels on in vitro fertilization cycles. Fertil Steril. 2004;81:1713-4.
95. Casson PR, Santoro N, Elkind-Hirsch K, et al. Postmenopausal dehydroepiandrosterone administration increases free insulin-like growth factor-I and decreases high-density lipoprotein: a six month trial. Fertil Steril. 1998;70:107-10.
96. Sunkara SK, Coomarasamy A. Androgen pretreatment in poor responders undergoing controlled ovarian stimulation and in vitro fertilization treatment. Fertil Steril. 2011;95:e73-e75.
97. Sunkara SK, Coomarasamy A, Arlt W, et al. Should androgen supplementation be used for poor ovarian response in IFV? Hum Reprod. 2012;27:637-40.
98. Weiner Z, Thaler I, Levron J, et al. Assessment of ovarian and uterine blood flow by transvaginal color Doppler in ovarian-stimulated women: correlation with the number of follicles and steroid hormone levels. Fertil Steril. 1993;59:743-9.
99. Bassil S, Wyns C, Toussaint-Demylle D, et al. The relationship between ovarian vascularity and the duration of stimulation in-vitro-fertilization. Hum Reprod. 1997;12:1240-5.
100. Pelicer A, Ballester MJ, Serrano MD, et al. Aetiological factors involved in the low response to gonadotrophins in infertile women with normal basal serum follicle stimulating hormone levels. Hum Reprod. 1994;9:806-11.
101. Battaglia C, Genazzani AD, Regnani G, et al. Perifollicular Doppler flow and follicular fluid vascular endothelial growth concentrations in poor respondents. Fertil Steril. 2000;74:809-12.
102. Rubinstein M, Marazzi A, Polak de Fried E. Low-dose aspirin treatment improves ovarian responsiveness, uterine and ovarian blood flow velocity, implantation, and pregnancy rates in patients undergoing in-vitro-fertilization: a prospective, randomized, double-blind placebo-controlled assay. Fertil Steril. 1999;71:825-9.
103. Nardo LF, Granne I, Stewart J. Medical adjuncts in IVF: evidence for clinical practice. Human Fertil. 2009;12:1-13.
104. Waldenstrom U, Hellberg D, Nilsson S. Low-dose aspirin in a short regimen as standard treatment in in-vitro-fertilization: a randomized, prospective study. Fertil Steril. 2004;81;1560-4.

105. Frattarelli JL, McWilliams GD, Hill MJ, et al. Low-dose aspirin use does not improve in-vitro-fertilization outcomes in poor responders. Fertil Steril. 2008;89:1113-7.
106. Urman B, Yakin K, Balaban B. Recurrent implantation failure in assisted reproduction: How to counsel and manage. B. Treatment options that have not been proven to benefit the couple. Reprod Biomed Online. 2005;11:382-91.
107. Hurst BS, Bhojwani JT, Marshburn PB, et al. Low-dose aspirin does not improve ovarian stimulation, endometrial response, or pregnancy rates for in-vitro-fertilization. J Experiment Clin Assist Reprod. 2005;2.
108. Revelli A, Dolfin E, Gennarelli G, et al. Low-dose acetylsalicylic acid plus prednisolone as an adjuvant treatment in IVF: a prospective, randomized study. Fertil Steril. 2008;90: 1685-91.
109. Gelbaya TA, Kyrgiou M, Li TC, et al. Low-dose aspirin for in-vitro-fertilization: a systematic review and meta-analysis. Hum Reprod Update. 2007;13:357-64.
110. Polyzos NP, Blockeel C, Verpoest W, et al. Live birth rates following natural cycle IVF in women with poor ovarian response according to the Bologna criteria. Hum Reprod. 2012;27:3481-6.
111. Ubaldi FM, Reinzi L, Baroni E, et al. Management of poor responders in IVF. Reprod Biomed Online. 2005;10:235-46.
112. Ubaldi FM, Reinzi L, Baroni E, et al. Hopes and facts about mild ovarian stimulation. Reprod Biomed Online. 2007;14:675-81.
113. Schimberni M, Morgia F, Colabianchi J, et al. Natural-cycle in-vitro fertilization in poor responder patients: a survey of 500 consecutive cycles. Fertil Steril. 2009;92:1297-301.
114. Ubaldi F, Anniballo R, Romano S, et al. Cumulative ongoing pregnancy rate achieved with oocyte vetrification and cleavage stage transfer without embryo selection in a standard infertility program. Hum Reprod. 2010;25:1199-205.
115. Practice Committees of American Society for Reproductive Medicine and Society for Assisted Reproductive Technology. Mature oocyte cryopreservation: a guideline. Fertil Steril. 2013;99:37-43.
116. Cobo A, Garrido N, Crespo J, et al. Accumulation of oocytes: a new strategy for managing low-responder patients. Reprod Biomed Online. 2012;24:424-32.
117. Noyes N, Porcu E, Borini A. Over 900 oocyte cryopreservation babies born with no apparent increase in congenital anomalies. Reprod Biomed Online. 2009;18:769-76.
118. Rienzi L, Cobo A, Paffoni A, et al. Consistent and predictable delivery rates after oocyte vitrification: an observational longitudinal cohort multicentric study. Hum Reprod. 2012;27:1606-12.

Endometrium and ART

35

Korsak Vladislav Stanislavovich, Samoylovich Yanina Andreevna

INTRODUCTION

A normal embryo can be implanted and a pregnancy can develop until full-term outside the uterus, for example, in the abdominal cavity. This is due to the ability of the tissues of mesenchymal origin for decidual transformation. This, however, does not change the physiological purpose of the uterus as a fetus receptacle and of the endometrium as the structure where an embryo should normally be implanted.

To date, it is a shared understanding that endometrial pathology is significant for the outcome of assisted reproductive technology (ART) programs.

CHRONIC INFLAMMATORY DISEASE OF THE UTERUS (CHRONIC ENDOMETRITIS)

Chronic endometritis (CE) is associated with a disorder of cyclic changes and receptivity of the endometrium. The diagnosis of CE is verified by detection of morphological and immunohistochemical signs of inflammation in the endometrium in the proliferative phase of the menstrual cycle.[1] The incidence of chronic endometritis in women with recurrent miscarriage ranges from 33–70%[1] and in patients with infertility it is 65.2%.[1] Chronic endometritis in women with tubal infertility is detected in 70% of cases.[2]

Complex etiopathogenetic therapy in patients with identified CE includes:

- *Stage I:* Elimination of the infectious agent from the endometrium (antibiotics and antiviral drugs).
- *Stage II:* Restoration of the endometrial morphofunctional potential, elimination of secondary damage, completion of regeneration, restoration of local hemodynamics and activity of the endometrial receptors (antioxidants/antihypoxants, nonsteroidal anti-inflammatory drugs, immunomodulators, fibrinolytics, physiotherapy, hormone therapy).

Stage I

Recommended regimens (no difference in efficacy between the recommended regimens has been demonstrated):

- *Outpatient regimens:*
  Intramuscular (IM) ceftriaxone 500 mg single dose followed by oral doxycycline 100 mg twice daily plus metronidazole 500 mg twice daily for 14 days (Evidence level Ia, A).
  - Oral ofloxacin 400 mg twice daily plus oral metronidazole 500 mg twice daily for 14 days (ofloxacin may be replaced by levofloxacin 500 mg once daily) (Evidence level Ib, A)
  - Oral moxifloxacin 400 mg once daily for 14 days (Evidence level Ia, A).
- *Inpatient regimens:*
  - Intravenous (IV)/IM ceftriaxone 1 g once daily plus IV doxycycline 100 mg twice daily (oral doxycycline may be used if tolerated) followed by oral doxycycline 100 mg twice daily plus oral metronidazole 500 mg twice daily to complete 14 days(Evidence level Ia, A).
  - IV clindamycin 900 mg three times daily plus IM/IV gentamicin (3–6 mg/kg as a single daily dose with renal monitoring) followed by either oral clindamycin 450 mg four times daily to complete 14 days or oral doxycycline 100 mg twice daily plus oral metronidazole 500 mg twice daily to complete 14 days (Evidence level Ia, A).

- Alternative regimens:
  The evidence for alternative regimens has been less robust than for the regimens above.
  - IV ofloxacin 400 mg twice daily plus IV metronidazole 500 mg three times daily for 14 days (Evidence level Ib, A).
  - IV ceftriaxone 500 mg single dose plus oral azithromycin 1 g single dose, followed by a second dose of oral azithromycin 1 g after one week (Evidence level Ib, A).

Where the above regimens are not available, antibiotic therapy should be given for 14 days and attempt to cover:

- *N. gonorrhoeae*, e.g. cephalosporins
- *C. trachomatis*, e.g. tetracyclines, macrolides
- Anaerobic bacteria, e.g. metronidazole.[3]

In women who are positive for *Mycoplasma genitalium*, treatment with moxifloxacin is recommended.[3]

For prevention of candidiasis, it is necessary to prescribe a systemic antifungal medication, fluconazole 150 mg twice during antibiotic therapy.[4]

Given the high incidence of pathogenic viruses in women suffering from miscarriage, antiviral drugs should be included in the complex therapy of pelvic inflammatory diseases.[5]

In order to reduce the recurrence of microbial biocenosis disturbances in patients with recurrent implantation failure (RIF) and CE, the vaginal microbiota must be restored by eubiotics administration.

Stage II

- Vitamins, antioxidants, hepatoprotectors, metabolic therapy and systemic enzyme therapy[6,7]
- Physiotherapy, which improves hemodynamics and microcirculation of the pelvic organs, stimulates functions of the receptors, accelerates the processes of endometrial regeneration, contributes to the destruction of fibrin overlays and enhances immune factors.[1]

"THIN" ENDOMETRIUM

Endometrial thickness is the distance between the echopositive boundaries at the junction of the endometrium and myometrium measured in the middle section by ultrasound.

The characteristics of "normal" and "thin" endometrium have not yet been determined. The endometrial thickness of 4–5 mm[8] does not exclude the possibility of pregnancy after embryo transfer, but the chances of pregnancy are significantly lower than with a higher value of this indicator. The maximum pregnancy rate for endometrial thickness >9 mm,[9] >10 mm,[10] or 9–14 mm[11] has been reported. To date, there is no common opinion in relation to endometrium being "too thick" (more than 14 mm).

The mechanism by which "thin" endometrium can affect implantation is unknown but it appears to be associated with a defect in endometrial vascularization.

Zhao et al.[12] showed that the structure of the endometrium can be considered as a prognostic parameter. In their study, in women with the three-layer endometrium, the pregnancy rate was significantly higher than in patients with isoechogenic or hyperechogenic endometrium (35.7% and 55.6% versus 31.9% and 50.2% versus 22.1% and 34.3% respectively).

Specific values of ultrasound markers predicting successful implantation have not been defined. However, when "thin" endometrium is detected during the ART cycle, physicians should inform patients about possible solutions to the problem. These include the cycle continuation after informing the patient of the potentially lower probability of pregnancy, the cycle discontinuation with embryo cryopreservation and subsequent transfer of embryos in cryocycles.[8]

Methods of the "thin endometrium" correction:

- High doses of estrogens in the cycle of ovarian stimulation or in a frozen embryo transfer cycle
- Drugs improving blood circulation and blood rheology in the cycle of ovarian stimulation or a frozen embryo transfer cycle
- Use of granulocyte colony-stimulating growth factor
- Autologous platelet-rich plasma infusion
- Endometrial scratching.

Estrogens

- Long or super long protocol of ovarian stimulation plus high doses of estrogens according to the scheme: 2 mg/day for transdermal application (4 mg of oral form) from day 7–8 of ovarian stimulation, ultrasound control of the endometrium on day 9 of ovarian stimulation, if necessary increasing the dose to 6 mg/day of the transdermal form (8 mg of the oral form) of the drug.
- The administration of high doses or a combination of transdermal forms and oral forms of estrogens do not increase the effectiveness of therapy but increases the risk of side effects[13]—level of evidence 1a.
- *Drugs improving blood circulation and blood rheology*—level of evidence 4.

- Pentoxifylline: 400 mg per day plus vitamin E 500 IU per day for 6 months,[14] 800 mg per day plus 1000 IU of vitamin E for 3 months[15]
- Sildenafil: During ovarian stimulation until the day of the trigger introduction, 25 mg 2–4 times a day vaginally,[16] 50 mg per day orally during the stimulation with gonadotropins or, in case of donor programs, with estrogen.[17]

- *Granulocyte colony-stimulating growth factor*—level of evidence 4.
  - 30 million IU per day of embryo transfer subcutaneously once.[18]
- *Autologous platelet-rich plasma infusion*—level of evidence 4.
  - Use in cryocycles on days 11–12 and 13–14 of the menstrual cycle; intrauterine administration of 0.5 mL.[19]
- *Endometrial scratching*—level of evidence 1.
  - An analysis of 5 randomized clinical trials, a single meta-analysis and a systematic review for 2014–2015 was performed; none of these studies reported any improvement in reproductive results in terms of live birth rate.[20]

ENDOMETRIAL POLYPS

Endometrial polyps (EPs) are benign overgrowths of the endometrium with a high incidence rate in women with unexplained infertility (15.6–32%),[21] endometriosis (36–46.7%)[22] and recurrent miscarriage (15–50%).[23]

Possible impacts of endometrial polyps on implantation:

- Large polyps are a mechanical obstacle to the "movement" of embryos[24]
- Implantation may be impaired due to the influence of immunological factors as a result of increased mast cell infiltration and inflammatory response[25]
- Increased expression of estrogen receptors and low expression of progesterone receptors are often observed against the background of polyps.[21] This can lead to impaired secretion of implantation markers,[26] insulin-like growth factor binding protein-1 (IGFBP-1) and osteopontin,[27] as well as the level of glycodelin, which inhibits the natural killer cell (NK) function[28]
- Increase of proliferative processes[29]
- Apoptosis is inhibited in the glandular epithelium of a polyp.[30]

Evidence of the effectiveness of polypectomy prior to an IVF cycle is insufficient and requires further research.[31] Many doctors in their daily practice consider hysteroscopic polypectomy before ART (without electrocoagulation) to be the best way to solve the problem.[32]

If an endometrial polyp is detected during an ART cycle, it is necessary to segment the IVF cycle with embryo cryopreservation, polypectomy and subsequent transfer of frozen embryos.[33]

INTRAUTERINE ADHESIONS

Asherman syndrome (AS) is a condition characterized by complete obliteration of the tubal ostia, uterine cavity and/or the cervical canal with adhesions. Intrauterine adhesions (IUAs) refer to a less severe disorder, in which endometrial walls are partially replaced with fibrotic tissue. The frequency of intrauterine adhesions according to different authors ranges from 0.3%–21.5%.

Although there are no studies analyzing how adhesions of uterine affect reproductive outcomes, they are believed to disturb endometrial receptiveness thereby impairing the implantation of the embryo and increasing the risk of miscarriage.[34]

The best way to prevent intrauterine synechia is to reduce the number of intrauterine interventions.

When intrauterine adhesions are detected in any form and any severity, first-line treatment should be hysteroscopic adhesiolysis using hysteroscopic scissors to avoid thermal damage to the endometrium associated with the use of electrical energy.[35]

The frequency of recurrence of Asherman syndrome after adhesiolysis remains high (3.1%–62.5%). Until now, methods used to rule out recurrences of intrauterine adhesions can only presumably prevent relapse. Surgical methods include insertion of an intrauterine device (IUD),[36] a Foley catheter balloon,[36] hyaluronic acid,[36] Hyalobarrier gel (Baxter, Pisa, Italy)[37] and polyethylene oxide-sodium carboxymethylcellulose gel.[38,39] Other preventive measures, such as antibiotics,[40] IUDs containing estrogens/cytokines[41] or stem cells[42] currently do not have sufficient evidence to allow them to be used in clinical practice.

CONCLUSION

The influence of each of the known endometrial pathologies on the effectiveness of ART cycles remains completely unclear. In addition, most of the published recommendations do not have a high level of evidence and effectiveness, which requires further well-organized research in this area.

REFERENCES

1. Suhih GT, Shurshalina AV. Hronicheskij endometrit [Chronic endometritis]. Moskva: «GJeOTAR-Media», 2010:P-72 (In Russian).
2. Korsak VC, Zabelkina OI, Isakova Je V. Issledovanie endometrija u pacientok s trubno-peritoneal'nym besplodiem na jetape podgotovki k JeKO [Study of the endometrium in patients with tuboperitoneal infertility at the stage of preparation for IVF]//Problemy reprodukcii. 2005;No 2:P.39 (In Russian).
3. Ross J, Guaschino S, Cusini M, et al. 2017 European guideline for the management of pelvic inflammatory disease. Int J of STD & AIDS. 2018,29(2):108-14.
4. Krasnopol'skij VI, Logutova LS, Zarochenceva NV. i dr. Pregravidarnaja podgotovka zhenshhin s nevynashivaniem beremennosti i hronicheskim jendometritom [Pregravid preparing of women with miscarriages and chronic endometritis.] Uchebnoe posobie. Moskva. 2014:P-32 (In Russian).
5. Ershov FI, Romancev MG. Lekarstvennye sredstva, primenjaemye pri virusnyh zabolevanijah: Rukovodstvo dlja vrachej [Medicines used for viral diseases: a guide for physicians] M.: GOJeTAR-Media. 2007:P. 363 (In Russian).
6. Sidorova IS, Makarov IO, Unanjan AL. Patogenez i patogeneticheski obosnovannaja terapija hronicheskogo jendometrita (klinicheskaja lekcija) [Pathogenesis and pathogenetic treatment of chronic endometritis (clinical lecture).]. Akusherstvo, ginekologija i reprodukcija. 2010;3:21-4 (In Russian).
7. Sidel'nikova VM, Suhih GT. Nevynashivanie beremennosti [Miscarriage]. Moskva: MIA. 2011:P. 300 (In Russian).
8. Check JH, Cohen R. Live fetus following embryo transfer in a woman with diminished egg reserve whose maximal endometrial thickness was less than 4 mm. Clin Exp Obstet Gynecol. 2011;38:330-2.
9. Richter K, Bugge K, Bromer J, et al. Relationship between endometrial thickness and embryo implantation, based on 1,294 cycles of in vitro fertilization with transfer of two blastocyst-stage embryos. Fertil Steril. 2007;87:53-9.
10. Rinaldi L, Lisi F, Floccari A, et al. Endometrial thickness as a predictor of pregnancy after in-vitro fertilization but not after intracytoplasmic sperm injection. Hum Reprod. 1996;11:1538-41.
11. Check JH, Dietterich C, Graziano V, et al. Effect of maximal endometrial thickness on outcome after frozen embryo transfer. Fertil Steril. 2004;81:1399-400.
12. Zhao J, Zhang Q, Li Y. The effect of endometrial thickness and pattern measured by ultrasonography on pregnancy outcomes during IVF-ET cycles. Reprod Biol Endocrinol. 2012;10:100.
13. Primenenie jestrogenov v programmah VRT. Nauchno-prakticheskie rekomendacii RARCh [The use of estrogen in ART programs. Scientific and practical recommendations RARCH]. 2015 (In Russian).
14. Lédée-Bataille N, Olivennes F, Lefaix J-L, et al. Combined treatment by pentoxifylline and tocopherol for recipient women with a thin endometrium enrolled in an oocyte donation programme. Human Reproduction. 2002;17(5):1249-53.
15. Turki F, Methni A, Balet R, et al. Effect of long term combined Pentoxifylline and Tocopherol administration on the endometrial proliferation: a prospective cohort study of 368 cases of thin endometrium. ESHRE Final Programme. 2015.
16. Sher G, Fisch JD. Effect of vaginal sildenafil on the outcome of in vitro fertilization (IVF) after multiple IVF failures attributed to poor endometrial development. Fertil Steril. 2002;78(5):1073-6.
17. Aisaka K, Ikezuki Y, Uemura H, et al. The Nevada Center for Reproductive Medicine, Reno, NV. 2005;84(1), S246 Abstracts.
18. Obidnjak DM, Gzgzjan AM, Niauri DA. Vlijanie granulocitarnogo koloniestimulirujushhego faktora rosta na jeffektivnost' programm VRT. Materialy konferencii RARCh [The effect of granulocyte colony-stimulating growth factor on the effectiveness of ART programs. Materials from the RAHR conference]. 2016 (In Russian).
19. Zadehmodarres S, Salehpour S, Saharkhiz N, et al. Treatment of thin endometrium with autologous platelet-rich plasma: a pilot study. JBRA Assist Reprod. 2017;1;21(1):54-6.
20. Santamaria X, Katzorke N, Simón C. Endometrial 'scratching': what the data show. Curr Opin Obstet Gynecol. 2016;28(4):242-9.
21. Hatasaka H. Clinical management of the uterine factor in infertility. Clin Obstet Gynecol. 2011;54:696-709.
22. Shen L, Wang Q, Huang W, et al. High prevalence of endometrial polyps in endometriosis-associated infertility. Fertil Steril. 2011;95(8):2722-4.
23. Varasteh NN, Neuwirth RS, Levin B, et al. Pregnancy rates after hysteroscopic polypectomy and myomectomy in infertile women. Obstet Gynecol. 1999;94(2):168-71.
24. Bosteels J, Weyers S, Puttemans P, et al. The effectiveness of hysteroscopy in improving pregnancy rates in subfertile women without other gynaecological symptoms: a systematic review. Hum Reprod Update. 2010;16(1):1-11.
25. El-Hamarneh T, Hey-Cunningham AJ, Berbic M, et al. Cellular immune environment in endometrial polyps. Fertil Steril. 2013;100(5):1364-72.
26. Rackow BW, Jorgensen E, Taylor HS. Endometrial polyps affect uterine receptivity. Fertil Steril. 2011;95(8):2690-2.
27. Ben-Nagi J, Miell J, Yazbek J, et al. The effect of hysteroscopic polypectomy on the concentrations of endometrial implantation factors in uterine flushings. Reprod Biomed Online. 2009;19(5):737-44.
28. Richlin S, Ramachandran S, Shanti A, et al. Glycodelin levels in uterine flushings and in plasma of patients with leiomyomas and polyps: implications and implantation. Hum Reprod. 2002;17:2742-7.
29. Vanni R, Dal Cin P, Marras S, et al. Endometrial polyp: Another benign tumor characterized by 12q13-q15 changes. Cancer Genet Cytogenet. 1993;68(1):32-3.
30. Taylor L, Jackson T, Reid J, et al. The differential expression of oestrogen receptors, progesterone receptors, Bcl-2 and Ki67 in endometrial polyps. BJOG. 2003;110(9):794-8.
31. Bosteels J, Kasius J, Weyers S, et al. Treating suspected uterine cavity abnormalities by hysteroscopy to improve reproductive

outcome in women with unexplained infertility or prior to IUI, IVF, or ICSI. Gynecol Surg. 2013;10(3):165-7.
32. Pellicano M, Guida M, Zullo F, et al. Carbon dioxide versus normal saline as a uterine distension medium for diagnostic vaginoscopic hysteroscopy in infertile patients: a prospective, randomised, multicenter study. Fertil Steril. 2003;79(2):418-21.
33. Galliano D, Bellver J, Díaz-García C. ART and uterine pathology: how relevant is the maternal side for implantation? Hum Reprod Update. 2015;21(1):13-38.
34. Schenker J.G. Etiology of and therapeutic approach to synechia uteri. Eur J Obstet Gynecol. Reprod Biol. 1996; 65: 109–113.
35. Roge P, Cravello L, D'Ercole C, et al. Intrauterine adhesions and fertility: results of hysteroscopic treatment. Gynaecol Endosc. 1997;6:225-8.
36. Lin X, Wei M, Li TC, et al. A comparison of intrauterine balloon, intrauterine contraceptive device and hyaluronic acid gel in the prevention of adhesion reformation following hysteroscopic surgery for Asherman syndrome: a cohort study. Eur J Obstet Gynecol Reprod Biol. 2013;170(2): 512-6.
37. Pabuccu R, Atay V, Orhon E, et al. Hysteroscopic treatment of intrauterine adhesions is safe and effective in the restoration of normal menstruation and fertility. Fertil Steril. 1997;68(6):1141-3.
38. Di Spiezio Sardo A, Spinelli M, Bramante S, et al. Efficacy of a polyethylene oxide-sodium carboxymethylcellulose gel in prevention of intrauterine adhesions after hysteroscopic surgery. J Minim Invasive Gynecol. 2011;18(4):462-9.
39. Fuchs N, Smorgick N, Ben Ami I, et al. Intercoat (Oxiplex/AP gel) for preventing intrauterine adhesions after operative hysteroscopy for suspected retained products of conception: double-blind, prospective, randomized pilot study. J Minim Invasive Gynecol. 2014;21(1):126-30.
40. Knopman J, Copperman AB. Value of 3D ultrasound in the management of suspected Asherman's syndrome. J Reprod Med. 2007;52(11):1016-22.
41. Tu CH, Yang XL, Qin XY, et al. Management of intrauterine adhesions: a novel intrauterine device. Med Hypotheses. 2013;81:394-6.
42. Cervello I, Mas A, Gil-Sanchis C, et al. Somatic stem cells in the human endometrium. Semin Reprod Med. 2013;31(1):69-76.

Thin Endometrium

36

Sathy M Pillai, KK Gopinath, Fessy Louis, KU Kunjumoideen

INTRODUCTION

The concept of the window of implantation (WOI) and endometrial receptivity is still a gray area due to the lack of knowledge regarding its role in infertility and implantation failure. In the ancient times, one of the first detailed descriptions of infertility treatment was given by Hippocrates (460-377 BC).[1] Later in the 20th century, Huhner described postcoital test and Aschheim-Zondek introduced pregnancy test for the diagnosis of infertility. Noyes in 1950 introduced endometrial histology as a diagnostic test for the evaluation of the endometrial factors which introduced endometrial dating in natural cycles. Later, Hertig and Rock in 1956, first suggested that WOI and endometrial receptivity played important roles in embryo implantation and pregnancy.[2,3]

PHYSIOLOGY OF ENDOMETRIUM

Human endometrium is controlled by hormones. It undergoes cyclic morphological and functional changes due to the hormones secreted by the hypothalamic-pituitary-ovarian (HPO) axis. These hormones prepare the endometrium to be receptive to the embryo and this occurs in the mid-secretory phase. This is known as the WOI or fertile window. WOI is personalized. It lasts from 12 hours to 2 days. In about 30% women, it is displaced, ranging from P+4 days to P+7 days (P—progesterone), in a hormone replacement therapy (HRT) cycle.[4]

BIOMARKERS OF ENDOMETRIAL RECEPTIVITY

The best biomarker is a blastocyst implantation and pregnancy.[5] Earlier, the appearance of ectoplasmic projections called pinopodes was thought to be important in establishing a diagnosis of a receptive endometrium.[6] Recently this has been disputed.[7,8] Human endometrium is composed of epithelial, stromal, vascular and immune cell compartments. The endometrial epithelium is the first structure which interacts with the embryo. Decidual reaction is a pregnancy-independent process. It occurs soon after closure of the WOI. The decidualization process initiates during the mid-secretory phase of the menstrual cycle due to elevated levels of estrogen and progesterone, independent of the presence of an implanting blastocyst.[9] It is necessary for the trophoblast invasion and placental formation. Decidual reaction is characterized by modification of the fibroblast endometrial stromal cells, into larger and rounder decidual cells. Along with this, secretory glands also develop and grow.

Embryoendometrial dialog is also mediated by secretion of molecules such as prolactin, Insulin-like growth factor-binding protein-1 (IGFBP-1) and extracellular materials such as laminin, type 4 collagen, fibronectin, heparin sulfate and proteoglycan. Biomarkers of endometrial receptivity are adhesion molecules (integrins, cadherins, adherens, selectins, immunoglobulins, mucins, cytokines), leukemia inhibitory factor (LIF), interleukins (IL-6, IL-11) and growth factors [vascular endothelial growth factor (VEGF), colony-stimulating factor (CSF), transforming growth factor-β (TGF-β) and prostaglandins]. There are many more which have not been identified. Endometrial immune cells also play an important role in preimplantation. They are uterine natural killer (uNK) cells, macrophages, dendritic and T cells.[10]

Proinflammatory T helper cell-1 (TH-1) and cytokines [LIF, IL-6, IL-8, tumor necrosis factor-α (TNF-α)] are present in the early stages of implantation.[11] Of these, uNK cells are found in plenty in the endometrium during WOI. But their exact role in implantation is still not clear.[12] uNK cells regulate invasion of the cytotrophoblast and have been found to infiltrate the endometrium and accumulate around the spiral arterioles and the decidualized stroma from luteinizing hormone (LH) + 3 days. Deregulations of these cells are found in unexplained infertility, recurrent pregnancy loss (RPL) and endometriosis. However, prognostic value of measuring uNK cells or peripheral NK cells parameters remains uncertain.

CAUSES OF DEFECTIVE ENDOMETRIAL RECEPTIVITY

- Endometrial polyps
- Fibroids
- Endometriosis
- Thin endometrium
- Endometrial atrophy
- Hydrosalpinx.

THIN ENDOMETRIUM

Incidence of thin endometrium varies according to the chosen cutoff. Bu et al. found the incidence of thin endometrium less than 7 mm, to be 1.49% in high responders and 2.5% in poor responders.

Causes

- Inflammatory
- Iatrogenic
- Idiopathic
- Hyperandrogenic state
- Older women (5% in <40 years and 25% in >40 years). This is probably due to the decreased endometrial vascularity.
- Controlled ovarian hyperstimulation (COH).

Inflammatory Causes

Infections, acute and chronic pelvic inflammatory disease (PID), will destroy the basal layer of the endometrium. The most common cause in India is Koch's disease. Fibrosis which occurs due to the healing will destroy the basal layer of the endometrium. So, the endometrium cannot regenerate during the menstrual cycle even under the effect of estrogen. This happens even after completion of the treatment of endometritis. This fibrosis also leads to the narrowing of the uterine cavity.

Idiopathic Causes

This may be due to the uterine architecture or due to the intrinsic property of the endometrium which will affect its growth. Stress and malposition of the uterus can impede the uterine blood flow and cause thin endometrium.[13]

Iatrogenic Causes

- Previous trauma of the uterus like cesarean section or repeated vigorous curettage will damage the basal layer of the endometrium.
- Removal of intracavitary polyps or myomas either through hysteroscopy or laparoscopy will destroy the endometrial lining leading to thin endometrium and intrauterine adhesions (Asherman's syndrome).
- Drugs like clomiphene (repeated use) can result in the development of thin endometrium due to its antiestrogenic effects.
- Controlled ovarian hyperstimulation and ovulation inductions.
- Antitumoral treatments like radical surgery, chemotherapy and radiotherapy can permanently affect both present and future reproductive function.[14] Patients are asymptomatic with a low radiotherapy dose (20 Gy),[15] while a prepubescent uterus or a very small uterus with an atrophic endometrium may be the result when exposed to higher doses (40 Gy).[16]

Hyperandrogenic State

Endometrium in women with polycystic ovary syndrome (PCOS) has an inverse relationship with the serum and total testosterone and a positive correlation with body mass index (BMI).

Controlled Ovarian Hyperstimulation

Controlled ovarian hyperstimulation has adverse effect on endometrial receptivity. So, freezing of embryos and transfer of frozen embryos in an HRT cycle is advocated. In HRT cycles, an endometrial thickness of 9–14 mm on the day of progesterone supplementation was associated with a higher pregnancy rate and implantation rate.[17]

In another study, pregnancy rate in patients with endometrial thickness less than 6 mm was low.[18] Three pregnancies occurred out of 35 embryo transfers (8.5%) and only two delivered (5.7%).

In another study,[19] which compared pregnancy rate, live birth rate (LBR) and implantation rate between fresh and frozen embryo transfers in an endometrium of less than 6 mm, the authors found implantation rate and LBR at 4–5 mm endometrium in fresh versus frozen embryo transfers were 10.6% versus 27.2% and 10% versus 36%, respectively. This study implies that HRT replacement can overcome the negative effect of COH in women with thin endometrium.

Why Thin Endometrium Affects Implantation?

In thin endometrium there is:

- Poor growth of glandular epithelium
- Decreased VEGF expression
- Poor vascular development
- High vascular impedance in blood flow in the radial arteries
- This again impairs growth of the glandular epithelium resulting in decreased VEGF levels in the endometrium.

This vicious cycle causes poor vascular development there by decreasing blood flow to the endometrium.

How is Endometrial Thickness Measured?

Endometrial thickness is measured by transvaginal sonography (TVS), as the maximal distance between the echogenic interfaces of the myometrium and endometrium, in the sagittal plane of the uterus. An endometrial thickness of more than 7 mm was found on the day of oocyte retrieval in women who conceived during that cycle.

A triple-line pattern of the endometrium on the day of trigger is called Grade-A endometrium (receptive endometrium), while a homogeneous appearance or nonmultilayered endometrium is called Grade-C endometrium. This is a nonreceptive endometrium. Progesterone causes changes in the endometrium, making it appear as homogeneous near the junctional zone and a well-defined central echogenic line. This pattern is called Grade-B endometrium.

What is Thin Endometrium?

A thin endometrium is an endometrial thickness of less than 7 mm on ultrasound.[20,21] But a range between 6 mm and 8 mm may be accepted.[22,23] A thin endometrium is associated with poor in vitro fertilization (IVF) success rates irrespective of the cause. But pregnancies have been reported with endometrial thickness of 4 mm and 5 mm.[24] This suggests that endometrial receptivity may not be related to endometrial thickness. Thin endometrium is usually seen in older women, probably because of the poor vascularity.

Three groups of women were studied, women with:

1. Endometrial thickness ≥4–5 mm
2. Endometrial thickness ≥5–6 mm
3. Endometrial thickness ≥6–7 mm.

Implantation rate and pregnancy rate did not show any difference between the three groups. Next this group was compared to 5,573 women who had embryo transfers and had an endometrium greater than or equal to 7 mm.

Clinical pregnancy rate (CPR) was 51% in the second group and 26% in the thin endometrium group, whereas miscarriage rate was 31% in the thin endometrium group and 17% in women with greater than or equal to 7 mm.[19]

Clinical pregnancy rate, implantation rate and LBR between the three groups of women with endometrium less than 7 mm were compared according to age, number of oocytes recovered and embryos transferred. Better results were obtained in women less than 35 years or if the number of retrieved oocytes were more than 5 or if the number of embryos transferred were 3 or more. So, the authors suggested that the embryos should be frozen if endometrial thickness at the time of OR is less than 7, unless the patient has more than 5 eggs and number of embryos available for transfer is 3 or more. This study shows that endometrial thickness is not the only determinant of a positive pregnancy after embryo transfer.

In another study,[25] the authors gave a contradictory opinion. They suggested that endometrial thickness cannot be used as a parameter to decide on cycle cancellation and freezing of all embryos. However, these women had a lower probability for CPR (23.3% vs 48.1%). The positive predictive value for the outcome of a clinical pregnancy was 77% and negative predictive value was 48%.

In some studies, endometrial thickness on the day before embryo transfer was nearly 2 mm thicker in women who conceived (10.2 mm) than in those who did not (8.6 mm).[26] Only two pregnancies were reported when endometrial thickness was less than 7.5 mm and no pregnancy was seen when endometrial thickness on day of embryo transfer was less than 5 mm.[26] According to another similar study, no difference was observed in endometrial thickness among women who conceived compared to those who did not.[27] However, when endometrial thickness was greater than 9 mm with a triple-line appearance, a favorable pregnancy outcome was observed.[28] In another retrospective study, pregnancy rate was significantly higher in women who had a triple-line pattern of the endometrium.[29] Such contradictory results show that ultrasonography (USG) using biophysical measures is not sensitive enough to predict endometrial receptivity. The exception is a strong negative correlation between thin endometrium and implantation rate.[30]

In oocyte donation cycles, Dain et al.[31] found no statistically significant difference in CPR (29.6% vs 30%) and LBR (16.7% vs 23.6%) in women with endometrium less than 6 mm compared with women with endometrium greater than 6 mm. However, more live births were found in the group with thicker endometrium. This may be due to the inability of the thin endometrium to sustain a pregnancy after implantation, which results in more abortions.

In the group of patients with endometrial thickness less than 6 mm, only few patients had Grade-A endometrial pattern, while more women had Grade-C endometrial pattern. A completely homogeneous endometrial pattern at trigger correlated with poor implantation rate.[22] Currently, there are no evidence-based data showing the positive predictive value of endometrial thickness on pregnancy rate after embryo transfer.[32] The only statistically significant evidence is that pregnancy is very unlikely when endometrial thickness is below 7 mm.

In 5% of cases taken up for IVF, fluid collection in the uterine cavity is noted during stimulation. In 2%, the fluid persists at the time of embryo transfer. Implantation rate and pregnancy rate in such women are markedly low.

Color Flow Doppler Ultrasonography

When pulsatility index (PI) of the uterine arteries were measured there were no pregnancies in women with high PI value.[33] Such high values indicate impedance to vascular flow in the uterine artery and is associated with a significantly low pregnancy rate.[34] Uterine artery resistance index (RI) measurement is not useful for predicting probability of pregnancy.[35] PI of greater than 3.3 and RI of greater than 0.95 before embryo transfer was associated with poor conception rate.[36] When color flow mapping is done, absence of detectable subendometrial blood flow is associated with failure of implantation.

When power flow Doppler USG was done, on women whose endometrial thickness was greater than or equal to 10 mm, and when the intraendometrial blood flow calculation indicated a vascular flow of less than 5 mm,[2] the pregnancy rate was low. Spiral arterial flow and uterine artery flow were not different between pregnancies and nonpregnant women. But if the spiral arterial flow was absent, no pregnancy occurred.[37] Also, an increased endometrial perfusion seen with three-dimensional (3D) USG indicated a more favorable endometrium.[38]

Three-dimensional Imaging of the Endometrium

Endometrial receptivity and probability of achieving implantation can now be predicted using 3D USG. Implantation rate and pregnancy rate were significantly low when the endometrial volume was less than 2 mL and no pregnancy occurred when the volume was less than 1 mL. But a contemporary study found no relationship between 3D volume of the endometrium and conception.[39] There was also no correlation between estradiol (E2) levels, endometrial thickness and endometrial volume indicating that endometrial volume would not predict conception. But endometrial perfusion measured by 3D power flow Doppler had some predictive value.[40] Spiral artery blood flow measurement in 3D had positive predictive value when performed on the first day of ovarian stimulation. Women who became pregnant had lower RI and higher 3D flow index than those who did not.[37]

TREATMENT OPTIONS

There are various treatment options to improve the endometrial thickness in women with thin endometrium **(Fig. 1)**.

- Extended use of exogenous estrogens[41]
- Aspirin[42]
- L-arginine[43]
- Tocopherol with pentoxifylline[43]
- Vaginal sildenafil citrate[44]
- Electroacupuncture[45]

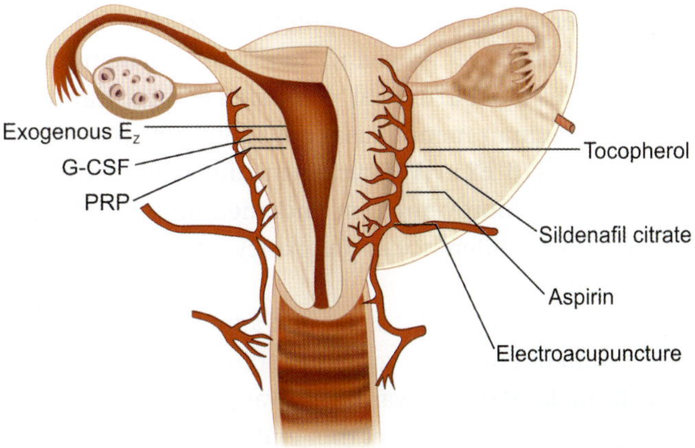

Fig. 1: Various treatment options to improve the endometrial thickness in women.

- Application of granulocyte colony-stimulating factor (G-CSF)[46]
- Using autologous platelet-rich plasma (PRP).[47]

Exogenous Estrogens

Frozen-thawed embryos or donor embryos may be transferred into the uterus in a natural cycle, hormone replacement cycle or stimulated cycle. Of this, hormone replacement cycle with exogenous E2 administration is recommended for older women, women without ovaries and women with regular irregular menstrual cycles. E2 is administered for 10–12 days in the standard regimen. In extended use, administration is given at a higher dose for a longer period. Vaginal administration of micronized E2 significantly increases serum E2 levels and endometrial E2 concentration.[48]

In a study by Chen et al., estrogen therapy was started on day 3 of the cycle and administration ranged from 14 days to 82 days. Mean endometrial thickness increased from 6.7 mm to 8.6 mm, with a pregnancy rate which also increased significantly (38.5% vs 4.3%).[41]

Tourgeman et al.[49] showed that extended use of vaginal E2 could achieve adequate endometrial lining. Fanchin et al.[50] showed that vaginal E2 administration improved endometrial thickness and uterine blood flow by acting on systemic and local level. Here the hormone concentration in higher when estrogens are administered by the vaginal route.

The presence of a healthy endometrium is necessary for this therapy. It will not act in women who have endometrial damage. Endometrial receptivity to estrogen requires stromal epithelial interaction together with adequate paracrine growth factor production.[51]

Poor endometrial development is thought to be the reason behind lower pregnancy rate in in vitro maturation (IVM) cycles too. Elizur et al. compared administration of low-dose human menopausal gonadotropin (hMG) and micronized 17β-E2 in IVM cycles with thin endometrium.[52] A significant improvement in endometrial thickness was noted with no difference in pregnancy rate between users of either drug.

Papanikolaou et al.[53] suggested administration of 150 IU of human chorionic gonadotropin (hCG) daily for 7 days from day 8 or 9 onward. This was given along with E2 in 17 patients with resistant thin endometrium. The mean endometrial thickness increased from 5.18 mm to 6.01 mm in 12 out of 17 patients. Seven out of these patients conceived. In five patients whose endometrium had not improved with hCG, two pregnancies occurred.

Aspirin

Aspirin has an antithrombotic and vasodilatory effect and improves uterine and ovarian vascularization.[54] But its effect on improving endometrial thickness is still controversial.[55] Aspirin improves the PI of the uterine artery, but considering the controversial results, it has been concluded that the outcome of IVF does not depend significantly on the PI of the uterine artery, and the blood flow enhancement due to aspirin does not improve the endometrial pattern.[42]

L-Arginine

Takasaki et al., in a study, gave L-arginine 6 g/day for women with thin endometrium and found that the RI of the uterine radial artery improved in eight out of nine patients and endometrial thickness also improved in six patients.[43] Nitric oxide (NO) is synthesized from L-arginine, which in turn causes relaxation of smooth muscles, by elevating cyclic guanosine monophosphate (cGMP) levels. L-arginine also has a direct effect on the uterine luminal epithelium causing proliferation of the endometrium, thus providing an adequate environment for embryo adhesion and implantation.

Tocopherol with Pentoxifylline

Tocopherol (vitamin E) has antioxidant properties and hence, is used to favor endometrial growth. Thin endometrium is the result of high blood flow impedance of the uterine radial arteries causing a decrease in VEGF expression. Low VEGF levels can cause poor vascular development decreasing the blood flow in the endometrium and compromising glandular epithelial proliferation. Tocopherol acts by preventing lipids hydrolysis of the red blood cell (RBC) membrane. This results in improved development of blood vessels and consequent growth of glandular parenchyma.[56] Takasaki et al.[43] showed that vitamin E improves uterine vascularization and endometrial thickness by increasing VEGF expression.

Cicek et al. showed that though there is an increase in endometrial thickness, there was no significant difference in implantation rate or pregnancy rate.[57]

Pentoxifylline, a methyl xanthine derivative, has not only vasodilating, antiaggregant and anticoagulant properties, but also anti-inflammatory and antifibrotic actions. It also antagonizes TNF-α production.

In a study by Lédée-Bataille et al.,[48] patients who were treated with a combination of 400 mg pentoxifylline and 500 IU vitamin E twice a day for 6 months showed significant improvement in endometrial thickness.

Higher TNF-α expression has been associated with implantation failure because of an inflammation like reaction.[58] So, pentoxifylline + vitamin E administration may be adequate in some cases of implantation failure but not in all cases of thin endometrium.[59]

Sildenafil

Sildenafil citrate acts by causing vasodilatation (relaxation of vascular smooth muscles through a cGMP mediated pathway). Vascular endothelium and the human endometrium and myometrium have inducible NO synthase isoforms. Sildenafil augments the vasodilatory effects of NO on vascular smooth muscle by preventing the degradation of cGMP. It also improves endometrial arterial blood flow. However, Check et al. found no significant difference in endometrial thickness in patients treated with vaginal sildenafil citrate.[60]

Electroacupuncture

Endometrial receptivity can be measured by measuring the PI of the uterine artery. If the PI value is more than or equal to 3 at the time of embryo transfer the pregnancy rate will be low.[32] Stener-Victorin et al.[61] found a reduction in the PI of uterine arteries following electroacupuncture in 10 infertile women with PI more than or equal to 3. But no significant difference in pregnancy rate and endometrial thickness has been found.[45]

Granulocyte Colony-stimulating Factor

Granulocyte colony-stimulating factor is a glycoprotein that carries out both cytokine and growth factor activities. Intrauterine instillation of G-CSF produced successful thickening of the endometrium, in patients previously resistant to other therapies.[46] However, some studies failed to show an improvement in pregnancy rate and implantation rate.[62]

Platelet-rich Plasma

Autologous PRP increased proliferation of not only cultured fibroblasts, but also of mesenchymal cells which are progenitors of different types of cells including endometrial cells. So, it is hypothesized that PRP stimulates cellular processes involved in endometrial regeneration.[63] Chang et al. reported for the first time[47] an improvement in the endometrial thickness after intrauterine instillation of autologous PRP. Pregnancy also occurred in all these patients. Another study[64] showed that PRP is effective in improving pregnancy outcome in recurrent implantation failure **(Fig. 2)**.

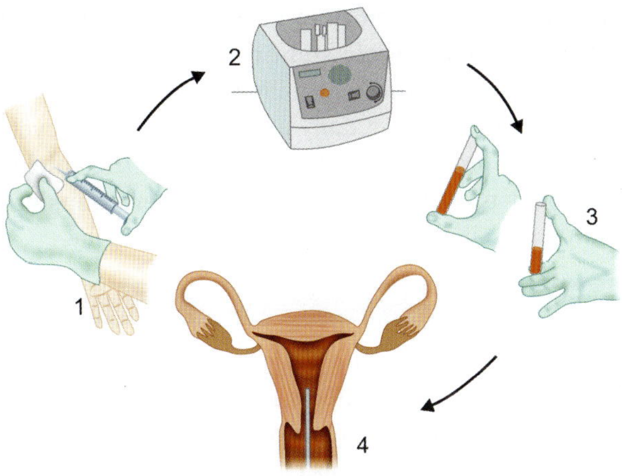

Fig. 2: Platelet-rich plasma treatment.

Relative contraindications for PRP instillation are:

- Platelet count less than 100,000/mm^3
- Hemoglobin less than 10 g/dL
- Presence of a blood tumor or metastatic disease or infection.

Platelet-rich plasma is introduced into the uterine cavity with a Tomcat catheter (0.5–1 mL). If necessary PRP infusion can be performed one to two times more, the last infusion being 48 hours before embryo transfer. Endometrial thickness can be reassessed 48–72 hours after the instillation.

Stem Cell Therapy

Endometrial stem or progenitor cells are found in the basalis and functionalis layers of the human endometrium.[65] Cervelló et al.[66] found out that human endometrial adult stem cells are able to generate human endometrium after transplantation in nonobese diabetic-severe combined immunodeficiency (NOD-SCID) mice renal capsules. Even hematopoietic and nonhematopoietic bone marrow-derived stem cells are recruited to the endometrium in response to the injury.[67] In 2011, in a case of thin endometrium (3.6 mm) secondary to Asherman's syndrome and which was refractory to E2 treatment, autologous endometrial angiogenic stem cells were infused into the uterine cavity. This was followed by high dose of E2 valerate, aspirin 75 mg daily and four cycles of cyclical estrogen and progesterone therapy. Endometrial thickness reached 7.1 mm. Three donor oocytes were transferred, resulting in a single viable intrauterine pregnancy.

CONCLUSION

The coexistence of a thin endometrium with absence of triple-line pattern reflects diminished endometrial responsiveness to ovarian hormones and also a diminished endometrial receptivity. This can lead to a low pregnancy rate. In such cases, cycle cancellation and frozen embryo transfer is recommended. However, endometrial thickness has a limited capacity to identify women with poor chances of conception after IVF. The cutoff of 7 mm is only related to a lower chance of pregnancy. Increasing the dose of E2 valerate, vaginal sildenafil and intrauterine G-CSF infusion is a treatment option. Tocopherol with/without pentoxifylline, aspirin and acupuncture can also be considered. Results obtained with autologous PRP are encouraging and it is now a new therapy for treatment of patients with thin endometrium.

REFERENCES

1. King H. Hippocrates' Women: Reading the Female Body in Ancient Greece. London and New York: Routledge; 1998. xvi; pp. 322.
2. Noyes RW, Hertig AT, Rock J. Dating of endometrial biopsy. Fertil Steril. 1950;1:3-7.
3. Hertig AT, Rock J, Adams EC. A description of 34 human ova within the first 17 days of development. Am J Anat. 1956;98(3):435-93.
4. Ruiz-Alonso M, Galindo N, Pellicer A, et al. What a difference two days make: "personalized" embryo transfer (pET) paradigm: a case report and pilot study. Hum Reprod. 2014;29(6):1244-7.
5. Klentzeris LD. The role of endometrium in implantation. Hum Reprod. 1997;12(11 Suppl):170-5.
6. Murphy CR. Understanding the apical surface markers of uterine receptivity: pinopodes or uterodomes? Hum Reprod. 2000;15(12):2451-4.
7. Lessey BA. Assessment of endometrial receptivity. Fertil Steril. 2011;96(3):522-9.
8. Quinn CE, Casper RF. Pinopodes: a questionable role in endometrial receptivity. Hum Reprod Update. 2009;15(2): 229-36.
9. Vinketova K, Mourdjeva M, Oreshkova T. Human decidual stromal cells as a component of the implantation niche and a modulator of maternal immunity. J Pregnancy. 2016; 2016:8689436.
10. Dekel N, Gnainsky Y, Granot I, et al. The role of inflammation for a successful implantation. Am J Reprod Immunol. 2014;72(2):141-7.
11. Van Sinderen M, Menkhorst E, Winship A, et al. Pre-implantation human blastocyst-endometrial interactions: the role of inflammatory mediators. Am J Reprod Immunol. 2013;69(5):427-40.
12. Moffett-King A, Entrican G, Ellis S, et al. Natural killer cells and reproduction. Trends Immunol. 2002;23(7):332-3.
13. Mahajan N, Sharma S. The endometrium in assisted reproductive technology: how thin is thin? J Hum Reprod Sci. 2016;9(1):3-8.
14. Madsen BL, Giudice L, Donaldson SS. Radiation-induced premature menopause: a misconception. Int J Radiat Oncol Biol Phys. 1995;32(5):1461-4.
15. Critchley HO. Factors of importance for implantation and problems after treatment for childhood cancer. Med Pediatr Oncol. 1999;33(1):9-14.
16. Fajardo L. Female reproductive organs. In: Fajardo L (Ed). Pathology of Radiation Injury. New York: Masson; 1982. pp. 108-28.
17. El-Toukhy T, Coomarasamy A, Khairy M, et al. The relationship between endometrial thickness and outcome of medicated frozen embryo replacement cycles. Fertil Steril. 2008;89:832-9.
18. Dix E, Check JH. Successful pregnancies following embryo transfer despite very thin late proliferative endometrium. Clin Exp Obstet Gynecol. 2010;37:15-6.
19. Check JH, Cohen R, Wilson C, et al. Very thin endometria in the late proliferative phase is more associated with poor pregnancy rates following controlled ovarian hyperstimulation than graduated estradiol regimens used for frozen embryo transfer. Fertil Steril. 2014;101:e21.
20. Kumbak B, Erden HF, Tosun S, et al. Outcome of assisted reproduction treatment in patients with endometrial thickness less than 7 mm. Reprod Biomed Online. 2009;18:79-84.
21. Richter KS, Bugge KR, Bromer JG, et al. Relationship between endometrial thickness and embryo implantation, based on 1,294 cycles of in vitro fertilization with transfer of two blastocyst-stage embryos. Fertil Steril. 2007;87:53-9.
22. Coulam CB, Bustillo M, Soenksen DM, et al. Ultrasonographic predictors of implantation after assisted reproduction. Fertil Steril. 1994;62:1004-10.
23. Gingold JA, Lee JA, Rodriguez-Purata J, et al. Endometrial pattern, but not endometrial thickness, affects implantation rates in euploid embryo transfers. Fertil Steril. 2015;104:620-8.e5.
24. Check JH, Dietterich C, Check ML, et al. Successful delivery despite conception with a maximal endometrial thickness of 4 mm. Clin Exp Obstet Gynecol. 2003;30:93-4.
25. Kasius A, Smit JG, Torrance HL, et al. Endometrial thickness and pregnancy rates after IVF: a systematic review and meta-analysis. Hum Reprod Update. 2014;20:530-41.
26. Evans GE, Phillipson GT, Sin IL, et al. Gene expression confirms a potentially receptive endometrium identified by histology in fertile women. Hum Reprod. 2012;27(9):2747-55.

27. Gregory PA, Bert AG, Paterson EL, et al. The miR-200 family and miR-205 regulate epithelial to mesenchymal transition by targeting ZEB1 and SIP. Nat Cell Biol. 2008;10(5):593-601.
28. Domínguez F, Avila S, Cervero A, et al. A combined approach for gene discovery identifies insulin-like growth factor-binding protein-related protein 1 as a new gene implicated in human endometrial receptivity. J Clin Endocrinol Metab. 2003;88(4):1849-57.
29. Altmäe S, Martinez-Conejero JA, Esteban FJ, et al. MicroRNAs miR-30b, miR-30d, and miR-494 regulate human endometrial receptivity. Reprod Sci. 2013;20(3):308-17.
30. Creighton CJ, Benham AL, Zhu H, et al. Discovery of novel microRNAs in female reproductive tract using next generation sequencing. PLoS One. 2010;5(3):e9637.
31. Dain L, Bider D, Levron J, et al. Thin endometrium in donor oocyte recipients: enigma or obstacle for implantation? Fertil Steril. 2013;100:1289-95.
32. Broekmans FJ. ESHRE'S 2016 annual meeting. Helsinki, Finland; 2016.
33. Steer CV, Campbell S, Tan SL, et al. The use of transvaginal color flow imaging after in vitro fertilization to identify optimum uterine conditions before embryo transfer. Fertil Steril. 1992;57(2):372-6.
34. Serafini P, Batzofin J, Nelson J, et al. Sonographic uterine predictors of pregnancy in women undergoing ovulation induction for assisted reproductive treatments. Fertil Steril. 1994;62(4):815-22.
35. Tekay A, Martikainen H, Jouppila P. Blood flow changes in uterine and ovarian vasculature, and predictive value of transvaginal pulsed colour Doppler ultrasonography in an in-vitro fertilization programme. Hum Reprod. 1995;10(3):688-93.
36. Cacciatore B, Simberg N, Fusaro P, et al. Transvaginal Doppler study of uterine artery blood flow in in vitro fertilization-embryo transfer cycles. Fertil Steril. 1996;66(1):130-4.
37. Schild RL, Knobloch C, Dorn C, et al. Endometrial receptivity in an in vitro fertilization program as assessed by spiral artery blood flow, endometrial thickness, endometrial volume, and uterine artery blood flow. Fertil Steril. 2001;75(2):361-6.
38. Bonilla-Musoles F, Raga F, Osborne NG, et al. Endometrial receptivity: evaluation with ultrasound. Ultrasound Q. 2013;29(1):3-20.
39. Raga F, Bonilla-Musoles F, Casañ EM, et al. Assessment of endometrial volume by three-dimensional ultrasound prior to embryo transfer: clues to endometrial receptivity. Hum Reprod. 1999;14(11):2851-4.
40. Wu HM, Chiang CH, Huang HY, et al. Detection of the subendometrial vascularization flow index by three-dimensional ultrasound may be useful for predicting the pregnancy rate for patients undergoing in vitro fertilization-embryo transfer. Fertil Steril. 2003;79(3):507-11.
41. Chen MJ, Yang JH, Peng FH, et al. Extended estrogen administration for women with thin endometrium in frozen-thawed in-vitro fertilization programs. J Assist Reprod Genet. 2006;23(7-8):337-42.
42. Khairy M, Banerjee K, El-Toukhy T, et al. Aspirin in women undergoing in vitro fertilization treatment: a systematic review and meta-analysis. Fertil Steril. 2007;88(4):822-31.
43. Takasaki A, Tamura H, Miwa I, et al. Endometrial growth and uterine blood flow: a pilot study for improving endometrial thickness in the patients with a thin endometrium. Fertil Steril. 2010;93(6):1851-8.
44. Sher G, Fisch JD. Effect of vaginal sildenafil on the outcome of in vitro fertilization (IVF) after multiple IVF failures attributed to poor endometrial development. Fertil Steril. 2002;78(5):1073-6.
45. Ho M, Huang LC, Chang YY, et al. Electroacupuncture reduces uterine artery blood flow impedance in infertile women. Taiwan J Obstet Gynecol. 2009;48(2):148-51.
46. Gleicher N, Vidali A, Barad DH. Successful treatment of unresponsive thin endometrium. Fertil Steril. 2011;95(6):2123.e13-7.
47. Chang Y, Li J, Chen Y, et al. Autologous platelet-rich plasma promotes endometrial growth and improves pregnancy outcome during in vitro fertilization. Int J Clin Exp Med. 2015;8(1):1286-90.
48. Lédée-Bataille N, Olivennes F, Lefaix JL, et al. Combined treatment by pentoxifylline and tocopherol for recipient women with a thin endometrium enrolled in an oocyte donation programme. Hum Reprod. 2002;17(5):1249-53.
49. Tourgeman DE, Slater CC, Stanczyk FZ, et al. Endocrine and clinical effects of micronized estradiol administered vaginally or orally. Fertil Steril. 2001;75(1):200-2.
50. Fanchin R, Righini C, Schönauer LM, et al. Vaginal versus oral E(2) administration: effects on endometrial thickness, uterine perfusion, and contractility. Fertil Steril. 2001;76(5):994-8.
51. Pierro E, Minici F, Alesiani O, et al. Stromal-epithelial interactions modulate estrogen responsiveness in normal human endometrium. Biol Reprod. 2001;64(3):831-8.
52. Elizur SE, Son WY, Yap R, et al. Comparison of low-dose human menopausal gonadotropin and micronized 17beta-estradiol supplementation in in vitro maturation cycles with thin endometrial lining. Fertil Steril. 2009;92(3):907-12.
53. Papanikolaou EG, Kyrou D, Zervakakou G, et al. Follicular hCG endometrium priming for IVF patients experiencing resisting thin endometrium. A proof of concept study. J Assist Reprod Genet. 2013;30:1341-5.
54. Rubinstein M, Marazzi A, Polak de Fried E. Low-dose aspirin treatment improves ovarian responsiveness, uterine and ovarian blood flow velocity, implantation, and pregnancy rates in patients undergoing in vitro fertilization: a prospective, randomized, double-blind placebo-controlled assay. Fertil Steril. 1999;71(5):825-9.
55. Hsieh YY, Tsai HD, Chang CC, et al. Low-dose aspirin for infertile women with thin endometrium receiving intrauterine insemination: a prospective, randomized study. J Assist Reprod Genet. 2000;17(3):174-7.
56. Chung TW, Yu JJ, Liu DZ. Reducing lipid peroxidation stress of erythrocyte membrane by alpha-tocopherol nicotinate plays an important role in improving blood rheological properties in type 2 diabetic patients with retinopathy. Diabet Med. 1998;15(5):380-5.

57. Cicek N, Eryilmaz OG, Sarikaya E, et al. Vitamin E effect on controlled ovarian stimulation of unexplained infertile women. J Assist Reprod Genet. 2012;29(4):325-8.
58. Hazout A. Tumor necrosis factor and underlying infection. Contracept Fertil Sex. 1995;23(10):631-4.
59. Acharya S, Yasmin E, Balen AH. The use of a combination of pentoxifylline and tocopherol in women with a thin endometrium undergoing assisted conception therapies—a report of 20 cases. Hum Fertil (Camb). 2009;12(4):198-203.
60. Check JH, Graziano V, Lee G, et al. Neither sildenafil nor vaginal estradiol improves endometrial thickness in women with thin endometria after taking oral estradiol in graduating dosages. Clin Exp Obstet Gynecol. 2004;31(2):99-102.
61. Stener-Victorin E, Waldenström U, Andersson SA, et al. Reduction of blood flow impedance in the uterine arteries of infertile women with electro-acupuncture. Hum Reprod. 1996;11(6):1314-7.
62. Barad DH, Yu Y, Kushnir VA, et al. A randomized clinical trial of endometrial perfusion with granulocyte colony-stimulating factor in in vitro fertilization cycles: impact on endometrial thickness and clinical pregnancy rates. Fertil Steril. 2014;101(3):710-15.
63. Aghajanova L, Houshdaran S, Balayan S, et al. Platelets for endometrial regeneration: a novel approach. Fertil Steril. 2016;106:e82.
64. Nazari L, Salehpour S, Hoseini S, et al. Effects of autologous platelet-rich plasma on implantation and pregnancy in repeated implantation failure: a pilot study. Int J Reprod Biomed (Yazd). 2016;14(10):625-8.
65. Gargett CE, Nguyen HP, Ye L. Endometrial regeneration and endometrial stem/progenitor cells. Rev Endocr Metab Disord. 2012;13(4):235-51.
66. Cervelló I, Mas A, Gil-Sanchis C, et al. Reconstruction of endometrium from human endometrial side population cell lines. PLoS One. 2011;6(6):e21221.
67. Taylor HS. Endometrial cells derived from donor stem cells in bone marrow transplant recipients. JAMA. 2004;292(1):81-5.

Endometrial Receptivity Analysis

37

Manish Banker, Poornima Nadkarni

INTRODUCTION

Since the first successful in vitro fertilization (IVF) birth, efforts are being made to improve results. A process of implantation of a good quality blastocyst over a healthy receptive endometrium is very complex. Endometrial receptivity (ER) is an important parameter for successful implantation, especially in IVF treatment where, in each cycle, embryo transfer is to be performed at a specific time depending on the stage of embryo development.[1] Finding a peak receptive endometrial window for an embryo has been a difficult task. Also, available tests to diagnose an ER (like ultrasound and histopathology) are less accurate and more subjective. After many years of research, decoding endometrial transcriptomics using next-generation sequencing (NGS) and thus objectively identifying the personalized window of implantation (pWOI) is now possible.[2] Thus, NGS technology has helped us to develop a molecular diagnostic tool called endometrial receptivity analysis (ERA) for the diagnosis of peak ER.

However, implantation stills remains uncertain and a challenge. The window of implantation (WOI) is not constant in all women, but rather personalized and even displaced in one out of four patients with recurrent implantation failure (RIF).[3,4]

Recurrent implantation failure is defined as the failure of three or more IVF cycles in which one or two morphologically good quality embryos are transferred.[4] Some common causes of RIF include pathological alteration of endometrial cavity (which are found in 18–27% of cases) such as submucous polyps/fibroids, endometritis, endometrial hyperplasia, and synechia;[5] embryonic chromosomal abnormalities;[6] hydrosalpinx (affecting either by a direct embryotoxic effect or by altering ER);[7] and hereditary or acquired thrombophilias.[8] Implantation of embryo is not always achieved after correcting the above-mentioned causes of RIF, which comes under the category of unexplained RIF.

The endometrial WOI is defined as the window of opportunity during which the endometrium becomes maximum receptive to the embryo. Histological, biochemical, and ultrasound markers of ER are operator-dependent and less accurate with low predictive value.[9] The ERA is a customized test to analyze 236 genes expressed at the various stages of the endometrial cycle in a given endometrial sample and matched by a computational predictor that is able to identify the receptivity status and diagnose the pWOI of a given patient. Compared to other methods, the accuracy of ERA test is much better (sensitivity of 0.997 and a specificity of 0.885) and the results are reproducible in the same patients 29–40 months after the first test.[10]

ENDOMETRIAL RECEPTIVITY ANALYSIS TEST PROCEDURE

ERA® test is a diagnostic molecular tool, patented by IGENOMIX in 2009, based on gene expression used to determine woman's ER. Microarray technique was used for ERA before the availability of more accurate NGS. Since 2017, NGS is used for ERA test. It analyzes the gene expression pattern of a given sample and compares with the 236 genes expressed in receptive endometrium by a computational predictor; and then classifies the sample as "receptive" or "nonreceptive (NR)" endometrium.[10]

ENDOMETRIAL PREPARATION AND BIOPSY

The first ERA® test can be performed in natural, modified natural cycle or hormone replacement therapy (HRT) protocol, according to the kind of cycle/protocol in which subsequent embryo transfer is going to be performed. ERA test should not be performed in stimulated cycles. An endometrial sample must be taken in similar conditions that will have the embryo transfer cycle (type of cycle, medications used, and route and dose of administration). This is very important in order to make the result reproducible.

- Endometrial biopsy in the natural cycle [at luteinizing hormone (LH)+7]:
  - Detection of LH surge: Ultrasound assessment of the ovarian follicle size from day 11, when the follicle size is 15 mm, LH surge will be searched for in the urine or blood.
  - The day of LH surge is LH+0 and the sample is taken 7 days (168 hours) after that (LH+7).
- Endometrial biopsy in the modified natural cycle [natural cycle with human chorionic gonadotropin (hCG)] (hCG+7):
  - Human chorionic gonadotropin will be administered as a routine when the follicle size becomes more than 17 mm.
  - The day of hCG injection is hCG+0, the biopsy will be taken on hCG+7.
- Endometrial biopsy in HRT protocol (P+5):
  - Preferable protocol for endometrial preparation because of its easy execution and lesser cancellation rates as compared to other protocol.
  - Estradiol tablets will be started from the 2nd/3rd day of the menses. Sonography will be performed on 9th/10th day of menses till a trilaminar endometrium more than 6 mm is reached. Then progesterone administration can be started (P+0).
  - Progesterone will be administered for 5 full days (120 hours) (P+5).
  - The day of progesterone start is P+0; the endometrial biopsy will be taken on P+5.

INTERPRETATION OF RESULTS

Two possible results: "receptive" or "nonreceptive":

- *Receptive (R)*: Suggests that the gene expression profile is similar to that of a normal receptive endometrium. Embryo transfer is recommended to be performed in the similar protocol in which the endometrial biopsy has been taken.
- *Nonreceptive*: Suggests that the gene expression profile is not similar to that of endometrium of receptive phase. To analyze and visualize the gene expression profile of NR samples, a principal component analysis (PCA) is to be performed against the sample training sets (prereceptive and postreceptive samples) used in the development of the ERA prediction profile.

Nonreceptive test results are usually reported as prereceptive or postreceptive and a recommendation is also to be given for a putative pWOI. In some cases, to validate this pWOI, a second endometrial biopsy and ERA analysis is performed as per the recommendation of the ERA classifier. The second endometrial biopsy should be performed with similar protocol and biopsy was taken on the recommended day. The recommended day for second biopsy is later than the previous biopsy day in case of prereceptive endometrium and some days earlier when the endometrium is reported as postreceptive the exact time of which is specified in the report.

PERSONALIZED EMBRYO TRANSFER

The blastocyst transfer is recommended to be performed in the same type of cycle and on the same day in which the biopsy result was receptive. A receptive result indicates the ideal day on which the blastocyst transfer should be performed. If the embryo is of day 3 embryo, it should be transferred 2 days earlier than what the ERA suggests **(Fig. 1)**.

CLINICAL APPLICATION OF ENDOMETRIAL RECEPTIVITY ANALYSIS

Indications

The ERA test is recommended in women with unexplained RIF with high grade embryos (three or more IVF cycles in which one or two good quality embryos). Women with a morphologically normal uterus with endometrial thickness of more than or equal to 6 mm can be taken for the test.

Clinical Outcome

Endometrial receptivity factor was neglected since many years and therefore a clinical personalized approach to improve assisted reproductive technology (ART) outcome, at the level of endometrium, was needed. ERA identifies the pWOI and recommends the best time to transfer embryo(s), thereby increasing the chances of a successful outcome.

According to Ruiz et al. (2013),[4] clinical outcome of the women in the control group (0.4 ± 0.5 previous failed cycles) was 81.8% pregnancy rate (PR) and 55.0% implantation rate (IR) versus 51.7% PR and 33.9% IR in the receptive RIF group with 4.8 ± 2.1 previous failed cycles **(Table 1)**. This finding suggests that after the ERA test and personalized embryo

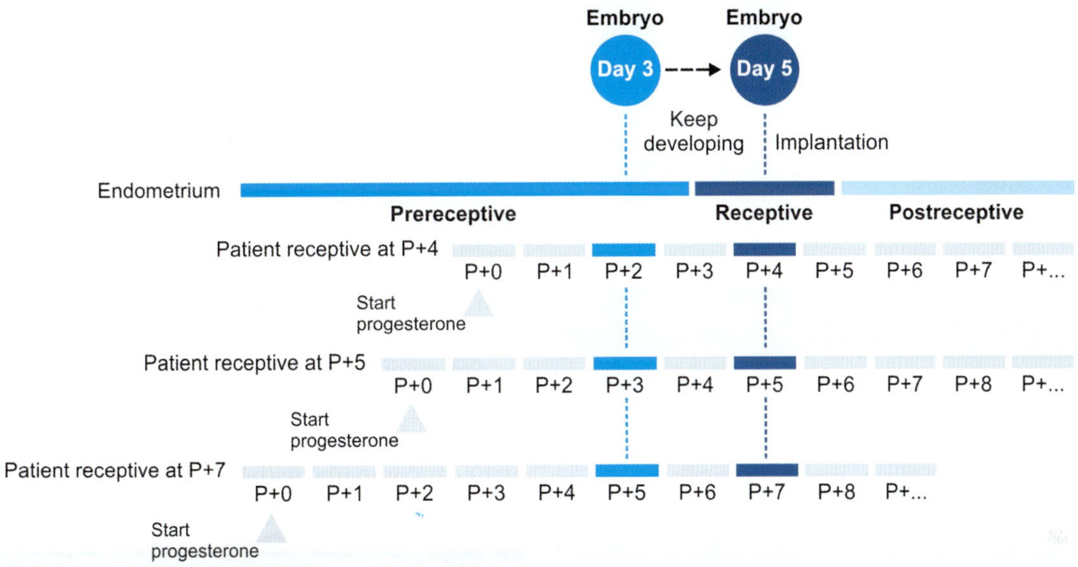

Fig. 1: Personalized embryo transfer recommendation based on endometrial receptivity analysis (ERA) results in hormone replacement therapy (HRT) protocol.[2]

Table 1: Clinical outcomes of recurrent implantation failure (RIF) and control group patients following the endometrial receptivity analysis (ERA) test.[4]

	RIF	*Control*
No. of patients	85	25
Age (years)	38.4 ± 4.7	39.9 ± 5.1
No. of receptive era®/total analyzed (%)	63/85 (74.1)	22/25 (88.0)
No. of previous failed cycles	4.8 ± 2.1	0.5 ± 0.5
Total patients with pET after receptive ERA®	29	11
Implantation rate after 1st pET (%)	19/56 (33.9)	11/20 (55.0)
Pregnancy rate after 1st pET (%)	15/29 (51.7)	9/11 (81.8)
Biochemical pregnancies (%)	3/15 (20.0)	2/9 (22.2)
Clinical abortions (%)	0/15 (0.0)	0/9 (0.0)
Ovum donation patients/Total (%)	22/63 (34.9)	13/22 (59.1)
Patients with pET after receptive ERA®	16	8
Implantation rate after 1st pET (%)	12/33 (36.4)	7/15 (46.7)
Pregnancy rate after 1st pET (%)	9/16 (56.2)	6/8 (75.0)
Biochemical pregnancies (%)	2/9 (22.2)	1/6 (16.7)
Clinical abortions (%)	0/9 (0.0)	0/6 (0.0)
IVF/ICSI patients/Total (%)	41/63 (65.1)	9/22 (40.9)
Patients with pET after receptive ERA®	13	3
Implantation rate after 1st pET (%)	7/23 (30.4)	4/5 (80.0)

Contd...

Contd...

	RIF	*Control*
Pregnancy rate after 1st pET (%)	6/13 (46.2)	3/3 (100.0)
Biochemical pregnancies (%)	1/6 (16.7)	1/3 (33.3)
Clinical abortions (%)	0/6 (0.0)	0/3 (0.0)
No. of receptive era®/total analyzed (%)	22/85 (25.9)	3/25 (12.0)
No. of previous failed cycles	5.0 ± 1.8	0.3 ± 0.6
Ovum donation patients/Total (%)	11/22 (50.0)	2/3 (66.6)
IVF/ICSI patients/Total (%)	11/22 (50.0)	1/3 (33.3)

(ICSI: intracytoplasmic sperm injection; IVF: in vitro fertilization; pET: personalized embryo transfer)

Table 2: Clinical outcome of NR RIF and comparison group patients that underwent pET.[4]

	Nonreceptive
No. of patients	25
No. of previous failed cycles RIF patients	5.0 ± 1.8
No. of previous failed cycles control patients	0.3 ± 0.6
ERA® Prediction	
Prereceptive	21/25 (84.0)
Postreceptive	4/25 (16.0)
2nd ERA® at the specified day (P+4; P+6; P+7; LH + 9)[a]	18
Months between 1st and 2nd ERA®	2.6 ± 2.8
2nd ERA® receptive at the specified day	15
Patients with pET[b] after 2nd receptive ERA®	8
Months between 2nd receptive ERA® and pET	1.8 ± 0.7
Implantation rate using pET	5/13 (38.5)
Pregnancy rate using pET	4/8 (50.0)
Biochemical pregnancies (%)	0/4 (0.0)
Clinical abortions (%)	0/4 (0.0)

[a]The specified day for the 2nd ERA® was calculated by ERA® Test according to the gene profile of each sample.
[b]pET implies to do the embryo transfer under the same conditions in which a Receptive ERA® was obtained in those which the 2nd ERA® was performed.
(NR: nonreceptive; pET: personalized embryo transfer; RIF: recurrent implantation failure)

transfer (pET), even in poor prognosis patient (RIF) group, clinical outcome was fairly good.

25.9% of the women with RIF were NR at the time when embryo transfer had previously failed. Only 12% women were NR in control group. This NR endometrium was classified by our computational predictor as prereceptive or postreceptive, which was further verified by a second ERA test. When pET was employed in these women with RIF with NR endometrium, IR and PR increased to the level of women with receptive endometrium **(Table 2)**.

Simon et al. (2016)[11] with his prospective randomized study, proved that after pET (based on ERA test results) PRs and ongoing PRs (85.7% and 55.1%) were significantly higher as compared with fresh embryo transfer (61.7% and 43.3%) or deferred embryo transfer (60.8% and 44.6%).

CONCLUSION

Endometrial receptivity analysis test is very accurate and sensitive in identifying genetic expressions of the endometrium to pinpoint embryo transfer timing. pET guided by ERA significantly improves PRs and IRs, especially in unexplained RIF cases. This provides us an objective diagnostic tool for pET and must be included in infertility workup, especially in cases of previous failed cycles when embryo factor is less likely.

REFERENCES

1. Díaz-Gimeno P, Ruíz-Alonso M, Blesa D, et al. Transcriptomics of the human endometrium. Int J Dev Biol. 2014;58(2-4):127-37.
2. Igenomix. (2009). ERA® Endometrial Receptivity Analysis. [online] Available from https://www.igenomix.com/hubfs/493037/.com/era_presentation.pdf?t=1519722655280 [Last accessed February, 2019].
3. Mahajan N. Endometrial receptivity array: Clinical application. J Hum Reprod Sci. 2015;8(3):121-9.
4. Ruiz-Alonso M, Blesa D, Díaz-Gimeno P, et al. The endometrial receptivity array for diagnosis and personalized embryo transfer as a treatment for patients with repeated implantation failure. Fertil Steril. 2013;100(3):818-24.
5. Demirol A, Gurgan T. Effect of treatment of intrauterine pathologies with office hysteroscopy in patients with recurrent IVF failure. Reprod Biomed Online. 2004;8(5):590-4.
6. Pehlivan T, Rubio C, Rodrigo L, et al. Impact of preimplantation genetic diagnosis on IVF outcome in implantation failure patients. Reprod Biomed Online 2003;6:232-7.

7. Meyer WR, Castelbaum AJ, Somkuti S, et al. Hydrosalpinges adversely affect markers of endometrial receptivity. Hum Reprod. 1997;12(7):1393-8.
8. Penzias AS. Recurrent IVF failure: other factors. Fertil Steril. 2012;97:1033-8.
9. Murray MJ, Meyer WR, Zaino RJ, et al. A critical analysis of the accuracy, reproducibility, and clinical utility of histologic endometrial dating in fertile women. Fertil Steril. 2004;81:1333-43.
10. Díaz-Gimeno P, Horcajadas JA, Martínez-Conejero JA, et al. A genomic diagnostic tool for human endometrial receptivity based on the transcriptomic signature. Fertil Steril. 2011;95:50-60.
11. Simon C, Vladimirov I, Castillon Cortes G, et al. Prospective, randomized study of the endometrial receptivity analysis (ERA) test in the infertility work-up to guide personalized embryo transfer versus fresh transfer or deferred embryo transfer. Fertil Steril. 2016;106(3):e46-7.

Recurrent Implantation Failure

38

Sulbha Arora, Mirudhubashini Govindarajan, Laxmi Shrikhande

INTRODUCTION

Assisted reproductive technologies have come a long way since the birth of the first in vitro fertilization (IVF) baby Louise Brown in 1978. Over the last 40 years, success rates have dramatically improved and the incidence of unwanted complications has reduced. This has largely been due to the advent of simpler, more patient-friendly stimulation protocols, along with advances in the embryology laboratory such as more efficient culture media, advanced cryopreservation techniques, and the ability to culture embryos to the blastocyst stage. This has enabled the reduction of the number of embryos being transferred and the improvement in the implantation rate of each individual embryo produced. Yet, we seem to hit a glass ceiling beyond which the implantation rates cannot be further improved. The 2016 report published by Society for Assisted Reproductive Technology (SART) quotes a live birth rate of 47.6% for women less than 35 years of age.[1] This implies that the majority of the embryos transferred do not seem to implant.

Human embryo implantation involves a complex cross talk between the maternal endometrium and the developing embryo. The embryo needs to hatch out of its protective shell or zona pellucida. Simultaneously, the endometrium needs to open its window of implantation. Multiple pinopodes appear at this stage that function to absorb uterine cavity fluid and bring the endometrium in close contact with the floating embryo. This is followed by the triad of apposition, adhesion, and invasion of the endometrium by the blastocyst, leading to successful implantation. Therefore, when the process of implantation fails, we are faced with the question—is it in the seed, or is it in the soil? The cause of failure may be an advanced maternal age, aneuploid gametes or embryos, uterine or tubal pathology, as well as a disruption of the endometrial receptivity. Diagnosing the exact cause of implantation failure can thus be difficult.

DEFINITION

For some women, the process of implantation may fail repeatedly. There is no consensus to the number of attempts or the number of transferred embryos required to qualify for a diagnosis of recurrent implantation failure (RIF). The difference of opinion stems from the number and stage of embryos being transferred. The 2005 European Society for Human Reproduction and Embryology (ESHRE) Preimplantation Genetic Diagnosis (PGD) Consortium defines RIF as failure to achieve a viable pregnancy, following "more than three embryo transfers with high quality embryos or the transfer of more than or equal to 10 embryos in multiple transfers; exact numbers to be determined by each center". However, in today's world and age where we are moving towards elective single embryo transfers at blastocyst stage, it is no longer practical to wait up to a failure of 10 such embryos before seeking answers. Orvieto et al. defined it as a failure to conceive after three transfers with good quality embryos.[2] Zeyneloglu's definition is similar, specifically adding two embryos of high quality.[3] Rinehart pointed out that maternal age and stage of embryos, whether cleavage or blastocyst, should be taken into consideration while defining RIF.[4] Coughlan et al. suggested a more working definition incorporating maternal age, the number of transfers, and the number of embryos.[5] As per their definition,

"Recurrent implantation failure refers to failure to achieve a clinical pregnancy after transfer of at least four good-quality embryos in a minimum of three fresh or frozen cycles in women under 40 years of age."

INCIDENCE

It is difficult to accurately calculate the incidence or prevalence of RIF due to differences in its definition. Added to that, some studies consider biochemical pregnancy to be an implantation whereas some consider only an ultrasound evidence of pregnancy to be an implantation. Most assisted reproductive technology (ART) clinics report an implantation rate of 40–60%,[4] however, due to differences in criteria for RIF, exact data on its incidence is lacking.

ETIOLOGY

Many factors can contribute to a negative result after an ART procedure including suboptimal ovarian stimulation, detrimental culture conditions or lack of quality control in the laboratory, and problems during the embryo transfer technique. However, these problems should cause low success rates for all patients attending a particular clinic. There are times when clinics with high overall success rates are also faced with patients in whom implantation repeatedly fails. In some of these cases, diagnosis of the exact cause may be often elusive. The problem may arise from the embryo, the uterus or it may be multifactorial.

Genetic Factors

Parental Abnormalities

Incidence of parental chromosomal abnormalities is reported to be 2.5%.[6] In extreme cases of RIF (>6 failed cycles or >15 transferred embryos), 15.4% of were found to have chromosomal translocations, mosaicism, inversions or deletions.[7] When balanced translocations are present in the parental chromosomes, the gametes produced by such individuals often contain chromosomal anomalies that are destined to lead to a range of failed outcomes, from abnormal gametogenesis[8] to recurrent pregnancy loss.[9]

Translocations are a variety of rearrangements between nonhomologous chromosomes. In reciprocal translocation, two nonhomologous chromosomes exchange segments. In Robertsonian translocations, two acrocentric chromosomes break at the centromere to fuse as a single large chromosome with loss of two short arms. Parental translocations, when present, may result in a variety of aneuploidies depending upon which chromosome is involved as well as the size of the rearrangements.

Due to these observations, it is recommended to study the parental karyotypes in couples with RIF. Cases where translocations are present should be offered the option of PGD of the embryos and selection of unaffected embryos for transfer.

Embryonic Aneuploidies

Chromosomal abnormalities in the embryos account for 30–40% of cases of RIF.[10] Rates of oocyte aneuploidies increase proportionately with the woman's age, and a sudden steep rise in the percentage of abnormal oocytes is seen in the late 30s and early 40s. Franasiak et al. observed that the rate of aneuploidy increases from 58% at the age of 40 years to 100% at the age of 47.[11] Thus, female age is the single most important determinant of the implantation potential of embryos. Aneuploid embryos often cannot be differentiated from euploid ones using standard morphological parameters that can be observed under the microscope.

Role of Aneuploidy Studies in Recurrent Implantation Failure

Over the last 2 decades, techniques have been developed to diagnose these chromosomal abnormalities in embryos before transfer. These techniques aim to aid in euploid embryo selection thereby not only increasing the chances of implantation but also reducing the incidence of spontaneous miscarriages and chances of having a live born child with genetic defects. Biopsy of the polar body for preimplantation genetic screening (PGS) was one such technique that was common earlier, however it analyses only maternal sources of aneuploidies and is therefore not preferred now. Biopsy of a day 3, 6–8 cells cleavage stage embryo with excision of a single blastomere from each embryo was the more commonly used technique till recently. However, it suffers from the drawback of misdiagnosing a mosaic embryo as either euploid or aneuploid. There is a tendency of a mosaic embryo to undergo autocorrection during subsequent development, where the aneuploid cells will either not multiply or be pushed to the trophectoderm. At blastocyst stage, therefore, such embryos may actually have a euploid inner cell mass, however might have been wrongly discarded after a day 3 biopsy reporting a diagnosis of aneuploidy. Also, as a blastomere is a single cell, sometimes the PGS reporting may not be possible if insufficient deoxyribonucleic acid (DNA) is detected. With recent advances in laboratory culture media, it is now possible to culture all embryos up to blastocyst stage and that is the preferred stage for biopsy. As a trophectoderm biopsy analyses multiple cells, the chances of missing mosaic embryos are reduced. Similarly, fluorescence in situ hybridization (FISH) techniques have been replaced with comparative genomic hybridization (CGH) and next-generation sequencing (NGS). These techniques allow scanning of the entire genome to pick up any variations in the DNA copy number. The embryos are reported as euploid, aneuploid or mosaic. Mosaic embryos are further analyzed to find out the degree of mosaicism. Low degree mosaic embryos with 30% or less aneuploid cells may be transferred. High degree mosaic embryos may be transferred after genetic counseling of the couple. As the biopsy is carried out at blastocyst stage, it necessitates freezing of all the embryos while the report is awaited. The embryos are then thawed and transferred in a remote cycle.

Many trials have analyzed the role of PGS in patients with RIF. In a 2003 study, Pehlivan et al. compared the outcome of 49 RIF patients undergoing PGS with that of controls. The blastomeres were extracted on day 3 and subjected to FISH analysis of chromosomes 13, 16, 18, 21, 22, X, and Y. They found higher rates of aneuploidy in patients with RIF than in the controls (67.4% vs 36.3%). The pregnancy rates in the RIF group after PGS (34%) was comparable to the controls (33.1%).[12] Gianaroli et al. found a directly proportionate relationship where couples with higher numbers of failed attempts had correspondingly higher ratios of aneuploid embryos.[13]

Data from prospective studies analyzing the benefit of PGS in patients with RIF is mixed, largely due to the use of older FISH techniques. Gianaroli et al. used day 3 biopsy and the FISH technique, and found a significant improvement in implantation rates (28.0% vs 11.9%) after PGS.[13] Their subsequent randomized trial on patients with three or more previous failed IVF cycles confirmed their findings once again.[14] On the other hand, Blockeel et al. found a lower live birth rate of 21% in the PGS-FISH group in his study, as compared to 39% in the control group.[15] A 2011 meta-analysis found lower live birth rates of between 13% and 23% in women of advanced maternal age undergoing PGS as compared to controls who had a live birth rate of 26% without PGS. They concluded the cause to be technical drawbacks and a high incidence of mosaic embryos. All nine randomized controlled trials (RCTs) included in this meta-analysis used FISH and all, but one performed the biopsy at cleavage stage.[16]

These negative outcomes, however, can be justified by the potential inaccuracy of the FISH technique and the damage caused to the embryo by performing the biopsy at the cleavage stage.[17-19] Trophectoderm biopsy has several advantages over blastomere biopsy, as outlined above. It has been recommended for women over the age of 40 years undergoing IVF with their own eggs.[20] More recently, Lee et al. conducted a retrospective study of women aged 40–43 years with RIF undergoing IVF with PGS. They found the live birth rate after PGS and subsequent frozen embryo transfer (45.5%) to be much higher than the live birth rates for fresh or frozen transfer of non-PGS embryos (15.8% and 19.0%, respectively).[21]

The same significant improvement in outcomes may not be seen in younger women with RIF, as we know aneuploidy rates increase with age, and in these women other factors must be ruled out as well. Also, for women of all age groups, it should be kept in mind that PGS would add to the treatment cost, would not increase the implantation potential of a euploid embryo, and even at blastocyst stage carries a small albeit persistent risk of discarding an embryo with an aneuploid trophectoderm but euploid inner cell mass. Thus, it should be judiciously used in selected cases and not as a blanket protocol for all.

The Sperm Factor

Routinely tested semen parameters such as sperm count, motility, and morphology may serve as a guideline for deciding between basic treatment options such as intrauterine insemination (IUI) and more advanced options such as intracytoplasmic sperm injection (ICSI). However, they do not predict the ability of the sperms to give rise to good quality embryos. Additionally, valuable information such as sperm aneuploidy and sperm DNA fragmentation, that may contribute to RIF, is not obtained from routine semen analyses.

A higher percentage of aneuploidies has been found in semen samples of men with abnormal semen parameters on routine analysis and also in samples of men with RIF, even when the paternal karyotype is normal. Burrello et al. conducted a five-probe FISH analysis of sperms from 48 men enrolled for ICSI.[22] They found higher implantation rates (34% vs 13%) and pregnancy rates (75% vs 34%), as well as lower miscarriage rates (11% vs 38%) in men who had higher percentage of euploid sperms. Unlike PGS of embryos, the individual tested sperms cannot themselves be used, so the clinical utility of sperm aneuploidy testing is limited. However, it does point to the potential benefit of PGS before transferring embryos formed using sperms samples from men with higher percentage of aneuploidy.

Several studies have shown that there is a higher incidence of chromosomal aneuploidies in embryos, lower chances of success, and a higher miscarriage rate in men with high amounts of sperm DNA fragmentation.[23-28] DNA fragmentation is lower in sperms surgically retrieved from the testes as compared to sperms that are ejaculated or retrieved from the epididymis.[29-31] In couples with RIF, with a high DNA fragmentation index (DFI), one treatment option is testicular sperm aspiration (TESA).[29,32] Greco et al. conducted a study on 18 couples who had at least two failed embryo transfers, with a DFI of more than 15% in the sperm samples.[29] They found significantly higher DFI in ejaculated sperms in these cases as compared to sperms extracted from the testes (23.6% vs 4.8%). Furthermore, the clinical pregnancy rate was 44.4% in subsequent cycles in these couples when testicular sperm was used.

Standard sperm wash techniques such as swim-up and density gradient filter sperms based on motility, but are unable to separate sperms with high DNA fragmentation. A number of techniques have been recommended to filter out these damaged sperms from an ejaculate. These include annexin V columns [magnetic-activated cell sorting (MACS)], sperm hyaluronic acid binding, confocal light absorption scattering spectroscopy, and selection of sperms for ICSI under high power microscopes [intracytoplasmic morphologically selected sperm injection (IMSI)].[33-36] The advantage of these techniques is that they are noninvasive as opposed to TESA.

Cells undergoing apoptosis start to lose membrane integrity early on in the process. This leads to externalization of phospholipid phosphatidylserine (a molecule with a high affinity for annexin V).[37]Annexin V beads conjugated with magnetic microspheres are mixed with the sperm sample. They attach to the apoptotic sperms. When these sperms are passed through a magnetic column, these apoptotic sperms are retained in it while unlabeled sperms with intact DNA flow out of it. This procedure is called MACS. Recent studies have found MACS to be beneficial regardless of the DFI, because DNA fragmentation is not the only cause of apoptotic sperms.[38] Monica Gil et al. performed a systematic review and meta-analysis of the available literature to summarize the results of using MACS as a sperm selection technique and determine its efficacy in improving ART success rates.[39] They found the technique led to an improvement in sperm quality and function. Several included studies reported improvements in fertilization rates and embryo quality. Most studies found that density gradient centrifugation (DGC) followed by MACS was the most ideal sperm selection method. They found MACS to be especially promising in improving the outcomes of couples with RIF and recommended its use for this indication.

Intracytoplasmic morphologically selected sperm injection has also been recommended for patients with RIF.[36,40-42] Presence of large vacuoles has been found to be associated with increased DNA defects.[43-46] Therefore, the use of IMSI to select sperms devoid of vacuoles has been postulated to improve embryo quality and pregnancy rates.[36,41] However, subsequent studies did not find an improvement in ongoing pregnancy, miscarriage or live birth rates with the use of IMSI.[47] One study of 200 RIF patients that specifically evaluated the role of IMSI (8,400X magnification) failed to find any significant improvements in fertilization, implantation or pregnancy rates with the use of this technique.[42]

Cleavage versus Blastocyst Stage Transfer

Blastocyst transfer has been proposed as a strategy to improve implantation rates and pregnancy rates in patients with RIF. Most embryos will reach the cleavage stage, however not all progress up to blastocyst stage even in optimum laboratory culture conditions. This is because most embryos that get arrested between cleavage and blastocyst stage are aneuploid embryos. Thus, a natural selection takes place that assists us in identifying embryos with the best implantation potential. It also enables us to reduce the number of embryos being transferred and aim for elective single embryo transfer, minimizing the risks associated with multiple pregnancy. This is a good approach even for patients who have only one or two embryos at cleavage stage and there is not much to choose from. This is because the blastocyst is a complex structure with a trophectoderm, a cavity and an inner cell mass. An embryo that appears to be of high quality on day 3, but shows absence of an inner cell mass on reaching an expanded blastocyst stage, would have led to a negative outcome or a miscarriage if it had been transferred at cleavage stage. Also, the development of an embryo up to the cleavage stage is controlled by maternal ribonucleic acid (RNA) transcripts.[48] Thereafter the switch to the embryonic genome occurs, that drives further development to blastocyst stage. Waiting up to blastocyst stage can help to differentiate between embryos that are of poor quality due to maternal or paternal factors and accordingly guide further cycles. Earlier monophasic culture media resulted in unsatisfactory blastulation rates, however the newer sequential culture media are well suited for long culture and facilitate the selection of embryos most ideal for transfer. Blastocyst transfer is also more physiological, as this is the stage when the embryo reaches the uterine cavity in a natural cycle. At cleavage stage it is still in the fallopian tube, which has a different environment than the uterus. The uterus may not meet the developmental needs of a cleavage stage embryo. Also, uterine contractions that may have been stimulated during the ovum pick-up process have had more of time to reduce by day 5. In cases of RIF if previous transfers have been at cleavage stage, it is recommended to wait up to blastocyst stage in the next attempt.

Zona Pellucida and Implantation

Elasticity and thinning of the zona pellucida are essential prerequisites for successful embryo hatching and implantation. The zona naturally hardens after fertilization. Increased zona hardening may occur in vivo with ageing and in vitro due to exposure to culture conditions or cryopreservation.[49,50] Failure of zona to rupture can theoretically cause implantation failure. Cleavage stage embryos with thin zonae have better implantation rates than those with thick zona. Moreover, only 25% of blastocysts hatch in vitro. Thus, assisted hatching was suggested as a means to facilitate the hatching process.[51-53] Various different techniques have been tried for assisted hatching. These include mechanical partial dissection of the zona, chemical exposure to acid Tyrode's solution, use of enzymes, laser-assisted hatching, and piezo micromanipulation.[54-59] In addition to facilitating implantation, these techniques may aid a two-way exchange of metabolites between the embryo and the culture medium.[60]

Selective assisted hatching may improve pregnancy rates in women over 38 years or thick zona pellucida more than 15 µm.[54] Evidence from literature does not support a benefit of applying this technique to all ART cycles, however it has been shown to be of benefit in cases of RIF.[57,61,62] Martins et al. conducted a meta-analysis examining data from five RCTs that included 561 patients.[63] They found a 73% higher clinical pregnancy rate in patients with RIF after the use of assisted hatching. However, unselected patients did not seem to benefit from it, and a Cochrane database systemic review that included 31 RCTs (5,728 women) found no significant increase in the odds of live birth in women undergoing assisted hatching.[64]

Uterine Factors

An evaluation of the uterine cavity by hysteroscopy is not recommended for all women prior to embryo transfer. The 2016 National Institute for Health and Care Excellence (NICE) guidelines recommend that hysteroscopy should not be offered on its own as part of the initial evaluation, unless clinically indicated, because there is no evidence of improved pregnancy rates after surgical treatment of uterine abnormalities.[65] However, uterine cavity evaluation is advisable in women with RIF. Uterine causes contributing to RIF include polyps, fibroids, adenomyosis, intrauterine adhesions, chronic endometritis, and Müllerian anomalies. These are usually diagnosed easily on ultrasound; however studies seem to indicate a range of 25–50% of RIF cases where previously undiagnosed pathology was detected on hysteroscopy.[66]

Endometrial Polyps

Intrauterine polyps are one of the commonest findings on hysteroscopy and can have a negative impact on implantation rates.[67] Even chances of spontaneous conception increase after excision of endometrial polyps.[68-70] A RCT of 215 women diagnosed with polyps found that women who had a polypectomy had 2.1 times higher chances of conceiving than women who had no intervention.[71]

Fibroids

Fibroids can reduce the chances of implantation in many ways. These include anatomical distortion, mechanical obstruction of the tubal ostia, changes in the uterine environment, chronic intrauterine inflammation, and increased uterine contractility. They may also have a negative effect on overlying endometrium and affect endometrial receptivity.[72-74] Their impact on fertility may depend on their size, location, and number. Subserous fibroids do not affect fertility and their removal is not mandatory. On the other hand, submucous fibroids reduce the chances of implantation, and also increase the miscarriage rates. Excision of submucous myomas usually restores implantation rates. For intramural myomas, the benefits of excision are debatable.[75,76] Eldar-Geva et al. found lower implantation and pregnancy rates in women with intramural fibroids even in the absence of a distortion of the cavity.[77] In the largest ever published meta-analysis on this pathology, Sunkara et al. found a 21% decrease in live birth rates in women with intramural fibroids even in the absence of any distortion of the cavity. However, the results were inconclusive about improvement in live birth rates after myomectomy.[78]

Congenital Anomalies

Congenital anomalies of the uterus can cause a range of reproductive disruption from decreased endometrial receptivity to recurrent miscarriages.[74] The most common anomaly is the septate uterus. Although an arcuate uterus may not have much of an impact on fertility, the presence of a septum may cause first and second trimester miscarriages, and also repeated implantation failure.[79,80] In light of this, resection of the septum is advisable to improve outcomes. On the other hand, women with bicornuate uteri usually do not face difficulty conceiving or carrying the pregnancy to term, and surgical correction is therefore not usually required.[81]

Adenomyosis

Adenomyosis is a condition where the glands of the endometrium invade the surrounding myometrium. It can potentially lead to RIF.[82] It may at times go undetected as it may be difficult to diagnose on ultrasound. Magnetic resonance imaging, especially with contrast, is a far superior diagnostic technique.[83-87] Adenomyosis may have an even greater impact on implantation rates, as it usually affects the junctional zone of the uterus immediately overlying the endometrium. Intramural fibroids, on the other hand, are some distance away from the endometrium. Ironically, this condition is more difficult to eliminate.[88,89] Surgical excision of adenomyosis is technically more difficult than fibroids as there is no defined capsule, and the procedure invariably involves removal of part of the normal myometrium. Downregulation with ultralong-acting gonadotropin releasing hormone agonist has been tried prior to IVF with limited success.[82] A newer technique that employs the use of magnetic resonance-guided focused ultrasound to noninvasively treat diffuse and focal adenomyosis as well as fibroids, without affecting fertility, has emerged as a promising option.

Intrauterine Adhesions

Intrauterine adhesions interfere with successful implantation of embryos by creating a hostile environment and preventing them from attaching to the endometrium. Their incidence in one study was found to be 8.5% of women with RIF.[90] Improved fertility outcomes after hysteroscopic adhesiolysis have been documented in many studies.[91-93]

The Endometrium

Implantation requires a functioning as well as receptive endometrium. During the menstrual cycle various morphological and biological changes occur that prepare the endometrium for implantation of the embryo. Only once the endometrium is receptive, will the embryo attach, invade, and finally implant. One of the diagnostic modalities that can be used to assess the endometrium and predict the likelihood of implantation is its ultrasound measurement in the follicular phase. There is no consensus on the minimal thickness of endometrium below which implantation is considered unlikely, and successful pregnancies have been reported with endometrial thickness as low as 5 mm. However, most studies appear to accept 7 mm on the day of human chorionic gonadotropin (hCG) administration as the ideal cutoff below which RIF is more likely. It suggests a lack of response of the endometrium to estrogenic stimulation, whether endogenous or exogenous. This is a challenging situation with many possible causes and limited treatment options. Sometimes it may result from congenital causes, Turner's syndrome, or a T-shaped uterus. Other causes, such as history of radiotherapy, pelvic tuberculosis, endometritis, and intrauterine adhesions need to be detected and treated before proceeding with an embryo transfer.

In frozen embryo transfer or recipient cycles, high doses of exogenously administered estrogen in the form of oral or vaginal tablets or transdermal gels may help in building up the endometrium. Adjuvants such as low dose aspirin and vaginal sildenafil have been tried with the aim of increasing endometrial blood flow. Other modalities such as intrauterine granulocyte-colony stimulating factor (G-CSF) and platelet rich plasma have been used, but still need larger RCTs to prove their efficacy.

Endometrial scratching in the cycle prior to embryo transfer may help in stimulating local inflammatory response and prepare the endometrium for implantation. If all else fails, surrogacy may become the only option.

Endometrial Scratching

The outcomes of using endometrial scratching to improve implantation rates have so far been mixed. It is postulated to cause a release of cytokines, immune modulators and other growth factors, and promote decidualization, which may aid the implantation process.[94,95] Barash et al. conducted a study of 134 women with RIF. 54 patients underwent endometrial biopsies in the cycle preceding IVF. He found a significantly higher implantation rate (27.7% vs 14.3%) in the biopsy group.[96] Subsequent studies seemed promising initially,[97] however later data has been mixed in outcomes.[98] Some studies have even shown a decrease in pregnancy rates in the group undergoing scratching,[99] whereas others have shown no significant difference with or without this technique.[100] Additionally, there are many unanswered questions regarding the optimal technique, the timing and frequency of endometrial injury, and the potential disadvantages, if any.[101] Therefore, it cannot be considered a recommended therapy until data from large scale RCTs has documented a benefit.

Chronic Endometritis

Chronic endometritis should be ruled out in patients with RIF where no other cause is found. Endometrial inflammation has been linked to RIF in many studies.[102-104] The incidence of chronic endometritis in RIF patients has been documented to be as high as 30.3% based on histologic findings. Implantation rates in these cases have been found to be lower.[105] Cicinelli et al. conducted a study to compare the pregnancy rates in women with RIF after successful treatment of endometritis versus those in whom endometritis persisted despite antibiotic therapy. Patients whose endometrial biopsy cultures were positive for Gram-negative bacteria were prescribed ciprofloxacin for 10 days. For Gram-positive cultures, a combination of amoxicillin and clavulanate was prescribed for 8 days. If there was histologic evidence of endometritis with a negative culture report, patients were treated with a single intramuscular administration of ceftriaxone, followed by a combination of doxycycline and metronidazole for 14 days. They found live birth rates of 60.8% in patients with successfully treated endometritis as opposed to 13.3% for women in whom it persisted even after three rounds of antibiotics.

Defective Endometrial Receptivity and the Endometrial Receptivity Array

Our deeper understanding of the endometrium has led us to a stage where we have learnt that it is not just the morphology of the endometrium on ultrasound that is essential for implantation but also its functionality. Microarray studies have broadened our insight and have resulted in the development of gene expression diagnostic techniques that are aimed at translating findings into clinical applications. These studies can potentially improve implantation and pregnancy rates. Intravenous infusion (IVI) has developed the ERA test or the endometrial receptivity array, a tool that studies 238 endometrial genes responsible for receptivity in both natural and hormone replacement cycles.[106] This array is more accurate than conventional histologic dating of the endometrium, and the test result for any given patient stays valid for up to 40 months after biopsy.[107] This test was designed to detect a shifted window of implantation, that may be either advanced or delayed, thus preventing implantation of a transferred embryo due to embryo-endometrial dyssynchronization. The endometrium is prepared using the identical protocol that is planned for the embryo transfer cycle. An endometrial biopsy is taken 5 days after starting luteal support and sent for the ERA analysis. The report is generated as either receptive or nonreceptive. A nonreceptive report indicates a shifted window which may be either prereceptive or postreceptive, and is accompanied by a recommendation for the precise duration of luteal support required for embryo transfer. 85 RIF and 25 controls underwent the ERA test. 88% of controls had a receptive report, whereas in RIF patients 74.1% had a receptive report. 15 RIF patients with a nonreceptive report subsequently had an embryo transfer done according to their personalized window of implantation, and 8 of them conceived.[108]

Thrombophilia

Thrombophilias, both inherited and acquired (antiphospholipid antibody syndrome) have been implicated in the etiology of recurrent pregnancy loss. The treatment of this condition with aspirin and heparin has been shown to significantly improve the outcome. However, there is controversy regarding the association between antiphospholipid antibodies and RIF. Some studies found a significant association,[109-111] whereas others could not confirm it.[112,113] Similarly, several studies have observed increased prevalence of inherited thrombophilias in women with RIF.[114,115] However, no association could be established between thrombophilia and IVF failure in a relatively large case-control study of 468 women undergoing IVF, although, the study population did not refer specifically to recurrent IVF failure.[116] A later study investigating the relationship of thrombophilia with repeated IVF failure, concluded that factor V Leiden, methylenetetrahydrofolate reductase mutations, and prothrombin gene mutations do not have a significant role in IVF embryo transfer implantation failure.[117] Overall, it remains to be determined whether thrombophilic conditions are a cause of RIF.

Immunological Factors

Decidualization is the process of differentiation of endometrial stromal cells, which is considered critical for the establishment and maintenance of pregnancy. Decidualized stromal cells develop the ability to regulate trophoblast invasion and to protect against local maternal immune responses.[118] Evidence in the literature on the value of various immunological investigations and treatments in women with RIF is conflicting.[119,120] There is no consensus on whether or not immunological testing should be carried out and whether immunological treatment is beneficial.

Tubal Pathology

Tubal pathology may also be a causative factor in RIF. A hydrosalpinx can have adverse effects on the fertility potential in multiple ways. Hydrosalpinx fluid that intermittently leaks into the uterine cavity may be directly embryotoxic. It may physically flush an embryo out of the uterine cavity. Lastly it may hamper endometrial receptivity.[5] A laparoscopic delinking of the hydrosalpinges is recommended before proceeding with embryo transfer to avoid its deleterious effects. If not done then live birth rates have been found to be reduced.[121-123] Seli et al. described a direct effect on the endometrium, where they found the expression of the endometrial cytokine leukemia inhibitory factor (LIF) was deranged in the presence of hydrosalpinges and restored back to normal after their excision.[124] Similarly, Bildirici et al. documented a restoration of Avb3 integrin expression after salpingectomy.[125] Strandell et al. conducted a prospective multicentre RCTs to evaluate the differences in outcome for women with hydrosalpinges undergoing IVF with or without a salpingectomy. They found pregnancy and live births rates of 36.6% and 28.6% respectively after salpingectomy, whereas without intervention the same were 23.9% and 16.3%, respectively.[122] The difference was especially more marked in women with ultrasound-visible hydrosalpinges. In women with RIF, the presence of hydrosalpinges must be ruled out as they can have a profound impact on implantation.

Embryo Transfer Technique

In addition to embryo quality and endometrial receptivity, the third variable determining the chances of implantation is the efficiency of the embryo transfer technique.[126] A Cochrane database review of 21 studies that incorporated data from 6,218 women, compared the outcomes using ultrasound guidance for embryo transfers versus clinical touch. They found that a live birth rate of 23% with clinical touch could be increased to 28% to 33% by adding ultrasound guidance during the transfer.[127] A trial embryo transfer should ideally be performed before transferring the embryos preferably in all patients, but especially for those with a history of a difficult transfer in the past. While this factor alone may not independently cause RIF, it does impact the outcomes and should be considered.

NOVEL THERAPIES

Low Molecular Weight Heparin

Heparin is postulated to aid the process of implantation by multiple direct effects on the blastocyst as well as the endometrium, apart from its anticoagulant effects. Its benefits in cases of acquired and inherited thrombophilias are well documented. Due to this reason, it has been attempted empirically in patients with RIF without thrombophilia as well. Recently, Khalife et al. performed a review to study the effect of heparin on the physiologic process of implantation and its use as an adjuvant treatment in patients with RIF with or without the presence of thrombophilia. They found that the evidence on the efficacy of heparin is conflicting due to the lack of knowledge and considerable heterogeneity in the studies. Further studies and larger RCTs are needed, as heparin appears to play a promising role in enhancing success rates in women with RIF. Based on current evidence, the use of low molecular weight heparin (LMWH) cannot be recommended as empirical treatment in all RIF patients. Indeed several studies have documented its benefit in a subset of patients who suffer from a thrombophilia mutation, thus the group of patients that might benefit needs to be identified.[128]

Intravenous Immunoglobulin

Intravenous immunoglobulin (IVIG) is a fat emulsion containing an immunoglobulin G antibody that promotes differential cell receptor expression, reduces natural killer (NK) cell activity, and regulates the T helper cell type 1/T helper cell type 2 (Th1/Th2) responses by increasing Th2 cell production, which is beneficial for clinical pregnancy. However, IVIG and immunologic tests are expensive interventions, the optimal protocol for the administration of IVIG is undefined and the overall benefits of IVIG are still controversial.

Intralipid Infusion

Intralipid infusion is a 20% fat emulsion that reduces the Th1/Th2 ratio and suppresses the abnormal NK cytotoxicity of peripheral NK cells, thereby increasing the likelihood of implantation and clinical pregnancy. Further studies are needed to determine the efficacy of intralipid infusion in women with RIF.

Co-culture

The IVF laboratory attempts to replicate in vivo culture conditions for optimal development of embryos, and yet many aspects of their growth and biochemical synthetic activity are poorly understood causing them to lag behind at times. In order to create a more supportive culture condition, co-culture of embryos with tubal epithelium, endometrial epithelium, granulosa or cumulus cells has been proposed.[129-132] Tubal cells have been obtained during hysterectomies or tubal ligations and harvested for this purpose.[129] Significant improvement in embryo quality was seen using this technique. Barmat Li et al. have developed a co-culture system where the patient's own endometrial cells are obtained by a midluteal phase biopsy in the preceding month. Glandular epithelial and stromal cells extracted from these specimens are added in equal measure to four-well tissue plates. The embryos are transferred to this system after fertilization and cultured in it till the day of transfer. The potential benefit seems to arise from the physiology of the complex crosstalk between the embryo and the endometrium that takes place in vivo, aiding in the process of implantation.[133] This technique was first described in 1995 by Jayot et al. who found a pregnancy rate of 21% as compared to 8% in previous cycles.[134] Nieto et al. found reduced fragmentation in cleavage stage embryos using autologous endometrial co-culture.[130] Simon et al. used this technique in 168 cycles of women with three or more previous failed transfers, and managed to achieve a 39.2% blastulation rate, 11.8% implantation rate, and 20.2% pregnancy rate.[135,136] Kattal et al. performed a meta-analysis of 17 studies and found significantly improved blastomere numbers, implantation, and pregnancy rates in cycles where co-culture systems were used. In spite of having proven benefits, co-culture is not universally practiced as it is time consuming and requires additional skills. At the same time, the development of better incubators and techniques such as culture at low oxygen tensions have shown promising results too, and may be preferred by laboratories in lieu of more demanding techniques like co-culture.

THIRD PARTY REPRODUCTION—DONOR GAMETES AND SURROGACY

Counseling plays a very important role while handling couples with RIF. They need to be dealt with a lot of empathy and proper guidance on the appropriateness of proceeding with several IVF attempts. If implantation fails to occur despite repeated treatment or if the prognosis of further IVF treatment is considered poor, alternative treatment options need to be discussed. If the likely source of the problem lies with the embryo, gamete donation needs to be considered. On the other hand, if the problem lies in the uterus, which has failed to respond to various treatment modalities available, surrogacy may be a better option.

CONCLUSION

Recurrent implantation failure is one of the most challenging and frustrating situations in the field of ART. Although repeated failures can be equally disappointing for clinician and patients alike, newer diagnostic techniques and therapies to improve the chances of success in this subset of patients continue to emerge. Chromosomal aneuploidies and suboptimal embryo development may play a major role. Optimal culture conditions and blastocyst transfer may result in better implantation and pregnancy rates. Emerging technologies, such as MACS or IMSI for better sperm selection and PGS for embryonic chromosomal aneuploidies may enable more comprehensive screening of embryos and better selection of the embryos with greatest implantation potential for transfer. Anatomical malformations or acquired uterine and tubal pathologies need to be identified and treated by operative laparoscopy where indicated, before proceeding with embryo transfer. A deeper understanding of not just the endometrial morphology but also its receptivity and therapies that may aid the implantation process is likely to lead to further improvement of success rates.

The safety, efficacy, and practicality of new emerging methods of treatment should be evaluated in prospective randomized clinical trials before being accepted into regular clinical practice.

REFERENCES

1. Society for Assisted Reproductive Technology. (2015). National Summary Report. [online] Available from https://www.sartcorsonline.com/rptCSR_PublicMultYear.aspx?ClinicPKID=0 [Last accessed February, 2019].
2. Orvieto R, Brengauz M, Feldman B. A novel approach to normal responder patient with repeated implantation failures—a case report. Gynecol Endocrinol. 2015;31(6):435-7.

3. Zeyneloglu HB, Onalan G. Remedies for recurrent implantation failure. Semin Reprod Med. 2014;32(4):297-305.
4. Rinehart J. Recurrent implantation failure: definition. J Assist Reprod Genet. 2007;24(7):284-7.
5. Coughlan C, Ledger W, Wang Q, et al. Recurrent implantation failure: definition and management. Reprod Bio Med Online. 2014;28(1):14-38.
6. Stern C, Pertile M, Norris H, et al. Chromosome translocations in couples with in-vitro fertilization implantation failure. Hum Reprod. 1999;14:2097-101.
7. Raziel A, Friedler S, Schachter M, et al. Increased frequency of female partner chromosomal abnormalities in patients with high-order implantation failure after in vitro fertilization. Fertil Steril. 2002;78:515-9.
8. Crosignani PG, Rubin BL. Genetic Control of Gamete Production and Function. New: York: Academic Press; 1982.
9. Campana M, Serra A, Neri G. Role of chromosome aberrations in recurrent abortion: a study of 269 balanced translocations. Am J Med Genet. 1986;24:341-56.
10. Plachot M. Chromosome analysis of oocytes and embryos. In: Verlinsky V, Kuliev A (Eds). Preimplantation Genetics. Boston, MA: Springer; 1991.
11. Franasiak JM, Forman EJ, Hong KH, et al. The nature of aneuploidy with increasing age of the female partner: A review of 15,169 consecutive throphectoderm biopsies evaluated with comprehensive chromosomal screening. Fertil Steril. 2014;101:656-63.e1.
12. Pehlivan T, Rubio C, Rodrigo L, et al. Impact of preimplantation genetic diagnosis on IVF outcome in implantation failure patients. Reprod Biomed Online. 2003;6:232-7.
13. Gianaroli L, Magli MC, Ferraretti AP, et al. Will preimplantation genetic diagnosis assist patients with a poor prognosis to achieve pregnancy? Hum Reprod. 1997;12:1762-7.
14. Gianaroli L, Magli MC, Ferraretti AP, et al. Preimplantation diagnosis for aneuploidies in patients undergoing in vitro fertilization with a poor prognosis: Identification of the categories for which it should be proposed. Fertil Steril. 1999;72:837-44.
15. Blockeel C, Schutyser V, De Vos A, et al. Prospectively randomized controlled trial of PGS in IVF/ICSI patients with poor implantation. Reprod Biomed Online. 2008;17:848-54.
16. Mastenbroek S, Twisk M, van der Veen F, et al. Preimplantation genetic screening: A systematic review and meta-analysis of RCTs. Hum Reprod Update. 2011;17:454-66.
17. Treff NR, Scott RT Jr. Methods for comprehensive chromosome screening of oocytes and embryos: Capabilities, limitations and evidence of validity. J Assist Reprod Genet. 2012;29:381-90.
18. Treff NR, Levy B, Su J, et al. SNP microarray-based 24 chromosome aneuploidy screening is significantly more consistent than FISH. Mol Hum Reprod. 2010;16:583-9.
19. Northrop LE, Treff NR, Levy B, et al. SNP microarray-based 24 chromosome aneuploidy screening demonstrates that cleavage stage FISH poorly predicts aneuploidy in embryos that develop to morphologically normal blastocysts. Mol Hum Reprod. 2010;16:590-600.
20. Fragouli E, Katz-Jaffe M, Alfarawati S, et al. Comprehensive chromosome screening of polar bodies and blastocysts from couples experiencing repeated implantation failure. Fertil Steril. 2010;94:875-87.
21. Lee HL, McCulloh DH, Hodes-Wertz B, et al. In vitro fertilization with preimplantation genetic screening improves implantation and live birth in women age 40 through 43. J Assist Reprod Genet. 2015;32:435-44.
22. Burrello N, Vicari E, Shin P, et al. Lower sperm aneuploidy frequency is associated with high pregnancy rates in ICSI programmes. Hum Reprod. 2003;18:1371-6.
23. Robinson L, Gallos ID, Conner SJ, et al. The effect of sperm DNA fragmentation on miscarriage rates: A systematic review and meta-analysis. Hum Reprod. 2012;27:2908-17.
24. Evenson DP, Larson KL, Jost LK. Sperm chromatin structure assay: Its clinical use for detecting sperm DNA fragmentation in male infertility and comparisons with other techniques. J Androl. 2002;23:25-43.
25. Bungum M, Humaidan P, Spano M, et al. The predictive value of sperm chromatin structure assay (SCSA) parameters for the outcome of intrauterine insemination, IVF and ICSI. Hum Reprod. 2004;19:1401-8.
26. Bungum M, Humaidan P, Axmon A, et al. Sperm DNA integrity assessment in prediction of assisted reproductive technology outcome. Hum Reprod. 2007;22:174-9.
27. Duran EH, Morshedi M, Taylor S, et al. Sperm DNA quality predicts intrauterine insemination outcome: A prospective cohort study. Hum Reprod. 2002;17:3122-8.
28. Muriel L, Meseguer M, Fernández JL, et al. Value of the sperm chromatin dispersion test in predicting pregnancy outcome in intrauterine insemination: A blind prospective study. Hum Reprod. 2006;21:738-44.
29. Greco E, Scarselli F, Iacobelli M, et al. Efficient treatment of infertility due to sperm DNA damage by ICSI with testicular spermatozoa. Hum Reprod. 2005;20:226-30.
30. Steele EK, McClure N, Maxwell RJ, et al. A comparison of DNA damage in testicular and proximal epididymal spermatozoa in obstructive azoospermia. Mol Hum Reprod. 1999;5:831-5.
31. Suganuma R, Yanagimachi R, Meistrich ML. Decline in fertility of mouse sperm with abnormal chromatin during epididymal passage as revealed by ICSI. Hum Reprod. 2005;0:3101-8.
32. Weissman A, Horowitz E, Ravhon A, et al. Pregnancies and live births following ICSI with testicular spermatozoa after repeated implantation failure using ejaculated spermatozoa. Reprod Biomed Online. 2008;17:605-9.
33. Jakab A, Sakkas D, Delpiano E, et al. Intracytoplasmic sperm injection: A novel selection method for sperm with normal frequency of chromosomal aneuploidies. Fertil Steril. 2005;84:1665-73.
34. Said TM, Grunewald S, Paasch U, et al. Advantage of combining magnetic cell separation with sperm preparation techniques. Reprod Biomed Online. 2005;10:740-6.
35. Sakkas D, Alvarez JG. Sperm DNA fragmentation: Mechanisms of origin, impact on reproductive outcome, and analysis. Fertil Steril. 2010;93:1027-36.
36. Bartoov B, Berkovitz A, Eltes F, et al. Pregnancy rates are higher with intracytoplasmic morphologically selected sperm injection than with conventional intracytoplasmic injection. Fertil Steril. 2003;80:1413-9.
37. Vermes I, Haanen C, Steffens-Nakken H, et al. A novel assay for apoptosis. Flow cytometric detection of phosphatidylserine

expression on early apoptotic cells using fluorescein labelled Annexin V. J Immunol Methods. 1995;184(1):39-51.
38. Romany L, Garrido N, Fernandez JL, et al. 28th Annual Meeting of the European Society on Human Reproduction and Embryology (ESHRE) Assisted reproduction results improvements due to magnetic activated cell sorting (MACS) depletion of apoptotic sperm is not mediated by sperm DNA fragmentation decrease. Hum Reprod. 2012; 27(suppl 2):ii121-50.
39. Gil M, Sar-Shalom V, Sivira YM, et al. Sperm selection using magnetic activated cell sorting (MACS) in assisted reproduction: a systematic review and meta-analysis. J Assist Reprod Genet. 2013;30(4):479-85.
40. Berkovitz A, Eltes F, Lederman H, et al. How to improve IVF-ICSI outcome by sperm selection. Reprod Biomed Online. 2006;12:634-8.
41. Nadalini M, Tarozzi N, Distratis V, et al. Impact of intracytoplasmic morphologically selected sperm injection on assisted reproduction outcome: A review. Reprod Biomed Online. 2009;19(3):45-55.
42. Oliveira JB, Cavagna M, Petersen CG, et al. Pregnancy outcomes in women with repeated implantation failures after intracytoplasmic morphologically selected sperm injection (IMSI). Reprod Biol Endocrinol. 2011;9:99.
43. Franco JG Jr, Baruffi RL, Mauri AL, et al. Significance of large nuclear vacuoles in human spermatozoa: Implications for ICSI. Reprod Biomed Online. 2008;17:42-5.
44. Oliveira JB, Massaro FC, Baruffi RL, et al. Correlation between semen analysis by motile sperm organelle morphology examination and sperm DNA damage. Fertil Steril. 2010; 94:1937-40.
45. Perdrix A, Travers A, Chelli MH, et al. Assessment of acrosome and nuclear abnormalities in human spermatozoa with large vacuoles. Hum Reprod. 2011;26:47-58.
46. Boitrelle F, Ferfouri F, Petit JM, et al. Large human sperm vacuoles observed in motile spermatozoa under high magnification: Nuclear thumbprints linked to failure of chromatin condensation. Hum Reprod. 2011;26:1650-8.
47. El Khattabi L, Dupont C, Sermondade N, et al. Is intracytoplasmic morphologically selected sperm injection effective in patients with infertility related to teratozoospermia or repeated implantation failure? Fertil Steril. 2013;100:62-8.
48. Telford NA, Watson AJ, Schultz GA. Transition from maternal to embryonic control in early mammalian development: A comparison of several species. Mol Reprod Dev. 1990;26: 90-100.
49. De Vos A, Van Steirteghem A. Zona hardening, zona drilling and assisted hatching: New achievements in assisted reproduction. Cells Tissues Organs. 2000;166:220-7.
50. Fehilly CB, Cohen J, Simons RF, et al. Cryopreservation of cleaving embryos and expanded blastocysts in the human: A comparative study. Fertil Steril. 1985;44:638-44.
51. Cohen J, Inge KL, Suzman M, et al. Videocinematography of fresh and cryopreserved embryos: A retrospective analysis of embryonic morphology and implantation. Fertil Steril. 1989;51:820-7.
52. Malter HE, Cohen J. Blastocyst formation and hatching in vitro following zona drilling of mouse and human embryos. Gamete Res. 1989;24:67-80.
53. Cohen J. Assisted hatching of human embryos. J In Vitro Fert Embryo Transf. 1991;8:179-90.
54. Cohen J, Alikani M, Trowbridge J, et al. Implantation enhancement by selective assisted hatching using zona drilling of human embryos with poor prognosis. Hum Reprod. 1992;7:685-91.
55. Khalifa EA, Tucker MJ, Hunt P. Cruciate thinning of the zona pellucida for more successful enhancement of blastocyst hatching in the mouse. Hum Reprod. 1992;7: 532-6.
56. Fong CY, Bongso A, Ng SC, et al. Blastocyst transfer after enzymatic treatment of the zona pellucida: Improving in-vitro fertilization and understanding implantation. Hum Reprod. 1998;13:2926-32.
57. Valojerdi MR, Eftekhari-Yazdi P, Karimian L, et al. Effect of laser zona pellucida opening on clinical outcome of assisted reproduction technology in patients with advanced female age, recurrent implantation failure, or frozen-thawed embryos. Fertil Steril. 2008;90:84-91.
58. Laufer N, Palanker D, Shufaro Y, et al. The efficacy and safety of zona pellucida drilling by a 193-nm excimer laser. Fertil Steril. 1993;59:889-95.
59. Nakayama T, Fujiwara H, Yamada S, et al. Clinical application of a new assisted hatching method using a piezo-micromanipulator for morphologically low-quality embryos in poor-prognosis infertile patients. Fertil Steril. 1999;71: 1014-8.
60. Hershlag A, Feng HL. Effect of pre-freeze assisted hatching on post-thaw survival of mouse embryos. Fertil Steril. 2005;84:1752-4.
61. Antinori S, Selman HA, Caffa B, et al. Zona opening of human embryos using a non-contact UV laser for assisted hatching in patients with poor prognosis of pregnancy. Hum Reprod. 1996;11:2488-92.
62. Chao KH, Chen SU, Chen HF, et al. Assisted hatching increases the implantation and pregnancy rate of in vitro fertilization (IVF)-embryo transfer (ET), but not that of IVF-tubal ET in patients with repeated IVF failures. Fertil Steril. 1997;67:904-8.
63. Martins WP, Rocha IA, Ferriani RA, et al. Assisted hatching of human embryos: A systematic review and meta-analysis of randomized controlled trials. Hum Reprod Update. 2011;17:438-53.
64. Carney SK, Das S, Blake D, et al. Assisted hatching on assisted conception (in vitro fertilization (IVF) and intracytoplasmic sperm injection (ICSI)). Cochrane Database Syst Rev. 2012;12:CD001894.
65. National Institute for Health and Care Excellence. (2017) Fertility problems: assessment and treatment. [online] Available from https://www.nice.org.uk/guidance/CG156 [Last accessed February, 2019].
66. Makrakis E, Pantos K. The outcomes of hysteroscopy in women with implantation failures after in-vitro fertilization: Findings and effect on subsequent pregnancy rates. Curr Opin Obstet Gynecol. 2010;22:339-43.
67. Richlin SS, Ramachandran S, Shanti A, et al. Glycodelin levels in uterine flushings and in plasma of patients with leiomyomas and polyps: Implications for implantation. Hum Reprod. 2002;17:2742-7.

68. Shokeir TA, Shalan HM, El-Shafei MM. Significance of endometrial polyps detected hysteroscopically in eumenorrheic infertile women. J Obstet Gynaecol Res. 2004;30:84-9.
69. Spiewankiewicz B, Stelmachów J, Sawicki W, et al. The effectiveness of hysteroscopic polypectomy in cases of female infertility. Clin Exp Obstet Gynecol. 2003;30:23-5.
70. Varasteh NN, Neuwirth RS, Levin B, et al. Pregnancy rates after hysteroscopic polypectomy and myomectomy in infertile women. Obstet Gynecol. 1999;94:168-71.
71. Perez-Medina T, Bajo-Arenas J, Salazar F, et al. Endometrial polyps and their implication in the pregnancy rates of patients undergoing intrauterine insemination: A prospective, randomized study. Hum Reprod. 2005;20:1632-5.
72. Buttram VC Jr, Reiter RC. Uterine leiomyomata: Etiology, symptomatology, and management. Fertil Steril. 1981;36:433-45.
73. Donnez J, Jadoul P. What are the implications of myomas on fertility? A need for a debate? Hum Reprod. 2002;17:1424-30.
74. Taylor E, Gomel V. The uterus and fertility. Fertil Steril. 2008;89:1-16.
75. Metwally M, Farquhar CM, Li TC. Is another meta-analysis on the effects of intramural fibroids on reproductive outcomes needed? Reprod Biomed Online. 2011;23:2-14.
76. Pritts EA, Parker WH, Olive DL. Fibroids and infertility: An updated systematic review of the evidence. Fertil Steril. 2009;91:1215-23.
77. Eldar-Geva T, Meagher S, Healy DL, et al. Effect of intramural, subserous, and submucosal uterine fibroids on the outcome of assisted reproductive technology treatment. Fertil Steril. 1998;70(4):687-91.
78. Sunkara SK, Khairy M, El-Toukhy T, et al. The effect of intramural fibroids without uterine cavity involvement on the outcome of IVF treatment: A systematic review and meta-analysis. Hum Reprod. 2010;25:418-29.
79. Fedele L, Arcaini L, Parazzini F, et al. Reproductive prognosis after hysteroscopic metroplasty in 102 women: life-table analysis. Fertil Steril. 1993;59(4):768-72.
80. Pabuccu R, Gomel V. Reproductive outcome after hysteroscopic metroplasty in women with septate uterus and otherwise unexplained infertility. Fertil Steril. 2004;81(6):1675-8.
81. Grimbizis GF, Camus M, Tarlatzis BC, et al. Clinical implications of uterine malformations and hysteroscopic treatment results. Hum Reprod Update. 2001;7(2):161-74.
82. Tremellen K, Russell P. Adenomyosis is a potential cause of recurrent implantation failure during IVF treatment. Aust NZ J Obstet Gynaecol. 2011;51:280-3.
83. Ascher SM, Arnold LL, Patt RH, et al. Adenomyosis: Prospective comparison of MR imaging and transvaginal sonography. Radiology. 1994;190(3):803-6.
84. Atzori E, Tronci C, Sionis L. Transvaginal ultrasound in the diagnosis of diffuse adenomyosis. Gynecol Obstet Invest.1996;42:39-41.
85. Bazot M, Darai E, Rouger J, et al. Limitations of transvaginal sonography for the diagnosis of adenomyosis, with histopathological correlation. Ultrasound Obstet Gynecol. 2002;20(6):605-11.
86. Bromley B, Shipp TD, Benacerraf B. Adenomyosis: Sonographic findings and diagnostic accuracy. J Ultrasound Med. 2000;19(8):529-34.
87. Reinhold C, McCarthy S, Bret PM, et al. Diffuse adenomyosis: comparison of endovaginal US and MR imaging with histopathologic correlation. Radiology. 1996;199(1):151-8.
88. Maheshwari A, Gurunath S, Fatima F, et al. Adenomyosis and subfertility: A systematic review of prevalence, diagnosis, treatment and fertility outcomes. Hum Reprod Update. 2012;18:374-92.
89. Sunkara SK, Khan KS. Adenomyosis and female fertility: A critical review of the evidence. J Obstet Gynaecol. 2012;32:113-6.
90. Demirol A, Gurgan T. Effect of treatment of intrauterine pathologies with office hysteroscopy in patients with recurrent IVF failure. Reprod Biomed Online. 2004;8(5):590-4.
91. Dawood A, Al-Talib A, Tulandi T. Predisposing factors and treatment outcome of different stages of intrauterine adhesions. J Obstet Gynaecol Can. 2010;32(8):767-70.
92. Katz Z, Ben-Arie A, Lurie S, et al. Reproductive outcome following hysteroscopic adhesiolysis in Asherman's syndrome. Int J Fertil Menopausal Stud. 1996;41(5):462-5.
93. Yasmin H, Nasir A, Noorani KJ. Hysteroscopic management of Ashermans syndrome. J Pak Med Assoc. 2007;57(11):553-5.
94. Finn CA, Pope M. Vascular and cellular changes in the decidualized endometrium of the ovariectomized mouse following cessation of hormone treatment: A possible model for menstruation. J Endocrinol. 1984;100:295-300.
95. Gnainsky Y, Granot I, Aldo PB, et al. Local injury of the endometrium induces an inflammatory response that promotes successful implantation. Fertil Steril. 2010;94:2030-6.
96. Barash A, Dekel N, Fieldust S, et al. Local injury to the endometrium doubles the incidence of successful pregnancies in patients undergoing in vitro fertilization. Fertil Steril. 2003;79:1317-22.
97. Karimzadeh MA, Ayazi Rozbahani M, Tabibnejad N. Endometrial local injury improves the pregnancy rate among recurrent implantation failure patients undergoing in vitro fertilization/intra cytoplasmic sperm injection: A randomised clinical trial. Aust NZ J Obstet Gynaecol. 2009;49:677-80.
98. Narvekar SA, Gupta N, Shetty N, et al. Does local endometrial injury in the nontransfer cycle improve the IVF-ET outcome in the subsequent cycle in patients with previous unsuccessful IVF? A randomised controlled pilot study. J Hum Reprod Sci. 2010;3:15-9.
99. Baum M, Yerushalmi GM, Maman E, et al. Does local injury to the endometrium before IVF cycle really affect treatment outcome? Results of a randomized placebo controlled trial. Gynecol Endocrinol. 2012;28:933-6.
100. Yeung TW, Chai J, Li RH, et al. The effect of endometrial injury on ongoing pregnancy rate in unselected subfertile women undergoing in vitro fertilization: A randomized controlled trial. Hum Reprod. 2014;29:2474-81.
101. Simon C, Beliver J. Scratching beneath 'The Scratching Case': Systematic reviews and meta-analyses, the back door for evidence based medicine. Hum Reprod. 2014;29:1618-21.
102. Strandell A, Waldenstrom U, Nilsson L, et al. Hydrosalpinx reduces in-vitro fertilization/embryo transfer pregnancy rates. Hum Reprod. 1994;9:861-3.
103. Feghali J, Bakar J, Mayenga JM, et al. Systematic hysteroscopy prior to in vitro fertilization. Gynecol Obstet Fertil. 2003;31:127-31.

104. Johnston-MacAnanny EB, Hartnett J, Engmann LL, et al. Chronic endometritis is a frequent finding in women with recurrent implantation failure after in vitro fertilization. Fertil Steril. 2010;93:437-41.
105. Cicinelli E, Matteo M, Tinelli R, et al. Prevalence of chronic endometritis in repeated unexplained implantation failure and the IVF success rate after antibiotic therapy. Hum Reprod. 2015;30:323-30.
106. Diaz-Gimeno P, Horcajadas JA, Martínez-Conejero JA, et al. A genomic diagnostic tool for human endometrial receptivity based on the transcriptomic signature. Fertil Steril. 2011;95:50-60.
107. Diaz-Gimeno P, Ruiz-Alonso M, Blesa D, et al. The accuracy and reproducibility of the endometrial receptivity array is superior to histology as a diagnostic method for endometrial receptivity. Fertil Steril. 2013;99:508-17.
108. Ruiz-Alonso M, Blesa D, Díaz-Gimeno P, et al. The endometrial receptivity array for diagnosis and personalised embryo transfer as a treatment for patients with repeated implantation failure. Fertil Steril. 2013;100:818-24.
109. Birkenfeld A, Mukaida T, Minichiello L, et al. Incidence of autoimmune antibodies in failed embryo transfer cycles. Am J Reprod Immunol. 1994;31:65-8.
110. Coulam C, Kaider B, Kaider AS, et al. Antiphospholipid antibodies associated with implantation failure after IVF-ET. J Assist Reprod Genet. 1997;14:603-6.
111. Kaider BD, Price DE, Roussev RG, et al. Antiphospholipid antibody prevalence in patients with IVF failure. Am J Reprod Immunol. 1996;35:388-93.
112. Qublan HS, Eid SS, Ababneh HA, et al. Acquired and inherited thrombophilia: implication in recurrent IVF and embryo transfer failure. Hum Reprod. 2006;21(10):2694-8.
113. Hill JA, Scott RT. Immunologic tests and IVF: 'Please, enough already'. Fertil Steril. 2000;74:439-42.
114. Hornstein MD, Davis OK, Massey JB, et al. Antiphospholipid antibodies and in vitro fertilization success: a meta-analysis. Fertil Steril. 2000;73(2):330-3.
115. Azem F, Many A, Ben Ami I, et al. Increased rates of thrombophilia in women with repeated IVF failures. Hum Reprod. 2004;19(2):368-70.
116. Martinelli I, Taioli E, Ragni G, et al. Embryo implantation after assisted reproductive procedures and maternal thrombophilia. Haematologica. 2003;88(7):789-93.
117. Simur A, Ozdemir S, Acar H, et al. Repeated in vitro fertilization failure and its relation with thrombophilia. Gynecol Obstet Invest. 2009;67(2):109-12.
118. Blois SM, Klapp BF, Barrientos G. Decidualization and angiogenesis in early pregnancy: unravelling the functions of DC and NK cells. J Reprod Immunol. 2011;88(2):86-92.
119. Clark DA, Coulam CB, Stricker RB. Is intravenous immunoglobulins (IVIG) efficacious in early pregnancy failure? A critical review and meta-analysis for patients who fail in vitro fertilization and embryo transfer (IVF). J Assist Reprod Genet. 2006;23(1):1-13.
120. Stephenson MD, Fluker MR. Treatment of repeated unexplained in vitro fertilization failure with intravenous immunoglobulin: a randomized, placebo-controlled Canadian trial. Fertil Steril. 2000;74(6):1108-13.
121. Camus E, Poncelet C, Goffinet F, et al. Pregnancy rates after in-vitro fertilization in cases of tubal infertility with and without hydrosalpinx: A meta-analysis of published comparative studies. Hum Reprod. 1999;14:1243-9.
122. Strandell A, Lindhard A, Waldenström U, et al. Hydrosalpinx and IVF outcome: A prospective, randomized multicentre trial in Scandinavia on salpingectomy prior to IVF. Hum Reprod. 1994;14:2762-9.
123. Zeyneloglu HB, Arici A, Olive DL. Adverse effects of hydrosalpinx on pregnancy rates after in vitro fertilization-embryo transfer. Fertil Steril. 1998;70:492-9.
124. Seli E, Kayisli UA, Cakmak H, et al. Removal of hydrosalpinges increases endometrial leukaemia inhibitory factor (LIF) expression at the time of the implantation window. Hum Reprod. 2005;20:3012-7.
125. Bildirici I, Bukulmez O, Ensari A, et al. A prospective evaluation of the effect of salpingectomy on endometrial receptivity in cases of women with communicating hydrosalpinges. Hum Reprod. 2001;16:2422-6.
126. Paulson RJ, Sauer MV, Lobo RA. Factors affecting embryo implantation after human in vitro fertilisation: a hypothesis. Am J Obstet Gynecol. 1990;163:2020-3.
127. Brown J, Buckingham K, Buckett W, et al. Ultrasound versus 'clinical touch' for catheter guidance during embryo transfer in women. Cochrane Database Syst Rev. 2016;3:CD006107.
128. Khalife D, Ghaziri G. Recurrent implantation failure and low molecular weight heparin. Open J Obstet Gynecol. 2018;8(2):146-62.
129. Yeung WS, Lau EY, Chan ST, et al. Co-culture with homologous oviductal cells improved the implantation of human embryos—A prospective randomized controlled trial. J Assist Reprod Genet. 1996;13:762-7.
130. Nieto FS, Watkins WB, Lopata A, et al. The effects of coculture with autologous cryopreserved endometrial cells on human in vitro fertilization and early embryo morphology: A randomized study. J Assist Reprod Genet. 1996;13:386-9.
131. Plachot M, Antoine JM, Alvarez S, et al. Granulosa cells improve human embryo development in vitro. Hum Reprod. 1993;8:2133-40.
132. Quinn P, Margalit R. Beneficial effects of coculture with cumulus cells on blastocyst formation in a prospective trial with supernumerary human embryos. J Assist Reprod Genet. 1996;13:9-14.
133. Cross JC, Werb Z, Fisher SJ. Implantation and the placenta: Key pieces of the development puzzle. Science. 1994;266:1508-18.
134. Jayot S, Parneix I, Verdagner S, et al. Coculture of embryos on homologous endometrial cells in patients with repeated failures of implantation. Fertil Steril. 1995;63:109-14.
135. Simón C1, Mercader A, Garcia-Velasco J, et al. Coculture of human embryos with autologous human endometrial epithelial cells in patients with implantation failure. J Clin Endocrinol Metab. 1999;84:2638-46.
136. Kattal N, Cohen J, Barmat LI. Role of coculture in human in vitro fertilization: A meta-analysis. Fertil Steril. 2008;90:1069-76.

Setting of an ART Laboratory

39

Rajul Tyagi, Meenu Handa, Sunita Arora, Kalyani Bade

INTRODUCTION

The assisted reproductive technology (ART) laboratory forms the most integral part of fertility practice. Before setting up the ART laboratory we must know the amount of patient load expected. Laboratory design and the equipment are taken depending upon the expected foot fall. At the same time we should consider space for the future expansion of the laboratory. Equipment and consumables used in in vitro fertilization (IVF) laboratory are an important component in setting up IVF laboratory for any fertility clinic. Provision of an optimal environment for the gametes and embryos is essential, but at the same time we have to keep in mind to provide a good working environment to the embryologist.

DESIGNING THE IN VITRO FERTILIZATION LABORATORY

The design of laboratory should consider the adjacent operation theater where ovum pickup will be done so both of them together form a single unit. Laboratory must have provision for an air handing unit. The importance of clean air free of volatile organic compound (VOC) cannot be over emphasized. In this regard, one can seek guidance from clean room experts and eliminate VOCs and chemical air contaminants (CACs) in the laboratory.[1] Structural design means details like layout of the laboratory and exact specifications with regards to the bench height, flooring, wall paint, and lighting. Design should be such that the ambient air quality must be optimum for procedures.

ASSISTED REPRODUCTIVE TECHNOLOGY LABORATORY LAYOUT

The layout should be planned and designed in such a way that it allows smooth running of routine procedures. The main laboratory consists of areas allotted for oocyte and embryo culture and a separate room for sperm preparation. Each workstation should contain a laminar flow hood, incubator, centrifuge machine, and microscope to prevent unnecessary movement of staff in the laboratory during procedures. It also decides the type of a laminar air flow unit which is based on quality of air present. A good high-efficiency particulate air (HEPA) filtration in the heating, ventilation, and air-conditioning (HVAC) can sometimes overcome the need for a laminar air flow unit. However, the need for laminar air flow unit in a certified cleanroom design makes it necessary. Separate areas will be needed for cryopreservation, record keeping, and for storage of consumables. Then coming to further design there are two possibilities. A situation where load is less and space is limited, the two rooms can be connected by a window for passing oocytes and embryos. In the other situation were there is no space constraint one can have a door between the operating room and the culture room and this allows a circulating operation theatre (OT) technician to carry follicular aspirates directly into the laboratory during the egg retrieval procedure. It also allows the embryologist to pass the embryo transfer catheter directly to the clinician for the embryo transfer procedure. The window maximizes space utilization and minimizes mixing of air between two rooms. This works well except in the situation where afterloading technique of catheter loading is used.[2,3]

The environmental lighting and air-conditioning must be adequate with proper humidity and temperature control.

Other Details

- Laboratory should be designed according to the flow of work. The place for the equipment should be marked considering the requirement of its use, like the nearest equipment to the pass window should be the laminar flow.
- The material of the inner lining of the room, flooring, and furniture should be such so as to emit minimal VOC.
- Laboratory should have preferably biometric lock so that only authorized personals are allowed. It also helps to check the timing of the duty staff.
- Changing room must be separate from the IVF laboratory.
- Facilities for washing hands should be available outside the laboratory.
- The area for cleaning and serialization should be separate from the laboratory.

The Room

In India where climate is hot and humid, it is better to avoid basement area for construction of IVF laboratory. Construction of the laboratory must be done using materials which are safe for the gametes and/or embryo viability. So it is important to select construction material for building the laboratory. Aim is to avoid materials that will release VOC gases, which are toxic for embryos. Laboratory validation is compulsory after completion of laboratory.

For flooring purpose choice is seamless sheet vinyl, which extends about 4 inches on the wall and the joint of floor and the walls, is rounded. Where pieces of flooring meet, the seam is sealed. Cleaning vinyl is easier than tile flooring and it prevents water seepage under the walls. Material of choice for walls is stainless steel since it is odorless, washable, and does not shed. Another options are plaster and plastic wallboard.

Ceiling again can be made of stainless steel in tile form, the joints are sealed to make it air tight and smooth surfaced. Air supply ducts with HEPA filters are placed in the ceiling and sealed. Most lights used in the ceiling are of short wavelength (470–480 nm), can be harmful to cell culture and embryo culture,[4-7] the light emitted from the microscopes may also be harmful, hence should be avoided.[6] Use of incandescent light bulbs or fluorescent lights with ultraviolet (UV) sleeve protection is recommended.[2]

Other Requirements in Laboratory

Laboratory will also need a gas storage room, a small conference room, at the same time special attention will have to be paid to the electrical, plumbing, and alarm systems.

Conference Room

It is preferred to have a conference room which can used to discuss the day-to-day problems of the laboratory with laboratory staff and also for class.

Gas Storage Room

This is the place where gas cylinders are stored. Present day incubators use triple gas mixtures which is supplied in premixed form and also mixtures can be prepared in required form by taking gases from different cylinders which is the preferred method. Besides this, there will also need for oxygen and nitrous for anesthesia purposes. Cylinders are heavy so this room can be far away from the laboratory from where cylinders can be transported in and out without much difficulty. One of the biggest benefits of building up a new IVF laboratory is to be able to give gas outlets throughout the laboratory for incubators and gassing devices.[8]

Plumbing System

The gases from the gas storage room are brought to the culture room in different pipe lines, CO_2 and N_2 should be placed near the incubators. With the advent of incubators that use premixed gas, the gas line should also be placed at each port.[9] Smaller laboratories may find this a costly affair, but the potential benefits outweigh the cost as it prevents contamination.

The gas storage room needs an oxygen alarm and automatic switching stainless steel gas panels. Number of couplings per panel per gas will depend on the number of incubators used, but normally it is two tanks per side. Stainless steel lines or copper lines can be used.[3]

Electrical System

Power system to the laboratory should be able to supply an uninterrupted power supply without any power surges or other fluctuations which my damage the equipment. It is better to have an online uninterruptible power supply (UPS) of a capacity calculated for the power load of lab. There will also be need for backup generators.

Alarm System

It is again *must have* for a good IVF laboratory. There must be a system that flashes a prompt notification in case of a device failure. There are alarm devices which send automatic notifications on cell phone, choice of the system can be tailored according to the needs of the laboratory.

Laboratory Air Quality

- Positive pressure is recommended for the laboratory to minimize air contamination.
- All the air coming to the laboratory should get filtered in a HEPA and VOC control system.
- Procedures which involve gamete or embryo manipulation must be performed in a controlled environment.
- National guidelines must be complied with to maintain air quality and regular monitoring should be done, processing of tissue and cell must be performed in a good manufacturing practice (GMP) Grade A environment. However, if it is detrimental or not feasible to carry out a specific procedure in a Grade A environment, it can be performed in at least a Grade D environment.[10]

Laboratory Equipment

- First of all, all equipment used in the laboratory should be calibrated and validated before it is put to use. Equipment should preferably be *CE*-marked.
- All essential items and disposables needed for IVF, in a quantity according to the workload must be made available.
- The incubators which are heart of the laboratory should be very carefully selected and placed at an appropriate position. Gametes and embryos should be distributed between incubators in such a way that numbers of door openings are minimized.
- Heating devices should be installed to maintain the temperature of media and reproductive cells during handling.
- The accepted reference range for all measured parameters must be determined and recorded. In case of any deviation from the normal range corrections must be done.
- The instruction manual must be available for every equipment in the laboratory.

CONCLUSION

The need of the hour is to regulate and recommend the construction of the ART laboratory in terms of its size, material used, the air quality, and the equipment so that one can work comfortably and at the same time provide a good environment for the embryos to grow.[11] As all this combined together will only give us good results and make our patients happy.

REFERENCES

1. IVF World. (2015). IVF/ICSI/IUI ART Lab Setup—Embryology—ART Technology in Fertility Clinic. [online] Available from https://ivfworld.wordpress.com/2015/06/22/ivf-icsi-iui-art-lab-setup-embryology-art-technology-in-fertility-clinic/ [Last Accessed February, 2019].
2. Boone WR, Higdon HL, Skelton WD. How to design and implement an assisted reproductive technology (ART) clean room. J Clin Embryol. 2007;10(4):5-15.
3. Cohen J, Gilligan A, Garrisi J. Setting up an ART laboratory. In: Gardner DK, Weissman A, Howles CM, Shoham Z (Eds). Textbook of Assisted Reproductive Techniques. New York: Taylor & Francis Group; 2004.
4. Korhonen K, Sjovall S, Viitanen J, et al. Viability of bovine embryos following exposure to the green filtered or wider bandwidth light during in vitro embryo production. Hum Reprod. 2009;24:308-14.
5. Oh SJ, Gong SP, Lee ST, et al. Light intensity and wavelength during embryo manipulation are important factors for maintaining viability of preimplantation embryos in vitro. Fertil Steril. 2007;88:1150-7.
6. Ottosen LDM, Hindkjaer J, Ingerslev J. Light exposure of the ovum and preimplantation embryo during ART procedures. J Assist Reprod Genet. 2007;24:99-103.
7. Takenaka M, Horiuchi T, Yanagimachi R. Effects of light on development of mammalian zygotes. Proc Natl Acad Sci USA. 2007;104:14289-93.
8. Boone WR, Johnson JE, Locke AJM, et al. Control of air quality in an assisted reproductive technology laboratory. Fertil Steril. 1999;71(1):150-4.
9. Meintjes M, Chantilis SJ, Douglas JD, et al. A controlled randomized trial evaluating the effect of lowered incubator oxygen tension on live births in a predominantly blastocyst transfer program. Hum Reprod. 2009;24:300-7.
10. Cooke S, Tyler JPP, Driscoll G. Objective assessments of temperature maintenance using in vitro culture techniques. J Assist Reprod Genet. 2002;19:368-75.
11. Practice Committee of the American Society for Reproductive Medicine, Practice Committee of the Society for Assisted Reproductive Technology, Practice Committee of the Society of Reproductive Biology and Technology. Revised minimum standards for practices offering assisted reproductive technologies: a committee opinion. Fertil Steril. 2014;102(3):682-6.

Quality Control and Quality Assurance

40

Alex C Varghese, Julia Szeptycki

INTRODUCTION

The birth of first test tube baby at Oldham, Cambridge in 1978 sent waves of joy and wonder around the world. Again in mid 90s, the news shook the world by the birth of twins born out of mixed race by in vitro fertilization (IVF) in Netherlands. This initiated the regulators and practitioners to look seriously into the practices done in the assisted reproduction laboratories.

That was just the tip of the iceberg as still we are getting news of IVF mix ups from different countries. According to the Human Fertilization and Embryology Authority (HFEA) report (2014), 1,679 mistakes were made in UK fertility clinics between 2010 and 2012[1] and that means about 500 to 600 incidents per year out of the 60,000 IVF cycles performed per year in UK. Since there is a system in place to report such incidents in these countries we come to know about these reports. What about the countless mistakes happening in countries where there is no reporting system?

Although the laboratories have written protocols in place and adhere to, mistakes happen with catastrophic consequence. Assisted reproduction laboratory protocols, by their very nature, require careful attention to detail. Any error will have far reaching effects and jeopardize the goodwill of the organization and agony to the couples.

Many countries have established assisted reproductive technology (ART) regulatory authorities and code of practice.[2] In the countries where there is still a lack of regulation and law, the moral and ethical views of the owner of the program dictates the code of practice. When the moral and ethical sanctity of the management combines with the state regulation, it leads to fare practice in the ART. Countries like India, which have more than 1,500 clinics, warrant utmost urgency in legislator and regulatory framework for the interest of the infertile couples.

Amongst the many requirements of the ART in a regulated environment are the optimal training of clinical and laboratory staff, written standard operating protocols (SOPs) in place, following the acceptable standards in designing the unit and procuring the equipment. In these scenarios, central inspection agency conducts assessment on an annual basis and a license to practice issued based on the code of practice. The extreme sensitivities of gametes and early embryos to physical and environmental factors highlight the potential compromise of the IVF laboratory in absence of strict controls. As such, attention to the general components of a quality control and quality assurance program are necessary for a repeatable process and as such total quality management (TQM) program must be stressed.

IN THE BEGINNING

Historically, quality management was to the discretion of a Laboratory Director and often developed based on individual quality improvement activities and statistical techniques. As reproductive technologies grew worldwide, disparities amongst laboratories practices warranted attention by clinicians and policy makers.

The advent of Clinical Lab Improvement Amendments of 1988 (CLIA'88) established standards of quality for all laboratories ensuring that the test results are accurate and reliable regardless of where the test was performed. Structural, regulatory bodies and multidisciplinary organizations operate to impose the regulatory standards of CLIA'88 regionally, nationally, and globally.

Governance of IVF laboratories based on established CLIA'88 regulations is hierarchical in both regulatory and nonregulatory aspects. In the US, the USA Food and Drug Administration and Centers for Disease Control are mandated to provide specific outcomes.

Collective organizations like Society for Assisted Reproductive Technologies (SART) and European Society of Human Reproduction and Embryology (ESHRE) act to advocate established regulations through monitoring and guidelines related laboratory performance compliance.

Membership organizations including American Society for Reproductive Medicine (ASRM) and Canadian Fertility and Andrology Society (CFAS) provide education, information, and advocacy of minimum standards and guidelines.

For Canadians specifically, the Assisted Human Reproduction (AHR) Act helps ensure the safe and ethical use of assisted reproductive technologies. Unlike the US and Europe, Canadian IVF laboratories, operating under the guidelines provided by the CFAS, are free to acquire accreditation status. A potentially cost-prohibitive undertaking those achieving accreditation status often use it as a marketing strategy in the increasingly competitive industry.

The complexity of regulatory and nonregulatory arms necessitates a comprehensive framework for engagement of essential quality management initiatives and their associated factors.

WHAT IS TOTAL QUALITY MANAGEMENT AND QUALITY MANAGEMENT CULTURE?

Quality controls as well as quality assurance are the two important parameters of the TQM system which helps to ensure the prevention of any defects by implementing correct approaches in process.

The quality control focuses on identifying defects and verifies that the products meet the set standard criteria. The over-simplified goal of TQM is to provide an optimal product with process efficiency. This is accomplished by identifying and eliminating problems in work processes and systems. Four major characteristics of healthcare practices are consumers (patients), product (specialized health services), staff (varied educational, experience and technical background), and owner (usually physician). The peculiar characteristics of IVF practices are that—(1) the patient population is knowledgeable about the treatment; (2) patients are highly motivated; (3) success rates are important in the choice of practice and clinician; and (4) patients have high expectations as they cover majority of treatment expenses.

Total quality management implementation involves satisfying customers, system/process, people, and improvement tools. These are further identified as the five pillars of TQM—product (service), process, organization, leadership, and commitment.[3,4]

Such an undertaking requires an organizational culture change involving a major training and learning of the staff followed by pilot quality initiatives in a number of major areas including human, financial, technological, and natural resources. Diverging from the traditional top-down approach, knowledge sharing is recognized as a key element in enhancing a company's capacity to be more responsive.[5] As such more personal involvement is required by top management to establish effective communication circles with personnel.[6]

In succeeding in building a quality culture in an organization three key steps are important—(1) involve everyone; (2) listen to everyone; and (3) show that you are listening.

IMPACT OF TQM ON REGULAR AND ROUTINE WORK IN THE ART LABORATORIES: ANDROLOGY, EMBRYOLOGY, AND CRYOBIOLOGY LABORATORIES

Several papers examine the complementary of TQM practices on management strategy and its impact on work life, quality, and performance. The results of TQM implementation are contradictory and inconclusive with the majority of UK and US companies revealing "zero competitive gain" or mixed findings if TQM's success is taken into consideration.[7]

Job content, job control, global participation, and social relations are the positive impacts of TQM.[8] The negative changes are also reported for workload such as lack of clarity of duties.[8] These discrepancies may be attributed to a gap about intentions and reality of implementation of TQM in the various subunits of the organization.

Total quality management programs are also charged with failing to create a significant change in organizations. Communication circles, thought to increase the innovativeness, and participation of personnel, reveal only acute, unsustainable effects in altering employees' attitudes and organizational culture. The importance of organizational culture and attitudes of work force cannot be understated as being conducive to TQM success.[9,10]

It should be understood that a quality management culture is not a goal, but an ongoing process that requires constant adaptability in human and/or financial resources. A shortage of either of these resources and/or opposition to adopting innovations is barrier to successful TQM implementation, even if their values seem positive for the organization.[11]

List of documents essential in a quality management system include:

- Quality manual
- System procedures
- Procedures and process maps
- Work instructions
- Forms
- Job descriptions.

Quality management activities requiring full traceability and documentation are labor-intensive. Lacking international standards, and of noteworthy mention, it is an important QC issue to have sufficient number of personnel to perform routine laboratory work without subjecting either personnel or patients to undue stress or risk. The number of personnel should be fixed for routine work, with additional personnel for more complex procedures.[12]

An organization's top management has a major role to play to promote quality culture across the departments. Successful TQM implementation will only persist in a climate of senior leadership capacity to institute an organizational-wide commitment to behavioral changes, cross-functional mechanisms, leadership skills, and dialogue needed to not only learn but enable further change.[13]

HOW TO COLLECT AND MANAGE THE DATA?

There is general consensus of the value in data reporting of national and clinic-specific outcomes. Performance can be monitored using a quality control system in simple tabulated form. For reproductive technologies, at a laboratory level, these may include—(1) fertilization rates; (2) cleavage/blastulation rates; and (3) embryo utilization rate. Efficacies as a function of primary endpoint may include rate of—(1) positive beta- human chorionic gonadotropin (β-hCG); (2) gestational sac development; (3) ongoing viable pregnancy (presence of a fetal heartbeat); and (4) live birth.

Data may be further analyzed per treatment—(1) initiation; (2) retrieval or (3) embryo transfer conventionally as a function of age range demographic.

In smaller data collections, direct cycle to cycle comparisons may pose little benefit as cell cycle specific factors including diagnosis, treatment, stimulation, number of cycles prior to achieving pregnancy, and accurate pregnancy outcome data are numerous and may dilute the observed trend.

Other end points including rates of ovarian hyperstimulation syndrome, miscarriage, multiple pregnancy, and ectopic pregnancy may lose value as patient-specific treatment and circumstances may vary.

Industry wide, arduous, and inefficient manual data collection is trending toward internet-based practice management software (e.g. eIVF, Baby Sentry) which integrates all aspects of practice management including treatment and inventory supply chain. Annual reports generated are based on the information collected and are pertinent to interpreting trends in the individual practice over time.

These data collections or registries, extend to regional (BORN, Ontario, Canada), national (CARTR Plus, Canada; SART, USA), and more sophisticated levels (EIM, Europe). On a global level, the World Reports of ICMART are providing the most comprehensive statistical census of ART quality, utilization, safety, and quality.[8] While this type of data is most desirable, it is expensive to collect and to control for accuracy. But they warn the data presented is reliant on the quality and completeness of data submitted.[8] Cloud-based paperless applications are getting introduced for the better management of the whole process. IVF quality control is such one with applications known as Generations, Reflection, and Kaleasy—for data management, laboratory quality control management, and patient appointments, respectively (www.ivfqc.com).

ART Clinic Management Systems

1.	Fertsoft	Fertsoft AB	*Sweden*
2.	IDEAS V.6	Mellonwood Medical	*Canada*
3.	BabySentry	Medical and Genetics Software Corp.	*USA*
4.	Babe IVF System	Cleodora Medical	*Finland*
5.	MediTex	CRITEX GmbH	*Germany*
6.	IVF Module of PALASH™	Palash IVF Solution	*India*
7.	Fertility EHR	Fertility EHR	USA
8.	Ankh Clinic & Lab E-suite	Ankh Data systems	USA
9.	E-IVF	Practicehwy	USA

INTERNAL AND EXTERNAL QUALITY CONTROL

Quality control includes establishing a standard for each aspect of a procedure that will result in a reliably reproducible result. In the case of diagnostic testing, the result may be a predictor of fertility or screening result. In other instances, successful rejuvenation of a cryopreserved sample or in the ART procedure, pregnancy is a measured outcome.

Internal quality control provides for full traceability and documentation including standardization of operating procedures with formal training programs for staff within a program.

On-going training, tools, and periodic assessments (QA) assure that laboratory- or technician-specific variations are within acceptable tolerance limits, corrected if needed, and that errors are not introduced over time. New tools (QI) including remote monitoring of environment (pH, temperature, humidity) and technological advancements aim to increase productivities or efficiencies.

In the laboratory, equipment is set at optimal performance, monitored, and recorded at regular intervals. Consumables (e.g. culture media, contact materials) are recorded as traceable by lot number and on a per patient basis. In principle, despite commercial availability of many products, periodic evaluation of all materials and their treatment before introduction into a laboratory is suggested.

Participation in an external quality assurance (EQA) program (e.g. College of American Pathologists) provides for international laboratories to assess accuracies in their methods, individual performance, and reporting.[14] This allows a laboratory to evaluate the same samples and procedures as other laboratories and to compare their performance against that of others. This will enable consistent quality improvement and better standard of care for the patients.

STANDARDIZED TRAINING PROGRAMS

Assisted reproductive technology is widely practiced worldwide and there is a lack of structured graduate/post graduate programs in this discipline in many countries. Appropriately, there is need for comprehensive training and continuing education for technicians of this highly skilled discipline.

Historically, training was performed in-lab with no specific educational requirements. Under CLIA'88 Andrology laboratories, but not Embryology laboratories, are required to comply with CLIA'88. Due to the multifaceted role of the technician, it is a common practice that all personnel achieve the same training and educational standards.

In general, the minimum educational requirement is a 4-year bachelor degree with advanced degree required for Supervisory, Managerial, and Director level roles. International and online distance learning programs exist such as the Masters in Clinical Embryology (UK, USA, Australia), although all are not accredited.

In Canada, there are currently no minimum educational requirements to work in ART and more specifically, no formal programs that provide specific learning in the laboratory aspects of ART. Post-secondary institutions are soon to offer advanced degree programs in the discipline and it is anticipated that a specific degree requirement will become the standard in the future.

While the educational requirements vary by country, established guidelines are designed to assist practices by setting criteria that meet or exceed the legislative requirements of each country. Countries lacking legislation may follow the standards established by ESHRE and ASRM.

Several organizations offer continuing education courses or certificates specializing in this discipline. The American Board of Bioanalysis (ABB), CFAS, and ESHRE are recognized certifying agencies for directors offering high complexity (HCLD), Embryology (ELD), and/or (ALD) Laboratory Directors. Working to standardize the theoretical knowledge and clinical skills of technicians may increase confidence in reliability and outcomes.

MONITORING KPIs

A key performance indicator (KPI) is a measured value evaluating performance outcomes.[15] Strategic goals and performance activities are aligned with a common goal of producing reliably improved outcomes. They must be specific, measurable, attainable, relevant, and time-bound (SMART) and will be short-lived unless they are (SMARTER) evaluated and re-evaluated.

In ART therapeutic procedures, monitoring pregnancy rates as a KPI ensures that pregnancy rates are maintained at an optimum level. IVF outcomes are monitored at specific time intervals, but this form of audit has major limitations: (1) the pregnancy rates are dependent on multiple factors and can be influenced by the underlying pathology of the patients; (2) the problem encountered at the time of treatment, usually a few weeks before, may result in drop in pregnancy rates; and (3) the root cause remains unrevealed.

Since the embryology laboratory is the epicenter of the IVF unit, the dependence of pregnancy outcome to a greater extend on the laboratory performance highlights the need for ensuring the quality of these services. It is therefore essential to lay down certain benchmarks to assess ART laboratory functions.

Any inherent deviation of a process from an established limit might lead to end product defect and in the medical field to defective care of patient.

Monitoring, which is a process able to identify deviations, and then being able to act should such deviation exceed certain limits, plays an important role in avoiding adverse outcomes. This in turn will maintain optimal performance.[16]

Many embryologists might recall the panic button getting on when the pregnancy rate dip in some months. The first thing many clinicians use to do is looking for an answer from the laboratory. The reason could well be due to factors extrinsic to the laboratory. Maintaining a KPI data including the fertilization rate, embryo utilization rate, blastulation rate, and implantation rate can be used to check the consistency of laboratory outcomes. Laboratory should make the habit of supplying the KPI data of each month to the clinical team to avoid any tussles that may arise from time to time.

The very recent international workshop at Vienna conjoined organized by ESHRE and Alpha Scientists in Reproduction (Alpha), designed to establish consensus on definitions and recommended values for the ART laboratory.[17] The expert committee is of the opinion that every ART laboratory need to build their own KPIs based on the organization and process structure. Each laboratory should develop an organized, transparent, and reliable way of data collection and investigation of KPIs.

Defining the Clinic's Success Rates in TQM and the Role of Statistics[18]

Performance indicators at the clinic as well as individual level should become an integral part of data management. Some clinics perform a negative analysis of each month's performance. This will help in discerning any adverse outcomes from any new drugs, procedures or individuals. Prior to any analysis, the input, process, and output quality of the data need to be investigated by proper auditing. Moreover, data on the functioning of equipment and culture systems, such as temperature, air quality, volatile organic compounds, and microbial count, must be collected and regularly audited. A graphical representation and analysis of performance indicators compared with the established limits is an easy way of detecting problems.

Many countries with strict ART regulations and published ART national registry help the intended couples to see the success rates of each IVF clinic in the web and choose the right clinic for treatment.

The problem here with individual clinic's web projection of their pregnancy statistics may be biased as there is a tendency to project the success from best IVF batches. However, a national registry (such as SART, HFEA) will invariably project truthful data from clinics.

Nonconformity in ART

In quality management, a nonconformity (or noncompliances) is a deviation from a specific expectation. A nonconformance could be identified through customer complaints, internal audits, external audits, incoming material inspection or simply during normal testing and inspection activities. ISO 9001:2008 requires that you document your nonconformance procedure and keep records of nonconformance issues you identify and the actions taken.[19]

Two types of noncompliances can be identified by inspection/auditing process—(1) those which need immediate preventive actions and may require immediate cessation of the service and (2) those which can be corrected in a stipulated time frame and does not require immediate action.

American Society for Reproductive Medicine guidelines on the disclosure of medical errors about human gametes and embryos state that—clinics have an ethical obligation to disclose errors out of respect for patient autonomy and in fairness to patients. Errors that affect the number or quality of gametes or embryos should be disclosed unless they clearly have a minimal effect on patient's interests.[20]

It is obligatory to disclose immediately errors in which the wrong sperm is used for insemination, or gametes or embryos are mistakenly switched resulting in embryo transfer, conception, or the birth of a child with a different genetic parentage than intended. Clinics should promote a culture of truth-telling and should establish written policies and procedures regarding disclosure of errors to patients. Fertility programs should have in place rigorous procedures to prevent the loss of gametes and embryos and to ensure proper identification of all gametes, embryos, and patients.

Honest full report of all adverse incidents is part of a proper TQM system. A "no-blame" and truth-telling culture should prevail it the IVF environment so that when a mistake is made it is not hidden but brought forward for preventive or corrective actions.

The electronic witness system (EWS) in the clinical practice is a recent innovation. Although embracing the electronic witnessing has been recommended to reduce the IVF mix-ups, the technology is implemented in only few IVF clinics all around the world.

Very few fertility clinics have a human double-checking approach as the usual norm of witnessing in IVF procedures. However, this mechanism of control has been shown to be vulnerable to human errors including: check omission, check incomplete, involuntary automaticity, and non-contemporaneous checking. Due to these reasons several alternative methods of witnessing have been developed devoid of human interventions. These includes systems based on—(1) barcode labels; (2) silicon barcodes that are incorporated directly into eggs or embryos, and (3) Radio Frequency Identification technology (RFID). The RFID has some proven advantages:

- Preventing embryologists accidentally working on multiple patient's eggs or sperm at a time.
- It marks each course step and prevents embryologists missing key tasks in the process. The use of these electronic systems is rapidly extending to fertility clinics worldwide. IVF Witness is an EWS (Cooper Surgicals, USA) based on RFID tags to track and record patients and samples during IVF. Using RFID tags, patient's identity is monitored at every stage of the treatment, and at the same time, the system captures information regarding the cycle progress and operator actions. Similar systems include IMT matcher (IMTinternational, UK), OctaxFertiproof (MTG, Germany), Gidget (GeneaBiomedix, Australia). The latter aids error prevention and enables a customized intelligent ART assistance for managing clinical work and trace patients by being available on any laboratory PC through the Gidget Web Application and also a dashboard available on a large wall mounted TV screen. Another tracking product in pipeline is the Bluechiip (Australia) which may aid in sample identification and tracking in cryogenic temperatures.

A recent questionnaire-based study evaluated the patient concerns regarding the IVF process errors and the client satisfaction if there is an electronic witnessing system in place. About 90.4% of patients were concerned relating to sample mix-up. The system of EWS reduced these in 92.1% of patients, 97.1% of which were particularly satisfied with the electronic traceability of their gametes and embryos in the IVF laboratory.[21]

It is not sufficient to just have quality control programs in place; they should also be audited to check how they are working in practice. An ART unit with TQM in place will subject its procedures to internal and external audit. The IVF programs can compile a checklist based on the clauses given on the TQM system being followed (e.g. ISO) and use this for the pre-assessment audit. Once all the requirements of the checklist are fulfilled the unit is ready for the first-line audit usually the internal audit.

Preparation, Implementation and Review of SOPs

An SOP is a document containing detailed written instructions elaborating the stepwise process and technique of performing the procedure in a laboratory.

Standard operating procedures represent the sequence of steps that have been standardized to execute a task and are used every time a given task is performed to ensure that it is executed in the same way every time and by each team member.

The main reasons why fertility centers need SOPs as integral elements of the quality control system are: (1) IVF work involving repetitive, complex critically important tasks; (2) variation must be controlled; (3) multiple people in same place often performing the same task; (4) safety risks are present; and (5) quality control must be ensured.[21] SOPs are dynamic and should be constantly reviewed/updated, based on new knowledge and variation/errors detected after implementation.

No deviation should be permitted in SOP and the SOP should be strictly followed. The authorized person with their qualification and training should be specified in SOP. It also provides safety instruction, troubleshooting, waste disposal, etc. The SOP should be available to the staff in the working area itself and should be reviewed periodically by competent personnel. SOPs are the preliminary documents sought during the inspection by accreditation agencies. There should be SOP for staff training, equipment care, operation and calibration, cleaning, sterilization and disinfecting procedures, handling and disposal of waste, internal audit, participation in quality control program, etc.

Monitoring the Laboratory Equipment and Air Quality: Temperature, Gases, pH, Particle Count, VOCs and Microbial Count, etc.

The implanting blastocyst derived in vivo from the human oocyte and sperm traverses the fallopian tube and uterine endometrium during its pre-implantation development.

A perfect homeostasis is provided by the in vivo micro environment during the course of blastocyst development. However, the scenario is of stark difference when the in vitro derived embryo develops in the confinement of a culture droplet in a Petri dish. Several physical parameters need to be controlled meticulously to obtain a healthy embryo in vitro. Physical parameters pertaining to preimplantation embryo development in vitro does not limit to the integrity and complexity of culture media or the type of the incubators.

The major parameters to be controlled are: temperature, pH, osmolarity, humidity, air quality etc. Even though several electronic gadgets are currently available to measure each of the parameters, devices used for checking physical parameters need proper quality control. **Table 1** shows a list of available gadgets for routine quality checks.

Maintaining the oocytes and embryos at a constant temperature is of vital importance for the successful outcome and health of implanting blastocysts.

Table 2 shows the devices/equipment which need to be maintained at a physiological temperature. Many laboratory accrediting agencies require a secondary validation of temperature and will not allow you to rely solely on a digital reading from the instrument itself. There exist several different temperature measuring devices on the market today, from electronic thermometers with thermocouples to data-loggers, temp-tracers, and continuous temperature monitoring probes that can be connected to a clinic's IT network and the internet for instant access and easy monitoring and adjustment.

Thermochrons are button-sized and stainless steel devices that can be placed directly into your testing environment without the need for external probes. The Thermochron devices are calibrated by Thermodata using a system accredited to ISO/IEC 17025 and traceable to National Institute of Standards and Technology (NIST) standards. The monitoring device was adapted for use in incubator environments to continually read temperature

Table 1: List of commercially available QC devices.

pH meter	Orion Star™ A111 pH Benchtop Meter (Thermo Fisher USA)	LAQUA PH1200 Bench top meter (Horiba Scientific, Japan)	pH Meter-3 (Real time pH measurement) (ORIGIO, Denmark)	PetriSense® - Single sensor for monitoring of pH or CO_2. (Planer PLC, UK)	pH Online™ (MTG, Germany)	IVF-Safe sens continuous pH monitoring system (Safe Sens, USA)
Temperature	RI-IVF Thermometer (ORIGIO, Denmark)	K-System thermometer (ORIGIO, Denmark)	Solid temperature sensor (ORIGIO, Denmark)	GMH 3230 electronic thermometer (MTG, Germany)		
VOC	RI- VOC meter (ppm measurement ORIGIO, Denmark)	Sparmed VOC meter (ppb measurement; Denmark)	Grey Wolf VOC meter (ppb measurement; USA)	VOC meter (ppm measurement; S-tech Associates, India)		
CO_2/O_2	G-100 (Geotech, UK)	InControl 1050 (Labotect, Germany)				
Microbial air sampling	MAS-100® Microbial Air Monitoring Systems and ICR/ICRplus Settle Plates (Merck Millipore)					

Table 2: Equipment requiring maintenance at 37°C.

IVF laboratory	Incubators	IVF workstation bench	Stereo zoom heat plates	ICSI workstation stage	Test tube warmer
Oocyte retrieval suite	Test tube warmer	Heated trolley top			
Andrology laboratory	Test tube warmer	Incubator			

(ICSI: intracytoplasmic sperm injection; IVF: in vitro fertilization)

and humidity in small areas. The continual monitoring allows the user to—validate the external display readings; assess incubator usage during the daytime so as to distribute usage more evenly over time; gauge recovery times of different types of incubators; challenge incubators with alterations in temperature to examine whether the Thermochron buttons detected any anomalies. Moreover, thermo coins are useful to monitor the temperature in actual working condition such as culture media.

Continuous temperature and humidity monitoring are critical for proper medical laboratory operation from a quality perspective. The information collected will facilitate strict quality control of routine IVF instrumentation and in particular benchtop incubators; provide the clinical user with a means for challenging the response time of incubators to fluctuations in environment; and can help to maintain a constant, regulated state of control for temperature sensitive areas.

Recently, preliminary data have suggested that even slight rises in pHe during brief manipulations outside the laboratory incubator can significantly impact mouse blastocyst development and hatching, as well as significantly alter gene expression profiles.[22] One manner in which pHe may be influencing the embryos is likely due, in part, to its impact on intracellular pH (pHi) and cellular resources expended in maintaining intracellular homeostasis. Various commercial media companies recommend differing pHe ranges, most within the range of 7.2–7.4. Historically, CO2 set-points in incubators are adjusted to attempt to create the ideal media pH environment for any development stage of embryos. CO_2 adjustments are generally done by spot checking the pH of equilibrated media once a month or once a week.

In addition to obtaining the ideal pH, maintaining a stable pH environment is important for embryo development. It has been observed that denuded mature oocytes lack robust mechanisms to regulate internal pH, cryopreserved/warmed embryos have a reduced ability to regulate internal pH for several hours, and cleavage stage embryos have reduced ability to regulate internal pH compared to post-compaction embryos. Additionally, changes in intercellular pH of embryos impact metabolic activity, can impact organelle localization, and can even influence resulting fetal development. Thus, maintaining a stable and appropriate external pH (media pH) is critical.

There are many gadgets for pH measurement for IVF culture systems. A benchtop pH meter can be used for the routine pH measurement with proper calibration buffers. However, it is essential to keep the certificate of analysis of the media being used handy to check the pH of the given media lot each time.

A new technology, SAFE Sens TrakStation, enables real time noninvasive pH monitoring within an incubator environment. Use of this technology can reveal incubator conditions which are not ideal for maintaining ideal pH levels.

Many recent studies have suggested an association between poor laboratory air quality conditions and impaired embryo development, resulting in decreased implantation and pregnancy rates. Once the clean room concept is implemented in the IVF program, rigorous quality control is required to maintain the clean air. Periodic checks on particle count, volatile organic compounds, filter integrity, and microbial count should be undertaken. Though the particle counts and filter integrity tests can be carried by certified vendors, it is ideal to monitor the volatile organic compound (VOC) levels and microbial counts regularly. VOCs can be measured either at ppb (Sparmed VOC meter, Grey Wolf VOC meter) or ppm level (ORIGIO Denmark, S-tech associates India). If you are using ppm-based VOC meter, the ideal measurement should be less than 0.5 ppm for the IVF laboratories. One ppm is 1 part in 1,000,000. The common unit mg/L is equal to ppm. For example, Four drops of ink in a 55-gallon (208 liters) barrel of water would produce an "ink concentration" of 1 ppm. One part per billion is 1 part in 1,000,000,000. One drop of ink in one of the largest tanker trucks used to haul gasoline would represent 1 ppb. Following is a conversion table of ppm to ppb:

PPM	***PPB***
1	1,000
2	2,000
3	3,000
4	4,000
10	10,000
15	15,000
20	20,000

Standard ppm (parts per million) VOC meters cannot detect low level of VOCs present in IVF laboratories (less than 500 parts per billion) which can negatively affect embryo development. Some high performing units with ISO 5 laboratory standards have shown to have total VOC in laboratory air of less than 2 $\mu g/m^3$ (~ 0.5 ppb).

Following major problems are observed with regard to air quality management in IVF laboratories in many Indian IVF units.

- Lack of proper designing of air handling unit and initial assessment of air quality
- Substandard activated carbon or VOC filtration systems
- Lack of maintenance and periodic checks of **AHU** units
- Lack of periodic replacement of filters
- Not adhering to clean room disciplines
- Incorporating VOC emitting materials and systems in laboratory and adjacent areas
- Hesitation of management to invest in air quality management systems due to lack of knowledge.

Some laboratories in Australia have altogether stopped using any kind of disinfectants in IVF or adjacent laboratories. Instead the use of hospital grade high duty steam mopping systems are very common as these are devoid of any VOC generation, and these are a powerful steam-based sterilizer too.

Since the box type incubators derive more than 90% of its gas content from the laboratory air, the better option for culturing the embryos is to use humidified bench top incubators as it derives all its gas from the gas bottles. There should be strict check on the quality of the gases being used in the incubators as these can be the major culprit in miscarriages. It is unfortunate that there is no regulation on medical grade gases in India. Hence periodical replacement of activated carbon inline filters in the gas line is mandatory.[23]

Microbial testing and monitoring should also be part of the routine quality maintenance of the IVF program. Even though regular screening is done on the patient's samples brought into the laboratory environment, the microbial contamination can happen from many other sources. It has been observed that the air handling ducting can become a breeding ground for many moulds and even the HEPA filters in the safety hoods and air handling systems can harbor microbes. It is ideal to change the HEPA type of filters (even that of safety hoods) at stipulated intervals especially in places with high humidity.

Passive microbial air monitoring with the help of settle plates or contact plates is a useful complement to active air sampling methods. Settle plates allow a semi-quantitative determination of microbial contaminations in the air. Since they are fairly small, they can also be used conveniently in confined spaces such as laminar air flow hoods. Alternatively, active air monitoring systems are available from many companies (LA 474, HiMedia Laboratories India).

IoT is the concept of Internet-of-things—the interconnection via the Internet of computing devices embedded in everyday objects, enabling them to send and receive data. This can be very helpful in quality control situations, especially monitoring laboratory conditions for performance-based laboratories such as IVF where the correct temperature, gas concentration, humidity and organic compounds (VOC) content present are critical to human embryo growth.

There are many monitoring systems available in the market **(Table 3)**. Many of these wireless monitoring systems that are easy to install, require no additional wiring, and can integrate into existing Wi-Fi network infrastructure of the unit. The monitoring software enables organizations to remotely monitor incubators, refrigerators, freezers, and other vital appliances throughout the facility in real-time, automates internal monitoring processes, records historical data and corrective actions associated with all alerts. Users can easily configure the monitoring software to provide automated reports and alarms. Advanced communication functionality of facility monitoring systems allows key

Table 3: Remote monitoring systems.

The XiltriX® laboratory monitoring system	IKS International	The Netherlands
LU 45 (for pathogens) and QA-20 (for VOCs)	NuWave Sensors	Ireland
Log and Guard	VitroLife	Sweden
Esco PROtect Wireless Monitoring System	Esco Global	Denmark
BioEase Inventory and Monitoring Software	Lab IVF	Singapore
Planer Monitoring systems	Planer PLC	UK
Monitoring systems	Mesa labs	USA
TSI FMS system	TSI	USA

personnel to view alerts on screen or receive alarm notifications through email or text messaging of incubator temperature, humidity, carbon dioxide and oxygen levels, cryo-storage vessels and fridges.

Cleanroom areas have independent pressure sensors and particle counting duties are performed by a TSI AeroTrak portable particle counter, which feeds data direct to the FMS system in real time.

Typical installations may include the following environmental sensors:

- Temperature
- Relative humidity
- Liquid nitrogen
- Oxygen
- Carbon dioxide
- Room pressure
- Differential pressure
- Open/closed doors
- Alarm state (Tri-gas incubators, time lapse incubators etc.)
- Airborne particulates.

Volatile organic compounds are known to affect the success rate of assisted reproductive techniques and continuous laboratory VOC monitoring as part of the FMS (Facility Monitoring systems) system may be useful. NuWave Sensors' LumAir is a patented rapid microbial detection sensor that facilitates remote monitoring of airborne pathogens (bacteria, yeasts, and moulds) and revolutionizes the approach to pathogen detection and control (www.nuwavesensors.com).

INCORPORATION QUALITY MANAGEMENT SYSTEMS IN NEW AND EXISTING ART UNITS

"The real voyage of discovery consists not in seeking new landscapes but in having new eyes"—Marcel Proust.

With the impending guidelines for ART clinics by the Government of India, it is apt to think first of implementing quality management systems whether it is new or existing unit. IVF programs are complex settings requiring the integration of multiple disciplines. ISO 9001:2008 is one quality management system that is readily adaptable to an ART program. Implementation of such TQM systems for the entire organization can bring in—(1) control of documents; (2) clear delineation of responsibilities of staff members; (3) documentation of the numerous processes and procedures; and (4) improvement in tracking and reducing errors and overall better control of systems. A quality ART program sets quality objectives and monitors their progress. ISO provides a sense of transparency within the organization and clearer understanding of how service is provided to patients. Most importantly, ISO provides the framework to allow for continual improvement.

Since 50% of the Indian IVF units are of batch IVF programs with either residential or visiting specialists to do the cases, implementation of the quality systems will be a tricky situation.[24]

Employing a sufficient number of qualified laboratory personnel to perform the work of the laboratory is essential. As per the ASRM guidelines, at a minimum, there should be two qualified embryologists.[25] **Table 4** provides minimum staff sizes for the volume of cycles (retrievals and cryopreservation cycles). Additional laboratory staff may be required if andrological and/or endocrinological duties are also assigned. Recent consensus meeting by Alpha recommended educational and staffing structure for an ART laboratory professionals **(Table 5)**. He/she must be either a medical graduate or have a post-graduate degree or a doctorate in an appropriate area of life sciences. (In the case of a clinic in existence for at least one year before the promulgation of these guidelines, a person with a B Sc or BVSc degree but with at least 5 years of first-hand, hands-on experience of the techniques mentioned below and of discharging the responsibilities listed below, would be acceptable for functioning as a clinical embryologist in the particular clinic. Such persons would also be eligible to take a test to be designed and conducted by an appropriate designated authority, to qualify for a position of a clinical embryologist in a new clinic.).

In vitro fertilization program cannot be run without employing an embryologist who is an integral part of the program.[27] Many start-ups major concern is who will be the embryologist. Since the ratio of qualified embryologists to the number of IVF clinics in India does not match, many programs utilizes the freelance embryologists, especially the clinics with IVF batching. Presently India has three Masters level clinical embryology courses and many post-graduate

Table 4: Minimum number of embryologists per cycles as per the ASRM guideline.

Number of laboratory cycles	*Minimum number of embryologists*
1–150	2
151–300	3
301–600	4
>600	1 additional embryologist per additional 200 cycles

Table 5: Alpha consensus meeting recommended educational qualifications for entry into each level of the basic staffing structure.

Basic staffing level	***Academic qualification***	***Relevant experience***
Assistance level	BSc or equivalent technical qualification	
Embryology level	BSc or equivalent academic or technical qualification	
Supervisory level	Ideally, MSc, but BSc at a minimum	5 years' clinical embryology laboratory experience
Direction level	Ideally, earned doctorate in biomedical science, but MSc at a minimum	*Doctorate:* 5 years' experience; *MSc:* 10 years' experience

Table 6: Process (Road map) to implement quality systems in new settings.

Process	***Comments***
Building and designing phase of new units	Make a visit to few clinics in India and abroad; do an extensive ground work by involving qualified engineers, designers, Laboratory directors/embryologists and consulting groups. Do not rely on turn-key projects.
Clean room construction	Involve clean room designers and MNCs having experience in air handling design. Since the clean room engineers have limited experience with VOC filtration systems, inputs should be given to them regarding the procurement of high-quality VOC filters (activated carbon, potassium permanganate and activated alumina, etc.)
Road map of all process	It is apt to put the quality systems from inception
Data management system	Both paper registry based and software data management system should be incorporated without any fail. This should be started with the clinical side as the infertility specialist may invariably start the OPD well ahead of the actual IVF cycle initiation
Standard operating procedures (SOPs)	Put the SOP of all the intended procedures from the initial days of operation. Technical SOP of each equipment also should be in place.
QC of equipment	Make QC sheets for each and every equipment including the physical parameters of laboratory QC and reviewed from time to time
Statistician	Either a full time or part time statistician can offer valuable contribution in the data management and analysis. They will be of much help in clinical trials, research activities, and in getting data analyzed for different purposes
The organization of laboratory staff	The Alpha consensus meeting[27] put forward roles and responsibilities of the various levels of staff within the clinical embryology laboratory, arranged using the PACER (Personal, Administration, Clinical, Education, Research) system. The consensus on the basic staffing structure in the clinical embryology laboratory is presented in Figure.

(IVF: in vitro fertilization; MNCs: multinational companies; OPD; out-patient department; QC: quality control; SOP: standard operating protocols VOC: volatile organic compound)

diploma courses. This will make sufficient professionals in near future. I have seen few new IVF clinics employing 2–3 Masters candidates in life sciences well in advance of start-up of the IVF program. They are then sponsored by the employer for 3–6 months training in advanced laboratories abroad. I have still seen them working in the same clinic even after 8–10 years. Hiring and maintaining an employee, especially an embryologist, is an asset and shows the integrity of the clinic's management. This model may be an option for upcoming centers. As the success in IVF results from a good team work, the team building should be a priority which also leads to overall quality improvements.

Table 6 with some modifications can be a guide for incorporation of the quality culture in the existing centers. However, the centers with batch IVF programs employing visiting clinical and laboratory experts may need rigorous overhauling of the current practices with regard to the quality assurance and quality control. Here too, the will of the management for stringent practice of data management of each and every patient and treatment, procedures will pave way for further incorporation of quality systems in place. Societies like ISAR through accreditation drive could make such clinics grow from "No data and fragmented data clinics to clinics of quality systems in place".

A Laboratory Director with ample experience and knowledge in ART is a must for complex laboratories like IVF laboratories. The Laboratory Director is responsible for the overall operation and administration of the laboratory. They coordinate activities of laboratory with clinical activities of department and devises strategies to improve the outcomes and maintain the consistency in results. They are also involved in overseeing as well as participating in laboratory procedures whenever necessary and monitor related quality assurance, quality control, and record-keeping. They ensure compliance with all regulatory requirements, medical and technical policies, and procedural guidelines applicable to the laboratory; reviews recommendations by medical and technical groups; and oversees any required licensing inspections. Once the ART guidelines are implemented in India, we may observe a drastic difference in the organizational and quality structure of the current programs.

"Nothing is impossible; there are ways that lead to everything, and if we had sufficient will we should always have sufficient means. It is often merely for an excuse that we say things are impossible."—Francois de La Rochefoucauld

It is better to initiate the culture of quality management right now rather than to wait for the regulator to come and teach what to be done or not to be done.

CONCLUSION

Quality management is a culture that need to be implemented at different levels in an organization to yield fruitful results. Introduction of few QC gadgets may not be itself ideal solution to obtain the results. Proper staff training, mind-set to instill TQM, continuous education, internal and external auditing of the process, implementation of ideal quality control strategies etc. will yield the desired outcomes.

REFERENCES

1. HFEA report 2014. Available from http://hfeaarchive.uksouth.cloudapp.azure.com/www.hfea.gov.uk/9017.html.
2. Johnson L. Regulation of assisted reproductive treatment (ART) in Australia & current ethical issues. Indian J Med Res. 2014;140(Suppl 1):S9-S12.
3. Rowitz L. Public Health Leadership-Putting Principles Into Practice, 2nd edition; 2003.
4. Rowitz L. Public Health Leadership: Putting Principles into Practice. J Healthc Qual. 2002;24(3):47.
5. Chua J, Eze U, Goh G. Knowledge sharing and Total Quality Management: A conceptual framework. 2010 IEEE International Conference on Industrial Engineering and Engineering Management. 2010;(DEC):1107-11.
6. Matejka K, Brooks V, Gates L. The Total Quality Journey: By Invitation Only? Management Decision. 1993;31(5).
7. Sohal AS, Terziovski M. TQM in Australian manufacturing: Factors critical to success. International Journal of Quality & Reliability Management. 2000;17:158-68.
8. Dyer S, Chambers GM, de Mouzon J, et al International Committee for Monitoring Assisted Reproductive Technologies world report: Assisted Reproductive Technology 2008, 2009 and 2010. Hum Reprod. 2016;31(7):1588-609.
9. DI Prajogo, McDermott CM. The relationship between total quality management practices and organizational culture. International Journal of Operations & Production Management. 2005;25:1101-22.
10. Kumar M, Sankaran S. Indian culture and the culture for TQM: A comparison. The TQM Magazine. 2007;19: 176-88.
11. Roldán JL, Leal-Rodríguez AL, Leal AG. The influence of organisational culture on the Total Quality Management programme performance. Investigaciones Europeas de Dirección y Economía de la Empresa. 2012;18:183-9.
12. Balaban B, Ubaldi FM. Total Quality Management in the ART Laboratory. Global Fertility Academy. Available from: https://media.reachmd.com/uploads/related_-_client_provided_materials/8586_total_quality_management_for_download.pdf
13. Beer M. Why Total Quality Management Programs Do Not Persist: The Role of Management Quality and Implications for Leading a TQM Transformation. Decision Sciences. 2003;34(4):623-42.
14. Matson P. Internal quality control and external quality assurance in the IVF laboratory. Hum Reprod. 1998; 13(suppl 4):156-65.
15. Klipfolio.com. 2018. What is a KPI? Definition, Best-Practices, and Examples [online]. Available from: https://www.klipfolio.com/resources/articles/what-is-a-key-performance-indicator.
16. Franco Jr JG, Petersen CG, Mauri AL, et al. Key performance indicators score (KPIs-score) based on clinical and laboratorial parameters can establish benchmarks for internal quality control in an ART program. JBRA Assist Reprod. 2017;21:61-6.
17. ESHRE Special Interest Group of Embryology, Alpha Scientists in Reproductive Medicine. The Vienna consensus: report of an expert meeting on the development of art laboratory performance indicators, Hum Reprod Open. 2017;2.
18. Germond M, Urner F, Chanson A, et al. What is the most relevant standard of success in assisted reproduction?: The cumulated singleton/twin delivery rates per oocyte pick-up: the CUSIDERA and CUTWIDERA. Hum Reprod. 2004;19(11):2442-4.
19. Bento FC, Esteves SC. Establishing a quality management system in a fertility center: experience with ISO 9001. MedicalExpress (São Paulo, online). 2016;3(3):M160302.

20. Disclosure of medical errors involving gametes and embryos. Fertil Steril. 2011; 96(6):1312-4.
21. Forte M, Faustini F, Maggiulli R, et al. Electronic witness system in IVF—patients perspective. J Assist Reprod Genet. 2016;33(9):1215-22.
22. Koustas G, Sjoblom C. Epigenetic consequences of pH stress in mouse embryos. Hum Reprod. 2011;26:i78.
23. Varghese AC, Palmer G. Clean room technology for low resource IVF units. In: Esteves S, Varghese AC, Worrilow K (Eds). Clean Room Technology In ART Clinics: A Practical Guide. CRC press: UK.
24. Ahemmed BP, Varghese AC. Batch IVF Programme in ART: Practical Considerations; In: Fleming S, Varghese AC (Eds). Organization and Management of IVF Units. USA: Springer; 2016. pp. 27-50.
25. The Alpha Consensus Meeting on the professional status of the clinical embryologist: proceedings of an expert meeting, Reprod BioMed Online. 2015;30(5):451-61.
26. Revised Guidelines for Human Embryology and Andrology laboratories. Fertil Steril. 2008;90(5):S45-S59.
27. Go KJ. By the work, one knows the workman': the practice and profession of the embryologist and its translation to quality in the embryology laboratory. Reprod Biomed Online. 2015;31(4):449-58.

Accreditation of the Assisted Reproductive Technique Laboratory

41

Surendra Pal Singh Virk, Arya Salaskar, Nilam Ghamne

INTRODUCTION

An assisted reproductive technique (ART) has specific requirements, which are essential for any in vitro fertilization (IVF) program to be successful. Dedication, knowledge and experience among the team members and the techniques performed in the laboratory, can set up a quality ART clinic. There is a need for transparency regarding the effectiveness, health outcomes and safety aspects of ART treatments.

Maintenance of quality control depends majorly upon coordination among the team members, care for the patients and strict supervision on factors such as power supply, air quality, medicines, culture media, disposables and equipment. The crucial step in the establishment of the best IVF laboratory is recruiting the right people for right job and also ensuring consistent and continuous education and training for them. Evaluation of the outcome, equipment, staff, research programs, and audit by an external central body at regular intervals improves the overall quality of the ART program.

Like other industries, ART clinics use quality management system (QMS) to meet the requirements and also to monitor the delivery of the services. Implementation of QMS is important for the planning, setting, and meeting improvement through documented processes, facilitating continuous improvement in the system.

ACCREDITATION

Accreditation is a process of auditing by an external professional, which is an independent accreditation body. It gives a formal acknowledgment that the laboratory is competent to render quality services compliant with rigorous professional standards.

International Standard and Accreditation for In Vitro Fertilization Centers

The main purpose of accreditation is to ensure that quality control standards are set high by quality assurance methods. This requires high laboratory standards with highly qualified staff and a defined quality management system.

ISO 9001:2008: It is the most widely used ISO certifications and a standard for a quality management system. It allows the organization to demonstrate that its services and products meet customer's requirements, and show the consistent improvement in the quality. An IVF center can have its QMS certified to ISO 9001-2008 to ensure it enhances customer satisfaction through continual improvement with adherence to applicable statutory and regulatory requirements.

ISO 14001:2004: ISO 14001:2004 is advertised by IVF clinics sometimes. This standard specifies requirements for an organization to implement a policy which respects legal obligations and other conditions relating to environmental aspects.

ISO 15189:2007: Most medical laboratories in Europe are accredited according to ISO 15189:2007 or 17025:2005. ISO 15189:2007 addresses the need for equivalency of quality management systems and competency requirements between laboratories. It focuses on patient outcome and the service provided by a medical laboratory.

ISO 17025:2005: It covers the technical part of the laboratory, validations of all the methods and calibration of the equipment.

An ISO certification is a good standard to possess by the field of ART. It demonstrates a professional and responsible approach. It is very important in the laboratory and for the whole ART clinic to be actively operating quality management principles and demonstrating a commitment to the continuous improvement. While some clinics are not yet ISO certified, all clinics must adhere to the regulations which their country lay down before being granted a license. Thus, the clinics can be confident that even without ISO, the clinics operate within a strictly defined set of regulations.

National/Regional Standards

While the ISO standards cover the fundamental needs for the quality systems in the IVF laboratory, many countries have specific laws, regulations, and guidelines.

Europe

In vitro fertilization laboratories located in the European Union (EU) have to adhere to the directive on setting standards of safety and quality for the testing, procurement, donation, storage, distribution and preservation of human cell and tissues, called the European Union Tissue and Cells Directive (EUTCD). The European Society of Human Reproduction and Embryology (ESHRE) has issued a paper on the EUTCD. However, each EU country interprets the directive differently but EUTCD demands a quality system.

Australia and New Zealand

In Australia, Reproductive Technology Accreditation Committee (RTAC) regulates IVF laboratories separately. It mandates the ART clinic to have QMS and various other requirements like risk management policies for procedures and review of the management. The requirement is quality policy. In the United Kingdom, the Human Fertilization and Embryology Authority (HFEA) license all the IVF clinics. There are further guidelines detailed in the HFEA Code of Practice (HFEA CoP) regulating the IVF laboratories. Specifically the CoP contains demands for risk management, sample identification and embryology staffs.

Russia

Russia has limited standards and regulations for IVF and separates between state and private clinics.

United States

In the United States, the guidelines for human andrology and embryology laboratories are made by the practice Committee of the Society of Assisted Reproductive Technology (SART) and the American Society of Reproductive Medicine (ASRM).

Middle East

Assisted reproductive technique in many of the Muslim countries is covered by a number of religious opinions called Fatwas, which are issued by the Islamic scholar. The core requirement is that the couple should be married and the use of donor sperm and donor oocyte is strictly prohibited.

India

In 2005, the Indian Council for Medical Research (ICMR) introduced national guidelines for the regulation of ART clinics. These guidelines were introduced for accreditation, regulation and supervision of ART clinics, but these are yet to be legislated.

Based on the availability of complexity of ART service, the infertility clinics are categorized in three levels as per ICMR guidelines. The guidelines also describe the minimum requirement regarding staff in infertility clinics and also about physical requirements of ART clinic. Following any ethical guidelines would mean that doctors would have to look critically at issues of screening donors, written informed consent, and ethical and legal issues including the misuse of sex—preselection technologies like preimplantation diagnosis. It remains to be seen how this will be implemented in India.

In developing country, like India, the problem of infertility, childbirth, motherhood, and issues surrounding pregnancy are very complicated and its consequences can be multiple.

REQUIREMENTS FOR AN ASSISTED REPRODUCTIVE TECHNIQUE CLINIC

Assisted reproductive technique clinics are basically divided into the clinical part and the embryology laboratory.

According to the ICMR guidelines, a nonsterile and a strictly sterile area is to be maintained by an ART clinic. The nonsterile area should have a reception area **(Fig. 1)**, patients waiting room, doctors consulting and examination rooms with ultrasound equipment facility, blood collection room, a general-purpose clinical laboratory, postoperative recovery rooms, semen collection room, nursing quarters, autoclave room, records storage and/or IT server room, etc. in addition other inhouse clinical facilities (e.g. staff meeting room, counseling rooms).

The sterile area should have the operation theater **(Fig. 2)**, separate room for IUI and embryo transfer procedure, and an embryology and sperm processing laboratory in the adjoining area. Entry to the sterile area must be strictly controlled by an area for changing into sterile garments and a scrub station, in addition to an anteroom for changing footwear.

The In Vitro Fertilization Laboratory

An ideal IVF laboratory plays an important role in the success of ART. To set up an efficient and safe ART laboratory, the three key areas to focus on are the location of the laboratory, the protocols or procedures and the embryologists. The primary function of any ART laboratory is to provide an optimal environment for gametes and embryos.

Essential Qualification of an Assisted Reproductive Technique Team

The ART practice requires a well-coordinated team work among the five major functional areas of an IVF clinic: clinical, counseling, embryology, nursing, and administration. The staff should processes standard qualifications in their area of responsibility and their actual performance should be monitored against set standards.

Location

The location of any IVF laboratory is very important and should be considered carefully, when setting up a laboratory to provide a safe, nontoxic, stable, and a pathogen-free environment. The IVF laboratory has to be designed in such a way that the outcome of the procedure is optimal and not affected by environmental factors. It is better to avoid locations around gasoline service stations, parking places, and construction area while establishing an ART laboratory. This will limit the adverse impacts of the pollutants on cell tissue culture.

Work Station and Laboratory Design

Laboratory should be in close vicinity to the procedure room or operating theater for oocyte retrieval and embryo transfer. Laboratory work stations must provide a heated surface and filtered air to maintain optimum temperature and avoid any contamination. The laboratory design with regards to the flooring, bench height, lighting and wall paint, etc. should be based on the layout of the laboratory and specifications. Care for elimination of volatile organic compounds (VOCs) and chemical air contaminants (CACs) should be taken in the laboratory. All equipment and processes must be checked and corrected before treatment of patients is commenced. Laminar flow hood, incubator, and microscope should be placed in a way to prevent unnecessary movement of staff in the laboratory during procedures **(Fig. 3)**. Micromanipulation procedures,

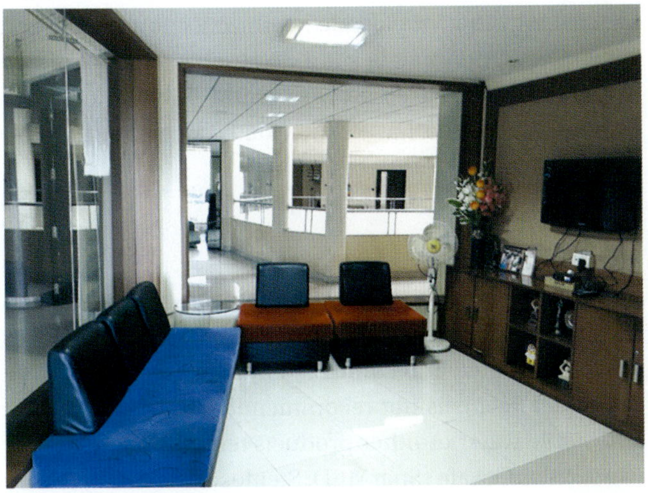

Fig. 1: Patient friendly reception area.

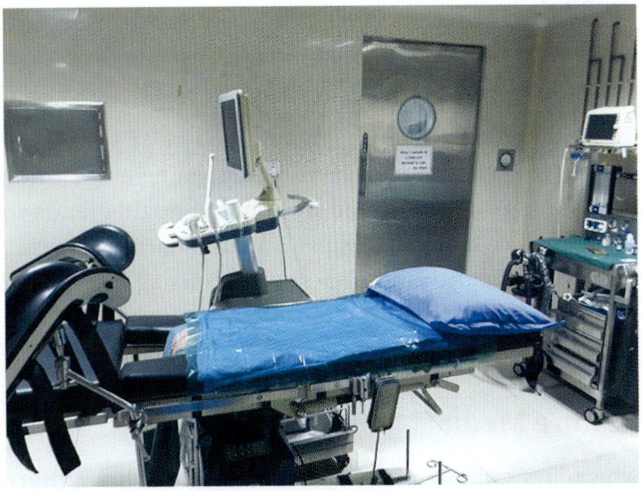

Fig. 2: Operation theater with connecting embryology laboratory.

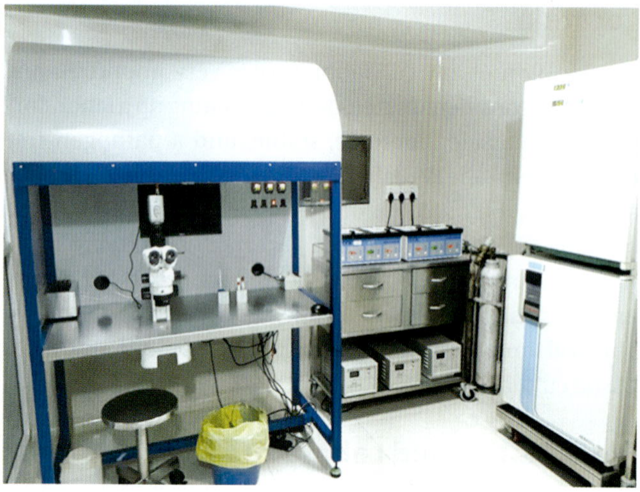

Fig. 3: Laminar air flow with stereo zoom microscopes and benchtop incubators in close proximity to the workstation.

cryopreservation, data or record keeping and storage area should have separate space in laboratory.

Air Quality in the Laboratory

The ambient air in the laboratory should be highly sterile and this can be achieved by a heating, ventilation, and air conditioning (HVAC) system, and an air handling unit that supplies only to the ART laboratory. Activated carbon filters and potassium permanganate filters should be placed next to the pre-filters at the supply inlet to absorb VOCs emitted from electrical equipment, new furniture, etc. High efficiency particulate air (HEPA) filters or ultra-low penetration air (ULPA) should be placed on the ceiling of the laboratory, and there should be at least 18 air exchanges per hour.

Incubators

The incubators should be maintained at 37°C and the pH has to be maintained. Frequent opening and closing of incubator doors should be avoided as this leads to fluctuation of temperature, pH, and osmolarity. Accuracy of the temperature should be checked by using a calibrated thermometer. Low oxygen tension has proven to be the preferred choice.

Culture Media

Nowadays commercially available high quality culture media are being used in laboratories and each lot of medium should have a certification of pH, osmolarity, endotoxin level testing, and mouse embryo assay (MEA) and sperm survival test. Each batch of media should have batch numbers, date of production and expiry dates written on the product container. Properly registered media should only be used for IVF procedures. The composition of the media should be well known to the embryologist that are being used. Most media are supplemented with serum; they should, therefore, be tested for antibodies to HIV 1 and 2, hepatitis B surface antigen and hepatitis C RNA.

Backup Power Supply

It is very important to have a power backup in infertility clinics in the form of a UPS system and/or a captive power generative system.

Temperature

Temperature maintenance during ART procedures is extremely important when handling oocytes and embryos. It has been shown that brief exposure of human oocytes to room temperature results in spindle disruption and microtubule disassembly. A laboratory without temperature control cannot be accredited.

Equipment and Consumables

All consumables that come in contact with gametes and embryos must be validated as nontoxic and safe for culture of human gametes and embryos. All plastic ware, such as test tubes, culture dishes, petri dishes, pipettes, embryo transfer catheters, and glass wares, injecting and holding needles for intracytoplasmic sperm injection (ICSI), and oocyte aspiration needles are disposables and for single use only. Powder-free gloves should only be used. All disposables should have expiry dates clearly written on them.

Cleanliness

An IVF laboratory should always be clean and it is recommended that documented frequent cleaning procedures are implemented and confirmed by active signatures. The use of detergents is not recommended, only 70% alcohol and sterile water or other products tested for embryology use such as Oosafe (SparMED, Stenlose, Denmark) can be used for cleaning.

EMBRYOLOGISTS: TRAINING AND ACCREDITATION

The skills and knowledge of the embryologists is the main contributor to IVF success. The laboratory should be led by a qualified, responsible, and experienced person with expertise in the field of embryology and should have a good background in reproductive biology or biological sciences. The embryologist should have sufficient knowledge of cell and reproductive biology to analyze and solve problems from basic physiological principles. The embryologist must write in a legible writing in order to author quality management documents. An embryologist needs to keep a routine check on equipment, consumables, and environmental conditions. There should be emphasis on the strict adherence of the standard operating procedure (SOP). Embryologist should be attending conferences and various academic events in order to increase their knowledge and competency.

STANDARD OPERATING PROCEDURES AND DOCUMENTATION

Laboratory protocols should be transposed into SOPs. All activities performed within the ART laboratory have to be clearly written with sufficient details on the techniques. The SOPs should be structured in a standardized format. All new methods should be checked and monitored in the current setup of laboratory before their implementation. The implantation rate is the most significant measure of the success in the ART laboratory than clinical pregnancy rates. Detailed records of procedures must be maintained for proper risk assessment and management in the clinic. Cross-checking and witnessing is extremely important when performing IVF procedures. There should be at least two individuals confirming, in writing, the identity of the specimen. This will minimize the risk of errors. When witnessing, both individuals should document the various steps during which, the witnessing was done on to the patients' record book.

AUDITS

An audit is a systematic independent examination of the entire quality management system. Internal and external audits can be done to assess and to maintain quality. Internal audits are a requirement of ISO 15189. Audits also help in assessing problems, taking corrective action and initiating preventive actions.

CONCLUSION

In ART program the goal of quality assurance is to improve patient care and satisfaction using a proactive strategy of ongoing evaluation and monitoring.

With the improvement in the ART technique and the expansion of indications, the number of ART treatment cycles undertaken worldwide is increasing and as a result more babies are born every year in IVF. This implies that, after 30 years of IVF, there is a diversification of technique with a consequent customization of treatment for every single category of patients. All IVF centers, striving for excellence, should consider a quality management system. Serious consideration needs to be given to introducing ISO standards to units providing infertility services worldwide. The major advantage of adaptation of an international standard to infertility treatment is being able to unify national guidelines and develop a consensus on what are important quality measurements in our field.

For a successful ART program, the ART laboratory should establish and maintain strict quality controls. The embryologists selected should be experienced and highly skilled and be able to deliver consistent results. Extensive research is necessary before admitting new procedures to standard technique protocols, which are routinely performed in IVF laboratories. Development of a quality program is time consuming and requires dedication and organization from every member of the ART program for it to succeed. By using a structured and comprehensive quality system, it is possible to ensure that the IVF program is successful and guarantees an optimal standard of treatment and care for its patients.

Finally, it is important to understand that quality assurance with 100% commitment to improve services, is the only way forward toward a future to assure safe and effective treatment for all patients.

SUGGESTED READING

1. Abramczul JW, Lopata A. Incubator performance in the clinical in vitro fertilization program: importance of temperature conditions for the fertilization and cleavage of human oocytes. Fertil Steril. 1986;46:132-4.
2. Alper MM, Brinsden PR, Fischer R, et al. Is your IVF programme good? Hum Reprod. 2002;17:8-10.
3. Boone WR, Johnson JE, Locke AJ, et al. Control of air quality in an assisted reproductive technology laboratory. Fertil Steril. 1999;71:150-4.
4. Clinical and laboratory guidelines for assisted reproductive technologies in the Nordic Countries: NFOG bulletin supplement. NFOG 1997;3.

5. Cohen J, Gilligan A, Esposito W, et al. Ambient air and its potential effects on conception in vitro. Hum Reprod. 1997; 12:1742-9.
6. Cohen J, Gilligan A, Willadsen S. Culture and quality control of embryos. Hum Reprod. 1998;13(Suppl):137-44.
7. Critchlow JD, Matson PL, Maureen CN, et al. Quality control in an in-vitro fertilization laboratory: Use of human sperm survival studies. Hum Reprod. 1989;4:545-9.
8. Dawson KJ. Quality control and quality assurance in IVF laboratories in the UK. Hum Reprod. 1997;12:2590-1.
9. Directive 2003/23/EC of the European Parliament and of the Council of 31 March 2004 on setting standards of quality and safety for the donation, procurement, testing, processing, preservation, storage and distribution of human tissues and cells. (2004). Official J Eur Union 2004; 102: 48-58. [online] Available from http:/Europa.eu.int/eur-lex/en/oj/ [Last accessed February, 2019].
10. ESHRE position paper on the EU Tissues and Cells Directive EC/2004/23, November, 2007. [online] Available from www.eshre.com/file.asp?filetype=doc/04/010/eshre_position_paper_on_the_eu_tissues_and_cells_directive_ec_final.pdf [Last accessed February, 2019].
11. Fertility Clinics Abroad. (2019). ISO Accreditation in IVF Clinics Abroad. [online]. Available from https://www.fertilityclinicsabroad.com/egg-donation-abroad-europe/iso-accreditation-ivf-clinics-abroad/ [Last accessed February, 2019].
12. Gianaroli I, Plachot M, Van Kooij R, et al. Guidelines for good practice in IVF laboratories. Hum Reprod. 2000;15:2241-6.
13. Hall J, Gilligan A, Schimmel T, et al. The origin, effects and control of air pollution in laboratories used for human embryo culture. Hum Reprod. 1998;13(Suppl):146-55.
14. Hazekamp JT. Current differences and consequences of legislation on practice of assisted reproductive technology in the Nordic countries. The Nordic Committee on Assisted Reproduction of the Scandinavian Federation of Societies and Gynecology. Acta Obstet Gynecol Scand. 1996;75:198-200.
15. Human Fertilisation and Embryology Authority (HFEA). (2009). Code of Practice, 8th edition, published 2009, revised 2011. [online] Available from http://www.hfea.gov.uk/code.html [Last accessed February, 2019].
16. Human Fertilisation and Embryology Authority (HFEA). (Available from: www.HFEA.gov.uk)
17. Indian Council of Medical Research, National Academy of Medical Sciences (India). (2005). National Guidelines for Accreditation, Supervision and Regulation of ART Clinics in India. [online] Available from https://www.icmr.nic.in/sites/default/files/guidelines/Guidline_content.pdf [Last accessed February, 2019].
18. Indian Council of Medical Research Drafting Committee. (2010). The Assisted Reproductive Technology (Regulation) Rules—2010; Draft; New Delhi. [online] Available from https://icmr.nic.in/sites/default/files/guidelines/ART%20REGULATION%20Draft%20Bill1.pdf [Last accessed February, 2019].
19. Inhorn MC. Making muslim babies: IVF and gamete donation in sunni versus shi'a islam. Cult Med Psychiatry. 2006;30: 427-50.
20. ISO/IEC Guide 2:2004. (2016). Standardization and related activities—General vocabulary. 2004 International Organization for Standardization. Geneva, Switzerland. [online] Available from https://www.iso.org/standard/39976.html [Last accessed February, 2019].
21. Jin M, Jin Z, Hyllner SJ, et al. Sensitivity evaluation of a mouse embryo assay (MEA) used for quality control of IVF culture media. Hum Reprod.1998;13:282.
22. Joint Commission International Accreditation Standards for Clinical Laboratories. Joint Commission International. 2nd edition, 2010. [online]. Available from www.jointcommissioninternational.org [Last accessed February, 2019].
23. Kastrop P. Quality management in the ART laboratory. Reprod Biomed Online. 2003;7:691-4.
24. Lieberman BA, Matson PL, Hamer F. The UK human fertilization and embryology Act 1990. How well is it functioning? Hum Reprod. 1994;9:1779-82.
25. Magli MC, Van den Abbeel E, Lundin K, et al. Revised guidelines for good practice in IVF laboratories. Hum Reprod. 2008;23:1253-62.
26. Meintjes M, Chantlis SJ, Douglas JD, et al. A controlled randomized trail evaluating the effect of lowered incubator oxygen tension on live births in a predominantly blastocyst transfer program. Hum Reprod. 2009;24(2):300-7.
27. Pickering SJ, Braude PR, Johnson MH, et al. Transient cooling to room temperature can cause irreversible disruption of the meiotic spindle in the human oocyte. Fertil Steril. 1990;54:102-8.
28. Pool TB. Practices contributing to quality performance in the embryo laboratory and the status of laboratory regulation in the US. Hum Reprod. 1997;12:2591-3.
29. Practice Committee of American Society for Reproductive Medicine; Practice Committee of Society for Assisted Reproductive Technology. Revised guidelines for human embryology and andrology laboratories. Fertil Steril. 2008;90:S45-59.
30. The Fertility Society of Australia. (2010). Code of practice for Assisted Reproductive Technology Units. Fertility Society of Australia Reproductive Technology Accreditation Committee (RTAC) revised October 2010. [online] Available from www.fertilitysociety.com.au/wp.../201011201-final-rtac-cop.pdf [Last accessed February, 2019].
31. The fertility Society of Australia. (2016). Reproductive Technology Accreditation committee RTAC Technical Bulletins. [online] Available from http://www.fertilitysociety.com.au/rtac/technical-bulletins/ [Last accessed February, 2019].

Culture Media

42

Prashant Patil, Jignasha Chauhan

INTRODUCTION

Louise Brown, first in vitro fertilization (IVF) baby of the world, was transferred as an eight cell at the time of embryo transfer.[1] Usually this implantation stage embryo stays in fallopian tubes. Such embryos expelled out when they are placed in uterus in case of other mammals. Transfer of early precompaction embryos to the uterus is seen to be successful only in humans. The successful of transfer of gametes [gamete intrafallopian transfer (GIFT)] and zygote [zygote intrafallopian transfer (ZIFT)] in fallopian tube by laparoscopy, had higher success rates than IVF in spite of IVF becoming a regular procedure. The success rate of IVF and intracytoplasmic sperm injection (ICSI) with uterine placement of early embryos gradually improved from approximately 10% to 20–25% when pregnancy rates for GIFT remained relatively constant at 20–25% over decade of the 1990s.[2] This was possible because of the gradual improvement in embryo culture. Due to improvement in culture media we have achieved pregnancy rate up to 48% per egg retrieval in patient age less than 35 year,[3] higher blastocyst formation and single embryo transfer (SET).

Physiology behind culture media before attempting to culture any cell type, be it embryonic or somatic, it is important to consider the physiology of the cell in order to establish its nutrient requirements. The mammalian embryo represents an intriguing situation in which significant changes in its molecular regulation, physiology, and metabolism occur during the period of preimplantation.

The preimplantation human embryo is a highly dynamic entity that changes its needs as development proceeds. Indeed, it goes from being one of the most quiescent tissues in the body (the oocyte) to being amongst the most metabolically active (the blastocyst) within just 4 days.[4] Interestingly, the pronucleate oocyte, like the metaphase II oocyte exhibits relatively low levels of oxygen consumption and has a preference for the carboxylic acid pyruvate as its primary energy source.[5]

Lactate can be utilized as the sole substrate from the two-cell stage, but glucose is only consumed and utilized in relatively small amounts by the early embryo.[6] Maintenance of metabolic homeostasis at these early stages is paramount for the maintenance of viability. Consequently, the environment of the early embryo provided by the culture media continues to be a major focus of the culture system in the laboratory. With development and cell multiplication energy demands increases.

After activation of embryonic genome there is increase in transcription and protein synthesis, and concomitant increase in glucose utilization. Blastocyst has high oxygen utilization and ability to utilize glucose. **Table 1** highlights some of the differences between the precompacted and postcompacted embryo.[7]

Within the human female reproductive tract, the nutrients available are according to the changing needs of nutrients of the embryo. When the embryo is situated in the fallopian tube, the fluid within is characterized by high concentrations of pyruvate (0.32 mM) and lactate (10.5 mM), and low concentration of glucose (0.5 mM). Uterine fluid contains low levels of pyruvate (0.1 mM) and lactate (5.87 mM), and a better concentration of glucose (3.15 mM), as per the changes in the embryo energy production.[8]

Table 1: Differences between precompaction embryo and postcompaction embryo.

Precompaction embryo	***Postcompaction embryo***
Low synthetic capacity	High synthetic capacity
Pyruvate used for nutrition	Glucose used for nutrition
Low QO_2	High QO_2
Requires specific amino acids including alanine, aspartate, glutamate, glycine, proline, serine, and taurine	Requirement of more comprehensive group of amino acids
Maternal genome	Embryonic genome
Individual cells	Multiple cells with transporting epithelium
One cell type	Two distinct cell types: inner cell mass and trophectoderm

COMPOSITION

The composition of the media in which embryos are cultured is supposed to have an impact on the quality of embryos generated in IVF/ICSI cycles eventually influencing implantation and pregnancy rates.

Understanding their effects on embryo physiology will greatly assist clinics to make a more informed decision regarding their choice of culture media. Carbohydrates (glucose) are the primary variables in sequential culture media. Cleavage stage embryos can use glucose in minimal amounts compared to oxidative substrates like pyruvate. Sequential media utilize reduced levels of glucose (0–0.5 mM) in the first step media and often include ethylenediaminetetraacetic acid (EDTA), further suppressing glycolysis.

Culture media devoid of glucose support high rates of human embryo development and pregnancy during the first 3 days of culture. Any minimal initial requirement for glucose may likely be obtained through initial exposure and carryover from handling media containing glucose or from internal stores of glycogen. Embryos mainly utilize glucose during compaction and blastocyst development. Hence, second media employed in sequential media, there is increased concentration of glucose (2.0 mM). Pyruvate utilization remains high throughout human preimplantation embryo development. Around the time of compaction, shift in preference from pyruvate to glucose occurs.

Only lactate does not support embryo development before the stage of two cells. Low levels of lactate can affect pyruvate metabolism and can acidify internal pH. Metabolically active L-lactate isomer should be included in culture media to avoid excess suppression of internal pH that occurs with use of both D and L isomers.[9]

Amino Acids

Amino acids serve as energy sources for developing embryos, maintain intracellular homeostasis by acting as zwitterions to buffer pH, antioxidants, and also acts as organic osmolytes to control cell volume.[10]

For the process of stimulation of cleavage rate, blastocyst formation and hatching nonessential amino acids (alanine, asparagine, aspartate, glutamate, glycine, proline, and serine), and glutamine are needed. The role of essential amino acids is to stimulate cleavage rates after the eight-cell stage and development of the inner cell mass (ICM) in the blastocyst.

The fluid in oviduct contains all 20 amino acids. The spontaneous breakdown of amino acids in the culture medium occurs when incubated at 37°C producing ammonium, which has hostile effects on embryo development. Solution to this is to replace the most labile amino acid, glutamine, with a dipeptide form such as alanylglutamine. This dipeptide does not break at 37°C. Therefore, media containing this stable form of glutamine produce significantly lower levels of ammonium.[11]

Protein Supplementation

Serum albumin is contaminated with fatty acids and other small molecules. In addition to these compounds, serum albumin preparations also contain variable levels of contaminants that include carbohydrates, amino acids, transition metals, growth factors, and microribonucleic acids (miRNAs). Recombinant human albumin eliminates the problems inherent with using blood-derived products and lead to the standardization of media formulations. Recombinant human albumin has now been shown to be as effective as blood-derived albumin in supporting fertilization and embryo development.[12] Embryos cultured in the presence of recombinant albumin has an increased tolerance to cryopreservation.[13]

Hyaluronan

The hyaluronan-enriched medium was found to have significant increases in implantation rates and clinical pregnancy rates in case of day-3 as well as day-5 embryo transfers. The positive impact was more significant effect in women who were more than 35 years of age with poor-quality embryos available for transfer or had previous implantation failures.

Cochrane report confirmed the improvement in pregnancy rates as well as take-home baby rates when hyaluronan was included in the transfer medium.[14] The reason was unclear for the fact that protein cannot penetrate zona pellucida to access the embryo and also that there are no receptors present on the zona pellucida. There may be direct uterine effects. Hyaluronan in the culture medium is beneficial for cryosurvival ability of cultured embryos.[15]

Osmolality

Osmolarity around the embryo in vivo is 280–290 mOsm/kg. Most of the culture media has osmolarity between 275 mOsm and 290 mOsm. Development occurs normally in media with lower osmolality (¼ 260 mOsm). The optimal value of osmolality required for human embryo culture is still not known.[16]

CULTURE SYSTEM

The embryo culture system consists of the media, gas phase, macromolecules, medium overlay, the culture vessel, the incubation chamber, ambient air quality, and even the embryologists themselves. The concept of an embryo culture system successfully highlights the interactions that exist not only between the embryo and its physical surroundings, but also between all parameters within the laboratory.

Incubator

Whatever incubation chamber is chosen, a key to successful embryo culture is to minimize perturbations in the atmosphere around the embryo. The two key perturbations to avoid are pH and temperature changes. This means that ideally the environment in which the embryo is placed should not be disturbed during the culture period. Incubators with infrared (IR), as opposed to thermocouple CO_2 sensors, are quicker at regulating the internal environment of the chamber. Therefore, incubators equipped with IR sensors will provide a more stable environment for embryo development. With regards to temperature changes, incubators with an air jacket are less susceptible to large temperature fluctuations than those with a water jacket. The use of inner doors will aid in minimizing environmental fluctuations within the chamber.

Alternatives to classic tissue culture incubators are bench top mini-incubators with constant flow chambers, which allow for direct heat transfer between the chamber and culture vessel. Such chambers also allow for a direct flow of premixed gas, therefore minimizing changes in pH. Consequently, this approach has been shown to have inherent advantages for embryo development by minimizing there handling and variations in temperature and pH.

It is important to consider the frequency of opening an incubator in a day and to keep this to a minimum. It is advisable to have separate incubators for media equilibration and for embryo culture to control the access to incubators containing embryos and minimize the contamination.[17]

pH and Carbon Dioxide

When discussing pH, it is worth considering that the pH of the embryo is around 7.2, while the pH of the media routinely ranges from 7.25 to 7.4. Specific media components, such as lactic and amino acids, directly affect and buffer pH, respectively. Of the two isomers of lactate, D-and L-lactate, only the L-lactate form is biologically active. However, both the D-and L-lactate forms decrease pH of the embryo.[9] Therefore, it is advisable to use only the L-isomer of lactate in a medium. Amino acids increase the intracellular buffering capacity and help maintain the pH at around 7.2. When using bicarbonate-buffered media, the concentration of CO_2 has direct effect on medium's pH. Most media work over a wide range of pH (7.2–7.4), pH should not go over 7.4. CO_2 concentration of between 6% and 7% yield a medium pH of around 7.3.

When using a CO_2/bicarbonate-buffered medium, it is essential to minimize the amount of time the culture dish is out of a CO_2 environment to prevent increases in pH. To facilitate this, modified pediatric isolettes designed to maintain temperature, humidity, and CO_2 concentration can be used. An oil overlay also reduces the speed of CO_2 loss and the associated increase in pH.

Oxygen

A human embryo has capacity to grow at atmospheric oxygen concentration (~20%) and give viable pregnancies. Hence, the optimal concentration of oxygen required for embryo culture is still unclear. Consequently, the validity of having to use a reduced oxygen concentration for human embryo culture is continually challenged. The continued use of 20% oxygen in a human IVF culture system is a good example of something that has been used for over 3 decades and does give results; however, the question remains: does 20% oxygen adversely affect the physiology of the developing embryo before implantation?

It was initially established in the mouse model that 20% oxygen impacts embryo development by as early as the first cleavage. Interestingly, it was determined that 20% oxygen is detrimental to embryo development at all stages, but with the greatest detrimental effects being imparted at the cleavage stages.

Clinical data, including a randomized controlled trial, support this move to more physiological conditions in showing that lower oxygen concentrations increase both implantation and live birth rates.[18]

CULTURE VESSEL

It includes different disposables and instruments in the assisted reproductive technology (ART) laboratory. All medical devices coming in contact with gametes and embryos such as ovum pick up (OPU) needles, embryo transfer catheters, test tubes, pipettes, petri dishes, denuding pipettes, etc. should be properly quality tested and must meet minimum quality assurance such as CE-marked, mouse embryo assay (MEA) tested, and Food and Drug Administration (FDA) cleared. It should be produced under ISO 13485 with lot traceability.

Temperature

During IVF procedures gametes and embryos may be exposed to varied temperatures while handling them at different stages which can again be a stress factor in developing embryo. Therefore, laboratories aim to have the temperature of 37°C in incubators as well as at work station like stages of laminar flow and micromanipulator which is based on human core body temperature. Exposure of oocytes and embryos to lower temperatures affects the microtubules, thus risking aneuploidy in resulting embryos.[19] Lower temperatures can result in increase in pH of certain media, thus monitoring temperature is also important for maintaining stability. Higher temperature can disrupt the microtubule organization. Exposure to suboptimal temperature can affect transmembrane transport and metabolism and thus slows down embryo development.

Maintaining the embryos at a constant temperature inside the incubators may be challenging due to various factors such as media volume, frequency of door openings, and incubator type. Therefore, great care must be taken to reduce temperature fluctuations by minimizing the working time outside incubator and using warm working stages and minimizing frequency of door opening.

Light

Embryos are exposed to light for various processes in laboratory. The indirect effect of light can be via photo oxidation where chemical reaction between light and components of culture medium and oil may occur. Light has also been linked for increases production of reactive oxygen species (ROS) which may lead to fragmented embryos and apoptotic processes.

Few authors has demonstrated that (1) plastic polystyrene dishes did reduce or absorb small amounts of energies in the 400–500 nm spectra, (2) inclusion of antioxidants and exclusion of photo-oxidative components in media reduces effect of oxidation, and (3) short wavelength filters applied to halogen bulb microscopes and room (background fluorescent and natural lighting) significantly reduced the light energies.

In conclusion, it is important and beneficial to reduce light intensity and time of exposure to light for the gametes and embryos.[20]

Air Quality

Another vital parameter for the success of IVF is air quality. Presence of volatile organic compounds (VOCs), microbes, and perfumes which may be present in air are harmful to embryo development in vitro.

Ambient air of IVF laboratories may carry harmful VOCs (e.g. styrene, formaldehydes, glutaraldehydes, toluene, etc.), malignant microbes, perfumes, deodorants, and even odors from the outside environment may affect embryonic development.[21,22] VOCs are emitted by various industries like vehicles, heat exhausts, as well as by a variety of cleaning products used in IVF laboratory and instruments, such as computers, microscopes, television monitors, and furniture. High levels of VOCs (over 1 ppm) are directly toxic to embryos.[23] In ideal situation, VOC levels should be below 0.2 ppm, but preferably zero.

How to Improve Air Quality?

Central air handling unit (AHU) which includes activated carbon prefilters, chemical filters, photocatalytic conversion, and high efficiency particulate air (HEPA) filters are important for the maintenance of air quality. Mobile filter units are also available which work efficiently by purification of the air and filtration of harmful volatile compounds, bacteria, and moulds.[24]

Compressed gas used in laboratory may have harmful compounds such as benzene, pentane, and isopropanol.[22] Medical grade N_2 and CO_2 should be used. The gases should be filtered to remove any lingering contaminants before they enter the incubators by gas line filters.

In incubators high levels of VOCs may be present. The existing air filtering systems inside may reduce the levels of VOC inside incubators themselves. Anesthetic gases use in oocytes retrieval may get mixed in the air, a suitable extraction system should be installed in the operation theatre. The shelves, tables, and cupboards in the laboratory should be replaced with stainless furniture and workbenches. No wooden furniture should be allowed.

Staff can be one of the contaminants. It is necessary to have good hygiene practice among the staff. Exhaled air from smokers contains residual tobacco particles (0.5 and 2 micron in size) that can remain indefinitely in the air or settle on surfaces and walls. Therefore, the staff should be nonsmokers as far as possible or at least prevent them from smoking on a working day.

Maintaining Good Air Quality

Good laboratory practice must be continued to maintain good air quality. The air flow parameters should be recorded regularly, e.g. filter integrity and daily positive pressure measurements. Regular servicing of equipment safeguards against drop in air quality and must be done without fail. Positive pressure in laboratory should be monitored by the pressure differential recorded by a simple pressure gauge to indicate filter efficiency. Validation of air quality can be done periodically by measuring particle count and VOC levels.

EMBRYO:VOLUME RATIO

Embryo cultured in drops of culture medium under an oil overlay is the preferred and effective method of culturing embryos. Physiologically the embryo is exposed to microliter volumes of fluid. In contrast, when the embryos are grown in vitro is subject to relatively large volumes of medium of up to 1 mL.

There may be dilution of any autocrine factor(s) produced by the developing embryo because of the larger volume of fluid. It has been demonstrated in the mouse that cleavage rate and blastocyst formation increase when embryos are grown in groups (of up to 10) or reduced volumes (around 20 μL).[25]

To increase the viability of the embryo, the incubation volume has to be minimum to increase ICM development.[26] In order to culture in such reduced volumes (of 20–50 μL), an oil overlay is required. Although the use of an oil overlay is time-consuming, it prevents the evaporation of media and increase in osmolality. It also reduces changes in pH.

Care must be taken in selecting and storing oil, which if done incorrectly will lead to it becoming toxic. Oil should be stored in the dark and in glass. It should not be stored for extended periods in the incubator. Oil should never be aliquoted into tissue culture flasks as these are styrene based and oils are able to leach styrene from such containers at high rates over time.

EMBRYOLOGIST

The embryologist maintains laboratory conditions most conducive for embryos to flourish. The skills required by an embryologist are complex, delicate, and require years of experience.

MONOCULTURE OR SEQUENTIAL CULTURE MEDIA

Embryo during development uses amino acids and produces ammonium. Medium should ideally be renewed/replenished at least every 48 hours to make sure that accumulation of embryotoxic ammonium is minimal irrespective of culture system used.[27]

In last few years, the sequential culture media is commonly used in which cleavage stage embryos are cultured in one media formulation for first 1–3 days, then subsequently cultured in a second media formulation for next 2–3 days.

The composition of these media varies to match the changing levels of glucose and other energy substrates as well as the complement of amino acids, chelators, and other components. This is to meet the changing needs of the embryo by attempting to mimic vivo, where the composition of oviductal fluid differs from that of uterine-fluid.[8] This approach is to ensure the adequate supply of substrates and removal of potentially harmful by-products, such as ammonia.

In contrast, monoculture media systems are designed for "letting the embryo decide" which components it prefers. In a number of laboratories, monoculture systems prove to be as efficient as sequential culture systems.[28]

Importantly, though many media are commercially available, their efficiency needs to be evaluated in the context of their use within a particular laboratory, in conjunction with the variety of other processes that makeup the complete culture system. Which culture system be used is depends usually on individual preferences, availability, and experiences.

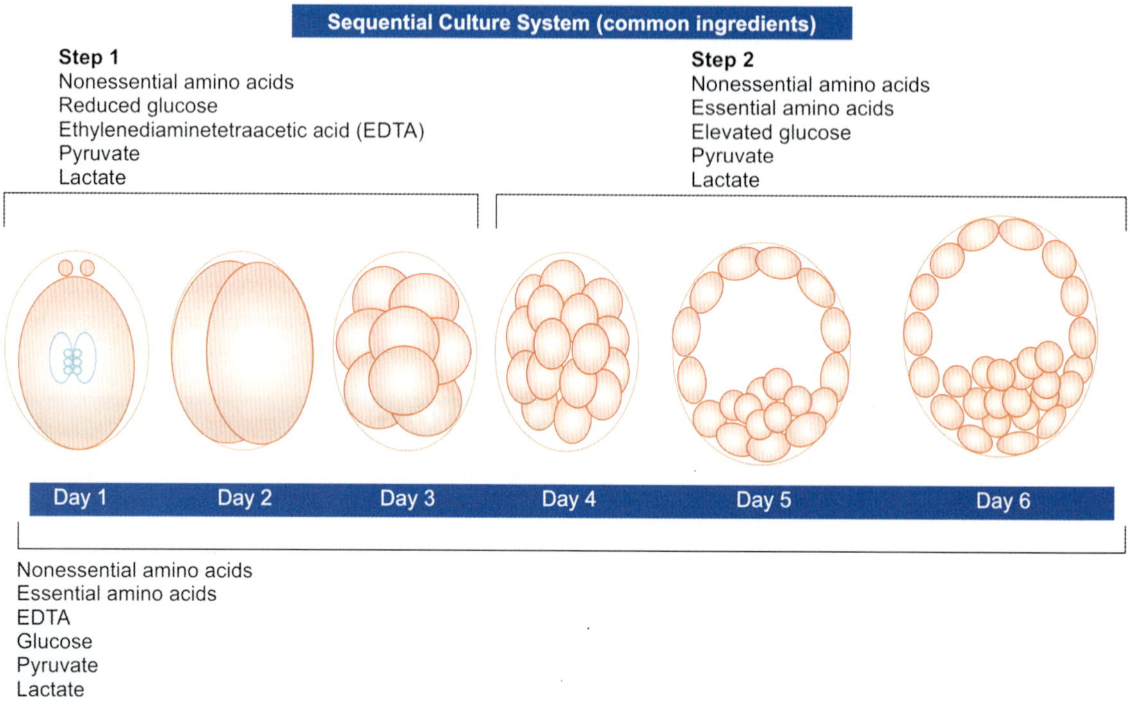

Monoculture (Common Ingredients)

With the advent of time-lapse microscopy, the emergence of media designed specifically for the purpose of uninterrupted embryo culture, with the aim of minimizing the build-up of ammonium.[29] These media have been shown to be effective, but further work is warranted in this area, such as the development of sequential media in situ, upon which existing media drops are not renewed but supplemented with a second formulation to give rise to a modified culture environment.

Handling Media and Buffers

Culture media formulations used within incubators have significantly improved our ability to produce better embryos in vitro when the composition of media used for manipulations outside the incubator is not given priority.

Oil overlay is important technique to prevent pH rise above 7.4.[30] Thus, for procedures such as oocyte retrieval, sperm processing, oocyte denuding, and ICSI it is recommended that special handling media be utilized that resists changes in pH.

Commonly used commercially available handling media for ART are 4-(2-hydroxyethyl)-1-piperazineethanesulfonic acid (HEPES) and 3-(N-morpholino) propanesulfonic acid (MOPS) and selected based on their pKa values, and their optimal buffering capacity.

The standard one is HEPES at -21 mM for IVF handling media. More recently, commercial companies also include MOPS in their IVF handling media. Both the buffer media are efficient and need not be equilibrated.

Progressive Media and Microfluidics

For the improvement of IVF culture media another technology is underdevelopment known as microfluidics. Nanosensors could theoretically detect changes in the growth environment or sense other clues from the developing cells and subsequently modify the culture environment. Hence, there is no need for removing dishes from the incubator or manually moving embryos. Microfluidics will be the future as it provides customized growth environment for the specific needs of the embryos.[31]

Medium Storage

When using culture media, they should be placed in the incubator for the minimum time required for equilibration, and they should certainly never be stored in the incubator. Vitamins are light sensitive and therefore care should be taken to minimize exposure to light by storing the culture media in the dark. Do not aliquot medium in test tube and then store these in the refrigerator until the day of use. It is not good practice because handing the media like this makes them prone to microbial contamination; pH will go up during the whole process.

CONCLUSION

Significant improvements in culture media formulations and embryo culture systems have conclusively provided better conditions for the human embryo to develop in the laboratory. The ability to culture embryos to the blastocyst stage has facilitated the introduction of the safer practice of SETs for an increasing number of patients, including those undergoing oocyte donation or who are less than 38 years of age and in their first cycle, and increasingly in conjunction with preimplantation genetic screening.

It is evident that culture conditions affect the ability of embryos to survive cryopreservation. As we move closer to the day when single-embryo/blastocyst transfer is considered the standard of care, it becomes more important than ever to ensure embryos are given the best chance of being cryopreserved for transfer at a later date, thereby increasing the efficiency of each oocyte retrieval procedure.

- Measure pH of each new lot of product received.
- Store media in dark place and maintain temperature between 2°C and 4°C.
- Equilibrate bicarbonate media for sufficient time—minimum of 4 hours but usually overnight at 37°C and 6% CO_2 (CO_2 concentration may change according to altitude of place from sea level, e.g. high altitude places will require higher concentration of CO_2).
- Buffers like HEPES or MOP should be used for procedures like oocyte retrieval, sperm processing, oocyte denuding, and ICSI. They do not require equilibration in CO_2 prior use.
- Renew the culture medium at least every 48 hours, or one can refresh the medium by adding more volume to dilute out the ammonium present.
- Use air jacket incubator with IR sensor and inner doors. Use two separate incubators, one for media equilibration and other for embryo culture. Keep door opening minimum. Use incubators providing 5% O_2.
- Culture embryo in group, usually three to four embryos in 50 μL of media. Use oil overlay.

REFERENCES

1. Steptone PC, Edwards RG. Birth after the reimplantation of a human embryo. Lancet. 1978;2:366.
2. Quinn P. The development and impact of assisted reproductive technologies culture media. Fertil Steril. 2004;8:27-9.
3. SART. (2015). National Summary Report. [online] Available from https://www.sartcorsonline.com/rptCSR_PublicMultYear.aspx?reportingYear=2015 [Last accessed February, 2019].
4. Gardner DK. Changes in requirements and utilization of nutrients during mammalian preimplantation embryo development and their significance in embryo culture. Theriogenology. 1998;49:83-102.
5. Leese HJ. Metabolism of the preimplantation mammalian embryo. Oxf Rev Reprod Biol. 1991;13:35-72.
6. Hardy K, Hooper MA, Handyside AH, et al. Noninvasive measurement of glucose and pyruvate uptake by individual human oocytes and preimplantation embryos. Hum Reprod. 1989;4:188-91.
7. Gardner DK, Wale PL. Analysis of metabolism to select viable human embryos for transfer. Fertil Steril. 2013;99: 1062-72.
8. Gardner DK, Lane M, Calderon I, et al. Environment of the preimplantation human embryo in vivo: Metabolite analysis of oviduct and uterine fluids and metabolism of cumulus cells. Fertil Steril. 1996;65:349-53.
9. Lane M, Gardner DK. Regulation of ionic homeostasis by mammalian embryos. Semin Reprod Med. 2000;18(2): 195-204.
10. Gardner DK, Lane M. Culture systems for human embryos. In: Gardner DK, Weissman A, Howles C, Zeev S (Eds). Textbook of Assisted Reproductive Technologies. Boca Raton: Informa UK Ltd; 2009. pp. 219-40.
11. Biggers JD, McGinnis LK, Lawitts JA, et al. Enhanced effect of glycyl-L-glutamine on mouse preimplantation embryos in vitro. Reprod Biomed Online. 2004;9(1):59-69.
12. Bungum M, Humaidan P, Bungum L. Recombinant human albumin as protein source in culture media used for IVF: A prospective randomized study. Reprod Biomed Online. 2002;4:233-6.
13. Lane M, Maybach JM, Hooper K, et al. Cryo-survival and development of bovine blastocysts are enhanced by culture with recombinant albumin and hyaluronan. Mol Reprod Dev. 2003;64:70-8.
14. Bontekoe S, Heineman MJ, Johnson N, et al. Adherence compounds in embryo transfer media for assisted reproductive technologies. Cochrane Database Syst Rev. 2014;2:CD007421.
15. Stojkovic M, Kolle S, Peinl S, et al. Effects of high concentrations of hyaluronan in culture medium on development and survival rates of fresh and frozen-thawed bovine embryos produced in vitro. Reproduction. 2002;124:141-53.
16. Dawson KM, Baltz JM. Organic osmolytes embryos: substrates of the Gly and beta transport systems protect

mouse zygotes against the effects of raised osmolarity. Bio Reprod. 1997;56:1550-8.
17. Wale PL, Gardner DK. The effects of chemical and physical factors on mammalian embryo culture and their importance for the practice of assisted human reproduction. Hum Reprod Update. 2016;22:2-22.
18. Wale PL, Gardner DK. Time-lapse analysis of mouse embryo development in oxygen gradients. Reprod Biomed Online. 2010;21:402-10.
19. Menezes J. Embryo culture systems. In: Nair MS (Ed). Insights into Infertility Management. New Delhi: Jaypee Brothers Medical Publishers; 2012.
20. SAGE Journals. (2012). The Effect of Light on Embryos and Embryo Culture. [online] Available from https://journals.sagepub.com/doi/abs/10.1177/205891581200300203 [Last accessed February, 2019].
21. Brown SK. Chamber assessment of formaldehyde and VOC emissions from wood-based panels. Indoor Air. 1999; 9:209-15.
22. Cohen J, Gilligan A, Esposito W, et al. Ambient air and its potential effects on conception in vitro. Hum Reprod. 1997;12:1742-9.
23. BioNews. (2010). Air pollution linked to lower IVF success. [online] Available from https://www.bionews.org.uk/page_92290 [Last accessed February, 2019].
24. Forman M, Polanski V, Horvath P. et al. Reduction in volatile organic compounds, adehydes, and particulate air contaminants in an IVF laboratory by centralized and standalone air filtration systems. Fertil Steril. 2004; 82(Suppl 2):S324.
25. Ahern TJ, Gardner DK. Culturing bovine embryos in groups stimulates blastocyst development and cell allocation to the inner cell mass. Theriogenology. 1998;49:194.
26. Lane M, Gardner DK. Effect of incubation volume and embryo density on the development and viability of mouse embryos in vitro. Hum Reprod. 1992;7:558-62.
27. Gardner DK, Lane M. Embryo culture systems. In: Gardner DK, Simon C (Eds). Handbook of In Vitro Fertilization, 4th edition. Boca Raton: CRC Press; 2017. pp. 205-244.
28. Macklon NS, Pieters MH, Hassan MA, et al. A prospective randomized comparison of sequential versus monoculture systems for in vitro human blastocyst development. Hum Reprod. 2002;17(10):2700-5.
29. Hardarson T, Bungum M, Conaghan J, et al. Noninferiority, randomized, controlled trial comparing embryo development using media developed for sequential or undisturbed culture in a time-lapse setup. Fertil Steril. 2015;104:1452-59. e1-4.
30. Steel T, Conaghan J. pH equilibration dynamics of culture medium under oil. Fertil steril. 2008;89 suppl 2:s27.
31. Angle M. Using two concurrent sequential culture media improves pregnancy outcomes. Clinical Embryologist. 2006;9(1):5-11.

Gamete and Embryo Morphology 43

Pinky Shah, Hima Shah

SPERM MORPHOLOGY

INTRODUCTION

The term spermatozoa is derived from the ancient Greek words "sperma" (meaning seed) and "zoon" (meaning living being). The first detailed description of sperm was done in 1677 by Antoni Van Leeuwenhoek.

The human sperm has specialized structure and plays an important role of transferring the paternal genome into the egg at the time of fertilization. Postfertilization, the male and female chromosomes with process of syngamy form the genetic constitution of zygote.

ULTRASTRUCTURE OF SPERM

The human spermatozoon is approximately 60 μm in length. A mature sperm cell is divided into three morphologic parts: head, neck (middle piece), and tail **(Fig. 1)**.

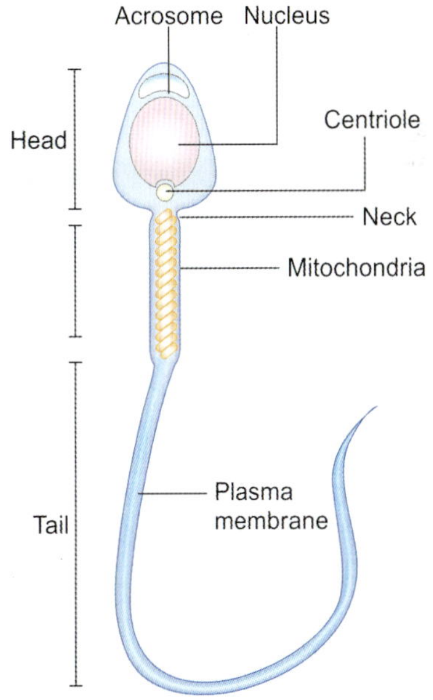

Fig. 1: Structure of sperm.

Head

Sperm head is plate-like structure. It is oval in shape and slightly tapered on the anterior side. The thickness of the head gradually increases from the apex towards the base, due to which, the sperm head appears pointed when viewed from the side and oval from the front. It is 3–5 μm in length and 2–3 μm in width. The ratio of the length/width is around 1.5–1.75.

The components of head are the nucleus, nuclear membrane, acrosomal cap, inner acrosomal membrane, outer acrosomal membrane, and plasma membrane **(Fig. 2)**.

The nucleus is highly compacted chromatin and the acrosome is membrane bound organelle which harbors enzymes that penetrates the outer layer of the egg prior to fertilization.

Acrosome constitutes about two-thirds of the anterior head area. It is formed from Golgi complex of the spermatid as it differentiates to spermatozoa. It is divided into a cap and an equatorial region. Acrosome contains hydrolytic enzymes like hyaluronidase, acrosin, and others.

The hyaluronidase enzyme assists the sperm to pass through the cumulus matrix while acrosin helps the sperm to penetrate ZP. The contents of acrosome are released

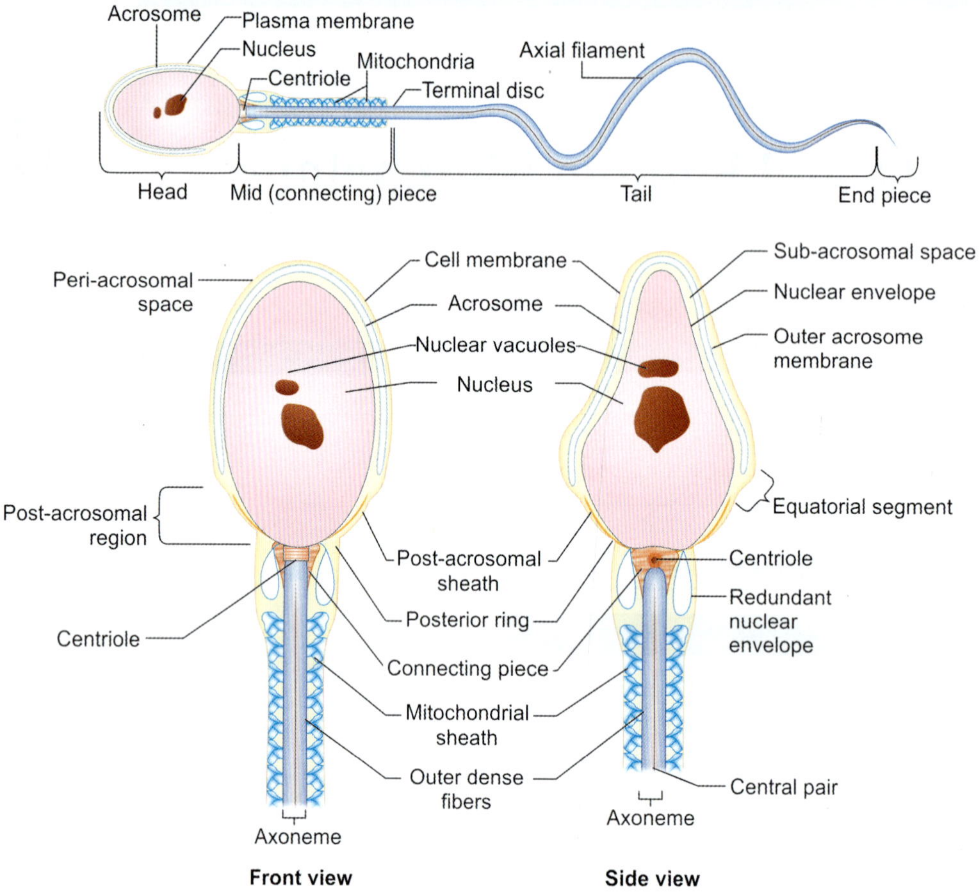

Fig. 2: Components of sperm.
Source: Williams PL, Warwick R (Eds). Gray's anatomy, 36th edition. Edinburgh: Churchill Livingstone; 1980.

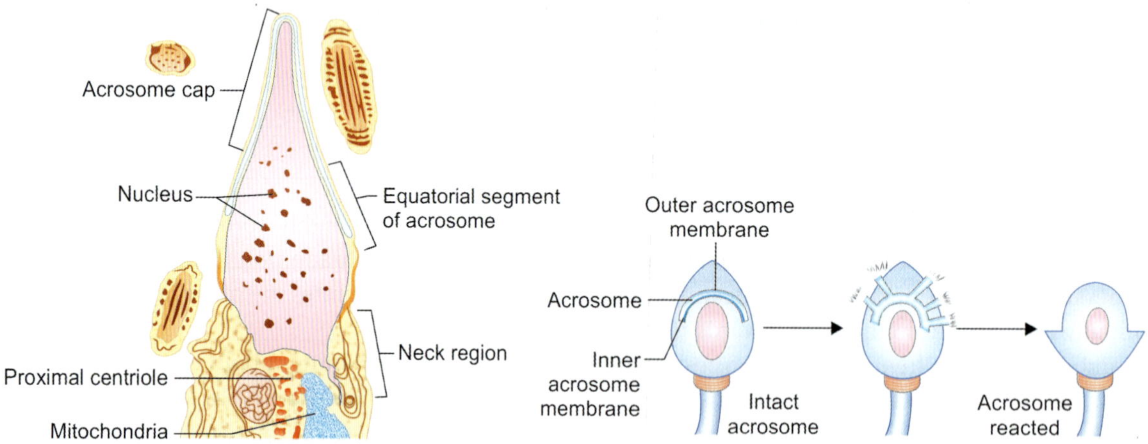

Fig. 3: Acrosome and acrosome reaction.

at the time of acrosomal reaction. The fusion of outer acrosomal membrane occurs with plasma membrane at multiple sites and anterior half of the head is then void of plasma and outer acrosomal membrane. The equatorial segment of the acrosome remains more or less intact (**Fig. 3**).

Postacrosomal Region

The postacrosomal region starts just after the equatorial region. The sperm egg membrane fusion occurs in this region usually. It is in this region where the sperm egg membrane fusion occurs usually.

Nucleus

The nucleus occupies the majority of the space in the head of the spermatozoa. It is the shape of the nucleus that decides the shape of the head. It contains proteins and deoxyribonucleic acid (DNA) as compact chromatin and is covered by nuclear membrane.

The genetic information conducted by the spermatozoa is coded and retained in the DNA molecule and the hereditary characteristics are passed by the sperm nucleus.

Neck

It is also called as the connecting piece as it unites the head and the tail of the spermatozoon. The plasma membrane that covers the head continues to surround the neck and tail.

The neck region encompasses the proximal centriole, distal centriole, and the basal body. The neck is connected to the basal plate proximally and to the middle piece distally.

In its proximal portion, the basal body has a plate like structure called "capitulum" which fits into the depression (implantation fossa) in the base of the nucleus. Nine segmented rod-like structures are seen in the neck region. Each of this segmented rod-like structure is continuous distally with the corresponding coarse fibril of the axial filament. The proximal centriole lies just below the implantation fossa. The axial filament begins just behind the proximal centriole from the posterior end knob that originates from the distal centriole of the spermatid. It passes through the middle piece and extends into the tail. At the junction of the middle piece and the principal piece the axial filament passes through a ring-like structure called the annulus. The proximal centriole is composed of nine triplets of microtubules which resemble a pin wheel, which is surrounded by pericentriolar material, and is concealed inside the vault of black box. The black box is composed of capitulum and nine segmented columns. These columns merge posteriorly with outer dense fibers of midpiece and tail.

Tail

The tail is around 50 µm in length. It consists of three parts—middle piece, principal piece, and the end piece. The midpiece and tail aid in sperm motility. These contain axoneme which comprises of nine doublets of microtubules, which surrounds a central doublet.

Middle Piece

It is a long cylindrical structure which consists of the central axial filament surrounded by the mitochondrial sheath and is covered by the cell membrane. The mitochondria of the spermatid are arranged in helical (spiral) manner in the mitochondrial sheath. There are 12 turns of mitochondrial helix. The mitochondrial sheath provides the sperm with energy for motility. The axial filament is made up of fibrous sheath, which surrounds several longitudinal fibrils in a particular manner. The fibrous sheath is composed of several branching and interlinking semicircular strands held together by their attachment to two longitudinal bars located at opposite sides. These longitudinal bars run along the tail.

Immediately inside the fibrous sheath is a layer of nine coarse fibrils. These fibrils are petal shaped and are of unequal size and are present in the middle piece and the principal piece of the tail, but are absent in the end piece.

Inside the layer of nine coarse fibrils is the layer of nine pairs of doublets of microtubules. Each pair of doublet of microtubule is situated on the inner side each coarse fibril. Finally, the core of the axial bundle consisting of a central pair of microtubules is present inside of the nine pair of doublets of microtubules. There are radial links from the coarse fibrils to the central pair of chromosomes **(Fig. 4)**.

Physiologically axoneme forms a motor assembly with 200–300 proteins. Main role is played by "9 + 2" pattern of microtubules. The dynein protein extends from one microtubule doublet to adjacent doublet. It thus forms both inner and outer arms of the axoneme.

Principal Piece

This part constitutes most of the length of the tail and is the motile part. It provides most of the propellant movement to the sperm.

The structure of the principal piece is similar to that of the middle piece. It is devoid of its mitochondrial sheath. The coarse nine fibrils in the middle piece gradually decrease in thickness and finally disappear leaving only the inner fibrils in the axial core for most of the length of

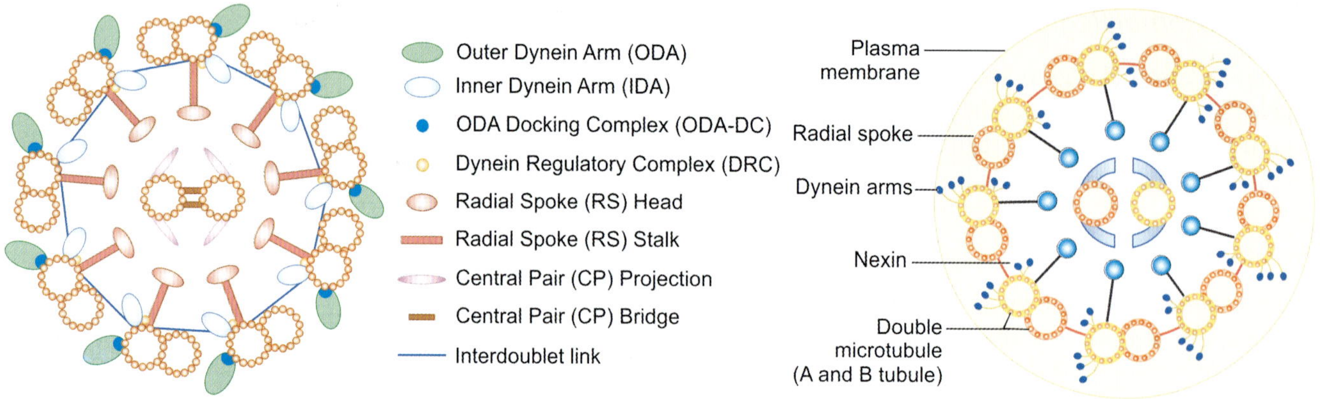

Fig. 4: "9 + 2" sperm axonemal structure.

the principal piece. Inside the layer of fibrous sheath there are nine coarse fibrils with numbers designated from 1 to 9 in clockwise manner. The line joining fibril 3 and 8 divides the tail into a major compartment containing 4 fibrils and minor compartment containing 3 fibrils. This line also passes through both the central microtubules and provides an axis for symmetrical sperm movements. Thus, this provides powerful stroke of the tail in one direction.

End Piece

The principal piece terminates in the end piece which is the most distal part of the sperm. It consists of the axial filament and the plasma membrane.

The Kruger's criteria for assessment of normal forms of the sperm:

- *Head*: Smooth; oval configuration; length, 5–6 µm diameter, 2.5–3.5 µm; and acrosome, must constitute 40–70% of the sperm head.
- *Midpiece*: Slender, axially attached; 50% of the size of the sperm head.
- *Tail*: Single, unbroken, straight, without kinks or coils approximately 45 µm in length.

GAMETE MORPHOLOGY

INTRODUCTION

Human reproduction is the union of the oocyte and the sperm resulting in a zygote, which eventually leads to a live birth.

The oocyte contributes the cytoplasm for early embryonic development, receives the sperm for fertilization, and also provides for half of the genome of the resulting zygote. The quality of an embryo and its development depends on the nature of the two gametes.

The morphological assessment of an oocyte depends on the external impression of the cumulus cells or the cumulus-oocyte complex (COC). Oocytes that are mature and might have a dynamic secretion of hyaluronic acid usually have an expanded cumulus complex. This active secretion appears to give the cumulus cells its fluffy appearance.

The oocytes can be evaluated better once the cumulus cells have been removed with the use of hyaluronidase. The morphology of the cytoplasm, stage of maturity, and the presence or absence of extracytoplasmic structures helps us in determining the quality of the oocyte. A normal, mature human oocyte ideally has a healthy cytoplasm, a polar body (PB), and an adequate perivitelline space (PVS) and a zona pellucida (ZP) of about 17.5 micron thickness.

The oocyte morphology alone does not provide enough insight into the fertilization potential or developmental capability of the zygote.

CORONA-CUMULUS COMPLEX

When a follicular antrum is formed, the granulosa cells (GCs) differentiate to form the cumulus cells which are usually seen around the oocyte and another layer of mural GCs which are found lining the follicular wall.

The cumulus cells provide nutrition to the oocyte during its development. The layer of cells immediately adjacent to the ZP is called corona radiata, which extend their cytoplasm towards the oocyte through the ZP.

Oocyte nuclear maturation is associated with an increased extension and mucification of the cumulus cells in a regular unstimulated cycle. However, during stimulated cycles this may be characterized by an asynchrony of these two processes. This was probably due to a difference in the responsiveness to the stimulants of the oocyte and the cumulus-corona.

Ng and team (1999), used a reformed grading method adapted by Wolf and his team (1988) **(Box 1)**, and showed that COCs that had reached maturity **(Fig. 5)** resulted in higher fertilization rates.

Box 1: Grading method for cumulus-oocyte complex (COC).

- Grade 1: Cumulus cells may not be present and very few corona cells can be seen.
- Grade 2: Compact cumulus and corona cells
- Grade 3: Extensive, fluffy cumulus and corona cells
- Grade 4: Scanty cumulus and corona cells

Source: Adapted from Wolf, 1988.

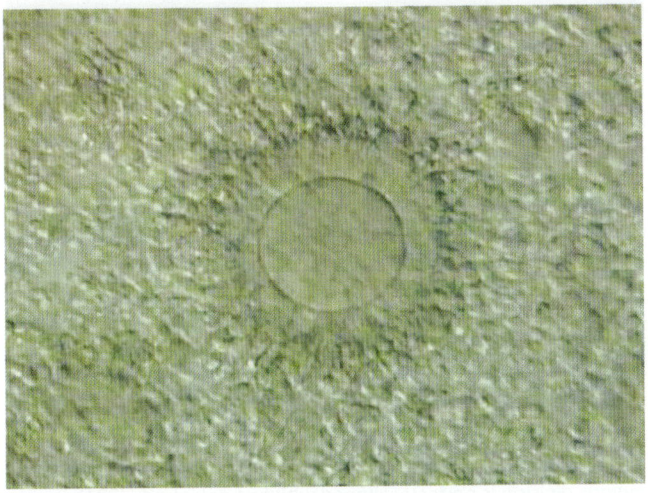

Fig. 5: Expanded cumulus-oocyte complex (COC) after ovarian stimulation. First polar body (PB1) can be seen at the 1 o'clock position.

Studies grade oocyte maturity based on the structure of the ooplasm and other factors such as cumulus mass, GCs, and the corona radiata **(Table 1)**.

A lot of studies show that metaphase II (MII) oocytes yield a higher rate of fertilization and the embryo quality tends to be better, whereas oocytes with a poor morphology yield a higher number of bad quality embryos.

Thus concluding that for in vitro fertilization (IVF), COC grading can help in predicting the oocyte maturity whereas for intracytoplasmic sperm injection (ICSI), such a scoring system is ineffectual since oocytes are denuded before insemination.

OOCYTE NUCLEAR MATURITY

The oocyte morphology and other extracellular and intracellular components can be observed only after denudation, i.e. the removal of the corona-cumulus mass with the help of hyaluronidase enzyme. A meiotically mature oocyte is arrested at MII stage and it completes maturation only after the entry of a sperm.

A mature oocyte is one which has a visible PB and no germinal vesicle (GV) **(Fig. 6)**.

An oocyte which is in the metaphase of the first meiotic division has no visible PB or GV. In vitro maturation can be performed for GVs **(Fig. 7)** and MI **(Fig. 8)** oocytes, but the fertilization rates are recorded to be much lower with a higher occurrence of genetic abnormalities.

The meiotic spindle (MS) plays a vital role in the accurate completion of meiosis and fertilization. The microtubules of the spindle being very sensitive to any physical variation such as change in temperature and any changes in the chemical composition such as pH which might occur during oocyte handling are known to have a serious effect on the chromosomal organizations.

Table 1: Grading of oocyte maturity.

Grade	*Cumulus*	*Corona Radiata*	*Zona Pellucida*	*Ooplasm*	*Granulosa Cells*
1 (Mature)	Expanded	Dispersed	Clear	Homogenous	Expanded and well aggregated
2 (Almost mature)	Expanded	Slightly dense	Clear	Homogenous	Expanded and well aggregated
3 (Immature)	Dense/Compact	Very adherent	Slightly thick	Germinal vesicle seen	Compact
4 (Postmature)	Clumped and expanded	Radiant and clumped	Thick and dark	Slightly heterogeneous	Nonaggregated
5 (Atretic)	Almost none	Clumped	Thick and dark	Deformed	Small clumps

Source: Adapted from Lin, 2003.

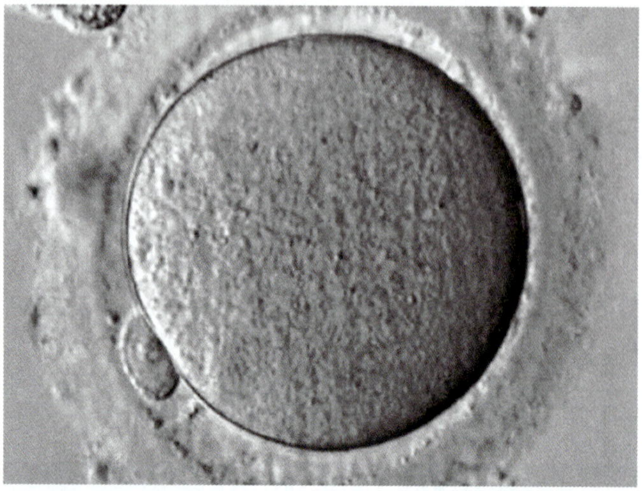

Fig. 6: Metaphase II (MII) oocyte with a polar body (PB) seen in the perivitelline (PV) space (400×).

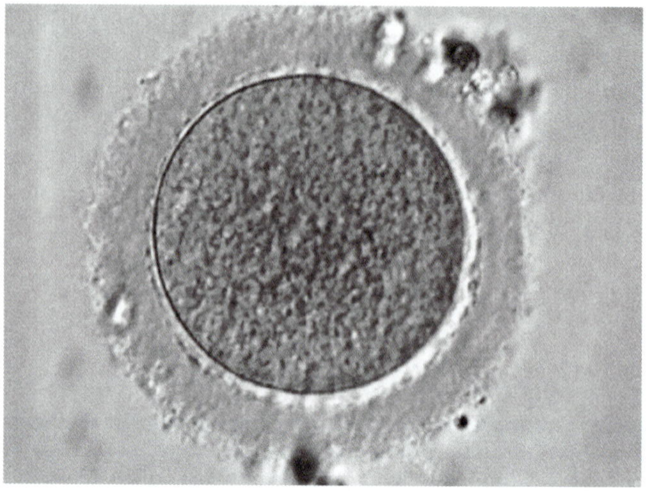

Fig. 8: Metaphase I (MI) oocyte. No visible nucleus or polar body (PB) (400×). Perivitelline space (PVS) is usually narrow.

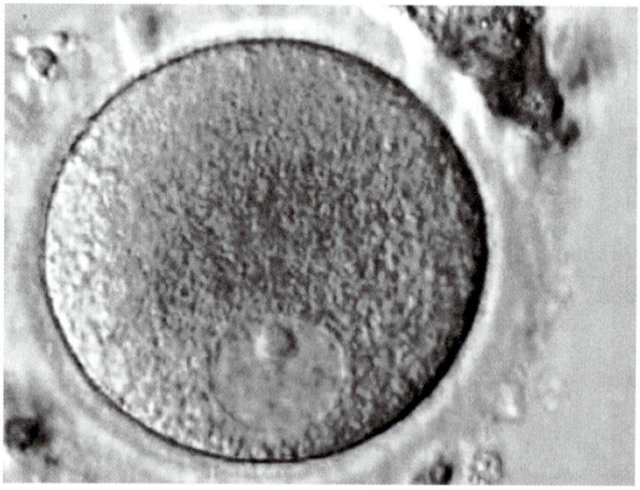

Fig. 7: Germinal vesicle (GV) oocyte with a nucleus off center and a distinguished single nucleolus (400×).

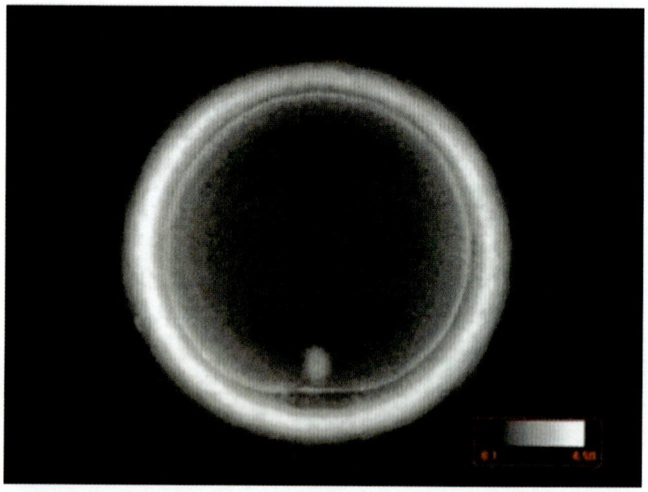

Fig. 9: Mature metaphase II (MII) oocyte (400×). Extruded polar body (PB) (6 o'clock position) and the meiotic spindle (MS) of the second meiotic division is perfectly aligned with first polar body (PB1).

The introduction of an orientation independent polarized light microscopy system (spindle view Pol-Scope system) coupled with an imaging software, allows the visualization of the MS **(Fig. 9)** in living oocytes. It is essential to have an observable MS in the oocyte before ICSI as shown in studies. The presence of a MS had a positive impact on the rate of fertilization and further embryo development.

Apart from its role in chromosomal segregation, the MS also plays a vital role in the formation of the PB1. Its position determines the orientation of the cleavage furrow and the site of extrusion of the PB1. However, the PB1 can be dislocated due to denudation.

Embryos that result in a high BC formation rate had an intact PB as compared to those with a fragmented PB. However, recent evidence suggests that it is not a dependable marker since its structure changes in culture.

OOPLASM

Severe abnormalities of the cytoplasmic homogeneity **(Fig. 10)** adversely affect the developmental and implantation potential of the embryo, but the different heterogeneities are still under research.

Granular cytoplasms **(Fig. 11)** are badly defined as of now. Smooth endoplasmic reticulum (SER) disks within

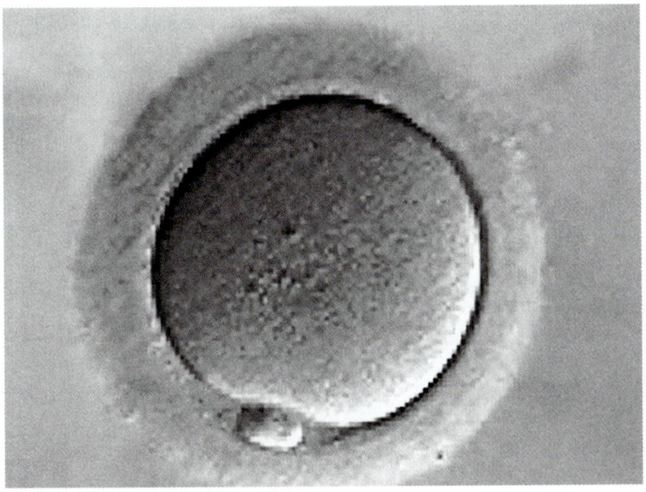

Fig. 10: Mature oocyte with a homogenous cytoplasm (400×).

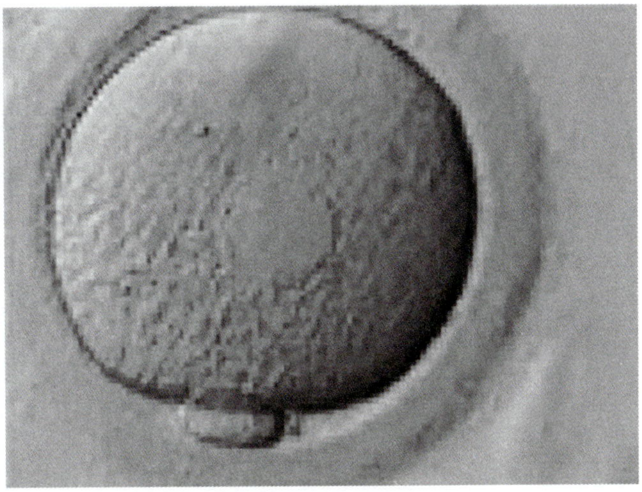

Fig. 12: Metaphase II (MII) oocyte showing smooth endoplasmic reticulum (SER) disks within the cytoplasm (400×).

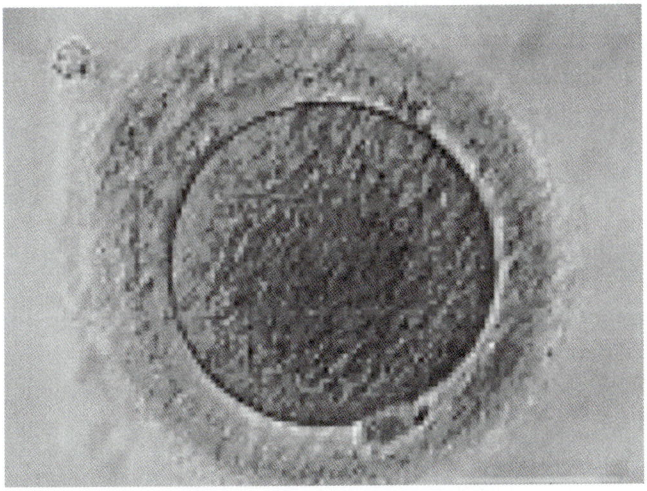

Fig. 11: Metaphase II (MII) oocyte with granular cytoplasm and a thicker zona pellucida (ZP) (400×).

the cytoplasm are the most striking abnormality of MII oocytes **(Fig. 12)**. It has been shown that that embryos formed from such oocytes are at a greater risk of severe abnormal outcomes (Balaban, Ebner, 2006). The cytoplasm may also contain vacuoles (fluid-filled complexes) of different sizes which may adversely affect the rate of fertilization (if > 14 μm).

Studies show that oocytes with a highly viscous cytoplasm result in a poor quality embryo and a lower pregnancy and implantation rate. Loutradis in 1999, showed that the degree of cytoplasmic defect (dark cytoplasm, vacuoles, and fragments) affects the overall formation and quality of an embryo.

ZONA PELLUCIDA AND PERIVITELLINE SPACE (FIGS. 13A AND B)

Montag (2008) and Ebner (2010) showed that the inner layer of the zona is highly ordered and embryos with a good prognosis in terms of blastocyst formation and implantation rate can be predicted while observing with a polarized light source.

Many authors suggested that a large PVS had a negative impact on overall fertilization rate and embryo quality. Also, granularities in the PVS could be a result of an overdose of gonadotropins (Hassan Ali et al., 1998), but the results showed no difference in implantation potential.

Xia et al. (1997) graded oocytes based on two extracytoplasmic (PB and PVS) and one cytoplasmic (inclusions) features. He extrapolated these results to see if it had any effect on the rate of fertilization or embryo quality. The results indicated that the oocytes with cytoplasmic inclusions but no extracytoplasmic defects showed a lower fertilization rate and a poor embryo quality. Whereas the group of oocytes without cytoplasmic inclusions but with extracytoplasmic deformities showed a minor decrease in overall embryo quality.

Therefore, the most important characteristic of an oocyte which determined the embryo development was the cytoplasmic integrity and composition rather than any extracytoplasmic abnormalities (Balaban et al., 1998).

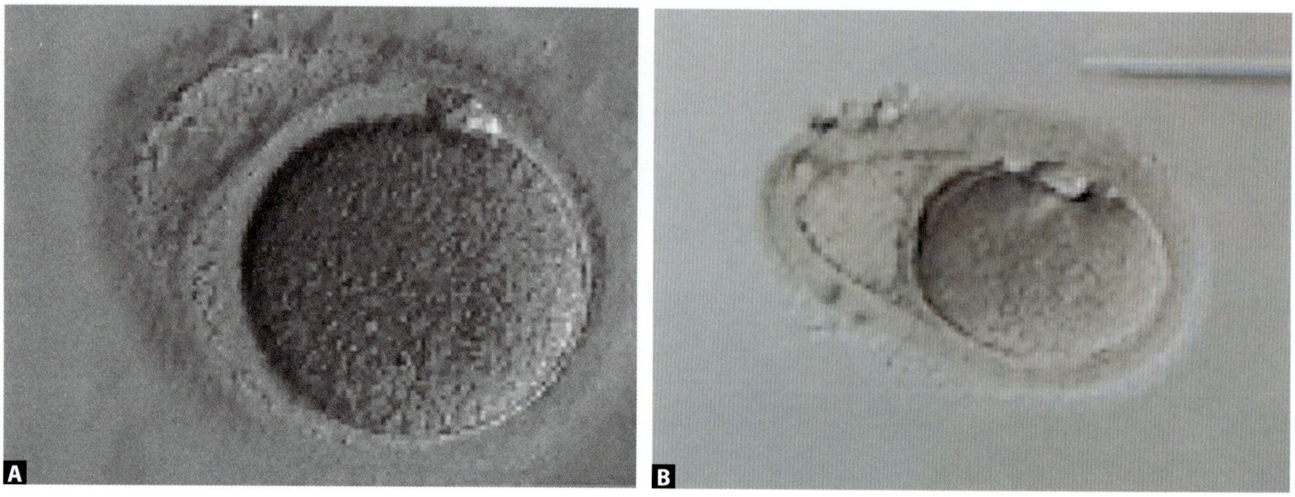

Figs. 13A and B: (A) Oocyte with a normal shape but an irregular zona pellucida (ZP) and a tear in the ZP; (B) Oocyte with an irregular shape and a torn ZP.

OOCYTE MORPHOLOGY, EMBRYO DEVELOPMENT, AND IMPLANTATION

De Sutter (1996), demonstrated that the number of deformities in an oocyte did not determine the embryo quality. Balaban et al. (1998) also demonstrated that the occurrence of two or three abnormalities together in a group of oocytes was 26% and 6%, respectively.

More recently Kahraman et al. (2000) showed that 53% of the embryos derived from the group of oocytes with centrally granulated cytoplasm were aneuploid and the fate of oocytes with any extracytoplasmic deformities is not known. It was recently demonstrated that, although the aneuploidy rate of the group of embryos derived from oocytes with extracytoplasmic abnormalities (46.7%) were similar to the group of embryos derived from oocytes with normal morphology (41.8%), the aneuploidy rate for the group of embryos derived from oocytes with cytoplasmic abnormality was higher (60.0%) when compared with the group of embryos derived from oocytes with extracytoplasmic abnormality and oocytes with normal morphology (Balaban et al., 2003).

CORRELATION BETWEEN OVARIAN STIMULATION, OOCYTE QUALITY, AND MORPHOLOGICAL APPEARANCE

Recent studies suggest that higher concentrations of luteinizing hormone (LH) during stimulation might adversely affect oocyte quality and thus the pregnancy rate (Howles et al., 1986). Most studies depend on nuclear maturity of the oocytes and not the morphology and a few handful of research articles take into consideration different protocols and gonadotropins and its effects (Imthurn et al., 1996).

Unfortunately there are no reliable articles that study the effect of different stimulation protocols and gonadotropin dosages on oocyte maturity.

Thus, concluding that oocyte morphology is one of the parameters that aid in determining embryo quality and implantation potential. Other parameters like the rate of blastocyst formation and other genetic screening tests along with oocyte and embryo morphology might help us decide the ideal embryo for transfer.

EMBRYO MORPHOLOGY

INTRODUCTION

The zygote is the first stage of embryonic development after fertilization. Early stage development markers like morphology and cleavage stage add some predictive value for the embryo's implantation potential.

The zygote scoring system attempts to differentiate normal embryos with more developmental potential from abnormal embryos by evaluating the pronuclei. However, no correlation between zygote morphology and implantation has been identified.

Clinical research has implied that early embryo morphology and cleavage can help in determining the implantation potential of an embryo. These criteria are based on embryo appearance, are considered to be the "gold standard" in assessing embryo development.

Zygotes ideally have the same number of small nucleolar precursor bodies distributed in the nucleus or large nucleolar precursor bodies with polar distribution between the pronuclei. Zygote abnormalities frequently observed can be a large, PVS, dark ZP, dark incorporations, spots, vacuoles, and irregular shape. The second criterion observed in the morphological analysis is the occurrence of meiotic division, which can be observed by the presence of two blastomeres. Continued morphological assessment relies on symmetry of blastomeres, cellular fragmentation, and developmental rate. While a number of studies support use of early embryo scoring systems, others cannot demonstrate a strong relationship between these measures and pregnancy.

Embryo quality evaluation all over the world includes morphological appearance of cleavage stage embryos and blastocysts thus making it a vital part of a successful IVF program.

Most classification systems are based on the analysis of the number of blastomeres, the amount of fragmentation, the structural similarities of the blastomeres, the presence of multinucleation, and the degree of compaction.

Cleavage stage embryos are those with 2 cells to about 8 to 16 cells (morula). This number is used as the main parameter to predict the quality of an embryo (Van Royen et al., 1999).

Normally, cell division in an embryo occurs every 18–20 hours with respect to the time of insemination. Embryos dividing at a significantly lower or higher rate may be the result of a metabolic and/or chromosomal defect.

During mitosis a part of the cytoplasm may be extruded, thus leading to fragments within the plasma membrane (Antczak and van Blerkom, 1999).

The amount of fragmentation is widely used to analyze the implantation potential embryos (Ebner et al., 2001). It is accepted that if the fragmentation is less than 10%, it does not seem to have an impact on the embryo's developmental potential (Van Royen et al., 2001).

Mitosis of the fertilized oocyte should produce two equally sized daughter cells. If the division is asymmetric, one of the cells of the next generation will inherit less than half the amount of cytoplasm from the parent blastomere thus leading to a defective lineage in the embryo.

An embryo ideally has four equally sized cells with a clear homogenous cytoplasm, forming a tetrahedron, with one nucleus each after two cleavages.

Compaction occurs at the 8-cell stage when the adherence between cells increases and reaches a point where the boundaries cannot be detected.

Multiple nuclei can be associated with various genetic abnormalities (Hardarson, 2001). Also during compaction if any cells are excluded it may lead to a poor quality blastocyst (Tao, 2002)

CELL NUMBERS

The development of an embryo, based on the number of cells (1 cell to 10 cells), on days 1, 2 or 3 after insemination is vital in predicting the implantation potential and thus pregnancy rates. The currently accepted optimal cleavage rate is as follows:

- *Day 1*: 2 cells (26–28 hours postinsemination—**Fig. 14**)
- *Day 2*: 4 cells (44 hours postinsemination—**Fig. 15**)
- *Day 3*: 8 cells (68 + 1 hour—**Fig. 16**)

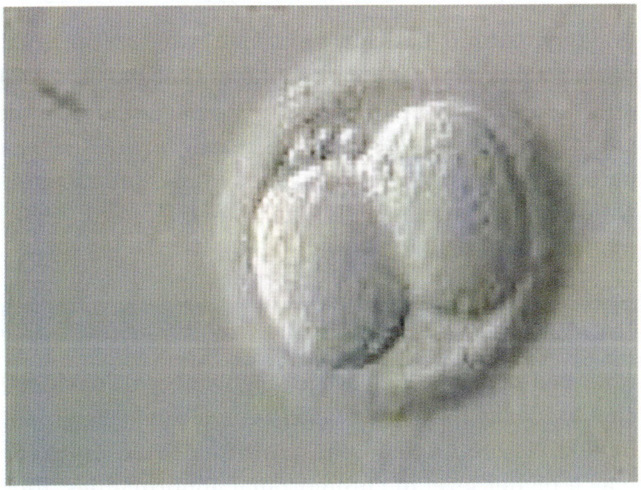

Fig. 14: 2-cell embryo.

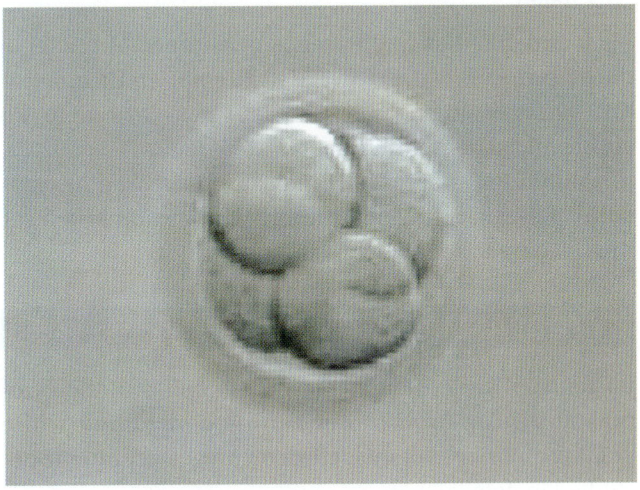

Fig. 15: 4-cell embryo arranged in a tetrahedron.

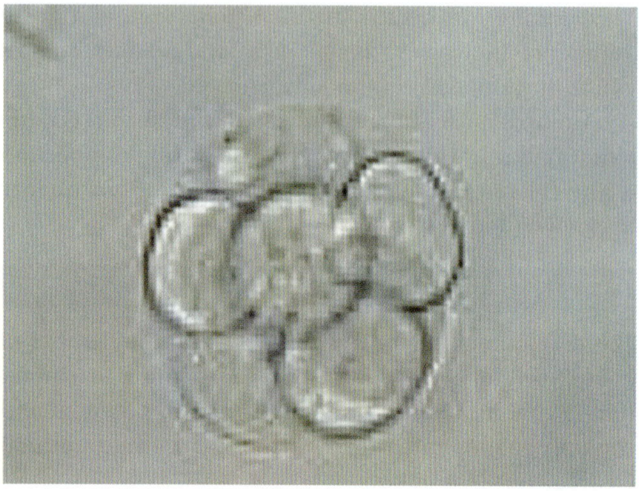

Fig. 16: 8-cell embryo.

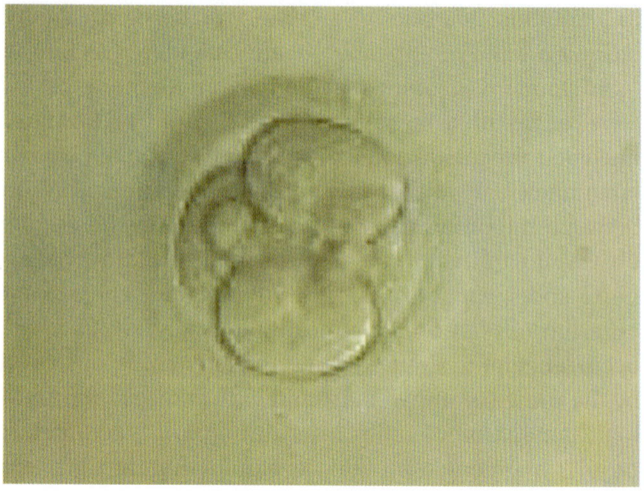

Fig. 17: Day 2 embryo with less than 10% fragmentation.

FRAGMENTATION (FIGS. 17 TO 19)

Fragmentation is basically anucleate structures formed during cell division of the blastomeres (Keltz et al., 2006) and the extent of fragmentation is a part of almost all embryo assessment systems. It is usually expressed as a percentage of the total cytoplasmic volume. The categorization of fragmentation is established as mild (10%), moderate (10–25%), and severe (25%).

NUCLEATION

After cell division of cleavage stage embryos, each cell should ideally have one nucleus. Anucleate cells do not have a visible nucleus and multinucleated embryos may a higher level of chromosomal abnormalities, thus resulting in a higher risk of spontaneous abortion (Scott et al, 2007).

It is defined as the presence or absence of nuclei in the blastomeres of the cleavage stage embryo. The nucleation status is either a single nucleus per blastomere, no visible nuclei or multinucleation.

Multinucleation usually indicates decreased implantation potential and a higher level of chromosomal defects, thus leading to spontaneous abortions

CYTOPLASMIC ANOMALIES

Presence of various anomalies like granules in the cytoplasm, pitting or vacuoles can be considered while grading embryos, but their effect on pregnancy rates is not studied in details.

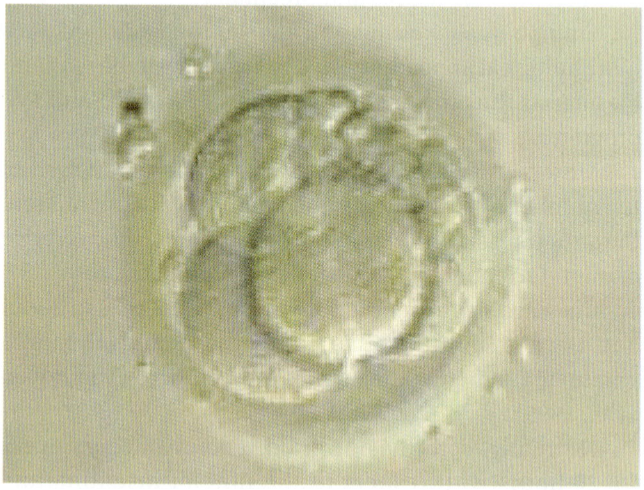

Fig. 18: Day 2 embryo with 10–20% fragmentation.

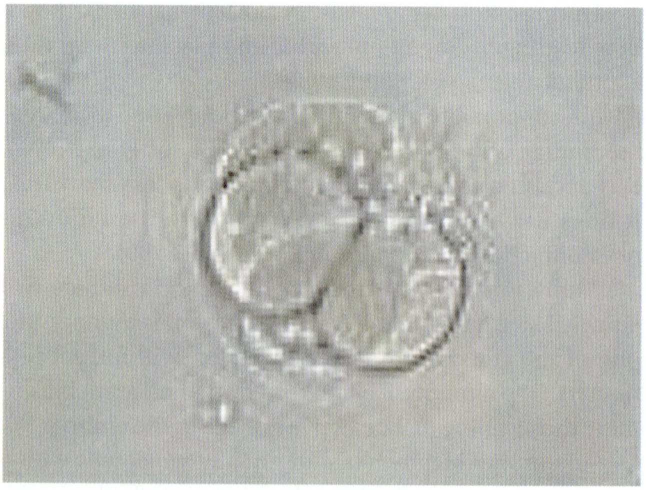

Fig. 19: Day 2 embryo with 15–20% fragmentation.

COMPACTION

Day 4 of development presents itself as a mass of cells termed as a morula (16 or more cells), all of which should be a part of the compaction process **(Fig. 20)** (Tao, 2002).

The Istanbul consensus has established that all blastomeres must be included in the morula on day 4, and usually the embryos that have any fragments left behind may have a lower rate of implantation.

THE BLASTOCYST

An embryo that reaches the blastocyst stage has proven more developmental competency over those that stall in early development. A blastocyst has proven ability to develop into a more organized structure than an embryo in the more primitive stages of development **(Table 2)**.

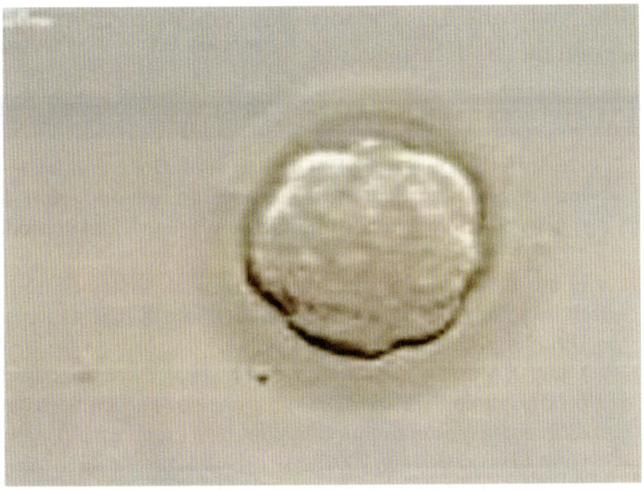

Fig. 20: Morula showing all blastomeres as one single mass.

Table 2: Embryo scoring based on blastocyst expansion grade (according to Gardner et al.).

Expansion grade	*Description*
1.	Blastocyst development and stage status
2.	Blastocoel cavity more than half the volume of the embryo
3.	Full blastocyst, cavity completely filling the embryo
4.	Expanded blastocyst, cavity larger than the embryo, with thinning of the shell
5.	Hatching out of the shell
6.	Hatched out of the shell

Blastocyst transfer also correlates more timely with the natural physiological timeline of implantation. It is logical to assume mimicking conditions found in nature will yield more successful outcomes. Research supports this theory, as blastocysts cultured in favorable conditions routinely result in successful implantation and pregnancy rates as high as 60%. It is important to remember all blastocysts are not of equal quality and only the highest quality blastocyst should be selected for transfer. Formation of a distinct blastocele, trophectoderm (TE), and tightly compacted inner cell mass (ICM) indicate high quality blastocyst with the TE grade being the strongest morphological predictor **(Tables 3 and 4)**. These visually apparent attributes are observed during morphological assessment.

EXPANSION OF THE EMBRYO

An important process in embryonic development is when fluid starts to collect in between the cells of the morula stage and as the levels of fluid increase it forms the blastocoel cavity and a rapid increase in the number of cells **(Fig. 21)**. These processes together cause a gradual enlargement of the blastocyst and slowly the ZP becomes thinner. Eventually, the blastocyst breaks out of the ZP and this process is called hatching **(Fig. 22)**.

INNER CELL MASS MORPHOLOGY

The outer cells lining the blastocyst are called TE cells and cells inside the cavity for the ICM at one side. The ICM eventually goes on to form the embryo and the extraembryonic structures.

The ICM is categorized depending on the number of cells and the tight bond between the cells.

Table 3: Blastocyst scoring based on inner cell mass (ICM) grade (according to Gardner et al.).

ICM grade	*ICM quality*
A	Many cells, tightly packed
B	Several cell, loosely grouped
C	Very few cells

Table 4: Blastocyst scoring based on trophectoderm (TE) grade (according to Gardner et al.).

TE grade	*TE quality*
A	Many cells, forming a cohesive layer
B	Few cells, forming a loose epithelium
C	Very few large cells

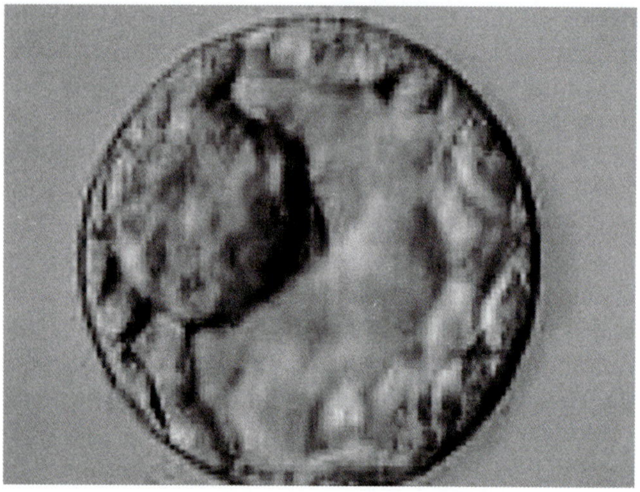

Fig. 21: Blastocyst with inner cell mass (10 o'clock).

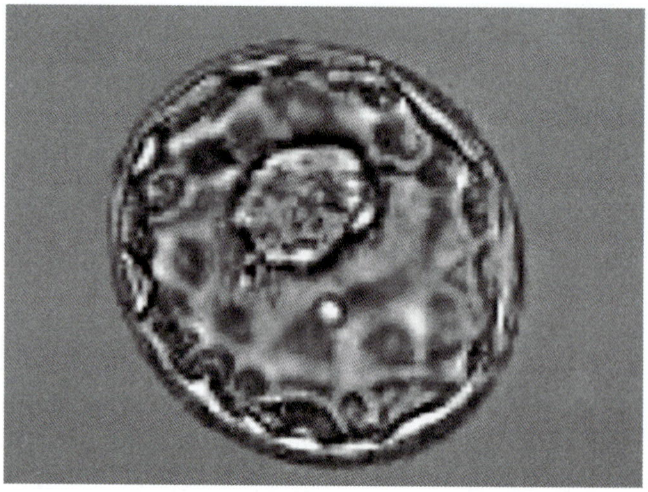

Fig. 23: Expanded blastocyst with a large inner cell mass (ICM).

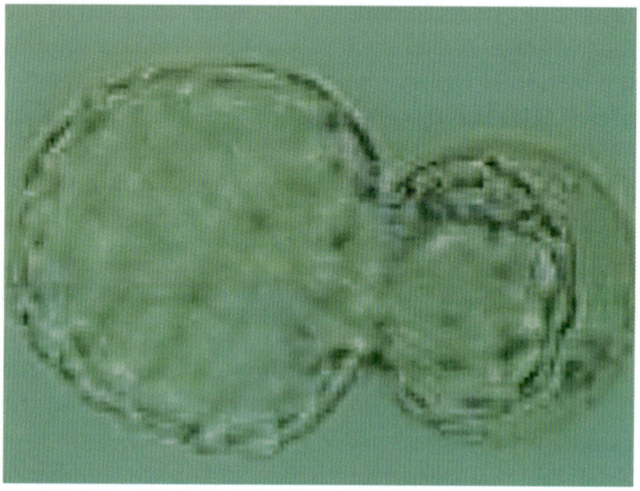

Fig. 22: Hatching blastocyst.

- It contains numerous cells that are tightly packed.
- It is composed of several cells that are loosely bound.
- It contains very few cells that are barely bound together.

Studies have shown that the larger the ICM the more chances of it resulting in a successful pregnancy **(Fig. 23)**. Thus the morphological appearance is supposed to be of considerable importance (Balaban, 2000).

TROPHECTODERM MORPHOLOGY

The TE cells are of paramount importance in defining the ICM and they allow the hatched blastocyst to embed itself into the endometrium by adhesion and invasion. They also help in the process of hatching out from the ZP. Ultimately, the TE cells form the fetal extraembryonic membranes and the placenta.

SUGGESTED READING

1. De Sutter P, Dozortsev D, Qian C, et al. Oocyte morphology does not correlate with fertilization rate and embryo quality after intracytoplasmic sperm injection. Hum Reprod. 1996;11(3):595-7.
2. Ebner T, Moser M, Sommergruber M, et al. First polar body morphology and blastocyst formation rate in ICSI patients. Hum Reprod. 2002;17(9):2415-8.
3. Ebner T, Moser M, Sommergruber M, et al. Selection based on morphological assessment of oocytes and embryos at different stages of preimplantation development: a review. Hum Reprod Update. 2003;9(3):251-62.
4. Gardner D, Lane M. Culture and selection of viable blastocysts: a feasible proposition for human IVF? Hum Reprod Update. 1997;3(4):367-82.
5. Gerris J, De Neubourg D, Mangelschots K, et al. Prevention of twin pregnancy after in-vitro fertilization or intracytoplasmic sperm injection based on strict embryo criteria: a prospective randomized clinical trial. Hum Reprod. 1999; 14(10):2581-7.
6. Hafez E. Human semen and fertility regulation in men. Missouri, United States: Mosby; 1976.
7. Hill MJ, Richter KS, Heitmann RJ, et al. Trophectoderm grade predicts outcomes of single-blastocyst transfers. Fertil Steril. 2013;99(5):1283-9.e1.
8. Kazuo I. Molecular Architecture of the Sperm Flagella: Molecules for Motility and Signaling. Zool Sci. 2003;20(9): 1043-56.
9. Kruger TF, Coetzee K. The role of sperm morphology in assisted reproduction. Hum Reprod Update. 1999;5(2):172-8.
10. Laufner N, Tarlatzis BC, DeCherney AH, et al. Asynchrony between human cumulus-corona cell complex and oocyte

maturation after human menopausal gonadotropin treatment for in vitro fertilization. Fertil Steril. 1984;42:366-72.
11. Laura R, Balaban B, Ebnerand T, et al. The oocyte. Hum Reprod. 2012;27: i2-21.
12. Maro B, Verlhac MH. Polar body formation: new rules for asymmetric divisions. Nat Cell Biol. 2002;4(12): E281-3.
13. Moon JH, Hyun CS, Lee SW, et al. Visualization of the metaphase II meiotic spindle in living human oocytes using the Polscope enables the prediction of embryonic developmental competence after ICSI. Hum Reprod. 2003;18(4):817-20.
14. Nagy ZP, Cecile J, Liu J, et al. Pregnancy and birth after intracytoplasmic sperm injection of in vitro matured germinal-vesicle stage oocytes: case report. Fertil Steril. 1996;65(5):1047-50.
15. Nashiri A, Eftekhari-Yazdi P. An overview of the available methods of morphological scoring of pre-implantation embryos in in vitro fertilization. Cell J. 2015;16(4):392-405.
16. Oldenbourg R, Mei G. New polarized light microscope with precision universal compensator. J Microsc. 1995; 180(Pt 2):140-7.
17. Rienzi L, Ubaldi FM, Martinez F, et al. Relationship between meiotic spindle location with regard to the polar body position and oocyte developmental potential after ICSI. Hum Reprod. 2003;18(6):1289-93.
18. Sathananthan AH (Ed). Visual Atlas of Human Sperm Structure and Function for Assisted Reproductive Technology. Melbourne: La Trobe and Monash Universities; Singapore: National University; 1996.
19. Sathananthan AH, Ratnasooriya WD, de Silva PK, et al. Characterization of human gamete centrosomes for assisted reproduction, Ital J Anat Embryol. 2001;106(2 Suppl 2):61-73.
20. Sathananthan AH, Trounson A, Freemann L, et al. The effects of cooling human oocytes. Hum Reprod. 1988;3(8):968-77.
21. Savitha P, Raja DR, Pandiyan R. Normal and abnormal oocytes observed during assisted reproductive technique (ART) procedures. Chettinad Health City Med J. 2012;1:4-11.
22. Swain JE, Pool TB. ART failure: ooctye contributions to unsuccessful fertilization. Hum Reprod Update. 2008;14(5): 431-46.
23. Testart L, Lassalle B, Frydman R, et al. A study of factors affecting the success of human fertilization in vitro. II. Influence of semen quality and oocyte maturation on fertilization and cleavage. Biol Reprod. 1983;28(2):425-31.
24. Ubaldi FM, Rienzi L. Micromanipulation techniques in human infertility: PZD, SUZI, ICSI, MESA, PESA, FNA and TESE. In: Revelli A, Tur-Kaspa I, Holte JG, Massobrio M (Eds). Biotechnology of Human Reproduction. Nashville, USA: Parthenon Publishing; 2002.
25. Wang WH, Meng L, Hackett RJ, et al. Developmental ability of human oocytes with or without birefringent spindles imaged by Polscope before insemination. Hum Reprod. 2001;16(7):1464-8.
26. Wein AJ, Kavoussi LR, Peters CA. Male reproductive physiology. Campbell-Walsh Urology. Amsterdam, Netherlands: Elsevier; 2016. 516-37.
27. Wittemer CK, Bettahar-Lebugle J, Ohl C, et al. Zygote Evaluation: An Efficient Tool for Embryo Selection. Hum Reprod. 2000;15(12):2591-7.

Sperm Preparation Techniques

44

Virendra Shah, Randhir Singh, Monica Singh, Anagha Deshpande

INTRODUCTION

Separation of sperms from seminal plasma is required for diagnostic as well as therapeutic purposes. For sperm function tests, the spermatozoa should be separated from the seminal plasma within an hour of ejaculation, to limit any damage from products of non-sperm cells.

Seminal plasma besides providing nutrition to the spermatozoa also helps it to penetrate the cervical mucus. However, various other components in seminal plasma like prostaglandins, zinc etc. cause hindrance to the achievement of pregnancy. The various semen preparation techniques involve separation of morphologically normal and motile sperms, free from debris, non-germ cells and dead spermatozoa, and are of utmost importance in clinical practice. The various sperm wash techniques include dilution and centrifugation, swim-up and density-gradient centrifugation (DGC).

CHOICE OF METHOD

The nature of the semen sample dictates the choice of sperm preparation technique. The direct swim-up technique is used when the semen samples are largely normal, whereas in cases of severe oligozoospermia, teratozoospermia or asthenozoospermia, density gradients are usually preferred because of the greater total number of motile spermatozoa recovered. Density gradients can also be altered to optimize handling of specific properties of individual samples. Volume of gradient material can be reduced, limiting the distance that the spermatozoa migrate and maximizing total motile sperm recovery, or the centrifugation time can be increased for specimens with high viscosity.

Each laboratory should determine the centrifugal force and centrifugation time necessary to form a manageable sperm pellet. When sperm numbers are extremely low, the centrifugal force and time can be modified in order to increase the chances of recovering the maximum number of spermatozoa. These modifications should be rigorously tested prior to clinical implementation. The most suitable method of preparation can be identified from the functional capacity of the prepared spermatozoa using zona free hamster oocyte penetration test.

EFFICIENCY OF SPERM SEPARATION FROM SEMINAL PLASMA AND INFECTIOUS ORGANISMS

The absolute sperm number, the number of motile spermatozoa, or numbers of morphologically normal motile spermatozoa are usually used to express the efficiency of sperm selection technique. Swim-up generally produces a lower recovery of motile spermatozoa (<20%) than DGC (>20%). Swim-up and DGC also produce different levels of in the final sperm preparation. Using zinc as a marker of soluble seminal components, it was demonstrated that swim-up preparations have greater contamination with seminal components compared to density-gradient preparation.

Semen samples may contain harmful infectious agents. Sperm preparation techniques are not 100% effective in removing infectious agents from semen, and so technicians should handle them as a biohazard with extreme care.[1] Safety guidelines should be strictly adhered to.

GENERAL PRINCIPLES

Semen should be collected in a sterile manner. Sterile materials and techniques are essential when applying a sperm preparation technique for therapeutic purposes. Three simple sperm preparation techniques are described in the following sections. Balanced salt solution supplemented with protein with a buffer suitable for environmental conditions is usually preferred culture medium. For advanced ART procedures like in-vitro fertilization (IVF), intracytoplasmic sperm injection (ICSI), artificial insemination (AI) or gamete intrafallopian transfer (GIFT), only commercially available human serum albumin which is highly purified and is free from bacterial, viral, and prior contamination should be used. If the samples are incubated in only atmospheric air at 37°C, the tubes should be tightly capped and HEPES buffered medium should be used. However, if the sample is incubated in atmosphere with 5% (v/v) CO_2 in air and the temperature is 37°C, the medium should be buffered with sodium bicarbonate, and the test tubes should be capped loose to allow gas exchange. Adherence to this will ensure that the culture pH is compatible with sperm survival. The final disposition of the processed spermatozoa will determine which buffered medium is appropriate. Sperm function assays in general will require a medium that supports sperm capacitation, and typically contains sodium bicarbonate (25 mmol/L).

TECHNIQUES OF SPERM PREPARATION

A large volume of assisted reproductive technology (ART) procedures now are done for male factor infertility. This led to numerous andrological researches so as to better understand the sperm physiology and develop more sophisticated techniques to separate functional spermatozoa from immotile, poor morphology sperms or sperms with poor capacitation.

The method used to prepare a semen sample depends on the following:

- Volume
- Viscosity
- Motile sperm count
- Presence of leukocytes, other cells and debris.

Preparation methods which do not use centrifugation are in general advantageous. A normal ejaculate contains a large number of defective spermatozoa and granulocytes which on centrifugation can generate a high number of reactive oxygen species (ROS) and damage the sperm DNA.[2] These ROS also attack the sperm plasma membrane, resulting in oxidative stress which can damage the sperm function. Therefore, depending on the ejaculate quality, different methods have different efficiency and areas of use.

The various sperm preparation techniques are as follows:

- *Swim up method* **(*Figs 1A to C*)**:
  1. Take one part of liquefied semen sample in test tube then add two part of culture media, gently mix and centrifuge at 1500 rpm for 10 minutes **(Fig. 1A)**.
  2. Removed supernatant from the tube, leaving the sperm pellet undisturbed at the bottom **(Fig. 1B)**.
  3. The pellet is then layered gently with 1 mL culture media without disturbing the pellet, and incubated at 37° in an incubator for 45 minutes **(Fig. 1C)**.
  4. 0.5 mL of supernatant is taken in a new tube and check for count and motility. The sample is ready for use.
     - *Advantages:*
       - Simple
       - Easy to perform

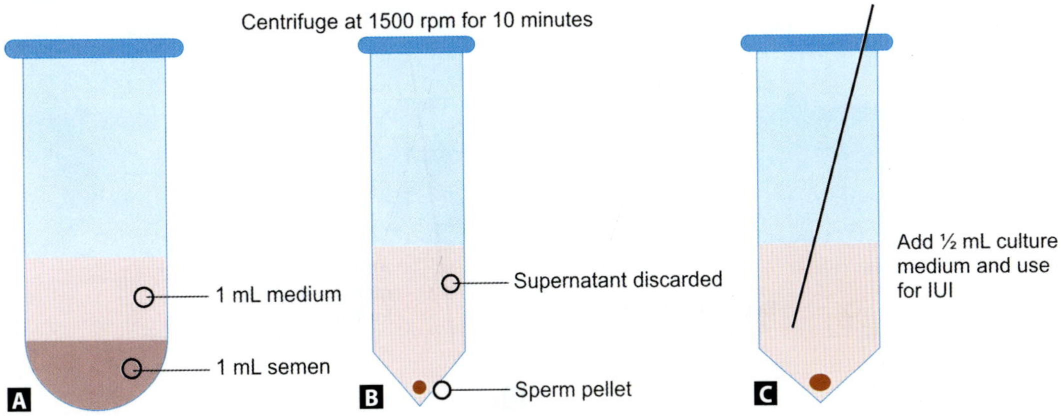

Figs. 1A to C: Swim-up method. Centrifuge at 1500 rpm for 10 minutes.

- Cost effective
- Good number of highly motile sperms are recovered.

– *Disadvantages:*
- Restricted for normal or marginally abnormal ejaculates.
- Does not separate morphologically normal sperms from abnormal ones.
- When cell pellet is too concentrated, some motile spermatozoa may be trapped in it and may not travel as far as the sperm cells at the edges of the pellet.
- Centrifugation which is performed to create pellet has been shown to generate ROS.

▪ *Layering Method* **(*Figs 2A to D*)** *(For normal semen samples):*
0.5 mL culture medium is placed in each of four test tubes (5 mL capacity). 0.5 mL of liquefied semen is then gently underlayered at the bottom of each tube **(Fig. 2A)**. This is then incubated at 37° in an incubator for 30 minutes. After 30 minutes, the supernatant from each tube is picked up and pooled together in a conical bottom centrifuge tube. This is then centrifuged at 1500 rpm for 10 minutes **(Fig. 2B)**. The medium is then removed from the tube leaving the sperm pellet undisturbed at the bottom. The pellet is resuspended in 0.5 mL culture medium and used **(Figs. 2C and 2D)**. This method makes use of the intrinsic motility of the sperm for the harvest. The sperm is not subjected to harsh centrifugal force (like in the conventional spin and swim up technique), thus there is no release of ROS and subsequent sperm damage.

♦ *Advantages*:
– Avoids centrifugation
– Useful for ejaculates with normal semen parameters.

♦ *Disadvantages*:
– Cannot be used for viscous sample.

▪ *Gradient Method* **(*Figs 3A to C*)** *(For oligoastheno-zoospermic sperm samples)*: Ready gradients 40% and 80% are commercially available. 1 mL of 40% gradient is placed at the bottom of a conical centrifuge tube. 1 mL of 80% gradient is gently underlayered at the bottom of the tube without disturbing the 40% gradient which rises to the top of the tube. 2 mL of liquefied semen is then gently overlayered above the two gradients **(Fig. 3A)**. The tube is then centrifuged at 2500 rpm for 20 minutes **(Fig. 3B)**. 2 mL of culture medium is placed in a new conical tube, the pellet is gently aspirated without disturbing the gradients and transferred the fresh culture media. This is then spun at 1200 rpm for 10 minutes. The supernatant containing traces of the gradient is removed and the sperm pellet is resuspended in 0.5 mL of fresh culture media and used for IUI, IVF, ICSI **(Fig. 3C)**. This method allows recovery of all sperms in the original semen sample without release of ROS and all components of

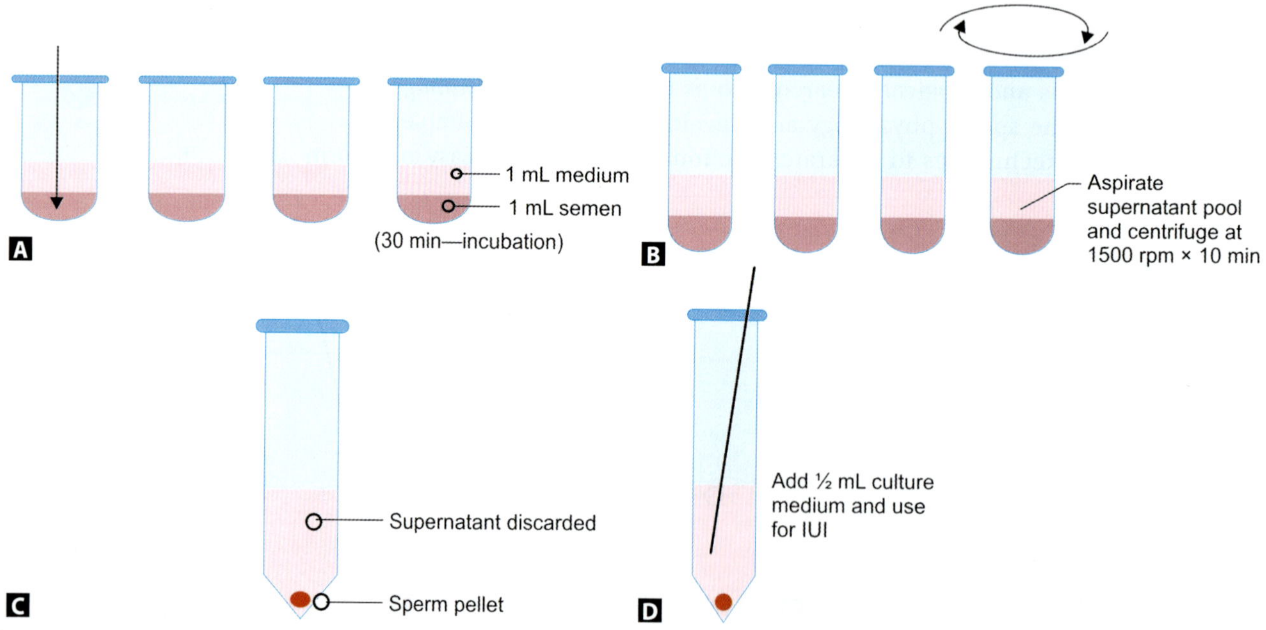

Figs. 2A to D: Layering method.

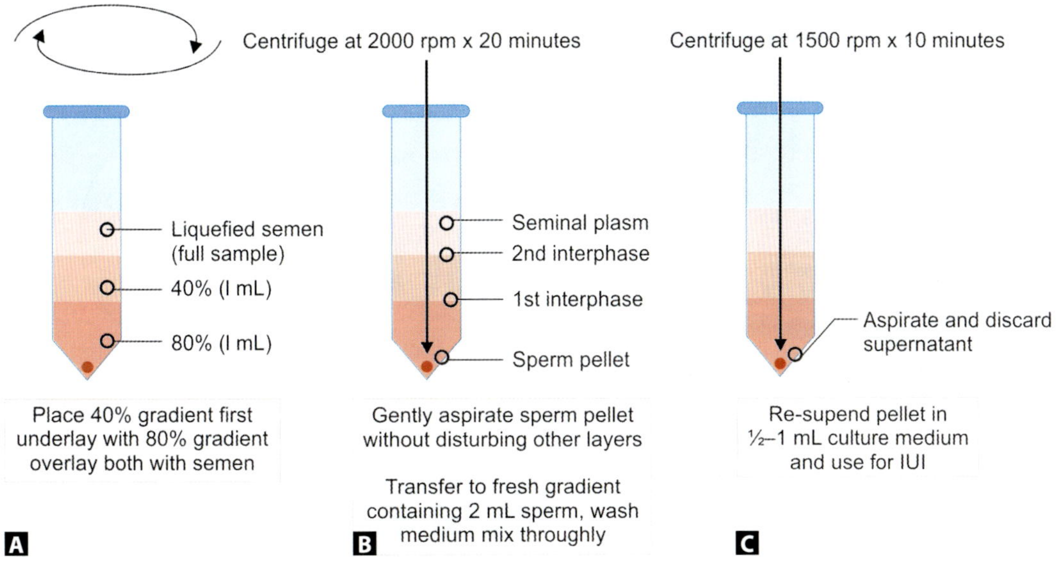

Figs. 3A to C: Gradient method.

semen are separated beautifully. It is extremely useful for male factor infertility.

- *Advantages:*
  - Separates leukocytes, cell debris and morphologically abnormal sperm with poor motility.
  - Produces higher recovery of motile spermatozoa.
  - Fast and easy to perform.
  - Consistent results and easy standardization.
- *Disadvantages*:
  - Production of good interphase between layers can take some time.
  - There is a risk of contamination with endotoxins.

- *Magnetic Activated Cell Sorting* ***(Fig. 4):*** Magnetic activated cell sorting (MACS) is a procedure for separating apoptotic from non-apoptotic sperms. It has been observed that phospholipid phosphatidylserine is one of the early markers of apoptosis, and this phospholipid is known to have high affinity for annexin V. Annexin V, conjugated with magnetic microspheres when exposed to a magnetic field in an affinity column can separate apoptotic from non-apoptotic sperms **(Fig. 4)**.
  - *Magnetic activated cell sorting procedure*:
    - Assess the sperm count and motility.
    - Use minimum 105 to maximum 108 spermatozoa for MACS separation.
    - Perform DGC.
    - After DGC, add 1 mL of 1 × MACS ART binding buffer to the pellet, mix well and centrifuge for 5 minutes at 300 g.
    - Remove all supernatant and add 100 µL of ART annexin V reagent.
    - Add 1 × MACS ART binding buffer to a final volume of 500 µL
    - Mix well and incubate for 15 minutes at room temperature.
    - Attach the MACS-ART separation unit to the MACS multistand.
    - Place the MACS-ART MS column in the MACS-ART separation unit.
    - Place a tube below the MACS-ART MS column to collect rinsing buffer.
    - Rinse column with 1 mL of 1X MACS ART binding buffer.
    - Discard effluent and place a new collection tube for the target cell fraction under the MACS-ART MS column.
    - Apply cell suspension prepared according to points above onto the column.
    - Collect the flow through fraction.
    - Wash the column with 500 µL of 1X MACS ART binding buffer.
    - Collect the flow through fraction in the same tube. The combined fraction represents enriched viable sperms.
    - Mix the cell suspension in equal volume of sperm wash media and centrifuge at 300 g for 5 minutes. Aspirate supernatant completely.
    - Resuspend the cells in sperm washing medium or culture for further use.

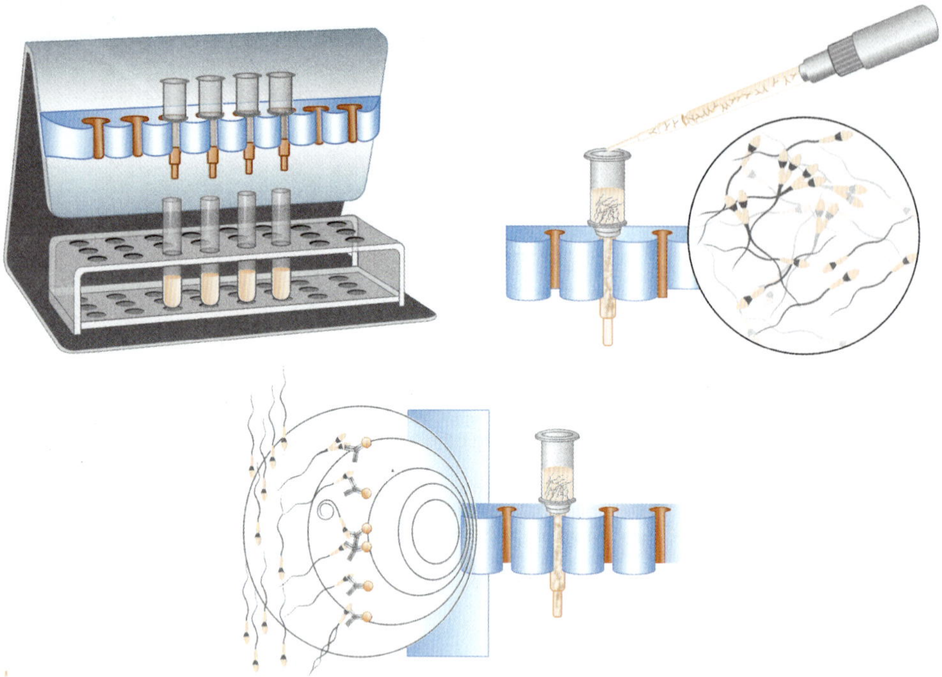

Fig. 4: Magnetic activated cell sorting.

- *Advantages:*
  - Noninvasive, rapid and convenient.
  - Only technique which separates apoptotic from non-apoptotic sperms an
  - Instead of relying on sperm density and motility, it acts at the molecular level.
  - Does not require bead detachment.
  - The results are consistent and reliable with optimal purity.
- *Disadvantages:*
  - Can only be used in conjugation with other techniques such as DGC to remove other substances (leukocytes and seminal plasma).

Advanced Methods for Sperm Preparation

There are mainly three groups of methods to facilitate selection of high quality sperm, based on *morphology*, *electrical charge*, and *sperm surface* maturity and organization **(Table 1)**:

- *Motile sperm organelle morphology examination*: Bartoov et al. in the year 2002 introduced this technique in which sperms are magnified to approximately 6,000X magnification, to check for subtle defects in sperm morphology. The most suitable sperms are then picked up for ICSI, and this modified ICSI technique is called *intracytoplasmic morphologically selected sperm injection (IMSI)*.[3] Several studies have reported that though the fertilization rates were similar with ICSI or IMSI, the implantation rates were higher and miscarriage rates lower in the IMSI group.[4] The method of sperm preparation technique (swim-up or density gradient) had no effect on the IMSI outcome.
- *Sperm birefringence:* The mature sperm nucleus has high intrinsic birefringence due to longitudinally orientated subacrosomal protein filaments. With the use of polarized light microscopy, sperm birefringence can be evaluated and a mature sperm selected.[5]
- *Sperm charge selection*: Normally differentiated sperm are charged electronegatively. The zeta potential of the sperm is the electrical potential between the sperm membrane and its surroundings, and this decreases with capacitation. Based on these, normally differentiated negatively charged sperm can be rapidly separated when semen is placed into an electrophoretic device and a current is applied.[6] The technique allows for sperm selection with strict normal morphology and DNA integrity. However, the total number of sperms recovered using this technique is very low. The procedure should be carried out immediately after sperm separation from seminal plasma, as sperms looses negative charge near capacitation.
- Hyaluronic acid (HA) or hyaluronan is a negatively charged glycosaminglycan present in the female reproductive tract and in the cumulus oophorus complex, and directs sperm binding to the zona pellucida. It has

Table 1: Grading of oocyte maturity.

Sperm selection approach	*Author (year)*	*Sperm selection method*	*Outcomes reported*
Selection based on surface charge	Ainsworth et al. (2007)	Electrophoretic separation	Fertilization and live birth
	Fleming et al. (2008)	Electrophoretic separation	FR (IVF) 62% versus 69% (NS) FR (ICSI) 64% versus 52% (NS) PR NA
	Kheirollahi-Kouhestani et al. (2009)	Zeta potential	FR 66% versus 52% (S) FR 54% versus 33% (NS) PR NA
Non-apoptotic sperm selection	Dirician et al. (2009)	DGC + MACS	FR 69% versus 70% (NS) PR 48% versus 37% (S)
Mature sperm selection	Ye et al. (2006)	HA binding	HBA score when FR >50 versus HBA score when FR <50%: 75% versus 69% (marginal S)
	Nasr-Esfahani et al. (2008)	HA binding	FR 79% versus 68% (S) PR 46% versus 40% (NS)
	Tarozzi et al. (2009)	HA binding	FR when HBA score ≥80% versus FR when HBA score when <80%: 86% versus 87% (NS) PR when HBA score ≥ versus PR when HBA score <80%: 36% versus 32% (NS)
	Van Den Bergh et al. (2009)	HA binding	FR 76% versus 70% (NS) PR NA
	Parmegiani et al. (2010a,b)	HA binding	FR 92% versus 70% (NS) PR 25% versus 21% (NS)
	Parmegiani et al. (2010a,b)	HA binding	FR 93% versus 87% (NS) PR 33% versus 22% (NS)
Selection based on ultramorphology	Bartoov et al. (2002)	MSOME	Normal nucleus by MSOME when FR >60% versus when FR <60%: 32% versus 22% (S)
	Bartoov et al. (2003)	IMSI	FR 63% versus 64% (S) PR 66% versus 30% (S)
	Berkovitz et al. (2005)	IMSI	FR 71% versus 50% (NS) PR 52% versus 18% (NS)
	Berkovitz et al. (2006a,b)	IMSI	FR 73% versus 69% (NS) PR 50% versus 18% (S)
	Berkovitz et al. (2006a,b)	IMSI	FR 67% versus 69% (NS) PR 48% versus 20% (S)
	Hazout et al. (2006)	IMSI	FR NA PR 38% versus 2% (S)
	Check et al. (2007)	IMSI	Fertilization
	Antinori et al. (2008)	IMSI	FR NA PR 39% versus 27% (S)
	Vanderzwalmen et al. (2008)	IMSI	FR NA PR NA
	Mauri et al. (2010)	IMSI	FR 71% versus 70% (NS)
	Glanaroli et al. (2008)	ICSI (Polarization microscopy)	FR 74% versus 72% (NS) PR 31% versus 21% (NS)
	Glanaroli et al. (2010)	ICSI (Polarization microscopy)	FR 69% versus 67% (NS) PR 55% versus 14% (S)

Source: Adapted from Lin, 2003.

been observed that sperms that bind to HA in vitro are of better quality in terms of nuclear maturation, membrane organization, remodeling and shaping than those who fail to bind to HA. The *physiological intracytoplasmic sperm injection (PICSI)* technique utilizes this fact. HA is utilized as a "physiological selector" of mature intact sperm. PICSI consists of a plastic culture dish with spots of HA attached to its base. When semen is added to these dishes, appropriate sperm get bound to HA and appear "slowed" and are selected.[7] SpermSlow is a viscous medium containing HA. Recent studies has demonstrated that HA-binding spermatozoa display higher pregnancy rates, better embryo quality and an overall better clinical outcome.

CONCLUSION

Each sperm selection modality utilizes different characteristics of sperm structure, physiology or function to promote selection of the most normal sperm. Selection of the most appropriate sperm for fertilization in vitro may help to improve fertilization and the quality of embryos created. Advanced sperm selection protocols aim to improve ART outcomes and may limit possible deleterious effects on offspring of using sperm with defective DNA.[8]

REFERENCES

1. Savasi V, Ferrazzi E, Lanzani C, et al. Safety of sperm washing and ART outcome in 741 HIV-1 discordant couples. Hum Reprod. 2007;22:772-7.
2. Aitken RJ, Clarkson JS. Significance of ROS and antioxidants in defining the efficacy of sperm preparation techniques. J Androl. 1988;9:367-76.
3. Bartoov B, Berkovitz A, Eltes F, et al. Real-time fine morphology of motile human sperm cells is associated with IVF-ICSI outcome. J Androl. 2002;23:1-8.
4. Bartoov B, Berkovitz A, Eltes F, et al. Pregnancy rates are higher with intracytoplasmic morphologically selected sperm injection than with conventional intracytoplasmic injection. Fertil Steril. 2003;80:1413-9.
5. Gianaroli L, Magli C, Cooldel G, et al. Sperm head's birefringence: a new criterion for sperm selection. Fertil Steril. 2008;90:104-12.
6. Ainsworth C, Nixon B, Aitken R. Development of a novel electrophoretic system for the isolation of human spermatozoa. Hum Reprod. 2005;20:2261-70.
7. Huszar G, Jakab A, Sakkas D, et al. Fertility testing and ICSI sperm selection by hyaluronic acid binding: clinical and genetic aspect. Reprod Biomed Online. 2007;14:650-63.
8. Aitken R, De lullis G. Origins and consequences of DNA damage in male germ cells. Reprod Biomed Online. 2007;14:727-33.

General Principles of Micromanipulation

45

Steven D Fleming

SUMMARY BOX

Micromanipulation enables microsurgery to be performed under high magnification with the unaided hand. This technique has provided the cornerstone for many advances in assisted reproduction including the alleviation of severe male infertility and preimplantation genetic testing. The general principles and applications of this technology are considered in this article, offering a glimpse into possible future developments in this field.

INTRODUCTION

In the context of assisted reproduction, micromanipulation is the general term that encompasses all techniques whereby micromanipulators and microinjectors are used to manipulate spermatozoa, oocytes, and embryos. In this respect, micromanipulation has been used to inseminate oocytes with spermatozoa, to biopsy embryos for genetic analysis, to improve the cytoplasmic quality of oocytes, and to avoid the inheritance of mitochondrial disease. The outcomes from these procedures have a direct impact upon the reproductive potential of infertile couples and those wishing to avoid conceiving a child affected by a serious genetic disease and, therefore, the principles underlying their use are of great importance.

HISTORY

Prototype micromanipulators were first designed by various pioneers during the 1920s, including Chambers, De Fonbrune, Emerson, May, and Taylor. One of the leading microscope companies at that time was Leitz, a company that was originally founded as the Optical Institute in Wetzlar by Carl Kellner in 1849, the company management being taken over by Ernst Leitz 20 years later. The original Leitz joystick micromanipulators, first released in 1952, were so well built that some remain in operation today. Leica Camera AG was founded by Ernst Leitz in 1914 and in 1986 Leitz changed its name to Leica.

Various companies began specializing in manufacturing micromanipulation equipment during the late 20th century. Research instruments were established by Mike Lee and Vince Grispo in 1963, developing a range of instruments including a triple axis, single lever mechanical micromanipulator released in 1964. Narishige Scientific Instrument Laboratory was established in Tokyo by Eiichi Narishige in 1958, producing their first single axis hydraulic micromanipulator in 1969. However, it was not until the early 1980s that Narishige manufactured a triple axis hydraulic micromanipulatior, necessary for proper microsurgery, Narishige Company Ltd being established in 1985 as a separate entity from Narishige Scientific. Eppendorf–Netheler–Hinz GmBH launched their microprocessor controlled TransferMan micromanipulator in 1995.

Micromanipulation was first demonstrated to be a feasible technique for fertilizing oocytes in the hamster.[1] Following the successful clinical application of in vitro fertilization in 1978, the need to overcome severe male infertility led to the development of various micromanipulation techniques in the late 1980s designed to bring spermatozoa and oocytes closer together **(Table 1)**.

A technique called microinjection sperm transfer, whereby spermatozoa were microinjected into the perivitelline space of the oocyte, was the first to demonstrate that fertilization could be achieved in cases of severe

Table 1: Chronological development of micromanipulation techniques for fertilization of human oocytes.

Micromanipulation technique	*First year of publication*
Microinjection sperm transfer	1987
Zona drilling	1988
Partial zona dissection	1988
Intracytoplasmic sperm injection	1988

Table 3: Chronological development of micromanipulation techniques for improving oocyte and embryo quality

Micromanipulation technique	*First year of publication*
Ooplasmic transfer	1997
Fragment removal	1999
Germinal vesicle transfer	1999
Pronuclear transfer	2010
Spindle transfer	2017

Table 2: Chronological development of micromanipulation techniques for biopsy of human oocytes and embryos.

Micromanipulation technique	*First year of publication*
Blastomere biopsy	1989
Trophectoderm biopsy	1990
Polar body biopsy	1990

male infertility[2] and was subsequently termed subzonal insemination (SUZI). Unfortunately, SUZI never became adopted as a routine micromanipulation procedure due to various limitations including high rates of polyspermy and its inability to achieve fertilization in those instances where spermatozoa fail to undergo a spontaneous acrosome reaction. These limitations were overcome with the development of the intracytoplasmic sperm injection (ICSI) technique.[3]

The next steps in the evolution of micromanipulation occurred in response to the desire to identify embryos free of known inherited genetic diseases **(Table 2)**.

By combining the micromanipulation techniques of zona drilling (ZD) with blastomere biopsy, it was first demonstrated that sex-linked diseases could be avoided by sexing embryos using DNA (deoxyribonucleic acid) amplification.[4] Subsequently, ZD was adapted as a means of assisted the hatching of embryos, following the observation that embryos of some patients fail to hatch spontaneously in vitro leading to repeated implantation failure.[5]

More recently, with advances in our understanding of oocyte quality and mitochondrial disease, micromanipulation techniques have been developed in an effort to resolve these problems, primarily using donor oocytes **(Table 3)**.

Initial attempts to treat patients deemed to have poor quality oocytes were made using micromanipulation to "rejuvenate" their oocytes via transfer of ooplasm from donor oocytes.[6] Subsequently, this concept was extended by using micromanipulation to transfer the germinal vesicle from patients' oocytes into enucleated immature donor oocytes.[7] Also, micromanipulation was applied to treat patients considered to have poor quality cleavage stage embryos by using fragment removal.[8]

The most recent clinical application of micromanipulation has been the use of pronuclear transfer as a form of mitochondrial replacement therapy (MRT) for those patients at risk of transmitting mutated mitochondrial DNA known to result in serious mitochondrial diseases.[9] Recently, the first live birth following spindle transfer as a micromanipulation approach to MRT has been reported.[10]

PRESENT SCENARIO

Nowadays, micromanipulation is a standard practice but general principles still apply. Early micromanipulators such as those produced by Leitz had a high mass in an attempt to isolate the micromanipulation tools from external vibration. Currently available micromanipulators have a low mass and, therefore, some form of antivibration is required, typically in the form of an antivibration table or plate placed underneath the inverted microscope **(Fig. 1)**.

Another general principle of micromanipulation is that of maintaining sterile conditions during procedures involving reproductive tissues that will be cultured and transferred to a patient. Though oil overlays provide a physical barrier to microbial contamination, the micropipettes are not always kept below the surface of the oil and have to be fitted in the open air. For that reason, it is preferable to perform micromanipulation procedures within a laminar flow workstation or high-efficiency particulate air (HEPA)-filtered biological cabinet **(Figs. 1 and 2)**.

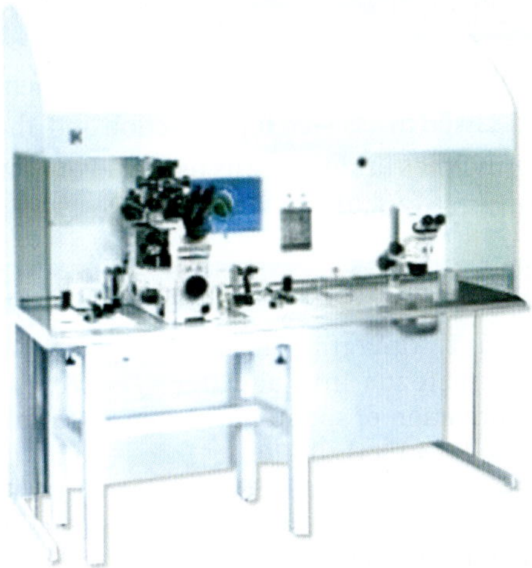

Fig. 1: Micromanipulation rig and inverted microscope suspended upon an antivibration table situated below the workstation.

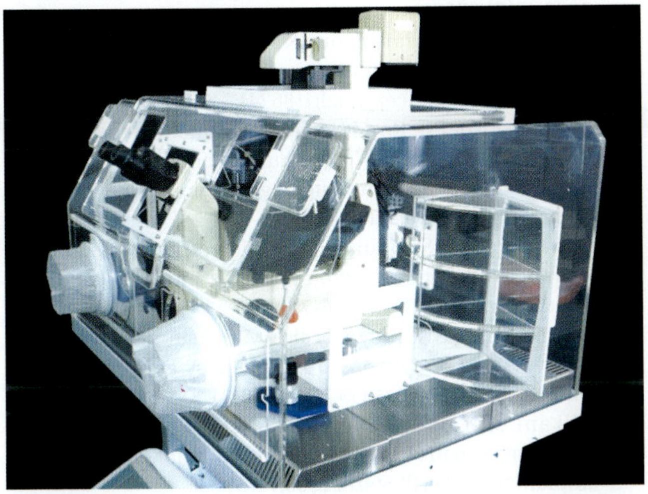

Fig. 2: Micromanipulation rig and inverted microscope suspended upon an antivibration plate within a HEPA-filtered biological cabinet. (HEPA: high-efficiency particulate air)

In addition to maintaining sterility, it is very important to maintain physiological temperature, especially when working with mature oocytes whose metaphase spindle is particularly vulnerable to depolymerization at temperatures below 35°C. One of the advantages of working within a biological cabinet is that temperature is more stable. On the contrary, when working within or outside of a workstation then maintenance of physiological temperature is entirely dependent upon the quality of the heated stage of the inverted microscope, as well as its proper calibration. Evidently, a metal-heated stage with a hole at its center for the light path of the inverted microscope is physically incapable of maintaining temperature at its center. Glass-heated stages overcome this problem to some extent but are still liable to variable heating across their surface due to the heat-sink effect of the underlying metal objective lens that tends to draw heat from the heated stage. Research instruments have overcome this issue by incorporating a Thermosafe™ warm air system that blows heated air between the heated stage and objective lens to counteract the heat-sink effect of the latter. Equally important is the correct setting of the heated stage relative to individual micromanipulation rigs. This can only be accurately determined using a thermocouple probe inserted into the media within the micromanipulation dish under working conditions and adjusting the temperature setting of the heated stage until a reading of 37°C is reached. Inevitably, the heated stage setting will be more than 37°C but, once calibrated, can be checked on a daily basis using a surface thermometer to ensure there has been no drift.

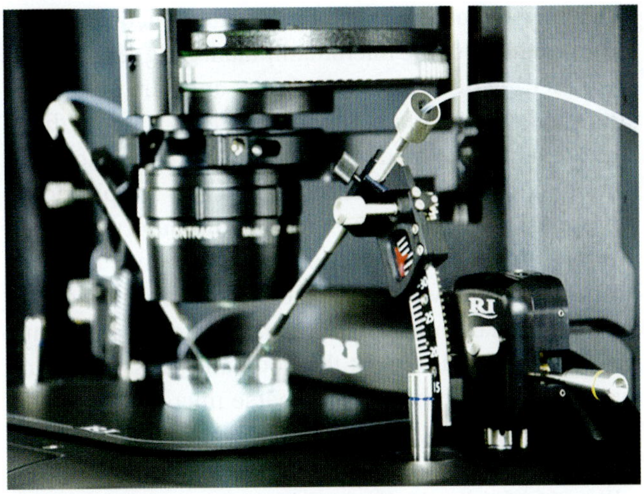

Fig. 3: PL3 tool holder that allows adjustment to micropipette bend angles from 16° and 43° "on the fly".

The angle at which the micropipettes are held by the tool holders is critical for some procedures, such as ICSI, where it is necessary to be able to effectively manipulate a spermatozoon and inject it into an oocyte while minimizing the shearing force that is exerted upon the oocyte, which increases as the angle of the microinjection pipette increases. Hence, there is a fine line between too flat an angle and too steep an angle, which has to be determined empirically by gradually increasing the tool-holder angle until it is possible to effectively manipulate spermatozoa. This task is made that much easier if the tip of the micropipette does not move during adjustment so that it does not have to be removed from the ICSI dish each time, allowing the tool-holder angle to be adjusted "on the fly" **(Fig. 3)**.

Other general principles of micromanipulation include the ergonomics of the micromanipulation rig setup, initial "zero" setting of micromanipulators and microinjectors, fitting and equilibration of micropipettes to stabilize them, and prevent unwanted capillary flow. Ergonomically, it is more comfortable if the microinjectors are placed on the opposite side from the micromanipulators to which they are attached, so that the operator's hands are used on their respective side of the microscope to control both micromanipulator and microinjector concurrently without any need to twist the body and cross one hand over the other. Both fine and coarse micromanipulators should be set to the middle of their vertical travel and left in their vertical positions prior to use to ensure their full range of operation is available. Likewise, air injectors should be set to their mid-point and oil injectors should be fully primed with oil before starting any procedures. Micropipettes should be primed with micromanipulation media or a 7–10% polyvinylpyrrolidone solution, adjusting the microinjectors as necessary to stabilize capillary flow. Operation of the micromanipulators and microinjectors should be smooth and slow to avoid unnecessary errors and all micromanipulation equipment should be regularly serviced.

FUTURE TRENDS

There has been some interest in the concept of performing micromanipulation without having to look down microscope eyepieces, observing a computer monitor instead, the image being relayed from the microscope via a camera. Also, in common with other laborious technical procedures, there is an incentive to make micromanipulation semi- or fully automated, not least because of the variability in practitioner competency and results. Indeed, robotic ICSI using computer algorithms has been developed previously but is yet to be incorporated into routine clinical practice.

CONCLUSION

Micromanipulation is now an integral component of various procedures used in assisted reproduction and, therefore, the general principles underlying its use need to be understood and uniformly applied.

REFERENCES

1. Uehara T, Yanagimachi Y. Microsurgical injection of spermatozoa into hamster eggs with subsequent transformation of sperm nuclei into male pronuclei. Biol Reprod. 1976;15(4):467-70.
2. Laws-King A, Trounson A, Sathananthan H, et al. Fertilization of human oocytes by microinjection of a single spermatozoon under the zona pellucida. Fertil Steril. 1987;48:637-42.
3. Lanzendorf SE, Maloney MK, Veeck LL, et al. A preclinical evaluation of pronuclear formation by microinjection of human spermatozoa into human oocytes. Fertil Steril. 1988;49(5):835-42.
4. Handyside AH, Pattinson JK, Penketh RJ, et al. Biopsy of human preimplantation embryos and sexing by DNA amplification. Lancet. 1989;1(8634):347-9.
5. Cohen J, Elsner C, Kort H, et al. Impairment of the hatching process following IVF in the human and improvement of implantation by assisting hatching using micromanipulation. Hum Reprod. 1990;5(1):7-13.
6. Cohen J, Scott R, Schimmel T, et al. Birth of infant after transfer of anucleate donor oocyte cytoplasm into recipient eggs. Lancet. 1997;350(9072):186-7.
7. Zhang J, Wang CW, Krey L, et al. In vitro maturation of human preovulatory oocytes reconstructed by germinal vesicle transfer. Fertil Steril. 1999;71(4):726-31.
8. Alikani M, Cohen J, Tomkin G, et al. Human embryo fragmentation in vitro and its implications for pregnancy and implantation. Fertil Steril. 1999;71(5):836-42.
9. Craven L, Tuppen HA, Greggains GD, et al. Pronuclear transfer in human embryos to prevent transmission of mitochondrial DNA disease. Nature. 2010;465(7294):82-5.
10. Zhang J, Liu H, Luo S, et al. Live birth derived from oocyte spindle transfer to prevent mitochondrial disease. Reprod Biomed Online. 2017;34(4):361-8.

IVF/ICSI/IMSI/PICSI

46

Sudesh A Kamat, Vrunda Kuchekar, Akanksha Mishra

IN VITRO FERTILIZATION

INTRODUCTION

The World Health Organization (WHO) defines infertility as the inability to conceive after 12 months of regular and unprotected intercourse. Assisted reproductive technologies (ARTs) refer to techniques and allied methods used to assist people in achieving a pregnancy. Simple techniques are ever so often attempted initially; they are less invasive and include ovulation induction and artificial insemination, which include intrauterine insemination and donor insemination. Advanced ART techniques include in vitro fertilization (IVF) and intracytoplasmic sperm injection (ICSI).

HISTORY

In vitro fertilization is a very well documented and popular technology today. However, its history, going back to about half a decade, is somewhat obscure. The first in vitro fertilization was performed on a rabbit leading to a live birth in 1959, by Min Chueh Chang at Worcester Foundation. This experiment inspired latter researchers to explore the possibility of in vitro insemination in humans. The first pregnancy achieved through IVF was, in fact, by a team from Monash, which unfortunately ended up being biochemical. Parallel efforts by the team led by Robert Edwards and Patrick Steptoe resulted in the famous birth of first IVF baby Louis Brown on July 25th, 1978, and not so famous first IVF boy, Alastair MacDonald born on January 14, 1979 in Glasgow.

Meanwhile, in India, the efforts of a relatively unknown physician, Dr Subhash Mukhopadhyay from Kolkata, bore fruit in the form of first IVF baby in India, Durga. However, he faced severe criticism and was ostracized from the society, which led him to commit suicide.

DESCRIPTION

The IVF is a process by which an egg is fertilized by sperm outside the body: in vitro. The process is carried out in a Petri dish containing culture medium, placed inside a CO_2 incubator in the IVF laboratory. The resulting zygote is further cultured to embryo or blastocyst stage and then transferred back to the patient's uterus with the intention of establishing a successful pregnancy. IVF as a technique was developed primarily to overcome female infertility predominantly addressing the shortcomings of the fallopian tube.

The basic steps in an IVF process are:

1. *Ovulation induction*: Ovulation induction can be performed using different protocols depending upon the stimulation used.

- *Natural cycle IVF*: It was natural cycle IVF, which gave us first ever IVF baby, Louise Brown, born in (1978). No fertility drugs are given during fertility treatment.
- *Mild IVF*: Mild IVF is performed in a woman's natural cycle without suppressing the natural cycle of the woman. Small dosages of fertility drugs are given aiming to produce high-quality eggs, not high quantity. Mild IVF shows comparable success rate to conventional IVF, and also adds the benefits of reducing the cost, fewer risks, and much fewer side effects.

- *Conventional IVF*: Conventional IVF is the most popularly practiced. This is done in order to obtain multiple oocytes, thus making available more embryos with which higher pregnancy rates can be achieved. The ovaries are usually downregulated about 10 days before the woman's natural menstrual cycle and this is followed by high dosages of fertility drugs in order to stimulate the growth of multiple follicles. The response to ovarian stimulation is monitored by serial determination of plasma estradiol levels and daily monitoring of ovarian follicular growth by ultrasonography.

2. *Ovum pick-up*: At the appropriate moment of follicular growth, the follicles are punctured and aspirated to obtain the oocytes. Oocytes are retrieved through a minor surgical procedure, under general anesthesia, that uses ultrasound imaging to guide a hollow needle through the pelvic cavity to remove the eggs.

3. *Scanning, identification, and grading of oocytes*: This step of the IVF procedure is carried out in the IVF laboratory. Prior to follicular aspiration, the following dishes are prepared and properly labeled:

- *Oocyte-scanning dish*: Center well dish (Falcon 3037) with 1-mL HEPES buffered medium in the inside well and 3-mL medium in the outside well. For handling of oocyte cumulus complexes outside the CO_2 incubator, commercially available HEPES-buffered flushing medium is widely used, as it maintains the physiological pH of the media between 7.2 and 7.4. Oocytes and embryos are cultured in bicarbonate-based IVF media inside the CO_2 incubator (5% CO_2, 37°C). All media and oil are equilibrated overnight in the CO_2 incubator.
- *Oocyte culture dish*: Center well dish with 1-mL IVF culture medium, overlaid with paraffin oil. A range of commercially available media can be used. The two most frequently used media are the sequential step media and the single step media.

Once the follicles are punctured, the follicular fluid is aspirated and collected in sterile 15 mL test tubes. The tubes are then passed to the IVF laboratory. Here, contents of the follicular fluid are poured out into plain sterile Petri dishes (Falcon 3652) and scanned under the stereo-zoom microscope. This procedure is carried out inside the laminar flow hood. Once the cumulus-oocyte complex (COC) is identified, it is picked up with a sterile transfer pipette (Falcon 7575), washed in HEPES buffered medium, in the outside well of the oocyte scan dish (center well), and then transferred to the central well. All the COCs are quickly identified and collected together. Once the ovum pick-up procedure is over, the washed COCs are transferred into the center well dish containing IVF culture media and placed back into the incubator.

- *Oocyte grading*: On finding a COC, its stage of maturity is assessed by taking note of the volume, density, and condition of the surrounding coronal and cumulus cells. When the egg is scanned, the presence of a single polar body signifies that it has reached the stage of metaphase II.

The following grading criteria are used routinely for assessment:

- *Germinal vesicle*: The oocyte is very immature. There is no expansion of the surrounding cells, which are tightly packed around the egg. A large nucleus (the germinal vesicle) is still present and may occasionally be seen with the help of an inverted microscope **(Fig. 1)**.
- *Immature metaphase I*: Immature metaphase I has a tightly apposed layer of corona cells around the oocyte and also has tightly packed cumulus approximately size of five egg diameters. Lack of germinal vesicle and absence of a polar body denotes that oocyte is in metaphase I **(Fig. 2)**.
- *Preovulatory metaphase II*: It is the optimum level of maturity, suitable for successful fertilization. One polar body has been extruded and though coronal cells are appear apposed to the egg, but are fully radiating, the cumulus has expanded into a fluffy mass and can be effortlessly stretched **(Fig. 3)**.
- *Postmature*: The postmature egg is often seen as a pale orb; slight coronal material is present and is dissociated from the egg. The cumulus is very profuse but is still cellular. However, the later events of this stage involve condensation of cumulus into small black (refractile) drops, if a tight corona is reforming around the egg **(Fig. 4)**.
- *Luteinized*: The egg is very pale and often is grueling to find. The cumulus has broken down and becomes a gelatinous mass around the egg. These eggs have a low-slung probability of fertilization **(Fig. 5)**.
- *Atretic*: Granulosa cells are fragmented and have a lace-like appearance. The oocyte is very dark and can be grim to identify **(Fig. 6)**.

4. *Sperm preparation for IVF*: The semen sample is collected in a wide mouth sterile container and allowed to liquefy for 20 minutes. The sperm parameters like count, motility, morphology are recorded. Add 2–3 mL of sperm preparation medium to the semen sample, mix and transfer

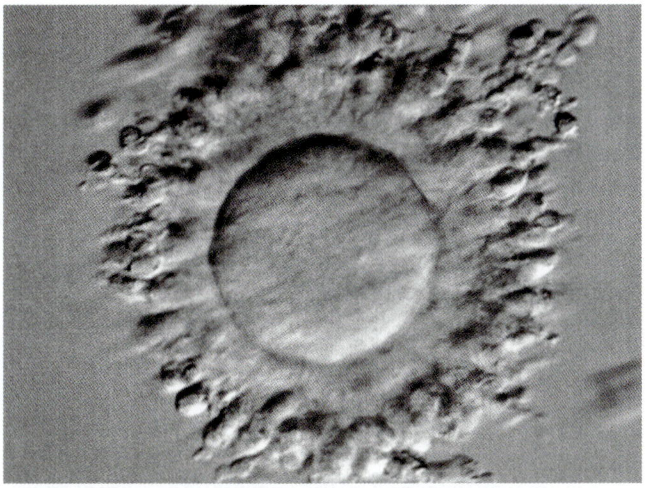

Fig. 1: Germinal vesicle (GV) is visible at 3 o'clock position.

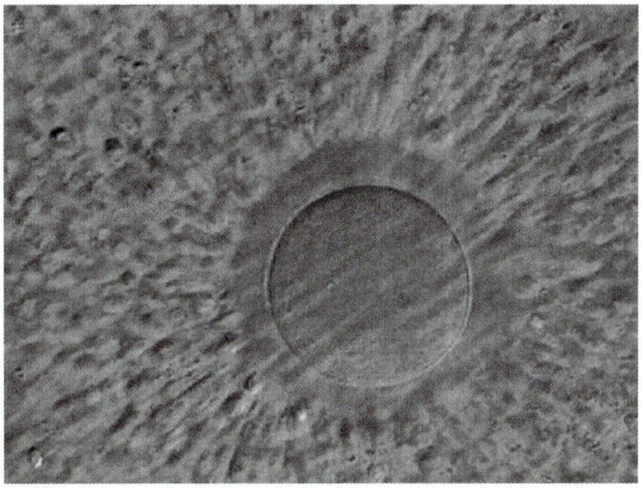

Fig. 2: Metaphase I: Polar body has not extruded out.

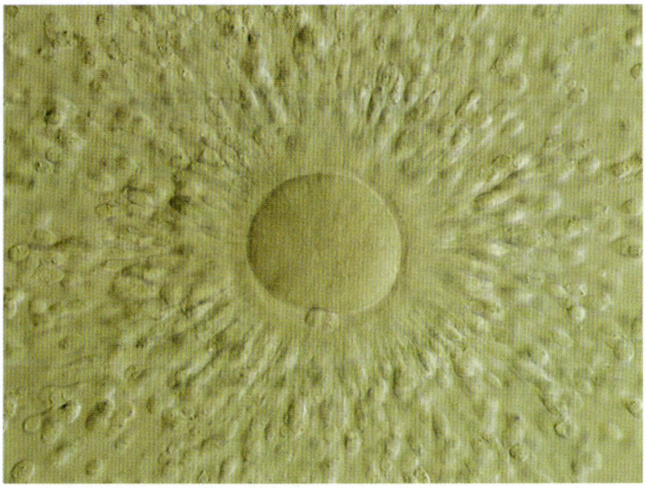

Fig. 3: Metaphase II COC: Polar body is seen at 6 O'clock position.

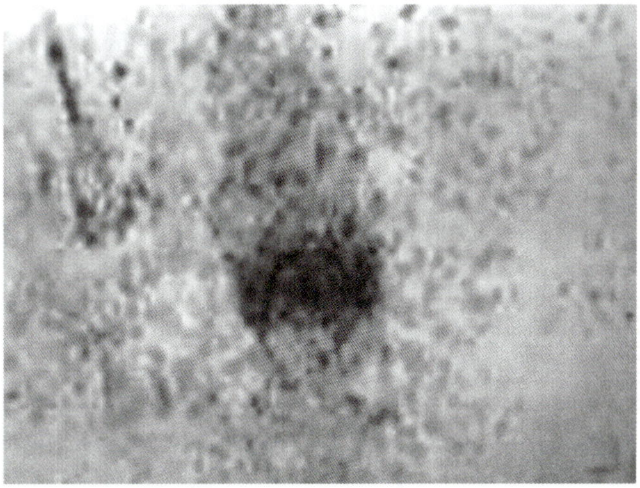

Fig. 4: Postmature oocyte.

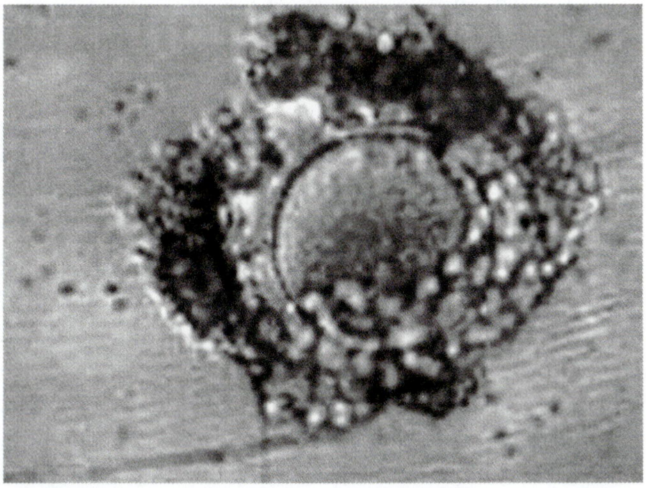

Fig. 5: Luteinized oocyte.

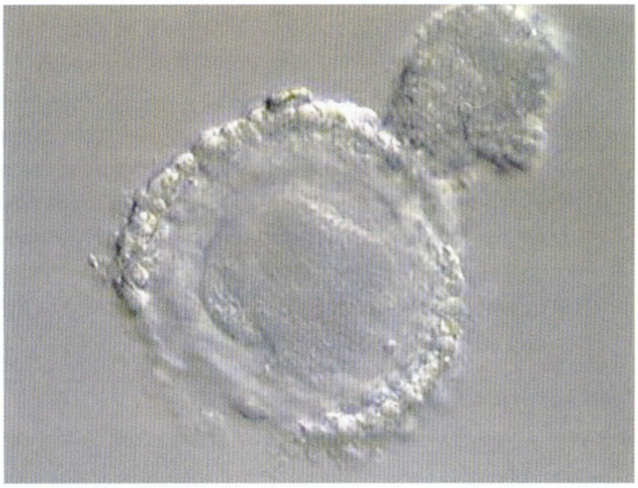

Fig. 6: Atretic oocyte.

into 6-mL round bottom tubes. The tubes are labeled and centrifuged at 1,500 rpm for 7 minutes. The supernatant is discarded and the pellet is gently layered with 0.3–0.5 mL of culture medium and placed in the incubator. Density gradient centrifugation method can also be used for sperm preparation.

5. *Insemination*: In this process, the sperm and eggs are mixed together and incubated to achieve fertilization. The eggs are checked after 18–20 hours for the presence of 2PN (pronuclei) to confirm that fertilization has taken place. The fertilized oocytes are called zygotes. Insemination is the most important step for successful fertilization in an IVF program and the success depends on a variety of factors:

- *Time of insemination*: Insemination is ideally done 2–4 hours after oocyte aspiration to allow the oocyte to equilibrate with the media and also help in final maturation of a few immature oocytes to metaphase II stage. However, prolonged (>4 hours) delay between oocyte retrieval and insemination is avoidable because the quality of both gametes will be negatively impacted after this period.[1]
- *Sperm concentration*: Optimum is about 80,000–100,000 progressively motile sperms/mL/oocyte provided there is no other significant male factor. The insemination should be added away from the eggs so that the sperm can gradually swim toward the eggs attracted by the chemotactic factors. Visualization of the sperms after insemination can be done using phase-contrast optics.
- *Media for insemination*: Glucose-containing media is used as it is the sperm's main energy source. Glucose improves sperm motility and has a role in sperm–oocyte fusion as well. There are various commercial media available for this purpose.
- *Duration of insemination*: Previously, a standard duration of insemination was considered to be 16–18 hours. This practice was followed by world-wide and for many years. Nowadays, however, there have been a few studies citing increased reactive oxygen species (ROS) production with prolonged incubation of sperms during insemination. This has persuaded embryologists to carry out a so-called "short insemination" during IVF in which sperms are coincubated with oocytes for periods as short as 1 hour.[2]

Methods of insemination:

- *Step 1—insemination plate for fertilization*: Different types of plates can be used depending on the incubator space or personal choice. Some use 60-mm falcon plate with 100 μL droplets of fertilization media, while some do it in a four-well plate where 0.5 mL (500 μL) media is used. A 35-mm falcon dish with 2 mL of fertilization media can also be used and 8–10 eggs can be inseminated in this plate. It is important that plates are prepared 1 day in advance to allow the media to equilibrate. It is also pertinent to overlay the media with mineral oil to avoid evaporation and consequent alterations in pH and osmolality.
- *Step 2—washing plate for the partially denuded oocytes*: Depending on whether one pursues a short or long incubation, the cumulus complexes are taken out of the incubator for denudation. A 300-μm Flexipet can be used gently to tease off the cumulus cells—which are anyway loosened by the enzymatic activity of sperm kept in the medium. It is important to be gentle and remove only that cumulus that comes off easily—there is no need to completely denude the egg. This partially denuded complex is washed thoroughly in culture media.
- *Step 3—culture plate after partial oocyte denudation*: Oocytes are now shifted to the culture media droplets covered with oil, for further incubation. Routine denudation is carried out at 18 hours along with fertilization check and then transferred to fresh culture plate for 24 hours.
  Droplet method: 100–150 μL drops (8–10 in number) are made in a 60-mm plate and covered with oil. One COC is placed per microdrop and then the sperm inseminate (a few μL only) is added. Denudation is carried out as with other methods.

6. *Embryo culture and embryo transfer*: The growing embryo is cultured for 2–5 days in the incubator, and different stages of the cleaving embryos and blastocysts are observed, graded, and finally transferred back into the patient's uterus, using an embryo transfer catheter. The spare embryos are cryopreserved and to be used in the next cycle.

IVF AND FERTILIZATION FAILURE

One of the major disappointments faced by the clinic and patients alike is failed fertilization of oocytes after an IVF procedure. It takes a financial and emotional toll on the couple. Among many reasons possible for failed fertilization, a common one is idiopathic sperm-egg recognition failure. Depletion of molecular chaperon HSPA2, which plays a key role in regulating the expression of sperm surface receptors, which are, in turn, responsible for sperm-egg recognition, causes fertilization failure. For such patients, probably IVF should be bypassed in favor of ICSI.[3]

Sperm oxidative stress, caused by increased ROS generation, was widely considered to be a significant contributory factor to sperm DNA damage/apoptosis/lipid peroxidation and reduced motility, which, in turn, increased the risk of male factor subfertility and also birth defects. Compared to IVF, ICSI has been known to minimize the exposure of gametes to endogenous sources of oxidative stress.[4]

Total failed fertilization can also be caused due to lack of oocyte activation factor in the sperm. This physiological factor is a novel phospholipase C (PLC) isoform, PLC zeta, that causes the calcium oscillations that precede oocyte activation. In the absence of this factor, there will be fertilization failures with even ICSI procedure because the sperm will fail to activate the oocyte. Some measures of success have been reported by injecting sperms during ICSI in a medium that contains calcium ionophores.[5,6]

INTRACYTOPLASMIC SPERM INJECTION

INTRODUCTION

The conventional IVF method usually produces a fertilization rate between 50% and 70%. However, in the case of infertility caused by a male factor, fertilization with conventional IVF can be severely compromised, if it occurs at all. Improving fertilization for male infertility was probably the first application of micromanipulation in ART.[7] The early micromanipulation techniques developed included zona drilling, partial zona dissection (PZD), and sub-zonal insemination (SUZI). However, the drawbacks of these techniques were lower or complete fertilization failure in male factor infertility or higher incidence of polyspermy (in SUZI). The breakthrough in the treatment of male infertility was in 1992, with the development of ICSI technique by Palermo et al. (Free University, Brussels). ICSI resulted in higher fertilization and pregnancy rates in patients with male factor infertility. Because ICSI is much more effective in fertilizing oocytes than other assisted reproductive techniques; today, it has become the ART of choice for male infertility.

In intracytoplasmic sperm injection (ICSI) technique, a single spermatozoon is injected directly into the cytoplasm of the oocyte in order to achieve fertilization.[8] Although ICSI is now considered a routine technique, it remains one of the most demanding techniques to master, due partly to its inherent technical difficulty and partly to the heterogeneity of the cases encountered for treatment (Fleming and King, 2003).

The ICSI is indicated predominantly for patients with male factor infertility (oligospermia, cryptozoospermia, asthenozoospermia, teratozoospermia, and globozoospermia). Surgical sperm retrieval techniques like percutaneous epididymal sperm aspiration (PESA) and testicular sperm extraction (TESE) can be used in conjunction with ICSI for patients with obstructive or nonobstructive azoospermia (hypospermatogenesis, Sertoli cell-only syndrome, and spermatogenic arrest). Patients with high titer of anti-sperm antibodies, poor cryopreserved sperm motility upon thawing, immotile cilia syndrome, ejaculatory dysfunction (anejaculation and retrograde ejaculation), unexplained infertility, fertilization failure with standard IVF (rescue ICSI) can be treated with ICSI. ICSI can also be carried out in patients with female factor where standard IVF has resulted in either poor fertilization or repeated high incidence of polyspermy.

The basic steps involved in an ICSI process, in the laboratory, include setting up the micromanipulator, preparation of dishes with culture media, sperm preparation, scanning, identification, and grading of the oocyte cumulus complexes (OCC), denuding the oocytes and the actual ICSI procedure.

MICROMANIPULATOR

The micromanipulator **(Fig. 7)** consists of an inverted microscope supported on a solid vibration-free table. The hydraulic manipulators are mounted on to the microscope pillars and bear micro-pipette holders that are connected to the micro-injector syringes. The coarse manipulators are motorized whereas the fine manipulators consist of hanging joysticks capable of moving in x, y and z-axis. Hoffman modulation contrast optics is employed and the temperature controlled microscope stage is maintained at 37°C to help maintain cell viability. The microscope is fitted with a video camera for viewing and recording the ICSI procedure.

The microinjector syringes are filled with oil, taking care to remove any air bubbles from the system. The holding pipette is usually fitted on the left-hand side holder and the microinjection pipette on the right-hand side. The pipettes are aligned, first under low power and then high power, parallel to the stage and facing each other so that under the microscope, it appears like a straight line **(Fig. 8)**. The holding pipette as an outer diameter of 80 μm and an inner diameter of 20 μm, whereas the microinjecting pipette has a tip diameter of 5 μm. The microinjection pipette has a sharp beveled end with or without a spike, to facilitate

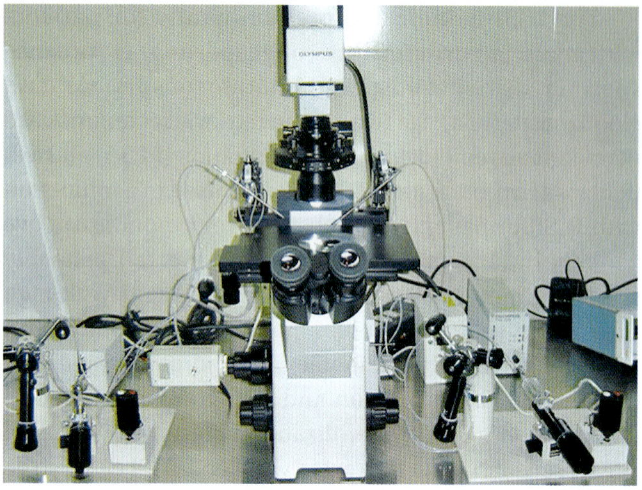

Fig. 7: Intracytoplasmic sperm injection (ICSI) micromanipulator.

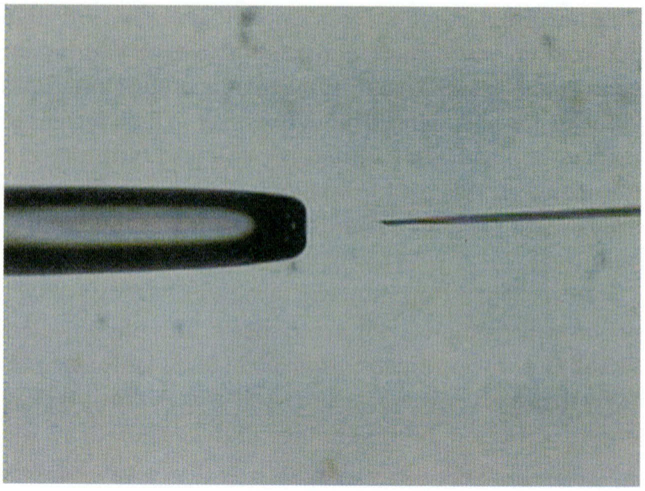

Fig. 8: Alignment of micropipettes. The holding pipette is on the left hand side and the microinjection pipette on the right hand side.

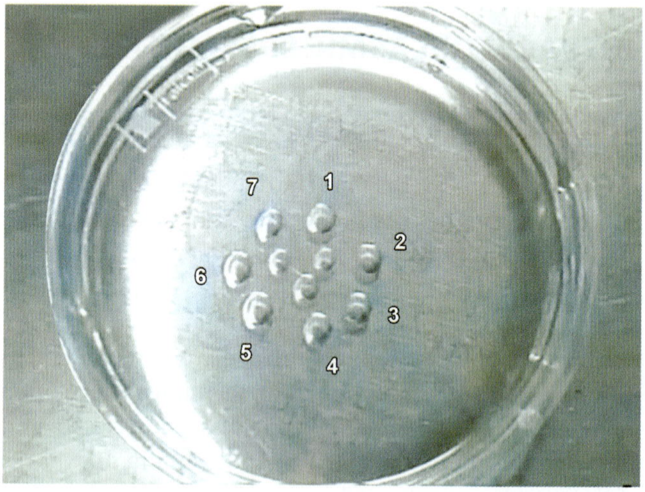

Fig. 9: *Intracytoplasmic sperm injection (ICSI) dish:* 3 central PVP droplets and 7 droplets of HEPES buffered flushing medium which are numbered and overlaid with paraffin oil.

easy penetration of the egg membrane. The micropipettes are angled at about 30–35° to ensure smooth manipulation without interference from the bottom surface of the Petri dish. The pipettes can be aligned just prior to the ICSI procedure.

PREPARATION OF DISHES

For manipulation of gametes outside the CO_2 incubator, commercially available HEPES buffered flushing medium is widely used, as it maintains the physiological pH of the media between 7.2 and 7.4. Oocytes and embryos are cultured in bicarbonate-based IVF media inside the CO_2 incubator (5% CO_2, 37°C). All media and oil are equilibrated overnight in the CO_2 incubator. The following dishes are prepared and properly labeled:

- *Oocyte scanning*: Center well dish (Falcon 3037) with 1-mL HEPES buffered medium in the inside well and 3-mL medium in the outside well.
- *Oocyte culture*: Center well dish with 1-ml IVF culture medium, overlaid with paraffin oil.
- *Oocyte denuding*: Center well dish with 0.5-mL hyaluronidase (80 IU/mL).
- *ICSI dish*: 2–3 droplets (10 µL each) of PVP (polyvinylpyrrolidone) are placed in the center of the ICSI dish (Falcon 1006). 7–8 droplets (10 µL each) of HEPES buffered flushing medium are then placed in a circle around the PVP droplets and overlaid with oil. The droplets are numbered on the back-side of the dish **(Fig. 9)**. The harvested sperms are placed in 10% PVP, which has a dual function. The viscous nature of PVP slows down the sperm movement making us easy to manipulate them. PVP enhances fine control aspiration and injection and also lubricates the inner wall of the microinjecting pipette thereby preventing sperm from sticking inside.

SPERM PREPARATION FOR ICSI

In the case of TESE, the seminiferous tubules are mechanically teased under the stereo-zoom microscope using two needles. The contents of the tubules are washed, centrifuged, and observed for spermatozoa. In case of viable immotile spermatozoa, the viable spermatozoa may be identified using the hypo-osmotic swelling test.

SCANNING, IDENTIFICATION, AND GRADING OF OOCYTES

The contents of the follicular fluid are poured out into a plain petri dish (Falcon 3652) and scanned under the stereo-zoom microscope. Once the oocyte cumulus complex is identified, it is picked up with a sterile transfer pipette (Falcon 7575), washed in HEPES buffered medium and transferred into the dish with IVF culture media, and placed back into the incubator. Based on the appearance of cumulus and corona cells, the OCCs are graded as immature, preovulatory, and hypermature.

DENUDING THE OOCYTES

The oocyte cumulus complexes **(Fig. 10)** are transferred from the culture medium and placed into the dish containing enzyme hyaluronidase. The denudation of oocytes relies upon the mechanical dispersal of the cumulus cells that comprise the corona radiata. The oocytes are gently aspirated in and out, using a 300 μm denuding pipette attached to a mouth tubing aspiration assembly, so as to loosen the cumulus cells. The oocytes should not remain in hyaluronidase for more than 1 minute. The partially denuded oocytes, with its corona radiata intact **(Fig. 11)**, are then transferred into droplets of flushing medium and denuded further using Flexipet of reducing diameters (170 μm and 140 μm). The oocytes are simultaneously washed repeatedly in different droplets of flushing medium till all the coronal cells are removed **(Fig. 12)**. The oocytes are then placed in the HEPES buffered medium in the ICSI dish and observed for different stages of oocyte maturity. The dish with the oocytes is placed back into the incubator. The denuded oocytes are classified as follows:

1. *Germinal vesicle*: The presence of a large nucleus inside the cytoplasm, absence of the polar body.
2. *Metaphase I*: Absence of germinal vesicle, an absence of the polar body.
3. *Metaphase II*: The presence of the polar body, no germinal vesicle present.

Metaphase II oocyte is a prerequisite for successful fertilization through ICSI. This ensures that they contain a haploid set of chromosomes, so that a normal diploid karyotype should be carried by the zygote following injection of another haploid set of chromosomes from the spermatozoa.

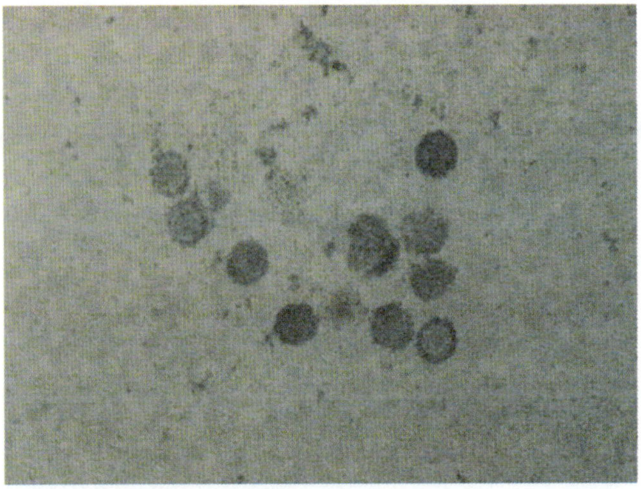

Fig. 11: The partially denuded oocytes, with its corona radiate intact.

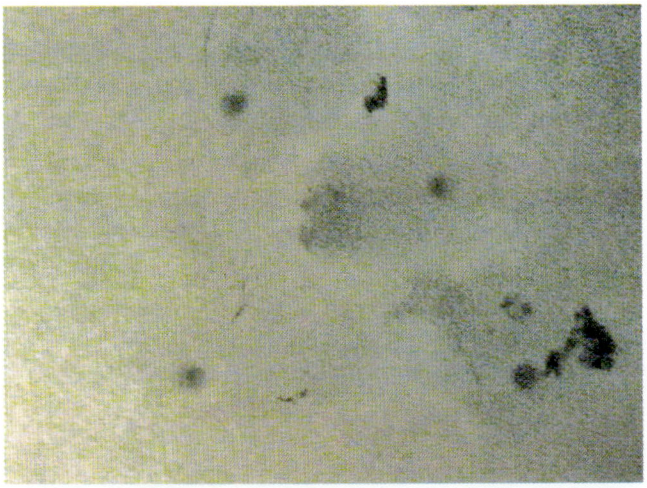

Fig. 10: The oocyte cumulus complexes in culture medium.

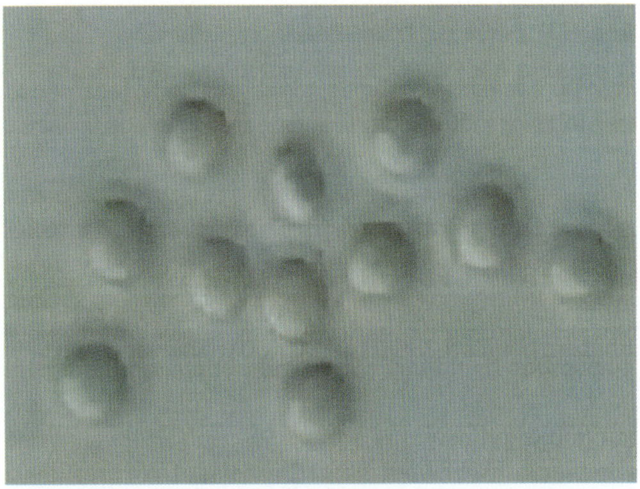

Fig. 12: Denuded oocytes with all the coronal cells removed.

ICSI TECHNIQUE (FIGS. 13 TO 28)

The ICSI involves the injection of a single spermatozoon into the cytoplasm of a mature metaphase II oocyte. The entire process is carried out in the ICSI dish containing oocytes and sperm placed in media droplets covered with oil. The holding and injection pipettes are properly aligned on the micromanipulator. The ICSI dish containing the oocytes is removed from the incubator and the washed sperm suspension is added to one of the droplets of PVP. The prepared ICSI dish is then placed on the heated stage of the micromanipulator.

The actual procedure of ICSI can be divided into two parts:

1. *Sperm selection and immobilization*: It is absolutely vital to damage the plasmalemma of the spermatozoon and so immobilize it to prevent undue disruption of the ooplasm and ensure oocyte activation. Oocyte activation is a prerequisite for decondensation of the sperm nucleus and formation of the male pronucleus. The aligned microinjection needle is gently lowered into the droplet of plain PVP. PVP will be sucked in by capillary action. The microinjection pipette is raised and then lowered into another droplet of PVP containing the sperm. The spermatozoa are first focused and then the

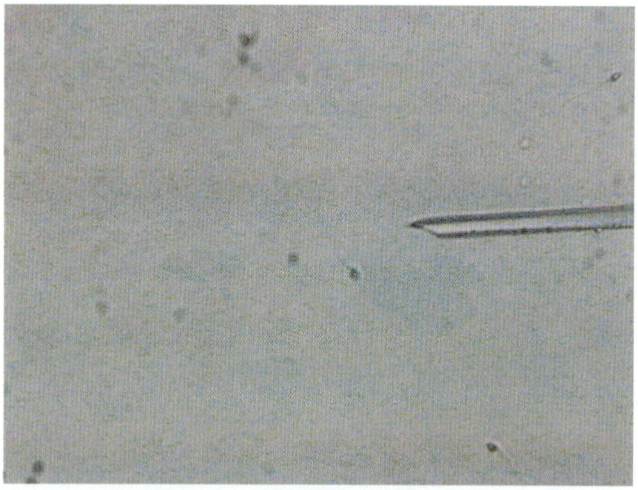

Fig. 13: A morphologically normal motile spermatozoon is selected and then the microinjection needle is adjusted so as to make sure they are in the same plane.

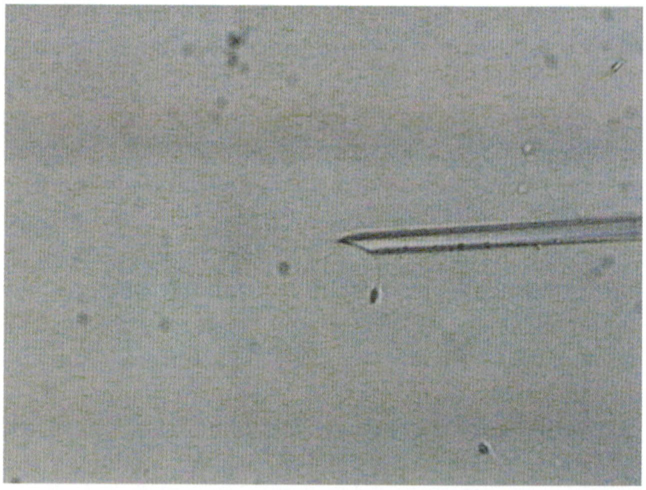

Fig. 14: The selected sperm is immobilized by hitting the sperm tail with the tip of the microinjection pipette.

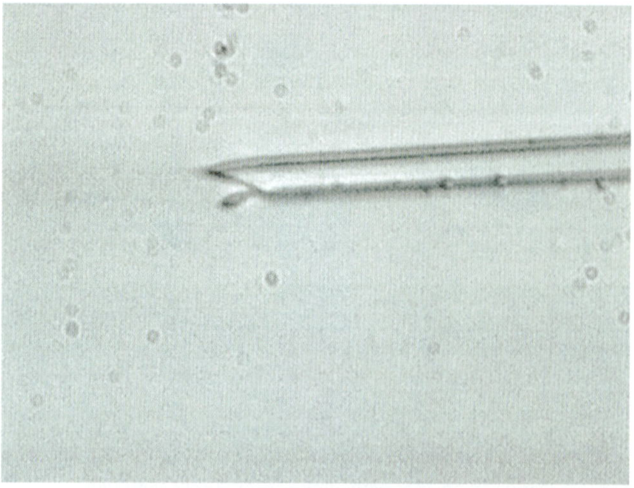

Fig. 15: The immobilized sperm is aspirated tail in first into the microinjection pipette.

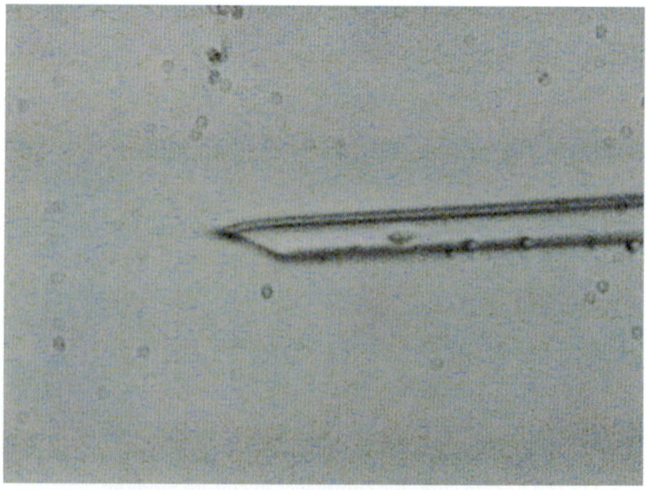

Fig. 16: The immobilized sperm is clearly visible at some distance away from the tip of the microinjection pipette.

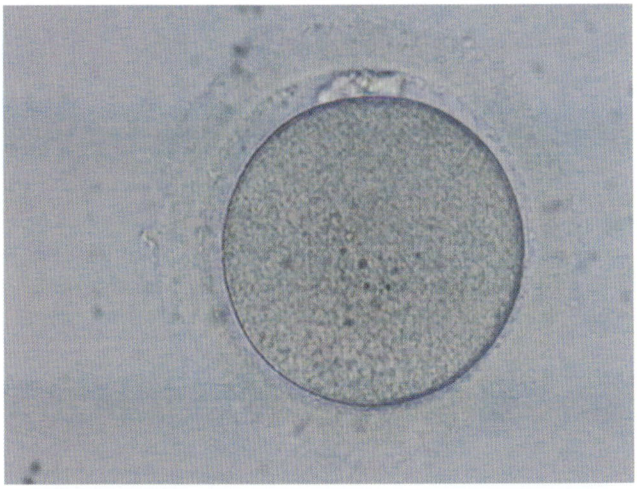

Fig. 17: A mature metaphase II oocyte with the polar body visible at 12 O'clock position.

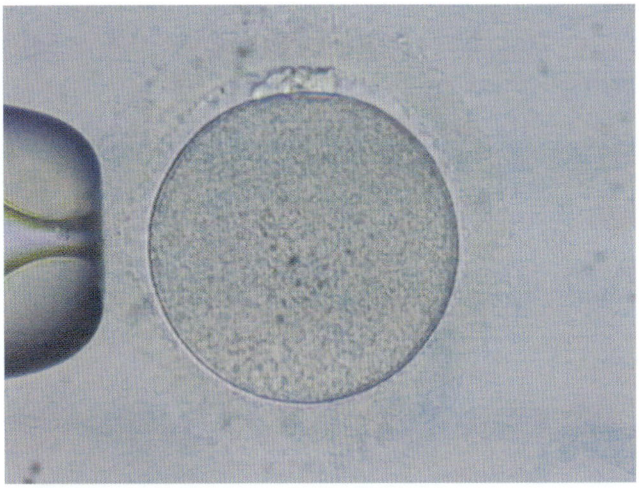

Fig. 18: The oocyte is fixed to the holding pipette, at 9 O'clock position, by aspirating or applying negative pressure.

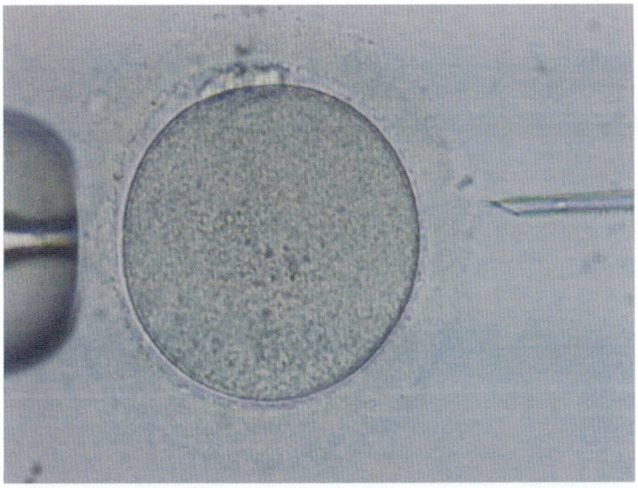

Fig. 19: The microinjection pipette is aligned close to the egg at the 3 O'clock position.

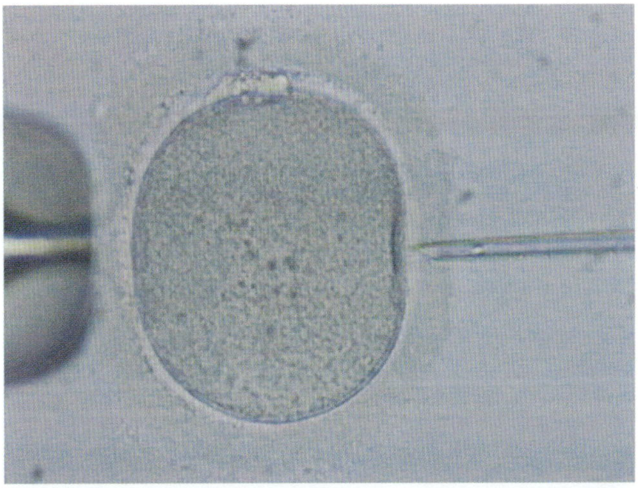

Fig. 20: The sperm is gently advanced forward toward the pipette tip and the pipette is slowly and steadily inserted through the zona pellucida.

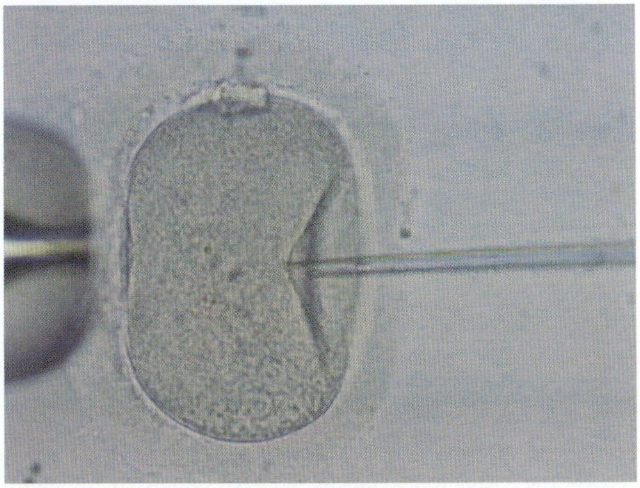

Fig. 21: The microinjection pipette has penetrated the zona pellucida and is gently advanced forward toward the oolemma.

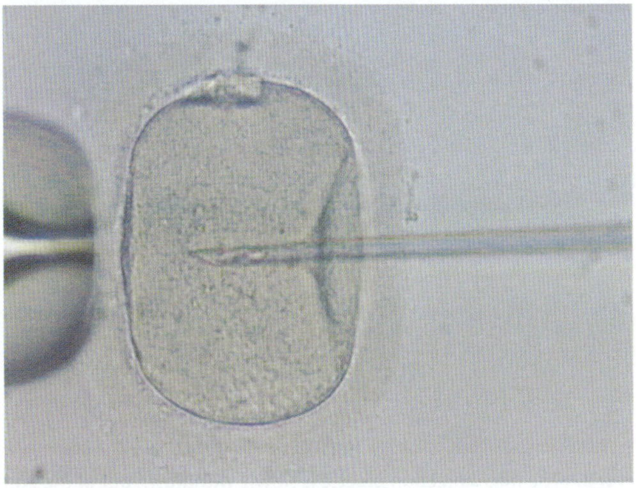

Fig. 22: The intact oolemma apparent by the invagination around the micropipette.

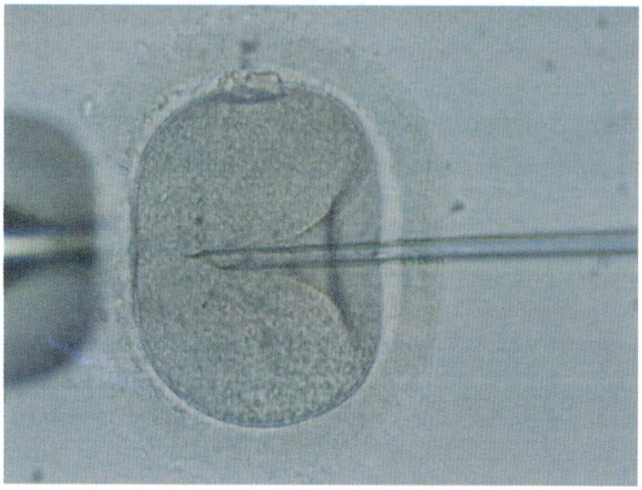

Fig. 23: A small quantity of ooplasm is then aspirated in the microinjection pipette.

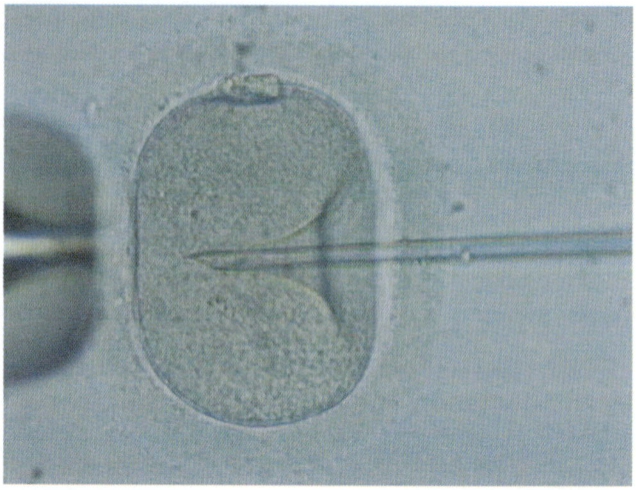

Fig. 24: The oolemma has ruptured, which is confirmed by the sudden free flow of the ooplasm.

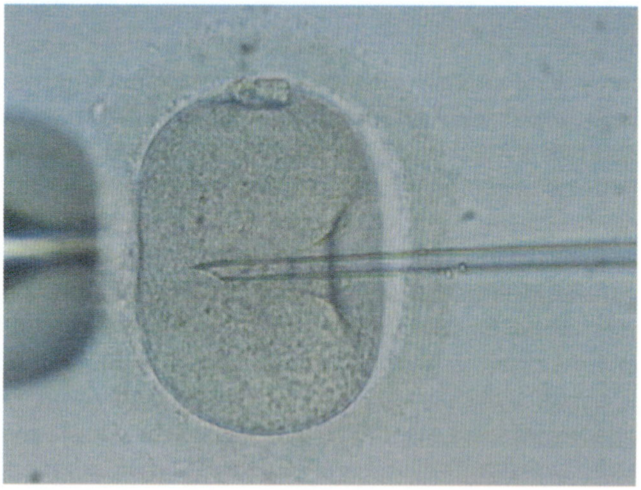

Fig. 25: The sperm is slowly released inside the oocyte.

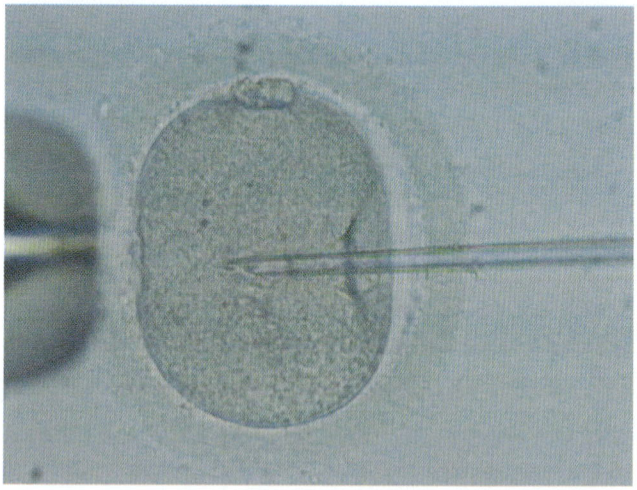

Fig. 26: The sperm can be seen deposited in the center of the oocyte.

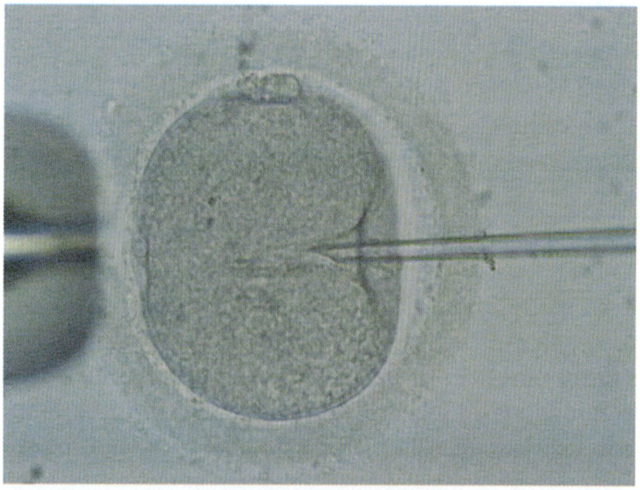

Fig. 27: The microinjection pipette is slowly withdrawn out of the egg as gently as possible making sure that the sperm remains inside.

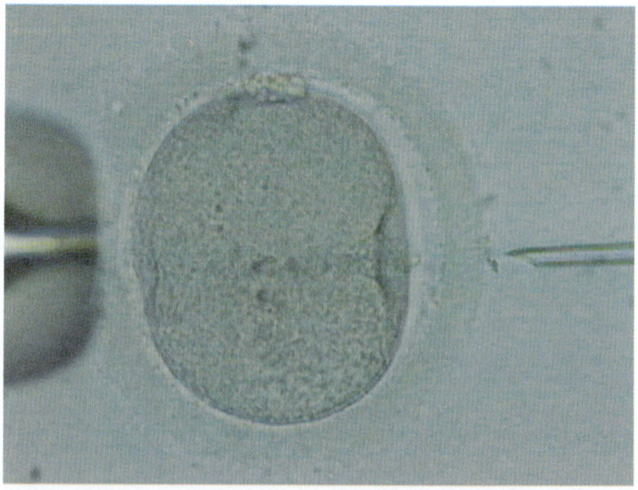

Fig. 28: The microinjection pipette has been completely withdrawn from the oocyte. The intracytoplasmic sperm injection (ICSI) procedure is over.

microinjection needle is adjusted so as to make sure they are in the same plane. A morphologically normal motile sperm is selected. The sperm is immobilized by hitting the sperm tail with the tip of the microinjection pipette. The immobilized sperm is then aspirated tail in first into the microinjection pipette. The pipette is then raised out of the PVP droplet.

2. *Ooplasmic penetration and sperm deposition*: A mature metaphase II oocyte is brought into focus using the moving stage. The holding pipette is next lowered into the droplet containing the mature egg. The egg is then rotated using the holding pipette, so as to bring the polar body either at 6 O'clock or 12 O'clock position. Placement of the polar body at 6 or 12 O'clock position ensures that the injection pipette does not penetrate the oocyte closer to where the spindle is presumed to lie. The oocyte is fixed to the holding pipette, at 9 O'clock position, by aspirating or applying negative pressure. The oocyte is again focused so that the plasma membrane is visible as a distinct line. The injection pipette is then gently lowered into the oocyte droplet and focused in the same plane as the oocyte. The sperm is then gently advanced forward toward the pipette tip, so that minimum amount of PVP (1–2 pL) would be pushed into the ooplasm. The microinjection pipette is then aligned close to the egg at the 3 O'clock position and slowly and steadily inserted through the zona pellucida and oolemma. The oolemma usually remains intact due to its inherent strength and elasticity, which is apparent by the fact that the oolemma remains invaginated around the micropipette. A small quantity of ooplasm is then aspirated in the microinjection pipette. Initially, the flow of ooplasm into the injection pipette will be slow as it is impeded by the intact oolemma. Eventually, however, the oolemma will rupture, which is confirmed by the sudden free flow of the ooplasm. Once the oolemma is ruptured and penetrated, the sperm is then slowly released and deposited in the center of the oocyte. The microinjection pipette is slowly withdrawn out of the egg as gently as possible making sure that the sperm remains inside. The oocyte is then released from the holding pipette. The procedure is repeated until all oocytes have been injected in a similar fashion. The injected oocytes are then transferred from the ICSI dish into IVF culture media dishes and placed back into the CO_2 incubator. The micropipettes are removed from the tool holder and discarded. Oocytes are assessed for evidence of fertilization 16–18 hours after ICSI.

INTRACYTOPLASMIC MORPHOLOGICALLY SELECTED SPERM INJECTION

In conventional in vitro fertilization, the zona pellucida prevents entry of abnormal sperm, so that only "normal" sperm can enter and fertilize the oocyte. Since ICSI bypasses the natural sperm selection process, there is an increased risk of genetic abnormalities being transmitted to the offspring. Hence, several sperm selection methods have been developed to select the most normal spermatozoa, prominent among, which is the intracytoplasmic morphologically selected sperm injection (IMSI) technique.

The ICSI is normally performed at a 200–400× magnification, which allows visualization of major sperm morphological defects, such as head abnormalities (round, tapering, etc.), mid-piece defects (bent neck and thick midpiece), tail defects (short stubby and double), whereas minor morphological defects, such as vacuoles in the sperm head, which may play a significant role in ICSI outcome, cannot be visualized **(Fig. 29)**.

The IMSI technique, developed by Bartoov et al.,[9,10] is the new modified version of ICSI, wherein the sperms are magnified to about 6,600 times and subjected to the MSOME criteria (Motile Sperm Organelle Morphology Examination) allowing us to select the most morphologically normal spermatozoa just prior to performing ICSI. The IMSI system consists of an inverted light microscope attached with high-power Nomarski optics enhanced by digital imaging to achieve a magnification of 6,600×. Using IMSI, the sperm is analyzed for nuclear integrity thereby allowing selection and injection of a normal sperm head free of vacuoles **(Fig. 30)**.

IMSI EQUIPMENT

The apparatus used for sperm evaluation comprises of:

- Inverted microscope (micromanipulator)
- Nomarski differential interference contrast (DIC) system
- Images are grabbed by a three charge-coupled device (CCD) video camera
- Monitor screen.

Once assembled, the equipment is capable of high magnification over 6,600×, required to achieve a detailed visualization of the sperm subcellular organelles.

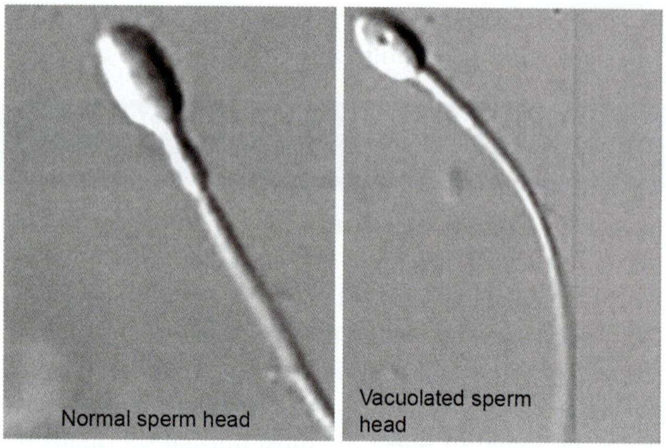

Fig. 29: Normal versus vacuolated sperm head.

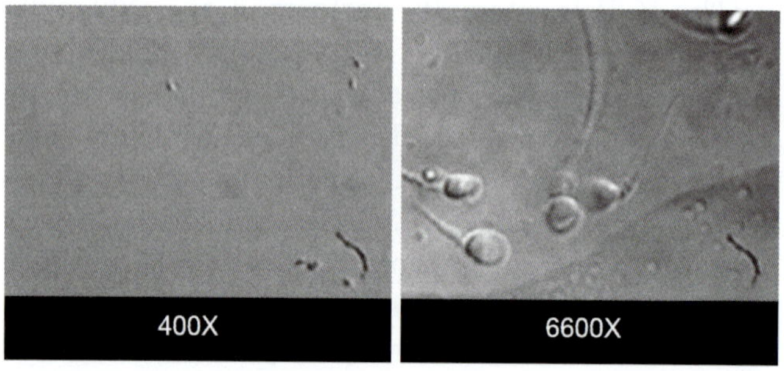

Fig. 30: Intracytoplasmic sperm injection versus intracytoplasmic morphologically selected sperm injection.

CALCULATION OF MAGNIFICATION

Calculation of the "total reached magnification" may vary depending upon the system components, but usually it is as follows:

Microscope Magnification (100× objective lens magnification × 1.5× magnification selector)

- Video coupler magnification (1×)
- Video magnification (CCD × monitor diagonal dimension) (44.45×).

Total magnification = 100 × 1.5 x 1 × 44.45 = 6,600×

MSOME CRITERIA FOR IMSI

The MSOME criteria are based on real-time high magnification (6,600×) morphological analysis of isolated motile spermatozoa. MSOME allows identification of both conventional morphological sperm defects as well as specific sperm vacuole nuclear defects. IMSI is basically a combination of MSOME criteria and the ICSI technique.

The MSOME criteria are performed on morphologically normal motile sperm, as morphologically abnormal sperm can be identified at low power and can be excluded. The sperm acrosome, post-acrosomal lamina, neck, mitochondria, tail, and nucleus are evaluated. Except for the sperm nucleus normality, the other sperm organelles do not seem to affect the ICSI fertilization outcome.

As per the MSOME criteria, a spermatozoon is classified as morphologically normal when the sperm head exhibits a normal nucleus shape (smooth, symmetric, and oval nucleus) and chromatin content (homogeneity of the chromatin mass containing no extrusion or invagination of nuclear chromatin). The criterion for normality of chromatin content is the absence of vacuoles occupying more than 4% of the sperm nuclear area. The average length and width limits are estimated to be 4.75 ± 0.28 and 3.28 ± 0.20 µm.

IMSI DISH PREPARATION

A glass bottom Petri dish is used for performing IMSI. Three droplets of polyvinylpyrrolidone medium (7% PVP) are placed in the center of the dish surrounded by 5–6 droplets of HEPES-buffered medium, the droplets are then covered with sterile liquid paraffin oil. The sperm suspension is loaded into the PVP droplets and denuded oocytes are placed in the peripheral HEPES media droplets.

MODIFIED IMSI TECHNIQUE

Morphological analysis mainly involves three elements such as the absence of sperm head vacuoles, sperm head size, and head shape. Selection of sperm according to these standards will take around 30–120 minutes. In order to minimize the time taken to perform the IMSI procedure, the Bloom IVF Center, Mumbai has modified the IMSI procedure. Two embryologists work together for analyzing the sperms to minimize the chances of human error. 20–30 morphologically normal motile sperm are selected and immobilized at 200× magnification. Sperms with obvious defects like pinhead, amorphous head, large midpiece, and double tail/head are not evaluated. To minimize the oocyte exposure outside the incubator, the IMSI dish contains only the spermatozoa and not the oocytes. The selected sperms are placed in a row one below the other in the microscopic field. They are then magnified real-time (6,000×) and then an image is clicked. With the help of the computer program, the measurement of the image of the sperm head is performed. The selected spermatozoa are subjected to the MSOME criteria, and the length and breadth of the sperm head are measured. Sperm, which fulfills the MSOME criteria, is magnified further to 6,600× and evaluated for the presence of vacuoles.

Based on the presence and size of sperm head vacuoles, the following grading system[11] can be applied:

- *Grade 1*: Absence of vacuole
- *Grade 2*: A maximum of two small vacuoles occupying less than 4% of the head surface
- *Grade 3*: At least one large vacuole
- *Grade 4*: A large vacuole with abnormal head shapes or other abnormalities.

The morphologically normal sperm, free of vacuoles is then used to perform ICSI at 200×.

INDICATIONS FOR IMSI

Following are the conditions that can be successfully treated using the IMSI sperm selection technique:

- Severe teratozoospermia
- Patients with high sperm DNA fragmentation index
- Previous ICSI failures
- Repeated poor-quality embryo development rate after ICSI cycle
- Unexplained infertility who failed in previous IVF attempts
- Surgically retrieved sperm from testis, especially micro-TESE
- Recurring abortion in the first trimester with MSOME showing nuclear defects.

SPERM MORPHOLOGY AND VACUOLES

Presence of nuclear vacuoles is associated with decreased fertility potential.[12] Several studies have shown that spermatozoa selected using the IMSI technique are positively associated with increased pregnancy rates in couples with previous and repeated implantation failures[13,14] suggesting that vacuolization reflects some underlying chromosomal DNA defects. Several studies have reported a lower miscarriage rate in the IMSI group,[15-17] others have reported that compared to ICSI, the IMSI procedure improved clinical pregnancy rates without compromising the aneuploidy rate.[18,19]

Garolla et al. demonstrated that sperm with vacuoles was related to the integrity of sperm DNA fragmentation, and abnormal chromosomes.[20] Recently, Hammoud et al. noted that the presence of large or multiple vacuoles was associated with a higher amount of DNA fragmentation in sperm than that which lacked vacuoles.[21] A recent study has demonstrated that morphologically normal spermatozoa, with an absence of vacuolization, selected using IMSI, are free of DNA damage, thereby establishing a direct relationship between a good morphological pattern on the sperm and good DNA quality. Furthermore, results showed spermatozoa presenting a normal morphology and no traces of vacuolization to be fully free of DNA damage. However, traces of vacuolization and more severe morphological alterations were accompanied by significant increase in the proportion of sperm containing a damaged DNA molecule.[22]

In a major study 1891, IVF-ICSI cycles were compared with 577 IVF-IMSI cycles. In first IVF cycles, either technique was equally effective in producing pregnancies and live births, so first cycles saw no difference. However, in second cycles after the first ICSI cycle failed, using IMSI to identify normal sperm showed a better pregnancy rate (56% vs 38% PRs) and delivery rates (28% vs 18%).[23] In another comparative study, IMSI resulted in better embryo quality and more number of blastocysts per cycle.[24]

In a retrospective study conducted at Bloom IVF Center, Mumbai, it was observed that in cases of recurrent implantation failures, there were significantly higher implantation and pregnancy rate in the IMSI group as compared to the ICSI group.[25]

CONCLUSION

Among the different malformations identified by MSOME, those affecting sperm nuclear structure, such as large vacuoles, have been demonstrated to be correlated to male reproductive impairment. Current literature agrees on the presence of higher decondensed DNA levels corresponding to vacuolated regions. Although IMSI is not an effective frontline treatment for all patients, it does allow real-time selection of the best available morphologically normal motile spermatozoa before oocyte injection. Only extensive use and availability of a large amount of data will help us to understand the feasibility, effectiveness, and safety of the IMSI technique.

PICSI

BACKGROUND

At ejaculation, millions of sperm are deposited by into the upper part of the vagina from where the sperm travel the female genital tract to reach the oocyte and fertilize.[26] In humans, only about 10% of the ejaculated spermatozoa will enter the cervix, 1% the uterus and 0.1% the fallopian tube, thus a diminutive percentage of the ejaculated sperm reach the oocyte. Eventually, a single spermatozoon fertilizes the egg.[26] This proves that the female genital tract plays an active and stringent role in selecting the best sperm essential for producing a healthy offspring.

Conventional semen preparation techniques (swim up, density gradient, etc.), bypass to varying extents the natural selection process taking place in the female genital tract. In the case of ICSI, all-natural barriers are bypassed, and the entire sperm is introduced into the oocytes. Since sperm DNA damage cannot be assessed real-time visually, there is a high chance of sperm with fragmented DNA being injected into the oocytes, subsequently leading to pregnancy loss.

Thus, conventional sperm preparation techniques might not necessarily select the most competent spermatozoa. To overcome this issue, advanced sperm selection techniques have been devised based on physiological selection procedures. One of these chief principles involves molecular binding.

Hyaluronic acid is a chief component of the extracellular matrix of the cumulus. In the human, plasma membrane remodeling is known to take place during the final stages of spermatogenesis that facilitates binding of the male germ cell hyaluronan and the zona pellucida. The human sperm has HA receptors, of which at least three hyaluronan binding proteins are involved in crucial steps like sperm maturation, acrosome reaction, motility, hyaluronidase activity, and sperm-zona binding.[27]

PICSI PROCEDURE

A Petri dish, with immobilized hyaluronic acid on it, comprises the PICSI dish. Prepared spermatozoa suspensions are placed over these spots of HA and incubated at 37°C for 15 minutes. Consequently, by gently rinsing the HA droplet, the freely moving spermatozoa are removed thus removing the unbounded sperm. The bound spermatozoa are picked with an ICSI injection pipette and injected into the oocytes.[28]

VERDICT

Although a number of studies claim to have improved embryo quality and development with the use of PICSI, there are quite a few that are not much in support of this procedure. The recent meta-analysis suggests that bigger and more adequately powered good quality-data is required before passing judgment on the efficacy of PICSI.[29]

REFERENCES

1. Hickman CFL. Optimising the timing between oocyte collection, cumulus removal and insemination by ICSI or IVF. Fertil Steril. 2011;96:S79.
2. Le Bras A, Hesters L, Gallot V, et al. Shortening gametes co-incubation time improves live birth rate for couples with a history of fragmented embryos. Syst Biol Reprod Med. 2017;63:331-7.
3. Ergur AR, Dokras A, Giraldo JL, et al. Sperm maturity and treatment choice of in vitro fertilization or ICSI: diminished sperm HSPA2 chaperone levels predict IVF failure. Fertil Steril. 2002;77:910-8.
4. Gupta S, Sekhon L, Kim Y, et al. The role of oxidative stress and antioxidants in Assisted Reproduction. Curr Women's Health Rev. 2010;6:227-38.
5. Nasr-Esfahani MH, Deemeh MR, Tavalaee M. Artificial Oocyte activation and intracytoplasmic sperm injection. Fertil Steril. 2010;94:520-6.
6. Bhattacharya S, Hamilton MP, Shaaban M, et al. Conventional in-vitro fertilization versus intracytoplasmic sperm injection for the treatment of non-male factor infertility: a randomized controlled trial. Lancet. 2001;357:2075-9.
7. Fleming S, King R. Micromanipulation in assisted conception. London (U.K.): Cambridge University Press. 2003.
8. Palermo G, Joris H, Devroey P, et al. Pregnancies after intracytoplasmic injection of single spermatozoon into an oocyte. Lancet. 1992;340:17-8.
9. Bartoov B, Berkovitz A, Eltes F. Selection of spermatozoa with normal nuclei to improve the pregnancy rate with intracytoplasmic sperm injection. N Engl J Med. 2001;345:1067-8.
10. Bartoov B, Berkovitz A, Eltes F, et al. Real-time fine morphology of motile human sperm cells is associated with IVF-ICSI outcome. J Androl. 2002;23:1-8.
11. Vanderzwalmen P, Hiemer A, Rubner P, et al. Blastocyst development after sperm selection at high magnification is associated with size and number of nuclear vacuoles. Reprod Biomed Online. 2008;17:617-27.
12. Bartoov B, Berkovitz A, Eltes F, et al. Pregnancy rates are higher with intracytoplasmic morphologically selected sperm injection than with conventional intracytoplasmic injection. Fertil Steril. 2003;80:1413-9.
13. Berkovitz A, Eltes F, Lederman H, et al. How to improve IVF-ICSI outcome by sperm selection. Reprod Biomed Online. 2006;12:634-8.
14. Hazout A, Dumont-Hassan M, Junca AM, et al. High-magnification ICSI overcomes paternal effect resistant to conventional ICSI. Reprod Biomed Online. 2006;12:19-25.
15. Souza Setti A, Ferreira RC, Paes de Almeida Ferreira Braga D, et al. Intracytoplasmic sperm injection outcome versus intracytoplasmic morphologically selected sperm injection outcome: a meta-analysis. Reprod Biomed Online. 2010;21:450-55.

16. Balaban B, Yakin K, Alatas C, et al. Clinical outcome od intracytoplasmatic injection of spermatozoa morphologically selected under high magnification: a prospective randomized study. Rep Biomed Online. 2011;22: 472-6.
17. Antinori M, Licata E, Dani G, et al. Intracytoplasmic morphologically selected sperm injection: a prospective randomized trial. Reprod Biomed Online. 2008;16: 835-41.
18. Figueira Rde C, Braga DP, Setti AS, et al. Morphological nuclear integrity of sperm cells is associated with preimplantation genetic aneuploidy screening cycle outcomes. Fertil Steril. 2011;95:990-3.
19. Luna D, Hilario R, Dueñas-Chacón J, et al. The IMSI Procedure Improves Laboratory and Clinical Outcomes without Compromising the Aneuploidy Rate when Compared to the Classical ICSI Procedure. Clin Med Insights Reprod Health. 2015;9:29-37.
20. Garolla A, Fortini D, Menegazzo M, et al. High-power microscopy for selecting spermatozoa for ICSI by physiological status. Reprod Biomed Online. 2008;17:610-6.
21. Hammoud C, Hassen MF, Albert F, et al. Can IMSI be efficient in a situation of ICSI failure and teratospermy, with a special study of macrocephaly? Fertil Steril. 2008;90:S192.
22. Gosálvez J. Single sperm selection and DNA fragmentation analysis: The case of MSOME/IMSI. Natural Sci. 2013;5: 7-14.
23. Klement AH, Koren-Morag N, Itsykson P, et al. Intracytoplasmic morphologically selected sperm injection versus intracytoplasmic sperm injection: a step toward a clinical algorithm. Fertil Steril. 2013;99:1290-3.
24. Knez K, Zorn B, Tomazevic T, et al. The IMSI procedure improves poor embryo development in the same infertile couples with poor semen quality: a comparative prospective randomized study. Reprod Biol Endocrinol. 2011;9:123.
25. Dalal R, Pai H, Palshetkar N, et al. Intracytoplasmic Morphologically selected Sperm Injection vs Intracytoplasmic Sperm Injection: A Retrospective Analysis. Int J Infertil Fetal Med. 2011;2:1-5.
26. Williams M, Hill CJ, Scudamore I, et al. Sperm numbers and distribution within the human fallopian tube around ovulation. Hum Reprod. 1993;8:2019-26.
27. Ranganathan S, Ganguly AK, Datta K. Evidence for the presence of hyaluronan binding protein on spermatozoa and its possible involvement in sperm function. Mol Reprod Dev. 1994; 38:69-76.
28. Parmegiani L, Cognigni GE, Bernardi S, et al. Physiologic ICSI": Hyaluronic acid (HA) favors selection of spermatozoa without DNA fragmentation and with the normal nucleus, resulting in improvement of embryo quality. Fertil Steril. 2010;93:598-604.
29. Henkel R. Sperm preparation: state-of-the-art—physiological aspects and application of advanced sperm preparation methods. Asian J Androl. 2012;14:260-9.

Assisted Hatching

47

Kanthi Bansal, Sugandha Goel, Hetal Patolia, Shilpa Damodar

INTRODUCTION

Assisted reproductive technique (ART) has had a leap and bound in advances of techniques. The rate of implantation and pregnancy rate still need more enhancements; there are 85% chances that the replaced embryos will not implant.[1] The embryonic development and implantation is dependent on chromosomal constitution and cytoplasmic structure.[2]

Studies showed that day 2 or 3 transfer has only 10–15% chances of implantation and 25% for blastocyst transfers. However a euploid embryo with full developmental potential and good endometrial receptivity fails to implant mainly due to disorders in hatching.[3,4]

Numerous approaches are being proposed to improve the implantation rate which involves techniques to improve endometrial receptivity, embryo transfer, and capacity to implant.[1,5,6] One of the technique to improve embryo's capacity to implant is assisted hatching (AH) which disrupt the zona pellucida (ZP) by artificial methods. AH was proposed for older patients, with frozen-thawed embryos in past but now is also used for recurrent implantation failure.[7-10] The various techniques used are chemicals, mechanical, and laser which work by making the zona thin or drilling the zona or breaching by creating a hole in the zona.[11] Cohen et al. reported the first pregnancy after AH in 1988.[12] Whether AH would increase the pregnancy rates or implantation is debated, some reports shows significant effect while other reports does not show any significant pregnancy rate improvement.[13-23]

Zona Pellucida

Zona pellucida is a thick acellular matrix, 13–15 μm in size which is present surrounding human oocyte and early embryo.[24] The main composition of ZP is of carbohydrates, ZP-specific protein and glycoproteins, bilayered with thicker outer wall and resilient inner.[5] ZP plays multiple roles in fertilization which is both structural and functional. It causes sperm binding, acrosomal reaction, fusion, and preimplantation development.[25] It also plays important role in preventing polyspermy, avoids dispersal of blastomeres, and facilitates transport of ovum through the fallopian tubes. It protects the embryo epithelial lining of the reproductive tract, leukocytes, and spermatozoa.[26] ZP maintains the integrity of embryo[27] and has a protective role against unfavorable uterine factors.[28] Trounson and Morre studied complete or partial ZP removal in degenerated sheep eggs.[29]

Hatching

Hatching is caused by blastocyst expansion and contraction which leads to thinning of zona. Cleaved embryo and uterus releases proteases which causes blastocyst phase by zona dissolution.[28-32] Zona thickness is reduced by embryonic mass by physical expansion and it is prepared for hatching.[31] There is interaction between trophectoderm and endometrial cells, and eventually implantation occurs.[33] The site of hatching is in close proximity to the inner cell mass (ICM) of blastocysts in humans as per two studies,[33,34] study by Hirotoshi et al. proposed that for proper hatching, the choice of AH site is important.[35]

Gordan and Dapunt showed that the escape of embryo from the ZP is independent of the pressure exerted by the expanding blastocyst and hatching is predominantly the result of ZP lysis.[36] A study on mouse blastocyst indicated that adequate number of cells constituting the embryo determines hatching in vitro. Hatching in vivo is differentiated from in vitro by uterine induced trophectoderm lytic factors.[37]

ASSISTED HATCHING

Implantation failure can be due to ZP hatching failure after blastocyst expansion. Thick ZP (>16 mm), high follicle stimulating hormone (FSH) levels and advanced age are possible reasons for a hatching failure. In vitro culture and treatment with hyaluronidase may leads to secondary hardening of the ZP.[38,39]

In 1990, the use of AH in human embryos was first published by Cohen et al.[46] This leads to prologue of AH in ART. Studies have shown that there are high rates of implantation by creating artificial gaps in zona with the use of micro surgical techniques.[40] The hypothesis states that there is good prognosis for implantation in embryos with reduced zona thickness.[41] There is variations in zona thickness at different stages of development of cleaved embryos as per study by Wright et al.[42] and there is no change in ZP thickness in embryos which did not cleave.[43] There is correlation between age and ZP thickness. Impaired hatching and when zona fails to rupture leads to low implantation rates.[44,45]

Few studies have proposed no correlation between the zona thickness and implantation, there may be other limiting factors which are required for successful hatching.[5,45] There is one more study which reports that the artificial formation of hole in ZP may improve the rate of implantation but removal of ZP has no impact on implantation.[17]

The intrinsic embryonic lysine which promotes hatching is coming up as an indicator for AH instead of zona thickness and zona hardness; this lysine produced causes the blastocyst to expand.[45] Thus, optimizing culture conditions will overcome all problems.[45]

Furthermore, experiments on mouse embryos have demonstrated that damaged blastomere have a toxic effect, and reduce the rate of hatching.[46] In human, with the removal of necrotic blastomeres which were partially damaged, a significant improvement in implantation rate was seen.[47]

Mechanism of Assisted Hatching

It has been also reported that the location of herniation of fresh, human hatched blastocysts can predict their implantation behavior.[48] Transferring of blastocysts that hatched close to the ICM showed significantly higher clinical pregnancy rates (72%) as compared to those that herniated from mural trophectoderm (51%). Applying AH at a specific site of the ZP may enhance vitrified blastocyst implantation.

The most important part of implantation is the implantation window which is the ideal receptive state of endometrium with complete synchronization between the embryo and the endometrium.[49] Early implantation has higher chances of viable pregnancy and delayed implantation has high incidence of abortion.[50] Embryos with artificial gap in ZP stimulate early hatching than zona intact embryos.[51] There is alteration in two-way transport of metabolites and growth factors across the ZP created by the artificial gap.[17,32] A study on mouse showed that embryo development and blastocyst formation is enhanced by artificial hatching as it opens the route for nutrients.[52]

Assisted Hatching Techniques

Mechanical methods were first used for AH.[53] Mechanical method of incising the zona followed this methodology.[51] The zona is also treated with acid medium and this method is known as chemical treatment for hatching.[54] Zona can be thinned by chemical method.[55] The hatching is also done by laser technique.[31] There is one more addition of piezo technology.[16]

For performing AH, technical expert is required who has extensive technical skill for making uniform, well controlled and standardized micro holes using mechanical and chemical methods with micropipettes mounted on micromanipulators. The embryo has to be at room temperature for as minimal time as possible to reduce pH and temperature variations or it can lead to detrimental effects on embryo development. The method of AH can be performed on day 2 or later on embryos as per the development.

Mechanical Techniques

Cohen et al. described partial zona dissection (PZD) which creates an artificial opening in the ZP of early cleaved embryos.[54] A microneedle is pushed tangentially through the space between the ZP and blastomeres for artificial piercing of ZP with pipette stabilizing the embryo. The parts of embryo trapped between the microneedle is recovered by gliding the microneedle with holding pipette. There is formation of a gap through which the portion is removed. PZD is quick mechanism to perform with holes of variable sizes.[56] A cross-shaped hole is made on the surface of the ZP with cuts in the ZP at right angle;[57] this advancement in the technique of PZD creates larger openings. ZP thickening is reduced by rubbing with a microneedle, as a result the risk of blastomere loss and invasion of microorganisms or immune cells is minimized with no gaps in the ZP. This technique was invented by Nijs et al.[58] but has the chances of multiple pregnancies.[59]

Expansion of zona pellucida-mechanical technique: Zone pellucida is expanded using hydrostatic pressure for embryo hatching. A study recently reported that the implantation rates increased in mechanically expanded ZP of frozen-thawed D3 embryos.[60] It is also reported that with same number of embryos transferred, AH had higher rates of implantation and clinical pregnancy rate. Henceforth ZP expansion using mechanical methods is both safe as well as effective to improve the outcome.[60]

Chemical Techniques

Cohen et al., did AH using acid Tyrode.[17] Microneedle is pierced through either empty perivitelline space or extracellular fragments (i.e. a blastomere-free area) of the ZP with embryo being secured with holding pipette. Preloaded Tyrode's acid in microneedle is inserted until the zona is breached. As soon as the breach is created, suction is applied to prevent entry of excess acid into ZP. Only trained expert with quick handling are required to prevent unnecessary exposure of the embryo to the acidic solution. As soon as the zona comes in contact with the acid, it starts to dissolve; thereafter the embryo is removed and washed to remove acid trace. The embryos are cleared from the acid.[5] The blastomeres near to the part drilled by acid may be affected.

Piezo Technology

The latest technique for ZP drilling using electric pulse[16] in which embryo is held by holding pipette and piezo-electric pulse will produce the vibratory movements. A conical area is carved in the ZP after 5–8 applications. It is regulated by a controller. It facilitates the complete hatching of blastocyst.

Laser-assisted Hatching

Tadir[61] and Palankar[62] first reported laser-assisted zona drilling in 1991. Laser beam is used in this technique which is directed using an optical lens or through an optical fiber. The contact approach was used with glass pipette delivering ultraviolet (UV) wavelength and quartz fiber delivering infrared (IR) wavelength.[63] Non-contact mode uses IR 1.48 μm (1,480 nm) diode laser[63,64] to thin the ZP without creating a hole and it significantly increased hatching in vitro. No ultrastructural degenerative alterations of the ZP of oocytes and embryos was seen following laser assisted zona drilling seen by both light electron microscopy (LEM) and scanning electron microscopy (SEM).[65] The type of AH performed by laser considered the best option as it has very high degree of accuracy and there is no side effect on the further development of the embryo. It is an easy, effective technique, time conserving, without any additional micromanipulations and performed in a sterile environment.[66-70]

CLINICAL APPLICATION OF ASSISTED HATCHING

Whether AH is actually beneficial or not is important to know. There are several studies reporting no increase in pregnancy rates with AH although there are groups of patients who have been benefitted from AH. In clinical practice these are the only indications for AH repeated IVF failure, thick zona, advanced age of patient and thawed embryo transfers. The various techniques used, patient selection and study designs made it difficult to compare between studies and pooled data.

Assisted Hatching in Recurrent In Vitro Fertilization Failure

In women with unexplained recurrent implantation failure, there is a significant increase in pregnancy and implantation rates by AH.[71] However, before unsuccessful in vitro fertilization (IVF) cycles it is important to identify patients who would benefit from AH.[72]

There has been a decline in IVF success rates with advancing maternal age.[73] Studies have shown that with increasing age, zona hardening occurs due to endocrinal changes and because of absence of lysins from surrounding tissues.[19,74] Therefore, AH has found to be beneficial in older women but still pregnancy rates are far lower than that seen in younger women.[75-77]

Frozen-thawed Embryos

Cryopreservation of embryos and the process of freeze-thaw induce the hardening of zona due to alteration in the glycoprotein matrix.[78] Check et al., found improvement in the rates of implantation and pregnancy by performing AH on embryos at stage of 6–8 cells.[79] and Tao and Tamis reported AH done on frozen-thawed two cell stage embryos was successful.[80]

Disadvantages of Assisted Hatching

Assisted hatching can lead to embryo blastocyst with reduction of embryo viability or even lethal embryos. It can also increase risk of monozygotic twinning.[81-85] The chances of contamination or infection increases due to hole in the ZP. ZP shields the embryos from any detrimental factors in the female reproductive tract such as toxins, microorganisms or immune cells. Blastomeres can get trapped in smaller holes of the ZP leading to incomplete hatching.[31] Larger holes can cause blastomeres to be lost as formation of tight junctions occurs later. This leads to monozygotic twins, embryonic death or even vesiculation.[54,81] In IVF patients the occurrence of monozygotic twins is more common,[86] found in eight (1.2%) of those in which AH was done as compared with none of the 559 embryos that were not hatched.[84] This higher incidence may result from—(1) a small narrow opening in the zona pellucida, may trap the hatching blastocyst and leads to formation of monozygotic twins[84] and (2) premature hatching of the blastomeres. After the 6-cell stage human blastomeres are joined with tight junctions.[87] There is increased risk of premature blastomere hatching due to larger opening in ZP suggesting that chemically AH needs to be used with caution.[88]

CONCLUSION

To prove the benefits and efficacy of AH several studies have been documented in different groups of patients using various methods. Patients with poor prognosis, including advanced age patients, patients with elevated concentrations of follicle stimulating hormone (FSH), patients with previous implantation failures, or patients with embryos with thick ZPs, constituted the majority in many of the studies, as a result contradictory results were obtained. One study included women with endometriosis not showing improvement after AH.[89] AH needs to be done in fresh, early cleavage stage embryos and vitrified warmed blastocysts.[90]

Assisted hatching significantly increase the implantation rates, pregnancy rates and ongoing pregnancy as per the study by Sallam et al., for patients with poor prognosis and with recurrent implantation failure.[72]

No evidence has been found for routine use of AH and its potential risks but some studies concluded that it can be performed in patients with a poor prognosis, including those with recurrent implantation failure, poor embryo quality and older women more than 38 years of age.

The variability of methodologies, study designs and groups of patients described in the published AH studies make it very difficult to come to a definitive conclusion on the possible effect of AH on clinical outcomes. Cochrane study concluded that a positive effect of AH on live birth rates was found.[91] On the other hand, a recent systematic review evaluating the effect of AH on ART outcomes concluded that AH was related to increased clinical pregnancy and multiple pregnancy rates in women with previous repeated failure or in frozen thawed embryo transfer.[92] Further, a retrospective study showed no increase in the risk of congenital abnormalities due to AH alone.[93]

The potential of AH in ART makes it imperative that more studies need to be undertaken to study the role. The various methods of AH needs to be applied at different development stages and sites of the embryo and in different subgroups of the population like women undergoing frozen embryos transfers elder age groups, repeated implantation failure, highly early proliferative phase serum FSH levels, and with embryos with thick or hardened ZPs or poor quality embryos. Studies need to be carried out in large scale to conclude the effect and affect of AH on implantation and pregnancy rates. Studies on whether different methods of AH yield similar or different outcomes and live birth rates are needed. Follow up of obstetric and post natal outcomes is mandatory.

REFERENCES

1. Edwards RG. Clinical approaches to increasing uterine receptivity during human implantation. Hum Reprod. 1995;10:60-6.
2. Huisman GJ, Fauser BC, Eijkemans MJ, et al. Implantation rates after in vitro fertilization and transfer of a maximum of two embryos that have undergone three to five days in culture. Fertil Steril. 2000;73:117-22.
3. Nehra A, Werner MA, Bastuba M, et al. Vibratory stimulation and rectal probe electroejaculation as therapy for patients with spinal cord injury: semen parameters and pregnancy rates. J Urol. 1996, 155:554-9.
4. Shah R. Ejaculatory and erectile dysfunctions in infertile men. In: Jansen R, Mortimer D (Eds). Towards Reproductive Certainty. New York: The Parthenon Publishing Group; 1999.
5. Tucker MJ, Luecke NM, Wiker SR, et al. Chemical removal of the outside of the zona pellucida of day 3 human embryos has no impact on implantation rate. J Assist Reprod Genet. 1993;10:187-91.
6. Antinori S, Panci C, Selman HA, et al. Zona thinning with the use of laser: a new approach to assisted hatching in humans. Hum Reprod. 1996;11:590-4.
7. Das S, Blake D, Farquhar C, et al. Assisted hatching on assisted conception (IVF and ICSI). Cochrane Database Syst Rev. 2009;(2):CD001894.

8. Practice Committee of Society for Assisted Reproductive Technology, Practice Committee of American Society for Reproductive Medicine. The role of assisted hatching in in vitro fertilization: a review of the literature. A Committee opinion. Fertil Steril. 2008;S196-8.
9. Margalioth EJ, Ben-Chetrit A, Gal M, et al. Investigation and treatment of repeated implantation failure following IVF-ET. Hum Reprod. 2006;21:3036-43.
10. Primi MP, Senn A, Montag M, et al. European multicentre prospective randomized study to assess the use of assisted hatching with a diode laser and the benefit of an immunosuppressive/antibiotic treatment in different patient populations. Hum Reprod. 2004;19:2325-33.
11. Valojerdi MR, Eftekhari-Yazdi P, Karimian L, et al. Effect of laser zona pellucida opening on clinical outcome of assisted reproduction technology in patients with advanced female age, recurrent implantation failure, or frozen-thawed embryos. Fertil Steril. 2008;90:84-91.
12. Cohen J, Malter H, Fehilly C, et al. Implantation of embryos after partial opening of oocyte zona pellucida to facilitate sperm penetration. Lancet. 1988;II:162.
13. Mansour RT, Rhodes CA, Aboulghar MA, et al. Transfer of zona-free embryos improves outcome in poor prognosis patients: a prospective randomized controlled study. Hum Reprod. 2000;15:1061-4.
14. Antinori S, Selman HA, Caffa B, et al. Zona opening of human embryos using a non-contact UV laser for assisted hatching in patients with poor prognosis of pregnancy. Hum Reprod. 1996;11:2488-92.
15. Magli MC, Gianaroli L, Ferraretti AP, et al. Rescue of implantation potential in embryos with poor prognosis by assisted zona hatching. Hum Reprod. 1998;13:1331-5.
16. Nakayama T, Fujiwara H, Yamada S, et al. Clinical application of a new assisted hatching method using a piezo-micromanipulator for morphologically low-quality embryos in poor-prognosis infertile patients. Fertil Steril. 1999;71:1014-8.
17. Cohen J, Alikani M, Trowbridge J, et al. Implantation enhancement by selective assisted hatching using zona drilling of human embryos with poor prognosis. Hum Reprod. 1992;7:685-91.
18. Demirel LC, Evirgen O, Al-Hasani S. The role of assisted hatching in human IVF. Middle East Fert Soc J. 2002;7:6-12.
19. Tucker MJ, Morton PC, Wright G, et al. Enhancement of outcome from intracytoplasmic sperm injection: does co culture or assisted hatching improve implantation rates? Hum Reprod. 1996;11:2434-7.
20. Chao KH, Chen SU, Chen HF, et al. Assisted hatching increases the implantation and pregnancy rate of in vitro fertilization (IVF)-embryo transfer (ET), but not that of IVF-tubal ET in patients with repeated IVF failures. Fertil Steril. 1997;67:904-8.
21. Frydman N, Madoux S, Hesters L, et al. A randomized double-blind controlled study on the efficacy of laser zona pellucida thinning on live birth in cases of advanced female age. Hum Reprod. 2006;21:2131-5.
22. Hurst BS, Tucker KE, Awoniyi CA, et al. Assisted hatching does not enhance IVF success in good-prognosis patients. J Assist Reprod Genet. 1998;15:62-4
23. Lanzendorf SE, Nehchiri F, Mayer JF, et al. A prospective, randomized, double-blind study for the evaluation of assisted hatching in patients with advanced maternal age. Hum Reprod. 1998;13:409-13.
24. Bleil JD, Wassarman PN. Structure and function of the zona pellucida: identification and characterization of the proteins of the mouse oocytes zona pellucida. Dev Biol. 1980;76:185-202.
25. Duin M, Polman JE, DeBreet IT, et al. Recombinant human zona pellucida protein zona pellucida3 produced by Chinese hamster ovary cells induces the human sperm acrosome reaction and promotes sperm-egg fusion. Biol Reprod. 1994;5:607-17.
26. Modliniski JA. The role of the zona pellucida in the development of mouse eggs in vivo. J Embryol Exp Morphol. 1970;23:539-51.
27. Trounson AO, Moore NW. The survival and development of sheep eggs following complete or partial removal of the zona pellucida. J Reprod Fertil. 1974;41:97-108.
28. Gordon JW, Dapunt U. A new mouse model for embryos with a hatching deficiency and its use to elucidate the mechanism of blastocyst hatching. Fertil Steril. 1993;59:1296-301.
29. Schiew MC, Araujo E, Asch RH, et al. Enzymatic characterization of zona pellucida hardening in human eggs and embryos. J Assist Reprod Genet. 1995;12:2-7.
30. Letterie GS. Assisted hatching: relative techniques and clinical outcomes. Assist Reprod Rev. 1997;8:116-25.
31. Cohen J. Assisted hatching of human embryos. J In Vitro Fertil Embryo Transf. 1991;8:179-90.
32. Cole RJ. Cinematographic observation on the blastocyst and zona pellucida of the mouse blastocyst. J Embryol Exp Morphol. 1967;17:481-90.
33. Veeck LL, Zaninovic N. Blastocyst hatching. In: Veeck LL, Zaninovic N (Eds). An atlas of human blastocysts. London: Informa Healthcare; 2003. pp. 159-71.
34. Gonzales DS, Jones JM, Pinyopummintr T, et al. Trophectoderm projections: a potential means for locomotion, attachment and implantation of bovine, equine and human blastocysts. Hum Reprod. 1996;11:2739-45.
35. Miyata H, Matsubayashi H, Fukutomi N, et al. Relevance of the site of assisted hatching in thawed human blastocysts: a preliminary report. Fertil Steril. 2010;94:2444-7.
36. Gordon J, Dapunt U. A new mouse model for embryos with a hatching deficiency and its use to elucidate the mechanism of blastocyst. Hum Reprod. 1996;11:2739-45.
37. Montag M, Koll B, Holmes P, et al. Significance of the number of embryonic cells and the state of the zona pellucida for hatching of mouse blastocysts in vitro versus in vivo. Biol Reprod. 2000;62:1738-44.
38. Morey AF, Deshon GE Jr, Rosanski TA et al: Technique of biopsy gun testis needle biopsy. Urology. 1993;42:325-26.
39. Friedler S, Raziel A, Strassburger D, et al: Testicular sperm retrieval by percutaneous fine needle aspiration compared

with testicular sperm extraction by open biopsy in men with non obstructive azoospermia. Hum Reprod. 1997;12: 1488-93.
40. Cohen J, Alikani M, Malter HE, et al. Partial zona dissection or subzonal sperm insemination: microsurgical fertilization alternatives based on evaluation of sperm and embryo morphology. Fertil Steril. 1991;56:696-706.
41. Cohen J, Inge KL, Suzman M, et al. Video cinematography of fresh and cryopreserved embryos: a retrospective analysis of embryonic morphology and implantation. Fertil Steril. 1989;51:820-7.
42. Wright G, Wiker S, Elsner C, et al. Observations on the morphology of human zygotes, pronuclei and nucleoli and implications for cryopreservation. Hum Reprod. 1990;5: 109-15.
43. Chan PJ. Developmental potential of human oocytes according to zona pellucida thickness. J In Vitro Fertil Embryo Transf. 1987;4:237-41.
44. Edwards R, Mettler LE, Walters DW. Identical twins and in vitro fertilisation. J In Vitro Fertil Embryo Transf. 1986;3:114-7.
45. Schiewe MC, Hazeleger NL, Sclinenti C, et al. Physical characterization of blastocyst hatching mechanisms by use of a mouse anti-hatching mode. Fertil Steril. 1995;63:288-94.
46. Alikani M, Olivienes F, Cohen J. Microsurgical correction of partially degenerate mouse embryos promotes hatching and restores their viability. Hum Reprod. 1993;8:1723-8.
47. Rienzi L, Nagy ZP, Ubaldi F, et al. Laser assisted removal of necrotic blastomeres from cryopreserved embryos that were partially damaged. Fertil Steril. 2002;77:1196-201.
48. Ebner T, Gruber I, Moser M. Location of herniation predicts implantation behavior of hatching blastocysts. J Turkish German Gynecol Assoc. 2007;8:184-8.
49. Liu HC, Cohen J, Alikani M, et al. Assisted hatching facilitates earlier implantations. Fertil Steril. 1993;60:871-5.
50. Liu HC, Rosenwaks Z. Early pregnancy wastage in in-vitro fertilization patients. J In Vitro Fertil Embryo Transf. 1990;8:65-72.
51. Malter HE, Cohen J. Blastocyst formation and hatching in vitro following zona drilling of mouse and human embryos. Gamete Res. 1989;24:67-80.
52. Hershlag A, Feng HL. The effect of pre-freeze assisted hatching on post-thaw survival of mouse embryos. Fertil Steril. 2005;84:1752-4.
53. Cohen JH, Mather H, Wright G, et al. Partial zona dissection of human oocytes when failure of zona pellucida penetration is anticipated. Hum Reprod. 1989;4:435-42.
54. Cohen J, Elsner C, Kort H, et al. Impairment of hatching process following IVF in the human and improvement of implantation by assisted hatching using micromanipulation. Hum Reprod. 1990;5:7-13.
55. Khalifa EAM, Tucker MJ, Hunt P. Cruciate thinning of the zona pellucida for more successful enhancement of blastocyst hatching in the mouse. Hum Reprod. 1992;7:532-6.
56. Cohen J, Feldberg D. Effects of the size and number of zona pellucida openings on hatching and trophoblast outgrowth in the mouse embryo. Mol Reprod Dev. 1991;30:70-8.
57. Cieslak J, Ivatchnenko V, Wolf G, et al. Three dimensional partial zona pellucida dissections for preimplantation genetic diagnosis and assisted hatching. Fertil Steril. 1999;71:308-13.
58. Nijs M, Vanderzwalman P, Bertin G, et al. Pregnancies obtained after zona softening of in vitro cultured or frozen-thawed human embryos. Hum Reprod. 1992;7:82.
59. Nijs M, Vanderzwalmen P, Segal-Bertina G, et al. A monozygotic twin pregnancy after application of zona rubbing on a frozen-thawed blastocyst. Hum Reprod. 1993;8:127-9.
60. Fang C, Li T, Miao BY, et al. Mechanically expanding the zona pellucida of human frozen thawed embryos: a new method of assisted hatching. Fertil Steril. 2010;94:1302-7.
61. Tadir Y. Ten years of laser-assisted gametes and embryo manipulation. Wyss P, Tadir Y, Tromberg BJ, Haller U (Eds). Photomedicine in Gynecology and Reproduction. Basel: Karger. 2000. pp. 326-39.
62. Palankar D, Ohad S, Lewis A, et al. Technique for cellular microsurgery using the 193 nm excimer laser. Laser Surg Med. 1991;11:580-6.
63. Rink K, Delacretaz G, Salathe RP, et al. Non-contact microdrilling of Mouse zona pellucida with an objective-delivered 1.48um Diode laser. Laser Surg Med. 1996;18:52-62.
64. Blake DA, Forsberg AS, Johansson BR, et al. Laser zona pellucida thinning—alternative approach to assisted hatching. Hum Reprod. 2001;16:1959-64.
65. Obruca A, Strohmer H, Blaschitz A, et al. Ultrastructural observations in human oocytes and preimplantation embryos after zona opening using an erbium:yttrium–aluminium Garnet Er: (YAG) laser. Hum Reprod. 1997;12:2242-5.
66. Hseih YY, Huang CC, Cheng TC, et al. Laser assisted hatching of embryos is better than the chemical method for enhancing the pregnancy rate in women with advanced age. Fertil Steril. 2002;78:179-82.
67. Makrakis E, Angeli I, Agapintou K, et al. Laser verus mechanical assisted hatching: a prospective study of clinical outcomes. Fertil Steril. 2006;86:1596-600.
68. Lanzendorf SE, Ratts VS, Moley KH, et al. A randomized, prospective study comparing laser-assisted hatching and assisted hatching using acidified medium. Fertil Steril. 2007;87:1450-7.
69. Sagoskin AW, Levy MJ, Tucker MJ, et al. Laser assisted hatching in good pronosis patients undergoing in vitro fertilization embryo transfer: a randomized controlled trial. Fertil Steril. 2007;87:283-7.
70. Huai L, Avner H, Gerald M, et al. A retroprospective study comparing three different assisted hatching techniques. Fertil Steril. 2009;91:1323-5.
71. Hellebaut S, DeSutter P, Dozortseu D, et al. Does assisted hatching improve implantation rates after in vitro fertilisation or intracytoplasmic sperm injection in all patients? A prospective randomised study. J Assist Reprod Genet. 1996;13:19-22.
72. Sallam HN, Sadek S, Agameya A. Assisted hatching—a meta-analysis of randomized controlled trials. J Assist Reprod Genet. 2003;20:332-42.

73. Lass A, Coucher C, Duffy S. 1000 initiated cycles of in-vitro fertilisation in women of 40 years old or more. Fertil Steril. 1998;70:1030-4.
74. Dokras A, Sargent IL, Ross C, et al. The human blastocyst: morphology and human chorionic gonadotrophin secretion in vitro. Hum Reprod. 1991;6:1143-51.
75. Schoolcraft WB, Schlenker T, Jones GS, et al. In vitro fertilisation in women aged 40 and older. The impact of assisted hatching. J Assist Reprod Genet. 1995;12: 581-3.
76. Bieder D, Liushits A, Yonish M, et al. Assisted hatching by zona drilling of human embryos in women of advanced age. Hum Reprod. 1997;12:317-20.
77. Edirisinghe WR, Ahnonkitpanit V, Promviengchai S, et al. A study failing to determine significant benefits from assisted hatching: patients selected for advanced age, zona thickness of embryos, and previous failed attempts. J Assist Reprod Genet. 1999;16:294-301.
78. Carroll J, Depypene H, Mathews CD. Freeze–thaw induced changes of the zona pellucida explains decreased rates of fertilisation in frozen–thawed mouse oocytes. J Reprod Fertil. 1990;90:547-53.
79. Check JH, Hoover L, Nazari A, et al. The effect of assisted hatching on pregnancy rates after frozen embryo transfer. Fertil Steril. 1996;65:254-7.
80. Tao J, Tamis R. Application of assisted hatching for 2-day-old, frozen-thawed embryo transfer in a poor-prognosis population. J Assist Reprod Genet. 1997;14:128-30.
81. Nagy ZP, Rienzi L, Iacobelli F, et al. Laser-assisted hatching and removal of degenerated blastomeres of frozen – thawed embryos improves pregnancy rates. Fertil Steril. 1999; S4.
82. Stein A, Rufas O, Amit S, et al. Assisted hatching by partial zona dissection of human pre-embryo in patients with recurrent implantation failure after in vitro fertilisation. Fertil Steril. 1995;63:838-41.
83. Montag M, Ven H. Laser-assisted hatching in assisted reproduction. Croat Med J. 1999;40:398-403.
84. Hershlag A, Paine T, Cooper GW, et al. Monozygotic twinning associated with mechanical assisted hatching. Fertil Steril. 1999;71:144-6.
85. Schieve LA, Meikle SF, Peterson HB, et al. Does assisted hatching pose a risk for monozygotic twinning in pregnancies conceived through in vitro fertilization? Fertil Steril. 2000;74:288-94.
86. Alikani M, Noyes N, Cohen J, et al. Monozygotic twinning in the human is associated with the zona pellucida architecture. Hum Reprod. 1994;9:1318-21.
87. Dale B, Gualtieri R, Talevi R, et al. Intercellular communication in the early human embryo. Mol Reprod Dev. 1991;29:22-8.
88. Tzong S, Su-Ru C, Heng-Kien A, et al. Herniated blastomere following chemically assisted hatching may result in monozygotic twins. Fertil Sterilt. 2001;75:442-4.
89. Nadir H, Bener F, Karagenc L, et al. Impact of assisted hatching on ART outcome in women with endometriosis. Hum Reprod. 2005;20:2546-9.
90. Rienzi L, Ubaldi F, Iacobelli M et al. Developmental potential of fully intact and partially damaged cryopreserved embryos after laser-assisted removal of necrotic blastomeres and post thaw culture selection. Fertil Steril. 2005;84:888-94.
91. Carney SK, Das S, Blake D, et al. Assisted hatching on assisted conception (in vitro fertilisation (IVF) and intracytoplasmic sperm injection (ICSI). Cochrane Database Syst Rev 2012;12:CD001894.
92. Martins WP, Rocha IA, Ferriani RA, et al. Assisted hatching of human embryos: A systematic review and meta analysis of randomized controlled trails. Hum Reprod Update. 2011;17:438-53.
93. Jwa J, Jwa SC, Kuwahara A, et al. Risk of major congential anomalies after assisted hatching. Analysis of three year data from the national assisted reproduction registry in Japan. Fertil Steril. 2015;104:71-8.

Day 3 versus Day 5 Embryo Transfer

48

Biswanath Ghosh Dastidar, Sudarsan Ghosh Dastidar, Geetha Haripriya

INTRODUCTION

Remarkable advancements have taken place in the field of IVF since the birth of Louise Joy Brown, the first IVF baby, in 1978. However, implantation rates remain low across the globe even today. Thus, intense research is being carried out globally to refine techniques and strategies for embryo culture, embryo assessment and embryo transfer, in order to improve IVF results for patients. Most IVF centers transfer fertilized embryos back into the uterus either at the day 3 following fertilization; or on day 5 or day 6 at the blastocyst stage. Both strategies are accompanied by their own set of advantages and disadvantages. Blastocyst transfers are associated with generally better implantation and pregnancy rates and make it more feasible to opt for single embryo transfer, thereby lowering multiple pregnancy rates. However, blastocyst culture is technically more challenging, expensive and associated with the risk of epigenetic modifications during in vitro culture. The field remains divided over which is the ideal embryo transfer strategy.

EARLY DEVELOPMENT AND IMPLANTATION OF THE HUMAN EMBRYO

The human embryo is formed when a diploid secondary oocyte with 46 chromosomes is fertilized by a haploid sperm cell, with 23 chromosomes, to result in a diploid zygote with the full complement of 46 chromosomes (after reduction division-extrusion of the second polar body). The first in vitro evidence of fertilization is the appearance of two pronuclei side by side within the oocyte, known as 2PN stage, usually seen after around 24 hours following fertilization. The diploid single cell embryo then undergoes a series of cleavage divisions to sequentially result in a 4 cell embryo on day 2 following fertilization, 8 cell embryo on day 3, a ball of cells called morula on day 4 and a specialized cavity containing structure called a blastocyst on day 5 after fertilization.

Fertilization takes place in the ampulla of the fallopian tube. Thereafter, the fertilized oocyte travels towards the endometrial cavity through the fallopian tube to reach it on day 4 following fertilization, at the morula stage. The morula further differentiates into a cavity containing structure called a blastocyst, lined by trophoectodermal (TE) cells which eventually contribute to placentation and an inner cell mass (ICM) which forms the true embryo and subsequently, fetus.

The blastocyst implants into the maternal endometrium between day 6 to day 9 following fertilization. This is achieved through a sequential series of steps which include orientation to the endometrium (ICM faces the endometrium), apposition and attachment to the endometrial epithelium (EE), adhesion and trophoblastic invasion into the decidua. This is a hormone regulated process facilitated by several molecular factors expressed both by the embryo and the endometrium which together establish an embryo-endometrial "cross talk" during the "implantation window"—the period of maximum endometrial receptivity.

INITIAL PHASE IN HUMAN IVF: EVALUATION AND TRANSFER OF DAY 3 CLEAVAGE STAGE EMBRYOS

Traditionally, since the beginning of human IVF, embryos were cultured in the laboratory for 2–3 days following

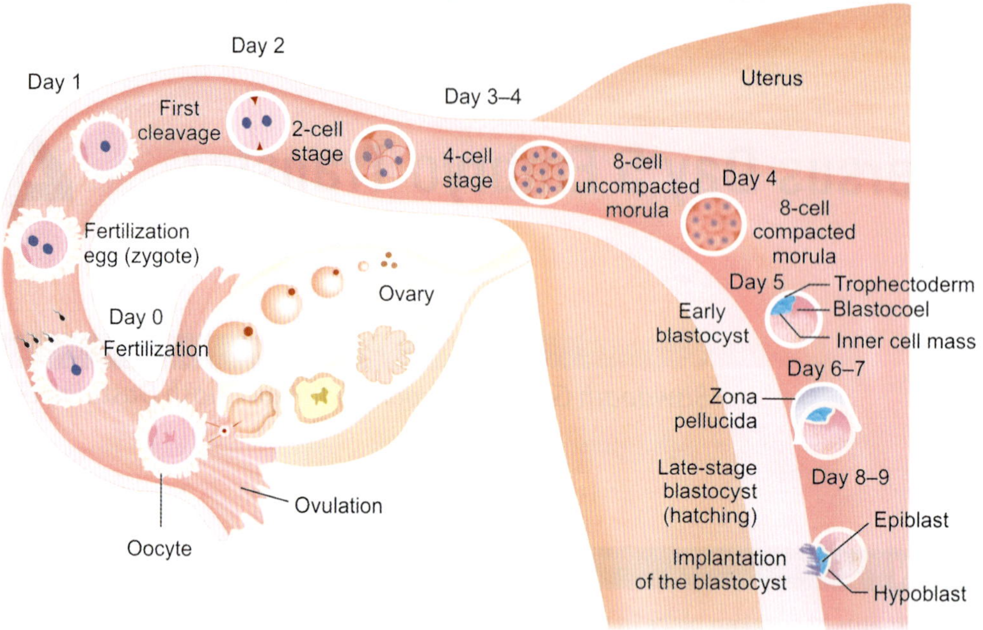

Fig. 1: Different stages of development of the embryo as it travel through the fallopian tube toward the endometrial cavity.

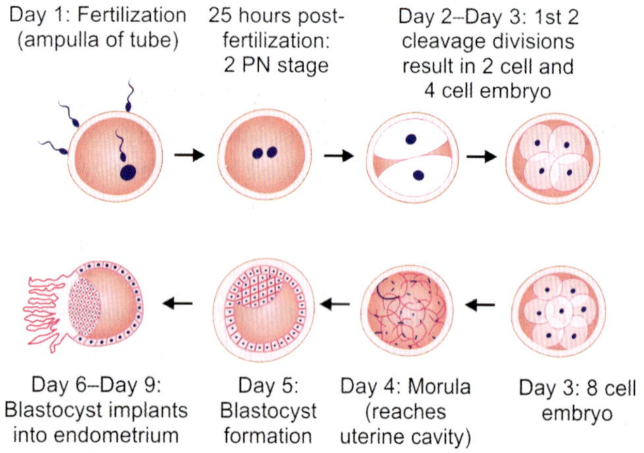

Fig. 2

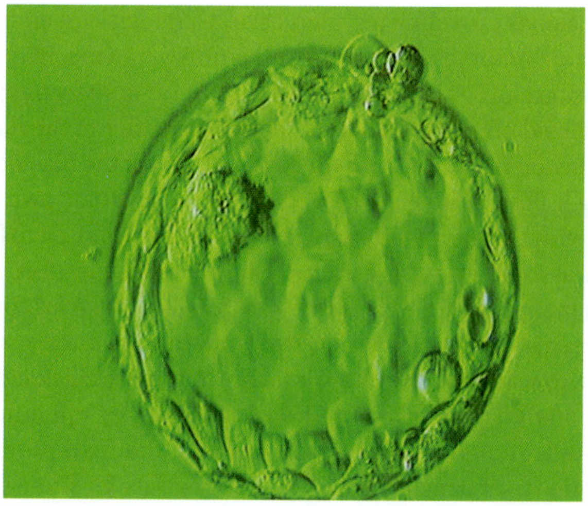

Fig. 3: Day 3 cleavage stage embryo showing 8 clear, uniform blastomeres at 2 visual planes, minimal fragmentation, and clear zona pellucida.

Source: Image used with permission from Ghosh Dastidar Institute for Fertility Research Pvt. Ltd.

fertilization and transferred into the patient's uterus on day 2 or 3. Day 2/day 3 transfers were considered advantageous because of many reasons. Embryos at the 4 cell and 8 cell stages on days 2 and 3 presented distinct morphological features which were convenient for visual evaluation in order to select the best quality embryos for transfer, compared to morula on day 4, which were difficult to separate from each other in terms of quality.[1] Moreover, it was technologically challenging and expensive to culture embryos successfully in vitro beyond 3 days when embryonic genome activation (EGA) takes place to result in maternal to embryonic transition (MET).[2] Furthermore, culture media sophisticated enough to support the more complex demands of blastocyst was yet to be developed.

Embryo selection on day 3 is routinely done based on morphological parameters which are thought to be highly indicative of pregnancy outcome.[3] Number of blastomeres, uniformity of size and compaction of blastomeres within the embryo, and degree of blastomeres fragmentation has been used as grading parameters for embryo selection. One of the most important parameters for day 3 embryo grading is the degree of fragmentation of blastomeres, and embryos may be classified into 4 grades based on percentage of fragmentation. As the grade increases, the quality of the embryo decreases.[4] Based on these parameters, embryos are assigned different grades and the best ones are selected for transfer back into the endometrial cavity.

ADVANTAGES OF DAY 3 ET

Adopting cleavage stage ET policy is likely to result in greater number of embryos being available for transfer on day 3 following IVF, and lesser incidence of cycle cancellation due to no embryos being available. In-vitro culture of embryos up to day 3 following fertilization is also technically simpler and more affordable. Moreover, replacing embryos back into the uterus after 3 days limits their exposure to an in-vitro environment, and thus reduces the odds of structural and epigenetic damage. One school of thought asserts that replacing embryos back into their natural in-vivo environment as quickly as possible gives them the best possible chance to result in a successful pregnancy because ultimately, the uterus is the best incubator available and no amount of technological advancement can match the ideal conditions for survival and growth which the maternal womb can offers. Such an ET strategy appears to be of particular merit when the couple is desperate for a pregnancy, when fewer oocytes/embryos are available, in centers where preimplantation genetic screening and diagnosis (PGS and PGD) are not available, or the couple in question is unsure of opting for extended culture and PGD/PGS due to financial constraints.

RECENT TRENDS: SHIFT TOWARDS DAY 5 BLASTOCYST TRANSFERS

However, with the recent development of more advanced blastocyst culture media capable of supporting the embryos in vitro beyond 3 days, as well as development of sequential media, it has become feasible to culture embryos up to blastocyst stage.[5] Growth up to blastocyst stage is in itself an indicator of the most developmentally competent embryos and thus a marker of embryo quality.[6] It is thought that only the most developmentally competent or viable embryos would survive the extended culture up to 5 or 6 days in vitro. Thus, in a blastocyst culture program, embryos which do survive the extended culture in order

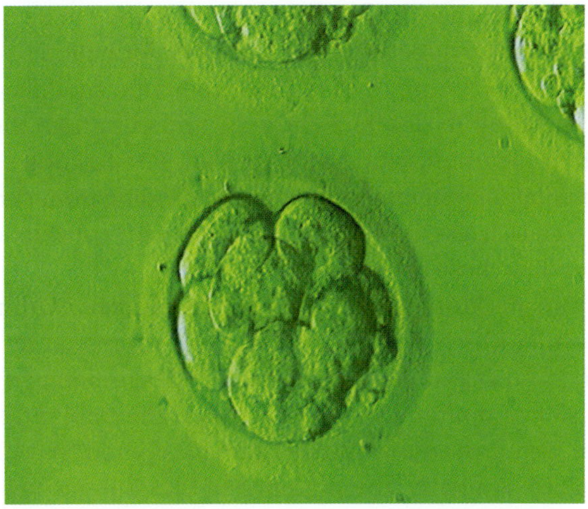

Fig. 4: Expanded blastocyst on day 5 following fertilization showing blastocoel cavities, uniform layer of trophoectoderm (TE) with many cells, and distinct inner cell mass (ICM).
Source: Image used with permission from Ghosh Dastidar Institute for Fertility Research Pvt. Ltd.

to develop to blastocyst are thought to be the best quality embryos. This process of "self-selection" means that any of these blastocysts are much more likely to implant into the maternal endometrium compared to day 3 embryos. Advent of sophisticated technology such as PGS has provided a potent tool for genetic screening of this blastocyst to determine the best quality embryos for transfer.[7] Thus, there has been recent advocacy to shift towards blastocyst transfers on day 5 or 6 following fertilization.

The development of time-lapse monitoring of embryos has recently opened up an array of predictive parameters for both embryo selection and rejection. Over the past few years, technological advancements have allowed the combination of embryo morphology assessment with kinetics, now named morphokinetics. This form of continuous surveillance of embryos in culture has opened up a new way of evaluating and selecting embryos for transfer. In addition, the fact that the embryos are left undisturbed during annotation has favored the growth of embryos to the blastocyst stage.

Currently, there are many automated time-lapse imaging systems available for embryo culture. Some include: The EmbryoScope^{TM,} Miri^{R}, Geri^{TM}, ProVision^{TM} and the Eeva^{TM} systems.[8] Published data have indicated that this new technology can pinpoint early predictors of embryos implantation. These are known as kinetic expressions and included: absolute cleavage timings, time intervals and time ratios. They are used as predictors of blastocyst formation. This new technology may alleviate the need for growing embryos past day three if kinetic expressions can be used as early as day three to predict blastocyst formation.

It is interesting to note that prediction models can also be used to deselect embryos and eliminate those with reduced implantation potential. For example, the implantation potential of an embryo dividing from two to three cells in less than 5 hours is considered [9] considerably lower than those with a normal pattern.

Morphokinetics can also provide image evidence of factors which are only momentarily expressed by the embryo such as multinucleation. In cycles resulting in the transfer of multinucleated embryos, [10] the implantation rates have been shown to be dramatically reduced (23.3 vs. 43.6). Similarly, the presence of blastomeres fusion, formerly known as reverse cleavage, has been shown to significantly compromise embryo development and thus reduce implantation potential.[11]

Recent publications have highlighted the high degree of imprecision of conventional morphological assessment methods in selecting euploid embryos.[12] In their study, 44.9% of aneuploidy was seen in blastocysts scored with a good prognosis of implantation potential. Thus, growing blastocysts and coupling it with preimplantation genetic diagnosis has the advantage of further selecting euploid embryos. In this scenario, a day 5 embryo transfer has a distinct advantage over a day 3 transfer.

In conclusion, morphokinetics is revolutionizing clinical embryology. It is envisioned that most IVF units will have this technology in use by the year, 2020. The advent of such technology favors the day 5 (blastocyst) transfers as it: alleviates the need to remove embryos out of the culture system, provides helpful kinetic markers which can predict blastocyst development/implantation and provided video proof of poor scenario markers such as multinucleation. In addition, this technology coupled with preimplantation genetic diagnosis at the blastocyst stage can further pinpoint aneuploidy embryos prior to embryo transfer. Time-lapse imaging of embryos thus leans towards the growth of embryos to the blastocyst stage (day 5).

THE CASE FOR BLASTOCYST CULTURE AND TRANSFER ON DAY 5

Two primary arguments support the culture of embryos to the blastocyst stage and transfer on day 5 or 6. The first is the issue of optimal timing for replacing embryos. Debate over the ideal timing for ET arose upon examining the differences between IVF and the natural in vivo reproductive process. There has been consensus that it is physiologically premature to expose cleavage stage embryos to the uterine environment. This is especially true following super ovulation and the resultant supraphysiological levels of estrogen to which the endometrium is subjected.[13] In the normal reproductive process, embryos traverse the fallopian tubes and only reach the uterus at the morula (16 cell compacted) stage,[14] corresponding to day 4 of in vitro culture. The uterine cavity provides a different nutritional environment from the fallopian tube; thus it is thought that this may result in stress to cleavage stage embryos leading to reduced implantation potential.[15] There is also gathering evidence of significantly reduced uterine pulsatility around day 5 and 6 when blastocysts are transferred, which may be beneficial for successful implantation.[16]

The other argument favoring blastocyst culture relates to their innately higher implantation potential in comparison to cleavage stage embryos. As a consequence of self-selection, it is believed that only the most developmentally competent embryos grow to blastocysts. Moreover, morphological criteria used to select embryos on day 2 to 3 are limited and correlation with pregnancy outcome is debatable.[17-22] Following the advent of PGD and PGS, it has come to light that a large proportion of morphologically normal day 3 embryos have chromosomal anomalies, thus explaining the 80% to 90% rates of implantation failure observed in cleavage stage ET.[23]

Although the transfer of day 5 blastocysts cannot guarantee the absence of any chromosomal abnormality,[24] Staessenand co-workers have shown that, at least in patients older than 36 years, the incidence of chromosomal anomalies can be reduced from 59% in cleavage stage embryos to 35% in day 5 blastocysts.[25]

BLASTOCYST CULTURE: ADVANCES IN DEVELOPMENT OF CULTURE MEDIA

Thus, the past few decades have witnessed a shift in approach to transfer embryos on day 5 or 6 at the blastocyst stage. This has been aided by the introduction of different preparations of sequential culture media in the late 1990s which were designed to support the embryo's changing nutritional requirements for extended culture to day 5 or day 6. Thus, there was rapidly growing interest in blastocyst culture with more and more academic IVF centers starting their own blastocyst transfer programs, resulting in a growing body of literature examining the merits and drawbacks of extended culture.

It should be borne in mind; however, that blastocyst culture is not novel. Indeed, the first reported IVF pregnancy was from a transferred blastocyst.[26] Yet, day 3 transfer was adopted as standard global practice in the early days of IVF for two reasons: the low rate of embryos successfully cultured past this stage; and the growing evidence that human embryos have a striking innate competency to survive when transferred prematurely into the uterus.[27]

However, as understanding of the metabolic requirements of the embryo advanced, so did the variety and availability of more advanced culture media[28] and co-culture techniques.[29-31] The most important development was the arrival of evidence that the in vitro environment best suited for blastocyst growth is different from that for a cleavage stage embryo. This discovery led to the evolution of stage-specific or sequential media (G1/G2) by Gardner in 1998.[32] In sequential culture, embryos are transferred on day 3 from a medium containing low concentrations of glucose and only one or a few amino acids to a more sophisticated medium with higher concentrations of glucose and a larger range of amino acids.[15] Cell compaction and genomic activation starts after day 3 so that the embryo is no longer being regulated by maternal RNA and transcripts.[33] Blastocyst development and implantation up to 60% to 65% have been reported employing these culture strategies.[34]

ELECTIVE SINGLE EMBRYO TRANSFER (ESET) AND MULTIPLE PREGNANCY REDUCTION

Changing regulatory environments globally have also led to rising popularity of blastocyst transfer. Initially, it was widely accepted that multiple embryo transfers offered a significant advantage in the pursuit of achieving high pregnancy rates.[35] However, public as well as expert opinion to reduce multiple pregnancies and higher order multiple births (triplets or more) have led to legislation in various countries to restrict the number of embryos replaced into the uterus. Elective single embryo transfers (eSET) for selected patients are now considered standard practice in many centers globally.[36] Thus, in view of restrictions regarding the number of embryos which may be transferred back into the uterus, it has become even more important to select the single most competent embryo for transfer. This had led to intensive research efforts to improve embryo assessment to select the best embryo. Blastocyst culture may be one such mechanism.[37,38] Advocates of blastocyst culture assert that only the most developmentally competent embryos will survive the extended culture to day 5 or 6. These would in turn have a higher probability of implantation and thus fewer embryos need to be transferred to achieve acceptable pregnancy rates, at the same time lowering multiple-birth rates.[39-41] Reports have shown that single blastocyst transfers can achieve pregnancy rates comparable to those achieved by transferring 2 day 3 cleavage stage embryos, while reducing the incidence of multiple births.[42]

DRAWBACKS WITH BLASTOCYST CULTURE AND TRANSFER STRATEGY

However, blastocyst culture is a more expensive procedure and technologically more challenging. Only a subset of day 3 embryos will go on to grow to blastocysts and so fewer embryos will be available for transfer on day 5 than on day 3. In many cases, none of a patient's embryos might survive the in vitro culture process up to day 5, resulting in there being no embryos available for transfer. Thus, day 5 embryo transfer strategy is associated with greater cycle cancellation rates due to unavailability of embryos for transfer when culturing to the blastocyst stage as only a percentage of day 3 embryos will successfully grow to blastocyst stage.[43]

This problem, however, may be circumvented by having clear cut practice policies laid out to determine minimum criteria for recruiting a patient into the blastocyst transfer group (in terms of minimum number of follicles, fertilized oocytes, 8-cell embryos on day 3 available) and group allocation late into the cycle only once these are met.[41]

Indeed, arguments against blastocyst culture and transfer are mainly related to this process of self-selection which puts couples undergoing blastocyst culture at risk of cycle cancellation due to failed embryo development[44] and of having fewer embryos cryopreserved.[45] Moreover, studies have shown that day 3 embryo transfers can be as effective as blastocyst transfers in terms of cycle results.[46]

Also, extended in vitro culture in the laboratory comes with its own set of disadvantages, the most important of which are the risk of inducing epigenetic modifications to the embryos due to culture in an artificial environment for a prolonged duration of time.[47] Furthermore, decision to culture to blastocyst stage necessitates initial availability of a large number of embryos, which necessitates strong ovarian stimulation initially, thus exposing the patient to greater adverse effects of hormonal hyperstimulation.[48]

Other adverse outcomes associated with blastocyst culture include monozygotic twinning and altered sex ratio favoring the male sex.[29] Monozygotic twinning is usually reported at around 1% in ART cycles,[49] whereas the rate of monozygotic twins in spontaneous conceptions is around 1 in 330. The phenomenon is associated with miscarriage, congenital anomalies, growth retardation and twin to twin transfusion syndrome (TTTS). Extended culture of embryos has been implicated to be one of the interventions responsible for an increase in the incidence of monozygotic twinning,[50-52] although there have also been reports showing that blastocyst transfers are not associated with increased rate of twinning when compared to day 3 transfers.[53] However, a recent report suggests that improved cell culture methods can result in a significant reduction in its incidence.[54] Similarly, identifying the underlying causative factors leading to such twinning, whether related to culture media constituents or embryo selection parameters, may rectify this imbalance.[55]

Thus, there has been recent advocacy to reconsider day 2 or day 3 transfers, based on the rationale that it may be best to return the embryo to their natural habitat, i.e. the mother's womb early, which may provide the best environment for their growth and support. As such, there is yet to be any consensus regarding which is the best embryo transfer policy and the verdict is still not in.

DAY 3 CLEAVAGE STAGE TRANSFERS VERSUS DAY 5 BLASTOCYST TRANSFERS

Conflicting results surface upon examining whether day 5 or day 6 blastocyst transfers offer significant advantages over day 2 or day 3 cleavage stage embryo transfers in IVF cycles. A Cochrane review done in 2016 by Glujovsky *et al* identified a total of 27 randomized controlled trials in the literature comparing cleavage stage versus blastocyst transfers which met their criteria for inclusion in the meta-analysis.

The meta-analysis concluded that although live birth rate and clinical pregnancy rates were higher in the blastocyst group, cumulative pregnancy rate with both fresh as well as frozen-thawed embryo transfers were higher in the day 3 cleavage stage embryo transfer group. Moreover, significantly larger number of embryos was available for freezing in the cleavage stage embryo transfer group, when compared to the blastocyst group. Furthermore, there was an increased likelihood of there being no embryos available for transfer when embryos were allocated for extended culture to day 5 and blastocyst transfer.[56] However, in good prognosis couples (who had a high number of good quality embryos), the likelihood of there being no embryos left for transfer was similar between two groups.

We conducted a study at Dr. DY Patil Hospital and Research Centre, Navi Mumbai, involving a total of 140 embryo transfer cycles including 108 patients who had day 3 transfers (Group A) and 32 patients undergoing day 5 transfers (Group B). Whereas 80.5% of oocytes developed to 8 cell embryos on day 3 in Group A, the blastocyst conversion rate from oocytes in Group B were significantly lower (54.3%). Thus, lesser embryos were available for transfer on day 5 compared to day 3 and an average of 2.4 embryos were transferred per patient on day 3 compared to 1.3 per patient on day 5 ($p < 0.01$). In the blastocyst group, implantation rate was higher (32.8% vs. 21.1%) and pregnancy rate lower (37.5% vs. 46.3%) than in the day 3 ET group. Neither of these two results was statistically significant. Incidence of multiple pregnancies and number of embryos available for cryopreservation were similar between the two groups.

Our results indicate that lesser number of blastocysts are likely to be available for transfer of day 5 following fertilization compared to availability of cleavage stage embryos on day 3. Moreover, although blastocysts are more likely to implant into the endometrium, pregnancy rates with day 3 transfers were similar, perhaps owing to greater number of embryos being transferred per patient.

CONCLUSION

Thus, the ideal embryo transfer strategy may vary based on the expertise and experience of the individual laboratory for extended embryo culture and embryo cryopreservation, availability of PGD/PGS, clinical scenario (number of oocytes/embryos that are available), national legislation, patient history of ART and genetic disease/carrier, patient affordability, as well as individual patient choice. The decision to opt for either strategy over the other must take all these factors into consideration and be taken in a team-based approached involving the clinician, embryologist, as well as taking into account the patient's choices.

REFERENCES

1. Stylianou C, Critchlow D, Brison DR, et al. Embryo morphology as a predictor of IVF success: An evaluation of the proposed UK ACE grading scheme for cleavage stage embryos. Hum Fertil (Camb).2012;15(1):11-7.
2. Telford NA, Watson AJ, Schultz GA. Transition from maternal to embryonic control in early mammalian development: A comparison of several species. Mol Reprod Dev. 1990;26(1):90-100.
3. De Placido G, Wilding M, Strina I,et al. High outcome predictability after IVF using a combined score for zygote and embryo morphology and growth rate. Hum Reprod. 2002;17(9):2402-9.
4. Racowsky C, Vernon M, Mayer J, et al. Standardization of grading embryo morphology. J Assist Reprod Genet. 2010;27(8):437-9.

5. Germond M, Wirthner D, Senn A, et al. Core data for assisted reproductive technology registers: Results of a consensus meeting. Reprod Biomed Online. 2008;17(6):834-40.
6. George K, Mangalraj A, Muthukumar K, et al. Blastocyst stage transfer vs cleavage stage embryo transfer. J Hum Reprod Sci. 2009;2(1):23-6.
7. Lagalla C, Barberi M, Orlando G, et al. A quantitative approach to blastocyst quality evaluation: morphometric analysis and related IVF outcomes. J Assist Reprod Genet. 2015;32(5):705-12.
8. Cetinkaya CP, Kahraman S. Morphokinetics of embryos-where are we now? J Reprod Biotechno Fertil.2016;5:1-8.
9. Ergin EG, Caliskan E, Yalcinkaya E, et al. Frequency of embryo multinucleation detected by time-lapse system and its impact on pregnancy outcome. Fertil Steril.2014;102(4): 1029-33.
10. Liu Y, Chapple V, Feenan K. Clinical significance of intercellular contact at the four cell stage of Human embryos, and the use of abnormal cleavage patterns to identify embryos with low implantation rate potential: a time-lapse study. Fertil Steril. 2015;103(6):1485-91.
11. Rubio I, Kuhlmann R, Agerholm I, et al. Limited implantation success of direct cleavage humanzygotes: a time-lapse study. Fertil Steril. 2012;98(6):1458-63.
12. Yang Z, Liu J, Collins GS, et al. Selection of single blastocysts for fresh transfer via standard morphology assessment alone and with array CGH for good prognosis IVF patients: results form a randomised pilot study. Mol Cytogenet.2012;5(1):24.
13. Valbuena D, Martin J, De Pablo JL, et al. Increasing levels of estradiol are deleterious to embryonic implantation because they directly affect the embryo. Fertil Steril. 2001;76(5):962-8.
14. Croxatto HB, Fuentealba B, Diaz S, et al. A simple nonsurgical technique to obtain unimplanted eggs from human uteri. Am J Obstet Gynecol. 1972;112(5):662-8.
15. Gardner DK, Leese HJ. Concentrations of nutrients in mouse oviduct fluid and their effects on embryo development and metabolism in vitro. J Reprod Fertil. 1990;88(1):361-8.
16. Fanchin R, Ayoubi JM, Righini C, et al. Uterine contractility decreases at the time of blastocyst transfers. Hum Reprod. 2001;16(6):1115-9.
17. Palmstierna M, Murkes D, Csemiczky G, et al. Zona pellucida thickness variation and occurrence of visible mononucleated blastomers in preembryos are associated with a high pregnancy rate in IVF treatment. J Assist Reprod Genet. 1998;15(2):70-5.
18. Puissant F, Van Rysselberge M, Barlow P, et al. Embryo scoring as a prognostic tool in IVF treatment. Hum Reprod. 1987;2(8):705-8.
19. Cai QF, Wan F, Huang R, et al. Factors predicting the cumulative outcome of IVF/ICSI treatment: a multivariable analysis of 2450 patients. Hum Reprod. 2011;26(9):2532-40.
20. Scott L, Alvero R, Leondires M, et al. The morphology of human pronuclear embryos is positively related to blastocyst development and implantation. Hum Reprod. 2000;15(11):2394-403.
21. Sjöblom P, Menezes J, Cummins L, et al. Prediction of embryo developmental potential and pregnancy based on early stage morphological characteristics. Fertil Steril. 2006;86(4): 848-61.
22. Steer CV, Mills CL, Tan SL, et al. The cumulative embryo score: a predictive embryo scoring technique to select the optimal number of embryos to transfer in an in-vitro fertilization and embryo transfer programme. Hum Reprod. 1992;7:117-9.
23. Magli MC, Gianaroli L, Munné S, et al. Incidence of chromosomal abnormalities from a morphologically normal cohort of embryos in poorprognosis patients. J Assist Reprod Genet. 1998;15(5):297-301.
24. Magli MC, Jones GM, Gras L, et al. Chromosome mosaicism in day 3 aneuploid embryos that develop to morphologically normal blastocysts in vitro. Hum Reprod. 2000;15(8):1781-6.
25. Staessen C, Platteau P, Van Assche E, et al. Comparison of blastocyst transfer with or without preimplantation genetic diagnosis for aneuploidy screening in couples with advanced maternal age: A prospective randomized controlled trial. Hum Reprod. 2004;19(12):2849-58.
26. Edwards RG. The history of assisted human conception with especial reference to endocrinology. Exp Clin Endocrinol Diabetes.1996;104(3):183-204.
27. Ezzati M, Djahanbakhch O, Arian S, et al. Tubal transport of gametes and embryos: a review of physiology and pathophysiology. J Assist Reprod Genet. 2014;31(10):1337-47.
28. Scholtes MCW, Zeilmaker GH. A prospective, randomized study of embryo transfer results after 3 or 5 days of embryo culture in in vitro fertilization. Fertil Steril. 1996;65(6): 1245-8.
29. Menezo YJ, Guerin JF, Czyba JC. Improvement of human early embryo development in vitro by coculture on monolayers of Vero cells. Biol Reprod. 1990;42(2):301-6.
30. Van Blerkom J. Development of human embryos to the hatched blastocyst stage in the presence or absence of a monolayer of vero cells. Hum Reprod. 1993;8(9):1525-39.
31. Yeung WS, Ho PC, Lau EY, et al. Improved development of human embryos in vitro by a human oviductal cell co-culture system. Hum Reprod. 1992;7(8):1144-9.
32. Sanchez T, Seidler EA, Gardner DK, et al. Will noninvasive methods surpass invasive for assessing gametes and embryos? Fertil Steril. 2017;108(5):730-7.
33. Braude P, Bolton V, Moore S. Human gene expression first occurs between the four- and eight-cell stages of preimplantation development. Nature. 1988;332(6163): 459-61.
34. Schoolcraft WB, Gardner DK. Blastocyst versus day 2 or 3 transfer. Semin Reprod Med. 2001;19(3):259-68.
35. Edwards RG, Steptoe PC. Current status of in-vitro fertilisation and implantation of human embryos. Lancet. 1983;322(8362):1265-9.
36. Hamberger L, Hardarson T, Nygren KG. Avoidance of multiple pregnancy by use of single embryo transfer. Minerva Ginecol. 2005;57(1):15-9.
37. Gardner DK, Surrey E, Minjarez D, et al. Single blastocyst transfer: A prospective randomized trial. Fertil Steril. 2004;81(3):551-5.
38. Milki AA, Hinckley MD, Westphal LM, et al. Elective single blastocyst transfer. Fertil Steril. 2004;81(6):1697-8.
39. Gardner DK, Schoolcraft WB, Wagley L, et al. A prospective randomized trial of blastocyst culture and transfer in in-vitro fertilization. Hum Reprod. 1998;13(12):3434-40.

40. Gardner DK, Vella P, Lane M, et al. Culture and transfer of human blastocysts increases implantation rates and reduces the need for multiple embryo transfers. Fertil Steril. 1998;69(1):84-8.
41. Milki AA, Fisch JD, Behr B. Two-blastocyst transfer has similar pregnancy rates and a decreased multiple gestation rate compared with three-blastocyst transfer. Fertil Steril. 1999;72(2):225-8.
42. Zander-Fox DL, Tremellen K, Lane M. Single blastocyst embryo transfer maintains comparable pregnancy rates to double cleavage-stage embryo transfer but results in healthier pregnancy outcomes. Aust New Zeal J Obstet Gynaecol. 2011;51(5):406-10.
43. Dessolle L, Fréour T, Barrire P, et al. A cycle-based model to predict blastocyst transfer cancellation. Hum Reprod. 2010;25(3):598-604.
44. Marek D, Langley M, Gardner DK, et al. Introduction of blastocyst culture and transfer for all patients in an in vitro fertilization program. Fertil Steril. 1999;72(6):1035-40.
45. Johnson N, Blake D, Farquhar C. Blastocyst or cleavage-stage embryo transfer? Best Practice and Research: Clinical Obstetrics and Gynaecology. 2007;21:21-40.
46. Hreinsson J, Rosenlund B, Fridström M, et al. Embryo transfer is equally effective at cleavage stage and blastocyst stage: A randomized prospective study. Eur J Obstet Gynecol Reprod Biol. 2004;117(2):194-200.
47. Fernández-Gonzalez R, Ramirez MA, Bilbao A, et al. Suboptimal in vitro culture conditions: An epigenetic origin of long-term health effects. Mol Reprod Dev. 2007;74(9): 1149-56.
48. Xin Z, Zhu H, Jin H, et al. Pregnancy outcomes of day 5 embryo transfer in patients at high risk of developing ovarian hyperstimulation syndrome and analysis of factors affecting blastocyst formation. J Int Med Res. 2013;41(4): 1127-34.
49. Sills ES, Tucker MJ, Palermo GD. Assisted reproductive technologies and monozygous twins: implications for future study and clinical practice. Twin Res. 2000;3:217-23.
50. Behr B, Fisch JD, Racowsky C, et al. Blastocyst-ET and monozygotic twinning. J Assist Reprod Genet. 2000;17(6): 349-51.
51. Cohen J. Assisted hatching of human embryos. J In Vitro Fert Embryo Transf. 1991;8(4):179-90.
52. de Felici M, Siracusa G. "Spontaneous" hardening of the zona pellucida of mouse oocytes during in vitro culture. Gamete Res. 1982;6(2):107-13.
53. Papanikolaou EG, Fatemi H, Venetis C, et al. Monozygotic twinning is not increased after single blastocyst transfer compared with single cleavage-stage embryo transfer. Fertil Steril. 2010;93(2):592-7.
54. Moayeri SE, Behr B, Lathi RB, et al. Risk of monozygotic twinning with blastocyst transfer decreases over time: an 8-year experience. Fertil Steril. 2007;87(5):1028-32.
55. Luna M, Duke M, Copperman A, et al. Blastocyst embryo transfer is associated with a sex-ratio imbalance in favor of male offspring. Fertil Steril. 2007;87(3):519-23.
56. Glujovsky D, Farquhar C, Quinteiro Retamar AM, et al. Cleavage stage versus blastocyst stage embryo transfer in assisted reproductive technology. Cochrane Database Syst Rev. 2016;(6):CD002118.

Time-lapse Monitoring

49

Hrishikesh D Pai, Nandita Palshetkar, Rushika Mistry, Rohan Palshetkar

INTRODUCTION

Recent advances in assisted reproduction have resulted in over a million babies born worldwide. The main aim of in vitro fertilization (IVF) programs is reducing multiple pregnancies while maintaining a good clinical outcome. Single embryo transfer is progressively becoming a reality which is the result of major improvements in the field of IVF. Concerns about multiple gestations have raised awareness of the risks not only to the mother (gestational diabetes, hypertension, and anemia) but also to the babies (extreme prematurity, low-birth weight, children with neurological damage). With major advances in the field, most recently, the introduction of time-lapse imaging systems allows us to assess embryos in a different way through their morphokinetics.

TIME-LAPSE IMAGING TECHNOLOGY

Time-lapse monitoring of human embryo development has been proposed as early as in the 1980s of the last century. However, the introduction of time-lapse monitoring systems into clinical routine has only recently been realized due to the availability of commercially ready to use time-lapse incubation systems. Since then, the possibility to track any morphological change during embryo development to the specific time when it occurred has enlightened our knowledge. Furthermore, we have been able to detect features of embryo development, which were so far unknown, like direct cleavage and reverse cleavage, both of which are compromising embryo viability. Through this approach, embryo categories are normally based on the number of blastomeres and nuclei, the percentage of fragments, cell symmetry, and the quality of the inner cell mass (ICM) and trophectoderm (TE). Through great knowledge achieved by this approach, it has been demonstrated that embryo status can markedly change within a few hours.[1-4] Also, inter- and intra-observer variability are commonly described problems due to subjective nature of traditional morphological assessment.[5] In theory, increasing the number of observations could provide better information on the development of an embryo and therefore improve its assessment.[3,6-10] At the same time, increased handling and higher evaluation frequency will expose the embryo to undesirable changes in temperature, humidity, and gas composition.[11-14]

Time-lapse monitoring systems provide a solution to this problem. The two main advantages of these systems are—(1) improved and stable culture conditions; and (2) the determination of objective and accurate markers, both qualitative and quantitative. In addition, it involves reduced handling and human risk; minimization of culture media, gas and oil, detection of abnormal events in embryo development and reduced number of hours required by the embryologists in the laboratory.[15]

Time-lapse monitoring enables morphokinetic analysis of embryos. It has been reported that some morphokinetic variables are correlated with the ability of the embryos to form a blastocyst or to implant. An embryo which falls within a favorable range of such a variable has a much higher implantation potential compared to one that is out of this range. Combining favorable ranges from several variables enables the creation of a prediction algorithm. Especially, this aspect of time-lapse monitoring systems attracts much attention and is controversially discussed among the embryological community.

On the other hand, time-lapse monitoring system is meanwhile an established topic at international conferences and dedicated time-lapse sessions confirm the importance of this relatively new technology. This is also reflected in publications that use time lapse for basic research and/or clinical routine for therapeutic as well as diagnostic purposes.

TIME-LAPSE STUDIES

The first experiments were aimed at validating the clinical utility of the time-lapse system as an incubator where it was introduced to study the kinetics of human embryonic development. In the initial studies, Meseguer et al. (unpublished) compared biochemical pregnancy rates (BPRs) and clinical pregnancy rates (CPRs) between cycles incubated in the embryoscope (ESD) and in a standard incubator (SI) in a retrospective match cohort study. No significant differences were observed for any of the variables studied between the two groups considered. Continuing to validate time-lapse technology for clinical use, Cruz et al. compared the blastocyst formation rate and the percentage of useful embryos (transferred + frozen) in a prospective study in which oocytes from the same patient were randomly split between an SI and the ESD after intracytoplasmic sperm injection (ICSI). No significant difference was observed for any of the variables studied (SI vs. ESD).[16] Further studies were aimed at determining specific time for kinetic parameters such as the first and second cleavage and for events related to intracellular dynamics including the extrusion of the second polar body, the appearance/disappearance of the pronuclei and the apposition and syngamy of the pronuclei.

MODELS AVAILABLE IN THE MARKET

There are different models of time-lapse systems available in the market. Some of them have all the items integrated into one single equipment [e.g. EmbryoScope® (VitriLife), Geri® (Genea Biomedx) and Miri® TL (Esco Medical)]. Others have the option of introducing a microscope inside an available incubator [e.g. Primo Vision® (VitroLife) and The Eeva™ Test (Merck-Serono)]. The technical and clinical features of all the time-lapse monitoring systems are described below:

- *EmbryoScope®:* The technical features of this system are—phase contrast microscopy, image capture frequency of every 10 min, 7 focal planes, the number of patients that can be observed at a time in the system is 6 with 12 embryos per EmbryoSlide dish. It has an integrated incubator. It has an accessory EmbryoViewer to analyze the data of annotation of each embryo. Data analysis is manual.
  The clinical features are that the system has no automatic assessment of the embryo quality. It is worker dependent, time consuming, embryo selection algorithm is set by the user, and no blastocyst formation prediction on day 3 of embryo development. Implantation prediction by day 3 is possible and prospective validation done **(Fig. 1)**.
- *Primo Vision®:* The technical features of this system are—phase contrast microscopy and image capture frequency of every 10 min. Focusing levels are several,

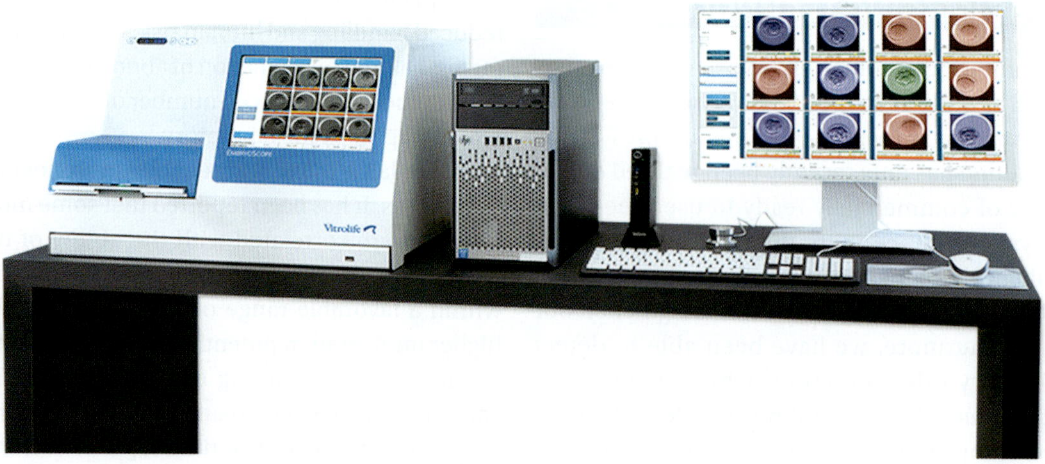

Fig. 1: EmbryoScope—time—lapse system.
Source: Vitrolife.

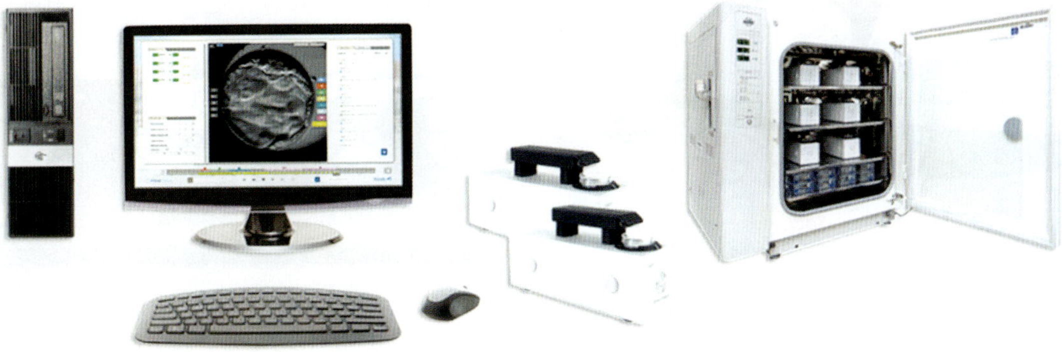

Fig. 2: Primo vision time lapse.
Source: Vitrolife.

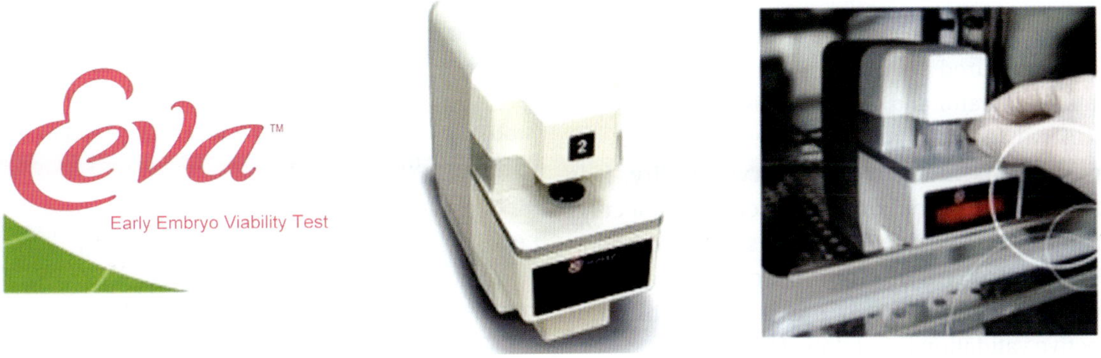

Fig. 3: Eeva—early embryo visibility test.
Source: Merck India Biopharma.

it can observe one patient at a time, and the number of embryos that can be cultured per dish are 16 per patient. It is placed within an incubator and data analysis is manual.

The clinical features are that the system has no automatic assessment of the embryo quality. It is worker dependent, time consuming, embryo selection algorithm is set by the user, and no blastocyst formation prediction on day 3 of embryo development. Implantation prediction by day 3 is possible and prospective validation is not done **(Fig. 2)**.

- *The Eeva™ test:* The technical features of this system are—dark field microscopy and image capture frequency of every 5 min. Focusing level is one, number of patients observed is one, and the number of embryos that can be cultured per dish are 12 per patient. It is placed within the incubator and the data analysis is real time.
  The clinical features are that the system has automatic assessment of the embryo quality. It is not worker dependent and since it is automatic, it is less time-consuming system. The embryo selection algorithm is preset, it can predict blastocyst formation on day 3 of embryo development and implantation prediction too. Prospective validation is done **(Fig. 3)**.
- *Geri®:* The technical features of this system are: phase contrast microscopy and image capture frequency of every 5 min. Focusing levels are several, it can observe six patients at a time and the number of embryos that can be cultured per dish are 16 per patient. It has integrated incubator and data analysis is manual.
  The clinical features are that the system has no automatic assessment of the embryo quality. It is worker dependent, time consuming, embryo selection algorithm is set by the user, and no blastocyst formation prediction on day 3 of embryo development. No implantation prediction by day 3 is possible and prospective validation is not done **(Fig. 4)**.
- *Miri® TL:* The technical features of this system are—phase contrast microscopy and image capture frequency of every 5 min. Focusing levels are several, it can observe

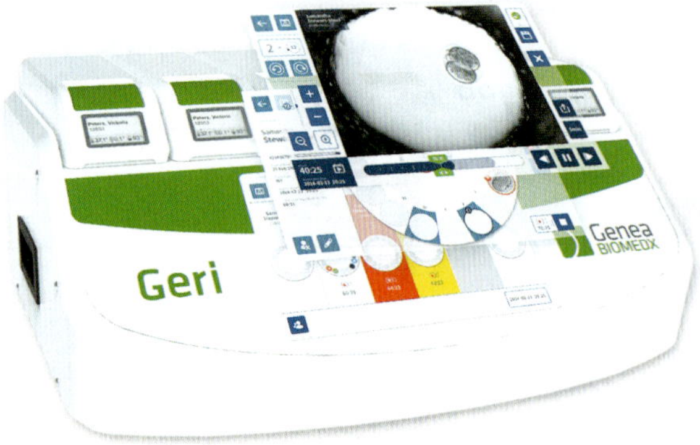

Fig. 4: Geri incubation system.
Source: GeneaBiomedix.

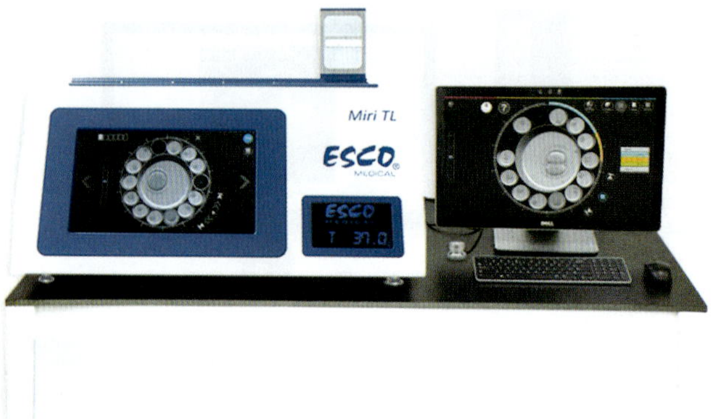

Fig. 5: Miri time—lapse incubator.
Source: ESCO medical.

six patients at a time, and the number of embryos that can be cultured per dish are 14 per patient. It has integrated incubator and data analysis is manual.

The clinical features are that the system has no automatic assessment of the embryo quality. It is worker dependent, time consuming, embryo selection algorithm is set by the user, and no blastocyst formation prediction on day 3 of embryo development. No implantation prediction by day 3 is possible and prospective validation is not done **(Fig. 5)**.[17]

KINETICS OF DEVELOPMENT AND KINETIC PARAMETERS

The selection of the embryo on the day of embryo transfer is dependent on morphological analysis established in the daily routine work of an IVF laboratory. However, the study of cellular activity during the early stages of embryonic development provides additional information that can later be used in the selection process. The time between fertilization and the first cleavage is an objective parameter that can easily be determined with certain predictive value of embryo viability.[18,19] Although the correlation between the number of cells and the embryo's development stage has been widely described, the assessment of early cleavage and its importance in embryo selection procedures is relatively recent.

As described in the proposed guidelines on the nomenclature and annotation of dynamic human embryo monitoring by a time-lapse user group, the following morphokinetic individual variables can be defined **(Table 1)**.[20]

Kinetic markers are associated with good quality prediction of formation of the blastocyst. This is supported by various studies carried by Wong et al., Hashimoto et al., Hinka et al., Cruz et al., Yang et al., Milewski et al., Motato et al. and many more researchers. In addition to blastocyst formation, kinetic markers are correlated to Implantation of embryo as the end point. This is supported by studies carried out by various researchers from the year 2008 (Lemen et al.) until recently by Goodman et al. in 2016.

Table 1: Kinetic markers.

t0	Time of IVF or mid-time of microinjection (ICSI/IMSI)
tpb2	The second polar body completely detached from the oolemma
tPN	Fertilization is confirmed
tPNa	Appearance of individual pronuclei
tPNf	Time of pronuclei disappearance
tZ	Time of PN scoring
t2 to t9	Time to 2 to 9 discrete cells
tSC	First evidence of compaction
tSB	Initiation of blastulation
tByz	Full blastocyst "y" corresponds to morphology of ICM "z" corresponds to morphology of TE cells

EMBRYO SELECTION ALGORITHM

Basile et al. correlated morphokinetics with embryo aneuploidy. The model identified t5-t2 (time to 5 cell stage—time to 2 cell stage) followed cc3 (cell cycle 3) as the most relevant variables related to chromosomally normal embryo **(Flowchart 1)**. An algorithm for selection of embryo based

Flowchart 1: Embryo selection algorithm.

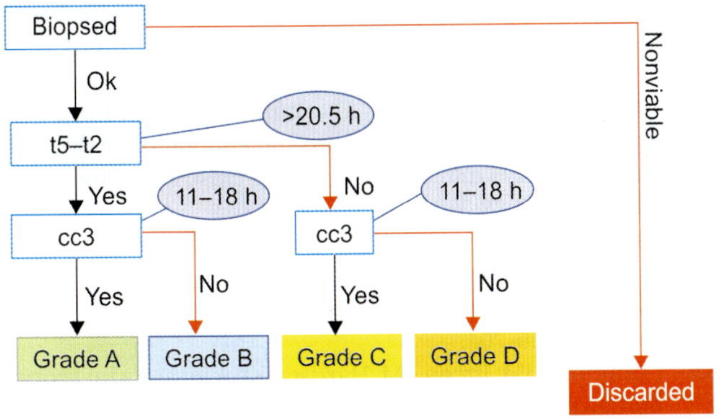

Source: Basile N, Nogales M del C, Bronet F, et al. Increasing the probability of selecting chromosomally normal embryos by time-lapse morphokinetics analysis. Fertil Steril. 2014;101:699-704.

Table 2: Grading of embryos on the basis of the algorithm.

t5- t2: Time interval between 5-cell and 2 cell (ideal >20.5 hrs)	
cc3: t5-t3 (ideal between 11 and 18 hrs)	
Grade A embryos	t5-t2 normal, cc3 normal
Grade B embryos	t5-t2 normal, cc3 abnormal
Grade C embryos	t5-t2 abnormal, cc3 normal
Grade D embryos	t5-t2 abnormal, cc3 abnormal

on these two variables classified embryos from A to D with significant differences in the percentage of normal embryos as we move from A to D. Specifically, A = 35.9%, B = 26.4%, C = 12.1%, and D = 9.8%($P < 0.001$).[21]

Table 2 explains the grading of embryos on the basis of the algorithm.

Grade A and B are 70% genetically normal and are found to give best results.

CONCLUSION

With the increasing pressure to reduce the number of embryos transferred to the uterus, there is development of new strategies which are aimed to optimize the predictive power of embryo viability. Cummings JM confirms the efficacy of combining a subjective score of embryo quality with the rate of development in culture to predict a possible pregnancy.[22] With the search of new markers for clinical use, the relationship between the kinetics of cleavage and the subsequent blastocyst formation rate helps in selection of embryos with higher implantation potential. The time-lapse monitoring systems along with molecular data correlate development from zygote to blastocyst stage and have proposed new specific markers for later stages of embryo development that can predict implantation.[23] Routine time-lapse monitoring of embryo development in a clinical setting provides numerous information about developmental parameters that differ between different types of embryos and help us select an embryo with higher implantation potential. Conventional morphological assessment can be performed on daily basis; however, if possible, it should be complemented with the detection of kinetic markers known to improve clinical results. This new approach will allow the embryologist to perform a more accurate and objective embryo selection and hence the goal of single embryo transfer (SET) slowly becomes possible.

REFERENCES

1. Meseguer M, Herrero J, Tejera A, et al. The use of morphokinetics as a predictor of embryo implantation. Hum Reprod. 2011;26:2658-71.
2. Mio Y, Maeda K. Time-lapse cinematography of dynamic changes occurring during in vitro development of human embryos. Am J Obstet Gynecol. 2008;199:660.e1-5.
3. Gardner DK, Meseguer M, Rubio C, et al. Diagnosis of human preimplantation embryo viability. Hum Reprod Update. 2015;21:727-47.
4. Alpha Scientists in Reproductive Medicine and ESHRE Special Interest Group of Embryology. The Istanbul consensus workshop on embryo assessment: Proceedings of an expert meeting. Hum Reprod. 2011;26:1270-83.
5. Baxter B, Allison E. Interobserver and intraobserver variation in day 3 embryo grading. Fertil Steril. 2006;86:1608-15.
6. Kaser DJ, Racowsky C. Clinical outcomes following selection of human preimplantation embryos with time-lapse monitoring: A systematic review. Hum Reprod Update. 2014;20:617-31.
7. Paternot G, Wetzels A, Thonon F, et al. Intra- and interobserver analysis in the morphological assessment of early stage embryos during an IVF procedure: A multicentre study. Reprod Biol Endocrinol. 2011;9:127.
8. Sundvall L, Ingerslev HJ, Breth Knudsen U, et al. Inter- and intra-observer variability of time-lapse annotations. Hum Reprod. 2013;28:3215-21.
9. Arce JC, Ziebe S, Lundin K, et al. Interobserver agreement and intraobserver reproducibility of embryo quality assessments. Hum Reprod. 2006;21:2141-8.
10. Scott L. The biological basis of non-invasive strategies for selection of human oocytes and embryos. Hum Reprod Update. 2003;9:237-49.
11. Meseguer M, Rubio I, Cruz M, et al. Embryo incubation and selection in a time-lapse monitoring system improves pregnancy outcome compared with a standard incubator: A retrospective cohort study. Fertil Steril. 2012;98:1481-9.
12. Kirkegaard K, Ahlstrom A, Ingerslev HJ, et al. Choosing the best embryo by time lapse versus standard morphology. Fertil Steril. 2015;103:323-32.

13. Zhang JQ, Li XL, Peng Y, et al. Reduction in exposure of human embryos outside the incubator enhances embryo quality and blastulation rate. Reprod Biomed Online. 2010;20:510-5.
14. Payne D, Flaherty SP, Barry MF, et al. Preliminary observations on polar body extrusion and pronuclear formation in human oocytes using time-lapse video cinematography. Hum Reprod. 1997;12:532-41.
15. Basile N, Caiazzo M, Meseguer M. What does morphokinetics add to embryo selection and in-vitro fertilization outcomes? Curr Opin Obstet Gynecol. 2015;27(3):193-200.
16. Cruz M, Gadea B, Garrido N, et al. Embryo quality, blastocyst and ongoing pregnancy rates in oocyte donation patients whose embryos were monitored by time-lapse imaging, J Assist Reprod Genet. 2011;28:569-73.
17. Herrero J, Meseguer M. Selection of high potential embryos using time-lapse imaging: The era of morphokinetics. Fertil Steril. 2013;99:1030-4.
18. Shoukir Y, Campana A, Farley T, et al. Early cleavage of in-vitro fertilized human embryos to the 2-cell stage: a novel indicator of embryo quality and viability. Hum Reprod. 1997;12:1531-6.
19. Sakkas D, Shoukir Y, Chardonnens D, et al. Early cleavage of human embryos to the two-cell stage after intracytoplasmic sperm injection as an indicator of embryo viability. Hum Reprod. 1998;13:182-7.
20. Ciray HN, Campbell A, Agerholm IE, et al. Proposed guidelines on the nomenclature and annotation of dynamic human embryo monitoring by a time-lapse user group. Hum Reprod. 2014;29:2650-60.
21. Basile N, Nogales M del C, Bronet F, et al. Increasing the probability of selecting chromosomally normal embryos by time-lapse morphokinetics analysis. Fertil Steril. 2014;101:699-704.
22. Cummings JM, Breen TM, Harrison Kl. A formula for scoring human embryo growth rates in in vitro fertilization: its values in predicting pregnancy and in comparison, with visual estimates of embryo quality. J In Vitro Fert Embryo Transf. 1986;3:284-95.
23. Meseguer M, Herrero J, Tejera A. The use of morphokinetics as a predictor of embryo implantation. Human Reprod. 2011;26:2658-71.

Newer Technologies in the IVF Laboratory

50

RB Agrawal, A Suresh Kumar, Madhuprita Agrawal

INTRODUCTION

The pioneering work of Steptoe and Edward, resulting in the birth of first in vitro fertilization (IVF) baby, Louise Brown in 1978, was a landmark in the management of infertile couples.[1] Since then, several technological advances have been introduced in this versatile field to enhance the success rates. The active research in both clinical [new drugs and regimens for stimulation, advanced ultrasonography, and embryo transfer (ET) techniques] as well as newer technologies in IVF laboratory [introduction of intracytoplasmic sperm injection (ICSI) and intracytoplasmic morphologically selecting sperm injection (IMSI), laser-assisted hatching (LAH), time-lapse monitoring system, preimplantation genetic diagnosis (PGD) and preimplantation genetic screening (PGS) using genetic and molecular platforms to select the euploid embryos for embryo transfer, etc.] have all increased pregnancy and take home baby rates. Now research aims more toward improving embryo viability and implantation rates as elective single embryo transfer (eSET) is the way forward to avoid complications due to multiple gestations.

Various aspects of embryological research both in technique and molecular biology will be reviewed in this chapter.

Firstly, micromanipulation procedures like ICSI[2] and IMSI have significantly improved the success rates in male factor associated infertility. The second major breakthrough is the ability to detect genetic disease and chromosomal disorders before the embryo transfer by PGD and PGS. Thirdly, the ultrarapid vitrification technique[3] allows efficient and long-term storage of unfertilized oocytes and embryos up to blastocyst stage both for IVF and somatic cell nuclear transfer. Fourthly, the largest new contribution may be from molecular biology focused on new noninvasive method for selecting viable embryo using molecular approaches.[4,5] Research in this field is still continuing.

TECHNOLOGICAL ADVANCES IN IVF LABORATORY

In the early 1980s when IVF was established as a mode of infertility treatment it was meant for female indications particularly tubal factor, but in case of male infertility and failed fertilization, there was no alternative approach, which was overcome after the advancement of ICSI technique. The development of ICSI was a major revolution in the field of assisted reproductive technique (ART) and especially for male infertility.

Intracytoplasmic Morphologically Selecting Sperm Injection

Palermo et al. introduced ICSI[2] in 1992. It is the treatment of choice in male factor infertility. The technique involves selection of a single spermatozoon under an optical magnification of 400×, which is then immobilized and injected into the oocyte cytoplasm with a micro-injection needle. This magnification enables the observation of major sperm morphological defects. However, minor morphological defects, which can affect the outcome, are often missed.[6] Even though the spermatozoon may appear morphologically normal, it may still harbor various structural abnormalities that can have deleterious effects on subsequent pregnancy outcomes.[7,8]

To overcome these limitations of ICSI, Bartoov et al. in 2002 introduced MSOME (motile sperm organellar morphology examination), a new method of visualizing unstained sperms in real time under high magnification of 6,600×. Inverted light microscope equipped with high power Nomarski differential interference contrast optics enhanced by digital imaging is used to achieve this magnification. The technique allows selection of sperms with strictly defined morphologically normal nucleus which can be used for ICSI. The procedure was named intracytoplasmic morphologically selected sperm injection by the original authors.[9] In patients with severe male factor infertility, IMSI has been shown to have better success rates in comparison to only ICSI.[10,11]

Use of Laser in ART (Assisted Hatching)

Over the last decade enormous number of attempts have been made to improve embryo implantation after IVF.

It was observed that implantation rates were better in embryos with thin zona. This led to the development of technique called assisted hatching. Hence it has been proposed that either an artificial opening or softening of the zona pellucida (ZP) might be able to promote the hatching process thereby improving the overall implantation and thus pregnancy rate after IVF-ET.[12,13]

Various methods have been tried for assisted hatching like mechanical hatching, chemical hatching (using acid tyrode's or pronase), and laser hatching. LAH is becoming the preferred method for assisted hatching, as it is simple, safe, reproducible, and accurate.[14] Holes with an unprecedented definition are obtained by laser-induced local thermal lysis of the glycoproteins matrix of the zona. The laser technique is also utilized for embryo biopsy procedures (polar body biopsy, blastomere or trophectoderm biopsy) for PGD.[15,16] However, concerns regarding the safety and efficacy of assisted hatching never allowed it to gain full access as a routinely used adjunct treatment to all cases undergoing ART. This technique is beneficial in cases: (1) Women age above 38 years; (2) Elevated follicle-stimulating hormone (FSH) levels; (3) Zona thickness greater than 18 μ; (4) Frozen-thawed embryos; (5) Repeatedly failed IVF cases. In addition, there have been very few reports to support the efficacy of assisted hatching after the initial randomized controlled trials published in 1992 by Cohen et al.[17] Other avenues need to be thought of where this powerful tool can further be used to improve the success rates.

Polarization Microscopy (Birefringence Imaging)

Polarization microscopy is another newer technology which can be an important tool in the ART laboratory for assessing the competence of eggs and sperms. A new type of polarization microscope utilizes liquid crystals to modulate the state of polarization.[18] With the current advancements in computer technology, this technique allows real-time visualization of birefringent structures and also real-time calculation of polarization parameters on a pixel-by-pixel basis. The spindle's architecture in live human oocytes can be studied noninvasively without any harmful effects.[19] In contrast to spindle imaging, polarization microscopy is an indirect method to measure oocyte quality.[20,21] The use of poloscope has also been extended during ICSI in the selection of viable sperm, as it has no adverse effect on sperm motility or membrane integrity,[22] it maximizes the viability of the resulting embryos thereby and significantly improving ART outcomes.[23]

LABORATORY ADVANCEMENT: BLASTOCYST CULTURE

The delivery of a single, healthy child is the desired outcome of an ART program. Multiple gestations are the most common side effect of IVF. Multiple pregnancies may be associated with severe obstetrics and neonatal complications. Hence, there is an increasing inclination toward minimum to eSET at various centres.[24] Various approaches have been tried for the selection of the best embryo for uterine transfer using blastocyst culture. However, preimplantation extended culture of embryos requires the use of hypoxic conditions. Ideally the use of benchtop incubators with low oxygen concentration, improved laboratory air quality, and the development of sequential media and single step media facilitate the development of the embryos up to the stage of blastocyst. The improved culture media takes into consideration the changes in the nutrient requirements and metabolism as the embryo development proceeds.[25] Transfer of blastocyst into the uterus would be closer to the in vivo situation. Secondly, culturing embryos for an extended period will select the developing embryos from those that have undergone developmental arrest. Guerif et al. reported high pregnancy rates following transfer of blastocysts.[26]

However, one should use extended culture to blastocyst only when there are multiple embryos at the cleavage stage available for transfer. As of now its routine application for ART in all cases does not seem justified.

LABORATORY ADVANCEMENTS: IN VITRO MATURATION OF OOCYTES

In vitro, two strategies have been tried to mature oocytes. In the first strategy oocytes collected from antral follicles, from a stimulated or an unstimulated cycle, are matured. In the second strategy primordial and preantral follicles are cultured in vitro. Though the second strategy is more challenging technically, it is potentially more beneficial.[27]

Historically, polycystic ovary syndrome (PCOS) patients were the selected group for in vitro maturation (IVM).[28] The advantages provided by IVM include reducing or curtailing the risk of ovarian hyperstimulation syndrome (OHSS) by reducing the requirement of gonadotropins and hence making the procedure cost-effective. For patients undergoing chemotherapy or radiotherapy which are gonadotoxic, fertility preservation becomes an important aspect. Cryopreservation of their immature oocytes followed by IVM years later has become a very important practical advantage of IVM.[27,28] The first birth after IVM of immature oocytes was reported in 1991 by Cha et al. [29] Though several studies have observed that oocyte maturation and fertilization rate are acceptable, the overall ART outcomes are not yet promising.[30] With new advancements in stimulation protocol, it can decrease or eliminate the risk of OHSS in conventional IVF cycles. The advantages of this technique are not yet clear and will need further optimization.

ADVANCES IN CRYOPRESERVATION TECHNIQUE

In recent year, the most significant advancement in IVF laboratory has been in the field of cryopreservation method. Embryo cryopreservation is now considered as an indispensable part of a successful IVF program.

Embryo cryopreservation enhances the cumulative pregnancy potential after performing an eSET and minimizes the risk of multiple gestations. The first successful pregnancy from a frozen human embryo occurred in 1983.[31] Currently, vitrification has been used widely for the cryopreservation of oocytes and embryos up to blastocyst stage using improved devices in humans.[32,33]

In contrast to the conventional method of slow freezing, vitrification is safe, simple, rapid, and inexpensive. The vitrification technique utilizes ultrarapid cooling with a very high concentration of cryoprotectants which totally eliminates formation of ice. The technique is highly effective for freezing early embryonic and blastocyst stage embryos.[33]

Cryopreservation of unfertilized oocytes presents more technical challenges than the embryos as the oocyte is a highly specialized cell. This new technique gives young girls and women the possibility of preserving fertility on demand and for medical indications.[34]

There are multiple indications for oocyte preservation like:

- Husband is unavailable or unable to provide semen sample on the day of egg harvesting
- Preservation of reproductive competence of young cancer patients who need pelvic radiation or chemotherapy
- Surgical intervention before or during the reproductive age involving removal of ovaries
- Patients at risk of loss of ovarian function with impending premature menopause.
- Ovarian hyperstimulation syndrome
- Cryobanking oocytes for egg donation programs or for research purposes
- When the women wish to delay motherhood due to personal reasons.

Human oocyte cryopreservation is performed either using conventional slow-rate freezing or vitrification. The first pregnancy resulting with use of cryopreserved oocytes was reported in 1986.[35] In 1999, the first birth following oocyte cryopreservation with the vitrification method was reported.[36]

With this technique of cryopreservation oocyte survival rates approached 90% by 2005. Pregnancy rates as good as fresh IVF cycles have been reported by many clinics after utilizing cryopreserved oocytes.[37]

Cryopreservation and transplantation of ovarian tissue are two emerging techniques for fertility preservation in cancer patients. Irrespective of age and marital status ovarian cortex can be obtained in any female cancer patient with the advantage of no delays in cancer therapy.[38] The preserved ovarian tissue can later be transplanted at orthotopic or heterotopic sites. A popular site for orthotopic transplantation is the existing menopausal ovary.[39]

Oktay and Karlikaya were the first to document in vivo restoration of ovarian function after autologous transplantation of cryopreserved ovarian cortex in the year 2000.[39]

Donnez et al. in the year 2004, reported the first live birth after the autologous orthotopic transplantation of frozen-thawed ovarian cortex[40] and since then more than 100 live births have been reported after replacing the frozen-thawed ovarian tissue.[41] First live birth of healthy twins after oocyte cryopreservation and bilateral ovariectomy in cancer patient was reported by Porcu E et al. in 2008.[42] These reports confirm ovarian tissue cryopreservation is a promising means of fertility preservation in patients fighting from cancer.

Cryopreservation of the whole ovary is challenging because as it involves large quantities of tissue and various biomolecules, followed by slow cooling. Although these advances are promising, cryopreservation of the intact ovary is still in experimental phase and has a long way to go before it can be routinely offered in clinical practice. Imhof et al. reported pregnancy and live birth by orthotopic microvascular reanastomosis of whole frozen-thawed sheep ovaries.[43]

TECHNOLOGIES EVALUATING EMBRYOS

Preimplantation Genetic Diagnosis

Preimplantation genetic diagnosis and preimplantation genetic screening are the invasive techniques used to analyze the genetic or chromosomal complement of human embryos developing in vitro with the aim of replacing embryos free from chromosomal abnormalities or genetic disease into the uterus of the patient (Handyside et al. 1990; Grifo et al. 1994: Munne et al. 1997). The couple needs to undergo the process of IVF, the embryos are subjected to single cell biopsy for PGD analysis, with genetic testing performed on cells from different stages of embryo development including polar body biopsy from the unfertilized and fertilized oocytes, biopsy of blastomere from day 3 cleavage-stage embryos,[44,45] and trophectoderm biopsy from blastocyst stage embryos.[46]

In case of cleavage stage biopsy only 1–2 blastomeres are available for establishing the genetic diagnosis while in blastocyst biopsy removal of a few trophectoderm cells is considered not to affect the development of the fetus. The clinical applications of blastocyst biopsy have been reported by de Boer et al. (2002)[47] and Kokkali et al. (2005).[48]

Preimplantation genetic diagnosis can be offered to both fertile and infertile couples who are at risk of passing on genetic disease such as thalassemia or cystic fibrosis, or to couples already undergoing infertility treatment for a variety of causes like (1) Aneuploidy analysis for poor embryo quality (selection against chaotic mosaicism); (2) Advanced maternal age (selection against Down syndrome, etc.); (3) Repetitive spontaneous pregnancy loss due to fetal chromosomal abnormalities; (4) Unexplained infertility; and (5) Severe male factor infertility.[49,50-52]

The technique is combined with two diagnostic methods: fluorescence in situ hybridization (FISH)[53] or polymerase chain reaction (PCR) analysis.[54] This technique can be used to diagnose chromosomal abnormalities or to sex the embryos in patients carrying X-chromosome-linked diseases. In contrast, PCR is useful in the diagnosis of single gene disorders like beta thalassemia, cystic fibrosis,[53,54] etc. In recent years, microarrays are being increasingly utilized for evaluation of all 24 pairs of chromosomes for aneuploidy or other chromosomal imbalances.[55]

Preimplantation Genetic Screening

Preimplantation genetic screening determines the chromosomal status of an embryo by screening all 23 chromosome pairs prior to transfer in an IVF cycle and leads to greater implantation rates and improved IVF outcomes.[55]

New diagnosis methods, such as array comparative genome hybridization (aCGH), single-nucleotide polymorphism (SNP) microarray, and next generation screening (NGS), introduced for screening of all 24 chromosomes aneuploidy. Microchips are now used for the screening of the most appropriate chromosomally normal embryos for uterine transfer.[55]

Cell extraction on day 5 has higher diagnostic value and does not practically present any additional risk for the embryo. The embryos are frozen using vitrification method and the transfer of the embryo is done in the next cycle after preimplantation analysis. Besides, we achieve the optimal preparation of the endometrium in this subsequent cycle, which results in a high success rate.[56]

The recent technological advances in preimplantation genetic testing suggest that there will be a wider implementation of PGD or PGS in the future. Technical limitations and mosaicism in the embryonic complex can confuse diagnostic results obtained through PGS or PGD. This poses a risk for which couples need to be appropriately counseled.

Time-Lapse Video Monitoring System for Assessing the Embryos

Recent advances in noninvasive assessment of embryos are the introduction of time-lapse monitoring system. Current method of embryo evaluation relies mainly on static observation of the morphology of the embryos.

These observations are inevitably restricted to specific times; several critical stages in between observations may go unnoticed. Therefore new markers that may add the selection of embryos with higher implantation probabilities are needed.[57,58]

Time-lapse video monitoring uses an IVF incubator with an in-built camera for automated time-lapse imaging of fertilized oocytes in a safe incubation environment beginning from fertilization until the time of transfer. Images of each embryo are automatically recorded at preset time intervals. All observations are performed inside the incubators so the embryos are never exposed to adverse growth conditions or temperatures. By evaluating specific growth patterns and cellular division patterns through these time-lapse camera-equipped incubators, the embryologists are enabled to select the best embryo for uterine transfer.[59,60]

The introduction of time-lapse equipment approved for use on human embryos offers novel clinical opportunities for continuous monitoring of embryos, enabling flexible evaluation of known morphological parameters, and potentially introducing new dynamic markers of viability. By allowing the most viable pre-embryos to be chosen for transfer, the technology will eventually increase the current success rate of infertility treatment.[61,62]

TECHNOLOGIES EVALUATING EMBRYOS: THE "OMICS"

"Omics" comprises of complementary platforms—proteomics, metabolomics, and genomics. Omics technologies including proteomics, metabolomics, and secretomes have already provided evidence that viable embryos possess unique molecular profiles with potential biomarkers that can be used for selection of the viable embryo for uterine transfer for increasing pregnancy rate.[63,64]

Metabolomics

The study of human embryo metabolism and metabolic profiling may also assist in the search for noninvasive methods to distinguish competent embryos in culture. In the early stages embryo requires lactate and pyruvate up to eight cell stage afterward glucose uptake is more from morula to blastocyst stage. Changes in pyruvate and glucose concentration in the culture medium can reflect the energy metabolism of the embryo, although their usefulness as a tool for prediction of embryo viability is not clear.[65]

The end products of embryo metabolism and cellular processes are low molecular weight molecules called metabolites that reflect the efficiency of the processes in response to a variety of nutrient or environmental changes that could represent potential biomarkers of embryo viability.[66]

Amino acids play a vital role during embryo metabolism and various studies have assessed their relationship to embryo viability using high performance liquid chromatography. Amino acids secreted and are taken up by human embryos, during various stages of preimplantation development, correlated to blastocyst development.[67]

One of the most common and widely used spectroscopic techniques for metabolomics is nuclear magnetic resonance spectroscopy.[68] This technology is costly and time consuming. Recently, most have used spectroscopy, especially near infrared spectroscopy which is very simple and less expensive for investigating possible links between the metabolome and embryo viability.[69] Metabolomic platforms have been shown in some studies to predict embryonic implantation potential.[66] It requires randomized trials and need to be confirmed by more studies.

Proteomics

The proteome represents all proteins translated from the specific gene expression products of a cell at a specific time. It is well known that blastocyst morphology could be recognized according to specific protein expression. It is proposed that embryos that are developmentally also possess a unique proteome profile with some of these expressed proteins secreted into surroundings environment. In proteomics (to a large extent also in metabolomics), mass spectrometry, coupled to a various separation techniques, is the key analytical tool, permitting rapid identification and quantization of proteins including low expression proteins.[63,70,71]

However, this application of proteomics is experimental and not yet widely utilized.

Secretome

Secretome refers to the proteins produced and secreted by the developing embryo. Analysis of the embryonic secretome is a noninvasive method suitable for clinical application.[72]

Several studies have shown that existence of soluble factor secreted by human embryo that could impart either or both developmental competence and implantation.

The human embryonic secretome involves targeted analysis of individual proteins and molecules.[72] It requires randomized trials and need to be confirm by more studies.

Genomics

Genomics studies the complete set of genes expression of certain cell types or tissues. The human genome comprises of approximately 25,000 genes. And the nucleotide sequence of all the human chromosomes can be traced to less than 3,00,000 nucleotides. Several studies using diverse microarrays have reported the characterization of transcriptome. Till date, it has been difficult to fully integrate the largest data which is provided by these studies, that assist in selection of best viable embryos for transfer due to numerous technical consideration.[73,74]

Stem Cells

Essentially, stem cells are uncommitted and undifferentiated parent cells of all human cells. Hence they are a part of every individual's biology. They are unique in their capacity to grow indefinitely in culture and renew themselves. They also have the capacity to multiline age differentiation, i.e. they can turn into any human cell type. A variety of stem cells with different origins and differentiation potency is expected to cure numerous degenerative diseases, chronic disease, and acute tissue injuries.[75]

Stem cells are found at all the stages of mammalian development and can be isolated from the embryonic, fetal, and the adult stage of human life.

Embryonic stem cells have the potential to contribute to all types of tissues in the body, i.e. they are pluripotent. Human embryonic stem cells are derived from the inner cell mass of the blastocyst stage embryo produced by IVF and donated after written informed consent. Embryonic stem cells, a powerful tool for developing cell populations, can be used for various clinical therapies. In addition, they have the potential to be genetically engineered giving them enormous therapeutic impact in transplantation medicine.[76]

Fetal stem cells are primitive cells types obtained from fetus, which can give rise to various organs in the body. Hematopoietic stem cells have been isolated from the fetal blood, spleen, liver, and from nonfetal tissue like umbilical cord and placenta. Stem cell enriched cord blood is used as a new therapy for treatment of β-thalassemia, leukemia, sickle cell anemia, and adjunct therapy for aggressive chemotherapy.[75,77]

Adult stem cells are undifferentiated cells, present in the differentiated tissues in the adult. They are found in mature tissues such as bone marrow, blood, skeletal muscle, dental pulp, liver, eye, brain, skin, etc. The adult stem cell can renew itself and can differentiate to yield some or all of the major specialized cell types of the tissue or organ.[75,78,79]

Recent advances in biological provide new avenue for pluripotent stem cells (PSCs) including embryonic stem cells (ESC), induces pluripotent stem cells (iPSC) which directly converted ordinary cells into stem cells, essential resources for the treatment of chronic diseases, drug screening, and cell therapeutics for regenerative medicines.[75,76]

Stem cells transplantation therapies may be possible in the future for various disorders like diabetes, neurodegenerative disorders (Parkinson's disease, muscular dystrophies, and atherosclerosis), spinal cord injury, etc.[79,80]

Controversies are much less about harvesting adult stem cells or collecting stem cells from the bone marrow. Ethics groups object to use of embryonic stem cells because it results in human embryos being destroyed.

Cloning

Cloning is commonly perceived as a means of generating genetically identical individuals, but it can also be used to obtain genetically matched embryo-derived stem cells, which could potentially be used in the treatment of the patient. The concept of cloning has fascinated both, the scientists and the general public, since the birth of Dolly, the sheep in 1996.[81,82]

Reproductive cloning involves transfer of somatic cell nucleus into an enucleated oocytes followed by creation of an embryo which can be transferred to uterus for achieving pregnancy. Therapeutic cloning involves somatic cell nuclear transfer to enucleated oocytes followed by development of embryos, which are used for the derivation of stem cells from the cloned embryo, which are antigenically identical to the donor and can be used in research into potential therapies for treating a wide variety of diseases.[83,84] In this way the stem cells or derived tissue such as neurons, muscle or blood cells would be immunologically identical with the patients and would not be subject to rejection.[85,86] The goal of therapeutic cloning is to produce a healthy copy of a sick person's tissue or organ for transplant. Recently, the researchers announced, creating specific cell lines out of skin cells of two adult men and have achieved first time therapeutic cloning of adult's skin cells.

This new technology heralds a new era of unparalleled advancement as the power to cure infertility. However, this technique has attracted a lot of criticism and much research is needed before it could be used for humans.[87]

CONCLUSION

There have been tremendous advances in the field of ART since the last three decades, particularly in the IVF laboratory. eSET, after selecting the viable embryo, has created the necessity to have an excellent freezing program in almost every IVF laboratory, as surplus embryos are available for embryo freezing. Embryo freezing by vitrification technique increases cumulative pregnancy rates, thus vitrification has pushed the technology to higher levels of clinical efficacy and utilization. Again genetic evaluation of chromosomally normal embryo by PGD and PGS technique including advance microarray technique and development of time-lapse system dramatically increased the IVF success and birth of a healthy child, thereby minimizing multiple pregnancies and associated complications.

Though the initial reports with proteomics and metabolomics seem promising, further prospective randomized control trials are required to prove their true clinical value. However, once their efficacy is proven, it will revolutionize the ART treatment by allowing for a noninvasive way of embryo selection and single embryo transfer. The potential of stem cell to treat the diseases is most exciting. Stem cell potential still requires much more continue research and one day it is going to be a common treatment for degenerative diseases.

REFERENCES

1. First test tube baby born, BBC, 25 July 1978, Retrieved 13 June 2009.
2. Palermo G, Joris H, Devroey P, et al. Pregnancies after intracytoplasmic injection of single spermatozoon into oocyte. Lancet. 1992;340:17-8.
3. Kuwayama M. Highly efficient vitrification for cryopreservation of human oocytes and embryos: the cryotop method. Theriogenology. 2007;67(1):73-80.
4. Petricoin EF, Liotta IA. Clinical application of proteomics. J Nutr. 2003;133:2476S-84S.
5. Botros L, Sakkas D, Seli E. Metabolomics and its application for non-invasive embryo assessment in IVF. Mol Hum Reprod. 2008;14(12):679-90.
6. Berkovitz A, Eltes F, Soffer Y, et al. ART success and in vitro sperm cell selection depend on the ultramorphological status of spermatozoa. Androlgia. 1999;31:1-8.
7. Tesarik J. Paternal effects on cell division in the human preimplantation embryo. Reprod Biomed Online. 2005; 10:370-5 .
8. Tesarik J, Greco E, Mendoza C. L late, but not early, paternal effect on human embryonic development is related to sperm DNA fragmentation. Hum Reprod. 2004;19:611-5.
9. Bartoov B, Berkovitz A, Eltes F, et al. Real-time fine morphology of motile sperm cells is associated with IVF-ICSI outcome. J Andro. 2002;23:1-8.
10. Bartoov B, Berkovitz A, Eltes F, et al. Pregnancy rates are higher with intracytoplasmic morphologically sperm injection than with conventional intracytoplasmic sperm injection. Fertil Steril. 2003;80:1413-9.
11. Balaban B, Yakin K, Alatas C, et al. Intracytoplasmic morphologically selected sperm injection: a prospective randomized trial. Reprod Biomed Online. 2008;16:835-41.
12. Cohen J, Elsner C, Kort H, et al. Impairment of the hatching process following IVF in the human improvement of implantation by assisted hatching using micromanipulation. Hum Repord. 1990;(1):7-13.
13. Tucker MJ, Cohen J, Massey JB, et al. Partial dissection of the zona pellucida of frozen thawed human embryos may enhance blastocyst hatching, implantation and pregnancies. Am J Obset Gynecol. 1991;165(2):341-4; discussion 344-5.
14. Antinori S, Panci C, Selman HA, et al. Zona thinning with the use of laser: a new approach to assisted hatching in humans. Hum Reprod. 1996;11(3):590-4.
15. Montag M, van der Ven K, Delacretaz G, et al. Laser-assisted microdissection of the zona pellucida facilitates polar body biopsy. Fertil Steril. 1998;69(3):539-42.
16. Phophong P, Doshi A, Harper JC. Comparison of embryonic development in cleavage stage mouse embryo biopsy between acid Tyrode's solution and laser assisted techniques. J Med Assoc Thai. 2001;84(8):1190-98.
17. Cohen J, Alikani M, Trowbridge J, et al. Implantation enhancement by selective assisted hatching using zona drilling of human embryos with poor prognosis. Hum Reprod. 1992;7(5):685-91.
18. Oldenbourg R, Mei G. New polarized light microscope with precision universal compensator J Microsc. 1995;180(Pt2):140-7.
19. Oldenbourg R. A new view on polarized microscopy. Nature. 1996;381(6585):811-2.
20. Liu L, Trimarchi JR, Oldenbourg R, et al. Increased birefringence in the meiotic spindle provides a new marker for the onset of activation in living human oocytes. Biol Reprod. 2000;63(1):251-8.
21. Keefe D, Tran P, Pellegrini C, et al. Polarized light microscopy and digital image processing identify a multilaminar structure of the hamster zona pellucida. Hum Reprod. 1997;12(6): 1250-2.
22. Gianaroli L, Magli MC, Ferraretti AP, et al. Birefringence characteristics in sperm heads allow for the selection of reacted spermatozoa for ICSI. Fertil Steril. 2010;93(3): 808-13.
23. Montag M, van der Ven H. Symposium: innovative techniques in human embryo viability assessment. Oocyte assessment

and embryo viability, prediction: birefringence imaging. Reprod Biomed Online. 2008;17(4):454-60.
24. Gardner DK, Lane M. Towards a single embryo transfer. Reprod Biomed Online 2003;6(4):470-81.
25. Balabain B, Urman B. Comparison of two sequential media for culturing cleavage-stage embryos and blastocysts: embryo characteristics and clinical outcome. Reprod Biomed Online. 2005;10(4):485-91.
26. Guerif F, Bidault R, Gasnier O, et al. Efficacy of blastocyst transfer after implantation failure. Reprod Biomed Online. 2004;9(6):630-6.
27. Russell JB, Knezevich KM, Fabian KF, et al. Unstimulated immature oocyte retrieval: early versus midfollicular endometrial priming. Fertil Steril. 1997;67(4):616-20.
28. Trounson A, Wood C, Kausche A. In vitro maturation and the fertilization and developmental competence of oocytes recovered from untreated polycystic ovarian patients. Fertil Steril. 1994;62(2):353-62.
29. Cha KY, Koo JJ, Ko JJ, et al. Pregnancy after in vitro fertilization of human follicular oocytes collected from nonstimulated cycles, their culture in vitro and their transfer in a donor oocyte program. Fertil Steril. 1991;55(1):109-13.
30. Buckett WM, Chain RC, Dean NL, et al. Pregnancy loss in pregnancies conceived after in vitro oocyte maturation, conventional in vitro fertilization, and intracytoplasmic sperm injection. Fertil Steril. 2008;90(3):546-50.
31. Trounson A, Mohr L. Human pregnancy following cryopreservation, thawing and transfer of an eight cell embryo. Nature. 1983;305:707.
32. Vajta G, Nagy ZP. Are programmable freezers still needed in the embryo laboratory? Review on vitrification. Reprod Biomed Online. 2006;12(6):779-96.
33. Kuwanama M. Highly efficient vitrification for cryopreservation of human oocytes and embryos: the cryotop method. Theriogenology. 2007;67:73-80.
34. Kuwayama M, Cobo A, Vajita G. Vitrification of oocytes: general considerations and the use of the cryotop method. In: Tucker MJ, Liebermann J (Eds). Vitrification in Assisted Reproduction. London: Informa Healthcare; 2007.
35. Craft I, Djahanbakhch O, McLeod F, et al. Human pregnancy following oocyte and sperm transfer to the uterus. Lancet. 1982;1(8280):1031-3.
36. Kuleshova L, Gianaroli L, Magli C, et al. Birth following vitrification of a small number of human oocytes: Case Report. Hum Reprod. 1999;14(12):3077-9.
37. Seki S, Mazur P. Ultra-rapid warming yields high survival of mouse oocytes cooled to-196^{0}C in dilutions of a standard vitrification solution. PLoS One. 2012;7(4):1-12.
38. Rao GD, Chian RC, Son WS, et al. Fertility preservation in women undergoing cancer treatment. Lancet. 2004; 363(9423):1829-30.
39. Oktay K, Karlikaya G. Ovarian function after transplantation of frozen, banked autologous ovarian tissue. N Engl J Med. 2000;342(25):1919.
40. Donnez J, Dolmans MM, Demyle D, et al. Rebirth after orthotopic transplantation of cryopreserved ovarian tissue. Lancet. 2004;364(9443):1405-10.
41. Bedaiwy MA, El-Nashar SA, El Saman AM, et al. Reproductive outcome after transplantation of ovarian tissue: a systematic review. Hum Reprod. 2008;23(12):2709-17.
42. Porcu E, Venturoli S, Damino G, et al. Healthy twins delivered after oocyte cryopreservation and bilateral ovariectomy for ovarian cancer. Reprod Biomed Online. 2008;17(2):265-7.
43. Imhof M, Bergmeister H, Lipovac M, et al. Orthotopic microvascular reanastomosis of whole cryopreserved ovine ovaries resulting in pregnancy and live birth. Fertil Steril. 2006;85(Suppl 1):1208-15.
44. Grifo JA, Boyle A, Fischer E, et al. Pre-embryo biopsy and analysis of blastomeres by in situ hybridization. Am J Obstet Gynecol. 1990;163(6 pt 1):2013-9.
45. Boada M, Carrera M, De La Iglesia C, et al. Successful use of a laser for human embryo biopsy in preimplantation genetic diagnosis: report of two cases. J Assist Reprod Genet. 1998;15:302-7.
46. Veiga A, Sandalinas M, Benkhalifa M, et al. Laser blastocyst biopsy for preimplantation diagnosis in the human. Zygote. 1997;5:351-4.
47. De Boer K, McArthur S, Murray C, et al. First live birth following blastocyst biopsy and PGD analysis. Reprod Biomed Online. 2002;4:35.
48. Kokkali G, Vrettou C, Traeger-Synodinos J, et al. Birth of a healthy following trophectoderm biopsy from blastocysts for PGD of beta-thalassaemia major. Hum Reprod. 2005;20(7):1855-9.
49. Handyside AH, Lesko LG, Tarin JJ, et al. Birth of normal girl after in vitro fertilization and preimplantation diagnostic testing for cystic fibrosis. N Engl J Med. 1992;327:905-8.
50. Munne S, Alikani M, Tomkin G, et al. Embryo morphology, developmental rates and maternal age are correlated with chromosome abnormalities. Fertil Steril 1995;64:382-91.
51. Wilding M, Forman R, Hogewind G, et al. Preimplantation genetic diagnosis for the treatment of failed in vitro fertilization-embryo transfer and habitual abortion. Fertil Steril. 2004;81(5):1302-7.
52. Gianaroli L, Magli MC, Ferraretti AP, et al. The role of preimplantation diagnosis for aneuploidies. Reprod Biomed Online. 2002;4(Suppl 3):31-6.
53. Munne S, Grifo J, Cohen J. Chromosome abnormalities in human arrested preimplantation embryos: A multiple probe FISH study. Am J Hum Genet. 1994;55:150-9.
54. Navidi W, Arnheim N. Using PCR in preimplantation genetic diagnosis. Hum Reprod. 1991;6:836-49.
55. Demko Z, Rabinowitz M, Johnson D. "Current Methods for Preimplantation Genetic Diagnosis". J Clin Embryol. 2010;13(1):6-12.
56. McArthur SJ, Leigh D, Marshall JT, et al. Pregnancies and live births after trophectoderm biopsy and preimplantation genetic testing of human blastocysts. Fertil Steril. 2005; 84(6):1628-36.
57. Kirkegaard K, Agerholm IE, Ingerslev HJ. Time-lapse monitoring as a tool for clinical embryo assessment. Hum Reprod. 2012;27(5):1277-85.
58. Wong CC, Loewke KE, Bossert NL, et al. Noninvasive imaging of human embryos before embryonic genome activation

predicts development to the blastocyst stage. Nat Biotechnol. 2010;28:1115-21.
59. Mio Y, Maeda K. Time-lapse cinematography of dynamic changes occurring during in vitro development of human embryos. Am J Obstet Gynecol. 2008;199(6):660, el-5.
60. Meseguer M, Rubio I, Cruz M, et al. Embryo incubation and selection in a time-lapse monitoring system improves pregnancy outcome compared with a standard incubator: a retrospective cohort study. Fertil Steril. 2012;98:1481-9.
61. Cruz M, Gadea B, Garrido N, et al. Ebmryo quality, blastocyst and ongoing pregnancy rates in oocyte donation patients whose embryos were monitored by time-lapse imaging. J Assist Reprod Genet. 2011;28(7):569-73.
62. Meseguer M, Hilligsoe KM, Pedersen KS, et al. Pregnancy rates after incubation in new time-lapse incubator (Embryoscope) providing detailed information about embryo development compared to incubation in a standard incubator. Fertil Steril. 2010;94(r suppl):S150.
63. Petricoin EF, Liotta LA. Clinical applications of proteomics. J Nutr. 2003;133:2476S-84S.
64. Botros L, Denny S, Emre S. Metabolomics and its applicable for non-invasive embryo assessment in IVF. Mol Hum Reprod. 2008;14(12):679-90.
65. Gott AF, Hardy K, Winston RM, et al. Noninvasive measurement of pyruvate and glucose uptake and lactate production by single human preimplantation embryos. Hum Reprod. 1990;5:104-8.
66. Singh R, Sinclair KD. Metabolomics: approach to assessing oocyte and embryo quality. Theriogenology. 2007;68 Suppl 1:S56-62.
67. Houghton FD, Hawkhead JA, Humpherson PG, et al. Noninvasive amino acid turnover predicts human embryo developmental capacity. Hum Reprod. 2002;17:999-1005.
68. Seli E, Botros L, Sakkas D, et al. Noninvasive metabolomic profiling of embryo culture media using proton nuclear magnetic resonance correlates with reproductive potential of embryos in women undergoing in vitro fertilization. Fertil Steril. 2008:90:2183-9.
69. Seli E, Sakkas D, Scott R, et al. Non-Invasive metabolomic profiling of human embryo culture media using Raman and near infrared spectroscopy correlates with reproductive potential of embryos in women undergoing in vitro fertilization. Fertil Steril. 2007;88:1350-7.
70. Dettmer K, Aronov PA, Hammock BD. Mass spectrometry-based metabolomics. Mass Spectrom Rev. 2007;26:51-78.
71. Pasikanti KK, Ho PC, Chan EC. Mass spectrometry in metabolic profiling of biological fluids. J Chromatogr B Analyt Technol Biomed Life Sci. 2008;871:202-11.
72. Katz-Jaffe MG, Schoolcraft WB, Gardner DK. Analysis of protein expression (secretome) by human and mouse preimplantation embyos. Fertil Steril. 2006;86:678-85.
73. Kimber SJ, Sneddon SF, Bloor DJ, et al. Expression of genes involved in early cell fate decisions in human embryos and their regulation by growth factors. Reproduction. 2008;135:635-47.
74. Ajjaye J. Whole genome approaches for large scale gene identification and expression analysis in mammalian preimplantation embryos. Reprod Fertil Dev. 2005;17:37-45.
75. Lavoir MC, Conghan J, Pedersen RA. Culture of human embryos for studies on the derivation of human pluripotent cells: A preliminary investigation. Reprod Fertil Dev. 1998;10(7-8):557-61.
76. Thomson JA, Itskovitz-Eldor J, Shapiro SS, et al. Embryonic stem cell lines derived from human blastocysts. Science. 1998;6:282(5391):1145-7.
77. Brustle O, Choudhary K, Karram K, et al. Chimeric brains generated by intraventricular transplantation of fetal human brain cells into embryonic rats. Nat Biotechnol. 1998;16(aa):1040-44.
78. Chiu RC. Bone-marrow stem cells as a source for cell therapy. Heart Fail Rev. 2003;8(3):247-51.
79. Reubinoff BE, Itsykson P, Turetsky T, et al. Neural Progenitors from human embryonic stem cells. Nat Biotechnol. 2001;19(12):1134-40.
80. Assady S, Maor G, Amit M, et al. Insulin production by human embryonic stem cells. Diabetes 2001;50(8):1691-97.
81. Brem G, Kiihholzer B. The recent history of somatic cloning in mammals. Cloning Stem Cells. 2002;4:57-63.
82. Campbell KH, McWhir J, Ritchie WA, et al. Sheep cloned by nuclear transfer from a cultured cell line. Nature. 1996;380: 64-6.
83. Kono T, Sotomaru Y, Sato Y, et al. Development of androgenetic mouse embryos produced by in vitro fertilization of enucleated oocytes. Mol Reprod Dev. 1993;34:43-6.
84. Holden C. Cloning. Carbon-copy clone is the real thing Science. 2002;295:1443-4.
85. Illmensee K, Levanduski M, Vidali A, et al. Human embryo twinning with applications in reproductive medicine. Fertil Steril. 2010;93:423-7.
86. Sung Ly, Chang CC, Amano T, et al. Efficient derivation of embryonic stem cells from nuclear transfer and parthenogenetic embryos derived from cryopreserved oocytes. Cell Reprogram. 2010;12:203-11.
87. de Wert GM, Geraedts JP. Cloning: Applications in humans II. Ethical considerations. Ned Tijdschr Geneeskd. 2000;144: 926-31.

Troubleshooting in the IVF Laboratory

51

Keshav Malhotra, Gaurav Majumdar

INTRODUCTION

Every once in a while things do start going south in the in vitro fertilization (IVF) laboratory and if we are not proactive then the results can be disastrous. Most of us believe that everything we do is right and this mindset is the one which can lead to more errors. There are basically three approaches to deal with problems: *remedial*—where we alleviate the symptoms; *corrective*—where we prevent recurrence; and *prevention*—where we prevent occurrence. Thus, being proactive in our approach is the best way to prevent any kind of mishap. But when should one initiate troubleshooting response. The key performance indicators (KPIs) in the laboratory help decide that. Each identifiable process can be monitored, but this would result in a very large set of KPIs. Thus, we need to identify a practical list of critical KPIs that will provide an adequate overview of the most important steps **(Table 1)**.[1]

CULTURE CONDITIONS

Most of the times poor outcomes in the form of poor fertilization, blastulation, and even pregnancy losses, are attributed to poor culture conditions. The culture media is the life support of the embryo. The media these days are designed in such a way that they not only suit embryo development but look after the growth of the developing embryo all throughout. Thus with the advent of newer media, blastulation rate has definitely increased[2] in the laboratory and more clinics are now confident in doing blastocyst transfers for their patients. So, if we were supplied with a good culture media and the media are quality tested, why do we still blame the culture media and culture conditions for our outcomes? The answer to this is very simple, even though we order a quality product, the way it is dealt with during transport or storage and even during use, determines how effective it will be in providing the best outcomes. As far as culture media are concerned, the two most important parameters are pH and osmolality.[2,3]

To ensure a stable pH and osmolality, please check **(Fig. 1)**:

- Whether the media was supplied with cold chain in place.
- Whether it was stored in the proper environment.
- Check the time taken to make the dishes as increased time can lead to evaporation of media especially from micro droplets.
- Check whether the CO_2 levels of the incubators are calibrated and set according to the media requirement.
- The number of door openings of the incubators and exposure of dishes should be restricted while the dishes are in use.

When in doubt about culture conditions, a simple pH test using a pH meter (not the pH strips) and the osmolality using the osmometer can be checked. If in doubt about the incubators, a dummy sigh with pH probes can be installed into the incubator for live readings.

TEMPERATURE

Temperature control for oocytes is crucial. Meiotic spindles are highly sensitive to temperature fluctuations. Abnormal spindles may result in aneuploidy, disruption of embryo development, and implantation; decreased pregnancy rates, thus making temperature control one of the most crucial elements in laboratory quality assurance. One of

Table 1: Key performance indicators (KPIs) in the in vitro fertilization (IVF) clinic.[1]

	IVF	*ICSI*
Laboratory	% mature COCs at OPU	% (mature) MIIs after stripping
	Fertilization rate (≥ 2 PNs)	Damage rate during ICSI
	Normal fertilization rate (2 PNs)	Degeneration rate on Day 1
	Low or failed fertilization rate	Normal fertilization rate (2PNs)
	Zygote cleavage rate	Zygote cleavage rate
	Day 2 embryo development rate (assess at 44 ± 1 hour)	
	Day 3 embryo development rate (assess at 68 ± 1 hour)	
	% good or better embryos on Day 3	
	Day 5 blastocyst development rate (assess at 116 ± 2 hour)	
	Utilization rate (embryos suitable for ET or cryopreservation)	
Clinic	Positive pregnancy test (+ve β-hCG)	
	Implantation rate per embryo transferred	
	Clinical pregnancy rate (fetal heart per ET)	
	Parameter	***Value to trigger action***
	Implantation rates	< 18%
	Clinical Pregnancy rate	>28%
	Biochemical rate	>10%
	Fertilization rates	<60%
	Cleavage rates	<85%
	Damage rate	>15%

(COCs: cumulus-oocyte complexes; ET: embryo transfer; hCG: human chorionic gonadotropin; ICSI: intracytoplasmic sperm injection; OPU: oocyte pick-up; PN: polar nuclei)

Developmental Stage:	pH Range—Lower	pH Range—Higher
Fertilization	7.3	7.4
Cleavage Stage	7.2	7.3
Blastocyst	7.3	7.4

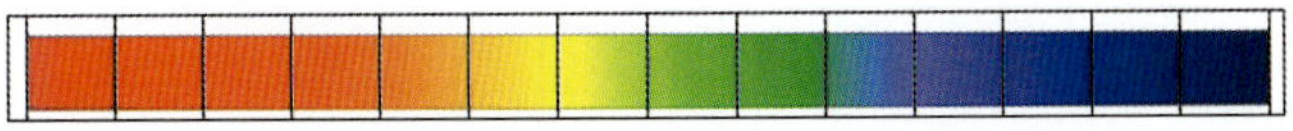

Fig. 1: pH requirements at different stages of development.[3]

the most crucial areas where temperature loss can occur is the incubator. Conventional box incubators have been researched in detail and studies have reported wide variations that occur in the incubator even when it is closed. When the lid is opened the temperature drops further and recovery time can be quite a tricky situation to handle when the number of cases being done in the laboratory are high and the equipment is not adequate enough to support it. Large incubators with multiple door openings will affect temperature—recovery may take up to 30 min. Increased door openings—temperature loss—increased miscarriage rates **(Fig. 2)**.[4,5]

Another place where temperature fluctuations are quite common is the micro-manipulator. Studies conducted by Cambridge IVF[6] have shown that there is quite significant temperature loss which occurs during intracytoplasmic sperm injection (ICSI) if caution is not observed. Spindle imaging has shown that when ICSI is done on a stage without the objective heater, the spindle was only observed 61.4% of the times and clinical pregnancy rates were significantly different from the eggs which were injected over an objective heater. They also compared outcomes from various heating stages available, i.e. the heated stage with aperture, the heated glass stage, and the heated stage with aperture and an air warming system **(Figs. 3 and 4)**.

It was observed that the stage with the air warming system had the most stable temperature and thus it may be concluded that this system is more suited for manipulation. Still further studies are needed to come to a definitive conclusion.[6]

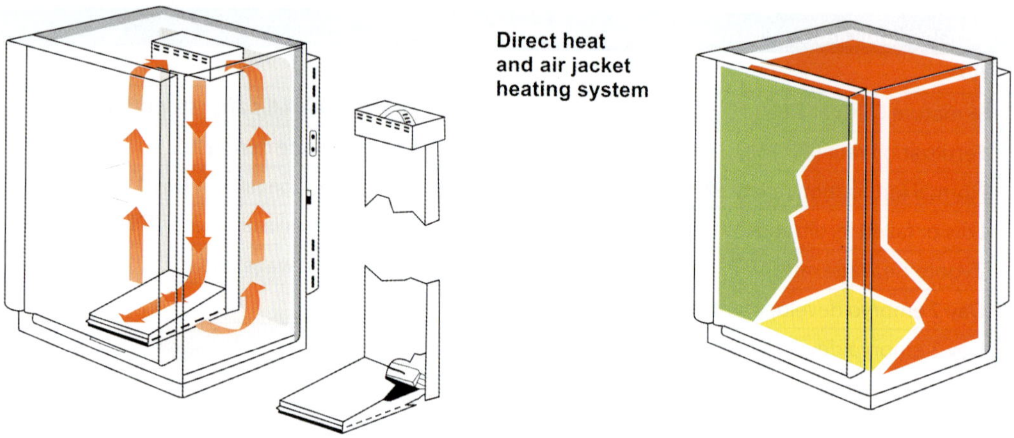

Fig. 2: Temperature fluctuations in a box incubator.

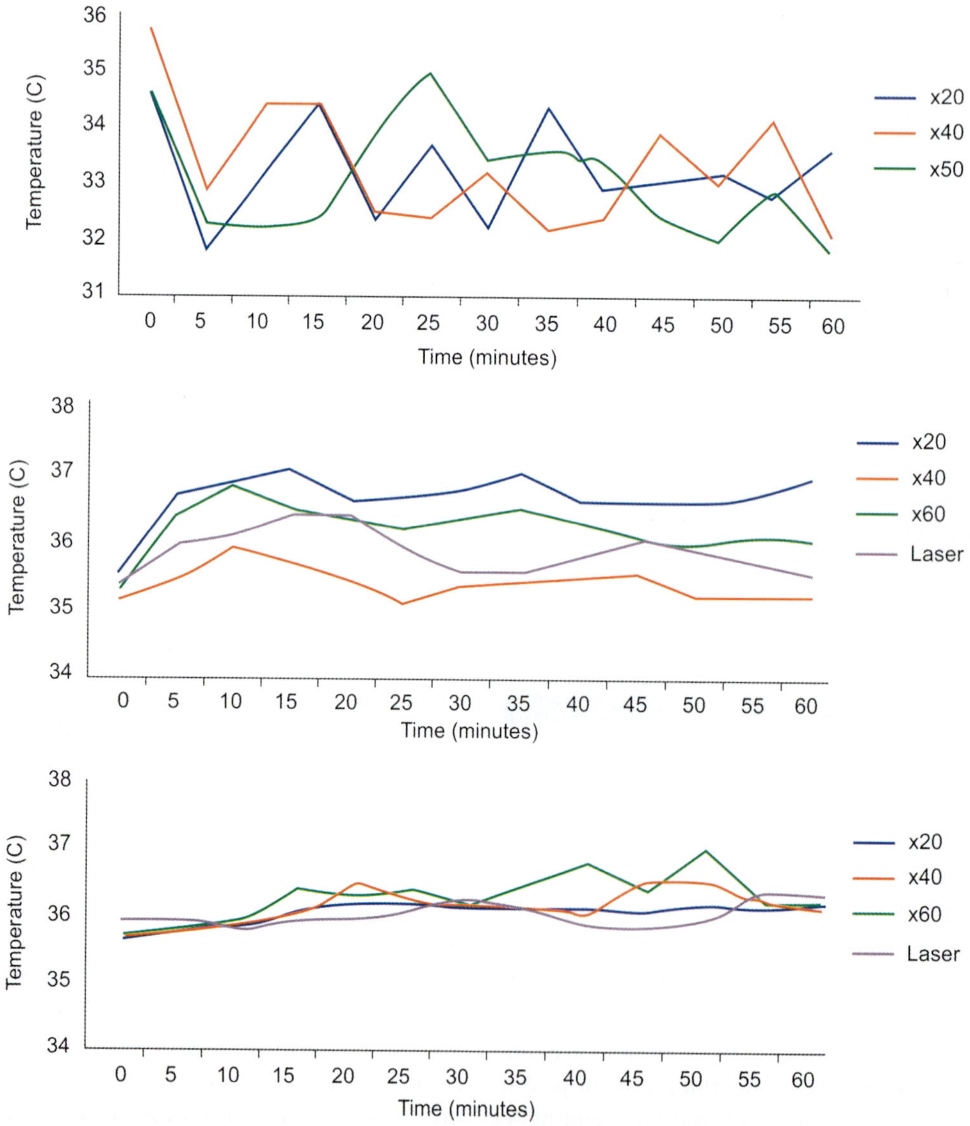

Fig. 3: Temperature fluctuations in different intracytoplasmic sperm injection (ICSI) manipulators.

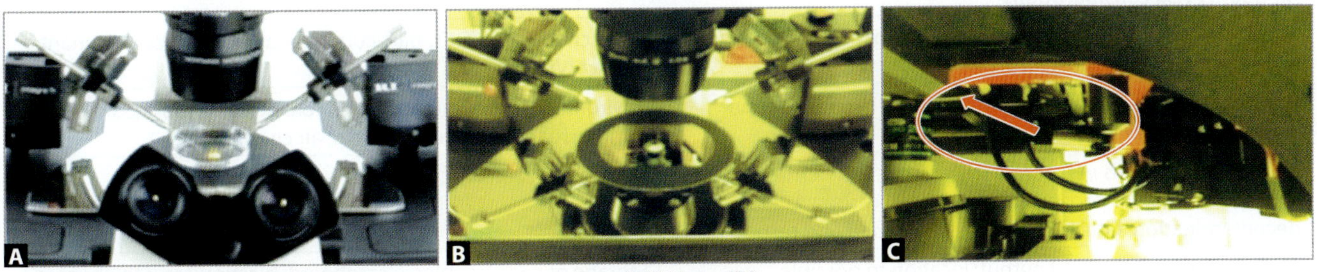

Figs. 4A to C: Different types of heated stages in an intracytoplasmic sperm injection (ICSI) manipulator.

INFECTION CONTROL

One of the major worries of any assisted reproductive technology (ART) laboratory is the risk of contamination and the transmission of infections within the laboratory. While most patients are screened for common communicable diseases like human immunodeficiency virus (HIV), hepatitis B, hepatitis C, venereal disease research laboratory (VDRL), and chlamydia, there is still a possibility that some diseases might go unnoticed. Thus, it becomes imperative for the staff to handle the gametes and body fluids taking all necessary precautions. It is also very important to have policies and standard operating procedure (SOPs) in place to handle infectious patients. Apart from the transmission of infection, another thing that worries laboratory directors is the contamination of dishes and even the equipment. As once contamination happens, it becomes very difficult to salvage that cycle. Therefore all sterile precautions in handling are absolutely necessary. Semen preparation, especially for infected samples by density gradient centrifugation, using sterile consumables, etc. are some of the ways in which a laboratory can prevent contamination.[7]

How to Implement Infection Control?

- Restrict entry in the laboratory.
- Positive pressure and high efficiency particulate air (HEPA) filters in the laboratory.
- Ensure ambient temperature 23–27°C with relative humidity 35–50%.
- Walls and floors to be made of materials which can be easily cleaned.
- All procedures to be done under the laminar hood.
- Regular replacements of laminar HEPA filters.
- Quarterly sterilization of incubators.
- Monthly cultures and colony forming unit (CFU) counts of the laboratory and equipment.
- Segregation of infected samples especially during cryopreservation.

Air Quality in the Laboratory

Air quality in the clinical embryology laboratory is one of the most crucial things[8] that determine the success of the laboratory. Both murine and human models have showed the association between the quality of air and the effect on embryo development, the negative effects of which have very well been established by numerous studies. However in our country, this parameter is mostly overlooked, and there is no regulatory authority that verifies the compliance of embryology laboratories with the standards of minimum care that have been mentioned in most international directives.[9] Richard Legro et al. (2010) noted the effects of declining air quality on reproductive outcomes after IVF are variable but increased nitrogen dioxide (NO_2) is consistently associated with lower live birth rates. Fine particulate matter ($PM_{2.5}$) in the IVF laboratory during embryo culture was associated with decreased conception rates. U.S. Environmental Protection Agency (US EPA) considers significant risk to humans and fertility following exposure to certain chemicals, volatile organic compounds (VOCs), and particulate matter. Sandro Esteves et al. suggested that particles between 0.1 µm and 10 µm are of interest in IVF laboratories. It is accepted that particles of 0.3 µm or larger should be targeted for particulate contamination control in ART as bacteria and other contaminants can attach to particles. Some considerations in regards to air quality are mentioned in **Table 2**.

Table 2: Air quality considerations.

Air quality risk considerations	
Age of laboratory—off gassing of equipment and construction materials	What chemicals, VOCs, particulates and microbial contaminants impact IVF outcomes?
Construction of laboratory—materials used in construction	Environmental pollution levels—coal burning; biomass burn off; mining; roads; freeways; heating; air conditioning
Air filtration systems in place—HEPA, potassium permanganate; activated carbon or coconut shell activated carbon; UV decontamination; filter replacement; validation and testing	Proximity to construction work—paints and glues; dust
Air flow ducts—input and output; location to possible contaminants	Storage of consumables—cardboard; plastic ware (Ethyibenzene and benzaldehyde); plasticizers (Phthalates)
Fragrances and cosmetics—may contain sodium, magnesium, silicon calcium, potassium or iron and may emit VOC	Cleaning products—alcohols; ammonia based; chemical composition
Disposable products utilized in laboratory—Styrene off gassing	Levels of halocarbons (isoflurane); In anesthesia—proximity to anesthetic gases
Air filtration systems in equipment	Air pressure of laboratory
Humidity, pressure and room temperature	Number of people in laboratory
Protective clothing and foot wear—tint and shedding	Benzene levels in CO_2 cylinders; in line gas filtes; cleaning of cylinders

Courtesy: Dr Adrian Pope/Pope consultancy.

Consumables

Each and every consumable that is intended to be used in an ART laboratory or will in any way come in contact with gametes/embryos must be certified as non-toxic. There are numerous instances which have been mentioned in various forums about how cheaper products have led to poorer outcomes and for an embryologist working in any ART setup it is of utmost importance to maintain quality and standards in the laboratory so that patient care is not compromised. There are a number of ways one can check for quality check (QC) standards for their consumables. Look for a Conformité Europèene (CE) certification on the product. CE is one of the most accepted certifications for any IVF product be it consumables or even media and it is one of the standards that most European clinics have to maintain and most manufacturers who want to sell in Europe have to ensure. Other things to look for are tests like sperm survival test or the mouse embryo assay.[1,2,6]

- Consumables should be CE certified for the purpose of IVF.
- Should be tested on mouse embryos and endotoxin free.
- Should have a quality control document in place.
- All seals and packagings should be checked before use.
- Each laboratory should have their own acceptance criteria and quality policy for their clinic.

The quality gadgets do not just cover the ART laboratory but also extend to the supplies department. The most important aspect in supply management is ensuring that cold chain is maintained throughout. Most companies nowadays supply data logging devices which help us in ensuring that quality products are delivered to our laboratories without fail.

TROUBLESHOOTING IN PROCEDURES

Intracytoplasmic Sperm Injection

Micromanipulation should be done in a stress-free environment with full focus on the work that is to be done. Ideally the ICSI station should be located in a silent area which is free from any vibrations and away from the hustle bustle of the lab. Antivibration tables and ergonomic seats can be bought for the comfort of the embryologist. Always ensure that critical parts are included in the machine like certain lenses, heating plates, etc. It is always beneficial to set up an annual maintenance contract with your service provider so that regular maintenance of the equipment is looked after.

It is very important to understand each and every part of the machine and how to assemble and dismantle if needed. Most of the emergencies which arise during ICSI are due to parts not working properly and most of these can be fixed by the in-house embryologist if he/she has a clear understanding of the parts and the mechanisms behind each, but there will be certain situations where the problem is not in the hands of the embryologist; therefore,

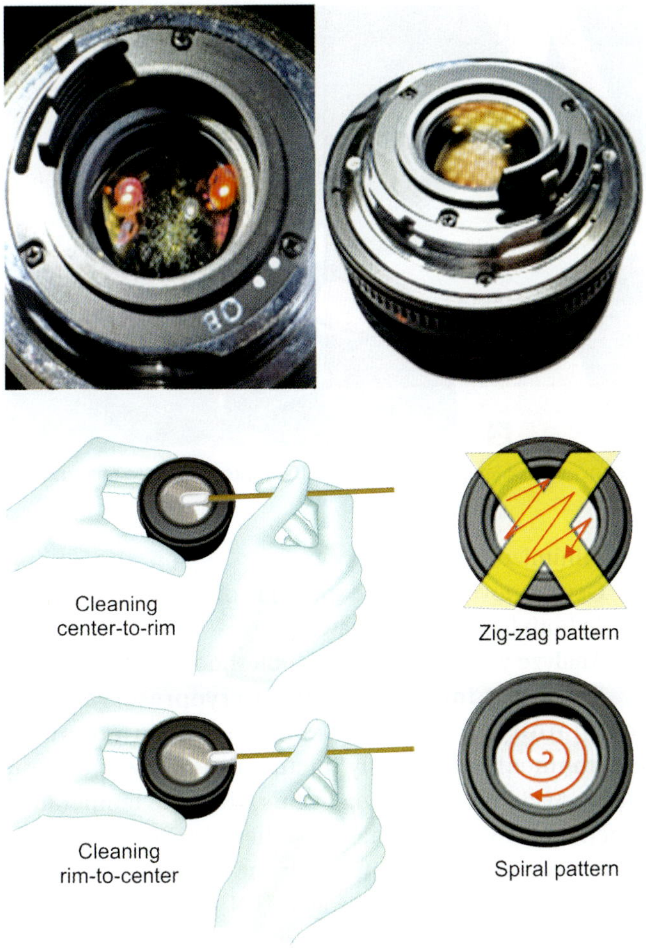

Fig. 5: Cleaning technique for intracytoplasmic sperm injection (ICSI) optics.

it is important to have a good understanding between service engineers for emergency visits also having spares for tubings, etc. can be beneficial in the long run.[1,2,6,9,10]

Optics

The micromanipulator machine has four major lenses 4X, 10X, 20X, and 40X and a laser lens if the center has one. For easier working, try and install the lenses sequentially so that you have a good ergonomic flow. Height adjustment and eyepiece adjustment are critical and differ from embryologist to embryologist. One of the major problems which embryologists face during ICSI is poor visualization and the most common cause for this is dirty optics. There can be dirt accumulation or fungal growth as shown in the **Figure 5**. These lenses can be cleaned in house using lens cleaning solutions but it is important to take precautions while cleaning as there is a chance of scratching the lens which can further deteriorate the vision.

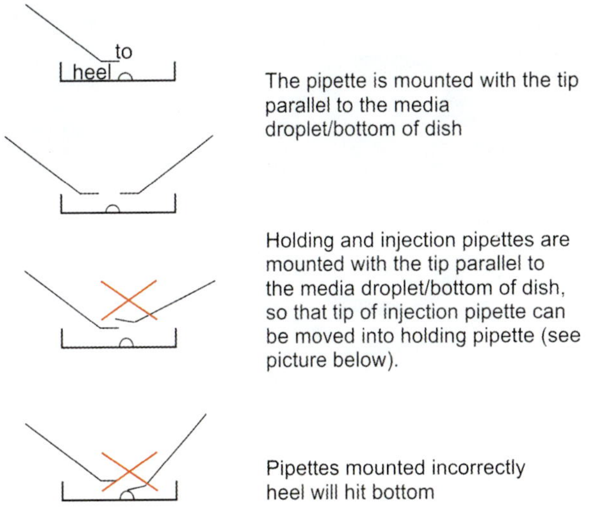

Fig. 6

Other common problem one has with ICSI is an increased degeneration rate especially for beginners. The most common reason for oocyte degeneration is improper alignment. The micromanipulation pipettes should be parallel to the surface so that once you inject the egg, the breach that is created is minimum and the chance of degeneration is the least. Another thing that disturbs the alignment if not done properly is the sperm immobilization. The injection technique itself is very important when ensuring better results.

Common causes of poor fertilization/no fertilization:

- Sperm did not penetrate the membrane.
- No sperm chromatin decondensation.
- Inherent patient factor.
- Check exposure time for oocytes during ICSI.

Air bubbles in the tubing/syringe can cause trouble in maintaining the pressure in the micropipettes **(Fig. 6)**.

Intracytoplasmic Sperm Injection Summary

- Dish should be prepared on the laminar with temperature switched off and flow switched off. This prevents evaporation of the microdroplets and ensures a stable droplet for ICSI.
- Do not incubate the dishes containing HEPES buffer unless the lid is tightly sealed.
- Do not overload the dish with a higher number of oocytes, time the micromanipulation for better consistent results.
- Always align the pipette according to the angle provided by the manufacturers; most pipettes have a 30–35° angle, so try and match that.

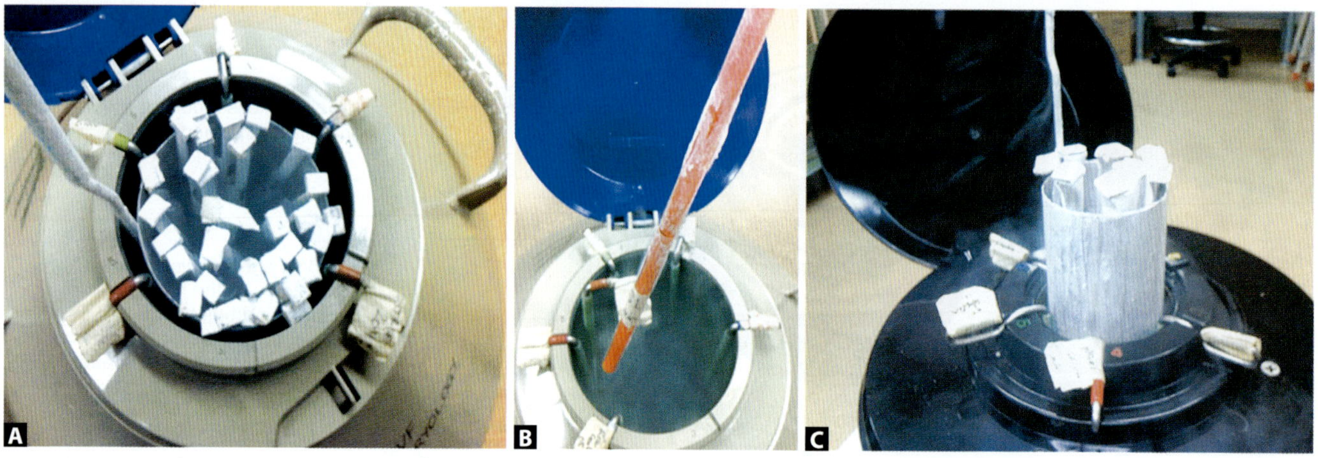

Figs.7A to C: (A) Correct way to identify the goblets to be taken out; (B) Improper way of labeling the goblets; (C) Improper way to taking of the goblets for thawing.

- If the pipette is stuck, try and check the lumen of the holder for any debris or broken glass.
- Ergonomics is very important so a chair with a good lumbar support is advisable.
- Center the manipulators before starting as if the range of movements is at its limit. The adjusting during the manipulation can lead exposing the gametes to sub-optimal conditions for a longer duration.
- If you are having difficulty in slashing the tail, check the focus and alignment.
- A properly slashed sperm should not retain motility, and an embryologist should not inject a motile sperm into an egg as the tail can disrupt the cytoplasm.
- Injection on the sperm into the oocyte should create a furrow, in some cases oocytes may be fragile so furrow may not be present, in other cases it can be due to improper alignment.
- Injecting the sperm head first is preferable.
- Polar body positioning at 6 or 12 o'clock is preferred to avoid spindle damage.
- Once injected, the oocytes should be shifted to fertilization media as soon as possible.

Cryopreservation (Figs. 7A to C)

We are in the age of vitrification, and with so many embryos being frozen, if care and attention is not given to this, it is a sure shot recipe to disaster.

Most embryologists are proficient in vitrification, but for the beginners some recommended tips are:

- Follow the protocol.
- Use the device and medium of your choice.
- Allow embryos/eggs to shrink and then expand completely.
- Minimize stress and aging.
- Gentle movements and speed are of utmost importance in both freezing and thawing.
- Analyze your results and troubleshoot.

The most important step in cryopreservation is maintaining those eggs/embryos in an adequate environment without any fluctuations and without any stress. Accidental warming occurs when the temperature reaches –12°C.[11] The main risk here is warming of the embryos which can be fatal for the embryos. The main culprits are low liquid nitrogen (LN_2) levels in the tank and lifting canister or cane above the neck. Good alarm systems or quality procedure in place can avoid incidents like accidental warming.

Tips to avoid maintenance issues with cryotanks:

- Check levels of the canisters regularly.
- Top-up the canisters regularly and maintain a control document so that it is done without fail.
- Alarm systems can be installed in the cans itself so as to avoid mishaps.
- Automatic filling mechanisms can also be installed to avoid manual labor.
- Handle the cans with utmost care as the cryocans are fragile.
- Even with all precautions, mechanical failure can still occur; therefore, consents covering the risk of mechanical failure to be taken from patients.

HOW TO CARRY OUT A TROUBLESHOOTING EXERCISE?

A troubleshooting exercise should be initiated when any of the parameters as mentioned in **Table 1** are below the average rates. The first thing to do in such a scenario is to segregate the good prognosis cases. These can be your patients who are young, first IVF cycles, tubal factor, normal semen parameters, good reserve, 10–12 oocytes collected, grade 1 embryos transferred, normal endometrial thickness.

Once the data for this subset is created, compare the rates in this group *which is number of* oocytes collected from follicles greater than 11 mm in size, maturity of the oocytes, fertilization rates, embryo development rates, clinical pregnancy rates, miscarriage rates, live birth rate, utilization rate, etc.[1,2,13]

If found skewed, try and control as many variables as possible for a few subsequent cases.

- Ensure lot numbers are recorded to eliminate any fluctuations in variables:
- Drug batches and expiry dates
- Culture medium
- Oil
- Culture dishes
- Oocyte pick-up (OPU) needles
- ET catheters
- Test tubes
- Pipettes
- Ovarian hyperstimulation protocols.
- Measure temperatures—try and map the fluctuations in temperature right from the oocyte collection to embryo transfer to see if any undesired extra exposure is being made.
- Ensure cold chain is maintained.
- Check the temperature fluctuations of the incubators and all heated surfaces using a thermocouple in culture medium drop under oil.
- pH can be checked using a pH meter.
- Osmolality can be checked using an osmometer.
- Assess any air quality issues should be checked and corrected things to look at are particulate matter and VOCs.
- Timing of procedures according to the guidelines.
- Embryotoxic products to be avoided especially alcohol.
- Validation, calibration, and servicing of equipment to be done.
- HEPA filter and activated charcoal replacement if not done in a long time.

Monitor the results in such a group. Repeat exercise if needed. Repeat exercise with an external auditor if required.[1]

REFERENCES

1. Mortimer ST, Mortimer D. Quality and Risk Management in the IVF Laboratory. Cambridge, UK: Cambridge University Press; 2015.
2. Gardner DK, Reed L, Linck D, et al. Quality control in human in vitro fertilization. Semin Reprod Med. 2005;23(4):319-24.
3. Swai JE. Is there an optimal pH for culture media used in clinical IVF? Hum Reprod Update. 2012;18(3):333-9.
4. Abramczuk JW, Lopata A. Incubator performance in the clinical in vitro fertilization program: importance of temperature conditions for the fertilization and cleavage of human oocytes. Fertil Steril. 1986;46(1):132-4.
5. Boone WR, Shapiro SS. Quality control in the in vitro fertilization laboratory. Theriogenology. 1990;33(1):23-50.
6. Elder K, Van den Bergh M, Woodward B. Troubleshooting ICSI procedures. Troubleshooting and Problem-Solving in the IVF Laboratory. Cambridge: Cambridge University Press; 2015. pp. 171-88.
7. Steyaert SR, Leroux-Roels GG, Dhont MARC. Infections in IVF: review and guidelines. Human Reprod Update. 2000;6(5):432-41.
8. Khoudja RY, Xu Y, Li T, et al. Better IVF outcomes following improvements in laboratory air quality. J Assist Reprod Genet. 2013;30(1):69-76.
9. Gianaroli L, Plachot M, van Kooij R, et al. ESHRE guidelines for good practice in IVF laboratories. Human Reprod. 2000;15(10):2241-6.
10. Go KJ, Pool TB. Troubleshooting in the IVF Laboratory. Principles of IVF Laboratory Practice: Optimizing Performance and Outcomes. Cambridge, UK: Cambridge University Press; 2017. p. 277.
11. Cobo A, Romero JL, Pérez S. Storage of human oocytes in the vapor phase of nitrogen. Fertil Steril. 2010;94(5):1903-7.
12. Lawsuit filed over lost eggs at San Francisco fertility clinic. Available from https://www.mercurynews.com/2018/03/13/lawsuit-filed-over-lost-eggs-at-san-francisco-fertility-clinic/.
13. Practice Committee of the American Society for Reproductive Medicine and Practice Committee of the Society for Assisted Reproductive Technology. Recommended practices for the management of embryology, andrology, and endocrinology laboratories: a committee opinion. Fertil Steril. 2014;102(4):960-3.

Preventing Mix Up in In Vitro Fertilization Laboratory

52

PM Gopinath, Parzan Mistry

INTRODUCTION

In vitro fertilization laboratories are set up as a very intricate environment in terms of technology and instrumentations required for its proper functioning. There is always a risk associated with the in vitro fertilization (IVF) cycles and is invariably correlated with the number of IVF cycles being performed. Evidently, mismatching incidents constitute a major threat in assisted reproductive technology (ART) program. Serious errors like gamete exchange or embryo mismatch can lead to complex litigations, financial expenses, reputational damage as well as have emotional and ethical consequences. Certain processes (e.g. mixing of eggs and sperm and transfer of embryos to the uterus) are seen as critical since they represent "the point of no return" in terms of being able to rescue the situation or ameliorate the incident.[1] There is no branch in medicine that is spared by human errors and so is this branch of infertility and hence it is always essential to be cautious and there should be a constant dialogue of the procedure as well as any errors encountered during or before the treatment and should be properly communicated to the organization as well as the patient.[2] Hence, electronic witnessing has made its way in the new IVF laboratories to prevent mix-ups.

HISTORY

The first assisted reproductive technology (ART) mix-up was reported in Manhattan, in the year 1987.[3] And since then many such mishaps have happened in several IVF centers across the world.[4] Human double-checking approach is the principal control measure directed to reduce such mix-ups, which was first recommended by the Human Fertilization and Embryology Authority (HFEA) and later by the European Society of Human Reproduction and Embryology (ESHRE).

PRESENT SCENARIO

The manual double-witnessing protocol is currently being used in most of the artificial reproduction techniques. International Authority Standards advises manual double witnessing (MDW) for all ART programs involving gametes or embryos to reduce the probability of the mix up of patient samples. Manual double witnessing can be defined as the "double checking performed on all clinical and laboratory procedures", and if the "operator" makes an error, it will be identified and sorted out by the other "witness".

Manual double witnessing protocols otherwise known as "independent double checks" have been widely questioned for its effectiveness. They are vulnerable to human errors and have possibility of common checking errors like check omission and check incomplete. Also, associated with other human error possibilities like involuntary automaticity and non-contemporaneous checking.[5]

Handwritten labeling of the samples has also identified as a potential source of error. Illegibility or imperfect spelling can add to errors, in spite of marking all the tubes and dishes. This may result in partial or total loss of biological material.[6,7]

Now, we have automated solutions for manual witnessing protocols. Electronic witnessing systems such as radiofrequency identification (RFID) based systems and barcoding of IVF specimens are the latest developments that could ensure more accurate identification and help avoid mix-ups.

BARCODE-BASED SYSTEMS

Special barcode-based system ensures control and traceability of all procedures in the IVF laboratory. It involves giving every patient taken for the IVF treatment, an individual barcode. Special printers are used for labeling dishes, tubes and other containers required in IVF process. Labels contain both the text name and birth date of the patient and a unique barcode identifying an individual container. Everything including actions, gametes, and embryos are documented. To prevent mistakes, the system blocks by itself if nonmatching containers are scanned **(Table 1)**.

RADIOFREQUENCY IDENTIFICATION SYSTEMS

RI-witness uses RFID (radiofrequency identification) to track samples at a defined procedural steps in IVF laboratories worldwide to prevent mix-ups. The commercially available RFID system—RI-witness—uses self-adhesive RFID microchips called "tags" that are placed on all the dishes and tubes containing gametes or embryos. All workstations should be equipped with readers and touchscreens that can register all tagged culture-ware and actions performed according to the tagged culture-ware present.

Radiofrequency identification technology maintains a time-stamped history of the tasks completed for patients by specific staff throughout the laboratory-based treatment process. The system is provided with an alarm which gives a visual and audible warning if a sample mismatch occurs within the working area and later this information is maintained in the records of the respective patients **(Fig. 1)**.

Radiofrequency identification systems have two major advantages over barcoding. First, RFID ensures that embryologists do not work on more than one sample at a time. Second, RFID ensures that embryologists do not omit any key steps in the process **(Table 2)**.

Though, electronic witnessing system (EWS) is in use in many centers worldwide, restrictions and challenges to practice still exist only because of mistaken perception of complicated usage and cost factors.

Table 1: Barcode-based systems.

Bar code based systems	
Advantages	***Disadvantages***
Provides IDC	Bar code readers require direct line of site to read
Do not require modifications of equipment	Process change required to incorporate scanning bar code
Provide additional management/QA information	Bar codes are ubiquitous
Less expensive	Bar codes have no read/write capabilities

PATIENTS CONCERNS ABOUT IN VITRO FERTILIZATION ERRORS AND ELECTRONIC WITNESSING SYSTEM SATISFACTION

Patient satisfaction is fundamental especially in fertility care. Study by Marina Forte et al. shows that 90.4% of IVF population in the study expressed significant concerns relating to sample mix-up. The use of EWS reduced these concerns in 92.1% of patients, 97.1% of patients felt highly comfortable with an IVF center equipped with an EWS.[7]

With reference to EWS it is essential to assess the reliability, safety, fitting into the laboratory dynamics, and the risks of introducing a new tracking platform is still ongoing. Even electronic systems need manual double witnessing.[1]

Hence, in order to eliminate the risk of any mix-up of gametes or embryos, IVF laboratories are strictly required to follow procedures in accordance with international standard best practices. For example,

- *One at a time*: Specimens of only one person or one couple will be processed at a time.
- *Labeling*: All labwares and instruments are labeled with the person or couple's name.
- *One for each use*: All disposables should be discarded after each use to avoid any contamination.
- *Counterchecking*: Fourth, a second operator should countercheck all critical steps and will ensure that the specimens are transferred to the correct receptacles.

FUTURE TRENDS

The necessity to develop a failsafe mechanism to prevent IVF mix-ups will ever exist and witness systems will continue to evolve.

Recently, an effective direct embryo tagging system which does not interfere with the in vitro and in vivo development of the tagged embryos has been developed by researchers using mouse model.[8] This system is also being tested in humans currently. It involves direct tagging based on lectin-biofunctionalized polysilicon barcodes of micrometric dimensions. Study conducted using donated fresh immature and mature fertilization-failed oocytes

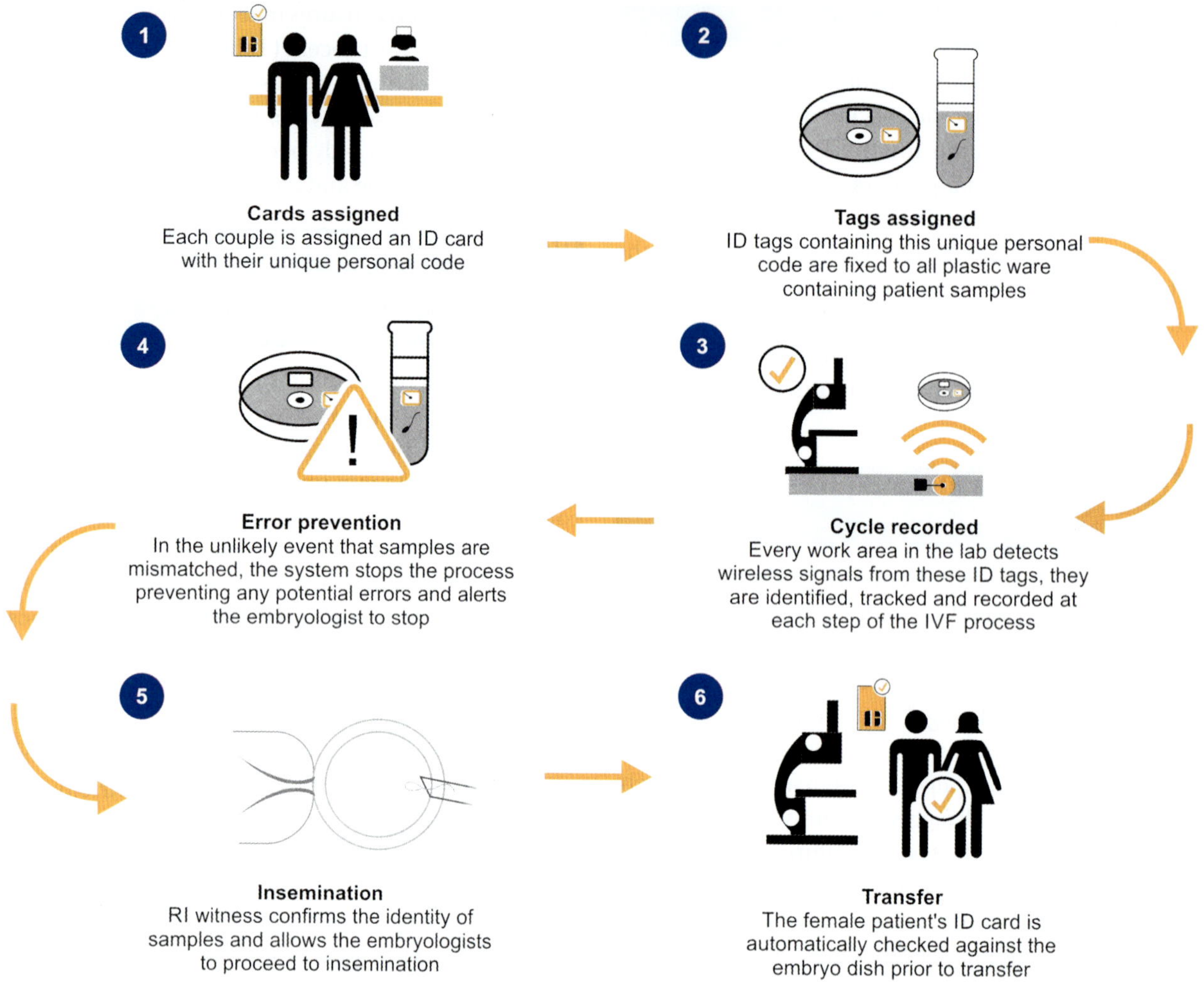

Fig. 1: Overview of radiofrequency identification (RFID) system.

Table 2: Radiofrequency identification (RFID) based systems.

RFID based systems	
Advantages	***Disadvantages***
Cannot be circumvented	Readers have to be installed on all working microscopes
No process change required for use	RFID frequency theoretically can be damaging to embryos
Labels have read/write capabilities	Cost
Multiple labels can be read at once	
Provide additional management/QA information.	

(RFID: radiofrequency identification)

and cryopreserved embryos produced by IVF or intracytoplasmic sperm injection (ICSI) concluded that it is simple, safe and highly efficient, allowing the identification of human oocytes and embryos during the various procedures typically conducted during an assisted reproduction cycle.[9] There are limitations to this tool as the direct embryo tagging system only allows the identification and traceability of oocytes destined for ICSI and embryos. Hence its application on the traceability of all reproductive samples (oocytes destined for IVF and sperm) is not yet ensured.[9]

These barcodes do not hamper embryo development, can be read by embryologists under a stereomicroscope, and seem to be compatible with cryopreservation protocols

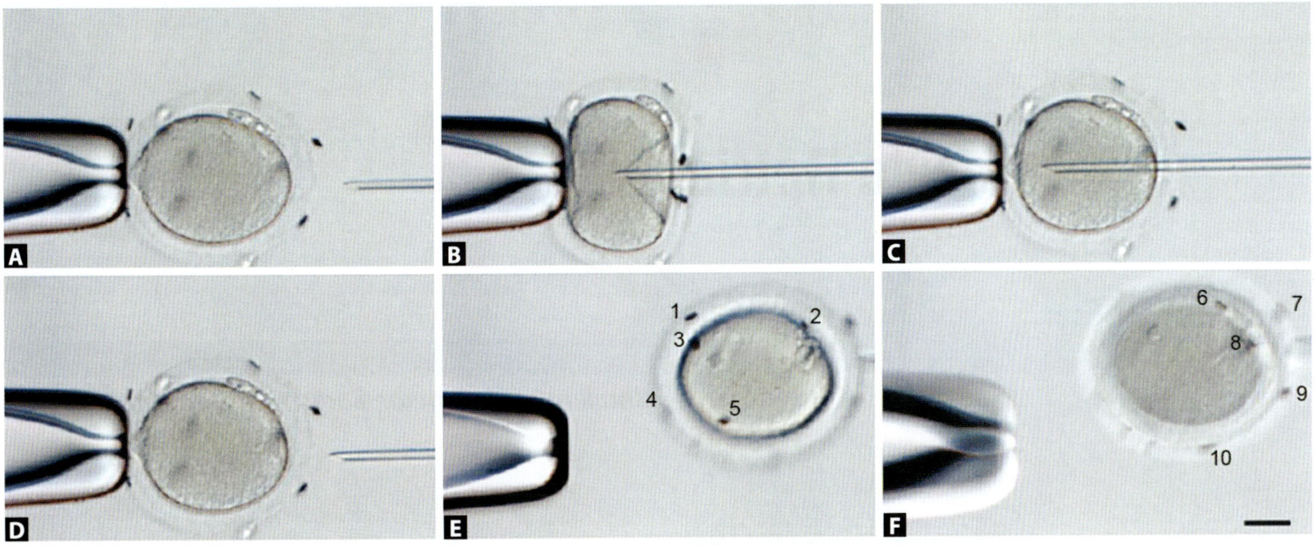

Figs. 2A to F: Barcodes in zona pellucida intracytoplasmic sperm injection [(ICSI) experiment].
Source: From Novo et al. 2014.

(Figs. 2A to F). However, this system has got its flaws not only in tagging oocytes and embryos, but also in the remaining identification steps (i.e. insemination, embryo freezing, ET).

For the current scenario, the direct introduction of silicon barcodes into eggs and embryos may be a complex and labor-intensive system and is not yet sufficiently validated in the clinical settings. It may have a future as a novel system of preventing mismatch errors in IVF.

CONCLUSION

In IVF laboratories if unnoticed misidentification occurs in a process involving gametes and embryos, the end result will be catastrophic for the patients. The introduction of recent innovation of the electronic witness system seems promising in improving traceability and reducing IVF mix-ups.

Having known the importance of identifiability of issues and given the availability of proven technology that eliminates the risks of mix-up incidents resulting from human error in the IVF laboratories, it is a mandatory requirement for current standard ART practice that we use electronic witnessing systems and not continue to take such avoidable risks.

SUMMARY

Proper patient and sample identification as well as traceability are fundamental steps during ART procedures. Electronic witnessing approaches include barcode identification and radiofrequency identification is increasing in popularity of use. Even EWS would need manual checking and human errors cannot be completely eliminated. There should be ample systems for documenting, identifying, analyzing and implementing improvements should be established and maintained.

REFERENCES

1. Thornhill AR, Brunetti XO, Bird S, et al. Reducing human error in IVF with electronic witnessing. Fertil Steril. 2011; 96(3):S179.
2. Sakkas D, Barrett CB, Alper MM. Types and frequency of non-conformances in an IVF laboratory. Hum Reprod. 2018;33(12):2196-204.
3. Liebler R. Are you my parent? Are you my child? The role of genetics and race in defining relationships after reproductive technological mistakes. DePaul J Health Care Law. 2002; 5:15-56.
4. Bender L. To err is human. ART mix-ups: a labor-based, relational proposal. J Race Gend Justice. 2006;9:443-508.
5. Maria José de los Santos, Amparo R. Protocols for tracking and witnessing samples and patients in assisted reproductive technology. Fertil Steril. 2013;100(6):1499-502.
6. Rienzi L, Bariani F, Dalla Zorza M, et al. Failure mode and effects analysis of witnessing protocols for ensuring traceability during IVF. Reprod BioMed Online. 2015;31:516-22.
7. Forte M, Faustini F, Maggiulli R, et al. Electronic witness system in IVF—patients perspective. J Assist Reprod Genet. 2016;33(9):1215-22.
8. Novo S, Barrios L, Santaló J, et al. A novel embryo identification system by direct tagging of mouse embryos using silicon-based barcodes. Hum Reprod. 2011;6(1):96-105.
9. Novo S, Nogues C, Penon O, et al. Barcode tagging of human oocytes and embryos to prevent mix-ups in assisted reproduction technologies. Hum Reprod. 2014;29(1):18-28.

Oocyte Retrieval

53

Shailendra Mahimkar, Suresh Kumar, Trupti Nagaria

INTRODUCTION

Oocyte retrieval, also commonly known as ovum pick-up (OPU), is an interventional procedure by which the oocytes are aspirated from the ovaries under ultrasound guidance **(Fig. 1)**.

In 1978, Steptoe and Edwards retrieved oocytes by laparoscopy for their first in vitro fertilization (IVF) conception. In the 1980s, a commercial OPU needle and pump became available and oocyte retrieval shot up to 90%. In 1983, Gleisher introduced (transvaginal sonography) TVS-guided oocyte retrieval technique, which is now followed as a standard procedure for oocyte retrieval. TVS-guided oocyte aspirations are much simpler, less invasive, with a shorter operation time and less morbidity. Comparisons were made between different methods of oocyte retrieval technique: laparoscopic harvesting, ultrasonic transabdominal-transvesical and ultrasonic transvaginal approach. The data demonstrated comparable success using an TVS-guided oocyte retrieval with a fixed needle guide and therefore this technique soon became the procedure of choice for all routine oocyte retrievals during in vitro fertilization (IVF) treatment.[1,2]

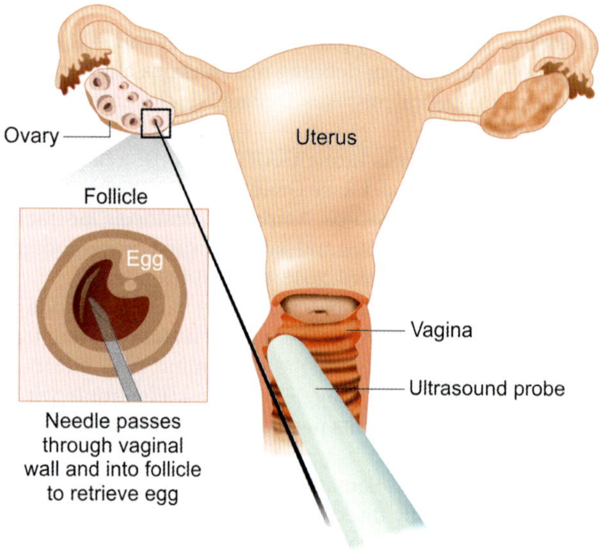

Fig. 1: Oocyte retrieval.

The oocyte yield and the fertilization rates were also found to be better with transvaginal approach.[3] Simultaneous ultrasound along with follicular aspiration ensures complete emptying of the follicles. It was observed that oocyte-cummulus complex often is likely to be aspirated when the follicle is nearly completely collapsed.

TYPES OF ANESTHESIA

Oocyte retrieval is the fundamental step during IVF. Though the transvaginal approach is less painful than laparoscopic approach, the procedure is quite painful and requires pain relief. Various types of pain relief procedures are used like conscious sedation and local, epidural, spinal and general anesthesia. Safe and effective analgesia facilitating optimum surgical conditions and a speedy post-operative recovery is the primary goal. There is also a concern about the potential effects of any drugs used on the reproductive outcome.[3]

In UK, two-thirds of OPU procedures are performed under intravenous anesthesia and remaining one-third OPU are performed under general anesthesia. In India, short general anesthesia with propofol is routinely used for oocyte retrieval. In Scandinavia, the OPU is performed under local anesthesia. A Cochrane review concluded that method of anesthesia should depend on the patient, clinician and the resources available, as no one method is superior to the other. Using more than one method of pain relief will be more effective. The regimen should ensure safety and efficacy with no adverse effects on respiratory or cardiovascular system and no adverse effects on oocytes.

PREREQUISITES

According to preconception and prenatal diagnostic techniques (PCPNDT) regulations, forms D/E/G have to be filled and signed by the surgeon. Do not forget to confirm the time of trigger with the patient before induction of anesthesia. Also clinicians to be clearly aware about patients and partners serology (human immunodeficiency virus (HIV), hepatitis B virus surface antigen (HBsAg), Hepatitis C virus (HCV), venereal disease research laboratory (VDRL)) marker status.

TIMING OF OOCYTE RETRIEVAL

Oocyte retrieval is a time bound procedure, i.e. done at 34 hr after the trigger in the antagonist cycle and 35 hr after trigger in the agonist cycle.

PREPARATION OF OVUM PICK-UP TROLLEY

The OPU trolley consists of a sponge holder, sponges, 10 cc syringe, normal saline, Sims speculum, camera cover, probe cover, Allis forceps, drapes, ultrasound jelly and sterile non-powdered gloves **(Fig. 2)**.

PREPARATION OF THE PATIENT

The procedure is done on empty bladder. Valid informed consent taken and PCPNDT forms are filled and signed.

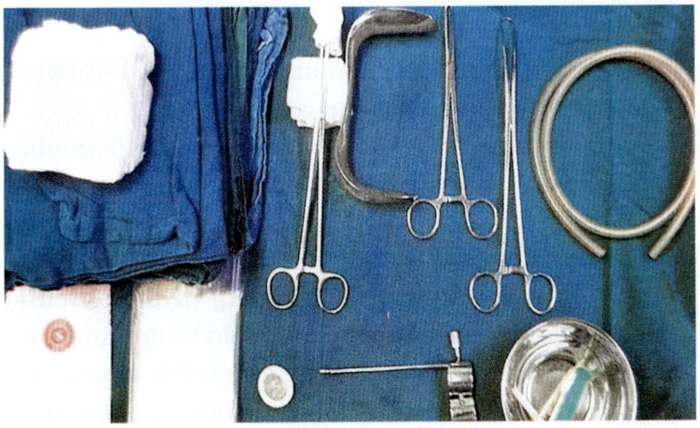

Fig. 2: Ovum pick-up trolley.

Short general anesthesia is given in the form of pre-medication and profofol. The procedure is done in lithotomy position. Vulva and perineum are cleansed with normal saline followed by irrigation of the vagina with normal saline. Use of povidone iodine 1% is discouraged unless increased risk of infection is expected (endometriosis, hydrosalpinx, PID). In such cases, cleansing of vagina with povidone 1% followed by vaginal irrigation with normal saline is done before the procedure.

PREPARATION BY THE GYNECOLOGIST

The hands are sterilized with alcohol and normal saline. Soap or povidone iodine should be avoided. The TVS probe is cleaned with alcohol and saline. The steel guide is sterilized by autoclaving and is flushed with saline prior to usage. The TVS probe is covered with non-toxic condom or probe cover and the guide is fixed to the probe.

INSTRUMENTATION

- USG machine with 5–6.5 MHz TVS probe and a guide.
- Ovum aspiration pump with a pressure setting at 110–150 mm Hg.
- OPU needle.
- Laboratory instruments: falcon tubes, warmer, work station, stereo zoom microscope, incubator, dishes for scanning the oocytes **(Fig. 3)**.

PROCEDURE

Before puncturing the vaginal wall, the entire pelvis is scanned to assess the ovaries, number of follicles, accessibility of the ovaries, their relation to the major vessels, free fluid in pouch of Douglas, endometriosis, hydrosalpinx, fibroids or any other pelvic pathology. During aspiration, the hand holding the probe should be steady and firm while the hand holding the needle should be gentle and soft. Once the needle is in the peritoneal cavity, the needle tip should always be seen at any given point. There should be minimum tissue between the probe surface and the ovary, i.e. a good approximation of probe is essential. Always enter the follicle at 90° and keep the tip at the center of the follicle during aspiration. It is advised to curette the follicle after the follicular fluid is completely aspirated. The needle is rotated gently and rapidly in a clockwise and counter-clockwise fashion inside the follicle. This increases the mature oocyte yield with no detrimental effect on oocyte quality or integrity and also reduces the risk of ovarian hyperstimulation syndrome (OHSS) as a larger number

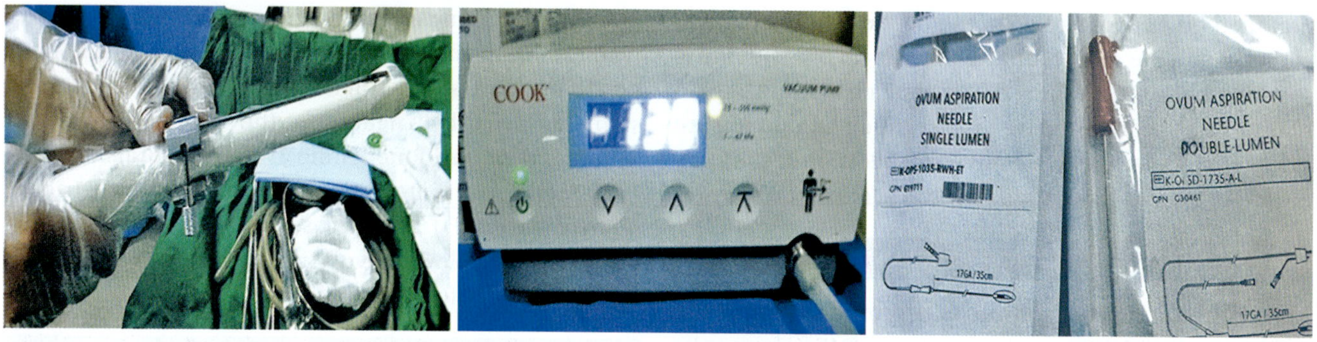

Fig. 3: Instruments used in the ovum pick-up procedure.

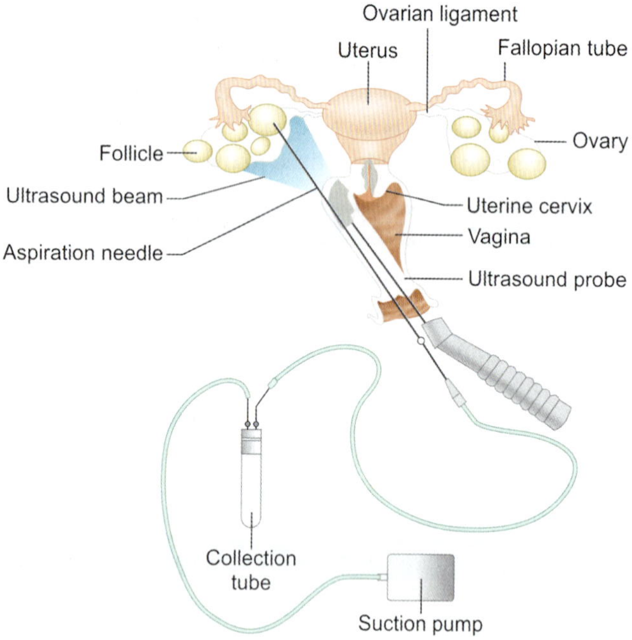

Fig. 4

of granulose cells are removed.[4] Aspirate the follicles from proximal to distal and from lateral to medial **(Fig. 4)**. Before changing planes, withdraw the needle a little to release the ovarian tissue before you enter adjacent follicle so as to prevent ovarian trauma. Take multiple vaginal punctures to reach follicles in different planes in order to avoid vaginal or ovarian surface tears. It is better to leave the odd difficult and inaccessible follicle. The pressure setting of the ovum aspiration pump should be at 110–150 mmHg. The vacuum should be deactivated before the needle is withdrawn from the follicles, otherwise air entry will create a turbulent cappuccino effect and lead to deleterious effect on the oocyte. After all the follicles are aspirated, the pelvis is re-scanned to look for any hematomas or collection in the POD. Another important point is to keep collection tubes in

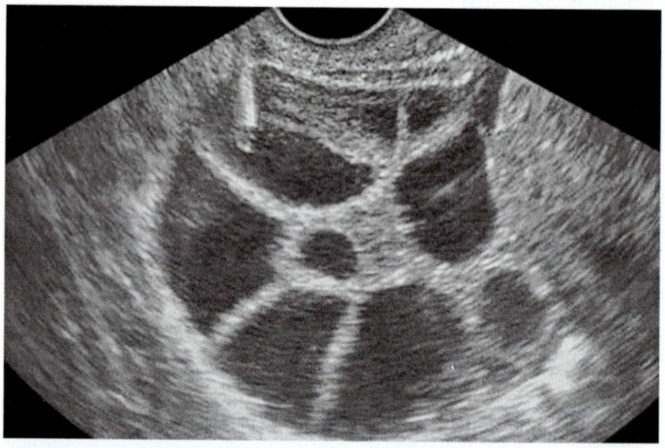

Fig. 5

test tube warmer while they are waiting to be connected to the collections system, in order to avoid damage to oocyte due to cooling effect **(Fig. 5)**.

DIFFICULT OVUM PICK-UP

Challenging OPU scenarios:

- Hyperstimulated enlarged ovaries.
- Poor responders: very few follicles.
- Highly placed ovaries.
- Mobile ovaries.
- Associated pathology: endometriomas, hydrosalpinx, multiple fibroids, frozen pelvis.
- Voluntary oocyte donor: fibrosed ovaries, hypermobile ovaries due to lax abdomen, lax vagina due to normal delivery, highly placed ovaries due to adhesions secondary to CS.

These should be anticipated during prior follicular monitoring scans and the patient should be appropriately counseled. Most ovaries become accessible after probe manipulation and with abdominal maneuvers. The cervix can be pulled with a vulsellum. Reverse Trendelenburg

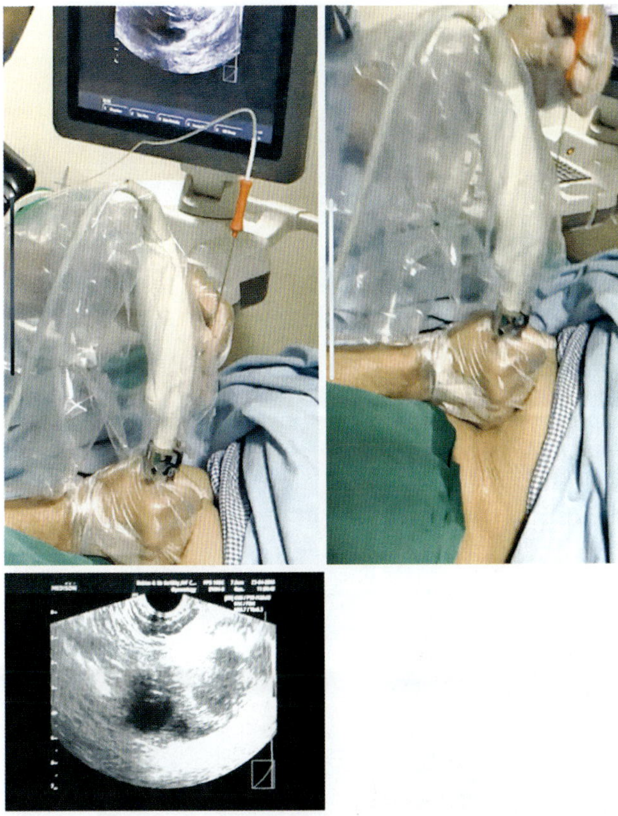

Fig. 6: Transabdominal OPU using TVS probe and guide for highly placed ovary. Not accessible vaginally.

position with lateral tilt of the table may help sometimes **(Fig. 6)**. In rare cases, transmyometrial aspiration may be needed. Transabdominal oocyte aspiration may be needed if the ovaries are highly placed. It has been observed that in women with significant ovarian displacement, transabdominal ultrasound-guided follicular aspiration with TVS probe is safe and efficacious.[5] Transabdominal ultrasound-guided aspiration with TVS probe should be the modality of choice when the ovaries are not accessible transvaginally **(Fig. 7)**.

COMPLICATIONS[6]

Complications with oocyte retrieval are rare, but several complications have been reported. The complications can either be anesthesia-related complications or they can be related to the procedure itself.

The most common problem associated with oocyte retrieval is minor vaginal hemorrhage which is reported in 3–6% of cases. However, in most cases, the blood loss is minor, and in only 0.8% of OPUs, the bleeding exceeds 100 mL and application of local pressure is required. In 0.11% of OPUs, a severe abdominal bleeding occurs.[7]

The second most common complication is pelvic infection. The infection can happen either due to direct inoculation by the needle through unsterile vagina or can be due to re-activation of latent infection. Patients with prior history of endometriosis, PID, pelvic adhesions are at high risk of pelvic infection. The incidence can be reduced by minimizing the number of vaginal punctures during the retrieval. The role of prophylactic antibiotics is controversial.

Other less common complications include damage to surrounding pelvic structures (bladder, bowel, iliac vessels).[8] Damage to the bowel is very rare and not easily detected as the damage is minor; hence, there is a delay in diagnosis. Only two cases of perforated appendicitis have been published in literature. Ureteric injury and consequent ureteric obstruction has also been described.[9] Other rare complications include vertebral osteomyelitis,[10] ovarian torsion and periumbilical hematoma.

Troubleshooting

Before commencing oocyte collection, the system should be tested by aspirating some culture medium. This also provides a column of medium into which to collect the follicular fluid, thus encouraging laminar flow.

Should suction then subsequently decrease or stop, the following steps should be undertaken:

- Ensure that the suction pump is turned on and that the suction pedal is functioning (many aspiration pumps have a light that goes on, and some have audible signals when the pump is activated).
- Check that all connections of tubing between the aspiration tube and the pump are tightly connected. Exclude any cracks in the aspiration test tube.
- Ensure that the collection tubing is not kinked or damaged.
- Rotate the needle within the follicle to ensure that it is not blocked by follicular wall tissue.
- If there is still no suction, remove the needle and perform a "retrograde flush" to clear any blockage.
- Before re-inserting the needle, re-check by aspirating some culture medium.

Failure to Get Oocytes

Check if human chorionic gonadotropin (hCG) has been given properly as ovulation trigger. Sometimes several

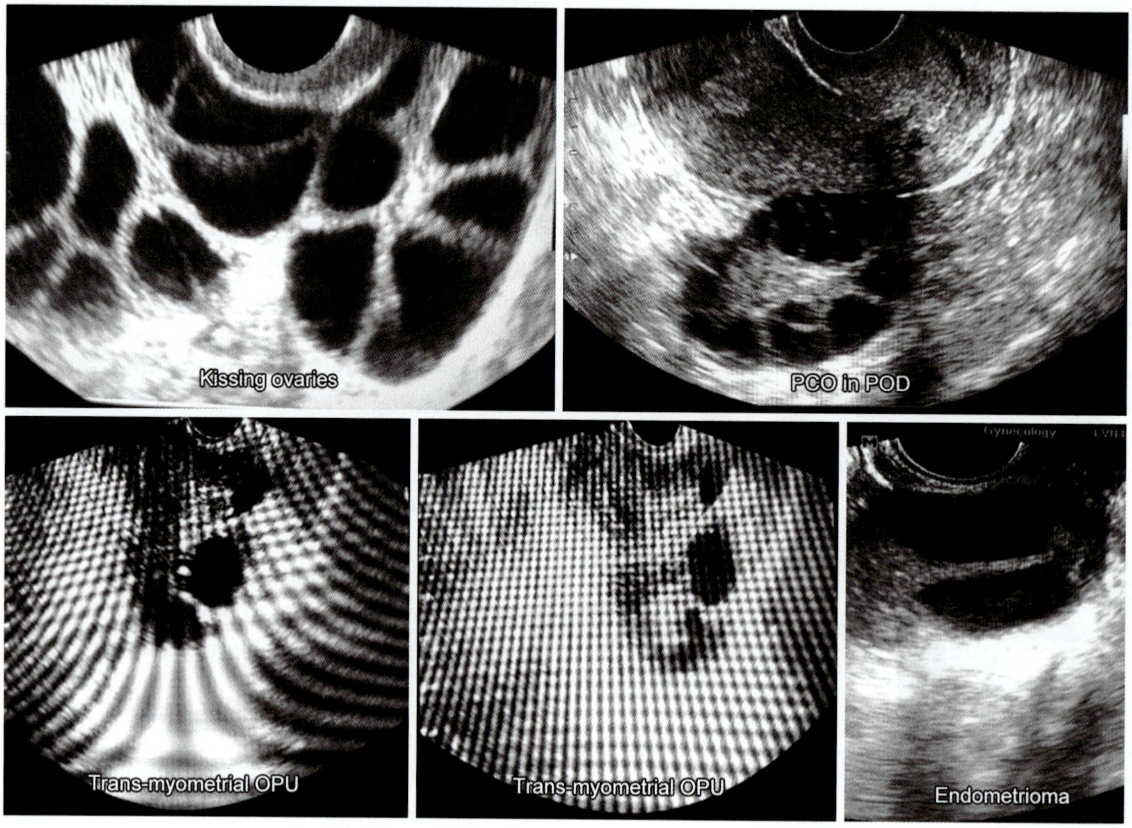

Fig. 7

follicles are aspirated and no oocytes are recovered. If the fluid collected is very clear and devoid of cells (granulosa and cumulus), it is possible that the patient has not had her trigger hCG. It is suggested that before follicles from the second ovary are aspirated, some of the follicular fluid is tested with a urinary pregnancy test strip. If the test is negative, it is possible to abandon the procedure, administer hCG, and defer the collection from the other ovary until about 36 hr later. In this way, it is still possible to salvage the cycle.

REFERENCES

1. Lenz S, Lauristen JG, Kjellow M. Collection of human oocytes for in vitro fertilization by ultrasonically guided procedure. Lancet. 1981;1:1163.
2. Seifer DB, Collins RL, Paushter DM, et al. Follicular aspiration: a comparison of an ultrasonic endovaginal transducer with fixed needle guide and other retrieval methods. Fertil Steril. 1988;49(3):462-7.
3. Kwan I, Bhattacharya S, Knox F, et al. Conscious sedation and analgesia for oocyte retrieval during IVF procedures: a Cochrane review. Hum Reprod. 2006;21(7):1672-9.
4. Dahl SK, Cannon S, Aubuchon M, et al. Follicle curetting at the time of oocyte retrieval increases the oocyte yield. J Assist Reprod Genet. 2009;26(6):335-9.
5. Barton SE, Politch JA, Benson CB, et al. Transabdominal follicular aspiration for oocyte retrievalin patients with ovaries inaccessible by transvaginal ultrasound. In: Proceedings of the 66th ASRM, Denver, Colorado, 2010.
6. Bennett SJ, Waterstone JJ, Cheng WC, et al. Complications of transvaginal ultrasound-directed follicle aspiration: A review of 2670 consecutive procedures. J Assist Reprod Genet. 1993;10:2-7.
7. Dessole S, Rubattu G, Ambrosini G, et al. Blood Loss following non-complicated transvaginal oocyte retrieval for in vitro fertilization. Fertil Steril. 2001;76(1):205-6.
8. Miller PB, Price T, Nichols JE, et al. Acute ureteral obstruction following transvaginal oocyte retrieval for IVF. Hum Reprod. 2002;17:137-8.
9. Jayakrishnan K, Raman VK, Vijayalakshmi VK, et al. Massive hematuria with hemodynamic instability—complication of oocyte retrieval. Fertil Steril. 2011;96:e22-4.
10. Almog B, Rimon E, Yovel I, et al. Vertebral osteomyelitis: a rare complication of transvaginal ultrasound-guided oocyte retrieval. Fertil Steril. 2000;73:1250-2.

Embryo Transfer

54

Sadhana Patwardhan, Mangala Ketkar

INTRODUCTION

In an in vitro fertilization (IVF) procedure, embryo transfer (ET) is not only the final but also the most crucial step. A good embryo transfer determines the probability of success of an IVF cycle and for this, clinicians and embryologists need to work in close collaboration. A perfect synchronization between the embryologist and clinician is needed to optimize embryo transfer. The embryologist needs to provide healthy good quality embryos and clinician needs to do flawless atraumatic transfer.

Review of literature supports that certain practices like an atraumatic transfer, an ultrasound guided transfer,[1-6] use of soft embryo transfer catheters,[7] depth at which the embryo is transferred,[8-10] and the experience of the clinician performing the embryo transfer,[11-13] all have a positive impact on the pregnancy and the implantation rates. Whereas techniques like trial transfer, aspiration of cervical mucus prior to transfer, timely completion of the embryo transfer procedure,[14] straightening of the uterocervical angle,[15] after loading technique for the embryo,[16] absence of bacterial contamination,[17] and the speed of injecting[18] hold questionable benefit and there is not enough evidence to support the inculcation of these techniques in regular practice to optimize cycle outcomes. Few things that are known to have a negative impact on the cycle outcomes are a difficult embryo transfer,[19-21] presence of blood on the catheter,[22-25] more than 120 seconds gap between loading the catheter and the embryo transfer,[26] contamination of the tip of the catheter, and stimulation of uterine contractions.[27,28]

The use of antibiotics prior to treatment,[29,30] immediate catheter withdrawal, air in the catheter,[31] performing two transfers in the same cycle, prolonged bed rest, sexual intercourse after embryo transfer or the use of sildenafil do not impact the outcome and the value of a mock transfer a few days before the actual procedure has been challenged as the position of the uterus may change.

The practice of assisted reproductive technology (ART) has experienced a shift toward single blastocyst embryo transfer recently as we strive toward decreasing the unpleasant complication of multiple pregnancies without compromising on pregnancy and live-birth rates and we owe to the every evolving culture systems along with refined methods to assess the developmental potential.[32-34] Hence, in lieu of the changing trend in the practice of ART, the technique of embryo transfer demands a detailed insight to optimize the pregnancy outcome.

THE LABORATORY PART OF EMBRYO TRANSFER

Embryo Quality and Selection

With elective single embryo transfer becoming the way forward in ART,[35,36] selection of the most viable embryo for transfer is of utmost importance. In recent years, with the improved understanding of embryonic development and advances in the field of assisted reproduction, the developmental stage at which an embryo can be transferred has become more advanced, and embryo selection criteria have evolved accordingly.

Morphological factors, along with metabolic, protein, and genetic markers in culture media aim to enhance embryo selection and IVF success rates.[37] Moreover, new technology for embryo selection, based on embryo developmental and morphological characteristics, using multilevel images combined with a computer-assisted scoring system (CASS), now has the potential to overcome the disadvantages with standard embryo evaluation and predict implantation and live-birth rates superior to that with the standard scoring system (SSS).[38] Image acquisition and the time-lapse analysis system make it possible to determine the exact timing of embryo cleavage and, possibly, estimate the time of implantation in a clinical setting.[39] Blastocyst culture is yet another means of evaluating the viability and developmental potential of the embryo. Enabling self-selection of embryos and improving uterine and embryonic synchronicity is the rationale behind moving to blastocyst culture which then translates into higher implantation rates.[40]

Time lapse observation now presents an opportunity for optimizing embryo selection based on morphological grading providing novel kinetic parameters which may further improve selection of viable embryo by identifying morphokinetics parameters. Meseguer et al. proposed a multivariate model based on these findings to classify embryos according to probability of their implantation. The efficacy needs to be evaluated by further randomized control trials (RCTs).

Selective single embryo transfer (SSET) is reported to yield a high rate of healthy baby per transfer in women less than 35 years of age. Enhanced selection by rapid PCR-based comprehensive chromosomal screening and trophectoderm biopsy prior to SET has increased ongoing pregnancy rate (55 vs. 41.8) and reduced miscarriage rates (24.8 vs. 10.5), eliminating the multiple gestation risk without compromising the clinical outcome per cycle **(Figs. 1A to D)**.

Loading the Catheter

The dynamics involved in the procedure of loading the embryo transfer catheter is not well understood. In a recent study, where an in vitro experimental model for embryo transfer simulations was used, Eytan and colleagues reported the importance of having a gas

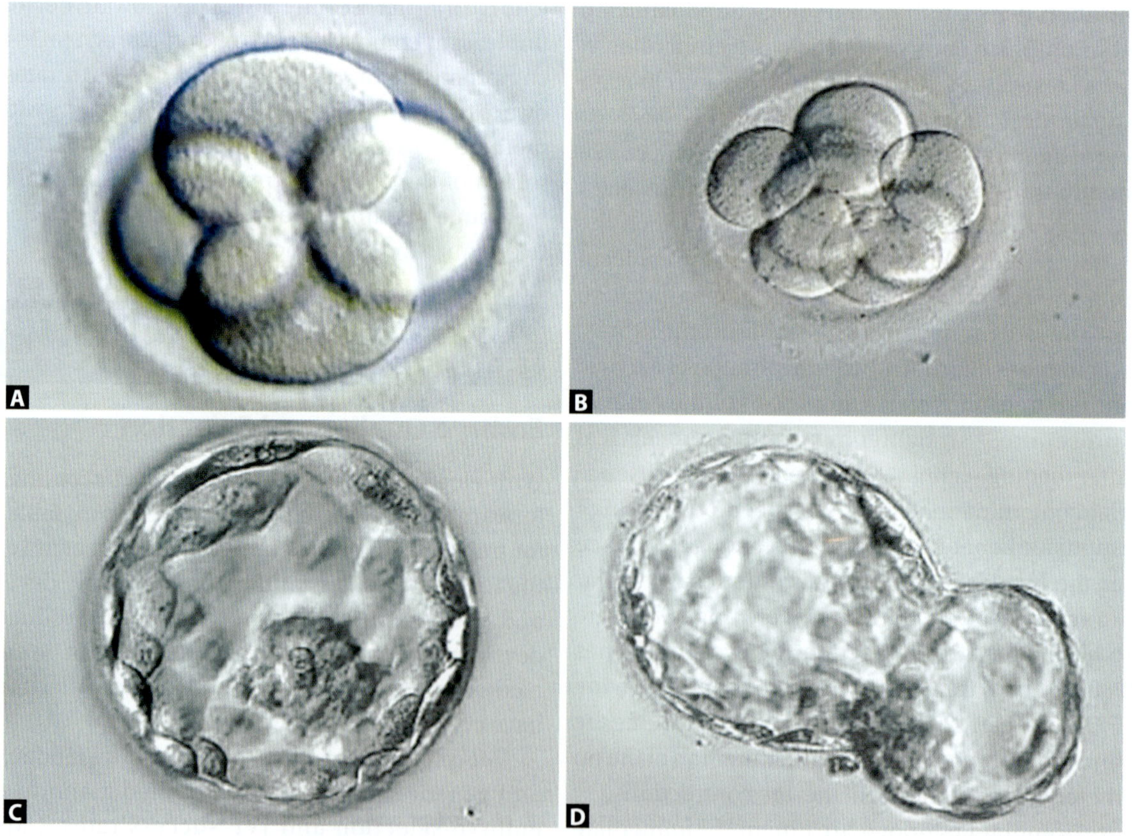

Figs. 1A to D

phase in the catheter load.[41] Within the uterus, the air bubbles were carried toward the fundal region, thereby dragging behind them the medium containing the embryos. Eytan and colleagues also found that the speed of injection upon the catheter load into the uterus could influence the results;a low speed generated several air bubbles, which led to more of the transferred media being carried toward the fundal end of the uterus and thereby a likely enhanced implantation rate. This syringe-catheter complex has also been studied clinically[42-44] as well as in a meta-analysis of Abou-Setta.[45] However, there is no consensus whether air or fluid-filled catheters provide better results. So far, the speed of injection has not been studied clinically.

Extended time between loading the catheter and deposition of the embryo(s) may have an effect on the pregnancy rate,[46] possibly influenced by light,[47] temperature,[48] and other environmental factors[49] in which detrimental effects seem to increase during the time the embryos spend from the incubator to the uterus.

Embryos may be retained, which necessitates re-transfer. In order to minimize the risk of retained embryos, a slow withdrawal of a transfer catheter is recommended **(Figs. 2A and B)**.[50]

CLINICAL PART OF EMBRYO TRANSFER

Experience of the Provider

The experience of the clinician in conducting an embryo transfer is, according to us, amongst the most significant factors that influences the clinical outcome and positively influences the success rates. In the hands of experienced, skilled operators, neither choice of transfer catheter and difficulty of transfer nor observations of blood on the transfer catheter caused any significant reduction in pregnancy outcomes.[51] Moreover, a significant difference in clinical pregnancy rates ($P \leq 0.01$) has been reported between different providers using the same method of loading embryos into the embryo transfer catheter and the same number of embryos (36.1% vs. 20.6%; $P \leq 0.01$), suggesting that the physician factor may be an important variable in embryo transfer technique.[52] Pregnancy rates, following embryo transfer, were shown to decrease when the technique was handled by less experienced providers: 29.9% for attending physicians (>20 years of experience), 28.2% for assistant physicians (2–5 years of experience), and 19.1% for resident physicians (<6 months of experience) ($P < 0.05$).

Routine Uterine Cavity Evaluation

A hysteroscopy or a three-dimensional (3D) saline sonohysterography as a routine pre-IVF evaluation of the uterine cavity gives a direct insight into the cavitary abnormalities that may interfere with embryo implantation and also provides an opportunity to correct the same. Studies have reported a 22.9% incidence of abnormality in the cavity following outpatient hysteroscopy in patients with pervious IVF failure and a benefit for resection of submucosal leiomyomas, adhesions and, at least, a subset of polyps. However, prospective randomized trials fail to clearly demonstrate that surgical removal of all abnormalities improve in IVF-ET outcomes.[53]

Gentle Atraumatic Transfer

This term refers to two important factors in optimizing the embryo transfer technique—namely, avoiding damage to

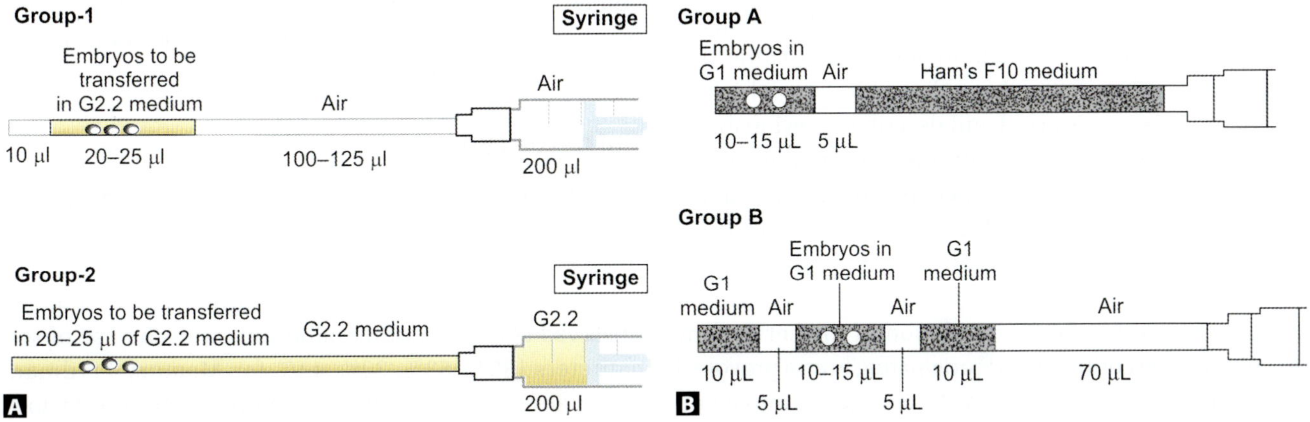

Figs. 2A and B

Source: Moreno V, Balasch J, Vidal E, et al. Air in the transfer catheter does not affect the success of embryo transfer. Fertil Steril. 2004; 81(5):1366-70.

the endometrium and unwanted uterine contractions both of which appear more often in so-called difficult transfer and also have a clear impact on the clinical pregnancy rate.[54,55] The term "gentle atraumatic transfer" also covers important clinical features,—i.e. a painless transfer with no problems passing the cervical canal and proper delivery of the embryo(s) within the uterine cavity—deposited at a level in accordance with the intention of the performer. A gentle atraumatic transfer is characterized by the lack of blood on the catheter tip, indicating bleeding from the endometrium.

Damage to Endometrium

A frequent injury left by difficult transfers or by transfers where a suboptimal technique is used is damaged to the endometrium with a subsequent negative impact on the receptivity of the endometrium and/or initiation of uterine contraction, which ultimately may displace or expel the embryos from the uterine cavity.[2] Damage to the endometrium is associated with a diminished implantation rate after embryo transfer and may be the result of several factors such as bleeding, inflammation, and plugging of the catheter tip, which in turn may retain the embryos within the catheter.[56,57]

Uterine Contractions

Uterine contractions are a physiological part of the activity in the uterine musculature.[58] During the menstrual period, the contraction form waves that can be directed toward the uterine cervix (anterograde). Successively, the direction of waves turns toward a fundal direction (retrograde), which is the most prominent during ovulation and the early luteal phase when implantation occur.[59]

The practical impact of this observation is the fact that anterograde contraction may be provoked during the transfer procedure. It is therefore logical to assume that transferred embryos may have the same fate, which in fact, has also been observed and described previously.[56,57] To prevent these unwanted uterine contractions, some precautions should be taken, such as using a soft transfer catheter,[60,61] avoiding touching the uterine fundus,[62] and manipulating gently while performing the transfer procedure.[60] Moreover, as far as possible, one should avoid using a tenaculum. Such stimulation of the cervix may provoke uterine contractions,[63] originating from a provoked release of oxytocin,[64] which may have negative impact on the final outcome of the treatment.

Atosiban was administered to women undergoing IVF-ET to improve pregnancy rate in certain studies. However, the results of this treatment need further trials for better results and safety. Thus far, vaginal progesterone, which resembles the hormonal sequence in a natural cycle, has been evaluated in regards to the initiation of the cycle.[65] Vaginal progesterone is a commonly used luteal phase support, where the eventual additional beneficial relaxant effect of progesterone is already being implemented in the treatment.[65]

Recommending bed rest after embryo transfer or advising sexual abstinence relies upon the same assumptions concerning uterine contractions. Two published studies have revealed no statistically significant differences between bed rest or an immediate mobilization after embryo transfer.[66,67] In one study, sexual intercourse after embryo transfer was actually found to increase pregnancy rates.[68]

Mock Embryo Transfer

The value of a trial transfer in a treatment cycle has also been evaluated.[69] Mansour and colleagues concluded that such a procedure would optimize the passage through the cervical canal, which in turn positively aids the implantation. It appears today, with improved ultrasound equipment, that this can be easily achieved by a careful examination of all levels of the uterus, including the optimal transfer depth.[70]

Performing a trial transfer at the time of oocyte retrieval 2–5 days before embryo transfer does not have a deleterious effect on the endometrium.[71] On the other hand, the value of a trial transfer ahead of the embryo transfer has been questioned,[72] due to the changed uterine anatomy between the trial and the real transfer.[73] Miller and Frattarelli found that uterine depth significantly differed between the blind pre-cycle trial transfer measurement and the ultrasound-guided embryo transfer measurement.[73] Many IVF centers have a practice of doing mock embryo transfer during the pre-treatment cycle.

Catheter Type

While some authors reported significantly higher pregnancy ($P < 0.0005$) and implantation rate ($P < 0.01$) with the ultrasoft catheter compared to the more rigid Frydman catheter,[18] others have reported significantly less frequently observed severe endometrial lesions with the use of soft catheters (85%, 53%, 32%, 11% for Memory Frydman, Frydman classic, Elliocath and In Vitro Fertilization Sydney Set, respectively; $P < 0.0001$).[7] The presence of blood on the catheter indicates severe endometrial lesions. They concluded that all embryo transfer catheters can lead to endocervical and endometrial damage but severe endometrial lesions were less frequent when soft catheters were used.[7,74] Echogenic catheters, such as the SureView™ catheter,[75] the echogenic Wallace catheter,[76] and the Cook Echo-Tip catheter,[76] offer several advantages such as better visualization owing to the ultrasonic contrast properties, minimizing the need for catheter movement to identify the tip and significantly shorter duration of the embryo transfer procedures thus simplifying ultrasound-guided embryo transfer, without a significant improvement in the clinical outcome in terms of pregnancy rates **(Figs. 3A to D)**.[75,76]

Ultrasound-guided Versus Clinical Touch

The ability to visually track the embryo transfer procedure to ensure an atraumatic delivery of embryos to the site of implantation is perhaps, a significant advance in the field of ART and an indispensable technology for ART practitioners, hard-pressed to improve the pregnancy rates. While a standard evidence-based protocol is still lacking, compared to clinical touch alone, embryo transfer done under transabdominal and transvaginal ultrasound guidance have been documented to significantly increase the chances of clinical pregnancy, embryo implantation, ongoing pregnancy, and live births.[1-3,77] Prospective randomized controlled trials comparing US-guidance with clinical touch embryo transfer have demonstrated significantly increased chances of live birth [odds ratio (OR) = 1.78], 95% confidence interval (CI) = 1.19–2.67, ongoing pregnancy (OR = 1.51, 95% CI =1.31–1.74), clinical pregnancy (OR = 1.50, 95%CI = 1.34–1.67), embryo implantation (OR = 1.35, 95% CI = 1.22–1.50), and easy transfer rates with US-guided

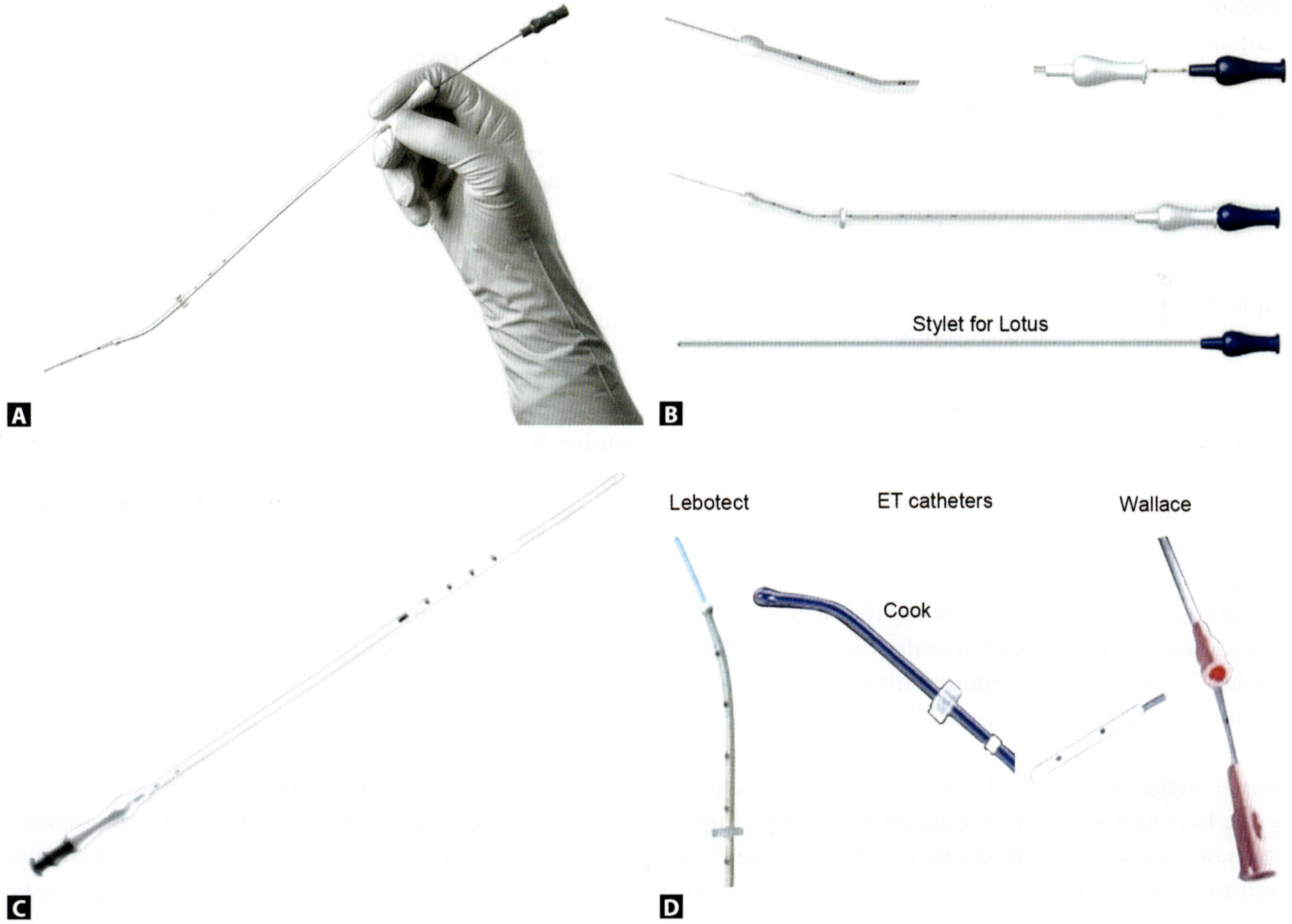

Figs. 3A to D: Types of catheters.

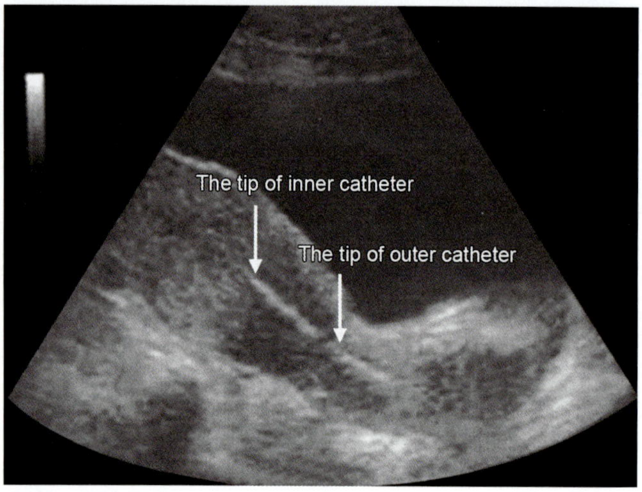

Fig. 4

embryo transfer compared with the clinical touch method in 5,968 embryo transfer cycles with no difference in multiple pregnancy, ectopic pregnancy, or miscarriage rates.[78,79] Compared to clinical touch method abdominal ultrasound-guided transfer has a better clinical pregnancy rate and ongoing pregnancy rate **(Fig. 4)**.

Depth of Embryo Transfer

The clinical pregnancy rate is reported to be significantly influenced by the TDF (difference between the cavity depth and depth of catheter insertion) after controlling for potential confounders, with the odds of clinical pregnancy increasing by 11% for every additional millimeter that the embryos are deposited away from the fundus.[4] Coroleu et al. reported a significantly higher (P <0.05) implantation rate when the transfer distance from the uterine fundus at the moment of the embryo deposition in the uterus was 15 ± 1.5 mm (31.3%) or 20 ± 1.5 mm (33.3%) compared to when it was10 ± 1.5 mm (20.6%).[9]

Amongst the largest recent study that included 5,055 ultrasound-guided embryo transfers in 3,930 infertile couples, Tiras et al.[80] also reported higher pregnancy and ongoing pregnancy rates when embryo were replaced at a distance more than 10 mm from the fundal endometrial surface suggesting that a distance 10–20 mm seems to be the best site for embryo transfer to achieve higher pregnancy rates. Hence, the depth of embryo transfer is an important variable in the embryo transfer technique that may influence the implantation rates.[81]

Cervical Mucus

Removing the cervical mucus prior to the embryo transfer has no positive effect on pregnancy rate. However, according to some reports, removal of cervical mucus during embryo transfer may increase pregnancy and implantation rates. The other school of thought is that cervical manipulation may cause unwanted uterine contractions.

Removing cervical mucus or flushing the cervical canal before embryo transfer has gained some focus in the literature. Hypothetically, two issues may be connected: first, the introduction of bacteria from the mucus into the uterine cavity during the transfer process; second, the possibility of the mucus covering the tip of the catheter causing interference with the deposition by retaining the embryos or dragging them into the cervix by the withdrawal of the catheter.

The cervical mucus represents a mechanical as well as an immunological barrier between the sterile uterine cavity and the bacterial colonized vagina, and the mucal concentrations of immunoglobins vary through the menstrual cycle. However, the reported studies[82] are not consistent with respect to the impact of removing cervical mucus or not.

AFTER EMBRYO TRANSFER

Catheter Removal

No difference has been noted between delayed versus immediate catheter removal following embryo transfer.[83]

Blood in Catheter

Studies have reported a significant concordance between the perceived difficulty of transfer, presence of blood on the catheter and the degree of endometrial damage (P < 0.05),[20] and a significant decrease in the pregnancy rates, implantation rates, and live-birth rates following the presence of blood on the catheter tip[22-24] or in the catheter[23] after the embryo transfer procedure. While documenting the significance of blood on the transfer catheter, in their retrospective analysis of 8,311 ultrasound-guided embryo transfers, performed in a single center, Tiras et al.[80] added that pregnancy rates were unaffected by mucus on the catheter that appeared to be as simple contamination,[80] though the association between macroscopic or microscopic presence of blood or mucus and pregnancy rates has not found support from others.[21]

Retained Embryos

In the absence of known risk factors, like blood and mucus in the transfer catheter, and other reported signs of difficult transfer,[84] immediate retransfer of embryos retained in the catheter following the initial transfer attempt has not been shown to have an adverse effect on pregnancy outcome in terms of pregnancy, implantation, and delivery rates per embryo transfer.[85] The type of embryo transfer catheter used did not show any difference in terms of embryo retention.[84] Provided there is no difficult transfer situation, the retained, embryos should be transferred back immediately.

Air Bubble Position

Air bubble location following embryo transfer is the presumable placement spot of embryos.[21] Though some authors have reported significantly higher pregnancy rates following observation of the relative position of the air bubbles in the fundal half of the endometrial plate compared with the lower half of the endometrial plate (43.0% vs. 24.4%, respectively, $P = .002$) following ultra sound-guided embryo transfer, and an absolute and relative position of the air bubbles significantly closer to the fundus in patients who became pregnant compared with those who did not,[84] recent large studies[86,87] failed to support this relation. Confine et al.[86] recorded the air bubble position immediately, 30 minutes later, and when the patient stood up after ultrasound-guided embryo transfer with a soft, coaxial end-opened catheter loaded with a single or double air bubble with the embryos. Bubble migration analysis supported a rather random movement of the bubble and possibly the embryos, even with the patient in the horizontal position following embryo transfer, suggestive of active uterine contractions, that horizontal rest post-embryo transfer may not be necessary, that gravity-related bubble motion was uncommon, and that, a very accurate ultrasound-guided embryo placement may not be mandatory.[86] Tiras et al.[80], in their large retrospective analysis of 7,489 ultrasound-guided embryo transfers, evaluated pregnancy outcomes in patients with no air bubble movement following embryo transfer, air bubble movement toward the uterine fundus spontaneously, a little time after transfer, and air bubbles movement toward the cervical canal. They reported higher pregnancy rates, higher miscarriage rates, and similar live-birth rates with air bubbles moving toward the uterine fundus with ejection compared to air bubbles remaining stable after transfer **(Fig. 5)**.[87]

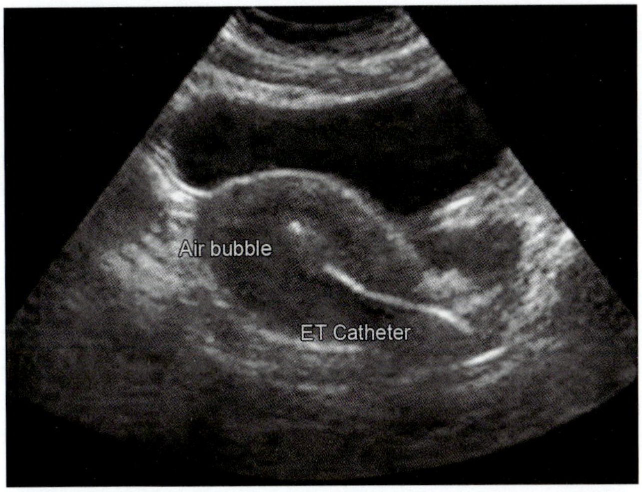

Fig. 5

RECENT ADVANCES

Recent advances in the area of embryo transfer address the influence of the variation in injection speeds in manual embryo transfer and pump-regulated embryo transfer (PRET) that generates a standardized injection speed with the aim to standardize the embryo transfer process. Seven laboratory technicians performed simulated transfers, using the conventional embryo transfer technique and compared their injection speeds with that of a PRET device. The results indicated that in manually performed transfers, even after standardization of the protocol, there is still a large variation in injection speed, while a PRET device generates a reliable and reproducible injection speed and therefore, brings new possibilities for further standardization of the embryo transfer procedure. Future research should reveal whether these experiments mimic real clinical circumstances and if a standardized injection speed results in more exact positioning of the transferred embryos and therefore, higher pregnancy rates.[88]

CONCLUSION

So far, the optimal embryo transfer protocol is not known. However, during the last few years, an increasing number of publications have led to a more optimal transfer technique that contributes to better pregnancy results. In several of the issues thought to have impact on the implantation rates, data are conflicting or well-designed prospective, randomized trials are lacking. Still, we need to learn more. However, what is well accepted today is the importance of a gentle atraumatic transfer where no damage to the endometrium and minimal uterine contractions are induced. In order to succeed, it is advisable to perform a trial transfer, using a soft catheter and ultrasound to find the correct deposition site, which is 2 cm below the fundus. Moreover, the collaboration between the clinician and the embryologist appears to be important. The time from the embryo leaving the incubator until it is deposited in the uterine cavity is of utmost importance. How to load the catheter, with air or fluid, the amount of volume, or whether the transfer media should be enriched are more controversial issues. Following embryo transfer, no particular factor other than progesterone luteal phase support has been shown to have a positive effect on pregnancy outcome.

PRACTICE COMMITTEE OF THE AMERICAN SOCIETY FOR REPRODUCTIVE MEDICINE GUIDELINES FOR PERFORMING THE EMBRYO TRANSFER

Good Evidence (Grade A)

- Ten RCTs to recommend ultrasound guidance during embryo transfer to improve clinical pregnancy rate and live birth rate.
- Use of a soft embryo transfer catheter to improve IVF-embryo transfer pregnancy rates.
- Data on live birth rates and specific types of soft catheters are limited.
- Not to recommend bed rest after embryo transfer.

Fair Evidence (Grade B)

- Acupuncture performed around the time of the embryo transfer does not improve live birth rates in IVF.
- There is fair evidence based on only one RCT that transcutaneous electrical acupoint stimulation (TEAS) improves IVF-embryo transfer outcomes. Given the lack of any other studies, recommendation for or against TEAS to improve IVF-embryo transfer outcomes cannot be made.
- Fair evidence based on a single RCT that an antibiotic regimen that includes amoxicillin and clavulanic acid given on the day before and the day of embryo transfer does not improve pregnancy rates.
- A benefit to removing cervical mucus at the time of embryo transfer to improve clinical pregnancy and live birth rates.
- Seven studies (three RCTs and four cohort studies) that placement of the catheter tip in the upper or middle (central) area of the uterine cavity, greater than 1 cm from the fundus for embryo expulsion, optimizes pregnancy rates.
- One RCT and one cohort study to recommend immediate withdrawal of the embryo transfer catheter after embryo expulsion.
- Retained embryos in the transfer catheter and immediate retransfer do not affect implantation, clinical pregnancy, or spontaneous abortion rates.

Insufficient Evidence (Grade C)

- Insufficient evidence to recommend for or against analgesics to improve IVF-embryo transfer outcomes.
- Routine anesthesia is not recommended to improve IVF-embryo transfer outcomes.
- Insufficient evidence for more specific recommendations regarding the positioning of the catheter at the time of embryo transfer.
- Insufficient evidence to conclusively state that the presence of blood on the catheter, once it is withdrawn, is associated with lower implantation or pregnancy rates.
- Insufficient evidence to recommend any specific injection speed of the catheter at the time of embryo transfer.

REFERENCES

1. Eskandar M, Abou-Setta AM, Almushait MA, et al. Ultrasound guidance during embryo transfer: aprospective, single-operator, randomized, controlled trial. Fertil Steril. 2008;90(4):1187-90.
2. Porter MB. Ultrasound in assisted reproductive technology. Semin Reprod Med. 2008;26(3):266-76.
3. Buckett WM. A meta-analysis of ultrasound-guided versus clinical couchembryo transfer. Fertil Steril. 2003;80(l):1037-41.
4. Matorras R, Urquijo E, Mendoza R, et al. Ultrasoundguided embryo transfer improves pregnancy rates and increases the frequency of easy transfers. Hum Reprod. 2002;17(7):I762-6.
5. Anderson RE, Nugent NL, Gregg AT, et al. Transvaginal ultrasound-guided embryo transfer improves outcome in patients with previous failed in vitro fertilization cycles. Fertil Steril. 2002;77(4):769-75.
6. Allahbadia GN. Ultrasonography-guided embryo transfer: evidence-based practice. In: Rizk BRMB (Ed). Ultrasonography in Reproductive Medicine and Infertility. Cambridge, UK: Cambridge University Press; 2010.
7. Poncelet C, Sifer C, Hequet D, et al. Hysteroscopic evaluation of endocervical and endometrial lesions observed after different procedures of embryo transfer: a prospective comparative study. Eur J Obstet Gynecol Reprod Biol. 2009;147(2):183-6.

8. Pope CS, Cook EK, Arny M, et al. Influence of embryo transfer depth on in vitro fertilization and embryo transfer out comes. Fertil Steril. 2004;81(l):51-8.
9. Coroleu B, Barri PN, Carreras O, et al. The influence of the depth of embryo replacement into the uterine cavity on implantation rates after IVF: a controlled, ultrasoundguided study. Hum Reprod. 2002;17(2):341-6.
10. Lambers Ml, Dogan E, Lens W, et al. The position of transfer red air bubbles after embryo transfer is related to pregnancy rate. Fertil Steril. 2007;88(I):68-73.
11. Angelini A, Brusco GF, Barnocchi N, et al. Impact of physician performing embryo transfer on pregnancy rates in an assisted reproductive program. J Assist Reprod Genet. 2006;23(7-8):329-32.
12. Desparoir A, Capellel I, Banet J, et al. Does the experience of the provider affect pregnancy rates after embryo transfer? J Reprod Med. 2011;56(9-10):437-43.
13. De Placido G, Wilding M, Stina I, et al. The effect of ease of transfer and type of catheter used on pregnancy and implantation rates in an I IVF program. J Assist Reprod Genet. 2002;19(1):14-8.
14. Mains L, Van Voorhis, BJ. Optimizing the technique of embryo transfer. Fertil Steril. 2010;94(3):785-90.
15. Derks RS, Farquhar C, Mol BW, et al. Techniques for preparation prior to embryo transfer. Cochrane Database Syst Rev. 2009;(4):CD007682.
16. Neithardt AB, Segars JH, Hennessy S, et al. Embryo after loading: a refinement in embryo transfer technique that may increase clinical pregnancy. Fertil Steril. 2005;83(3):710-4.
17. Selman H, Mariani M, Barnocchi N, et al. Examination of bacterial contamination at the time of embryo transfer, and its impact on the IVF/pregnancy outcome. J Assist Reprod Genet. 2007;24(9):395-9.
18. Grygoruk C, Pietrewicz P, Modlinski JA, et al. Influence of embryo transfer on embryo preimplantation development. Fertil Steril. 2012;97(6):1417-21.
19. Tiboni GM, Colangelo EC, Leonzio E, et al. Assisted reproduction out comes after embryo transfers requiring a mall eablesty let. J Assist Reprod Genet. 2012;29(7):585-8.
20. Cevrioglu AS, Esinler I, Bozdag G, et al. Assessment of endocervical and endometrial damage inflicted by embryo transfer trial: a hysteroscopic evaluation. Reprod Biomed Online. 2006;13(4):523-7.
21. Spitzer D, Haidbauer R, Corn C, et al. Effects of embryo transfer quality on pregnancy and live birth delivery rates. J Assist Reprod Genet. 2012;29(2):131-5.
22. Sallam HN, Agameya AF, Rahman AF, et al. Impact of technical difficulties, choice of catheter, and the presence of blood on the success of embryo transfer-experience from a single provider. J Assist Reprod Genet. 2003;20(4):135-42.
23. Munoz M, Meseguer M, Lizan C, et al. Bleeding during transfer is the only parameter of patient anatomy and embryo quality that affects reproductive outcome: a prospective study. Fertil Steril. 2009;92(3):953-5.
24. Tiras B, Korucuoglu U, Polar M, et al. Effect of blood and mucus on the success rates of embryo transfers. Eur J Obstet Gynecol Reprod Biol. 2012;165(2):239-42.
25. Moragianni VA, Cohen JD, Smith SE, et al. Effect of macroscopic or microscopic blood and mucus on the success rates of embryo transfers. Fertil Steril. 2010;93(2):570-3.
26. Sallam HN. Embryo transfer: factors involved in optimizing the success. Curr Opin Obstet Gynecol. 2005;17(3):289-98.
27. Levi Setti PE, Albani E, Cavagna M, et al. The impact of embryo transfer on implantation-a review. Placenta. 2003;24(SupplB):S20-6.
28. Schoolcraft WB, Surrey ES, Gardner DK. Embryo transfer: techniques and variables affecting success. Fertil Steril. 2001;76(5):863-70.
29. Kroon B, Hart RI, Wong BM, et al. Antibiotics prior to embryo transfer in ART. Cochrane Database Syst Rev. 2012;3:CD008995.
30. Brook N, Khalaf Y, Coomarasamy A, et al. A randomized controlled trial of prophylactic antibiotics (co-amoxiclav) prior to embryo transfer. Hum Reprod. 2006;21(11):2911-5.
31. Moreno V, Balasch J, Vidal E, et al. Air in the transfer catheter does not affect the success of embryo transfer. Fertil Steril. 2004;81(5):1366-70.
32. Zander-Fox DL, Tremellen K, Lane M. Single blastocyst embryo transfer maintains comparable pregnancy rates to double cleavage-stage embryo transfer but results in heal their pregnancy out comes. Aust NZ Obstet Gynaecol. 2011;51(5):406-10.
33. Marsh CA, Farr SL, Chang J. et al. Trends and factors associated with the Day 5 embryo transfer, assisted reproductive technology surveillance, USA, 2001-2009. Hum Reprod. 20l2;27(8):2325-31.
34. Kresowik JD, Stegma1m BJ. Sparks AE, et al. Five-years of a mandatory single-embryo transfer (mSET) policy dramatically reduces twinning rate without lowering pregnancy rates. Fertil Steril. 2011;96(6):1367-9.
35. Vilska S, Tiitinen A, Hyden-Granskog C, et al. Elective transfer of one embryo results in an acceptable pregnancy rate and eliminates the risk of multiple birth. Hum Reprod. 1999:14:2392-5.
36. Hamberger L, Hardarson T, Nygren KG. Avoidance of multiple pregnancy by use of single embryo transfer. Minerva Ginecol. 2005:57:15-9.
37. Wang SX. The past, present, and future of embryo selection in in vitro fertilization: Frontiers in Reproduction Conference, Yale. J Biol Med. 2011;84(4):487-90.
38. Paternot G, Debrock S, D'Hooghe T, et al. Computerassisted embryo selection: a benefit in the evaluation of embryo quality? Reprod Biomed Online. 2011;23(3):347-54.
39. Meseguer M, Herrero J, Tejera A, et al. The use of morpho kinetics as a predictor of embryo implantation. Hum Reprod. 2011;26(10):2658-71.
40. Glujovsky D, Blake D, Farquhar C, et al. Cleavage stage versus blastocyst stage embryo transfer in assisted reproductive technology. Cochrane Database Syst Rev. 2012;7:CD002118.
41. Eytan O, Elad D, Jaffa AJ. Evaluation of the embryo transfer protocol by a laboratory model of the uterus. Fertil Steril. 2007:88:485-93.
42. Meldrum DR, Chetkowski R, Steingold KA, et al. Evolution of a highly successful in vitro fertilization-embryo transfer program. Fertil Steril. 1987:48:86-93.

43. Kovacs GT. What factors are important for successful embryo transfer after in vitro fertilization? Hum Reprod. 1999:14:590-2.
44. Schoolcraft VB, Surrey ES, Gardner DK. Embryo transfer: techniques and variables affecting success. Fertil Steril. 2001:76:863-70.
45. Abou-Setta AM. Air fluid versus fluid-only models of embryo catheter loading: a systematic review and meta-analysis. Reprod Biomed Online. 2007:14:80-4.
46. Matorras R, Mendoza R, Exposito A, et al. Influence of the time interval between embryo catheter loading and discharging on the success of IVF. Hum Reprod. 2004:19:2027-30.
47. Smith LC. Membrane and intracellular effects of ultra violet irradiation with Hoechst 33342 on bovine secondary oocytes matured in vitro. J Reprod Fertil. 1993:99:39-H.
48. Rocha A, Randel RD, Broussard JR, et al. High environmental temperature and humidity decrease oocyte quality in *Bos taurus* but not in *Bos indicus* cows. Theriogenology. 1998:49:657-65.
49. Cohen J, Gilligan A, Esposito W, et al. Ambient air and its potential effects on conception in vitro. Hum Reprod. 1997:12:1742-9.
50. Mansour RT, Aboulghar A. Optimizing the embryo transfer technique. Hum Reprod. 2002:17:11-9
51. De Placido G, Wilding M, Stina I, et al. The effect of ease of transfer and type of catheter used on pregnancy and implantation rates in an IVF program. J Assist Reprod Genet. 2002;19(1):14-8.
52. Angelini A, Brusco GF, Barnocchi N, et al. Impact of physician performing embryo transfer on pregnancy rates in an assisted reproductive program. J Assist Reprod Genet. 2006;23(7-8):329-32.
53. Surrey ES. Should diagnostic hysteroscopy be performed before in vitro fertilization-embryo transfer? JM Invasive Gynecol. 2012;19(5):643-6.
54. Sallam HN. Embryo transfer: factors involved in optimizing the success. Curr Opin Obstet Gynecol. 2005:17:289-98.
55. Abusheikha N, Lass A, Akagbosu F, et al. How useful is cervical dilatation inpatients with cervical stenosis who are participating in an in vitro fertilization-embryo transfer program? The Bourn Hall Experience. Fertil Steril. 1999:72:610-2.
56. Woolcott R, Stanger F. Potentially important variables identified by transvaginal ultrasound-guided embryo transfer. Hum Reprod. 1997;12:963-6.
57. Lesny P, Killick SR, Tetlow RL, et al. Embryo transfer-can we learn anything new from the observation of junctional zone contractions? Hum Reprod. 1998:13:1540-6.
58. Abramowicz JS, Archer DF. Uterine endometrial peristalsis-a transvaginal ultrasound study. Fertil Steril. 1990;54:451-4.
59. Lyons EA, Taylor PJ, Zheng XH, et al. Characterization of sub endometrial myometrial contractions throughout the menstrual cycle in normal fertile women. Fertil Steril. 1991:55:771-4.
60. Buckett WM. A review and meta-analysis of prospective trials comparing different catheters used for embryo transfer. Fertil Steril. 2006:85:728-34.
61. Abou-Setta AM. Al-lnany HG. Mansour RT, et al. Soft versus firm embryo transfer catheters for assisted reproduction: a systematic review and meta-analysis. Hum Reprod. 2005:20:3114-21.
62. Frankfurter D, Trimarchi JB, Silva CP, et al. Middle to lower uterine segment embryo transfer improves implantation and pregnancy rates compared with fundal embryo transfer. Fertil Steril. 2004:81:1273-7.
63. Lesny P, Killick SR, Robinson J, et al. Junctional zone contractions and embryo transfer: is it safe to use at enaculum? Hum Reprod. 1999:14:2367-70.
64. Dorn C, Reinsberg J, Schlebusch H, et al. Serum oxytocin concentration during embryo transfer procedure. Eur J Obstet Gynecol Reprod Biol. 1999:87:77-80.
65. Fanchin R, Righini C, de Ziegler D, et al. Effects of vaginal progesterone administration on uterine contractility at the time of embryo transfer. Fertil Steril. 2001:75:1136-40.
66. Sharif K, Afnan M, Lashen H, et al. Is bed rest following embryo transfer necessary? Fertil Steril. 1998:69:478-81.
67. Botta G, Grudzinskas G. Is a prolonged bed rest following embryo transfer useful? Hum Reprod. 1997:12:2489-92.
68. Tremellen KP, Valbuena D, Landeras J, et al. The effect of inter course on pregnancy rates during assisted human reproduction. Hum Reprod, 2000:15:2653-8.
69. Mansour R, Aboulghar M, Serour G. Dummy embryo transfer: a technique that minimizes the problems of embryo transfer and improves the pregnancy rate in human in vitro fertilization. Fertil Steril. 1990:54:678-81.
70. Knutzen V, Stratton CJ, Sher G, et al. Mock embryo transfer in early luteal phase. The cycle before in vitro fertilization and embryo transfer: a descriptive study. Fertil Steril. 1992:57:156-62.
71. Katariya KO, Bates GW, Robinson RD, et al. Does the timing of mock embryo transfer affect in vitro fertilization implantation and pregnancy rates? Fertil Steril. 2007:88:1462-4.
72. Stafford-Bell MA. Which factors are important for successful embryo transfer after in-vitro fertilization? Hum Reprod. 1999;14:2678-9.
73. Miller KL, Frattarelli JL. The pre-cycle blind mock embryo transfer is an inaccurate predictor of anticipated embryo transfer depth. J Assist Reprod Genet. 2007:24:77-82.
74. Coroleu B, Barri PN, Carreras O, et al. Effect of using an echogenic catheter for ultrasound-guided embryo transfer in an IVF programme: a prospective, randomized, controlled study. Hum Reprod. 2006; 21(7):1809-15.
75. Allahbadia GN, Kadam K, Gandhi G, et al. Embryo transfer using the Sure View catheter-beacon in the womb. Fertil Steril. 2010;93(2):344-50.
76. Karande V, Hazlett D. Vietzke M, et al. A prospective randomized comparison of the Wallace catheter and the Cook Echo-Tip catheter for ultrasound-guided embryo transfer. Fertil Steril. 2002;77(4):826-30.
77. Kably Ambe A, Campos Canas JA, Aguirre Ramos G, et al. Evaluation of two transfer embryo systems performed by six physicians[Article in Spanish] Ginecol Obstet Mex. 2011;79(4):196-9.

78. Abou-Setta AM, Mansour RT, Al-lnany HG, et al. Among women undergoing embryo transfer, is the probability of pregnancy and live birth improved with ultrasound guidance over clinical touch alone? A systemic review and meta-analysis of prospective randomized trials. Fertil Steril. 2007;88(2):333-41.
79. Brown J, Buckingham K, Abou-Setta AM, et al. Ultrasound versus 'clinical touch' for catheter guidance during embryo transfer in women. Cochrane Database Syst Rev. 2010;(1):CD006107
80. Tiras B, Polat M, Korucuoglu U, et al. Impact of embryo replacement depth on in vitro fertilization and embryo transfer out comes. Fertil Steril. 2010;94(4):1341-5.
81. Pacchiarotti A, Mohamed MA, Micara G, et al. The impact of the depth of embryo replacement on IVF outcome. J Assist Reprod Genet. 2007;24(5):189-93.
82. Visschers BA, Bots RS, Peeters MF, et al. Removal of cervical mucus: effect on pregnancy rates in IVF/ICSI. Reprod Biomed Online. 2007:15:310-5.
83. Sroga JM, Montville CP, Aubuchon M, et al. Effect of delayed versus immediate embryo transfer catheter removal on pregnancy outcomes during fresh cycles. Fertil Steril. 2010;93(6):2088-90.
84. Vicdan K, Isik AZ, Akarsu C, et al. The effect of retained embryos on pregnancy outcome in an in vitro fertilization and embryo transfer program. Eur J Obstet Gynecol Reprod Biol. 2007;134(1):79-82.
85. Lee HC, Seifer DB, Shelden RM. Impact of retained embryos on the outcome of assisted reproductive technologies. Fertil Steril. 2004;82(2):334-7.
86. Confine E, Zhang J. Risquez F. Air bubble migration is a random event post embryo transfer. J Assist Reprod Genet. 2007;24(6):223-6.
87. Tiras B, Korucuoglu U, Polar M, et al. Effect of air bubble localization after transfer on embryo transfer outcomes. Eur J Obstet Gynecol Reprod Biol. 2012;164(1):52-4.
88. Groeneveld E, de Leeuw B, Vergouw CG, et al. Standardization of catheter load speed during embryo transfer: comparison of manual and pump-regulated embryo transfer. Reprod Biomed Online. 2012;24(2):163-9.

Frozen Embryo Transfer

55

Jatin P Shah

INTRODUCTION

In vitro fertilization (IVF) has been performed for more than 35 years, and it is estimated that in developed countries, more than 1% of all births are with the help of ART. Rapid improvements made in cryopreservation techniques (vitrification) have led to few or no detrimental effects to the embryo and have resulted in no consequences to the offspring when compared to fresh embryos. This inspired the concept of the freeze-all policy (when all viable embryos are electively cryopreserved in the fresh cycle and transferred in a remote cycle).

Controlled ovarian stimulation (COS) is considered an essential step during IVF treatment, its main objective being to induce the development of multiple follicles, more number of viable oocytes and embryos, and maximize the chances of a positive outcome. Although fresh embryo transfer (ET) has been the norm, there are many concerns about the possible adverse effects of COS on endometrial receptivity and the uterine environment. COS may contribute to modifications in the endometrium (by way of the supraphysiologic levels of estradiol and progesterone), which might be related to poorer outcomes when fresh ET is performed.[1] Despite rapid advances in laboratory technology, incubators, culture media, and recombinant gonadotropins, live birth rates with fresh ET have remained in the range of 18–42% with an average of 32%. Also, in cycles with fresh ET, there is still a risk for the development of late onset and often severe ovarian hyperstimulation syndrome (OHSS), which is an iatrogenic, serious, and potentially life-threatening complication of COS.[2,3] Furthermore, there is data to suggest that pregnancies from fresh ET are more prone (owing to COS and supraphysiologic hormonal levels) to early pregnancy losses, ectopic pregnancies, pregnancy-induced hypertension, low-birth weight (LBW), abnormal placentation, and accidental hemorrhage.[4,5]

In the freeze-all strategy, the entire cohort of embryos is vitrified (not just the "surplus") and the best embryos are transferred in a subsequent cycle with a more physiologic endometrium.[6] In the past few years, the freeze-all strategy has emerged as a safer and more successful alternative to conventional fresh ET during IVF/intracytoplasmic sperm injection (ICSI) cycles. Data suggest that live birth rates are higher and obstetric and perinatal outcomes in pregnancies resulting from frozen embryo transfer (FET) are better than those from fresh ET.[7-13] There is concern; however, about macrosomia and long-term implications of vitrification on the babies born.[14]

At the same time, although the principle that COS may cause a less physiological milieu for embryos to implant, we must establish when and for whom this freeze-all approach is appropriate. How can we balance better implantation rates against the possible unnatural changes that we may be causing to the embryo as a result of freezing? Is it time now to reconsider our freeze-all strategies and establish protocols for individualized segmented IVF and FET?

HOW DID THE "FREEZE-ALL" STRATEGY BEGIN?

Freeze-all was first proposed for patients of polycystic ovary syndrome (PCOS) who are invariably prone to moderate or severe OHSS with COS protocols. Despite anticipation of OHSS [polycystic ovaries, high-anti-Müllerian hormone (AMH) levels] and adjustment of the follicle-stimulating hormone (FSH) dose (use of lower doses of FSH such as 100–112.5 IU), the incidence of moderate to severe OHSS requiring hospitalization is as high as 30–40%. Extremely elevated estradiol levels result in a nonreceptive endometrium and exaggerated uterine contractions with subsequent lower implantation rates. Studies have found that uterine contractility is much higher in stimulated cycles than in natural cycles.[15-17] Fresh ET in patients with PCOS is also associated with higher risks of abnormal placentation [elevated E2 and vascular endothelial growth factor (VEGF)] resulting in greater placental weight, placenta previa, pregnancy-induced hypertension (PIH) and obstetric complications such as preterm delivery, LBW, and higher lower segment cesarian section (LSCS) rate. Also, weaker implantation contributes to a higher rate of early pregnancy loss in these patients. Use of the antagonist instead of agonist helps reduce, but not eliminate, the risk of OHSS in these patients. The antagonist brings with it the ability to use an agonist trigger [avoiding human chorionic gonadotropin (hCG) as trigger eliminates the risk of OHSS] albeit with a deficient luteal phase and extremely low-pregnancy rates. Efforts have been made to rescue the luteal phase with high doses of exogenous estradiol-progesterone support often with add back low-dose hCG but pregnancy rates remain disappointing. The "freeze-all" strategy with replacement of embryos in a subsequent estradiol-progesterone primed cycle gives extremely encouraging results.[18] One of the initial reports by Atkinson showed a 50% cumulative pregnancy rate after two FET cycles employing the freeze-all strategy in patients with PCOS.

In a trial by the author, 127 patients with elevated AMH levels and PCOS were subjected to a standard antagonist protocol using a starting dose of 150 IU of rFSH. Final oocyte maturation was triggered with 0.2 mg decapeptyl, oocytes were retrieved at 36 hours and embryos were vitrified at the 4-cell stage. FET was done with thawed 8-cell stage embryos in a subsequent downregulated estradiol-progesterone primed cycle. The clinical pregnancy rate in the first FET was 56.6% and after allowing for early pregnancy losses, the on-going pregnancy rate was 48.03%. Antagonist cycles with agonist trigger, "freeze-all" of all embryos and FET seems to be the most successful treatment for moderate to severe PCOS with a zero incidence of OHSS and excellent perinatal and obstetric outcomes on par with non-PCOS patients undergoing IVF.[19-21] Elective cryopreservation and subsequent FET also reduces the odds of small for gestational age (SGA) babies and PIH as compared to fresh ET in PCOS patients with elevated peak serum E2 levels (>3,450 pg/mL).

Other Indications for "Freeze-all"

- *Patients with elevated serum progesterone levels (>1.5 ng/mL) on day of hCG*: It has been shown that patients with premature progesterone rise (PPR) are prone to endometrial advancement and lower pregnancy rates with fresh ET. Pregnancy rates are decreased from 31% to 19% in patients with PPR in both agonist and antagonist cycles. An endometrial advancement of more than 3 days is associated with a zero pregnancy rate.[22-24] Also, it is interesting to note that it is only the endometrial receptivity and not oocyte quality that is affected by PPR as reflected in oocyte donation programs where elevated progesterone in the donor does not reduce pregnancy rates in the recipient. Freeze-all and thaw transfer in a subsequent cycle is extremely successful for patients with PPR.
- *Patients with very low serum progesterone levels (<0.5 ng/mL) on day of hCG*: Very low levels of serum progesterone have been associated with significantly lower pregnancy rates (17% vs. 30% as compared to patients with normal progesterone) with fresh ET. Freeze-all is preferred for these patients.[25]
- *Patients of endometriosis*: It has always been proposed that patients of endometriosis do better with downregulation protocols. It is the author's experience that a majority of these patients have an already depleted ovarian reserve and low AMH levels especially after single/multiple laparoscopic surgeries. Studies have shown that it is better to avoid downregulation (for a better ovarian response in patients with reduced AMH levels) and use an antagonist protocol for the initial controlled ovarian hyperstimulation (COHS) cycle to get more oocytes and embryos and then downregulate the patient for the embryo transfer cycle. Freeze-all and FET in a downregulated cycle, in patients with moderate to severe endometriosis, increase the pregnancy rates from 12% to 28%.[26]
- *Patients with thin endometrium*: There are many patients who have a thin endometrium on the day of hCG (<8 mm) and would have lower pregnancy rates with fresh ET. Freeze-all is recommended for these patients as there would be ample time in a frozen-thaw transfer cycle to prepare the endometrium with gonadotropin-releasing hormone (GnRH) agonist downregulation, high doses and prolonged administration of estradiol valerate, vaginal sildenafil, aspirin, low-molecular weight (LMW) heparin, and intrauterine instillation of granulocyte-colony stimulating factor (G-CSF).

Measures to improve the endometrial thickness in a fresh cycle usually prove inadequate owing to a shortage of time in terms of days available for implementing these measures.

- *Patients of repeated implantation failures with fresh ET*: COHS results in supraphysiologic levels of estradiol and progesterone which impair endometrial receptivity and reduce pregnancy rates in fresh ET. Many of these failures are unexplained and occur in the presence of a normal looking endometrium and good quality embryos. A significant number of these patients achieve pregnancy with FET (owing to a more conducive uterine environment).
- *Endometrial polyp*: Often, endometrial polyps/septum/thin endometrium/adhesions are diagnosed during the course of ovarian stimulation creating a dilemma about ET. In these cases, it is advisable to freeze all the embryos, perform an operative hysteroscopy concurrent with the ovum pick-up (OPU) procedure to correct the pathology and then do a FET in the next cycle. FET can be done as early as 35 days from the date of OPU with optimal pregnancy rates.[27]
- *Low responders*: Patients with a poor ovarian response can benefit from accumulation of embryos over repeated COS cycles allowing them to achieve better pregnancy rates. FET is done once 3–4 good quality embryos have been obtained. Success rate of 20–30% have been reported with freeze-all and embryo accumulation in poor responders.
- *Patients of advanced maternal age*: Freeze-all is also attractive for patients of advanced maternal age who, in addition to being low responders, require pre-implantation genetic screening. Nowadays, there is a trend toward performing the PGS in the blastocyst stage with 24-chromosome screening. There is growing evidence showing higher implantation and delivery rates following the 24-chromosome screening when compared to preimplantation genetic screening with fluorescence in situ hybridization (FISH-PGS).[28] The use of comprehensive chromosome screening (CCS) in blastocyst stage with elective single ET is as effective as double ET of unscreened embryos and dramatically reduces the risk of twins.[29] The embryos that undergo biopsy on day 6 are not eligible for fresh transfer due to an asynchrony between the embryo and endometrium. In these cases, it is necessary to perform the cryopreservation of all embryos and a posterior frozen-thawed ET.[30]
- *Patients with history of ectopic pregnancy/biochemical pregnancy/early pregnancy loss in a previous IVF cycle (with fresh embryo transfer):* IVF with fresh ET is associated with a higher risk of ectopic pregnancy owing to increased uterine contractility and supraphysiologic hormonal levels during COS.[31] There is a significant reduction in the incidence of ectopic pregnancies (by more than 50%) with freeze-all as compared to fresh ET.[32-34]
- *Normo-responders with normal progesterone levels*: The debate about whether freeze-all benefits normo-responders began with a recent meta-analysis which concluded that pregnancy rates and obstetric/perinatal outcomes are better with FET as compared to fresh ET even in normal responders with normal serum progesterone levels.[10] However, this meta-analysis includes only three small studies and controversy still exists when it comes to normo-responders. A recent study revealed no difference in terms of ongoing pregnancy and live birth rates between normo-responder patients who underwent fresh and deferred embryo transfers. This was a retrospective study which included 882 patients, aged 20–44 who underwent their first or second IVF/ICSI cycle, in which a normal oocyte yield (4–20) was obtained. The raw analysis showed that ongoing pregnancy (36.2 vs. 33.8%, P = 0.51) and live birth (33.2 vs. 32.9%, P = 0.94) rates for freeze-all versus fresh cycles, respectively were similar.[35] Normo-responders can face situations in which freeze-all may apply, such as those who undergo genetic screening, or present highprogesterone levels, impaired endometrium, etc.
- *Social egg/embryo freezing*: Freeze-all allows women to preserve their fertility today, the so-called "social freezing" enabling them to have the same success rates as fresh ET at a later date in life.[36]

A recent SWOT analysis (strengths, weaknesses, opportunities and threats with freeze-all) by Christophe Blockeel[37] summarized the strengths, weaknesses, opportunities, and threats of the freeze-all policy as described here.

Strengths

- *Establishing an OHSS-free clinic*: Elimination of OHSS and enhanced maternal safety (antagonist protocols, agonist trigger, and freeze-all).
- *Improved pregnancy rates as compared to fresh ET*: Reported by some but needs to be evaluated in more detail.

- *Better obstetric and perinatal outcomes*: FET pregnancies are significantly less likely to be complicated by perinatal mortality, SGA, LBW and antepartum hemorrhage (APH) as compared to fresh ET. The differences were even stronger when analyzing pregnancies within a single individual who conceived successive children with fresh and frozen ET. This proves that it is the "peri-implantation environment" created after COHS that is responsible for these changes.
- *Lower incidence of biochemical pregnancies*: Gonadotropins cause alterations in endometrial gene and protein expression which might compromise the ability of embryos to develop once implanted, possible increasing the biochemical pregnancy rate with fresh ET.
- *Lower ectopic pregnancy rate*: Most centers report ectopic pregnancies in fresh ET cycles in the range of 3–7%. The risk factors are longer stimulation, elevated estradiol, and progesterone causing abnormal tubal and uterine contractions. FET cycles have a lower incidence of ectopic pregnancies (2.2% vs. 5%), the incidence being lowest in blastocyst transfer cycles.

Weaknesses

- Increase in costs.
- Increased treatment duration time (2–3 months for one cycle).
- Patient disappointment for not having a fresh ET.
- Not enough randomized controlled trials (RCTs) comparing fresh and FET. Results of five major trials are awaited at the time of writing this chapter. Preliminary results from a Vuong (Vietnam) indicate no difference in pregnancy rate between fresh and FET (although PCOS was excluded from that study).
- Evidence of improved pregnancy rates in three RCTs only. Most studies are limited to high responders and elimination of OHSS.

Opportunities

- Elimination of hormone monitoring and patient friendliness (can do away with cumbersome estimations of estradiol-progesterone).
- More oocytes with delayed triggering (no concern about the implantation window).
- Scheduling possibilities.

Threats

- Available evidence for superiority of freeze-all is only for patients of PCOS.
- Extrapolation of these results to all IVF patients should be done with caution.
- There are reports of large for GA and macrosomic babies with FET (babies being heavier by 160 g) which warrants confirmation.
- Long-term implications of vitrification and FET on the babies are not known and need to be studied.

CONCLUSION

Freeze-all seems to be promising for numerous reasons. There are confirmed reports of better obstetric and perinatal outcomes with significant reduction in incidence of early pregnancy losses, ectopic pregnancies, biochemical pregnancies, preterm labor, SGA, PIH, abnormal placentation, and LBW babies with the use of FET as compared to fresh ET. The author's own experience has been extremely fulfilling especially in high responders, poor responders (with embryo accumulation), endometriosis, PCOS, thin endometrium, inadvertent diagnosis of an endometrial polyp during the course of COS, repeated implantation failures, and low- or high-serum progesterone levels on the day of hCG.

Whether "Freeze-all" should be applied to all IVF patients (especially normo-responders without any complicating factors) is still under study. There is no concrete evidence to support this at the current moment. It is necessary to have the "best" laboratory and vitrification "technique" to successfully implement a freeze-all program. Reports of macrosomic fetuses and long-term implications on the baby need to be studied in more detail.

AUTHOR'S RECOMMENDATIONS

Freeze-all (segmented IVF) seems to be ideal for patients with PCOS, poor responders, endometriosis, repeated implantation failures, thin endometrium, and those having very low- or elevated serum progesterone levels on the day of the hCG trigger.

Freeze-all is associated with a reduced risk of OHSS, improved endometrial receptivity, and higher implantation rates. Also, the risk of ectopic pregnancy, biochemical pregnancy, early miscarriage, placenta previa, pre-term birth, SGA, and perinatal mortality is significantly reduced.

For a successful freeze-all program, it would be mandatory to have the "best" laboratory and vitrification technique to implement freeze-all on a routine basis. The potential disadvantages of a freeze-all policy are an increased (yet unconfirmed) risk of macrosomia, increased costs, not enough RCTs to prove its efficacy for all patients (especially normo-responders), and no data on poor responders. Although there are many potential advantages in performing FET over fresh ET, it seems that the freeze-all strategy is not designed for all IVF patients. There are a large number of patients that get pregnant and do not have any obstetric/perinatal complications even after fresh ET. A recent study by Roque et al. (presented at ESHRE, 2017) showed that there is no benefit with freeze-all in cycles where 4–9 oocytes are retrieved. Also, there is no benefit in poor responders (not undergoing embryo accumulation) where 1–3 oocytes are retrieved. However, the study showed that for patients with more than 10 oocytes, freeze-all gives a higher live birth rate. The need of the hour is therefore, to individualize our clinical decisions (for normo-responders) on the basis of number of oocytes retrieved and to develop a noninvasive test to evaluate the endometrial receptivity during a fresh cycle that will allow the selection of patients that would benefit from fresh embryo transfer or freeze-all.

REFERENCES

1. Roque M. Freeze-all policy: is it time for that? J Assist Reprod Genet. 2015;32:171-6.
2. Nastri CO, Ferriani RA, Rocha IA, et al. Ovarian hyper stimulation syndrome: pathophysiology and prevention. J Assist Reprod Genet. 2010;27:121-8.
3. Youssef MA, van Wely M, Hassan MA, et al. Can dopamine agonists reduce the incidence and severity of OHSS in IVF/ICSI treatment cycles? A systematic review and meta-analysis. Hum Reprod Update. 2010;16:459-66.
4. Pandey S, Shetty A, Hamilton M, et al. Obstetric and perinatal outcomes in singleton pregnancies resulting from IVF/ICSI: a systematic review and meta-analysis. Hum Reprod Update. 2012;18:485-503.
5. Pindborg A, Wennerholm UB, Romundstad LB, et al. Why do singletons conceived after ART have adverse perinatal outcomes? Systematic review and meta-analysis. Hum Reprod Update. 2013;19:87-104.
6. Shapiro BS, Daneshmand ST, Garner FC, et al. Clinical rationale for cryopreservation of entire embryo cohorts in lieu of fresh transfer. Fertil Steril. 2014;102:3-9.
7. Maheshwari A, Pandey S, Shetty A, et al. Obstetric and perinatal outcomes in singleton pregnancies resulting from the transfer of frozen thawed versus fresh embryos generated through IVF treatment: a systematic review and meta-analysis. Fertil Steril. 2012;98:368-77.
8. Ishihara O, Araki R, Kuwahara A, et al. Impact of frozen-thawed single-blastocyst transfer on maternal and neonatal outcome: an analysis of 277,042 single-embryo transfer cycles from 2008 to 2010 in Japan. Fertil Steril. 2014;101:128-33.
9. Wennerholm UB, Henningsen AK, Romundstad LB, et al. Perinatal outcomes of children born after frozen-thawed embryo transfer: a Nordic cohort study from the CoNARTaS group. Hum Reprod. 2013;28:2545-53.
10. Roque M, Lattes K, Serra S, et al. Fresh embryo transfer versus frozen embryo transfer in IVF cycles: a systematic review and meta-analysis. Fertil Steril. 2013;99:156-62.
11. Aflatoonian A, Oskouian H, Ahmadi S, et al. Can fresh embryo transfers be replaced by cryopreserved-thawed embryo transfers in assisted reproductive cycles? A randomised controlled trial. J Assist Reprod Genet. 2010;27:357-63.
12. Shapiro BS, Daneshmand ST, Garner FC, et al. Evidence of impaired endometrial receptivity after ovarian stimulation for IVF: a prospective randomised trial comparing fresh and frozen-thawed embryo transfer in normal responders. Fertil Steril. 2011;96:344-8.
13. Shapiro BS, Daneshmand ST, Garner FC, et al. Evidence of impaired endometrial receptivity after ovarian stimulation for IVF: a prospective randomised trial comparing fresh and frozen-thawed embryo transfers in high responders. Fertil Steril. 2011;96:516-8.
14. Pinborg A, Henningsen AA, Loft A, et al. Large baby syndrome in singletons born after frozen embryo transfer: is it due to maternal factors or the cryotechnique. Hum Reprod. 2014;29:618-27.
15. Fanchin R, Righini C, Olivennes F, et al. Uterine contractions at the time of embryo transfer alter pregnancy rates after IVF. Hum Reprod. 1998;13:1968-74.
16. Fanchin R, Ayoubi JM, Oliviennes F, et al. Hormonal influence on the uterine contractility during ovarian stimulation. Hum Reprod. 2000;15(Suppl 1):90-100.
17. Zhu L, Li Y, Xu A. Influence of controlled ovarian stimulation on uterine peristalsis in infertile women. Hum Reprod. 2012;27:2684-9.
18. Devroey P, Polyzos NP, Blockeel C. An OHSS-free clinic by segmentation of IVF treatment. Hum Reprod. 2011;26:2593-7.
19. Kol S, Humaidan P. GnRH agonist triggering: recent developments. Reprod Biomed Online. 2013;26:226-30.
20. Fatemi HM, Popovic-Todrovic B, Humaidan P, et al. Severe OHSS after GnRH agonist trigger and "freeze-all" approach in GnRH antagonist protocol. Fertil Steril. 2014;101:1008-11.
21. Ling LP, Phoon JW, Lau MS, et al. GnRH agonist trigger and OHSS: relook at 'freeze-all' strategy. Reprod Biomed Online. 2014;29(3):392-4.
22. Humaidan P, Bungum L, Bungum M, et al. Reproductive outcome using a GnRH antagonist for luteolysis and follicular synchronisation in poor responder IVF/ICSI patients treated with a flexible GnRH antagonist protocol. Reprod Biomed Online. 2005;11:679-84.
23. Develioglu OH, Hsiu JG, Nikas G, et al. Endometrial estrogen and progesterone receptor and pinopode expression in stimulated cycles of oocyte doors. Fertil Steril. 1999;71:1040-7.
24. Kolibianakis E, Bourgain C, Albano C, et al. Effect of ovarian stimulation with recombinant FSH, GnRH antagonists, and HCG on endometrial maturation on the day of oocyte pick-up. Fertil Steril. 2002;78:1025-9.
25. Santos-Ribeiro S, Polyzos NP, Haentjens P, et al. Live birth rates are IVF are reduced by both low and high progesterone levels on the day of HCG administration. Hum Reprod. 2014;29(8):1698-705.

26. Mohamed AM, Chouliaras S, Jones CJ, et al. Live birth rate in fresh and frozen embryo transfer cycles in women with endometriosis. Eur J Obstet Gynecol Reprod Biol. 2011;156:177-80.
27. Ozgur K, Bulut H, Berkkanoglu M, et al. Concurrent oocyte retrieval and hysteroscopy: a novel approach in assisted reproduction freeze-all cycles. Reprod Biomed Online. 2016;33:206-13.
28. Scott Jr RT, Franasiak JM, Forman EJ. Comprehensive chromosome screening with synchronous blastocyst transfer: time for a paradigm shift. Fertil Steril. 2014;102:660-1.
29. Forman EJ, Hong KH, Ferry KM, et al. IVF with single euploid blastocyst transfer: a randomised controlled trial. Fertil Steril. 2013;100:100-7.
30. Rubio C, Rodrigo L, Mir P, et al. Use of array comparative genomic hybridisation (array-CGH) for embryo assessment: clinical results. Fertil Steril. 2013;99:1044-8.
31. Shapiro BS, Daneshmand ST, De Leon L, et al. Frozen-thawed embryo transfer is associated with a significantly reduced incidence of ectopic pregnancy. Fertil Steril. 2012;98:1490-4.
32. Fang C, Huang R, Wei LN, et al. Frozen-thawed day 5 blastocyst transfer is associated with a lower risk of ectopic pregnancy than day 3 transfer and fresh transfer. Fertil Steril. 2015;103(3):655-61.
33. Li Z, Sullivan EA, Chapman M, et al. Risk of ectopic pregnancy lowest with transfer of single frozen blastocyst. Hum Reprod. 2015;30(9):2048-54.
34. Ishihara O, Kuwahara A, Saitoh H. Frozen-thawed blastocyst transfer reduces ectopic pregnancy risk: an analysis of single embryo transfer cycles in Japan. Fertil Steril. 2011;95:1966-9.
35. Celada P, Bosch E, De Los Santos MJ, et al. Elective frozen embryo transfer does not improve reproductive outcome in normo-responder patients. Hum Reprod. 2015;30 (Suppl 1):i112.
36. Petropanagos A, Cattapan A, Baylis F, et al. Social egg freezing: risk, benefits and other considerations. CMAJ. 2015;187: 666-9.
37. Christophe B, Drakapoulos P, Ribeiro SS, et al. A fresh look at the freeze-all protocol: a SWOT analysis. Hum Reprod. 2016;31:491-97.

Elective Single Embryo Transfer

56

Gautam Khastgir

INTRODUCTION

The first successful in vitro fertilization and embryo transfer (IVF-ET) treatment was done in a natural cycle, where only one egg was collected and a single embryo was transferred.[1] However, in order to improve the success rate of IVF-ET, controlled ovarian hyperstimulation (COH) has been practiced to develop multiple oocytes. This has resulted in multiple embryos available for transfer, leading to higher incidence of iatrogenic twins, and higher-order multiple pregnancies. Over the period of years, it has been well accepted that the price one pays for higher success of any assisted reproductive treatment (ART) is increased maternal risk and poor perinatal outcome, mainly due to complications of twins and triplets. To avoid the problems of higher-order multiple pregnancies, clinicians often had no option other than to perform an invasive procedure like selective fetal reduction and accept its associated complications of pregnancy loss.

In spite of the fact that many twins are delivered healthy and the advances in neonatal medicine have decreased mortality and morbidity of premature babies, there still remains a significantly poor perinatal outcome with multiple pregnancies following ART. The risks related to multiple pregnancies include pregnancy-induced hypertension, gestational diabetes, pre-term delivery, low-birth weight, higher incidence of birth defects, and increase in the relative risk of neurological problems like cerebral palsy.[2] These complications lead to significant rise in the average healthcare cost of pregnancy, delivery, and neonatal care. It has been estimated that overall expenditure of multiple pregnancy is increased by 3–15 folds as compared to that of singleton pregnancies.[3-5] In addition, there are reports of severe stress experienced by the parents of multiples and lifelong support needed for mildly or severely disabled children.[6-9] As a result, there has been raving criticisms questioning the justification of entrusting the responsibility of our children's health in the hands of those involved with ART.[10,11] Hence, many reproductive scientists and clinicians from different parts of the world have voiced their opinions and convictions on elective single embryo transfer (eSET), in order to eliminate the problem of iatrogenic twin and higher-order multiple pregnancies.

RISKS OF MULTIPLE PREGNANCIES FOR CHILDREN

The main cause of morbidity and mortality in children born after ART is the higher incidence of premature births in twin pregnancies, not to mention the higher-order multiples. Data from Sweden during period 1982 to 1995 showed that the incidence of multiple births after ART was much higher (27%) than the general population (1%). There were also a significantly higher incidence of preterm births (30.3% vs. 6.3%), low-birth weight (<2.5 kg) babies (27.4% vs. 4.6%), and perinatal mortality (1.9% vs. 1.1%) among ART babies in contrast to that in the controls. The higher frequency of multiple births as well as maternal characteristics such as advanced age, associated medical problems, and obesity were regarded as the main factors for adverse outcome, and not the ART treatment itself.[12] Further analysis of this data showed that abnormalities detected in ART children in contrast to the control population were ever more alarming. The risk of neurological diagnosis was much higher among twins in comparison to the singletons born after ART, but interestingly, the risk did not differ from that of control non-ART twins. The most common neurological problem detected was cerebral palsy, for which all ART babies including twins had a risk ratio of 3.7 (95% CI 2.0–6.6) whereas in the singletons it was 2.8 (95% CI 1.3–5.8). In addition, the risk of developmental delay was four times higher among ART children in contrast to that in the controls.[13]

A similar population-based study in Denmark compared the risks between twins and singletons born after ART. The risk of prematurity was 10 times higher before 37 weeks and 7.4 times higher before 32 weeks in twins as opposed to that in singletons.[14] In addition, congenital anomalies are also more common in twin pregnancies. The total malformation rate (minor + major) in twins (73.7/1,000) was significantly higher than that in singletons (55.0/1,000).[14] Other studies have also shown a higher prevalence of major malformations (9.3%) among ART infants when compared with the control infants. Of the ART infants with malformations, 70% were born from twin or triplet pregnancies.[15,16] Congenital heart disease is more common among twins than in singletons. Patent ductus arteriosus, typical of pre-term births, was found to be very common among twins.[17,18] An increased risk of anencephaly was also evident among twin infants born after ART.[19] Other perinatal complications typical of a twin pregnancy also occur in ART twin pregnancies.

The risk of premature birth with multiple pregnancies is further enhanced in conditions associated with prematurity such as uterine malformations, cervical incompetence, hypoplastic uterus as in Turner syndrome, and previous history of premature delivery. Therefore, multiple pregnancies should not be induced among individual who has any increased risk factor of premature delivery. It has been confirmed that pregnancy complications like intrauterine growth retardation and prematurity even in singleton pregnancies are caused by the condition called vanishing twin syndrome, which is actually a consequence of an ART twin pregnancy.[20,21]

RISKS OF MULTIPLE PREGNANCIES FOR MOTHER

Multiple pregnancy is a very high-risk factor for mother too, since it is associated with many obstetric complications. The risks of pregnancy-induced hypertension, pre-eclampsia, eclampsia, impaired glucose tolerance, pregnancy-induced diabetes, placental abruption, and placenta previa are much higher in twins than among the singletons.[22-24] All these conditions have adverse effects on maternal health in addition to increasing chances of operative delivery resulting in infection and blood loss leading to higher incidence of maternal morbidity and mortality.[14] Women who are already suffering from essential hypertension, heart disease, kidney problem, and diabetes are more likely to develop complications in pregnancy and therefore should avoid multiples by all means in order to prevent an alarmingly high-risk situation. Obesity further increases the risk of pregnancy-induced hypertension and gestational diabetes.[25] Therefore, increasing the risk of complications, with a twin pregnancy by transferring more than one embryo, is not desirable in these high-risk individuals.

Women with Turner syndrome suffer from primary ovarian failure and need ART with donor oocytes.[26-28] These women often have associated cardiac anomaly and suffer from essential hypertension. The most dangerous complication in Turner syndrome is aortic dissection and several such cases have been reported in pregnancy.[29] It is therefore justified not to increase the risk in pregnancy by transferring more than one embryo at a time. Women requiring ART with donor oocytes for other indications are likely to be of advanced age and have a higher risk of all medical complications in pregnancy. Since oocyte donation ART gives a much higher pregnancy rate it is prudent to transfer only one embryo to avoid the additional risks of multiple pregnancy in these relatively elderly women.[30-32]

OUTCOME OF ELECTIVE SINGLE EMBRYO TRANSFER

Several prospective randomized trials have been published to identify the difference in the pregnancy rates between one or two embryos of high-implantation potential in a homogenous group of ideal patients, i.e. younger than 35 years, first or second IVF/ICSI cycle. The embryos were transferred on day 2 in two studies,[33,34] on day 3 in two other studies,[35,36] and on day 5 in blastocyst stage in only one study.[37] In these studies taken together, the mean pregnancy rate after elective single embryo transfer (eSET) was 31.3% with 1.58% twins, whereas that after double embryo transfer (DET), the rates were 47.6% with 29.8% twins **(Table 1)**. A formal Cochrane meta-analysis came to similar conclusion.[38] Out of these randomized trials, in two studies, patients were randomized to receive one excellent fresh embryo followed by one frozen/thawed embryo (1+1), just in case the fresh attempt proved unsuccessful, versus two fresh embryos.[2] With the strategy of fresh plus frozen transfer, the cumulative pregnancy rate of 39.7% did not differ when compared to 43.5% when two embryos were transferred together. Data for fresh embryo transfers only,

Table 1: Randomized and cohort studies comparing the pregnancy rates (PR) and twins with single embryo transfer (SET) and double embryo transfer (DET).

Author (year)	*SET PR (%)*	*Twins (%)*	*DET PR (%)*	*Twins (%)*
Randomized trials				
Gerris et al. (1999)[35]	38.5	10	74	30.0
Martikainen et al. (2001)[36]	32.4	4.17	47.1	18.2
Gardner et al. (2004)[37]	60.9	0	76	47.4
Thurin et al. (2004)[33]	27.6	1.10	43.5	36.1
van Montfoort et al. (2006)[34]	33	0	47.4	17.8
Total	31.3	1.58	47.6	29.8
Cohort studies				
Gerris et al. (2002)[39]	35.1	0.81	36.2	35.6
De Sutter et al. (2003)[40]	28.2	0.61	31.7	30.4
Tiitinen et al. (2003)[41]	34.5	1.23	36.7	30.1
Catt et al. (2003)[42]	44.1	2.04	58.8	44.1
Gerris et al. (2004)[43]	40.3	0	40.4	30.8
Martikainen et al. (2004)[44]	34.7	0.93	31.8	n.a.
Total	33.9	1.0	35.0	32.6

the pregnancy rates were lower for eSET versus DET (27.6% vs. 43.5%). Most importantly, twinning rate after eSET was significantly lower.[33] In the other study, the cumulative pregnancy rates after fresh and frozen embryo transfers were 47.3% after SET and 58.6% after DET but in the latter group there was a large number (39%) of twins.[36]

However in cohort studies,[39-44] the mean pregnancy rate after eSET was 33.9% with 1% twin versus 35% after DET with 32.6% multiple pregnancies **(Table 1)**. In most of these studies, SET was elective, which means that it was performed when an excellent quality embryo was available from a cohort of several embryos. Thus, taken together, these data suggest that eSET yields the same pregnancy rate as non-elective DET. The differences in the outcome of SET versus DET between randomized and cohort studies could be anticipated. In the randomized trials, all embryos were of good-quality, transferred in selected cases with good prognosis, and cryopreserved for future use; obviously two good quality embryos yielded more pregnancies with an increased risk of twining than the "best" embryo. However, in the real-life cohort studies, there were no differences in the outcome because SET meant elective transfer of a highly selected embryo of predictable implantation potential, whereas DET resulted in transfer of a mixture of embryos of excellent, intermediate or poor implantation potential. In addition, the significant difference found in the randomized trials disappears when one cryopreservation cycle is added to the fresh eSET cycle.[33] An effective and active cryopreservation policy along with eSET protocol increases pregnancy rates per oocyte retrieval.[45] The policy of eSET even in the frozen-thawed treatment cycles obviously reduces the incidence of multiple pregnancies without affecting the pregnancy rates.[46] One of the benefits of eSET is an increase in the number of embryos available for cryopreservation that increases the cumulative pregnancy rate per oocyte harvest. It also gives an option of a second baby which is actually a "delayed twin" after the success in the first attempt **(Table 2)**.[47,48]

In spite of the evidence supporting eSET, some authors have conveyed their reservation about this approach arguing that the benefits are limited to only good prognosis patients, which actually constitutes only a small minority of ART patients in clinical practice. They suggested that the argument in favor of indiscriminate eSET is unrealistic and should be reconsidered.[51,52] Others have stressed the importance of counseling and educating patients as well as members of the staff, since both are hankering after a higher success of ART for obvious reasons.[53] It is true that overzealous and indiscriminate use of eSET, without any option of embryo and patient selection, would damage the interest of the patients by significantly lowering the success rate of ART. Therefore, judicious application of eSET should

Table 2: Pregnancy rates (PR) with fresh and frozen assisted reproductive treatment (ART) cycles with single embryo transfer (SET) and double embryo transfer (DET).

	Fresh cycles PR (%)		***Fresh + Frozen cycles PR (%)***	
Author (year)	SET	DET	SET	DET
Tiitinen (2003)[41]	38.6	–	62.4	–
Thurin (2004)[33]	27.6	43.5	39.7	–
van Montfoort (2004)[49]	24	34	36	38
Catt (2003)[42]	44	59	74	70
Uchiyama (2004)[50]	44.9	–	72.4	–

be adopted with a balanced view about the benefits and limitations. Several reviews have given balanced arguments to optimize, not maximize, ART results by selective use of eSET.[54,55]

Many early studies demonstrated the difference in the pregnancy rates between nonelective and elective SET. If only one embryo was available for transfer, the pregnancy rate was 20% per transfer, but if an elective SET was carried out in a nonselected population, a pregnancy rate of 29.7% was achieved, which was similar to that in a non-selective two-embryo transfer (29.4%).[56] However, recent prospective randomized trials and cohort studies have confirmed that in a selected population of patients, when top or good quality embryos are available, elective SETs result in much better pregnancy rates than non-selective SETs and that such pregnancy rates are similar to those achieved by the transfer of two embryos.[57,58] Similarly, pregnancy outcome was not affected when blastocyst-stage embryos were transferred resulting in a live birth rate of 53.8% after eSET and 54.4% after DET with a twin rate of 3.1% and 51%, respectively.[59]

The practice of eSET has proved to be a successful method by which the incidence of multiple pregnancies can be reduced without affecting the overall pregnancy rates.[41] In real life, it has not only been equally affective but also, economically, substantially cheaper than DET with all its complications.[43,60] However, in order to be as effective as DET, there has to be some criteria to select the patients suitably for eSET because in a nonselected population eSET resulted in a lower pregnancy rate.[61] There are now data from Sweden and Belgium, which have laws and guidelines for regular SET, to support the fact that pregnancy rates have remained similar, while the rates of multiple pregnancies have dropped significantly when compared before and after adopting the practice of eSET.[62,63]

CRITERIA FOR ELECTIVE SINGLE EMBRYO TRANSFER

The essential prerequisites of introducing SET in an ART center are reasonably good ongoing pregnancy rate of the existing treatment protocol along with a compellingly highmultiple pregnancy rate, and presence of an efficient cryopreservation program. In order to achieve similar pregnancy rates between single and double embryo transfers, some kind of selection process must be there to balance the likelihood of pregnancy and minimize the risk of twins.[61] The criteria used in the majority of the studies include age of the female partner, absence of tubal pathology, endometriosis and severe male factor subfertility, fewer number of earlier unsuccessful cycles, non-ongoing pregnancy in the first cycle, good ovarian response with lower dose of FSH stimulation, adequate number of oocytes collected, fertilized 2-polar nuclei (PN) stage zygotes available and embryo quality.[64-67] Different authors have taken different values for some of these parameters but currently recommended criteria for eSET are: (1) age of the female partner between 35 and 39 years or less; (2) the number of previous unsuccessful ART cycles up to 2–3; and (3) most importantly, selection from at least two good quality embryos. By strictly following these criteria, there has been reports of unchanged pregnancy rates along with a twin pregnancy rate of less than 5%.[63]

Elective single embryo transfer implies that the choice of selection of only one embryo from among two or more good quality embryos. However, if only one embryo is available, obviously that is not elective but compulsory SET. Since the majority of these cycles occur in poor prognosis patients, i.e. older women, poor responders to ovarian stimulation, severe male factor subfertility, and intrinsic fertilization defects, the only available embryo may be of poor quality resulting in low implantation and live birth rates of 10–19% and 9–15%, respectively.[40,41] Therefore, in such patients, if two or more embryos of suboptimal quality are available, then eSET should be avoided to improve the pregnancy rate.

In a subpopulation of women multiple pregnancies substantially increase the risk of premature delivery. Congenital uterine anomaly, previous mid-trimester miscarriage due to cervical incompetence, past history of severe prematurity even with singleton pregnancy, previous loss of twin pregnancy, bad obstetrical history and severe systemic disease, i.e. essential hypertension, heart disease, kidney problems, and insulin-dependent diabetes constitute absolute contraindication against more than one embryo transfer. This is referred to medically indicated SET. Such contraindications are more relevant both in young women with Turner syndrome as well as in elderly women, since both groups of patients are at a greater risk of medical complications and also require oocyte donation which has much higher success rate of ART with an increased rate of pregnancy as well as multiples.

IMPROVED OUTCOME EVEN IN SINGLETONS WITH ELECTIVE SINGLE EMBRYO TRANSFER

It is interesting to note that eSET gives not only less twins but also better singletons. The outcome of singletons in a standard two-embryo transfer ART program is worse than naturally conceived singletons but such difference is not seen between ART and natural twins.[68,69] However, singletons after eSET do not compare unfavorably with spontaneously conceived singletons.[70] It has also been reported that ongoing ART pregnancies showing first-trimester blood loss had an inferior obstetrical and neonatal outcome than when no first-trimester blood loss occurred. The complications included antepartum hemorrhage, intrauterine growth retardation, preterm delivery, low-birth weight, preterm pre-labor rupture of membranes, increased cesarean sections, greater need for neonatal intensive care units (NICU) admission, respiratory distress syndrome, necrotizing enterocolitis, and higher-perinatal mortality. Interestingly, there was almost a linear relationship between the number of embryos transferred and the incidence of first-trimester blood loss.[40] Many of these singleton pregnancies after ART resulted in a vanishing twin manifested with first-trimester bleeding.[71] The association between the number of embryos transferred, first-trimester bleeding, and adverse pregnancy outcome provides a further argument in favor of eSET. Studies suggest that the birth weight of singletons born after eSET (3,324.6 ± 509.7 g) was lower than that after two-embryo transfer (3,204.3 ± 617.5 g). SET in comparison to DET shows lower incidence of low-birth weight (<2,500) (4.2% vs. 11.6%). The incidence of prematurity less than 37 weeks was 6.2% for singleton after SET versus 10.4% after DET.[72] eSET does not only prevent the well-known and documented complications of twin pregnancies, but actually improves the outcome of singleton pregnancies.

HEALTH ECONOMIC ASPECTS OF SINGLE EMBRYO TRANSFER

Although the main reason for adopting the practice of eSET is the good health of children at the beginning of their life, it is also true that the financial considerations are of great significance. The increased cost for the babies born after ART are mainly due to higher utilization of hospital care as a consequence of multiple pregnancies.[7] It has been calculated that the estimated cost for a twin pregnancy was 3 times and that of a triplet pregnancy was 15 times as expensive as a singleton pregnancy after ART.[4,5] However, health economic models have shown that eSET and DET are financially equivalent per live born child since eSET needs more cycles for successful outcome and yields less child per cycle but DET requires less number of cycles in achieving pregnancy with higher obstetrics plus neonatal costs per child and these effects balance out each other.[73,74] The financial burden imposed by multiple pregnancy would suffice to finance additional ART cycles.[75] Similarly, another study confirmed that multiple pregnancies after ART are associated with higher cost to the National Health System (NHS) and utilization of money saved by implementation of a mandatory two-embryo transfer policy could double the number of NHS-funded ART cycles at no extra cost; further saving could be made if good prognosis is less than 35 year age, SET policy were to be adopted.[3] In countries where patients self-fund their ART cycles, proper counseling is needed to convince them that the pregnancy rate would not decline with eSET if combined with cryopreservation. The acceptance of eSET would be higher if results are expressed and patients are charges per oocyte harvest and not per cycle or transfer. Patients are often happy with the prospect of twins and are keen to have more embryo transfer without any idea of higher obstetric and perinatal risks. As regards the higher cost of neonatal care with multiple pregnancies, the patient awareness can be increased by arranging group discussions for prospective parents with those who have already had such experiences.

CONCLUSION

To improve the success rates in ART, the clinicians have induced COH toward multifollicular development leading to in vitro fertilization of several oocytes and transfer of multiple embryos per cycle. This has resulted in an undesirable but expected side effect of twin and higher-order multiple pregnancies which increase the health risk of both mothers and their children. The problems are largely due to the higher chance of premature births and are also caused by the increased incidence of congenital anomalies among multiple pregnancies. With evolving embryo culture techniques even transfer of a single embryo of good quality now results in a pregnancy rate comparable to that of natural conception. Although the pregnancy rates of ART can be improved tremendously by increasing the number of embryos transferred, but sadly enough, the prices to be paid are the maternal and neonatal sufferings due to multiple pregnancies. Hence, it is prudent not to transfer more than one embryo to eliminate the possibilities of multiple pregnancies. Therefore, decreasing the prevalence of multiple pregnancies, while maintaining or improving overall success rates of ART, remains the most significant contemporary goal of infertility research.

In order to obtain equal pregnancy rates between single and double embryo transfer, certain criteria have been used for patient selection for ART. In women under the age of 40 years, during her first three ART cycles, and with good quality embryos, a reasonable success rate with a twin rate of less than 5% can be achieved. However, two embryos need to be transferred in women who do not fulfill these criteria. If the embryo is intact after thawing, only a single frozen-thawed embryo should be transferred. Irrespective of women's age, the number of earlier cycles or the embryo quality, single embryo should be transferred in women known to have a high risk of premature birth such as congenital uterine anomaly, cervical incompetence or hypoplastic uterus. The same is true as regards the maternal contraindications for multiple pregnancies, such as hypertension, cardiac problem, diabetes, and obesity. With increasing maternal age or Turner syndrome, in addition to maternal contraindication, a better success rate with ART using oocyte donation, single embryo transfer is considered more suitable.

The mainstay of eSET depends upon selection of the most appropriate embryo to be transferred to achieve pregnancy. Analysis of embryo morphology and development of suitable grading systems have helped in identification of most suitable embryo for transfer. As regards the criteria of good quality embryos, the features are early cleavage by 25 hours, four cells on day 2, eight cells on day 3, no multinucleated blastomere, less than 20% fragmentation, embryo within an even zona pellucida. An exception of one of these parameters still counts a good-quality embryo. In the blastocyst stage, an expanded blastocyst with compacted inner cell mass and cohesive trophectoderm epithelium on day 5 indicate good quality. The introduction of eSET compels the embryologists to optimize their embryo selection procedure. It appears that the decision may be made in the cleavage-stage selection, and in certain circumstances blastocyst culture may facilitate identification of the most suitable embryo to maximize results without increasing the risk of twin pregnancy. In frozen embryo transfer cycles, an intact embryo after thawing is indicative for eSET suitability.

In a number of developed countries, the problems associated with multiple pregnancies have been eliminated by legal restrictions on the number of embryos that can be transferred in one ART cycle. In other parts of the world, where no legal bindings exists, the onus is on the individual clinician as well as the patient to limit the number of embryos transferred, so that an acceptable balance can be achieved between the risks associated with multiple pregnancies and a reasonable pregnancy rate with ART. It is expected that the clinics in countries lacking legislation will be compelled by medicolegal, financial, and moral obligations to restrict the number of embryos transferred in order to minimize the risks of multiple pregnancy.

REFERENCES

1. Steptoe PC, Edwards RG. Birth after reimplantation of a human embryo. Lancet. 1978;2:366.
2. Adashi EY, Barri PN, Berkowitz R, et al. Infertility therapy-associated multiple pregnancies (births): an ongoing epidemic. Reprod Biomed Online. 2003;7:515-42.
3. Ledger WL, Anumba D, Marlow N, et al. The costs of to the NHS of multiple births after IVF treatment in the UK. BJOG. 2006;113:21-5.
4. Hidlebaugh DA, Thompson IE, Berger MJ. Cost of assisted reproductive technologies for a health maintenance organizations. J Reprod Med. 1997;42:570-4.
5. Wolner-Hanssen P, Rydhstroem H. Cost-effectiveness analysis of in-vitro fertilization: estimated costs per successful

pregnancy after transfer of one or two embryos. Hum Reprod. 1998;13:88-94.
6. Ellison MA, Hall JE. Social stigma and compound losses: equality-of-life issues for multiple-birth families. Fertil Steril. 2003;80:405-14.
7. Ericson A, Nygren KG, Otterblad Olausson P, et al. Hospital care utilization of infants born after IVF. Hum Reprod. 2002;17:929-32.
8. Glazebrook C, Sheard C, Cox S, et al. Parenting stress in first-time mothers of twins and triplets conceived after in vitro fertilization. Fertil Steril. 2004;81:505-11.
9. Ostfeld BM, Smith RH, Hiatt M, et al. Maternal behavior toward premature twins: implications for development. Twin Res. 2000;3:234-41.
10. Pennings G. Multiple pregnancies a test case for the moral quality of medically assisted reproduction. Hum Reprod. 2000;15:2466-9.
11. ESHRE Task Force on Ethics and Law. Ethical issues related to multiple pregnancies in medically assisted procreation. Hum Reprod. 2003;18:1976-9.
12. Bergh T, Ericson A, Hillensjo T, et al. Deliveries and children born after in-vitro fertilization in Sweden 1982-95: a retrospective cohort study. Lancet. 1999;354:1579-85.
13. Stromberg B, Dahlquist G, Ericson A, et al. Neurological sequelae in children born after in-vitro fertilization: a population-based study. Lancet. 2002;359:461-5.
14. Pinborg A, Loft A, Nyboe Andersen A. Neonatal outcome in a Danish national cohort of 8602 children born after in vitro fertilization or intracytoplasmic sperm injection: the role of twin pregnancy. Acta Obstet Gynecol Scand. 2004;83:1071-8.
15. Sperling L, Kiil C, Larsen LU, et al. Detection of chromosomal abnormalities, congenital abnormalities and transfusion syndrome in twins. Ultrasound Obstet Gynecol. 2007;29:517-26.
16. Merlob P, Sapir O, Sulkes J, et al. The prevalence of major congenital malformations during two periods of time, 1986-1994 and 1995-2002 in newborns conceived by assisted reproduction technology. Eur J Med Genet. 2005;48:5-11.
17. Caputo S, Russo MG, Capozzi G, et al. Congenital heart disease in a population of dizygotic twins: an echocardiographic study. Int J Cardiol. 2005;10:293-6.
18. Hajdu J, Beke A, Marton T, et al. Congentital heart diseases in twin pregnancies. Fetal Diagn Ther. 2006;21:198-203.
19. Ben-Ani I, Vaknin Z, Reish O, et al. Is there an increased rate of anencephaly in twins? Prenat Diagn. 2005;25:1007-10.
20. Spellacy WN. Antepartum complications in twin pregnancies. Clin Perinatol. 1988;15:79-86.
21. Pinborg A, Lidegaard O, Freiesleben NC, et al. Vanishing twins: a predictor of small for-gestational aging IVF singletons. Hum Reprod. 2007;22:2707-14.
22. Duckitt K, Harrington D. Risk factors for pre-eclampsia at antenatal booking: systematic review of controlled studies. BMJ. 2005;330:565.
23. Erez O, Vardi IS, Hallak M, et al. Preeclampsia in twin gestations: associations with IVF treatments, parity and maternal age. J Matern Fetal Neonatal Med. 2006;19:141-6.
24. Allen VM, Wilson RD, Cheung A, et al. Pregnancy outcomes after assisted reproductive technology. J Obstet Gynaecol Can. 2006;28:220-50.
25. Dokras A, Baredziak L, Blaine J, et al. Obstetric outcomes after in vitro fertilization in obese and morbidly obese women. Obstet Gynecol. 2006;108:61-9.
26. Khastgir G, Abdalla H, Thomas A, et al. Oocyte donation in Turner's syndrome: an analysis of the factors affecting the outcome. Hum Reprod. 1997;12:279-85.
27. Foudila T, Soderstrom-Anttila V, Hovatta O. Turner's syndrome and pregnancies after oocyte donation. Hum Reprod. 1999;14:532-5.
28. Hovatta O. Pregnancies in women with Turner's syndrome. Ann Med. 1999;31:106-10.
29. Bondy CA, Turner's Syndrome Study Group. Care of girls and women with Turner's syndrome: a guideline of the Turner Syndrome Study Group. J Clin Endocrinol Metab. 2007;92:10-25.
30. Soderstrom-Anttila V, Vilska S, Makinen S, et al. Elective single embryo transfer yields good delivery rates in oocyte donation. Hum Reprod. 2003;18:1858-63.
31. Soderstrom-Anttila V, Vilska S. Five years of single embryo transfer with anonymous and non-anonymous oocyte donation. Reprod Biomed Online. 2007;15:428-33.
32. Soderstrom-Anttila V, Tiitinen A, Foudila T, et al. Obstetric and perinatal outcome after oocyte donation: comparison with in-vitro fertilization pregnancies. Hum Reprod. 1998:483-90.
33. Thurin A, Hausken J, Hillensjo T, et al. Elective single embryo transfer in IVF, a randomized study. N Engl J Med. 2004;351:2392-402.
34. van Montfoort APA, Fiddelers AAA, Janssen JM, et al. In unselected patients, elective single embryo transfer prevents all multiples, but results in significantly lower pregnancy rates compared with double embryo transfer: a randomized control trial. Hum Reprod. 2006;21:338-43.
35. Gerris J, De Neubourg D, Mangelschots K, et al. Prevention of twin pregnancy after in-vitro fertilization or intracytoplasmic sperm injection based on strict embryo criteria: a prospective randomized clinical trial. Hum Reprod. 1999;14:2581-7.
36. Martikainen H, Tiitinen A, Tomas C, et al. One versus two embryo transfers after IVF and ICSI: randomized study. Hum Reprod. 2001;16:1900-3.
37. Gardner DK, Surrey E, Minjarez D, et al. Single blastocyst transfer: a prospective randomized trial. Fertil Steril. 2004;81:551-5.
38. Pandian Z, Templeton A, Serour G, et al. Number of embryos for transfer after IVF and ICSI: a Cochrane review. Hum Reprod. 2005;20:2681-7.
39. Gerris J, De Neubourg D, Mangelschots K, et al. Elective single day-3 embryo transfer halves the twinning rate without decrease in the ongoing pregnancy rate of an IVF/ICSI programme. Hum Reprod. 2002;17:2621-6.
40. De Sutter P, Van Der Elst J, Coetsier T, et al. Single embryo transfer and multiple pregnancy rate reduced after IVF/ICSI: a 5-year appraisal. Reprod Biomed Online. 2003;18:464-9.

41. Tiitinen A, Unkila-Kallio L, Halttunen M, et al. Impact of elective single embryo transfer on the twin pregnancy rate. Hum Reprod. 2003;18:1449-53.
42. Catt J, Wood T, Henman M, et al. Single embryo transfer in IVF to prevent multiple pregnancies. Twin Res. 2003;6:536-9.
43. Gerris J, De Sutter P, De Neubourg D, et al. A real-life prospective health economic study of elective single embryo transfer versus two-embryo transfer in first IVF/ICSI cycles. Hum Reprod. 2004;19:917-23.
44. Martikainen H, Orava M, Lakkakorpi J, et al. Day 2 elective single embryo transfer in clinical practice. Hum Reprod. 2004;19:1364-6.
45. Tiitinen A, Hyden-Granskog C, Gissler M. What is the most relevant standard of success in assisted reproduction? The value of cryopreservation on cumulative pregnancy rates per single oocyte retrieval should not be forgotten. Hum Reprod. 2004;19:2439-41.
46. Hyden-Granskog C, Undila-Kallio L, Halttunen M, et al. Single embryo transfer is an option in frozen embryo transfer. Hum Reprod. 2005;20:2935-8.
47. De Neubourg D, Mangelschots K, Van Royen E, et al. Impact of patients' choice for single embryo transfer of a top quality embryo versus double transfer in the first IVF/ICSI cycle. Hum Reprod. 2003;17:2621-5.
48. Gerris J, De Neubourg D, De Sutter P, et al. Cryopreservation as a tool to reduce multiple birth. Reprod BioMed Online. 2003;7:286-94.
49. van Montfoort APA, Janssen JM, Fiddelers AAA, et al. Single versus double embryo transfer: a randomized study. Hum Reprod. 2004;19(Suppl. 1): i134.
50. Uchiyama K, Aono F, Kuwayama M, et al. The efficacy of single embryo transfer with vitrification. Hum Reprod. 2004;19(Suppl. 1), i135.
51. Flisser E, Licciardi F. One at a time. Fertil Steril. 2006;85:555-8.
52. Gleicher N, Barad D. The relative myth of elective single embryo transfer. Hum Reprod. 2006;21(6):1337-44
53. Wang J, Lane M, Norman RJ. Reducing multiple pregnancy from assisted reproduction treatment: educating patients and medical staff. Med J Aust. 2006;184:180-1.
54. Bergh C. Single embryo transfer: a mini review. Hum Reprod. 2005;20:323-7.
55. El-Toukhy T, Khalaf Y, Peter Braude. IVF results: optimize not maximize. Am J Obstet Gynacol. 2006;194:322-31.
56. Vilska S, Tiitinen A, Hyden-Granskog C, et al. Elective transfer of one embryo results in an acceptable pregnancy rate and eliminates the risk of multiple birth. Hum Reprod. 1999;14:2392-5.
57. Croucher CA, Lass A, Margara R, et al. Predictive value of the results of a first in-vitro fertilization cycle on the outcome of subsequent cycles. Hum Reprod. 1998;13:403-8.
58. Henman M, Catt JW, Wood T, et al. Elective transfer of single fresh blastocysts and later transfer of cryostored blastocysts reduces the twin pregnancy rate and can improve the in vitro fertilization live birth rate in younger women. Fertil Steril. 2005;84:1620-7.
59. Fiddelers AA, Severens JL, Dirksen CD, et al. Economic evaluations of single-versus double embryo transfer in IVF. Hum Reprod Update. 2007;13:5-13.
60. Van Montfoort AP, Fiddelers AA, Land JA, et al. eSET-irrespective of the availability of a good-quality embryo in the first cycle only is not effective in reducing overall twin pregnancy rates. Hum Reprod. 2007;22:1669-74.
61. Styer AK, Wright DL, Wolkovich AM, et al. Single-blastocyst transfer decreases twin gestation without affecting pregnancy outcome. Fertil Steril. 2008;89:1702-8.
62. Van Landuyt L, Verheyen G, Tournaye H, et al. New Belgian embryo transfer policy leads to sharp decrease in multiple pregnancy rate. Reprod Biomed Online. 2006;13:765-71.
63. Karlstrom PO, Bergh C. Reducing the number of embryos transferred in Sweden: impact on delivery and multiple birth rates. Hum Reprod. 2007;22:2202-7.
64. Shapiro BS, Harris DC, Richter KS. Predictive value of 72-hour blastomere cell number on blastocyst development and success of subsequent transfer based on the degree of blastocyst development. Fertil Steril. 2000;73:582-6.
65. Shapiro BS, Richter KS, Harris DC, et al. Dramatic declines in implantation and pregnancy rates in patients who undergo repeated cycles of in vitro fertilization with blastocyst transfer after one or more failed attempts. Fertil Steril. 2001;76: 538-42.
66. Strandell A, Bergh C, Lundin K. Selection of patients suitable for one-embryo transfer may reduce the rate of multiple births by half without impairment of overall birth rates. Hum Reprod. 2000;15:2520-5.
67. Bates GW, Ginsburg. ES Early pregnancy loss in in vitro fertilization (IVF) is a positive predictor of subsequent IVF success. Fertil Steril. 2002;77:337-41.
68. Helmerhorst FM, Perquin DAM, Donker D, et al. Parinatal outcome of singletons and twins after assisted conception: a systematic review of controlled studies. BMJ. 2004;328:261-4.
69. Jackson RA, Gibson KA, Wu YW, et al. Perinatal outcome in singletons following in vitro fertilization: a meta-analysis. Obstet Gynecol. 2004;103:551-63.
70. De Neubourg D, Gerris J, Magelachots K, et al. The obstetrical and neonatal outcome of babies born after single-embryo transfer in IVF/ICSI compares favourably to spontaneously conceived babies. Hum Reprod. 2006;21:1041-6.
71. Pinborg A, Lidegaard O, La Cour Freiesleben N, et al. Consequences of vanishing twins in IVF/ICSI pregnancies. Hum Reprod. 2005;20:2821-9.
72. De Sutter P, Delbaere I, Gerris J, et al. Birth weight of singletons in ART is higher after single than after double embryo transfer. Hum Reprod. 2006;21(10):2633-7.
73. De Sutter P, Gerris J, Dhont M. A health-economic decision analytic model comparing with single embryo transfer in IVF/ICSI. Hum Reprod. 2002;17:2891-6.
74. De Sutter P, Gerris J, Dhont M. A health-economic decision analytic model comparing double with single embryo transfer in IVF/ICSI: a sensitivity analysis. Hum Reprod. 2003b;18:1361.
75. Ombelet W, De Sutter P, Van der Elst J, et al. Multiple gestation and infertility treatment: registration, reflection and reaction-the Belgian project. Hum Reprod Update. 2005;11:3-14.

Luteal Phase Support

57

BN Chakravarty, Sunita Sharma

INTRODUCTION

Luteal phase reflects the quality of the corpus luteum.[1] Normal corpus luteum function needs optimal development of follicle followed by adequate LH surge leading to rupture of follicle, and luteinization of granulosa cells. Continuous tonic LH pulses maintain the function of corpus luteum during the luteal phase. The life span of corpus luteum is 14 ± 2 days formed after[2] rupture of follicle. The primary objective of normal luteal phase is to build up an optimally receptive endometrium to allow a mature blastocyst implantation and its growth, under the influence of estrogen and progesterone. Luteal phase-deficiency (LPD) was first described by Georgeanna Jones[3] in 1949. It is inadequate functional secretory change of the endometrium due to inadequate endogenous progesterone synthesis causing infertility and also recurrent pregnancy loss.[4,5] Currently, there is no clinically reproducible standard test to diagnose LPD to distinguish fertile from infertile women.

Luteal phase deficiency is an unavoidable consequence of all stimulated assisted reproductive technology (ART) cycles but seen in only 8.1% natural cycle.[6] Supraphysiological steroids after controlled ovarian hyperstimulation (COS) inhibit LH both in frequency and amplitude[7] which impairs the corpus luteum ability to produce sufficient progesterone. Edwards and Steptoe were the first to suggest that luteal phase support (LPS) was an essential step for outcome of in vitro fertilization (IVF) treatment.[8] LPS causes significant improvement in pregnancy rates compared to IVF cycles without luteal support.[9] There is now a general consensus that administration of progesterone is essential in ART, especially during the first few weeks after oocyte retrieval.[1]

Other indications of luteal phase support are—infertility, threatened miscarriage, and recurrent miscarriages. Assuming that, in the absence of a definite diagnostic test available for diagnosis of LPD, use of LPS for these indications is still empirical. The question is, which agent (s) should be used for LPS both in terms of efficacy and safety. hCG, progesterone, and estrogen have been used. After nearly 40 years of extensive trial, undoubtedly *progesterone* has become the drug of choice. Though in the initial years of ART treatment, hCG was used either alone or in combination, its limitation has now been well realized. Estrogen as luteal support along with progesterone has also been used sporadically though its exact efficacy and role is yet to be ascertained.

This chapter will highlight the evidence-based indications of luteal support and different drugs used for luteal phase-deficiency.

EVIDENCE-BASED USE OF LUTEAL PHASE SUPPORT IN CLINICAL PRACTICE

As there is no reliable test to diagnose luteal phase insufficiency, its treatment is either correction of any underlying condition, otherwise LPS is used as empirical treatment.[10] The clinical situations where LPS is used by clinician are listed below:

- Threatened miscarriage or recurrent miscarriage.
- Ovulation induction with clomiphene (CC)/letrozole/gonadotropins

- Controlled ovarian hyperstimulation (COH) with gonadotropins for IVF cycles with GnRH agonist/antagonist
- Luteal phase support after GnRh-agonist trigger.

Threatened Miscarriage or Recurrent Miscarriage

Though LPS is used for these conditions, Cochrane meta-analysis did not demonstrate any benefit of progesterone support in threatened miscarriage but some benefit was shown in patients with recurrent miscarriage. In our unit, we routinely support patients of recurrent miscarriage with progesterone. In unstimulated cycles, luteal phase support is not useful.[10]

Ovulation Induction with Clomiphene/Letrozole/Gonadotropins

Clomiphene is commonly used for ovulation induction. Luteal phase insufficiency was observed in 50% cycles with CC stimulation[11,12] due to its antiestrogenic effect on endometrium and inhibition of steroidogenesis in granulosa and lutein cells.[13] Literature review does not support use of LPS after CC use as there is no difference in clinical pregnancy rate and also the miscarriage per cycle.[14] A recent study from our unit observed that LPS is useful in decreasing miscarriage in polycystic ovary syndrome (PCOS) after CC induction.[15]

Letrozole is recently being used in PCOS women for ovulation induction. Though literature suggests there is no antiestrogenic effect of letrozole and it upregulates endometrial estrogen receptor, Montville et al. showed higher pregnancy rates in PCOS women using LPS after letrozole induction. Gonadotropin itself and along with hCG trigger inhibits LH secretion. 20% of these cycles are short cycles leading to luteal insufficiency.[16] Systematic review and meta-analysis suggest improvement of reproductive outcome with luteal phase progesterone supplementation after gonadotropin-stimulated intrauterine insemination (IUI) cycles.[17]

Controlled Ovarian Hyperstimulation with Gonadotropins for IVF Cycles with GnRH Agonist/Antagonist

In IVF cycles, GnRH agonist or antagonist along with high dose of gonadotropins (Gn) are used GnRH as ovarian stimulation protocol. These protocols are associated with multi-follicular development which invariably cause luteal phase insufficiency.

Why Luteal Phase Support is required in ART Cycles?

- Gonadotropin stimulation
- hCG-suppressing LH activity
- Removal of granulosa cells during oocyte retrieval and/or damage of granulosa cell
- High level of estrogen and progesterone-suppressing LH activity?
- Use of GnRH agonist or GnRH antagonist.

GnRh-agonist[18] and antagonist[19] usage can also lead to luteolysis. So it is recommended that LPS is mandatory in ART cycles.[10]

Luteal Phase Support after GnRH-agonist Trigger

In antagonist protocol, if women develop multiple follicles and are at high risk for OHSS, GnRH agonist trigger followed by a "freeze-all" policy is usually done. But if there is low risk of OHSS, fresh embryo transfer can be performed by modified luteal support (hCG rescue bolus after oocyte retrieval) which showed good pregnancy rates.[20,21] Some studies also suggest dual trigger which can avoid intensive LPS.

DRUGS USED FOR LUTEAL SUPPORT

- Progesterone
- hCG injections alone or in combination
- Estrogen in combination with progesterone
- GnRH agonist.

Progesterone

Currently, progesterone is the gold standard drug used as LPS for the following reasons:[22]

- Progesterone transforms the proliferative endometrium into secretory phase.
- It improves the endometrial receptivity by regulating window of implantation (WOI).
- Progesterone induces endometrial nitric oxide synthase (eNOS) expression causing increased vascularization and improvement of uterine blood flow and therefore may be used to ameliorate embryonic growth retardation and help in stable implantation.[23]

Flowchart 1: Embryo protective immunomodulation.

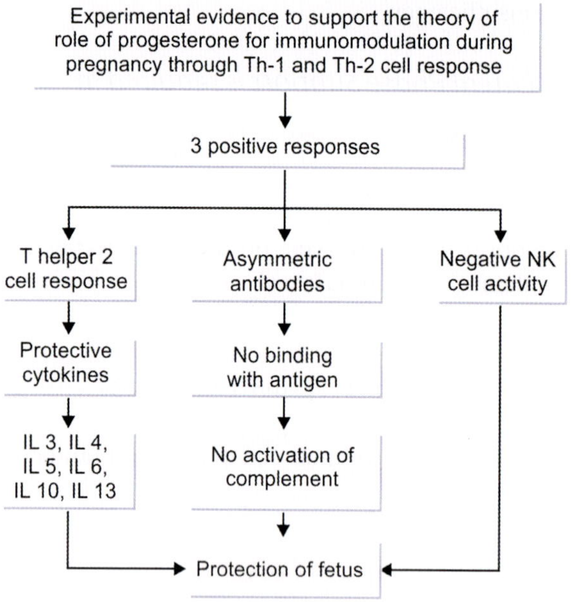

(IL: interleukin; NK: natural killer)

Flowchart 2: Immunologic protection of fetus through production of progesterone-induced blocking factor (PIBF).

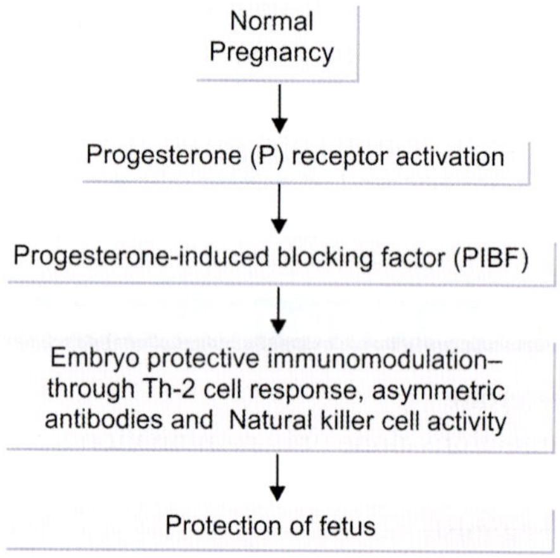

- Acts as immunomodulator which favors implantation and maintenance of pregnancy **(Flowcharts 1 and 2)**.
- Reduces uterine contractions during the period of implantation.

Routes of Progesterone Administration

Routes of administration of progesterone commonly used in practice are presented in the **Figure 1**.

Use of Natural Micronized Progesterone as LPS

This formulation was first marketed in France in 1980; extracted from soybeans or yam-roots (a Mexican Tree), and is identical to progesterone of ovarian origin. Different routes of administration have been depicted in the **Figure 1**.

Oral micronized progesterone,[24] is not a good drug for LPS because of poor bioavailability (6–8%)[25] due to intense hepatic metabolism during first "hepatic-pass" effect and is not able to produce sufficient pre-decidual changes in the endometrium.[26] Moreover, it has side effects of inducing drowsiness and gastric irritation. In spite of these limitations, recently oral "sustained release" formulation of these drugs with high protein binding of 90–99% has been introduced. This formulation allows once a day dosage which is convenient with minimum side effects. Efficacy of this formulation is yet to be approved in ART cycles.

For contraception, transdermal form of synthetic progestins exists but is not available for LPS in ART.

Vaginal progesterone is highly effective in inducing pre-decidual changes in endometrium, despite relatively low-serum levels and used for LPS and frozen embryo transfer (FET) treatment in ART cycles worldwide. Some women; however, report being distressed by the vaginal leakages encountered and/or wish to avoid vaginal application due to personal or cultural reason.

Injectable Progesterone Preparation

Progesterone in oil for daily intramuscular injection was found to be effective for LPS in ART and, in case of complete absence of endogenous progesterone, in donor egg[27] and FET models.[28] Serum concentration is higher than through vaginal route application. But pregnancy rates have been found similar in both with IM as with vaginal route administration.

Subcutaneous injectable aqueous formulation of progesterone is a newly introduced formulation of NMP which minimizes the side effects like pain and local inflammation seen with oil preparation. Two phase-III trials reported comparable efficacy of *subcutaneous injectable aqueous preparation* (25 mg) and vaginal progesterone preparations for LPS in ART.[29,30]

Types of Intravaginal Progesterone Used

Three types of intravaginal progesterone are used:

- *Capsules*: e.g. utrogestan, orgagest, microgest, etc.
- *Gel*: e.g. crinone 8.0%, susten 8.0%
- *Pessaries*: e.g. cyclogest.

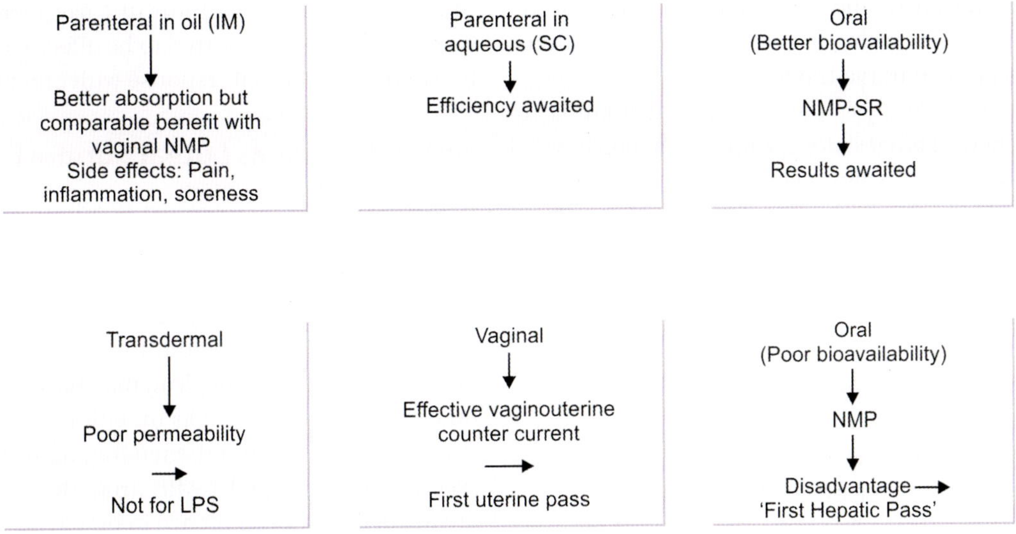

Fig. 1: Routes of administration of progesterone commonly used in practice.
(LPS: luteal phase support

Manufacturing procedure and pharmacological action, differences between capsules/pessaries and gel:

- *Progesterone capsules and pessaries are in oil emulsion:* Progesterone in the oily phase has to be dissolved in vaginal aqueous secretion for absorption. Abnormal vaginal discharge will interfere with absorption.
- *Progesterone gel:* Oil in water emulsion, on a polycarbophil base, ensures adhesion to vaginal epithelium. Oil in water emulsion guarantees controlled and continuous release. "Progesterone" in aqueous phase is first absorbed in tissues followed by replenishment from the oily phase depot. Polycarbophil maintains a vaginal pH 4.5 resulting in acidity of vaginal flora—acts against infection.

Advantages of gel over capsules and pessaries: Patient compliance is more with gel than with capsules or pessaries because:

- It is easier to handle.
- Less time-consuming.
- Less pain.
- Single application.

Overall advantage of one variety over the other: In spite of these differences in all vaginal applications, "first uterine pass" affects endometrial preparation and pregnancy rates are similar with each preparation.

Dydrogesterone, which is structurally and pharmacologically similar to natural progesterone, has improved bioavailability compared with micronized oral progesterone. It was shown to be as effective as other progesterone but has better tolerability and can be considered for luteal support in ART.[31,32]

A brief report of our study is given below: Our results suggest that oral dydrogesterone is as effective as micronized progesterone for LPS in women undergoing IVF. Several potential benefits of dydrogesterone have led us to believe that this drug may be considered as an alternative to vaginal progesterone for LPS. Dydrogesterone, an optical isomer of progesterone, has a high affinity for P receptors, and its conformational structure makes it a metabolically stable and orally effective drug. In patients diagnosed with LPD, dydrogesterone has been successfully used to induce normal endometrial maturation.[33,34] It is hypothesized that dydrogesterone, through its preferential affinity for progesterone receptor A, has a better potentiality to generate endothelial nitric oxide synthase and release nitric oxide, thereby enhancing endometrial vascularity.[35] It is also suggested that dydrogesterone restores normal concentration of progesterone-induced blocking factors in T lymphocytes and endometrial cells, which induces a favorable immunologic environment for implantation.[36]

Optimal Dose, Ideal Time to Start, and Duration of Progesterone Supplementation

Up till now, there is no uniformity of opinion regarding the exact starting day of progesterone administration following oocyte retrieval. There is now a general agreement for starting progesterone on the day of oocyte retrieval or the next day. Rationale of starting early LPS is to make the uterus quiescent on day of embryo transfer.

A recent meta-analysis concluded that there is no additional benefit of progesterone supplementation beyond the first positive hCG value—showing no difference in live birth, ongoing pregnancy, and miscarriage rates.[37] But in practice, most of the clinics continue progesterone supplementation till 8–12 weeks of gestation.[38] Doses of different progesterone formulations are:

- IM: 50–100 mg/day, subcutaneous 25–50 mg/day
- Vaginal capsules: 200 mg BID or TID
- Vaginal gel: 90 mg once or twice daily
- Vaginal tab: 200 mg BID or TID
- Dydrogesterone: 10 mg BID or TID.

SUMMARY

Literature has reported comparable efficacy with different routes of administration in terms of clinical pregnancy miscarriage and live birth. Though some studies showed better pregnancy with intramuscular progesterone compared to vaginal route, patient acceptability is low because of painful injections. So the choice of progesterone depends on side effects, acceptability, and availability.

hCG As Luteal Support

Human chorionic gonadotropin was shown to be superior or similar in efficacy to progesterone in terms of pregnancy outcome,[9] but use of hCG as luteal support has been abandoned because of increased risk of OHSS and progesterone is preferred for LPS.

Human chorionic gonadotropin as luteal support in our unit is occasionally used in combination with progesterone in poorly responding women where number of eggs retrieved is less than five and terminal estradiol is less than 700 pg/mL on day of hCG. The dose and protocol of hCG is as follows—2,000 IU on alternate day for 4 days following embryo transfer and the schedule is continued for 8 weeks if βhCG is positive.

Estrogen as Luteal Support

The corpus luteum produces both estrogen and progesterone. Addition of estrogen (E2) with progesterone can be beneficial for LPS. However, Cochrane 2011 review failed to show any beneficial effect of this combination in LPS. E2 can be administered orally, vaginally or transdermally. Estrogen pretreatment is essential part of endometrial preparation in frozen transfer cycles.[39] Non-oral route are reported to be effective in women who had poor endometrial response with oral estrogen.

GnRH Agonist as Luteal Support

A single dose GnRH agonist is administered 5–6 days following oocyte retrieval along with progesterone as LPS. The rationality of this supplementation is based on the fact that GnRH will induce LH release from pituitary which will maintain corpus luteum function. But it should also be remembered that the drug may have an adverse effect on endometrium as well as on embryos.[40] Though earlier studies[41-47] have reported encouraging results in subjects receiving GnRH agonist with progesterone, more studies are needed for its acceptance in practice.

But in spite of this encouraging report,[41-47] additional studies are required before this practice is *widely used as luteal phase support in ART cycles.*

Luteal Support in Frozen Embryo, or Donor-recipient Transfer Cycle

In these treatment protocols, normal cyclicity of the woman is either suppressed or absent. There is no formed corpus luteum and therefore there is no source of endogenous progesterone production. In these women, proliferative phase is artificially created with estrogen supplementation and then exogenous progesterone is added to induce secretory changes in the endometrium to create WOI.

After adequate endometrial preparation with estrogen, the duration of progesterone exposure of endometrium before embryo transfer is important. Nawroth and Ludwig[48] after reviewing the literature concluded that cleaving stage embryos should be transferred between 3 days and 4 days of progesterone treatment[49,50] *whereas blastocyst should be transferred on the 5th or 6th day of progesterone administration.*

TAKE HOME MESSAGE

- Luteal phase reflects the functional quality of the corpus luteum which is maintained by tonic luteinizing hormone pulses.
- Inadequate functional secretory changes of the endometrium can lead to infertility and recurrent pregnancy loss.
- Inadequate secretion of steroid hormones from corpus luteum causes inadequate functional secretory changes

of the endometrium leading to infertility and recurrent miscarriage.

- Since there is no reliable diagnostic test for luteal phase insufficiency, its treatment is also controversial in infertility and recurrent miscarriage.
- Luteal phase defect is an unavoidable consequence following ART protocols.
- Progesterone is the drug of choice for luteal phase support.
- Human chorionic gonadotropin, estrogen, and GnRH agonist may have a limited role.
- Different pharmacological preparations and routes of administration have been suggested for use of progesterone.
- Micronized progesterone through vaginal route is the preferred choice.
- Oral progesterone preparations except dydrogesterone has limited role.
- Efficacy of intra-muscular and vaginal micronized progesterone is similar but except the pain associated with intramuscular injection.
- Aqueous formulation of micronized vaginal progesterone is a recent introduction. Its efficacy and safety are yet be ascertained.

REFERENCES

1. Baird DT, Baker TG, McNatty KP, et al. Relationship between the secretion of the corpus luteum and the length of the follicular phase of the ovarian cycle. J Reprod Fertil. 1975;45(3):611-9.
2. Smith SK, Lenton EA, Landgren BM, et al. The short luteal phase and infertility. Br J Obstet Gynaecol. 194;91(11):1120-2.
3. Jones GES. Some newer aspects of management of infertility. JAMA. 1949;141:1123-9.
4. Siklósi GS, Bánhidy FG, Ács N. Fundamental role of folliculo-luteal function in recurrent miscarriage. Arch Gynecol Obstet. 2012;286(5):1299-305.
5. Sonntag B, Ludwig M. An integrated view on the luteal phase: diagnosis and treatment in subfertility. Clin Endocrinol (Oxf). 2012;77(4):500-7.
6. Tavaniotou A, Smitz J, Bourgain C, et al. Ovulation induction disrupts luteal phase function. Ann NY Acad Sci. 2001;943:55-63.
7. Tavaniotou A, Smitz J, Bourgain C, et al. Comparison between different routes of progesterone administration as luteal phase support in infertility treatments. Hum Reprod Update. 2000;6:139-48.
8. Buvat J, Marcolin G, Guittard C, et al. Luteal support after luteinizing hormone-releasing hormone agonist for in vitro fertilization: superiority of human chorionic gonadotropin over oral progesterone. Fertil Steril. 1990;53:490-4.
9. van der Linden M, Buckingham K, Farquhar C, et al. Luteal phase support for assisted reproduction cycles (Review). Cochrane Database Syst Rev. 2011;(10):CD009154.
10. Practice Committee of the American Society for Reproductive Medicine; 2015
11. Cook CL, Schroeder JA, Yussman MA, et al. Induction of luteal phase defect with clomiphene citrate. AJOG. 1984;149(6):613-6.
12. Balasch J, Vanrell JA, Durán M, et al. Luteal phase evaluation after clomiphene-chorionic gonadotrophin-induced ovulation. Int J Fertil. 1983;28(2):104-6.
13. Palomba S. Aromatase inhibitors for ovulation induction. J Clin Endocrinol Metab. 2015;100(5):1742-7.
14. Hill MJ, Whitcomb BW, Lewis TD, et al. Progesterone luteal support after ovulation induction and intrauterine insemination: a systematic review and meta-analysis. Fertil Steril. 2013;100:1373-80.
15. Sharma S, Geeta Rani BS, Bathwal S, et al. Progesterone supplementation in PCOS women undergoing clomiphene citrate stimulated IUI may improve pregnancy. Annals Int Med Dental Res. 2017;3(4).
16. Grazi RV, Frances MD, Taney H, et al. The luteal phase during gonadotropin therapy: effects of two human chorionic gonadotropin regimens. Fertil Steril. 1991;55(6):1088-93.
17. Miralpeix E, González-Comadran M, Solà I, et al. Efficacy of luteal phase support with vaginal progesterone in intrauterine insemination: a systematic review and meta-analysis. J Assist Reprod Genet. 2014;31:89.
18. Casper RF, Yen SS. Induction of luteolysis in the human with a long-acting analog of luteinizing hormone-releasing factor. Science. 1979;205:242-53,64.
19. Mais V, Kazer RR, Cetel NS, et al. The dependency of folliculogenesis and corpus luteum function on pulsatile gonadotropin secretion in cycling women using a gonadotropin-releasing hormone antagonist as a probe. J Clin Endocrinol Metab. 1986;62:1250-5.
20. Humaidan P, Polyzos NP. Human chorionic gonadotropin vs. gonadotropin-releasing hormone agonist trigger in assisted reproductive technology–"the king is dead, long live the king!". Fertil Steril. 2014;102:339-41.
21. Humaidan P, Alsbjerg B. GnRHa trigger for final oocyte maturation: Is hCG trigger history? Reprod Biomed Online. 2014;29:274-80.
22. Fatemi HM, Popovic-Todorovic B, Papanikolaou E, et al. An update of luteal phase support in stimulated IVF cycles. Hum Reprod Update. 2007;13(6):581-90.
23. Grazul-Bilska AT, Navanukraw C, Johnson ML, et al. Expression of endothelial nitric oxide synthase in the ovine ovary throughout the estrous cycle. Reproduction. 2006;132:579-87.
24. De Ziegler D, Fanchin R. Progesterone and progestins: applications in gynecology. Steroids. 2000;65:671-9.
25. Bruno de Lignières MD. Oral micronized progesterone. Clin Ther. 1999;21(1):41-60.
26. De Ziegler D, Fanchin R, Massonneau M, et al. Hormonal control of endometrial receptivity. The egg donation model

and controlled ovarian hyperstimulation. Ann N Y Acad Sci. 1994;734:209-20.
27. Navot D, Laufer N, Kopolovic J, et al. Artificially induced endometrial cycles and establishment of pregnancies in the absence of ovaries. N Engl J Med. 1986;314: 806-11.
28. Casper RF, Yanushpolsky EH. Optimal endometrial preparation for frozen embryo transfer cycles: window of implantation and progesterone support. Fertil Steril. 2016;105:867-72.
29. Lockwood G, Griesinger G, Cometti B, et al. Subcutaneous progesterone versus vaginal progesteronegel for luteal phase support in in vitro fertilization: A non-inferiority randomized controlled study. Fertil Steril. 2014;101:112-9.e3.
30. Baker VL, Jones CA, Doody K, et al. A randomized, controlled trial comparing the efficacy and safety of aqueous subcutaneous progesterone with vaginal progesterone for luteal phase support of in vitro fertilization. Hum Reprod. 2014;29:2212-20.
31. Chakravarty BN, Shirazee HH, Dam P, et al. Oral dydrogesterone versus intravaginal micronised progesterone as luteal phase support in assisted reproductive technology (ART) cycles: results of a randomised study. J Steroid Biochem Mol Biol. 2005;97(5):416-20.
32. Ganesh A, Chakravorty N, Mukherjee R, et al. Comparison of oral dydrogestrone with progesterone gel and micronized progesterone for luteal support in 1,373 women undergoing in vitro fertilization: a randomized clinical study. Fertil Steril. 2011;95(6):1961-5.
33. Balasch J, Vanrell JA, Marquez M, et al. Dehydrogesterone versus vaginal progesteronein the treatment of the endometrial luteal phase deficiency. Fertil Steril. 1982; 37:751-4.
34. Jacobs MH, Balasch J, Gonzalez-Merlo JM, et al. Endometrial cytosolic and nuclear progesterone receptors in the luteal phase defect. J Clin Endocrinol Metab. 1987;64:472-5.
35. Simunic V, Tomic V, Tomic J, et al. Comparative study of the efficacy and tolerability of two vaginal progesterone formulations, crinone 8% gel and utrogestan capsules, used for luteal support. Fertil Steril. 2007;87:83-7.
36. Szekeres-Bartho J, Polgar B. PIBF: the double edged sword. Pregnancy and tumor. Am J Reprod Immunol. 2001;64:77-86.
37. Liu XR, Mu HQ, Shi Q, et al. The optimal duration of progesterone supplementation in pregnant women after IVF/ICSI: a meta-analysis. Reprod Biol Endocrinol. 2012;10(1):107.
38. Vaisbuch E, de Ziegler D, Leong M, et al. Luteal-phase support in assisted reproduction treatment: real-life practices reported worldwide by an updated website-based survey. Reprod Biomed Online. 2014;28(3):330-5.
39. Hancke K, More S, Kreienberg R, et al. Patients undergoing frozen-thawed embryo transfer have similar live birth rates in spontaneous and artificial cycles. J Assist Reprod Genet. 2012;29:403-7.
40. Pirad C, Donnez J, Loumaye E. GnRH agonist as novel luteal support: results of a randomized, parallel group, feasibility study using intranasal administration of buserelin. Hum Reprod. 2005;20(7):1798-804.
41. Oliveira JB, Baruffi R, Petersen CG, et al. Administration of single-dose GnRH agonist in the luteal phase in ICSI cycles: a meta-analysis. Reprod Biol Endocrinol. 2010;8(1):107.
42. Tesarik J, Hazout A, Mendjoza-Tesarik R, et al. Beneficial effect of luteal-phase GnRH agonist administration on embryo implantation after ICSI in both GnRH agonist-and antagonist-treated ovarian stimulation cycles. Hum Reprod. 2006;21(10):2572-9.
43. Ata B, Yakin K, Balaban B, et al. GnRH agonist protocol administration in the luteal phase in ICSI-ET cycles stimulated with the long GnRH agonist protocol: a randomized. Controlled double blind study. Hum Reprod. 2008;23(3):668-73.
44. Isik AZ, Caglar GS, Sozen E, et al. Single-dose GnRH agonist administration in the luteal phase of GnRH antagonist cycles: a prospective randomized study. Reprod Biomed Online. 2009;19(4):472-7.
45. Razieh DF, Maryam AR, Nasim T. Beneficial effect of luteal-phase gonadotropin-releasing hormone agonist administration on implantation rate after intracytoplasmic sperm injection. Taiwan J Obstet Gynecol. 2009;48(3): 245-8.
46. Ata B, Urman B. Single dose GnRH agonist administration in the luteal phase of assisted reproduction cycles: is the effect dependent on the type of GnRH analogue used for pituitary suppression? Reprod Biomed Online. 2010;20(1): 165-6.
47. Van der Linden M, Buckingham K, Farquhar C, et al. Luteal phase support for assisted reproduction cycles. Cochrane Database Syst Rev 2011;10:CD009154.
48. Nawroth F, Ludwig M. What is the "ideal" duration of progesterone supplementation before the transfer of cryopreserved-thawed embryos in estrogen/progesterone replacement protocols? Hum Reprod. 2005;20(5):1127-34.
49. Gibbons WE, Toner JP, Hamacher P, et al. Experience with a novel vaginal progesterone preparation in a donor oocyte program. Fertil Steril. 1998;69(1):96-101.
50. Haddad G, Saguan DA, Maxwell R, et al. Intramuscular route of progesterone administration increases pregnancy rates during non-downregulated frozen embryo transfer cycles. J Assist Reprod Genet. 2007;24(10):467-70.

Ovarian Hyperstimulation Syndrome 58

Anupam Gupta, Pooja Mehta

INTRODUCTION

Ovarian hyperstimulation syndrome (OHSS) is by far the most serious complication of ovulation induction which results in wide spectrum of clinical and laboratory signs and symptoms. It occurs as a hyper response to ovulation induction in patients undergoing assisted reproduction. The overall incidence is 2–3%; however, severe OHSS is seen rarely these days.

PATHOGENESIS OF OVARIAN HYPERSTIMULATION SYNDROME (FLOWCHART 1)

Enlarged ovaries and increased capillary permeability are main features of OHSS.

Following mediators are thought to be responsible for increased vascular permeability:

- Vascular endothelial growth factor (VEGF): This is the principle mediator which increases the capillary permeability. Human chorionic gonadotropin (hCG) causes rising VEGF levels.
- *Estrogen:* High levels of vascular steroids and estrogen were found in ascitic fluid but role is uncertain.[1]
- *Prostaglandin:* Only animal studies are available and role is not proven.[2]
- *Renin-angiotensin (RA) system:* Some of the characteristics can be explained by this. But it is not clear whether it can trigger OHSS or is merely secondary reaction.[3]
- *Histamine:* Role of histamine is not proven.[4]
- *Interleukins:* Some interleukins (IL6, IL8, IL1) are known to be altered in OHSS. They can also cause hypoproteinemia.[5]

Flowchart 1: Pathophysiology of ovarian hyperstimulation syndrome (OHSS).

Multiple luteinized cysts in the ovaries, increased estradiol levels

↓

Vascular endothelial growth factor and other vasoactive mediators from ovary

↓

Increased vascular permeability, fluid shift into third space

↓

Intravascular hypovolemia

↓

Hemoconcentration

↓

Hypercoagulable state

↓

Electrolyte imbalance

↓

End-organ damage

These factors cause extravascular fluid accumulation and intravascular hypovolemia, hemoconcentration. VEGF is a potent vasoactive protein, elevated levels were found in ascitic fluid and serum, but according to some studies, follicular fluid VEGF was 100 times more than serum and peritoneal levels.[6] Abramov and colleagues integrated the role of VEGF in OHSS samples received from therapeutic ascitic tap, in which VEGF was a major factor. It was found that adding specific antibodies against VEGF neutralizes

70% of capillary permeability activity. Hence, it was concluded that VEGF is major trigger for OHSS.[7]

Human Chorionic Gonadotropin

Both exogenous in the form of trigger and/or endogenous HCG during early pregnancy can lead to OHSS. It is attributed to long half-life of hCG as compared to luteinizing hormone (LH). hCG is considered to be the principle factor causing OHSS. Though it may not be sufficient alone as a causative factor, some cases of OHSS have been reported in spontaneous conceptions.

CLASSIFICATIONS

Ovarian hyperstimulation syndrome has been classified into various stages and grades according to the clinical symptoms, signs, ultrasonographic findings, and laboratory parameters. In general, mild and moderate forms of OHSS can be treated expectantly on out-patient department (OPD) basis (Table 1). Those with severe form should be admitted and those with critical OHSS are best managed in consultation with other specialist in intensive care setting. Fortunately, with the current treatment protocols, the incidence of severe and critical OHSS is negligible.

Type of Ovarian Hyperstimulation Syndrome

- Early: Within 5–7 days of hCG trigger
- Late: Observed once pregnancy occurs.

RISK FACTORS FOR OVARIAN HYPERSTIMULATION SYNDROME

Various factors have been identified to help define patients at high risk of ovarian hyperstimulation syndrome:[8]

- Age less than 30 years.
- Polycystic ovarian disease (PCOD), especially lean PCO
- Serum estradiol (E2) level greater than 3,500 pg/mL
- High baseline anti-Müllerian hormone (AMH) levels[9-11]
- High antral follicle count on D2/3 scan
- Previous history of OHSS
- Large number of small follicles (8–12 mm) during stimulation
- Use of hCG for trigger and/or luteal support
- Large number of oocytes retrieved (>25).

PREVENTION

According to ASRM recommendations (2016):[11]

- *Stimulation protocol affects the risk of ovarian hyperstimulation*: A Cochrane review which included data from 29 randomized controlled trials (RCTs) that evaluated live birth, showed a statistically significant lower incidence of OHSS in gonadotropin-releasing hormone (GnRH) antagonist group. As we can use GnRH agonist trigger in antagonist protocol, it brings down risk of OHSS significantly. This is the major advantage of antagonist protocol in hyper-responders. According to some studies, there is no difference in live birth rate (LBR) compared with GnRH agonist group;[12] whereas some studies have reported lower pregnancy rates with agonist trigger in fresh embryo transfer cycles. However, it is unclear whether clomiphene, as a part of GnRH antagonist protocol, has any role in influencing the risk of OHSS.[13]
- *Use of aspirin in ovarian hyperstimulation*: Increased platelet activation due to VEGF levels may lead to release of substances histamine, serotonin, platelet-derived growth factors, thus initiate the cascade of OHSS. Low-dose aspirin from beginning of stimulation till pregnancy test and prednisolone at various doses (10–30 mg) have been shown to reduce incidence of OHSS.

  Single RCT comparing aspirin alone versus no treatment and another study comparing aspirin along with steroid versus no treatment have supported role of aspirin in OHSS prevention.[14,15]

Table 1: Classification of ovarian hyperstimulation syndrome (OHSS).

Mild	*Moderate*	*Severe*	*Critical*
Mild abdominal distention, discomfort, bloating Ovarian size <8 cm	Nausea ± vomiting Moderate abdominal pain Ultrasound suggestive of ascites Ovarian size 8–12 cm	Clinical evidence of ascites Oliguria Hematocrit >45% Hypoproteinemia Ovarian size >12 cm	Hematocrit >55% Tense ascites or hydrothorax WBC >25,000/mL Oliguria/Anuria Thromboembolism ARDS (acute respiratory distress syndrome)

- *Metformin:* Metformin is an insulin-sensitizing drug, used for those with type 2 diabetes and also for PCOS patients.

  Metformin is shown to affect ovarian response by reducing the number of nonperiovulatory follicles thus estradiol secretion. Hence, metformin reduces the risk of OHSS in PCOS patients.[16]
- *Coasting:* Coasting is practice of withholding gonadotropins toward the end of controlled ovarian stimulation, which may be extended for up to 4 days to reduce OHSS risk. It causes atresia of small follicles without affecting large follicles.

  A systemic review of four RCTs concluded that coasting does not reduce the risk of OHSS, but is associated with lesser number of oocytes being retrieved. Hence, the evidence is not sufficient to support coasting for prevention of OHSS.[17]
- *Choice of trigger for final oocyte maturation:* hCG used as a trigger for ovulation mimics the endogenous preovulatory LH surge. But since hCG has very long half-life, there is LH-like activity postretrieval, which can lead to OHSS.

  Lowering the dose of hCG was tried with conflicting results. But it may or may not result in reduction in OHSS.[18]

  A Cochrane review published in 2014 which combined results of 17 RCTs assessed GnRH agonist as compared to hCG trigger in OHSS.[19] The incidence of OHSS was significantly low in agonist group, but at same time it was associated with reduced live birth rate in a fresh cycle ET. The mechanism due to which pregnancy rate is lower in agonist group is rapid decline of LH support in luteal phase. No cases of moderate or severe OHSS are seen if hCG is totally eliminated. An RCT found if GnRH agonist trigger is combined with a single bolus of 1,500 IU of hCG after oocyte retrieval, it reduces risk of OHSS in high-risk patients.[20] There is a fair evidence that reproductive outcomes are better with low-dose hCG when co-administered at the time of agonist trigger for luteal support, but it will carry small risk of OHSS too.
- *Dopamine agonist:* The sequence of events occurring in OHSS is largely attributed to increased vascular permeability of ovarian and peritoneal capillaries, which is in turn effect of ovarian hypersecretion of VEGF. It has been suggested that use of cabergoline which is dopamine receptor agonist, reduces VEGF activity and thus OHSS.[21]
- *Albumin*: Albumin increases the plasma oncotic pressure, thus binds to vasoactive substances, like factors related to renin-angiotensin system and VEGF. But albumin is a blood-derived product, there can be allergic or anaphylactic reactions.

In a Cochrane review of nine RCTs, albumin has been shown to decrease the odds of OHSS.[22] Some studies have concluded that risk of OHSS was comparable in patients using albumin versus coasting.[23] So the data is insufficient to conclude that albumin reduces OHSS.

- *Calcium*: Studies have shown that use of IV calcium infusion (10 mL of 10% calcium gluconate in 200 mL NS) on the day of ovum pick-up and days 1, 2, 3 after that, can reduce risk of OHSS.[24] Mechanism of action being increase in calcium cyclic adenosine monophosphate (cAMP)-stimulated renin secretion reduces angiotensin 2 synthesis, VEGF, thus reducing OHSS.

So there is fair evidence in support of calcium reducing OHSS risk.

- *Cryopreservation of embryos*: Since pregnancy increases risk of late OHSS, it is often prudent to postpone the embryo transfer to subsequent cycle.

  In a Cochrane database of 2007, which is supported by ASRM guidelines of 2016, there is fair evidence that cryopreservation prevents OHSS.[25]
- *Miscellaneous:* Use of luteal antagonist, letrozole, methyl prednisolone, IM progesterone, and ketoconazole *do not* have significant data to make any recommendations.

Thus, prevention of OHSS is one of the most important challenges in assisted reproductive technology (ART).

It needs special attention for primary prevention by identifying patients at risk, using GnRH antagonist protocol, GnRH agonist for trigger, coasting, cryopreservation (vitrification), cycle cancellation. IV albumin, dopamine agonist are definitely of use.

Follicular Aspiration

Many authors are of opinion that follicular aspiration for IVF does not have role in prevention of OHSS. Target serum E2 levels in conventional ovulation induction should not exceed 1,200–1,700 pg/mL. Proper induction of ovulation should rarely require E2 values to rise above 1,400 pg/mL.[26] However, occasionally severe OHSS with life-threatening complications may occur with E2 values less than 1,000 pg/mL.

One study has directly demonstrated the protective value of follicular aspiration on OHSS outcome. Laufer and colleagues[27] demonstrated in IVF cycles where OHSS occurred with ovulation induction, with subsequent follicular aspiration it was avoided in the same patients. Although severe OHSS can occur despite follicular aspiration, it usually occurs when E2 target values of greater than 6,000 pg/mL are reached. These values are several fold higher than permissible without follicular aspiration. Ovarian hyperstimulation syndrome occurred in IVF cycles mostly when, either extremely high E2 values were encountered, hCG boosting was used, or disproportionately few oocytes were retrieved. In patients who are prone to severe OHSS, two therapeutic modifications may reduce the severity of OHSS. First, an ovulation induction IUI cycle may be converted to IVF if hCG was inadvertently administered at E2 values and follicular parameters exceeding the safety limits. Second, aspiration of all follicles should be meticulously performed during OPU. It is clear that follicular aspiration and intrafollicular hemorrhage following that have a negative impact on function of corpus luteum.[28] Hence, the intraovarian mechanism leading to OHSS can be modified by surgical follicular aspiration. The ovarian renin-angiotensin system plays a major role in the pathogenesis of OHSS and surgical follicular aspiration may have a negative impact on this system as well.

Flowchart 2: Algorithm for treatment of severe and critical ovarian hyperstimulation syndrome (OHSS).

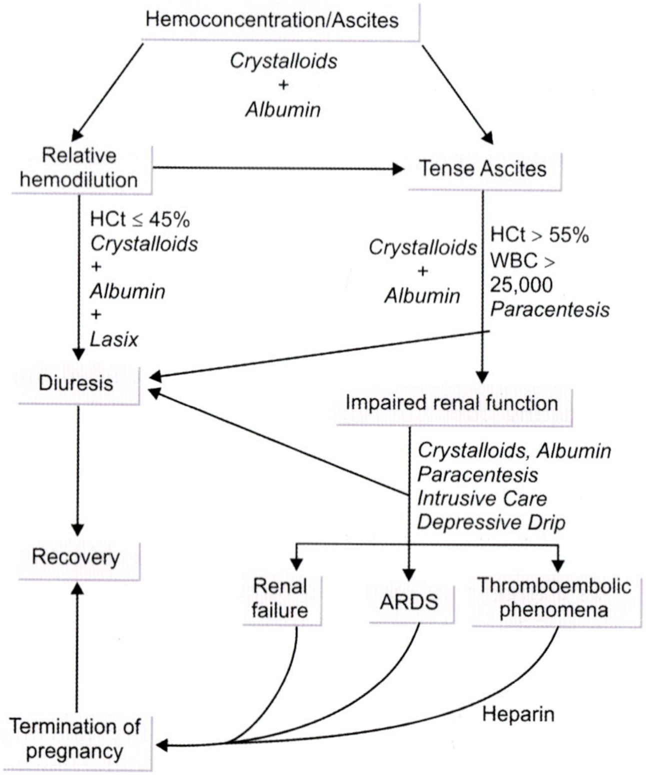

TREATMENT

Since the pathogenesis of OHSS is not clearly elucidated, treatment remains largely empirical. In patients having mild to moderate OHSS, bed rest, abundant liquid intake, and analgesics is the first-line of treatment. The symptoms of intravascular volume depletion and hyponatremia can be treated by balanced salt solution. If there is massive ascites and hemoconcentration, it means that OHSS is in the severe phase and hospitalization with intravenous (IV) fluid therapy is essential. Two important parameters: (1) laboratory signs of hemoconcentration; and (2) gradually accumulating ascites producing clinical symptoms should be monitored.

Algorithm

The algorithm for treatment of OHSS is described in **Flowchart 2.**

Hemoconcentration appears to best correlate with severity of OHSS.[29] Its level directly shows intravascular volume loss and blood viscosity. This, in turn, will influence kidney perfusion and the tendency for thromboembolic phenomenon. Another way to quantitatively measure hemoconcentration is the degree of leukocytosis; white blood cell (WBC) counts up to level of 35,000/mm have been observed. This severe neutrophilia can be result of generalized stress reaction. Therefore, the dual etiology of an elevated WBC count (stress and hemoconcentration) becomes very helpful in clinical assessment of OHSS. Electrolyte levels, renal function tests, levels of liver enzymes, and coagulation profile should be measured periodically. The daily volume replacement required can vary from 1.5 L to more than 3 L.

The five basic parameters to be monitored while maintaining the fluid balance are urine output, body weight, hematocrit, abdominal girth, and fluid input/output. Intravenous mode is preferred as it allows improvement in renal perfusion before it escapes into the peritoneal and/or pleural cavities. However, hemodilution achieved is at the cost of increasing ascites to some extent.

Ascites

There is a reciprocal relationship between hemoconcentration and the extravascular volume accumulation. At a relatively advanced stage of OHSS, which can occur after crystalloid and colloid therapy, gradual hemodilution is accompanied by a tightening abdominal wall secondary to the rapid accumulation of ascitic fluid. At this stage of intravascular volume expansion and improved renal perfusion, frequently there is a paradoxical situation characterized by oliguria, raised creatinine levels, and rapidly declining creatinine clearance. The probable cause for this effect is the intra-abdominal pressure produced by tense ascites. The increased intra-abdominal pressure may adversely affect renal venous outflow, thus leading to renal edema, congestion, and thrombosis. This problem can be dealt medically or surgically.

When hemodilution has been achieved, yet oliguria persists, furosemide at 10 mg or higher dose may be an effective form of treatment.[30,31]

Paracentesis stands the single most important treatment modality in life-threatening OHSS which is not responding to medication. It is indicated for symptomatic relief, in those with tense ascites, oliguria, increasing creatinine levels, and hemoconcentration not responding to medical therapy. Paracentesis should not be performed if the patient is hemodynamically unstable, or there is suspicion of hemoperitoneum. It should be performed under fully aseptic conditions. Z puncture in the abdominal wall is recommended to prevent continuous leakage of abdominal fluid. Ultrasound guidance during the procedure and careful monitoring of hemodynamic stability is mandatory. Up to 4 L of fluid can be removed by slow drainage to gravity.[31,32] Recently, Aboulghar and colleagues[33] and Rizk and Aboulghar[34] have suggested that transvaginal ultrasonically guided aspiration of ascitic fluid is also an effective and safe method.

Severe/Critical Ovarian Hyperstimulation

The most severe form of OHSS can lead to multi-organ failure. The major complications of OHSS are renal failure, thromboembolism, and acute respiratory distress syndrome (ARDS). It is very important to look for signs of impending renal failure and hypercoagulability. Those with such severe OHSS should be monitored in an intensive care unit. The first signs of impending renal failure are oliguria, gradually declining creatinine clearance, and increase in serum creatinine levels. These signs are usually accompanied by rapidly accumulating tense ascites. When all medications have failed to improve renal perfusion, dopamine drip can be used as last resort.[35] Intensive monitoring in the form of central venous pressure and pulmonary wedge pressure is indicated for monitoring hemodynamic balance.[36] The contracted intravascular volume would be expected to be accompanied by very low CVP.[36] Once stage of renal failure ensues, hemodialysis may be necessary, and at this stage, the painful alternative of interruption of pregnancy should be carefully considered.[35]

SUMMARY

Prevention

The primary way of preventing OHSS is identification of a high-risk patient. The patients who are most prone to develop OHSS have certain epidemiologic, hormonal, and ultrasonographic characteristics that should be at the back of mind of every clinician. A typical patient is usually young, with lean habitus, and PCOD-like hormonal composition, and a pathognomonic necklace sign on ultrasonography. During ovarian stimulation, if a patient has very high E2 levels in range of 4,000–6,000 pg/mL and multiple small, intermediate follicles are seen on sonography, the clinician should be on a high alert.[34] Whenever a patient is at high risk, hCG trigger should be withheld or GnRH agonist trigger should be used. Withholding hCG might cancel the cycle if required. Although follicular aspiration and in vitro maturation without hCG administration has been attempted, the clinical yield of such a strategy has not been established. Alternately, hCG may be administered in a lesser dose (i.e. 5,000 IU), oocyte retrieval performed, and embryo replacement deferred to a later date when the cryopreserved embryos can be thawed and transferred in subsequent cycle.

Treatment

Treatment of severe OHSS is to be conducted during hospitalization with meticulous monitoring of hemodynamic stability, plasma electrolytes, kidney and liver functions, coagulation profile, and most importantly hemoconcentration. Blood hemoconcentration is the single most important measure of both severity of the syndrome and the individual's response to treatment. An hematocrit of greater than 45% or greater than 30% increment over baseline are serious warning signs, whereas a hematocrit of greater than 55% signals a life-threatening situation. At this critical stage, leukocytosis may be in excess of 15,000–35,000 because of hemoconcentration and a generalized stress reaction. To correct for the contracted vascular space and electrolyte imbalance, a graduated approach is suggested. Initially, crystalloids are transfused at a rate of 100–150 mL/h. If hemoconcentration is not corrected or if oliguria ensues, human albumin is added to the IV regimen in doses of 100 g every 2–12 h. If diuresis is not induced; however, hematocrit is reduced and blood pressure maintained, and IV furesimide may be added to the regimen. Tense ascites with oliguria requires paracentesis. Impending renal failure and unrelenting hemoconcentration demand admission in intensive care unit and dopamine drip if needed. For thromboembolic phenomena, heparin should be started. Conditions like ovarian torsion, rupture of cyst, or ectopic (heterotopic) gestation would warrant surgical intervention. Lastly, therapeutic termination of an early gestation may be lifesaving if all other measures fail.

RECOMMENDATIONS[11] OF PRACTICE COMMITTEE OF THE AMERICAN SOCIETY FOR REPRODUCTIVE MEDICINE

- Women with PCOS, elevated AMH values, and elevated antral follicle count (AFC) may benefit from ovarian stimulation protocols that reduce the risk of OHSS (Grade B).
- Ovarian stimulation protocols using GnRH antagonists are preferable in women at high risk of OHSS (Grade A).
- The use of a GnRH agonist to trigger oocyte maturation prior to oocyte retrieval is recommended to reduce the risk of OHSS if peak estradiol levels are high or multifollicular development occurs during stimulation (Grade A).
- Low-dose hCG co-trigger, luteal hormonal support, or cryopreservation of embryos are strategies that may improve pregnancy rates in this setting (Grade B).
- Dopamine agonist administration starting at the time of hCG trigger for several days also may be used to reduce the incidence of OHSS (Grade A).
- Additional strategies to prevent OHSS which may be helpful include the use of metformin in PCOS patients (Grade A), aspirin administration (Grade A), and cryopreservation of embryos (Grade B).
- The mainstay of OHSS treatment includes fluid resuscitation and prophylactic anticoagulation. Paracentesis or culdocentesis may be recommended for management of OHSS when a large amount of ascites is present (Grade B).

REFERENCES

1. Meirow D, Schenker JG, Rosler A. Ovarian hyperstimulation syndrome with low oestradiol in non classical 17 alpha-hydroxylase. Hum Reprod. 1996;11(10):2119-21.
2. Schenker JG, Pollishuk WZ. The role of prostaglandins in OHSS. Eur J Obstet Gynecol Reprod Biol. 1976;6:47-52.
3. Abramov Y, Fatum M, Abrahamov D, et al. Hydroxyethylstarch versus human albumin for the treatment of severe ovarian hyperstimulation syndrome: a preliminary report. Fertil Steril. 2001;75(6):1228-30.
4. Erlik Y, Naot Y, Friedman M, et al. Histamine levels in ovarian hyperstimulation syndrome. Obstet Gynecol. 1979;53(5); 580-2.
5. Luke B, Brown MB, Morbeck DE, et al. Factors associated with ovarian hyperstimulation syndrome (OHSS) and its effect on assisted reproductive technology (ART) treatment and outcome. Fertil Steril. 2010;94:1399-404.
6. Jayaprakasan K, Herbert M, Moody E, et al. Estimating the risks of ovarian hyperstimulation syndrome (OHSS): implications for egg donation for research. Hum Fertil (Camb). 2007;10:183-7.
7. Levin ER, Rosen GF, Cassidenti DL, et al. Role of vascular endothelial cell growth factor in ovarian hyperstimulation syndrome. J Clin Invest. 1998;102:1978-85.
8. Lee TH, Liu CH, Huang CC, et al. Serum anti-Mullerian hormone and estradiol levels as predictors of ovarian hyperstimulation syndrome in assisted reproduction technology cycles. Hum Reprod. 2008;23:160-7.
9. . Practice Committee of the American Society for Reproductive Medicine. Prevention and treatment of moderate and severe ovarian hyperstimulation syndrome: a guideline. Fertil Steril. 2016;106:1634-47.
10. Ashrafi M, Bahmanabadi A, Akhond MR, et al. Predictive factors of early moderate/severe ovarian hyperstimulation syndrome in non-polycystic ovarian syndrome patients: a statistical model. Arch Gynecol Obstet. 2015;292:1145-52.
11. Ocal P, Sahmay S, Cetin M, et al. Serum anti-Mullerian hormone and antral follicle count as predictive markers of OHSS in ART cycles. J Assist Reprod Genet. 2011;28:1197-203.
12. Al-Inany HG, Youssef MA, Aboulghar M, et al. Gonadotrophin-releasing hormone antagonists for assisted reproductive technology. Cochrane Database Syst Rev. 2011:CD001750.
13. Gibreel A, Maheshwari A, Bhattacharya S. Clomiphene citrate in combination with gonadotropins for controlled ovarian stimulation in women undergoing in vitro fertilization. Cochrane Database Syst Rev. 2012;11:CD008528.
14. Vanagy A, Bodis J, Manfai Z, et al. Low-dose aspirin therapy to prevent ovarian hyperstimulation syndrome. Fertil Steril. 2010;93:2281-4.
15. Revelli A, Dolfin E, Gennarelli G, et al. Low-dose acetylsalicylic acid plus prednisolone as an adjuvant treatment in IVF: a prospective, randomized study. Fertil Steril. 2008;90:1685-91.
16. Huang X, Wang P, Tal R, et al. A systematic review and metaanalysis of metformin among patients with polycystic ovary syndrome undergoing assisted reproductive technology procedures. Int J Gynaecol Obstet. 2015;131:111-6.
17. D'Angelo A, Brown J, Amso NN. Coasting (withholding gonadotrophins) for preventing ovarian hyperstimulation syndrome. Cochrane Database Syst Rev. 2001:CD002811.
18. Lin H, Wang W, Li Y, et al. Triggering final oocyte maturation with reduced doses of hCG in IVF/ICSI: a prospective,

randomized and controlled study. Eur J Obstet Gynecol Reprod Biol. 2011;159:143-7.
19. Youssef MA, Van der Veen F, Al-Inany HG, et al. Gonadotropin-releasing hormone agonist versus HCG for oocyte triggering in antagonist-assisted reproductive technology. Cochrane Database Syst Rev. 2014:CD008046.
20. Humaidan P, Polyzos NP, Alsbjerg B, et al. GnRHa trigger and individualized luteal phase hCG support according to ovarian response to stimulation: two prospective randomized controlled multi-center studies in IVF patients. Hum Reprod. 2013;28:2511-2.
21. Leitao VM, Moroni RM, Seko LM, et al. Cabergoline for the prevention of ovarian hyperstimulation syndrome: systematic review and meta-analysis of randomized controlled trials. Fertil Steril. 2014;101:664-75.
22. Youssef MA, Al-Inany HG, Evers JL, et al. Intra-venous fluids for the prevention of severe ovarian hyperstimulation syndrome. Cochrane Database Syst Rev. 2011:CD001302.
23. Chen CD, Chao KH, Yang JH, et al. Comparison of coasting and intravenous albumin in the prevention of ovarian hyperstimulation syndrome. Fertil Steril. 2003;80:86-90.
24. Gurgan T, Demirol A, Guven S, et al. Intravenous calcium infusion as a novel preventive therapy of ovarian hyperstimulation syndrome for patients with polycystic ovarian syndrome. Fertil Steril. 2011;96:53-7.
25. D'Angelo A, Amso N. Embryo freezing for preventing ovarian hyperstimulation syndrome. Cochrane Database Syst Rev. 2007:CD002806.
26. Navot D, Rosenwaks Z. A systematic approach to ovulation induction. Contemp Obstet Gynecol. 1987;30:113-30.
27. Laufer N, Grunfeld L, Garrisi GJ. In vitro fertilization. In: Leibel MM (Eds). Infertility: A Comprehensive Text. Norwalk (CT): Appleton-Lange; 1990. pp. 481-511.
28. Dlugi AM, Laufer N, DeCherney AH, et al. The periovulatory and luteal phase of conception cycles following in vitro fertilization and embryo transfer. Fertil Steril. 1984;41:530-7.
29. Borenstein R, Elhalah U, Lunenfeld B, et al. Severe ovarian hyperstimulation syndrome: a re-evaluated therapeutic approach. Fertil Steril. 1989;51:791-5.
30. Belaisch-Allart J, Carmona F, Llach J, et al. Acute pre-renal failure and liver dysfunction in a patient with severe OHSS. Hum Reprod. 1990;5:348-51.
31. Padilla SL, Zamaria S, Baramki TA, et al. Abdominal paracentesis for the ovarian hyperstimulation syndrome with severe pulmonary compromise. Fertil Steril. 1990;53:365-7.
32. Thaler I, Yoffe N, Kaftory JK, et al. Treatment of ovarian hyperstimulation syndrome: the physiologic basis for a modified approach. Fertil Steril. 1981;36:110-3.
33. Aboulghar MA, Mansour RT, Serour Gl. Ovarian superstimulation in the treatment of infertility due to peritubal and periovarian adhesions. Fertil Steril. 1989;51:834-7.
34. Rizk B, Aboulghar MA. Modern management of ovarian hyperstimulation syndrome. Hum Reprod. 1991;6:1082-7.
35. Reed A, Tausk H, Reynolds H. Anesthetic considerations for severe ovarian hyperstimulation syndrome. Anesthesiology. 1990;73:1275-7.
36. Kirshon B, Doody MC, Cotton DB, et al. Management of ovarian hyperstimulation syndrome with chlorpheniramine maleate mannitol, and invasive hemodynamic monitoring. Obstet GynecoI. 1988; 71:485-7.

Adjuvant Therapies in ART

59

Surekha Kadam, Kinjal R Shah

INTRODUCTION

Adjuvants play a supportive role in each step of assisted reproductive technology (ART) cycle. Optimization of in vitro fertilization (IVF) process is extremely distressing for couples and presents a significant challenge to clinicians. Couples faced with unsuccessful IVF cycles may feel desperate to try anything to assist their chance of conception. This vulnerable population may eagerly utilize adjuvant therapies despite little evidence available to support their use. There are many adjuvant therapies to IVF with wide variety of different mechanism of action.

Success of IVF is determined by embryo quality and endometrial receptivity.

We can discuss adjuvants in ART in two groups:

1. First—adjuvants used during and before: Ovarian stimulation to enhance ovarian response, i.e. optimal folliculogenesis and oocyte maturation, e.g. growth hormone (GH), dehydroepiandrosterone (DHEA), coenzyme Q10 (CoQ10), letrozole, glucocorticoids, testosterone gel, etc.
2. Second—peri-implantation to increase embryo implantation, e.g.
   - Filgrastim [granulocyte colony-stimulating factor (GCSF)]
   - Aspirin
   - Low-molecular-weight heparin (LMWH)
   - Glucocorticoids
   - Intralipids
   - Platelet-rich plasma (PRP).

PRETREATMENT OF IN VITRO FERTILIZATION, INTRACYTOPLASMIC SPERM INJECTION

- Pretreatment of couples undergoing IVF with CoQ, antibiotics, metformin for polycystic ovary syndrome (PCOS) patients, have shown significant improvement in implantation rate.
- Pretreatment of poor responders with DHEA, testosterone gel, CoQ-10, etc. are commonly used by clinicians to improve embryo quality.

CoQ 10

- Coenzyme Q10 is a powerful antioxidant. It is found in every cell of the body, and is a part of the electron transport chain which is responsible for generating energy in our cells and is important for energy metabolism and preventing oxidative damage to cell membranes. COQ has shown to improve both sperm and egg quality.
- Coenzyme Q10 levels show declining trend with increasing age, which can lead to mitochondrial dysfunction and reduced oocyte quality and quantity. CoQ deficiency in male lead to not only DNA damage and but also low motility. Supplementation of CoQ in IVF in poor responders has shown higher ovarian responsiveness but without difference in birth rate.
- The suggested daily dose of CoQ for the average person is 100 mg/day.

- For elderly patients and patients with low CoQ levels we can start with 200–300 mg per day for 2 weeks then can be shifted to 100 mg daily for maintenance.

DHEA

- Androgen and their ovarian receptors have been shown to play an important role in ovarian physiology and follicular growth. Main androgen treatments involve direct androgen supplementation (DHEA and transdermal testosterone gel) and indirect increase of intraovarian androgen levels through aromatase inhibitors like anastrozole and letrozole
  Wiser et al. documented a beneficial effect of dehydroepiandrosterone supplementation on ovarian reserve.
- Dehydroepiandrosterone used in decreased ovarian reserve (DOR) patients have:
  1. Improved oocyte (ova, egg) production
  2. Improved embryo quality
  3. Both improved egg production and embryo quality in women aged 40–47 years
  4. Natural conception
  5. Considerable improvement in intrauterine insemination (IUI) and IVF outcome, as well as pregnancy outcome
  6. Reduced miscarriage risk.
- Women with PCOS are advised to avoid DHEA as their bodies often already have elevated levels of androgens.
- Most studies to date looking at the effects of DHEA on IVF outcome were based on retrospective or observational data and the results were not free from bias. Recent studies have found no difference in ovarian response in poor responder patients who received 12 weeks pre-IVF supplementation of DHEA vs placebo.

Testosterone Gel

- Patient compliance with testosterone gel is better due to convenience and it is painless. It is free of first pass effect liver metabolism.
- Experimental studies demonstrated that treatment with testosterone increased follicle-stimulating hormone (FSH) receptor expression in granulosa cells, promoting the initiation of primordial follicle growth and improving the number of growing preantral and small antral follicles.
- 12.5 mg TTG applied daily for 21 days in the cycle preceding COS for IVF, results in fewer days and total dose of recombinant human FSH used. The numbers of oocytes retrieved, mature oocytes, fertilized oocytes, and good-quality embryos are significantly higher in the TTG pretreatment patients. Embryo implantation rate and clinical pregnancy rate per cycle initiated also were significantly higher in the women pretreated with TTG. No patient reported adverse effects attributed to TTG use. TTG pretreatment might be beneficial in improving both response to COS and IVF outcome in low responders undergoing IVF or ICSI.
- However, heterogeneity is still encountered including: the dose and duration of the transdermal testosterone used. Further good quality randomized controlled trials (RCTs) are required to provide more *robust evidence and ensure more reliable conclusions in the future.*

Antibiotics

- Antibiotics have been shown to improve endometrial receptivity by reducing negative impacts of microbial colonization.
- The presence of infection has been suggested to negatively impact the likelihood of implantation and it has been demonstrated that antibiotics are effective in significantly reducing genital tract colonization.

Growth Hormone

- Poor responder patients show slight improvement in pregnancy rates with use of GH.
- Growth hormone is one such therapy. GH can be used in conjunction with gonadotropins, clomiphene, letrozole during ovarian stimulation.
- Growth hormone is produced not only by the pituitary but also locally by the ovary. It binds to GH receptors on granulosa, the thecal, and the luteal cells, thus promoting steroidogenesis and gametogenesis. GH, insulin-like growth factor 1 (IGF-1), and growth hormone-releasing hormone, all increase the sensitivity of ovaries to gonadotropin stimulation and enhance follicular development. GH also enhances aromatase and 3-β-hydrogenase activity, thus increasing the conversion of androgen into estrogens in females. This effect on the ovarian steroidogenic enzymes occurs through a direct and/or IGF-1-mediated mechanism. GHs, IGF-1, and IGF-2, all affect the maturation of the follicle and gamete as well.

- In hypogonadotropic hypogonadism role of GH in combination with human menopausal gonadotropin (hMG) and human chorionic gonadotropin (hCG) has evoked interest. This can reduce gonadotropin dose requirement, reduce duration of hMG treatment, and improve success rates.
- The Cochrane review of Harper and colleagues in 2003 showed the increase in IVF live birth rates in poor responders receiving GH adjuvant therapy.
- Meta-analysis and the updated Cochrane review have shown improved success rate of IVF in patients with GH.
- Recent reviews have listed the doses of GH used by various workers. Doses used in recent reports have ranged from 0.9 mg/week to 1.8 mg/week, administered until pregnancy is proven. Previously, higher doses have been used.
- Good patient selection has been shown to improve results of GH cotherapy for female infertility. Eugonadotrophicnormoprolactinemic patients with long-standing infertility and documented GH deficiency or pan hypopituitarism respond well to this treatment.

However, it cannot be recommended indiscriminately in every patient undergoing ovarian stimulation or assisted reproductive technology.

SECOND GROUP

Second group adjuvants used during peri-implantation to improve embryo implantation are described here.

Aspirin, Heparine, and Glucocorticoids

- Use of LMWH should be assessed and applied with counseling in patients with recurrent implantation failure after testing for inherited and acquired thrombophilia.
- Aspirin may enhance uterine perfusion and improve uterine receptivity.
- Low-molecular-weight heparin may have additional effects on embryo implantation and invasion of the endometrium.
- *Glucocorticoids:* Immune modulator, alters cytokine expression and excess natural killer (NK) cell activity, reduce endometrial inflammation

Aspirin and Heparin

- Aspirin may enhance uterine perfusion and it's anti-inflammatory, vasodilatory and anti-platelets properties. This improves endometrial receptivity.
- Dosage of aspirin used is typically between 50 mg and 100 mg daily, however there are wide variation in commencement and duration of aspirin. Literature includes many articles with mixed results concerning effect of this adjuvant. Five meta-analyses have been conducted investigating use of aspirin, in some studies aspirin is started on day of embryo transfer and in others it is started on day of downregulation. Four studies shown that it is not significant. Aspirin is also associated with vaginal bleeding and miscarriage. Thus despite of its theoretical potential or however, the use of aspirin as an adjuvant in ART remains controversial.
- Heparin: It may have effect on embryo implantation and invasion of the endometrium. It improves endometrial environment by activation of growth factors like IGF-1, cytokine expression, heparin-binding endometrial growth factor. This help in trophoblast invasion and proliferation, promoting embryo implantation. LMWH is derived from heparin by polymerization which shows increased bioavailability and half-life. LMWH is started on day of embryo transfer. Recent Cochrane review included three RCT, which showed peri-implantation heparin was associated with significant improvement in live birth rate than placebo.

Corticosteroids

Glucocorticoids have been found to have immuno-modulatory properties and alter NK cell activity[7] which provide optimal implantation conditions and protect against miscarriage. Varieties of drugs are used from embryo transfer to early placentation phase including prednisolone and dexamethasone. However dose schedules and duration of treatment vary enormously. Glucocorticoids used in ART are category D drug by FDA, which indicate routine administration is not indicated. The latest Cochrane review concerning the use of corticosteroids in ART was published in 2012 which shows inconclusive results, so more well-designed randomized studies are required to demonstrate efficacy of peri-implantation glucocorticoid therapy in IVF.

Endometrial Scratching

- Endometrial scratching prior to embryo transfer has shown beneficial effect on endometrial receptivity.
- Mechanical manipulation of endometrium induces secretion of proimplantation chemical factors like interlukin-1, epidermal growth factor (EGF)-like growth factor, and leukemia inhibitory factor. These factors

stimulate decidual reaction. It is done by introducing pipelle vaginally till uterine fundus and rotating within the uterine cavity.

- Karow et al. published initial studies on potential benefits of endometrial biopsy. 2015 Cochrane review on effectiveness and safety of endometrial scratching analyzed 14 trials. In the studies comparing endometrial injury performed between day 7 of the previous cycle and day 7 of the embryo transfer cycle, the intervention was associated with an increase in live birth or ongoing pregnancy rate in women with previous implantation failures. On the contrary, results from the only RCT comparing endometrial injury on the day of oocyte retrieval versus intervention, reported no significance.

GCSF

- In vitro fertilization success depends upon good quality embryo and receptive endometrium. Endometrial thickness is an important indicator evaluating endometrial receptivity and successful embryo implantation. Recently GCSF has been used in treatment of thin endometrium.
- First successful application of GCSF in the treatment of thin endometrium was reported by Gleicher and coauthors in 2012. Recently many researchers have found role of GCSF in female reproductive system from follicular development, ovulation, implantation, to maintenance of pregnancy. Suggested mode of actions are as follows:
  - *First:* Direct effect on endometrial proliferation by stimulating endometrial stem cells.
  - *Second:* GCSF has been shown to induce trophoblast proliferation and invasion for maintenance of pregnancy.
  - *Third:* Women with recurrent implantation failure (RIF) have low levels of GCSF receptors at feto-maternal interface, and GCSF administration increases the expression of GCSF receptors.
  - *Four:* GCSF has immune modulatory role. It enhances expression of CD16, CD56, and LIF. It switches the T cell cytokine secretion profile to the Th-2, and promotes differentiation of regulatory T cells.

  GCSF can be given as either subcutaneous injection or intrauterine infusion.
- Several studies have been conducted to study role of GCSF on outcome of ART. In meta-analysis by Zhao and Zhang et al in May 2016, GCSF has shown positive effects on clinical pregnancy outcome.

Intralipids

- Maternal and fetal immunology plays an important role in infertility, recurrent IVF failures, and recurrent pregnancy loss. Imbalanced cytokine network, aberrant immune response may be responsible for this.
- Patients with RIF, repeated IVF failures should be tested for thrombophilias, and if these tests are normal then they should be tested for immunological cause. Increase in levels of CD56 (dim) cells and NK cell cytotoxicity in peripheral blood may be contributing factors for RIF and IVF failures. Intralipid has been suggested to suppress NK cell activity, thus improves uterine receptivity.
- Intralipid is a fat emulsion constituting soy bean oil, egg phospholipids, and glycerine that has been shown to have immunosuppressive properties.
- Mode of administration—20% intralipid intravenous (IV) (9 mg/mL total blood volume—corresponding to 2 mL of intralipid 20% diluted in 250 mL saline; or 18 mg/mL—corresponding to 4 mL of intralipid 20% diluted in 250 mL saline), second infusion 2–3 weeks later.
- Studies suggest that intralipid may enhance implantation and maintenance of pregnancy when the patient has an abnormal NK cell activity. Larger studies are required to prove beneficial use of intralipids.

PRP

- Successful implantation of good quality embryo in IVF depends upon endometrial receptivity. Minimal endometrial thickness required for embryo transfer is 7 mm. Thin endometrium results in cycle cancellation and unplanned embryo freezing.
- Many strategies have been used for treatment of thin endometrium, which include exogenous estrogen, aspirin, vaginal sildenafil, VITE, GCSF, and electro-puncture.

  But many patients do not respond to conventional therapy. Intrauterine PRP infusion represents a new mode of treatment for the thin endometrium with poor response to conventional therapy.
- Platelet-rich plasma is prepared from centrifugation of autologous blood so that it contains concentration of platelets 4–5 times above normal. Platelets activate secretions of vascular endothelial growth factor

(VEGF), transforming growth factor (TGF), platelet-derived growth factor (PDGF), and EGF, which regulate endometrial proliferation and differentiation, and promote extracellular matrix accumulation.

- Platelet-rich plasma is prepared from centrifugation of autologous blood, and 0.5 mL to 1 mL is infused in the uterine cavity.
- If endometrial thickness did not improve in 72 hours, second instillation is done.
- A few studies so far have evaluated the role of intra-uterine instillation of autologous PRP in suboptimal endometrium.
- A single study by Chang et al. published in 2015 evaluated the role of autologous PRP in thin endometrium in five patients undergoing frozen embryo transfer cycles. It showed that all patients had increase in endometrial thickness more than 7 mm after 72 hours of PRP installation. All the five patients were pregnant. One of the patients had a missed miscarriage secondary to a chromosomally abnormal fetus, whereas the other four had viable intrauterine pregnancies, followed up till the first trimester.
- A review article by Garcia-Velasco et al. published in 2016 also cites the use of autologous PRP as a potential method of improving embryo transfer in women with refractory endometrium.
- To conclude PRP appears to be a promising tool in treatment of resistant poor endometrium where all routine therapies are ineffective. But more studies with better number and longer study duration are required before a strong recommendation of this therapy in future.

CONCLUSION

- For all adjuvant therapies, further investigation of their impact on the success of embryo transfers is needed with high-quality study designs.
- Couples faced with unsuccessful IVF cycles may feel desperate to try anything to assist their chance of conception. This vulnerable population may eagerly utilize adjuvant therapies despite little evidence available to support their use. Many of the interventions investigated in multiple studies fail to significantly demonstrate any effects of adjuvants on the success of embryo transfer. Continuous use of these adjuvants is not advisable until further high-quality trials with adequate sample sizes are performed.

SUGGESTED READING

1. Akhtar MA, Sur SD, Raine-Fenning N, et al. Heparin for assisted reproduction. Cochrane Database Syst Rev. 2013;(8):CD009452.
2. Aligeti S, Kirma NB, Binkley PA, et al. Colony-stimulating factor-1 exerts direct effects on the proliferation and invasiveness of endometrial epithelial cells. Fertil Steril. 2011;95:2464-6.
3. Boomsma CM, Keay SD, Macklon NS. Peri-implantation glucocorticoid administration for assisted reproductive technology cycles. Cochrane Database Syst Rev. 2007;(1):CD005996.
4. Chang Y, Li J, Chen Y, et al Autologous platelet-rich plasma promotes endometrial growth and Improves pregnancy outcome during in vitro fertilization. Int J Clin Exp Med. 2015;8(1):1286-90.
5. Dentali F1, Ageno W, Rezoagli E, et al. Low-dose aspirin for in vitro fertilization or intracytoplasmic sperm injection: a systematic review and a meta-analysis of the literature. J Thromb Haemost. 2012;10(10):2075-85.
6. Dirckx K, Cabri P, Merien A, et al. Does low-dose aspirin improve pregnancy rate in IVF/ICSI? A randomized double-blind placebo controlled trial. Hum Reprod. 2009;24(4):856-60.
7. Eftekhar M, Sayadi M, Arabjahvani F. Transvaginal perfusion of G-CSF for infertile women with thin endometrium in frozen ET program: A non-randomized clinical trial. Iran J Reprod Med. 2014;12:661-6.
8. Ferrario M, Secomandi R, Cappato M, et al. Ovarian and adrenal androgens may be useful markers to predict oocyte competence and embryo development in older women. Gynecol Endocrinol. 2015;31(2):125-30.
9. Gat I, Mejia BS, Balakier H, et al. (2015). The use of coenzyme Q10 and DHEA during COH and IVF cycles in patients with decreased ovarian reserve (DOR). [online] Available from https://doi.org/10.1016/j.fertnstert.2015.07.1015 [Last Accessed February, 2019].
10. Groeneveld E, Broeze KA, Lambers MJ, et al. Is aspirin effective in women undergoing in vitro fertilization (IVF)? Results from an individual patient data meta-analysis (IPD MA). Hum Reprod Update. 2011;17(4):501-9.
11. Kim CH, Howles CM, Lee HA. The effect of transdermal testosterone gel pretreatment on controlled ovarian stimulation and IVF outcome in low responders. Fertil Steril. 2011;95:679-83.
12. Kroon B, Hart RJ, Wong BM, et al. Antibiotics prior to embryo transfer in ART. Cochrane Database Syst Rev. 2012;(3):CD008995.
13. Ledee N, Lombroso R, Lombardelli L, et al. Cytokines and chemokines in follicular fluids and potential of the corresponding embryo: the role of granulocyte colony-stimulating factor. Hum Reprod. 2008;23:2001-9.
14. Nastri CO, Lensen SF, Gibreel A, et al. Endometrial injury in women undergoing assisted reproductive techniques. Cochrane Database Syst Rev. 2012;(7):CD009517.

15. ResearchGate. The effect of transdermal testosterone gel pretreatment on controlled ovarian stimulation and IVF outcome in low responders. [online] Available from https://www.researchgate.net/publication/46035741_The_effect_of_transdermal_testosterone_gel_pretreatment_on_controlled_ovarian_stimulation_and_IVF_outcome_in_low_responders [Last Accessed March, 2018].
16. Roussev RG, Acacio B, Ng SC, et al. Duration of intralipid's suppressive effect on NK cell's functional activity. Am J Reprod Immunol. 2008;60(3):258-63.
17. Roussev RG, Ng SC, Coulam CB. Natural killer cell functional activity suppression by intravenous immunoglobulin, intralipid and soluble human leukocyte antigen-G. Am J Reprod Immunol. 2007;57(4):262-9.
18. Siristatidis CS, Basios G, Pergialiotis V, et al. Aspirin for in vitro fertilisation. Cochrane Database Syst Rev. 2016; 11:CD004832.
19. Turi A, Giannubilo SR, Brugè F, et al. Coenzyme Q10 content in follicular fluid and its relationship with oocyte fertilization and embryo grading. Arch Gynecol Obstet. 2012;285(4):1173-6.
20. Vendola KA, Zhou J, Adesanya OO, et al. Androgens stimulate early stages of follicular growth in the primate ovary. J Clin Invest. 1998;101:2622-9.
21. Weil SJ, Vendola K, Zhou J, et al. Androgen receptor gene expression in the primate ovary: cellular localization, regulation, and functional correlations. J Clin Endocrinol Metab. 1998;83:2479-85.
22. Zeyneloglu HB, Onalan G. Remedies for recurrent implantation failure. Semin Reprod Med. 2014;32(4):297-305.

Optimize Oocyte Yield to Maximize Live Birth in Assisted Reproductive Technology

60

Sandros C Estevas

INTRODUCTION

In our society, the proportion of women with advanced female age and diminished ovarian reserve seeking fertility treatment is increasing steadily. Female age and oocyte number are the most robust predictors for pregnancy success in the in vitro fertilization (IVF) setting. It is, therefore, crucial to use the right ovarian stimulation (OS) protocol to secure the optimal oocyte yield. Flexibility in OS is critical because patients respond differently to exogenous gonadotropins. Recently, the POSEIDON criteria were proposed as a new and more detailed stratification system for infertility patients with "expected" or "unexpected" impaired ovarian response to exogenous gonadotropins. Furthermore, the POSEIDON group introduced a new measure of clinical success, namely, the ability to retrieve the number of oocytes needed to obtain, theoretically, at least one euploid blastocyst for transfer in each patient. Using the POSEIDON criteria, the clinician will, first of all, classify patients who have low prognosis in assisted reproductive technology (ART) and secondly, prepare an individualized stimulation plan aiming at achieving the number of oocytes that will increase the probability of generating at least one euploid blastocyst for transfer in each of the four POSEIDON patient categories. It is anticipated that the new POSEIDON concept of low prognosis will help improve counseling and management of challenging patients undergoing ART, ultimately maximizing success and shortening the time to live birth.

PRESENT SCENARIO

A current problem for clinicians working with reproductive medicine is that the proportion of patients of advanced age is increasing steadily. It is well-known that pregnancy rates are lower in these women than in their younger counterparts. However, it is also important to realize that the repetition of IVF treatments using a trial and error approach does not seem to help these patients much, since the gap between older and younger patients concerning cumulative pregnancy success actually increases after multiple IVF cycles.[1] In the era of personalized medicine, success in IVF goes far beyond pregnancy. It should be redefined taking into account other quality dimensions, without overlooking the patient perspective.[2,3] At Androfert Fertility Center, our approach includes the provision of proper evaluation, counseling about the chances of success, and development of a time-limited treatment plan taking in full consideration what patients' values and preferences are.[4]

Along these lines, ovarian biomarkers, like anti-Müllerian hormone (AMH) and antral follicle count (AFC), are now widely used for predicting ovarian response to gonadotropin stimulation. Despite their clear clinical value in that regard, we should not use their results to counsel our patients about their chances of achieving a pregnancy in IVF.[5,6] What became clear though over the last years is that if we want to maximize live births, we should optimize oocyte yields.[7-9] However, oocyte number should be combined with female age since the likelihood of achieving a live birth among patients with similar oocytes yield ultimately depends on female age. Thus, the number of oocytes needed to maximize live births should be individualized taking into account female age, and more importantly, patient-oriented strategies can be used to achieve the individualized oocyte number.

The abovementioned make the foundations of the novel POSEIDON criteria for low prognosis patients undergoing ART (www.groupposeidon.com).[10-12] The POSEIDON criteria propose a shift from the current terminology of poor ovarian response (POR) to the concept of low prognosis. The low prognosis patients are classified into four groups according to the results of ovarian markers (AMH, AFC, or both), female age, and the number of oocytes retrieved in previous stimulation if that information is available **(Fig. 1)**. Patients fitting the POSEIDON criteria have low prognosis owing to a decreased number of oocytes, a condition that can be further aggravated by aging and will affect cumulative live birth rates.[13] However, the prognosis of POSEIDON patients differs according to subgroup as it is affected by female age and the number of oocytes retrieved. In our institution, the proportion of patients classified as "POSEIDON patients" is approximately 50%.

According to the POSEIDON classification, patients are classified as groups 1 and 3 if younger than 35 years, and as groups 2 and 4 if older than that. Female age is a critical element because it is related to embryo ploidy. In a study by the POSEIDON group, we calculated the probability of a blastocyst being euploid as a function of female age.[14] This probability sharply declines after the age of 34 years and is lower than 50% overall in older patients **(Fig. 2)**. This phenomenon, in combination with the already reduced ovarian reserve in older patients, leads to an increased risk of having no euploid embryos for transfer. Moreover, the percent decline in blastocyst euploid probability progresses with every year of age, thus complicating matters further **(Fig. 3)**. In young women, the loss is low from 1 year to the next, but it increases remarkably as the patient ages.[14] In the study mentioned earlier, we also noted that the older the patient, the higher the number of embryos—and therefore, oocytes—needed to increase the chances of having at least one euploid embryo within the patient embryo cohort.

Overall, POSEIDON patients can be summarized as follows—(i) in groups 1 and 3, patients are young and therefore, the risk of embryo aneuploidy is relatively low. By contrast, (ii) in groups 2 and 4, patients are older, thus increasing the risk of embryo aneuploidy **(Fig. 4)**. As a result, the number of embryos generated is likely to be low in all categories, thus affecting the cumulative live birth rate. However, the prognosis of POSEIDON patients differs according to the group category.

Big data indicates that oocyte number to maximize cumulative live births should be higher than 15.[13] Although this number gives us general guidance, it might be hard to

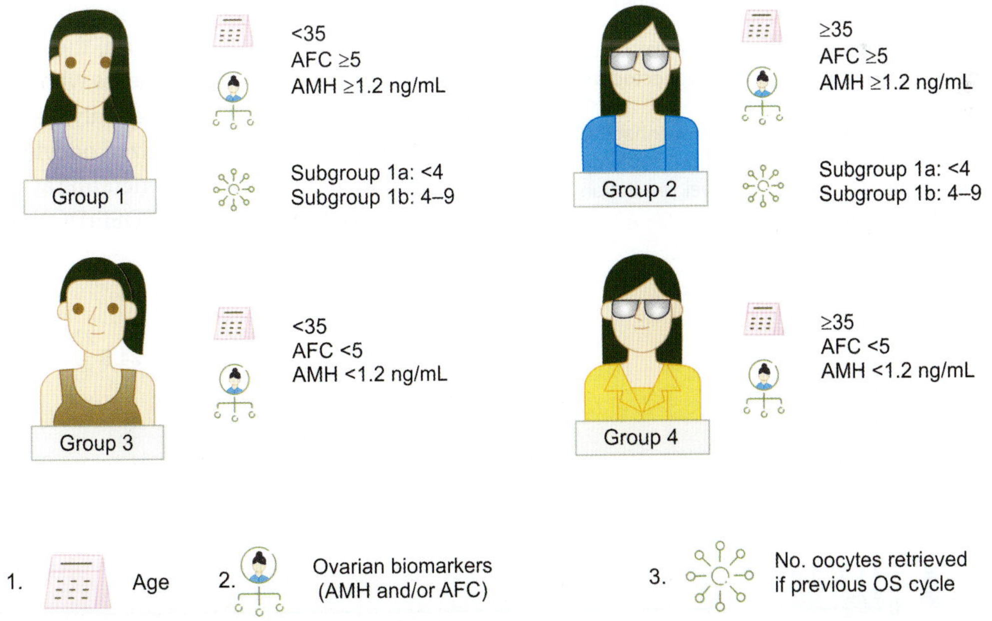

Fig. 1: The POSEIDON criteria of low prognosis patients in assisted reproductive technology (ART). Four distinct groups of low prognosis patients can be established based on quantitative and qualitative parameters, namely—(1) The age of the patient and the expected embryo aneuploidy rate; (2) Ovarian biomarkers [antral follicle count (AFC) and/or anti-Müllerian hormone (AMH)]; and (3) The ovarian response of the patient in terms of oocyte quantity provided a previous cycle of stimulation was carried out.
Source: Chloé Xilinas, EXCEMED, Rome, Italy.

achieve in POSEIDON patients. To help solve this issue, the POSEIDON initiative introduced a new metric of success in ART, namely, the ability to retrieve the number of oocytes needed to obtain at least one euploid blastocyst for transfer in each patient. The transfer of euploid embryos is associated, at any given age, with implantation rates in the range of 50–60%, thus markedly reducing the age-related decrease in implantation rates. Indeed, the POSEIDON marker of success seems to be a logical endpoint for clinicians providing care to infertility patients.

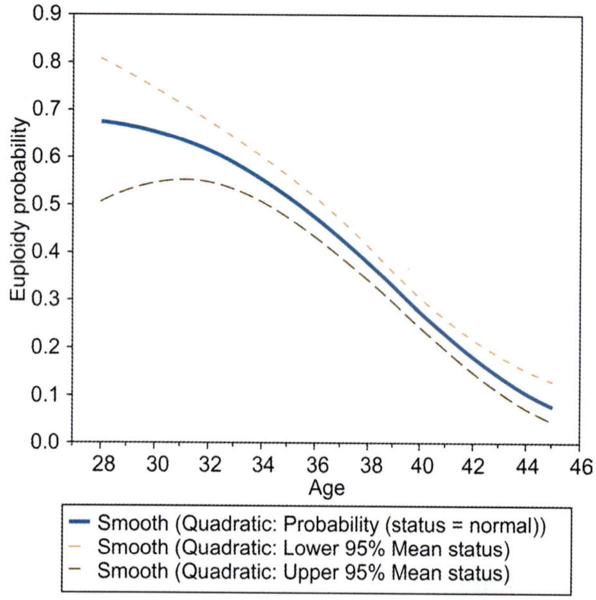

Fig. 2: Fitted probabilities (with 95% confidence intervals) of blastocyst euploidy as a function of female age following trophectoderm biopsy and next generation sequencing (NGS) analysis.
Source: Adapted from Esteves SC, Carvalho JF, Martinhago CD, et al. Estimation of age-dependent decrease in blastocyst euploidy by next generation sequencing: development of a novel prediction model. Panminerva Med. 2019;61(1):3-10.

Recently, a novel calculator, named as the "ART Calculator" was developed to predict the POSEIDON marker.[15] The predictive model used logistic regression analysis to select the relevant parameters affecting blastocyst euploidy. Female age, sperm source used for intracytoplasmic sperm injection (ICSI), and the number of mature (metaphase II) oocytes were the significant predictors. After internal validation, the model was used to calculate the individualized probability of blastocyst euploidy per mature retrieved oocyte and the minimum number of mature oocytes required to obtain more than or equal to one euploid blastocyst—with their 95% confidence interval (CI)—for different probabilities of success. The ART Calculator makes two types of predictions automatically, one using pretreatment information to estimate the minimum number of mature oocytes to achieve more than or equal to one euploid blastocyst, and another based on the actual number of mature oocytes collected/accumulated to estimate the chances of having a euploid blastocyst using that oocyte cohort for IVF/ICSI **(Figs. 5A and B)**. The new ART Online Calculator can be found at http://www.members.groupposeidon.com/Calculator/; it may assist in clinical counseling and individualized treatment planning regarding the number of oocytes required for at least one euploid blastocyst in IVF/ICSI procedures.

Using the POSEIDON criteria, the clinician can, first of all, identify and classify patients who are likely to have reduced success in ART, and secondly, develop a treatment plan to achieve the individualized oocyte number related to the optimal probability of generating at least one euploid blastocyst for transfer in each POSEIDON patient category.

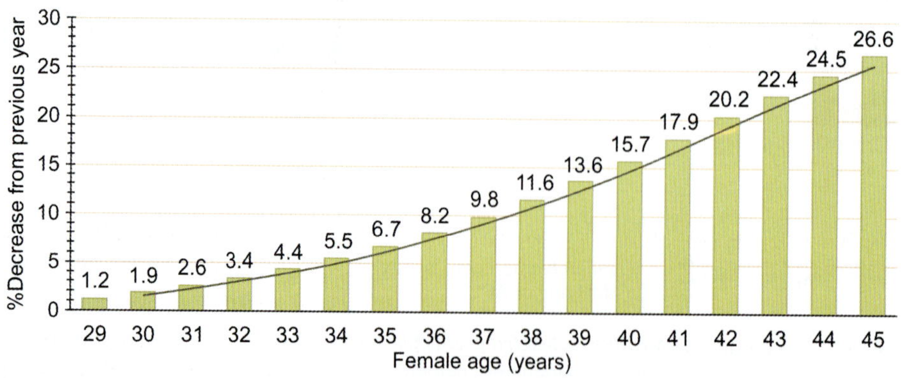

Fig. 3: The percent decrease in the probability of a blastocyst being euploid increases progressively with every year of female age.
Source: Adapted from Esteves SC, Carvalho JF, Martinhago CD, et al. Estimation of age-dependent decrease in blastocyst euploidy by next generation sequencing: development of a novel prediction model. Panminerva Med. 2019;61(1):3-10.

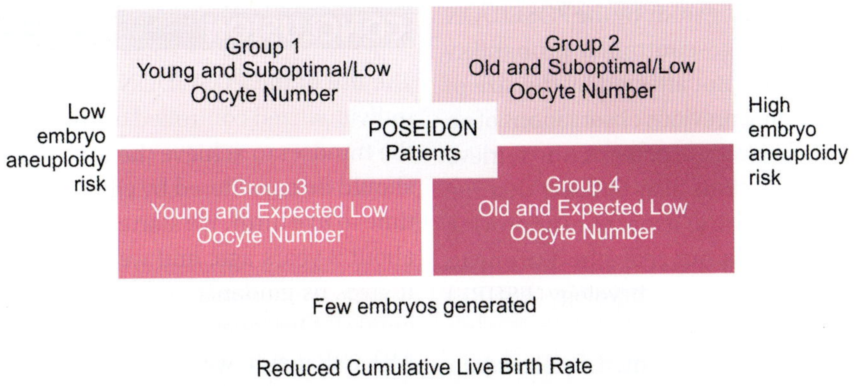

Fig. 4: The POSEIDON subgroups of low prognosis patients in assisted reproductive technology (ART). Due to low oocyte numbers, the POSEIDON patients are likely to have reduced pregnancy success. However, the prognosis is differentially affected by female age as it relates to risk of embryo aneuploidy.

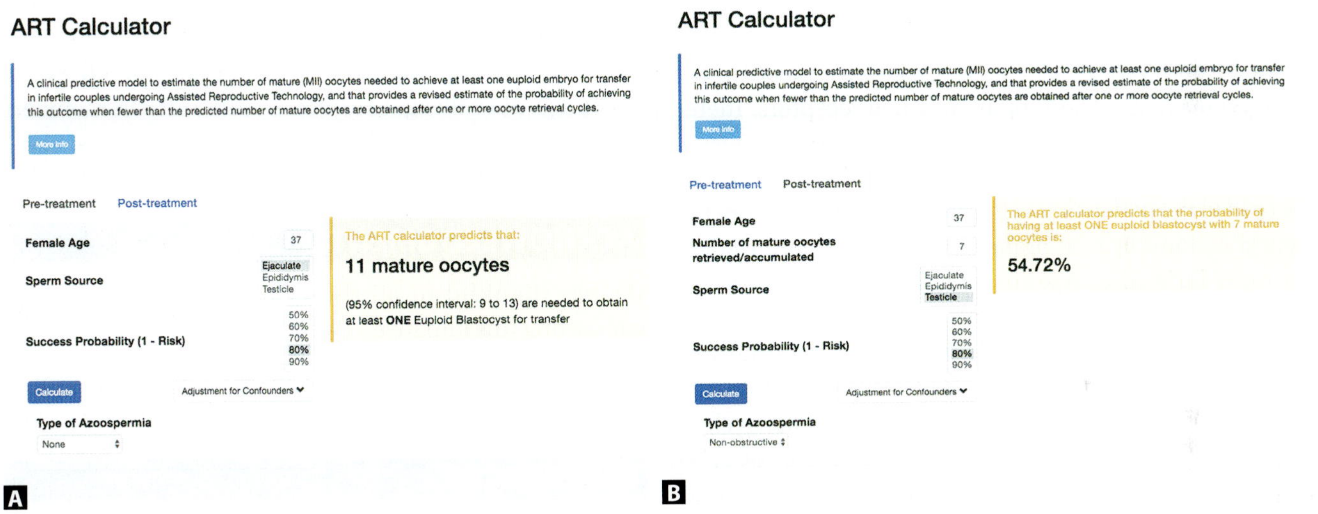

Figs. 5A and B: ART Online Calculator to predict the minimum number of mature oocytes required to obtain at least one euploid blastocyst for transfer in infertile patients undergoing IVF/ICSI cycles. (A) Pretreatment, clinicians should input the patient age and the sperm source to be used for IVF/ICSI, and choose the risk of predictions. The predicted minimum number of mature oocytes needed for obtaining at least one euploid blastocyst, with its 95% confidence interval, is displayed; and (B) Posttreatment, i.e. when fewer than the predicted number of mature oocytes are obtained after one or more oocyte retrieval cycles, the calculator estimates the prediction of achieving more than or equal to one euploid blastocyst with the available number of mature oocytes. (ART: assisted reproductive technology; ICSI: intracytoplasmic sperm injection; IVF: in vitro fertilization).

The novel POSEIDON classification of low prognosis patients in ART may help improve patient counseling and management, ultimately maximizing success and shortening the time to live birth.

FUTURE TRENDS

In practical terms, the individualized oocyte number can be achieved using patient-oriented strategies. For instance, gonadotropin starting dose and regimen can be tailored according to the POSEIDON stratification.[16-18] A crucial decision-making aspect regarding gonadotropin choice is that the number of competent follicles at the end of stimulation depends on the number of follicles attaining follicle-stimulating hormone (FSH) sensitivity.[17] In this regard, overwhelming evidence indicates oocytes yield is optimized by the use of recombinant FSH.[19-23]

Importantly, patient-oriented gonadotropin doses aimed at retrieving more oocytes that do not affect embryo genetic competence. In an ongoing study by the POSEIDON group, we observed that the age-controlled probability of a blastocyst being euploid is not affected by the size of embryo cohort, thus confirming previous observations of no detrimental effect on embryo ploidy in patients who retrieve more oocytes.[14,24] Our observations also indicate that the use of minimal or mild stimulation as a means of improving embryo genetic competence is not real [the European Society of Human Reproduction and Embryology (ESHRE) 2019, submitted]. In reality, what matters concerning embryo ploidy is female age and not the intensity of ovarian stimulation.

On the contrary, the use of low gonadotropin doses might result in hyporesponse and retrieval of fewer than expected oocyte number.[17,18] This phenomenon is seen in POSEIDON groups 1 and 2 patients, who despite adequate prestimulation ovarian parameters end up having poor or suboptimal oocytes yield, probably due to inappropriate low gonadotropin dose or presence of genetic polymorphisms affecting gonadotropins and their receptors. Therefore, proper patient evaluation is critical to help the clinician identify the low prognosis patient and plan a treatment tailored to the patient's specific needs. Naturally, use of the right gonadotropin starting dose and the possibility to adapt the dose during the cycle are essential to optimize oocytes yield while securing patient's safety.

In our practice, we routinely use individualized ovarian stimulation regimens. Different gonadotropin starting doses are chosen and adapted during the cycle—whenever needed—to optimize the number of oocytes retrieved and at the same time minimize risks such as ovarian hyperstimulation syndrome (OHSS) and cycle cancellation.[25,26] We apply the same reasoning concerning luteinizing hormone (LH) supplementation, trigger methods, and luteal phase support.[25-29] Notwithstanding, even using the best protocol, the optimal individualized oocyte number might be difficult to achieve in single ovarian stimulation, in particular, among POSEIDON groups 3 and 4 patients. In such cases, treatment should be planned to keep in mind that the number of oocytes needed to achieve at least one euploid blastocyst is lower in younger than in older patients. Hence, consecutive ovarian stimulation in the follicular phase and the luteal phase, known as DuoStim, is an attractive strategy to be considered in patients of POSEIDON groups 3 and 4.[30] The target oocyte number might be reached quicker, thus increasing the likelihood of having at least one euploid embryo in the resulting embryo cohort.

CONCLUSION

The use of the POSEIDON-based stratification along with individualized controlled ovarian stimulation (iCOS), with the mindset to achieve the individualized oocyte number, should be considered by clinicians aiming at reducing the time to live birth. We started using this system in our clinic about 2 years ago, and we are delighted with the results. It gives us guidance on how to most optimally treat each patient. Moreover, using the POSEIDON criteria and the ART Calculator, we have been able to provide transparent information, which helps our patients prepare both emotionally and financially for the treatment journey.

We invite our colleagues to learn more about the POSEIDON initiative and the ART Calculator at www.grouposeidon.com and https://www.frontiersin.org/research-topics/6849/poseidons-stratification-of-low-prognosis-patients-in-art-the-why-the-what-and-the-how. The POSEIDON group is also open for new members; we encourage our colleagues to join us as POSEIDON members (please find out more at http://www.groupposeidon.com/member-benefits/).

ACKNOWLEDGMENTS

We are thankful to all the POSEIDON members for supporting this initiative.

Conflict of interest: The author declares receipt of lecture fees from Merck, Besins, Gedeon-Richter, and Lilly.

REFERENCES

1. Smith AD, Tilling K, Nelson SM, et al. Live-Birth Rate Associated With Repeat In Vitro Fertilization Treatment Cycles. JAMA. 2015;314(24):2654-62.
2. Dancet EA, Van Empel IW, Rober P, et al. Patient-centred infertility care: a qualitative study to listen to the patient's voice. Hum Reprod. 2011;26(4):827-33.
3. Mainz J. Defining and classifying clinical indicators for quality improvement. Int J Qual Health Care. 2003;15(6):523-30.
4. Bento FC, Esteves SC. Establishing a quality management system in a fertility center: experience with ISO 9001. Medical Express. 2016;3(3):M160302.
5. Broer SL, Mol BW, Hendriks D, et al. The role of antimullerian hormone in prediction of outcome after IVF: comparison with the antral follicle count. Fertil Steril. 2009;91(3):705-14.
6. Broer SL, Dólleman M, Opmeer BC, et al. AMH and AFC as predictors of excessive response in controlled ovarian hyperstimulation: a meta-analysis. Hum Reprod Update. 2011;17(1):46-54.
7. McLernon DJ, Steyerberg EW, Te Velde ER, et al. Predicting the chances of a live birth after one or more complete cycles

of in vitro fertilisation: population based study of linked cycle data from 113,873 women. BMJ. 2016;355:i5735.
8. Sunkara SK, Rittenberg V, Raine-Fenning N, et al. Association between the number of eggs and live birth in IVF treatment: an analysis of 400,135 treatment cycles. Hum Reprod. 2011;26(7):1768-74.
9. De Geyter C, Fehr P, Moffat R, et al. Twenty years' experience with the Swiss data registry for assisted reproductive medicine: outcomes, key trends and recommendations for improved practice. Swiss Med Wkly. 2015;145:w14087.
10. Poseidon Group (Patient-Oriented Strategies Encompassing IndividualizeD Oocyte Number), Alviggi C, Andersen CY, et al. A new more detailed stratification of low responders to ovarian stimulation: from a poor ovarian response to a low prognosis concept. Fertil Steril. 2016;105(6):1452-3.
11. Humaidan P, Alviggi C, Fischer R, et al. The novel POSEIDON stratification of 'Low prognosis patients in Assisted Reproductive Technology' and its proposed marker of successful outcome. F1000Res. 2016;5:2911.
12. Esteves SC, Roque M, Bedoschi GM, et al. Defining Low Prognosis Patients Undergoing Assisted Reproductive Technology: POSEIDON Criteria-The Why. Front Endocrinol (Lausanne). 2018;9:461.
13. Drakopoulos P, Blockeel C, Stoop D, et al. Conventional ovarian stimulation and single embryo transfer for IVF/ICSI. How many oocytes do we need to maximize cumulative live birth rates after utilization of all fresh and frozen embryos? Hum Reprod. 2016;31(2):370-6.
14. Esteves SC, Carvalho JF, Martinhago CD, et al. Estimation of age-dependent decrease in blastocyst euploidy by next generation sequencing: development of a novel prediction model. Panminerva Med. 2019;61(1):3-10.
15. Esteves SC, Carvalho JC, Bento FC, et al. A novel predictive model to estimate the number of mature oocytes required for obtaining at least one euploid blastocyst for transfer in couples undergoing in vitro fertilization/intracytoplasmic sperm injection: The ART Calculator. Front Endocrinol. [Epub ahead of print].
16. Haahr T, Esteves SC, Humaidan P. Individualized controlled ovarian stimulation in expected poor-responders: an update. Reprod Biol Endocrinol. 2018;16(1):20.
17. Alviggi C, Conforti A, Esteves SC, et al. Understanding Ovarian Hypo-Response to Exogenous Gonadotropin in Ovarian Stimulation and Its New Proposed Marker—The Follicle-To-Oocyte (FOI) Index. Front Endocrinol (Lausanne). 2018;9:589.
18. Conforti A, Esteves SC, Cimadomo D, et al. The management of women with an unexpected low ovarian response to gonadotropin. Front Endocrinol. [Epub ahead of print].
19. Lehert P, Schertz JC, Ezcurra D. Recombinant human follicle-stimulating hormone produces more oocytes with a lower total dose per cycle in assisted reproductive technologies compared with highly purified human menopausal gonadotrophin: a meta-analysis. Reprod Biol Endocrinol. 2010;8:112.
20. Devroey P, Pellicer A, Nyboe Andersen A, et al. A randomized assessor-blind trial comparing highly purified hMG and recombinant FSH in a GnRH antagonist cycle with compulsory single-blastocyst transfer. Fertil Steril. 2012;97(3):561-71.
21. Bosch E, Vidal C, Labarta E, et al. Highly purified hMG versus recombinant FSH in ovarian hyperstimulation with GnRH antagonists—a randomized study. Hum Reprod. 2008;23(10):2346-51.
22. Hompes PG, Broekmans FJ, Hoozemans DA, et al. Effectiveness of highly purified human menopausal gonadotropin vs. recombinant follicle-stimulating hormone in first-cycle in vitro fertilization-intracytoplasmic sperm injection patients. Fertil Steril. 2008;89(6):1685-93.
23. Andersen AN, Devroey P, Arce JC. Clinical outcome following stimulation with highly purified hMG or recombinant FSH in patients undergoing IVF: a randomized assessor-blind controlled trial. Hum Reprod. 2006;21(12):3217-27.
24. Ata B, Kaplan B, Danzer H, et al. Array CGH analysis shows that aneuploidy is not related to the number of embryos generated. Reprod Biomed Online. 2012;24(6):614-20.
25. Fischer R, Nakano FY, Roque M, et al. A quality management approach to controlled ovarian stimulation in assisted reproductive technology: the "Fischer protocol". Panminerva Med. 2019;61(1):11-23.
26. Roque M, Haahr T, Geber S, et al. Fresh versus elective frozen embryo transfer in IVF/ICSI cycles: a systematic review and meta-analysis of reproductive outcomes. Hum Reprod Update. 2019;25(1):2-14.
27. Conforti A, Esteves SC, Di Rella F, et al. The role of recombinant LH in women with hypo-response to controlled ovarian stimulation: a systematic review and meta-analysis. Reprod Biol Endocrinol. 2019;17(1):18.
28. Alviggi C, Conforti A, Esteves SC, et al. Recombinant luteinizing hormone supplementation in assisted reproductive technology: a systematic review. Fertil Steril. 2018; 109(4):644-64.
29. Haahr T, Roque M, Esteves SC, et al. GnRH Agonist Trigger and LH Activity Luteal Phase Support versus hCG Trigger and Conventional Luteal Phase Support in Fresh Embryo Transfer IVF/ICSI Cycles-A Systematic PRISMA Review and Meta-analysis. Front Endocrinol (Lausanne). 2017;8:116.
30. Ubaldi FM, Capalbo A, Vaiarelli A, et al. Follicular versus luteal phase ovarian stimulation during the same menstrual cycle (DuoStim) in a reduced ovarian reserve population results in a similar euploid blastocyst formation rate: new insight in ovarian reserve exploitation. Fertil Steril. 2016;105(6):1488-95.e1.

Pregnancy after Assisted Reproductive Technology

61

Vijay Nahata, Arun Baruah

INTRODUCTION

Since the birth of the first in vitro fertilization (IVF) baby in 1978,[1,2] innumerable pregnancies have been achieved by this techniques now commonly known as assisted reproductive technology (ART). In United States, ART babies constitute approximately 1.5% of all births.[3] With a better understanding of the procedure and new technological advancements, the success rates have improved tremendously in past few years.

OBSTETRIC COMPLICATIONS AFTER ASSISTED REPRODUCTIVE TECHNOLOGY

Most obstetric complications following ART are associated with multiple gestations, though even singleton gestations are at slightly increased risk of antenatal complications. It was observed that pregnancies after frozen embryo transfers (FETs) were associated with decreased risk antepartum hemorrhage, suggesting that the endometrial condition at the time of implantation may play a role in the pathogenesis of these complications.[4]

- In a meta-analysis conducted by Masoudian et al. which included 19 retrospective studies, it was observed that the risk of hypertensive disease in pregnancies was higher in donor oocyte conceptions compared to pregnancies achieved by other methods of assisted reproduction or by natural conception. The pregnancies achieved with OD had more than double the risk of preeclampsia when compared with ART and a more than fourfold increased risk compared with natural conception [odds ratio (OR) 2.54, 95% confidence interval (CI) 1.98–3.24 and OR 4.34, 95% CI 3.10–6.06, respectively]. The risk of gestational hypertension in OD pregnancies was three times higher compared with other ART pregnancies and nearly eight times higher compared with naturally conceived pregnancies (OR 3.00, 95% CI 2.44-3.70 and OR 7.94, 95% CI 1.73–36.36, respectively).[5]
- In a retrospective cohort study of over 1 million deliveries between 2008 and 2012, it was observed that severe maternal morbidity was nearly two times more in pregnancies conceived with ART after controlling for maternal age, parity, comorbid conditions, history of prior cesarean delivery, and year of delivery. Even women with singleton pregnancies were observed to be at increased risk; however, these rate has been decreasing since 2008.[6]
- Another cohort study of more than 500,000 women, observed a small increased risk of preeclampsia in women undergoing ART in their second and third pregnancies compared with women who did not require ART, after adjusting for maternal age, interbirth interval, and presence of new partner (OR 1.2 for second pregnancy and 1.8 for third pregnancy). They concluded that ART increases the risk of preeclampsia and the risk may increase with parity. Advanced maternal age and interbirth intervals may be responsible to some extent for this increased risk; however no association was seen with change of partner or smoking.[7]

PREGNANCY OUTCOME

As with all normally conceived pregnancies, complications may occur following IVF treatment. Various studies and beliefs have raised concern that children born after IVF are at increased risk of early pregnancy loss, ectopic pregnancy, congenital malformations, prematurity, low birth weight

(LBW) neurological deficits and genetic abnormalities; and this risk cannot be solely attributed to multiple gestations.

Early Pregnancy Loss and Ectopic Pregnancy

Rate of early spontaneous pregnancy loss is similar for pregnancies conceived naturally and with ART. But, the rate of loss is more for multifetal pregnancy than singleton pregnancy.[8,9]

The spontaneous abortion rate is almost 16% of all pregnancies. The spontaneous abortion rates are strongly influenced by the age of the egg provider and to a lesser extent affected by the underlying cause of infertility.[10]

Approximately 0.7% of total ART cycles result in an ectopic pregnancy.[10] The risk of ectopic pregnancy after ART procedures depends on the type of procedure (higher with zygote intrafallopian transfer or ZIFT), the indication for ART treatment (higher with tubal factor infertility) and estimated embryo implantation potential.[11]

Proportion of Singleton and Multifetal Pregnancy

The rates of singleton and multifetal births following ART varies around the world. In United States in the year 2014, 60% of all ART births were singleton, compared with a nearly 80% singleton rate reported by 16 European countries in 2010.[12,13] When nearly 40% of ART infants were part of a multiple birth, the incidence of multiple gestations in naturally conceived infants was only 3.5%.[12]

Although multizygotic gestations are result from transfer of multiple embryos, the frequency of monozygotic twins was also increased from approximately 0.4% to 1–5% of pregnancies.[14] In one large study series, the frequency of monochorionic-diamniotic implantations was increased, but the frequency of monochorionic-monoamniotic twins was almost static.[15]

Preterm Birth and Low Birth Weight

The incidence of preterm birth and LBW (≤2,500 g) babies was higher in singleton IVF pregnancies compared to spontaneously conceived pregnancies.[16]

A population-based data from over 42,000 infants conceived with ART from 1996 to 1997 and 3 million births in the general population showed that LBW was significantly more common among term singleton, but not in twin infants conceived by ART compared with the spontaneously conceived pregnancies [for singletons 6.5% vs 2.5%; risk ratio (RR) 2.6, 95% CI 2.4–2.7]. Preterm LBW was also significantly more common among singleton, but not twin, infants conceived by ART (for singletons 6.6% vs 4.7%; RR 1.4, 95% CI 1.3–1.5).[16] These data may also support the contention that an increase in adverse outcomes among singletons is due to the "vanishing twin" phenomenon.

One extended follow-up study included over 62,000 singleton infants from ART procedures from 1996 to 2000. There was a decline in LBW deliveries, but no significant change in the rate of preterm birth.[17]

Chromosomal and Genetic Abnormalities

Multiple studies have not observed any higher incidence of karyotypic abnormalities (including mosaicism) in offspring of ART conceived pregnancies than in naturally conceived pregnancies, and prenatal diagnosis is not typically offered for this indication alone.[18,19]

Perinatal Outcomes

A higher incidence of preterm labor, spontaneous preterm delivery, placenta previa, gestational diabetes, preeclampsia, and neonatal intensive care admission is observed in pregnancies after ART.[20] Patients undergone ART should be advised of the increased risk for adverse perinatal outcomes. Obstetricians should not only manage these as high risk pregnancies but also avoid iatrogenic harm caused by preterm labor induction or cesarean section.

Cancer

A systematic review and meta-analysis including 25 case-control and cohort studies reported an association between fertility treatment with ART and cancer in offspring.

The offspring born after ART were at increased risk for all cancers (RR = 1.33; 95% CI, 1.08–1.63) and for hematological cancers (RR = 1.59; 95% CI, 1.32–1.91) and other solid cancers (RR = 2.19; 95% CI, 1.26–3.80). Specifically, increased risks for leukemias (RR = 1.65; 95% CI, 1.35–2.01), neuroblastomas (RR = 4.04; 95% CI, 1.24–13.18), and retinoblastomas (RR = 1.62; 95% CI, 1.12–2.35) associated with ART.[21] These associations do not establish causality.

Long-term Issues

Outcomes among ART babies up to 28 years of age have been reported, and are generally reassuring. In a study comparing 253 ART-conceived adolescents with case-matched controls, there were no detectable differences between groups for general health, mental health, or cognitive ability upon review of military pre-induction screening records (performed at ages 16–17 years). However, further studies with larger cohorts are required to confirm these results.[22]

CONCLUSION

Pregnancy after ART is at slightly higher risk of antenatal complications compared to natural conception, and so preconception counseling is very important. With improved ART success rates and expansion in indications of these procedures, both short- and long-term outcomes of ART pregnancies have been studies and the results are quite reassuring in some aspects and inconclusive for certain others for which further studies may be needed. However, the research in this field is complicated because of many confounding factors. These outcomes are also influenced by technological changes in ART procedures, as well as changes in obstetrical and neonatal care, over time.

REFERENCES

1. Steptoe PC, Edwards RG. Reimplantation of a human embryo with subsequent tubal pregnancy. Lancet. 1976;1(7965): 880-2.
2. Steptoe PC, Edwards RG. Birth after the reimplantation of a human embryo. Lancet. 1978;2(8085):366.
3. Ory SJ. The national epidemic of multiple pregnancy and the contribution of assisted reproductive technology. Fertil Steril. 2013;100(4):929-30.
4. Maheshwari A, Pandey S, Shetty A, et al. Obstetric and perinatal outcomes in singleton pregnancies resulting from the transfer of frozen thawed versus fresh embryos generated through in vitro fertilization treatment: a systematic review and meta-analysis. Fertil Steril. 2012;98(2):368-77.
5. Masoudian P, Nasr A, de Nanassy J, et al. Oocyte donation pregnancies and the risk of preeclampsia or gestational hypertension: a systematic review and metaanalysis. Am J Obstet Gynecol. 2016;214(3):328-39.
6. Martin AS, Monsour M, Kissin DM, et al. Trends in Severe Maternal Morbidity After Assisted Reproductive Technology in the United States, 2008-2012. Obstet Gynecol. 2016;127(1):59-66.
7. Tandberg A, Klungsøyr K, Romundstad LB, et al. Pre-eclampsia and assisted reproductive technologies: consequences of advanced maternal age, interbirth intervals, new partner and smoking habits. BJOG. 2015;122(7):915-22.
8. La Sala GB, Nucera G, Gallinelli A, et al. Spontaneous embryonic loss following in vitro fertilization: incidence and effect on outcomes. Am J Obstet Gynecol. 2004;191(3):741-6.
9. Dickey RP, Taylor SN, Lu PY, et al. Spontaneous reduction of multiple pregnancy: incidence and effect on outcome. Am J Obstet Gynecol. 2002;186(1):77-83.
10. Centers for Disease Control and Prevention. (2016). Assisted reproductive technology success rates. [online]. Available from http://www.cdc.gov/art/ARTReports.htm [LAst accessed February, 2019].
11. Clayton HB, Schieve LA, Peterson HB, et al. Ectopic pregnancy risk with assisted reproductive technology procedures. Obstet Gynecol. 2006;107(3):595-604.
12. Kupka MS, Ferraretti AP, de Mouzon J, et al. European IVF-Monitoring Consortium, for the European Society of Human Reproduction and Embryology, Assisted reproductive technology in Europe, 2010: results generated from European registers by ESHRE†. Hum Reprod. 2014;29(10):2099-113.
13. Sunderam S, Kissin DM, Crawford SB, et al. Assisted Reproductive Technology Surveillance—United States, 2014. MMWR Surveill Summ. 2017;66(6):1-24.
14. Derom C, Vlietinck R, Derom R, et al. Increased monozygotic twinning rate after ovulation induction; Lancet. 1987;1(8544):1236-8.
15. Knopman J, Krey LC, Lee J, et al. Monozygotic twinning: an eight-year experience at a large IVF center. Fertil Steril. 2010;94(2):502-10.
16. Schieve LA, Meikle SF, Ferre C, et al Low and very low birth weight in infants conceived with use of assisted reproductive technology. N Engl J Med. 2002;346(10):731-7.
17. Schieve LA, Ferre C, Peterson HB, et al. Perinatal outcome among singleton infants conceived through assisted reproductive technology in the United States. Obstet Gynecol. 2004;103(6):1144-53.
18. Shevell T, Malone FD, Vidaver J, et al. Assisted reproductive technology and pregnancy outcome. Obstet Gynecol. 2005;106(5 Pt 1):1039-45.
19. Conway DA, Patel SS, Liem J, et al. The risk of cytogenetic abnormalities in the late first trimester of pregnancies conceived through assisted reproduction. Fertil Steril. 2011;95(2):503-6.
20. Jackson RA, Gibson KA, Wu YW, et al. Perinatal outcomes in singletons following in vitro fertilization: a meta-analysis. Obstet Gynecol. 2004;103(3):551-63.
21. Hargreave M, Jensen A, Toender A, et al. Fertility treatment and childhood cancer risk: a systematic meta-analysis. Fertil Steril. 2013;100(1):150-61.
22. Fruchter E, Beck-Fruchter R, Hourvitz A, et al. Health and functioning of adolescents conceived by assisted reproductive technology. Fertil Steril. 2017;107(3):774-80.

First and Second Trimester Screening 62

Selvapriya Saravanan

INTRODUCTION

Everyone wants the best!!!

Prenatal screening in pregnancy has become as important and as stressful as delivering a baby.[1] The reason is because not only every parent dreams of a safe delivery alone anymore; they also want the healthiest form of their offspring in all ways. So it becomes the duty of obstetricians to perform everything what takes to make sure they deliver the healthiest form of baby to each and every patient.

Science has developed and reached miraculous heights. Gone are the days where only making sure that the baby in structurally normal was considered important. Now the functional capacity of the baby is also challenged.

So to convert the wrinkles on the patients' forehead into smiles on their face becomes the most challenging job for the obstetrician.

ROLE OF ULTRASOUND IN SCREENING

With the revolution happening in "imaging science", we are not only able to study the structures we are able to assess many of the functional status but also study the fetal tendency and psychology.

The sense of fear and pain has been demonstrated acceptably in fetuses undergoing medical termination.

Similarly happy rolling movement of the fetuses with touch therapy has also been acclaimed.

Music enhances fetal growth which is an accepted fact, similarly stress interrupts with the baby's growth that is also a proven fact.

Ultrasound henceforth is able to provide more predictive details and functional details than ever before. But the importance of sequential screening should also be emphasized to the patients. One ultrasound report showing the fetus to be normal at that period is not sufficient to ensure the fetus status till the end of pregnancy. "Quality of Scanning" is another major point to be emphasized. A scan report should have enough details to ensure that no corners have been left unnoticed.

Documenting every detail that has been screened is important. Documenting detail about what could not be seen also becomes important for certain times. Quality scanning with dedication and no compromise should be the concern of any one, be it the fetal medicine specialist or sonologist who puts the ultrasound probe on the pregnant mother.

SCREENING IN PREGNANCY

The "pyramid of screening" of the fetus in pregnancy has shifted itself upside down. The base of the pyramid which needs more frequent testing of the baby and mother falls now in early weeks of pregnancy. This shows how crucial the initial phase of pregnancy is to make sure that the baby is healthy.

Terminologies

The following terminologies are used for better understanding of "screening in pregnancy".

Birth defects: Any type of functional or structural abnormality determined largely by factors operating before birth, *in utero* or in the immediate postnatal period.

Congenital malformations: These are structural abnormalities present at birth and may or may not have a genetic component.[2]

Genetic disorders: DNA defects play a major role causing genetic disorders. Genetic disorders can either be inherited or sporadic **(Table 1)**. Some conditions are of late onset, but once detected in the index case, it can be diagnosed in utero as early as 10 weeks.

Genetic disorders are classified as:

Chromosomal abnormalities: There are 23 chromosomal pairs in the body of which 22 are autosomes and 1 pair is sex chromosomes—XX in females and XY in males. Any alteration in the number or structure of chromosomes can lead to chromosomal abnormalities. They are mainly caused by random errors of cell division in gamete formation or are sporadic and can be transferred to the next generation.

Single gene disorders: Mutation in a single major gene can lead to this manifestation which is variable depending on the ability of the normal gene. These are inherited as recessive, dominant, autosomal or X-linked inheritance.

Multifactorial conditions: This is due to the mutation and interaction of multiple genes and/or environmental factors.

Environmentally influenced conditions: These are birth defects caused due to interference of the environmental factors with normal embryogenic or fetal development. These include physical agents, chemicals and infections.

Table 1: Prevalence of genetic disease at birth in India.

Disorder	*Incidence*	*Estimated cases/year*
Congenital malformations	1 in 50	495,506
G6PD deficiency	1:35 to 1:10 (M)	390,000
Down syndrome	1:1,139	21,412
β-thalassemia	1:2,700	9,000
Sickle-cell disease	1:1,200	5,200
Amino acid disorders	1:2,347	9,760
Other metabolic disease	1:2,500	9,000
Duchenne muscular dystrophy	1:5,000 (M)	2,510
Spinal muscular atrophy	1:10,000	2,510

COMPONENTS OF GENETIC SERVICE

Genetic services have following integral components: Carrier screening, facilities for genetic counseling and facilities for sound diagnosis and establishment of laboratories for confirmation of the diagnosis. These need to be developed as a composite unit for effective genetic services. In order to ensure minimum work load, quality monitoring and cost effectiveness, there needs to be a setup of centralized special laboratories for genetic diagnosis. The biggest challenge is the establishment of laboratories for molecular genetics, cytogenetics, biochemical genetics and immunogenetics for analysis of parent as well as fetal samples.

CHALLENGES OF PRENATAL DIAGNOSIS

A couple want a healthy baby, but 2–3% of children is born with a birth defect which is a universal fact. Two basic questionnaires are required to be answered.

Can we offer prenatal diagnosis to all pregnant women?

- 90% of structural and chromosomal abnormal fetus are born to "low-risk women"
- Maternal age alone is "poor screening tool" [deters 30% of all Down syndrome cases **(Table 2)**]
- "Acceptance and tolerance of genetic risk" differ between elderly primigravida and multigravida
  - Birthing trend in society (1–2 children norm)
  - 1970: 5% birth to women over 35 years
  - 1990: 10% birth to women over 35 years
  - 2015: 15% birth to women over 35 years.

If abnormality is detected by screening test then what?

Further confirmatory testing is required (CVS/amniocentesis).

Referral to tertiary care center.

- Genetic counseling and altered obstetric management (MTP/NICU care).
  - Preparation for special needs for neonatal or child management.

Table 2: Aneuploidies interpretation.

Aneuploidies	*AFP*	*Estriol*	*hCG*	*Inhibin A*	*Mnemonic*
Doer's syndrome	Low	Low	High	High	High
Turner syndrome	Decreased	Decreased	Very high	Very high	High
Edwards syndrome	Unchanged	Low	Very low	Unchanged	Low
Patau syndrome	Increased	Normal	Normal	Normal	High

(AFP: alpha fetoprotein; hCG: human chorionic gonadotropin)

PRENATAL DIAGNOSIS

It is defined as the method of detection of structural or functional abnormalities in the developing fetus including genetic disorders and congenital malformations detected by biochemical markers or by ultrasound.

Indications for prenatal testing:
- Hereditary condition in one or both parents
- Infertility for long period of time
- History of recurrent pregnancy loss
- Strong family history of hereditary conditions
- Population group with a high frequency of certain genetic diseases (ethnic or geographic region)
- A consanguineous marriage
- Advanced age.

Samples collected via amniocentesis or chorionic villus sampling can be used for prenatal diagnosis of aneuploidy as well as single gene disorders. However, there is a risk to the fetus and/or mother during these procedures. Recently there has considerable advancement in the field of prenatal diagnostics to make these procedures noninvasive.

One of the major causes of perinatal death and childhood handicap is aneuploidies. Invasive prenatal diagnostic tests are required to detect chromosomal disorders. Screening tests such as dual and quadruple marker with ultrasound examination set risk ratio for Down syndrome,[3] trisomy 18, and open neural tube defects. The screening is considered positive if the disorders fall above a designated cut-off. It is important to counsel the patient and provide further confirmatory tests when a screen is positive.

Maternal risk factors:
- Age more than 35 years
- History of congenital malformation in previous pregnancy
  - Chromosomal anomaly in previous issue
- Family history of NTDs or familial genetic diseases
- One or both partners are a carrier of chromosomal disorder
- History of recurrent abortions
  - Patient belonging to any particular community with prevalence of any certain disease.

Antenatal risk factors in current pregnancy:
- Intake of teratogenic drugs or exposure to environmental teratogens
- Uncontrolled maternal diabetes in periconceptional period or raised glycosylated hemoglobin
- Amniotic fluid abnormalities like oligohydramnios or polyhydramnios
- Severe symmetrical fetal growth restriction
- Decreased fetal activity.

Various Noninvasive Prenatal Diagnostic Methods

- Detailed history, pedigree tree
- Maternal serum biochemistry.

Maternal serum alpha fetoprotein (MSAFP): Alpha fetoprotein (AFP) is the main glycoprotein produced by fetal liver which increases steadily in fetal serum and amniotic fluid until 13 weeks after which levels decrease rapidly. It crosses into maternal serum **(Table 3)**.

Maternal serum alpha fetoprotein rises steadily throughout pregnancy after 12 weeks

Clinical Significance

- Measured between 16 weeks and 20 weeks in ng/mL values at 2.5 multiples of the median (MOM) is considered upper limit of normal. Raised levels can detect 90% cases of anencephaly and 80% cases of open spina bifida.[2]

Human chorionic gonadotropin
- Secreted by placenta with maximum levels at 8–10 weeks
- Raised levels seen in trisomy 21 and Turner syndrome
- Low levels seen in Edwards syndrome.

Unconjugated estriol
- Produced by fetoplacental unit with levels gradually rising in pregnancy
- Maternal serum levels are lower[4] in Down, Turner and Edwards syndrome.

Table 3: Conditions associated with abnormal MSAFP levels.

Elevated levels	***Low levels***
Neural tube defects	Trisomy 21
Abdominal wall defects	Trisomy 18
Esophageal/duodenal atresia	Overestimated gestational age
Renal anomalies (polycystic kidneys, absent kidneys)	High maternal weight
Cystic hygroma, sacrococcygeal teratoma	Gestational trophoblastic disease
Multiple pregnancy	
Intrauterine death	
Low maternal weight	

(MSAFP: maternal serum alpha fetoprotein)

Inhibin A levels

- Produced by syncytiotrophoblast
- Raised levels seen in Down syndrome.[5]

Pregnancy-associated plasma protein A (PAPP-A)

- Secreted by syncytiotrophoblast
- Levels reduced in Down syndrome.

FIRST TRIMESTER SCREENING

Uses *PAPP-A* and *free β-human chorionic gonadotropin (hCG)* between 11 weeks and 14 weeks. It can detect 62% Down syndrome pregnancies with 5% false positive rate. Serum markers when combined with nuchal translucency measurement comprise *combined test* which has a detection rate of 79–87% with a 5% false-positive rate for Down syndrome.[4] Trisomies 18 and 13 can be screened with 90% sensitivity and 1% false-positive rate.[5]

SECOND TRIMESTER SCREENING

- Done between 15 weeks and 20 weeks
- Accurate gestational age is essential.

Triple Test—Maternal Serum Alpha Fetoprotein, Human Chorionic Gonadotropin and Unconjugated Estriol

- Down syndrome—Unconjugated estriol (uE3) and MSAFP levels are lower and hCG is higher
    - Edwards syndrome (trisomy 18)—levels of all three markers are low.
- Turner syndrome—picture similar to Down syndrome
    - Detection rate: 60–69%, and false positive rate: 5%.

Quadruple Test—Maternal Serum Alpha Fetoprotein, Human Chorionic Gonadotropin, Unconjugated Estriol and Inhibin A

- Raised inhibin A is seen in Down syndrome
- Detection rate: 67–81%, false-positive rate: 5%.[6]

Risk ratios with a cut-off of 1:250 are taken as screen positive requiring amniocentesis for confirmation of diagnosis.

Integrated Screening

Combines results of both the first and second trimester, screening tests into a single risk.[7,8]

- Highest Down syndrome detection: 94–96%

Stepwise Sequential Screen—First Trimester Screen and Quad Test[9]

- 1% offered diagnostic test after first-trimester screen
- 99% proceed to Quad test, results withheld until Quad test completed[4]
- Detection rate: 90–95%.

Contingent Sequential Screen

- 1% offered diagnostic test after first-trimester screen
- 15% proceed to Quad test, results withheld until Quad test completed
- 84% have no additional test after first-trimester screen
- *Detection rate*: 88–94%.

Screening for Down Syndrome

Newer Noninvasive Methods

- *Fetal cells from maternal circulation*: Fetal cells isolated from maternal blood by density gradient, fluorescence and other methods. It is useful in screening for aneuploidies because the number of cells in maternal blood increases sixfold. Using fluorescence in situ hybridization many gene defects can be detected, but this method is still under research.
- *Fetal cells in endocervical mucus:* It can be obtained in up to 50% of cases. However, this method too is under study.
- *Noninvasive prenatal testing (NIPT)*: Maternal plasma DNA is used NIPT to detect several conditions. NIPT has been used by obstetricians for many years to guide the management of rhesus D (RhD)-negative women whose fetuses are at risk of hemolytic disease of the fetus and newborn (HDFN).[10] Sex determination of fetuses with high risk sex-linked disorders is also an established practice. Using NIPT, testing for aneuploidy and Down syndrome is also possible. Although this test is more accurate, it is not diagnostic.

Until recently, invasive diagnostic sampling tests were required for genetic and aneuploidy diagnosis. However they carried a small but significant risk for miscarriage. The discovery of cell-free fetal DNA (cffDNA) in the maternal circulation in 1997 revolutionized prenatal diagnostics. cffDNA is detected from the first trimester and is cleared from maternal circulation rapidly postdelivery. Hence maternal blood is a good source for prenatal diagnosis. However there is a mixture with the maternal cell free

DNA. Currently there is not any technology that allows complete separation. Therefore, the first applications of this phenomenon focused on the detection, or exclusion of, paternally-inherited fetal DNA sequences that are not present in the mother, such as Y chromosome sequences in pregnancies with a male fetus or RhD sequences in women who are RhD-negative. However, with recent advancements in DNA sequencing technology, it is possible to get a precise but relative quantification of DNA fragments. Therefore, the detection of surplus material form fetal chromosome trisomy within the maternal plasma DNA can now be carried out in a robust manner.

Second Trimester Biochemical Screening Options

- AFP—malformations
- AFP + hCG + uE3 (triple test)
- AFP + hCG + uE3 + Inhibin A (Quad test)—preferred one

Alpha-fetoprotein (AFP) was the first serum marker to be used in screening programs for trisomy 21. AFP is a fetal-specific protein that is produced initially by the fetal yolk sac and subsequently by the fetal liver. Pregnancies with fetal Down syndrome are characterized by lower maternal serum AFP levels—approximately 0.7 MoM, higher hCG levels—approximately 2.0 MoM, and lower unconjugated estriol levels—approximately 0.8 MoM.[2] This triple test can detect 61–70% of Down syndrome cases as shown in (Alldred, 2012). Levels of all three markers are decreased in the setting of trisomy 18, with a detection rate similar to that for Down syndrome at a false-positive rate of only 0.5%.[2] Levels of a fourth marker—dimeric inhibin alpha—are elevated in Down syndrome, with an average value of 1.8 MoM (Spencer, 1996). The addition of dimeric inhibin to the other three markers is the quadruple or quad test, which has a trisomy 21 detection rate of approximately 80% at a false-positive rate of 5%. As with first-trimester screening, aneuploidy detection rates will be slightly lower in younger women and higher in women older than 35 years at delivery. If second-trimester serum screening is used in twin pregnancies, aneuploidy detection rates are significantly lower.[11-13] The quad test is the most commonly used second-trimester serum screening test for aneuploidy. As a stand-alone test, it is generally used if women do not begin care until the second-trimester or if first-trimester screening is not available. As subsequently discussed, combining the quad test with first-trimester screening yields even greater aneuploidy detection rates.

Combined First- and Second-trimester Screening

Combined screening strategies enhance aneuploidy detection. For this reason, the American College of Obstetricians and Gynecologists (2013c) recommends that a strategy incorporating both first- and second-trimester screening should be offered to women who seek prenatal care in the first trimester.

Three types of screening strategies are available:

Integrated screening: It combines results of first- and second-trimester tests. This includes a combined measurement of fetal NT and serum analyte levels at 11–14 weeks' gestation plus quadruple markers at 15–20 weeks. An aneuploidy risk is then calculated from these seven parameters. As expected, integrated screening has the highest Down syndrome detection rate—94–96% at a false-positive rate of 5%. If NT measurement is not available, serum integrated screening includes all six serum markers to calculate risk. This screening, however, is less effective.

Sequential screening: It discloses the results of first-trimester screening to women at the highest risk, who are then offered invasive testing with chorionic villus sampling or amniocentesis. There are two testing strategies in this category:

1. *Stepwise sequential screening*: Women with first-trimester screen results that confer risk for Down syndrome above a particular threshold are offered invasive testing, and the remaining women receive second-trimester screening. The threshold is set at approximately 1%, because in a screened population, the 1% at highest risk includes approximately 70% of Down syndrome pregnancies. This method of screening may achieve up to a 95% detection rate.
2. *Contingent sequential screening*: Women are divided into high-, moderate-, and low-risk groups. Those at the highest risk, for example, the top 1%, are offered invasive testing. Women at moderate risk, who comprise 15–20% of the population, undergo second-trimester screening. The remaining 80–85%, who are at or below a 1:1,000 risk, receive negative screening test results and have no further testing. Thus, most of those screened are provided with results almost immediately while still maintaining a high detection rate. This rate ranges from 88% to 94%. This option is also more cost-effective because a second-trimester test is obviated in up to 85% of patients. Integrated and sequential screening strategies require coordination between the provider

Table 4: Sequential screening policies: predicted detection rate for a given false-positive rate.

First trimester combination with second trimester AFP, Free β-hCG, uE3, and inhibin	***Early detection rate***	***Second trimester tests***	***False–positive rate***		
			1%	***3%***	***5%***
Integrated test					
PAPP-A and NT	0%	100%	85%	91%	93%
Stepwise test					
PAPP-A, free β-hCG, and NT	70%	99%	85%	93%	95%
Contingent test					
PAPP-A, free β-hCG, and NT	70%	15%	85%	92%	94%

(AFP: alpha fetoprotein; hCG: human chorionic gonadotropin; NT: nuchal translucency; PAPP-A: pregnancy-associated plasma protein A; uE3: unconjugated estriol)

and laboratory to ensure that the second sample is obtained during the appropriate gestational age window, sent to the same laboratory, and linked to the first-trimester results **(Table 4)**.[14-16]

TAKE HOME MESSAGE

Over the last 3–4 decades, there have been rapid advancements in the field of prenatal diagnostics. However, there has been a controversy in every step as to the best methods to employ.

Patient counseling is very important and screening should be opt-in procedure, patient should make aware by information brochures, videos and wormed consent, discussion and patient decision should be documented.

- There is a very high detection rate in the first trimester with the combined test for an acceptable false positive rate.
- Second-trimester screening has a much lower detection rate. This may lead to emotional stress to the pregnant patient. Some of these women have a baby bump; they are able to perceive fetal movements. Therefore, undergoing a second trimester abortion due to the detection of an anomaly can be quite distressing.
- In order to get the best possible detection rate, sequential screening must be done in both trimesters. The most efficient method is the contingent test. Obstetricians with adequate training and experience with ultrasound markers such as nasal bone hypoplasia should consider carrying out the contingent test within the 1st trimester.

Although comprehensive national data are not available, there is a continuing shift toward screening in the first trimester. Only the exact components and timing remain to be determined.

REFERENCES

1. American College of Obstetricians and Gynecologists: Screening for fetal chromosomal abnormalities. Practice Bulletin No. 77, January 2007.
2. Alldred SK, Deeks JJ, Guo B, et al. Second trimester serum tests for Down's syndrome screening. Cochrane Database Syst Rev. 2012;6:CD009925.
3. Cuckle H, Benn P, Wright D. Down syndrome screening in the first and/or second trimester: model predicted performance using meta-analysis parameters. Semin Perinatol. 2005;29(4):252-7.
4. Dugoff L, Hobbins JC, Malone FD, et al. Quad screen as a predictor of adverse pregnancy outcome. Obstet Gynecol. 2005;106(2):260-7.
5. Wapner R, Thom E, Simpson JL, et al. First-trimester screening for trisomies 21 and 18. N Engl J Med. 2003;349(15):1471-3.
6. Cuckle H. Biochemical screening for Down syndrome. Eur J Obstet Gynecol Reprod Biol. 2000;92(1):97-101.
7. Spencer K, Souter V, Tul N, et al. A screening program for trisomy 21 at 10-14 weeks using fetal nuchal translucency, maternal serum free beta-human chorionic gonadotropin and pregnancy-associated plasma protein-A. Ultrasound Obstet Gynecol. 1999;13(4):231-7.
8. Goetzl L, Krantz D, Simpson IL, et al. Pregnancy-associated plasma protein A, free beta-hCG, nuchal translucency, and risk of pregnancy loss. Obstet Gynecol. 2004;104(1):30-6.
9. Nicolaides KH. Nuchal translucency and other first-trimester sonographic markers of chromosomal abnormalities. Am J Obstet Gynecol. 2004;191(1):45-67.
10. Benn PA, Leo MV, Rodis JF, et al. Maternal serum screening for fetal trisomy 18: a comparison of fixed cutoff and patient-specific risk protocols. Obstet Gynecol. 1999;93(5 Pt 1): 707-11.
11. Nuchal Translucency Quality Review Program: Nasal bone education. (2013). [online] Available at https://www.ntgr.org/SM/ wfNasalBoneInfo.aspx. [Accessed February, 2013].
12. Greene MF, Haddow JE, Palomaki GE, et al. Maternal serum alpha-fetoprotein levels in diabetic pregnancies. Lancet. 1988;2(8606):345.

13. Lehmann S, Delaby C, Vialaret J, et al. Current and future use of "dried blood spot" analyses in clinical chemistry. Clin Chem Lab Med. 2013;51(10):1897-909.
14. Dugoff L, Hobbins JC, Malone FD, et al. First-trimester maternal serum PAPP-A and free-beta subunit human chorionic gonadotropic concentrations and nuchal translucency are associated with obstetric complications: a population-based screening study (The FASTER Trial). Am J Obstet Gynecol. 2004;191(6):1446-51.
15. Dugoff L, Society for Maternal-Fetal Medicine. First- and second-trimester maternal serum markers for aneuploidy and adverse pregnancy outcomes. Obstet Gynecol. 2010;115(5):1052-61.
16. Greene MF, Haddow JE, Palomaki GE, et al. First-trimester or second-trimester screening, or both, for Down's syndrome. N Engl J Med. 2005;353(19):2001-11.

Recurrent Miscarriage

63

Mala Arora

INTRODUCTION

Recurrent miscarriage (RM) is a profound personal tragedy experienced by couples seeking parenthood and is an equally challenging task for the attending obstetrician. Miscarriage is defined as the spontaneous loss of pregnancy before the fetus reaches viability and therefore includes all pregnancy losses from the time of conception until 20 weeks of gestation.[1] Recurrent miscarriage may also be referred as recurrent pregnancy loss (RPL) and recurrent spontaneous miscarriage (RSM).

DEFINITION

Royal College of Obstetricians and Gynecologists (RCOG, UK) defines recurrent miscarriage as three or more consecutive pregnancy losses at 20 weeks or less or with fetal weight of less than 500 g.[2] ACOG defines it as two or more spontaneous miscarriages for clinical purposes.[3] American Society of Reproductive Medicine (ASRM) defines recurrent pregnancy loss as two or more failed clinical pregnancies, which should be documented by either ultrasound or histopathological examination. None of the definitions include biochemical pregnancies, ectopic pregnancies or pregnancy of uncertain location.[4]

Sporadic miscarriages occur in 25% of pregnancies. A woman may have three sporadic miscarriages during her obstetric career, but if these are interspersed with viable births they are not classified as recurrent miscarriages.

Primary aborters are women who have no previous pregnancy that progressed to viability and *secondary aborters* are women who have one or more pregnancies that have proceeded beyond 20 weeks' gestation.

For research purposes, the definition of RM is three or more consecutive losses and RCOGrecommends investigations after three consecutive losses. However, ASRM practice guidelines state that in the clinical scenario, evaluation should be considered following two consecutive miscarriages, especially with advanced maternal age more than 35 years.[5] In patients that conceive with assisted reproductive technology (ART) procedures, early investigations are warranted. One sporadic miscarriage does not warrant detailed investigations as the chances of a subsequent normal birth are high.

INCIDENCE

Although spontaneous abortion occurs in around 15–25%[6] of pregnancies, recurrent miscarriages (as per definition of three or more consecutive pregnancy losses) affects 0.4–1% of couples and as per two consecutive losses affects 5% of couples.[7]

RECURRENCE RISK

The risk of recurrence is influenced by various factors, which includes maternal age, parental and fetal karyotypes, gestation age of previous loss and various laboratory parameters. The risk of miscarriage is higher (25–57%) in less than 6 weeks gestation and reduces to 2–3% in gestation above 10 weeks.[8] Chromosomal analysis offers an explanation in 50% of cases.[9] The risk of miscarriage with number of prior miscarriages is shown in **Table 1**.

ETIOLOGY

The causes of recurrent miscarriage are listed in **Box 1**.[10] The list is exhaustive and investigations are expensive. More

Table 1: Risk of miscarriage with number of prior miscarriages.

	Number of prior miscarriages	*Risk of recurrence in next pregnancy (%)*
Women with one liveborn infant	0	12
	1	24
	2	26
	3	32
	4 or more	40–50
Women with no live infant	2 or more	40–45

Box 1: Causes of recurrent miscarriage.

Life Style factors
- Maternal age > 35 years.
- Maternal obesity BMI > 30.
- Paternal age

Immunological: Auto immune
- Primary antiphospholipid syndrome
- Secondary antiphospholipid syndrome: SLE, autoimmune thyroiditis

Immunological: Alloimmune (Classified as Unexplained)
- Abnormalities of cytokine production: lack of shift of Th1 to Th 2 response
- Lack of alpha V beta 3 integrin
- Increased levels of tumor necrosis factor-alpha (TNFα) in the endometrium
- Increased uterine natural killer cells
- Abnormal timing and duration of Implantation window

Genetic
- Fetal trisomy, polyploidy, monosomy
- Parental balanced translocations, inversions, deletions, duplications
  - Skewed inactivation of X-chromosome
  - Single gene defects, e.g. alpha thalassemia major, Retts syndrome, etc.

Hormonal
- Polycystic ovarian syndrome
- Luteal phase defects
- Hyperandrogenism
- Hypothyroidism/hyperthyroidism
- Hyperprolactinaemia
- Low AMH /poor ovarian reserve
- Adrenal hyperplasia/Addison's disease
  - Deficiency of vitamin D
  - Uncontrolled diabetes mellitus

Anatomical
- Müllerian abnormalities, septate uterus
- *Fibroids:* Submucous, intramural
- Uterine synechiae and polyps
- T-shaped uterus
- Cervical incompetence

Contd...

Contd...

Inherited thrombophilia
- Antithrombin III deficiency
- Deficiency of protein C and protein S
  - Activated protein C resistance
- Factor V Leiden mutation
- Methyl tetrahydrofolate gene homozygosity and hyperhomocysteinemia
- Prothrombin gene mutation
  - Plaminogen activator inhibitor

Semen factors
- High sperm DNA fragmentation index
- Male urogenital infections

Infections
- Genital bacterial vaginosis, tuberculosis
- Systemic syphilis, Lyme's disease, toxoplasmosis, brucellosis

Systemic conditions:
- Hypertension
- Chronic renal disease
- Chronic pulmonary disease
- Heart disease
- Severe rhesus sensitization

Miscellaneous
- Endocrine disrupters
  - Smoking, alcohol, drugs
- Exposure to irradiation
- Exposure to environmental toxins, pesticides, DDT, dry-cleaning chemicals
- Exposure to anesthetic gases

Idiopathic
- Cytokine abnormalities
- Increased uterine natural killer cells
- Epigenetic modifications of the embryo

than one factor may operate in successive pregnancies, e.g. early miscarriages due to any cause may be coupled with a late miscarriage due to cervical incompetence. On the other hand, early miscarriages may be coupled with a late fetal demise in patients with either congenital or acquired thrombophilia.

Figure 1 shows percentage-wise distribution of etiology of recurrent miscarriages.

TREATMENT

Anatomical Causes

The treatment often involves corrective hysteroscopic surgery. Resection of the septum may be done with the use of cautery or rarely with hysteroscopic scissors. Excision of submucous myoma is performed with the resectoscope. Adhesion bands and polyps are excised with the help of hysteroscopic scissors. Rarely correction of bicornuate uterus requires a Strassman operation. Repeated

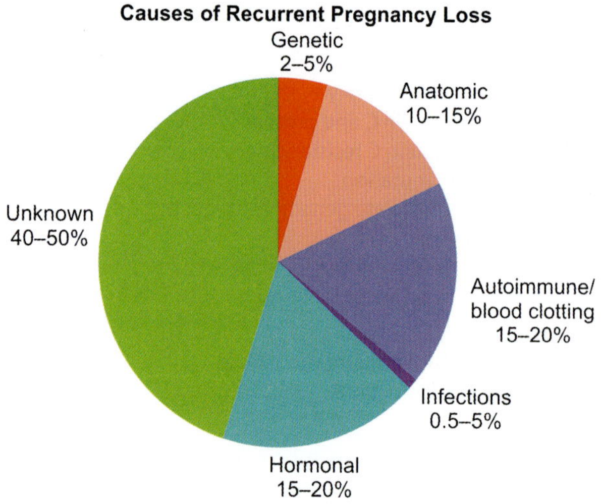

Fig. 1: Percentage-wise distribution of etiology of recurrent miscarriages.

implantation in the smaller horn of a bicornuate uterus may require excision of the rudimentary horn by laparoscopy/laparotomy. Disabling implantation in a rudimentary horn by placing an intrauterine contraceptive device (IUCD) in it may also be a viable noninvasive treatment option to prevent miscarriages.[11]

Cervical Insufficiency

Prenatal diagnosis can be done with a hysterosalpingogram. Serial cervical sonographic surveillance should be offered in the pregnant women with history of second trimester pregnancy loss and a cervical length of less than 25 mm is considered significant. Progesterone therapy (vaginal or parenteral) is recommended and cervical cerclage may be offered if cervical length is less than 1.5 cms.[12] However, there is no conclusive evidence that prophylactic cerclage reduces the risk of pregnancy loss and preterm delivery in women at risk of preterm birth or mid-trimester loss due to infective causes or multiple gestations. Most often cervical dilatation may be the result of a sterile inflammatory response (SIRS) at the decidual membrane interface that causes release of prostaglandins. Cervical dilatation may be prevented by diagnosing and treating subclinical endocervical infections as well as bacterial vaginosis. Probiotics may be more effective than antibiotics in many instances as there is an overgrowth of vaginal commensals that do not grow on routine cultures.

Hormonal Causes

Luteal Phase Deficiency

There is controversy whether this entity actually exists. Absence of corpus luteum formation at the 6 weeks scan is sometimes documented. Earlier the diagnosis is based on result of a phased endometrial biopsy; however, this is not recommended as a diagnostic modality any more. Poor echogenic change in the endometrium, low levels of serum progesterone in the mid luteal phase (<10 ng/mL) is considered diagnostic. A recent Cochrane review evaluating 15 trials concluded that routine administration of progesterone to all women with RPL had considerable benefit.[13] However, recently concluded randomized multicentric PROMISE study concluded that pregnancy outcome was not affected by progesterone administration.[14]

Thyroid Dysfunction

The American Thyroid Association recommends serum thyroid stimulating hormone (TSH) measurement for targeted screening and includes history of preterm delivery or miscarriage as one of the indication. TSH values greater than 2.5 IU/L is considered abnormal during pregnancy. The Endocrine Society recommends that patients with RPL be treated to maintain TSH levels between 1.0 and 2.5 mIU/mL in first trimester and upto 3 and 3.3 mIU/mL in second and third trimester, respectively. For TSH levels between 2.5 and 10 mIU/mL, levothyroxine is recommended in the starting dose of 50 µg/day.[15] The mechanism of pregnancy loss may be autoimmune rather than a hormonal deficiency.[16]

Abnormal Glucose Metabolism

Screening with HbA_{1c} levels is recommended for all women with recurrent miscarriages. This has replaced the oral glucose tolerance test in the first trimester. Weight reduction, diet alteration and life style modification are first steps in the management. Oral hypoglycemic agents like metformin are safe to prescribe during pregnancy in borderline cases. However, strict glycemic control is required in the first trimester to prevent congenital anomalies and insulin is often required. Patient education and counseling and initiation of self-blood glucose monitoring (SBGM) along with self-injections of insulin improves pregnancy outcome. Maintaining a diary of weekly blood sugar series fasting and post prandial with insulin dosage administered helps the clinician fine tune the glycemic control.

Strict glycemic control is desirable prior to pregnancy with HbA1c levels less than 7 in patients with overt diabetes.

Table 2 shows frequency of abnormal tests in RPL.[17]

Infections

The role of infection in recurrent pregnancy loss is unclear. Toxoplasmosis, rubella, cytomegalovirus, herpes and

Table 2: Frequency of abnormal tests in recurrent pregnancy loss (RPL).[17]

Frequency of abnormal tests in 1020 women with RPL					
Control	***Number of prior losses***	***2 N = 447***	***3 N = 343***	***≥4 N = 230***	***P Value 2, 3, or 4***
0.4 %	Parental genetics	2.8%	5.4%	5.2%	NS
7.5%	Anatomy	18.7%	18.2%	16.7%	NS
0.5%	Lupus anticoagulant	5.0%	2.9%	1.9%	NS
6.7%	Anti-cardiolipin	15.6%	13.1%	17.1%	NS
3.9%	TSH	8.1%	6.5%	6.2%	NS
6.9%	HbA1c	14.1%	16.3%	17.4%	NS

listeria infections are not implicated in recurrent pregnancy loss and hence routine TORCH test is not recommended. Most patients with RPL are not benefited by extensive work up for detecting infective etiology. Bacterial vaginosis is a risk factor for preterm delivery and a strong risk factor for late miscarriages. In symptomatic women, testing and treatment of bacterial vaginosis is indicated by checking the vaginal pH, which will be greater than 6 and looking for clue cells in vaginal secretions. The results of screening and treatment trials in asymptomatic women however are inconsistent.

Genetic Causes

Most early miscarriages show genetic abnormalities in the implanting embryo. Although this may be a sporadic event in embryogenesis and is not often repeated, patients with advanced maternal age and poor ovarian reserve will benefit by fast tracking to IVF with the possibility of trophectoderm biopsy of the blastocyst which will confirm the genetic make up of the embryo. Chromosomal analysis may be performed with fluorescent in-situ hybridization (FISH) for five chromosomes (13, 18, 21, X & Y), complete genomic hybridization (CGH) for all 23 chromosomes or next generation sequencing (NGS) can be performed for quicker results.

In cases where there are no normal embryos formed, the option of donor oocytes or embryos should be explored. In cases of balanced translocations in the parents, substitution with donor gametes may be required, although many cases of spontaneous normal embryogenesis and pregnancy are reported after multiple miscarriages.

Unexplained Recurrent Miscarriage

A significant proportion of cases of recurrent miscarriage remain unexplained despite detailed workup. Supportive care without pharmacological intervention in a dedicated RPL care offers an excellent prognosis for future pregnancy outcome for women with unexplained recurrent miscarriage. These women can be reassured that the prognosis for a successful future pregnancy with supportive care alone is in the region of 75%. The value of psychological support in improving pregnancy outcome cannot be overemphasized.[10]

Immune potentiation may be achieved by the following methods:

- *Lymphocyte immune therapy (LIT):* This involves injection of husband's/third party leucocytes subcutaneously in the mother. This therapy does not have the approval of US FDA and its benefits are to date unproven. Besides it carries the potential hazard of transmitting communicable diseases as well as a small risk of graft versus host reaction. Hence, LIT therapy is not recommended.
- *Correction of low-vitamin D levels:* Vitamin D deficiency is endemic in India. Besides contributing positively to bone health, vitamin D is a potent immune-potentiator, hence its deficiency should be corrected in all individuals.[18]
- *Intravenous immunoglobulins (IVIG):* In women with isolated IgG subclass 1–4 deficiency, these were measured in 160 patients of RM and 160 controls. In the RM group, 16 patients showed a deficiency of IgG which when corrected with IgG administration 200 mg/kg/month throughout pregnancy. This resulted in a successful pregnancy outcome in more than 90% of cases.[19] Use of IVIG in other autoimmune/alloimmune conditions is largely empirical.
- *Intralipids:* Is an extract of soy lecithin that was developed in Sweden for total parenteral nutrition. It demonstrated effective immune modulation in mice and has been used in a small number of humans with

recurrent implantation failure and idiopathic RM with promising results.[20] However, there are no randomized controlled trials as yet to prove its superiority over placebo.

A Cochrane review of immunotherapy for RM by Porter, which was conducted in 2006, and included 28 trials of high quality, that used paternal cell immunization, third party donor leucocytes, trophoblast membrane and intravenous immunoglobulins, concluded that various forms of immunotherapy did not show significant benefit over placebo.[21] There has been no review on vitamin D and intralipid use.

- *Granulocyte colony stimulating factor (GCSF):* In a randomized controlled trial, subcutaneous administration of GCSF in a dose of 1 µg/kg body weight/day administered from 6th post ovulatory day and repeated every alternate day has shown to improve clinical pregnancy rates in unexplained recurrent miscarriages.[22]
- *TNF-alpha blockers:* Although the diagnostic test for high TNF alpha levels as the cause of miscarriage is not robust, some people have tried using TNF alpha blockers with a variable response in patients with RM associated with high TNF alpha levels in the peripheral blood. These are expensive molecules with no data on fetal safety as yet and need to be used with extreme caution. However, in patients with rheumatoid arthritis with high TNF alpha levels these drugs have been used successfully. Ratio of interferon (IFN)-beta to IFN alpha, if high will predict a poor response to TNF-alpha inhibitors.[23] These are classified as category B drugs in pregnancy.

  The molecules that have been used during pregnancy are:
  - Infliximab.
  - Etanercept.
  - Adalimumab.
  - Cetrolizumab.

However, its use in pregnancy is limited to a few patients suffering from severe inflammatory bowel disease. Certolizumab is used and its use is stopped in the second trimester as it crosses the placenta and will cause IUGR.[24]

In a review of use of anti TNF alpha blockers during pregnancy of rheumatology patients, 58 case reports/ case series were analyses and the review concluded that the use of TNF alpha blockers does not increase the rate of congenital malformations nor does it increase the chances of any other adverse pregnancy outcomes.[25]

REFERENCES

1. Royal College of Obstetricians and Gynecologists. The investigation and treatment of couples with recurrent first-trimester and second-trimester miscarriage. Green-top Guideline No.17; April 2011. www.rcog.org.uk.
2. Bhattacharya S. Recurrent miscarriage: should the definition be revised? In: Arora M (Ed). World Clinics Obstetrics & Gynecology, vol. 1. New Delhi: Jaypee Brother Medical Publishers; 2011.
3. ACOG; 2013 FAQ 100 www.acog.org.
4. Practice Committee of the American Society for Reproductive Medicine. Definitions of infertility and recurrent pregnancy loss. Fertil Steril. 2008;89:1603.
5. Practice Committee of the American Society for Reproductive Medicine. Aging and infertility in women. Fertil Steril. 2006;86(5 Suppl):S248-52.
6. Stirrat GM. Recurrent miscarriage. Lancet. 1990;336:673-5.
7. Salat-Baroux J. Recurrent spontaneous abortions. Reprod Nutr Dev. 1988;28:1555-68.
8. Wilcox AJ, Weinberg CR, O'Connor JF, et al. Incidence of early loss of pregnancy. N Engl J Med. 1988;319(4):189-94.
9. Lathi RB, Gray Hazard FK, Heerema-McKenney A, et al. First trimester miscarriage evaluation. Semin Reprod Med. 2011;29:463-9.
10. Arora M, Konje J (Eds). Recurrent Pregnancy Loss. New Delhi: Jaypee; 2007.
11. Arora M, Basu HK. Non-surgical management of uterus didelphys. Saudi Med J. 1989:10(1):141-2.
12. O'Brien J. Cervical causes of preterm labor. In: In: Arora M (Ed). World Clinics Obstetrics & Gynecology, vol. 2. New Delhi: Jaypee Jaypee Brother Medical Publishers; 2012.
13. Haas DM, Ramsy PS. Progestogen for preventing miscarriage. Cochrane Database Syst Rev 2008;(2):CD003511.
14. Coomarasamy A, Williams H, Truchanowicz, E, et al. PROMISE trial: A randomized trial of progesterone in women with recurrent miscarriages. N Eng J Med. 2015:373; 2141-8.
15. De Groot L, Abalovich M, Alexander EK, et al. Management of thyroid dysfunction during pregnancy and postpartum: An Endocrine Society clinical practice guideline. J Clin Endocrinol Metab. 2012;97:2543-65.
16. Lata K, Dutta P, Sridhar S, et al. Thyroid autoimmunity and obstetric outcomes in women with recurrent miscarriages: a case control study. Endocr Connect. 2013;22;2(2):118-24.
17. Jaslow CR, Kutteh WH. Effect of prior birth and miscarriage frequency on the prevelance of acquired and congenital uterine anomalies in women with recurrent miscarriages: a cross sectional study. Fertil Steril. 2013;99(7):1916-22.
18. Ota K, Dambaeva S, Han AR, et al. Vit D deficiency may be a risk factor for recurrent pregnancy losses by increasing cellular immunity & autoimmunity. Hum Reprod. 2014;29(2):208-19.
19. Manfredi G, Dell A, Ligouri R. Overcoming RSM in women suffering from IgG subclass defeciency: high efficacy of low dose IVIG treatment. Eur Ann Allergy Clin Immunol. 2015;(4793):91-4.

20. Clark DA. Intralipid as treatment for recurrent unexplained abortion? Am J Reprod Immunol. 2013;32(4):290-3.
21. Porter TF, La Coursiere Y, Scott JR. Immunotherapy for recurrent miscarriage. Cochrane Database Syst Rev. 2006; 2:CD000112.
22. Scarpellini F, Sbracia M. Use of granulocyte colony stimulating factor for the treatment of unexplained recurrent miscarriage: a randomized controlled trial. Hum Reprod. 2009;24(11):2703-8.
23. Harrison P. Blood test predicts TNF inhibitor response in RA patients. Am Coll Rheumatol. 2014 Annual Meeting.
24. Gispert JP, Chaparro M. Safety of anti TNF agents during pregnancy and breast feeding in women with inflammatory bowel disease. Am J Gastroenterol. 2013;108(9): 1426-38.
25. Nielson OH, Loftus Jr EV, Jess T, et al. Safety of TNF alpha inhibitors during IBD pregnancy: a systematic review. BMC Med. 2013;11:174.

Ectopic Pregnancy

64

Suneeta Mittal, Sarita Sukhija, Laxmi Goel

INTRODUCTION

When a fertilized egg implants anywhere except the uterine lining, it is called an ectopic pregnancy. The worldwide reported incidence of ectopic pregnancy is 1–2%.[1] Although, the incidence has remained stable in the last two decades, but a six times rise was seen between 1972 and 1992. Amongst the various factors which led to this rise were increased use of assisted reproductive technology (ART), pelvic inflammatory disease, and smoking amongst women. It is one of the most common causes of morbidity and mortality of women of reproductive age contributing to 3.5–7% maternal mortality rates in developing countries including India.[2]

Fallopian tubes are the most common part of the uterus where ectopic pregnancies occur. It account to almost 95%. Prior pelvic or abdominal surgery and history of pelvic infections are important risk factor for the ectopic pregnancy in fallopian tube. Chlamydia trachomatis attributes to 30–50% of all ectopic pregnancies.[3] 30% of all ectopic pregnancies have been seen to be associated with smoking. Ectopic pregnancy is commonly seen in women seeking ART treatment for infertility. Women with a past history of ectopic pregnancy have more chances of ectopic pregnancies in subsequent conception. The increase in risk is directly proportional to the number of previous ectopic pregnancies.[4]

DIAGNOSIS

Ectopic pregnancy may be asymptomatic in 9% of cases or it may present with amenorrhea, abdominal pain and vaginal bleeding, although the classical triad is not seen in the majority of the cases. Ectopic pregnancies can be mostly diagnosed between 6 weeks' and 10 weeks' gestation. Symptoms may vary from nonspecific complaints, unaware of an ongoing pregnancy to persistent severe pain radiating to shoulder. Ruptured ectopic pregnancy may present with signs of hemodynamic instability (low blood pressure, increased heart rate, and respiratory distress) and syncope.

The bimanual examination should be done cautiously and gently as this may exacerbate bleeding. 50% of the cases present with palpable adnexal mass and almost one-third of cases present with cervical motion tenderness.[5]

Transvaginal ultrasonography and serum beta human chorionic gonadotropin (β-hCG) levels are the important tools of investigations.

Visualization of a gestational sac outside the uterus, with yolk sac and/or fetal node with or without cardiac activity on transvaginal ultrasound (TVS) is the definite diagnosis of ectopic pregnancy. If on TVS, there is an inhomogenous or noncystic adnexal mass that moves separate to ovary ("Blob" sign) or an empty extrauterine sac-like structure ("Bagel" sign) in the absence of intrauterine gestational sac, then there is probability of ectopic pregnancy.

If serum β-hCG is below 1,000 IU/L, even intrauterine pregnancy (IUP) cannot be seen in TVS. When hCG is above 1,000 IU/L, if on TVS, eccentrically positioned hyperechogenic ring-like structure with yolk sac or fetal node is seen, a diagnosis of intrauterine pregnancy is confirmed.[6] A "pseudosac" can be seen in up to 16.6% cases of ectopic pregnancy, there can be a collection of fluid which is centrally located in the endometrial cavity. Appearance of free fluid in pouch of Douglas in TVS with adnexal mass suggests ruptured ectopic pregnancy.

However, in many women, TVS fails to identify the exact location of pregnancy, and these are labeled as having a "pregnancy of unknown location" (PUL). Although on follow-up, many of these women are found to have viable or nonviable intrauterine pregnancies. Barnhart et al reported that 7–20% of PUL will be diagnosed with an ectopic pregnancy.[7] It is of importance to understand that any diagnosis of PUL should prompt additional investigative workup and the patient should be strictly kept on follow-up until the definite result of PUL is known.

Serial β-hCG concentrations over time are used to predict the end result of PULs. Kadar and Romero reported that the minimum rate of rise in serum β-hCG concentration is 66% in 48 hours during a normal ongoing pregnancy.[8] In a study by Seeber et al., the minimum rise in β-hCG for a viable IUP was 24% at 24 hours and 53% at 48 hours.[9] In a viable IUP, the β-hCG levels usually double in 2 days, but sometimes it increases to only 35% of the first value in 48 hours even in normal cases. About 20% of all ectopic pregnancies show twofold increase of β-hCG in 48 hours. An expeditious descent in the β-hCG values over 48 hours, by 21–35% or more, suggests a spontaneous abortion or a dissolving ectopic pregnancy.[10]

ECTOPIC PREGNANCY: SURGICAL TREATMENT

INTRODUCTION

A pregnancy that implants outside the normal uterine cavity, it is considered as ectopic pregnancy. The most common extrauterine pregnancies occur in fallopian tubes (84%),[11] but can occur in ovary, cervix, tubal cornua (interstitial pregnancy), uterine scar or abdominal cavity. Rarely, there may be heterotopic pregnancy, i.e., both intra- as well as extrauterine implantation of multiple gestations.

Several technological advances in ultrasound imaging, magnetic resonance imaging (MRI) in select cases and highly sensitive β-hCG assay have resulted in early diagnosis of ectopic pregnancy. Accordingly management can be expectant, medical or surgical. Quite a few ectopic pregnancies, which would not have been diagnosed earlier, resolve spontaneously, thus are left for expectant management based on specific criteria. Almost one-third cases can be successfully managed medically, while remaining would require surgery.[12] How and when to choose surgical treatment and different surgical modalities will be discussed here.

INDICATIONS FOR SURGICAL TREATMENT

1. Ruptured ectopic with hemoperitoneum
2. Hemodynamically unstable patient
3. Large ectopic
4. Coexisting pathology requiring surgery, e.g. ovarian cyst, hydrosalpinx, etc.
5. Patient preference for surgery or not able comply with follow-up on medical management
6. Contraindications to medical management (sac size >4 cm or hCG >5,000 IU)
7. Contraindication to methotrexate—liver, kidney, hematological, immune disorder or respiratory disease
8. Failure of medical treatment
9. Select cases of ectopic pregnancy at sites other than fallopian tube.

SURGERY FOR TUBAL ECTOPIC

Surgical approach for tubal pregnancy can be radical, i.e., salpingectomy (removal of the fallopian tube) or conservative, i.e. salpingostomy (incising the tube to remove the tubal gestation but leaving the remainder of the tube intact).[13] The choice is based on tubal status and the age and parity of woman. With conservative surgery there is a small risk of retained trophoblastic tissue and having a repeat ectopic in the diseased tube.

CHOICE OF SURGERY

Salpingostomy versus Salpingectomy

If tube is ruptured already and other tube looks healthy, the standard treatment is salpingectomy. Usually patient undergoing salpingectomy is relatively older,[14] however overall fertility outcome does not differ much when salpingostomy is compared with salpingectomy.

If the tube containing pregnancy is ruptured beyond repair, or there is uncontrolled bleeding salpingectomy is done irrespective of the status of other tube, as conception will still be possible with IVF.

Salpingectomy is also preferred in women with completed fertility goals and those with contraindications to methotrexate therapy, as following salpingostomy sometimes persistent or residual trophoblastic disease may require additional medical treatment. Women undergoing salpingostomy should be followed up with hCG level. Salpingostomy is preferred if future childbearing is desired and other tube is absent or damaged, as despite its availability, in India many women do not have access to IVF or cannot afford it. Salpingectomy has been shown to reduce risk of ovarian cancer, thus, bilateral salpingectomy is a good option for women wanting permanent sterilization.

Laparoscopy versus Laparotomy

In current era laparoscopic surgery is the standard surgical approach for ectopic pregnancy and there is a rising trend toward laparoscopic management in most units.[15] A systemic review of randomized trials comparing laparoscopy with laparotomy for salpingostomy has demonstrated a significantly shorter operating time, lesser blood loss, shorter hospital stay, and earlier recovery with laparscopy.[13] A recent randomized comparative study of laparoscopy versus laparotomy in women with ruptured ectopic comprising of 140 women, confirmed the same advantages of laparoscopy over laparotomy and estimated that a significantly larger number (25.5% vs. 14.5%) required blood transfusion in laparotomy group.[16] With a large bore suction cannula most ectopics even with gross hemoperitoneum can be managed successfully with laparoscopy. However, in an unstable patient with active bleeding sometimes laparotomy is preferred. A surgeon with limited expertise in laparoscopy should prefer laparotomy.

Surgical Procedures

Salpingostomy

After identifying the pregnancy, the tube is immobilized with laparoscopic forceps and 2–5 mL vasopressin solution (0.2 IU/mL) is injected in the tubal wall to decrease blood loss. A longitudinal incision is made over the gestation sac with cautery and products are evacuated and collected for pathological examination. Hemostasis is obtained with thorough irrigation and cauterization. The incision can be left open. The adhesion formation and subsequent fertility are same with or without closure.[17,18]

Salpingectomy

Salpingectomy may be partial or total depending on the patient's age, site of ectopic, condition of tube and plan for future pregnancy.

Laparoscopic salpingectomy may be carried out using a pretied surgical loop or using electrocautery or harmonic along the mesosalpinx to seal the vessels followed by cutting and removing the tube.

If laparotomy is performed, for total salpingectomy, a clamp is put from the lateral end on mesosalpinx close to the tube and another one at the corneal end. The tube is excised over the clamps and pedicles are ligated with 2-0 vicryl. For partial salpingectomy, the clamps are placed proximal and distal to the ectopic gestation and in between portion containing pregnancy is removed. The two remaining segments of tube can be anastomosed in future.

SURGERY FOR NONTUBAL ECTOPICS

Cervical Pregnancy

Cervical pregnancy is uncommon accounting for less than 1% of total ectopics;[19,20] however, it is more common following IVF. Approximately 0.1% of in vitro fertilization pregnancies and 3.7% of IVF ectopic gestations are reported to be cervical pregnancies.[21] A correct diagnosis is important to avoid serious blood loss.

Hemodynamically stable women with cervical pregnancy are treated medically with methotrexate and/or intra sac KCl. Intrasac injection is preferably done in the operating room as sudden bleeding may be precipitated. Some women may require intra-arterial embolization to control hemorrhage.

The traditional treatment of cervical pregnancy is dilation and evacuation under ultrasound guidance, with hysterectomy if there is uncontrolled hemorrhage. Preoperative uterine artery embolization,[22] transvaginal ligation of the cervical branches of the uterine arteries, cervical cerclage, or intracervical vasopressin injection can reduce the risk of bleeding significantly during dilatation and evacuation. Sometimes balloon tamponade for 24–48 hours may help control bleeding and prevent hysterectomy.[23]

Hysterectomy is done electively in women who have completed family or have some other uterine pathology. Isolated case reports also describe hysteroscopic resection of cervical pregnancy.[24]

Interstitial Pregnancy

Earlier interstitial pregnancy was mostly managed surgically by cornual resection or hysterectomy, as diagnosis was mostly delayed.[25] Currently, with early diagnosis both medical and conservative surgical management are possible.[26] Both laparoscopic cornulostomy after vasopressin injection and removal of gestation sac or corneal resection are feasible options.[27]

A case series of four cases describes management using single dose methotrexate, laparotomy, hysteroscopy and vacuum aspiration and vacuum aspiration under laparoscopic guidance,[28] suggesting that the management has to be highly individualized.

A recent case report describes temporary clamping of uterine and ovarian vessels at laparoscopy and managing a corneal pregnancy safely and efficiently.[29] Multilayer suturing of uterine cornua and myometrium needs to be carried out after removing the gestation products to prevent uterine rupture in subsequent pregnancy.

Cesarean Scar Pregnancy

Pregnancy in a previous cesarean scar occurs in about 1 in 2,000 pregnancies and accounts for 6% of ectopic pregnancies among women with a prior cesarean delivery.[30,31] The optimal treatment for a cesarean scar pregnancy is still debatable and tailored according to clinical presentation. If early diagnosis is made medical management is feasible. Surgical intervention is required if patient is bleeding and ranges from dilatation and evacuation, hysteroscopy guided evacuation after uterine artery embolization,[32] laparoscopic resection of ectopic and repair of scar dehiscence,[33] wedge resection of ectopic pregnancy via laparoscopy or laparotomy and rarely hysterectomy. A recent review of concluded that hysteroscopy or laparoscopic-guided evacuation of ectopic is best first-line approach for cesarean scar pregnancy and prior uterine artery embolization helps in reducing the blood loss significantly.[34]

Abdominal Pregnancy

Abdominal pregnancy, a rare occurrence (1per 10,000 births),[35] may be primary or secondary implanting over omentum, pelvic sidewall, broad ligament, posterior cul-de-sac, abdominal organs (e.g. spleen, bowel, liver), large pelvic vessels, diaphragm, and the uterine serosa. It can even take place after hysterectomy.[36,37]

There is a case report of abdominal pregnancy after in vitro fertilization (IVF) in a patient probably due to uterine perforation by the IVF transfer catheter.[38]

If the abdominal pregnancy is diagnosed early, operative laparoscopy is done. At any stage of pregnancy removal of placenta is a problem and may involve excision of abdominal organ involved, e.g. splenectomy.[39] Residual placenta is managed with postoperative methotrexate. In elective cases preoperative embolization helps to reduce blood loss.

Ovarian Pregnancy

Ovarian pregnancy occurs in 1/2,100 to 1/60,000 pregnancies and accounts for 1–3% of ectopic pregnancies.[40] Clinical or ultrasound diagnosis is difficult and is typically made only on surgery. Even on laparoscopy it may be confused with a hemorrhagic cyst. Strict histopathological criteria are used to confirm ovarian pregnancy. Surgical management ranges from wedge resection to excision of involved ovary.[41]

Rudimentary Horn Pregnancy

Rudimentary uterine horn pregnancy is actually an intrauterine pregnancy; however, clinical manifestation is like an ectopic pregnancy. Incidence is very low and mostly diagnosis is made after rupture of horn or failure to evacuate in a case of missed abortion. Early diagnosis and planned surgical removal of rudimentary horn is advocated.[42]

Heterotopic Pregnancy

Heterotopic pregnancy is two simultaneous pregnancies at different sites. Most often it is a combination of intrauterine and ectopic pregnancies.[43] Incidence was low earlier (1 in 30,000), but is on rise (1 in 3,900) currently due to IVF.[44] An analysis of IVF pregnancies reported an incidence of 1.5 per 1,000 ART pregnancies.[45] Usually diagnosis is made on laparoscopy for acute pain. Medical management is contraindicated and every effort is made at surgery to not disturb the intrauterine sac.

Salpingectomy is the standard surgical approach for tubal pregnancy. For other sites selective fetal reduction may be carried out.

SUMMARY

Laparoscopic surgery is the standard surgical approach for tubal ectopic pregnancy with no significant difference in outcome with salpingectomy or salpingostomy. Most ectopic pregnancies, even in the presence of hemoperitoneum, may be treated with minimal invasive surgery, however, with acute bleeding, some surgeons prefer laparotomy. Current evidence supports surgery as the primary treatment for ovarian, abdominal scar and interstitial pregnancy, however, a combined approach is being increasingly used with good outcome. The crux is early diagnosis. Elective uterine artery embolization has significant role in selected cases in reducing intraoperative blood loss.

MEDICAL MANAGEMENT OF ECTOPIC PREGNANCY

INTRODUCTION

The surgical treatment to remove the ectopic pregnancy has been in place since a long time but now a days, a more conservative approach has been established by offering medical management by using methotrexate (MTX) injections under supervision in selected patients which has been shown to treat the ectopic pregnancy with equally good success rates, if diagnosed, at an early stage so that surgery can be completely avoided. Systemic MTX is the drug of choice for medical treatment of ectopic gestation. There have been lots of studies comparing medical management with the surgical treatment and successful management with MTX, which has encouraged clinicians to use it judiciously in certain patients. Clinician should assess the initial β-hCG levels, the signs and symptoms of the patient, and explain in detail the advantages and disadvantages of both medical and surgical methods and then only should one take a final call as to which treatment is suited best for that particular patient.

PHARMACOKINETICS OF METHOTREXATE

Methotrexate is a folate antagonist which interrupts the synthesis of purine nucleotides and amino acids by binding to the catalytic site of dihydrofolate reductase, thus interfering with deoxyribonucleic acid (DNA) synthesis and repair and cell replication. Proliferating tissues like bone marrow, respiratory epithelium, buccal and intestinal mucosa, malignant cells, and trophoblastic tissue are directly affected by methotrexate. It has been used to treat gestational trophoblastic disease since 1956 and was first used to treat ectopic pregnancy in 1982.[46]

How to select patients for medical management?

- Hemodynamically stable
- Blood hCG levels less than 1,500 are preferred. However, levels up to 5,000 IU/L can also be taken up for medical management under adequate supervision
- Absent cardiac activity
- No intrauterine pregnancy on ultrasonography (USG) scan
- Patient willing for regular follow up
- No known sensitivity to MTX.

According to NICE guidelines,[47] methotrexate should be the first-line of treatment for women with unruptured ectopic pregnancy with no significant pain, with serum β-hCG between 1,500 and 5,000 IU/L, gestational sac or mass size smaller than 3.5 cm; no visible cardiac activity, and who can comply with regular follow ups. There should be no intrauterine pregnancy.

Women with pregnancy of unknown location (PUL) who full fill the inclusion criteria as listed above can also be offered medical treatment with MTX.

Serum β-hCG levels should be monitored serially before the decision for giving MTX is taken. If initial β-hCG levels are in lower range than expected, it raises a strong suspicion of ectopic pregnancy, but if the β-hCG titers are showing rising trend then a repeat scan should be advised to rule out intrauterine pregnancy, as methotrexate will have adverse effects on intrauterine gestation.

CONTRAINDICATIONS TO METHOTREXATE THERAPY

- *Absolute contraindications*:
  - Hemodynamically unstable
  - Known sensitivity to MTX
  - Presence of intrauterine pregnancy
  - Breastfeeding
  - Unwilling for regular follow-up
  - Chronic hepatic disease
  - Immunocompromised patients
  - Blood disorders
  - Peptic ulcer disease
  - Active pulmonary disease.
- *Relative contraindications*:
  - If fetal cardiac activity is seen on ultrasound
  - High initial β-hCG levels should not be taken up for MTX unless β-hCG levels repeated after 48 hours show low titers
  - If the ectopic pregnancy size is more than 4 cm on transvaginal ultrasonography
  - If the patient refuses to take blood transfusion if required.

INVESTIGATIONS

The following investigations must be performed before giving MTX:

- Blood group and hemoglobin
- Bleeding and clotting time
- Activated partial thromboplastin time (aPTT) and international normalized ratio (INR)
- Renal and liver function tests

- Viral markers and β-hCG levels.

The tests should be repeated as and when required.

METHOTREXATE REGIMENS IN PRACTICE

The various protocols used for the administration of MTX include:

- Single-dose protocol
- Two-dose protocol
- Fixed multiple-dose protocol.

Methotrexate can be administered systemically as:

- Single-dose regimen [MTX 1.0 mg/kg or 50 mg/m^2 intramuscular (IM) without folinic acid] or
- Multiple-dose regimen [MTX 1.0 mg/kg IM daily 0, 2, 4, 6 alternating with folinic acid 0.1 mg/kg orally on days 1, 3, 5, 7].[48]

The single-dose regimen is the simplest of all, but if the follow up β-hCG shows rising titers, then an additional dose may be required in some patients.[49,50] The two-dose regimen adheres to the same β-hCG monitoring schedule as the single-dose regimen, but a second dose of MTX is given on day 4 of treatment.[51]

Multiple-doses Regimen

In multiple-dose regimen, injection MTX 1.0 mg/kg IM is given on day 1, 2, 4 and 6 alternating with the folinic acid 0.1 mg/kg, rescue dose on days 1, 3, 5 and 7, so as to minimize the side effects of MTX.[52]

Resolution of an ectopic pregnancy depends on the MTX treatment regimen used and the initial hCG level. Approximately 70(95% will show resolution of the ectopic pregnancy without the need for surgery. Though there is no clear consensus regarding the optimal MTX regimen, single-dose regimen is preferred for patients with a relatively low initial hCG level, while two-dose or multiple-dose regimens is preferred for patients with high hCG titers

Single-dose versus Multiple-dose

Various observational studies have observed that multiple-dose regimen is more effective but has higher incidence of adverse effects when compared to the single-dose regimen.[49,53,54] However, a randomized controlled trial (RCT) conducted by Yang et al. showed that both regimens are equally effective, the risk of side effects is higher with multiple-dose regimen.[50] The two-dose and single-dose protocols were found to have similar resolution rates and comparable risk of adverse effects

Methotrexate Treatment Protocols

Single-dose Regimen

After administering single dose methotrexate, hCG levels are monitored on post treatment day 4 and day 7. If β-hCG levels decreases by more than 15%, then hCG is measured weekly, till it reaches non-pregnant. However, if the decrease is less than 15%, MTX is readministered at a dose of 50 mg/m^2 IM and hCG level are repeated. It advisable to consider surgery, If hCG does not decrease even after two doses. If hCG levels plateaus or increases during follow-up, MTX should be administered for treatment of a persistent ectopic pregnancy.

Two-dose Regimen

Methotrexate 50 mg/m^2 IM is administered on day 1 and day 4. β-hCG levels should be done on post-treatment day 4 and 7. If the levels decrease by more than 15%, hCG is measured weekly, till it reaches nonpregnant levels. If decrease is less than 15%, MTX is readministered on day 7 and hCG levels checked on day 11. If hCG levels decrease 15% between day 7 and day 11, it is monitored weekly until it reaches non pregnant levels. If the decrease is less than 15% between day 7 and day 11, MTX 50 mg/m^2 IM is re-administered on day 11 and hCG checked on day 14. Surgical management should be considered if hCG does not decrease even after four doses.

Fixed Multiple-dose Regimen

Human chorionic gonadotropin levels are measured on MTX dose days and continued until hCG has decreased by 15% from its previous measurement. If the decrease is greater than 15%, MTX administration is discontinued and hCG levels are measured weekly until nonpregnant levels are reached (may ultimately need one, two, three, or four doses). If hCG does not decrease after four doses, consider surgical management. If hCG levels plateaus or increases during follow-up, consider administering MTX for treatment of a persistent ectopic pregnancy.

Monitoring of Patients after Giving Methotrexate

Beta-hCG levels should be serially monitored until a non-pregnancy level (based upon the reference laboratory assay) is reached. Transvaginal sonography (TVS) should be done to make sure that the trophoblastic activity has disappeared completely and there is no persistent ectopic tissue left. β-hCG levels might increase to higher levels initially after first few days when MTX is administered but then β-hCG levels decrease progressively to reach non-pregnant normal level. If initial hCG levels are high then success rates are low. Resolution of serum hCG levels after medical management is usually completed in 2–4 weeks but can take up to 8 weeks.

ADVERSE EFFECTS OF METHOTREXATE THERAPY

Adverse effects of MTX usually are dependent on protocol and duration of management. The most common side effects are gastrointestinal problems, (e.g., nausea, vomiting, and stomatitis), more commonly seen after multiple-dose regimen, as MTX affects rapidly dividing tissues.[9] Abdominal pain is observed due to cytotoxic effect of the drug on the trophoblastic tissue.

Transient elevation of liver enzymes, pneumonitis and alopecia are other rare side effects.

Heterotrophic Pregnancy

Methotrexate should be avoided in cases of heterotopic pregnancy as it can have adverse effects on the intrauterine gestation.[55]

In case of interstitial, cervical and cesarean scar pregnancy, local Injection of hyperosmolar glucose into the extrauterine sac, or injection potassium chloride into either the fetal pole or the sac and aspiration of contents of sac can be done to minimize the risks to the coexisting intrauterine pregnancy by surgical approaches.

Follow-up with USG is essential to make sure that ectopic has resolved completely.[56,57]

Anti-D Prophylaxis in Ectopic Pregnancy

All Rh D-negative women should receive Anti-D prophylaxis after treatment of ectopic pregnancy as alloimmunization has been reported following ectopic pregnancy.

EFFECTS OF ECTOPIC PREGNANCY MANAGEMENT ON FUTURE FERTILITY

There is no difference in the fertility rate, the risk of future tubal ectopic pregnancy or tubal patency rates when medical or surgical management were compared. Expectant or medical management has better reproductive outcomes in future compared with surgical treatment. Long term studies have shown recurrent ectopic rate to be 18.5%.[58,59] Patency rates seen by hysterosalpingogram (HSG) were found to be similar in women who were managed medically or expectantly in either ipsilateral tube or in the contralateral tube.[60] No adverse effect has been seen on ovarian reserve of the patients after receiving the MTX.[61,62] Many RCTs have shown no difference in fertility outcomes whether women are managed with medical treatment or surgical treatment.

The oocyte recovery might be lower if fertility treatment is started within 180 days of giving MTX, so patients may be advised to use some kind of contraception and not plan pregnancy till 180 days of MTX.[63]

POST MEDICAL MANAGEMENT OF ECTOPIC PREGNANCY ADVISE TO THE PATIENTS

Conception should be avoided for at least 3 months after MTX administration as the drug remains in the system and can affect fetal development and can cause congenital malformations. However, if a woman does get pregnant within 3 months of MTX, then it should not be an indication for termination of pregnancy.[64]

MEDICAL VERSUS SURGICAL MANAGEMENT

Medical management of ectopic pregnancy is preferred option in selected cases, as it avoids the inherent risks of surgery and anesthesia. However, it demands longer surveillance, more visits, and the anxiety levels are high. Various randomized trials have shown that significant lower success rate are observed with the use of single dose MTX compared to laparoscopic salpingostomy, however the difference was not statistically significant with the use of multi-dose MTX.[65] Surgical management of ectopic pregnancy is more cost effective if time to resolution is expected to be prolonged, or there is a relatively high chance of medical management failure, such as in cases with high or increasing hCG values or when embryonic cardiac activity is detected.[66,67]

REFERENCES

1. Panti A, Ikechukwu NE, Lukman OO, et al. Ectopic pregnancy at Usmanu Danfodiyo University Teaching Hospital Sokoto: A ten year review. Ann Niger Med. 2012;6(2):87.
2. Shah P, Shah S, Kutty RV, et al. Changing epidemiology of maternal mortality in rural India: time to reset strategies for MDG-5. Trop Med Int Health. 2014;19(5):568-75.

3. Akande V, Turner C, Horner P, et al; British Fertility Society. Impact of Chlamydia trachomatis in the reproductive setting: British Fertility Society Guidelines for practice. Hum Fertil (Camb). 2010;13(3):115-25.
4. Shaw JL, Oliver E, Lee KF, et al. Cotinine exposure increases Fallopian tube PROKR1 expression via nicotinic AChRalpha-7: a potential mechanism explaining the link between smoking and tubal ectopic pregnancy. Am J Pathol. 2010;177(5):2509-15.
5. Tay JI, Moore J, Walker JJ. Ectopic pregnancy. BMJ. 2000; 320 (7239):916-9.
6. Kirk E, Bottomley C, Bourne T. Diagnosing ectopic pregnancy and current concepts in the management of pregnancy of unknown location. Hum Reprod Update. 2014;20(2):250-61.
7. Barnhart K, van Mello NM, Bourne T, et al. Pregnancy of unknown location: a consensus statement of nomenclature, definitions, and outcome. Fertil Steril. 2011; 95(3):857-6.
8. Romero R, Kadar N, Jeanty P, et al. Diagnosis of ectopic pregnancy: value of the discriminatory human chorionic gonadotropin zone. Obstet Gynecol. 1985; 66(3):357-60.
9. Seeber BE, Sammel MD, Guo W, et al. Application of redefined human chorionic gonadotropin curves for the diagnosis of women at risk for ectopic pregnancy. Fertil Steril. 2006; 86(2):454-9.
10. Barnhart KT, Sammel MD, Rinaudo PF, et al. Symptomatic patients with an early viable intrauterine pregnancy: hCG curves redefined. Obstet Gynecol. 2004;104(1):50-5.
11. Bouyer J, Coste J, Fernandez H, et al. Sites of ectopic pregnancy: a 10 year population-based study of 1800 cases. Hum Reprod. 2002;17:3224.
12. Van Den Eeden SK, Shan J, Bruce C, et al. Ectopic pregnancy rate and treatment utilization in a large managed care organization. Obstet Gynecol. 2005;105:1052.
13. Hajenius PJ, Mol F, Mol BW, et al. Interventions for tubal ectopic pregnancy. Cochrane Database Syst Rev. 2007:CD000324.
14. Chen L, Zhu D, Wu Q, Yu Y. Fertility outcome after laparoscopic salpingectomy or salpingostomy for tubal ectopic pregnancy: a retrospective cohort study of 95 patients. Int J Surg. 2017;48:59-63.
15. Paul C, Robson SJ. Hospital admission and surgical approach to tubal ectopic pregnancy in Australia 2000-2014: a population based study. Aust N Z J Obstet Gynecol. 2018;58(2):234-8.
16. Snyman L, Makulana T Makin JD. A randomized trial comparing laparoscopy with laparotomy in the management of women with ruptured ectopic pregnancy. S Afr Med J. 2017;107:258-63.
17. Tulandi T, Guralnick M. Treatment of tubal ectopic pregnancy by salpingotomy with or without tubal suturing and salpingectomy. Fertil Steril. 1991;55:53.
18. Fujishita A, Masuzaki H, Khan KN, et al. Laparoscopic salpingotomy for tubal pregnancy: comparison of linear salpingotomy with and without suturing. Hum Reprod. 2004;19:1195.
19. Yankowitz J, Leake J, Huggins G, et al. Cervical ectopic pregnancy: review of the literature and report of a case treated by single-dose methotrexate therapy. Obstet Gynecol Surv. 1990;45:405.
20. Bouyer J, Coste J, Fernandez H, et al. Sites of ectopic pregnancy: a 10 year population-based study of 1800 cases. Hum Reprod. 2002;17:3224.
21. Karande VC, Flood JT, Heard N, et al. Analysis of ectopic pregnancies resulting from in-vitro fertilization and embryo transfer. Hum Reprod. 1991;6:446.
22. Ushakov FB, Elchalal U, Aceman PJ, et al. Cervical pregnancy: past and future. Obstet Gynecol Surv. 1997;52:45.
23. Fylstra DL. Cervical pregnancy: 13 cases treated with suction curettage and balloon tamponade. Am J Obstet Gynecol. 2014;210:581.e1.
24. Ash S, Farrell SA. Hysteroscopic resection of a cervical ectopic pregnancy. Fertil Steril. 1996;66:842.
25. Moawad NS, Mahajan ST, Moniz MH, et al. Current diagnosis and treatment of interstitial pregnancy. Am J Obstet Gynecol. 2010;202:15.
26. Tulandi T, Al-Jaroudi D. Interstitial pregnancy: results generated from the Society of Reproductive Surgeons Registry. Obstet Gynecol. 2004;103:47.
27. Soriano D, Vicus D, Mashiach R, et al. Laparoscopic treatment of cornual pregnancy: a series of 20 consecutive cases. Fertil Steril. 2008;90:839.
28. Kahramanoglu J, Mammadov Z, Turan H, et al. Management options for interstitial ectopic pregnancies: a case series. Pak J Med Sci. 2017;33:476-82.
29. Yang H, Song T. Temporary simultaneous 2 arterial occlusions during laparoscopic management of cornual ectopic pregnancy. J Min Inv Gynecol. 2018;25(6):961-2.
30. Lee CL, Wang CJ, Chao A, et al. Laparoscopic management of an ectopic pregnancy in a previous Caesarean section scar. Hum Reprod. 1999;4:1234.
31. Rotas MA, Haberman S, Levgur M. Cesarean scar ectopic pregnancies: etiology, diagnosis, and management. Obstet Gynecol. 2006;107:1373.
32. Chen ZY, Li XY, Zhao D, et al. Clinical analysis on hysteroscopic surgery for treatment of type II ceasarean scar pregnancies in first trimester. Zhonghua Fu Chan Ke Za Zhi. 2017;52(10): 669-74.
33. Mahgoub S, Gabriele V, Faller B, et al. CS scar ectopic pregnancy: laparoscopic resection and total scar dehiscence repair. J Minim Invasive Gynecol. 2018;25(2):297-8.
34. van der Voet LF, Vervoort AJ, Veersema S, et al. Minimally invasive therapy for gynaecological symptoms related to a niche in the caesarean scar: a systematic review. BJOG. 2014;121(2):145-56.
35. Atrash HK, Friede A, Hogue CJ. Abdominal pregnancy in the United States: frequency and maternal mortality. Obstet Gynecol. 1987;69:333.
36. Fader AN, Mansuria S, Guido RS, et al. A 14-week abdominal pregnancy after total abdominal hysterectomy. Obstet Gynecol. 2007;109:519.
37. Fisch B, Peled Y, Kaplan B, et al. Abdominal pregnancy following in vitro fertilization in a patient with previous bilateral salpingectomy. Obstet Gynecol. 1996;88: 642.

38. Binder DS. Thirteen-week abdominal pregnancy after hysterectomy. J Emerg Med. 2003;25:159.
39. Greenbaum A, Miskmins R, Coffman B, et al. Management of splenic ectopic pregnancy presenting with massive haemoperitoneam. BMJ Case Rep. 2016:218291.
40. Comstock C, Huston K, Lee W. The ultrasonographic appearance of ovarian ectopic pregnancies. Obstet Gynecol. 2005;105:42.
41. Tabassum M, Atmuri K. The unexpected ovarian pregnancy at laparoscopy: a review of management. Case Rep Obstet Gynecol. 2017:9856802.
42. Yassin A, Munaza S, Mohammed A. Tale of rudimentary horn pregnancy: case reports and literature review. J Mater Fetal Med. 2019;32(4):671-6.
43. Reece EA, Petrie RH, Sirmans MF, et al. Combined intrauterine and extrauterine gestations: a review. Am J Obstet Gynecol. 1983;146:323.
44. Rojansky N, Schenker JG. Heterotopic pregnancy and assisted reproduction--an update. J Assist Reprod Genet. 1996;13: 594.
45. Clayton HB, Schieve LA, Peterson HB, et al. A comparison of heterotopic and intrauterine-only pregnancy outcomes after assisted reproductive technologies in the United States from 1999 to 2002. Fertil Steril. 2007;87:303.
46. Tanaka T, Hayashi H, Kutsuzawa T, et al. Treatment of interstitial ectopic pregnancy with methotrexate: report of a successful case. Fertil Steril. 1982;37:851-2.
47. Bourne T, Barnhart K, Benson CB, et al. NICE guidance on ectopic pregnancy and miscarriage restricts access and choice and may be clinically unsafe. BMJ. 2013;346: f197.
48. Stovall TG, Ling FW. Single-dose methotrexate: an expanded clinical trial. Am J Obstet Gynecol. 1993;168:1759-62.
49. Barnhart KT, Gosman G, Ashby R, et al. The medical management of ectopic pregnancy: a meta-analysis comparing "single dose" and "multidose" regimens. Obstet Gynecol. 2003;101:778-84.
50. Yang C, Cai J, Geng Y, et al. Multiple-dose and double-dose versus single-dose administration of methotrexate for the treatment of ectopic pregnancy: a systematic review and meta-analysis. Reprod Biomed Online. 2017;34:383-91.
51. Barnhart K, Hummel AC, Sammel MD, et al. Use of "2 dose" regimen of methotrexate to treat ectopic pregnancy. Fertil Steril. 2007;87:250.
52. Rodi IA, Sauer MV, Gorrill MJ, et al. The medical treatment of unruptured ectopic pregnancy with methotrexate and citrovorum rescue: preliminary experience. Fertil Steril. 1986;46:811-3.
53. Lipscomb GH, Givens VM, Meyer NL, et al. Comparison of multidose and single-dose methotrexate protocols for the treatment of ectopic pregnancy. Am J Obstet Gynecol. 2005;192:1844-7.
54. Dasari P, Sagili H. Life-threatening complications following multidose methotrexate for medical management of ectopic pregnancy. BMJ Case Rep. 2012;2012.
55. Habana A, Dokras A, Giraldo JL, et al. Cornual heterotopic pregnancy: contemporary management options. Am J Obstet Gynecol. 2000;182:1264-70.
56. Wang Y, Ma CH, Qiao J, et al. Efficacy of local aspiration in the conservative treatment of live interstitial pregnancy coexisting with live intrauterine pregnancy after in vitro fertilization and embryo transfer. Chin Med J. 2012;125: 1345-8.
57. GungorUgurlucan F, Bastu E, Dogan M, et al. Management of cesarean heterotopic pregnancy with transvaginal ultrasound-guided potassium chloride injection and gestational sac aspiration, and review of the literature. J Minim Invasive Gynecol. 2012;19:671-3.
58. van Mello NM, Mol F. Salpingotomy versus salpingectomy in women with tubal ectopic pregnancy, a randomised controlled trial. Hum Reprod. 2012;27(2):ii734.
59. Helmy S, Sawyer E, Ofili-Yebovi D, et al. Fertility outcomes following expectant management of tubal ectopic. 2007;30(7):988-93.
60. Elito Junior J, Han KK, Camano L. Tubal patency following surgical and clinical treatment of ectopic pregnancy. Sao Paulo Med J. 2006;124:264-6.
61. Boots CE, Gustofson RL, Feinberg EC. Does methotrexate administration for ectopic pregnancy after in vitro fertilization impact ovarian reserve or ovarian responsiveness? Fertil Steril. 2013;100:1590-3.
62. Singer T, Kofinas J, Huang JY, et al. Antimullerian hormone serum levels and reproductive outcome are not affected by neither methotrexate nor laparoscopic salpingectomy for the treatment of ectopic pregnancy in IVF patients. J Minim Invasive Gynecol. 2011;18(1):S46.
63. Ohannessian A, Loundou A, Courbiere B, et al. Ovarian responsiveness in women receiving fertility treatment after methotrexate for ectopic pregnancy: a systematic review and meta-analysis. Hum Reprod. 2014;29:1949-56.
64. Hackmon R, Sakaguchi S, Koren G. Effect of methotrexate treatment of ectopic pregnancy on subsequent pregnancy. Can Fam Physician. 2011;57:37-9.
65. Hajenius PJ, Mol F, Mol BW, et al. Interventions for tubal ectopic pregnancy. Cochrane Database of Systematic Reviews 2007;24(1):CD000324.
66. Morlock RJ, Lafata JE, Eisenstein D. Cost-effectiveness of single-dose methotrexate compared with laparoscopic treatment of ectopic pregnancy. Obstet Gynecol. 2000;95: 407-12.
67. Sowter MC, Farquhar CM, Gudex G. An economic evaluation of single dose systemic methotrexate and laparoscopic surgery for the treatment of unruptured ectopic pregnancy. BJOG. 2001;108:204-12.

Fetal Reduction

65

Devika Gunasheela, Ashwini M

INTRODUCTION

Assisted reproductive technology has contributed significantly to increasing the chances of conception and live births but parallelly there has been an increase in the incidence of multifetal pregnancies. The twin birth rate increased from 18.9 to 33.3 per 1,000 live births (76%) between the years 1980 and 2009. It has since 2009 stabilized and is currently 33.5 twins per 1,000 live births. Between 1980 and 1998, the birth rate for higher-order multiples increased more than 400% (1.935 per 1,000 births).[1] The deliveries of higher-order multiples decreased to 1.036 per 1,000 births in 2015 because of the stringent methods and policies regarding embryo transfer adopted by the in vitro fertilization (IVF) clinics and governing bodies.[2]

HISTORY OF FETAL REDUCTION

The first baby to be born through IVF was Louise Brown in July 1978. Since then, around millions of IVF babies have been born and the most common side effect of infertility treatments has been a higher incidence of multiple gestations.[2] In the USA, the incidence of twins from 1/90 in the preinfertility treatment era has been increased to nearly 1/30 now.[3] A woman with twins has a nearly 70% chance of having achieved that pregnancy with medical assistance.[4]

In 1980s, few clinicians from both the USA and Europe attempted to reduce the untoward consequences of multifetal pregnancies by selectively terminating or reducing the number of fetuses. Dumez and Oury[5] from Europe and Evans and Hanft[6] from America were the first to report on fetal reduction as a surgical approach to improve the outcome.

Dr Mark Evans, a physician at Hutzel Hospital in Detroit, was a pioneer in fetal reduction. He was known for his work in genetics, prenatal screening and diagnosis, and the selective reduction of pregnancies. Data from physicians performing fetal reductions at six medical centers was analyzed, and it was found that 40% of the mothers undergoing fetal reduction were carrying no more than triplets. They concluded that reduction of triplets to twins was an effective option compared to expectant management.[6] He quoted, "When reducing from 1 to zero is acceptable in this society, then why not from 2 to 1?"

PROBLEMS WITH MULTIPLE PREGNANCIES

Medical Complications

Multiple pregnancies are likely to be associated with an increase in adverse maternal and neonatal outcomes. The maternal complications include an increase in risk of abortions, ante-partum hemorrhage, preterm deliveries, preterm prelabor rupture of membrane, preeclampsia, etc. along with an increase need for operative deliveries, prolonged hospital stay and blood transfusions.[7] The neonatal complications encountered include prematurity, fetal growth restriction and growth discordancy, need for neonatal intensive care unit (ICU) care and all the other complications associated with preterm babies. An article from ACOG in 2003 showed about 20% of babies born at less than 750 g develop cerebral palsy.[8] Another study by Petterson et al showed that rate of cerebral palsy was 4.6 times higher for twins than singletons per live births.[9] In a study by Pharoah and Cooke, the cerebral palsy rates per 1,000 was 2.3 for singleton, 12.6 for twins, and 44.8 for triplets.[10,11] Monochorionicity has specific complications such as twin-to-twin transfusion syndrome, selective fetal growth restriction, single fetal demise, twin reversed arterial perfusion and conjoined twins.

Social and Economic Implications

The costs of multiple pregnancies to parents and society are quadrupled for twins and 10-fold higher for triplets along with additional childcare, greater household and medical expenditures, and the higher chances that one of the parents will be unable to return to the workforce.[12] John et al study in 2000 when analyzing US data, found that there were profound public health implications with regards to prematurity and showed that of USD 10.2 billion spent per year on initial newborn care. Fifty seven percent of the money was spent on the 9% of babies that was born at less than 37 weeks of gestation.[13]

In 2003, Cuevas[14] showed that more than USD 10 billion was spent on the 12.3% of babies born preterm. Studies have shown that parents are at an increased risk of severe stress and a compromised quality of life.[15] Maternal depression and child abuse have been reported in families particularly when one or more of the children had special needs and increased the rates of divorce among parents.[16]

FETAL REDUCTION

Multifetal pregnancy reduction is a procedure designed to decrease the number of live fetuses in higher-order multiples to improve the outcomes of pregnancies.[17] The term "multifetal pregnancy reduction" has been widely accepted and has been adopted in the most recent committee opinion of the American College of Obstetricians and Gynecologists on the subject, and it is believed that it should be used whenever the reduction of an apparently normal fetus is performed in an attempt to reduce the risk of premature delivery of other fetuses in the same uterus.[18]

WHEN TO PERFORM FETAL REDUCTION?

Based on the gestational age at reduction, it can be classified as:

- First trimester reduction
- Second trimester reduction.

First Trimester Reduction

This is fetal reduction being performed between 8 weeks and 12 weeks. It can be further classified into early or late based on the gestational age when it is performed.

Early First Trimester Fetal Reduction

It is when the procedure is performed between 8 and 10 weeks of gestational age. The advantages of early reductions are that it is a technically easy procedure and can be done through transvaginal route. But doing an early fetal reduction misses the chance of allowing a spontaneous miscarriage or spontaneous reduction of the fetus. There is also a real danger of reducing a normal fetus and leaving behind an abnormal one as most of the morphological abnormalities show up only at a later stage.

Late First Trimester Reduction

It is when the procedure is performed around 11–12 weeks of gestational age. The advantages are that it can be done after NT/NTD scan, which provides additional information about an abnormal fetus and also allows time for spontaneous reduction. However, late reductions are difficult and time consuming. A collaborative study in 2001 on late trimester reduction demonstrated that outcome of triplets reduced to twins, and quadruplets reduced to twins, performed essentially as if they started as twins.

Second Trimester Reductions

These are done by transabdominal route either mechanically or with potassium chloride (KCl) or sodium chloride (NaCl).

Ideal time to perform fetal reduction is between 11weeks and 12 weeks of pregnancy, as by this time, the spontaneous fetal demise should have occurred and early anomalies can be ruled out with a nuchal translucency scan, thus enabling the surgeon to choose the abnormal fetus for reduction.

PREREQUISITES

- A detailed written and verbal consent needs to be taken from the patient after explaining the detailed procedure, chances of complete loss of pregnancy, preterm labor, premature prelabor rupture of membranes (PPROM), chorioamnionitis.
- A detailed ultrasound examination for assessment of total number of fetuses, chorionicity, accessibility of the fetus and detection of fetal anomalies is a must before attempting fetal reduction as it would help to plan the procedure.
- Urine and vaginal swab cultures can be taken and are to be treated, if positive for infection.
- Prophylactic antibiotics are usually started a day prior to the procedure and continued after the procedure for 5–7 days.

- Progesterone depot injection and prophylactic tocolysis are given to reduce the post-procedure uterine irritability.

ROUTES AND METHODS OF FETAL REDUCTION

Multifetal pregnancy reduction can be performed under ultrasound guidance by transcervically, transvaginally or transabdominally.

Transcervical Aspiration

Transcervical method was first discovered in early 1980s by Martene Duplan.

Procedure

The procedure is carried out under general anesthesia, with the help of ultrasound guidance using an abdominal probe. The patient is placed in lithotomy position; the cervix and vagina are thoroughly cleaned. The cervix is mechanically dilated using Hegar's dilator followed by embryonic aspiration with Karman's cannula or metal cannula. The embryo close to the internal os is aspirated.

Disadvantages

Increased risk of chorioamnionitis, miscarriage and spotting/bleeding per vagina. Hence, this method is obsolete now-a-days.[5]

Transabdominal Reduction

The procedure is ideally performed between 10 and 13 weeks. It is technically more difficult to perform transabdominal procedures before 10 weeks, because the uterus is confined to the pelvis and a greater distance involved in reaching the fetuses from maternal abdominal wall. The fundally placed embryos are easily reduced when compared to the lower ones.

Procedure

Under ultrasound guidance with full aseptic precautions and local anesthesia, a 20 gauge sterile needle is inserted via the maternal abdomen into the fetal thorax. The position of the needle is confirmed and 1-2 mL of potassium chloride is injected, making sure the needle point does not move. The fetal cardia is observed for asystole and complete cessation of cardiac activity. Earlier, the fetal demise was achieved by injecting air or mechanical trauma but the success rate was low.

Disadvantages

Compared to transvaginal route, this method requires more skill especially in the earlier part of the learning period and an increase in miscarriage rate (loss rates were 16.7% in transabdominal vs. 10.9% in transvaginal).

Transvaginal Technique

The transvaginal technique is performed between 7 and 11 weeks, by injecting NaCl or KCl solution into the fetal thorax or repeated intra-cardiac punctures under ultrasound guidance. With strict aseptic precautions, a 20 gauge sterile needle is inserted into the targeting fetus through a guide attached to a vaginal probe. The position of the needle is confirmed, 2–3 cc of hypertonic KCl is injected, and the asystole is observed over 3–5 minutes. Alternatively, asystole can also be obtained by intra-cardiac punctures without aspiration of embryonic contents or amniotic fluid.

Potassium Chloride versus No Potassium Chloride

Potassium chloride is the most commonly used pharmacological agent in fetal reduction. It acts by causing fetal asystole followed by complete cessation fetal cardiac function. The injection of such substances into the embryo or fetal thorax, is not a risk-free procedure as cases of anencephaly, limb amputation has been described.[19]

If KCl is not strictly limited to fetal heart, it can diffuse into the amniotic sac, adjacent gestational sac and result in total loss of pregnancy. KCl can induce release of tissue plasminogen activator in the hypo-thalamo-neuro-hypophyseal system and up regulation in MMP-9 activity in the retina, which promotes retinal damage. By inducing matrix degrading enzymes in the uterus and inducing cytokines, KCl can cause pregnancy loss, preterm delivery and PPROM. Iberico et al in 2000 showed transvaginal intra-cardiac puncture till asystole without aspiration of embryonic parts or amniotic fluid between 7 and 9 weeks, achieved a mean gestational age at delivery of 35 weeks, take home baby rate of 89%, less inflammation due to less trophoblastic detachment, less post-operative infection and spotting. The method was less time consuming.[20]

A prospective controlled study by Mansour et al., which included 75 patients with higher-order pregnancies from assisted reproduction technique, used a modified method by aspirating either partially or completely the embryonic parts and avoiding aspiration of amniotic fluid showed that miscarriage rates was lower.[21]

In a retrospective study by Lee et al which compared the outcomes of different methods of fetal reduction (KCl vs. no KCl) showed a significantly higher take home baby rate with non-potassium chloride groups (86.1% vs. 69.7%, $P = 0.045$). In the potassium chloride group, the rates of extreme prematurity and PPROM were significantly higher. Early non-potassium chloride group had a significantly lower immediate loss rate, pregnancy loss rate and PPROM rate and higher take home baby rate. Thus, concluded the best method of fetal reduction is early non-KCl transvaginal approach.[22,23]

Postprocedure Care and Follow-up

The patient is hospitalized for observation during which if any bleeding is noticed, treated with hemostatics. The woman can be discharged on the next day after confirmation of number of viable fetus and no retro-placental bleeding on ultrasound. The patient is asked to review immediately if any bleeding per vagina, leaking per vagina, foul smelling discharge, fever and lower abdominal pain.

Complications

- Risk (1–2%) of complete pregnancy loss, even with experienced hands, due to accidental entry of KCl into non-targeted sacs.
- Threatened abortions, premature labor or PPROM, chorioamnionitis.
- Failed reduction is not uncommon; hence, careful mapping of fetus is crucial during the procedure to confirm the asystole.

Our Experience at Gunasheela

Between October 2010 and Feb 2018, the outcomes of multifetal pregnancy reduction was studied at the Gunasheela Surgical & Maternity Hospital, Bangalore. All patients with twins, triplets and higher-order multiples were counseled in detail about the procedure, type and duration of anesthesia, possible complications, chance of success and possible need for follow up therapy, psychological and economic aspects.

A detailed written and verbal consent was obtained from all participating couples. Detailed history, general examination, obstetric examination and bimanual examination, ultrasound to confirm number of fetuses, period of gestation, chorionicity, fetal heartbeat, any anomalies, and routine blood investigations was done for all patients.

Under spinal anesthesia, patients were placed in lithotomy position. The vagina was cleaned with 10% povidone iodine followed by normal saline. A routine transvaginal ultrasound confirming the number of fetuses, cardiac activity and the accessibility of the fetus to the ultrasound probe, was assessed before the procedure. All procedures were done between 10 and 12 weeks with ALOKA SSD 3500 ultrasound machine equipped with transvaginal transducer and puncture guide

A 16 gauge, 12-inch long oocyte pick-up (OPU) needle was introduced through a guide attached to the ultrasound. The most easily accessible fetus was selected and intracardiac puncture was done with OPU needle. Manual aspiration with 20 cc syringe was done till asystole was confirmed. Use of potassium chloride or sodium chloride solution into the sac was avoided. Those in whom NaCl or KCl was used were excluded from the study. Time factor did not matter in our study. All the procedures were over between 20 and 30 min. Once the asystole was confirmed and the viability of remaining fetuses was checked, the OPU needle was withdrawn. All women were given IV prophylactic antibiotics before the procedure and post procedure with oral antibiotics for 6 days. Women were discharged from the hospital on the next day after the check scan for number of viable fetuses and retroplacental bleeding. Follow up scan was done after a week. The patients were asked to review if any leak or watery discharge, bleeding per vagina, fever, lower abdomen pain, foul smelling discharge, uterine tenderness. The obstetric complications and medical illness were noted, and treated accordingly.

Total 129 women underwent the procedure, of which 5 were twins, 110 were triplets, 12 were quadruplets, 2 were quintuplets.

Of the 129 pregnancies, 2.32% were spontaneous pregnancies, 6.20% were ovulation induction pregnancies, 20.15% were intra-uterine insemination (IUI) pregnancies, followed by 50.38% with in vitro fertilization/intracytoplasmic sperm injection (ICSI), 8.52% with in vitro maturation (IVM), 8.52% with frozen embryo transfer (FET), 3.87% with donor embryo transfer (DET) **(Table 1)**.

Of the total 129 pregnancies that underwent fetal reduction, 14.4% had miscarriage (<24 weeks), 2.65% delivered between 24 and 28 weeks, 6.19% between 28 and 30 weeks, 7.07% between 31 and 32 weeks, 19.46% between 33 and 36 weeks, majority greater than 36 weeks, i.e. 43.36% and 6 pregnancies are ongoing. Two patients out of 16 patients who miscarried developed chorioamnionitis **(Tables 2 and 3)**.

Table 1: Mode of conception.

S. No.	Mode of conception	No. of pregnancies	Percentage
1	Spontaneous	3	2.32%
2	Ovulation induction + timed intercourse	8	6.20%
3	IUI	26	20.15%
4	IVF/ICSI	65	50.38%
5	IVM	11	8.52%
6	FET	11	8.52%
7	DET	5	3.87%

(IVM: in vitro maturation; DET: donor embryo transfer; FET: frozen embryo transfer; ICSI: intracytoplasmic sperm injection; IVF: in vitro fertilization; IUI: intra-uterine insemination).

Table 2: Outcome of fetal reduction.

S. No.	Period of gestation	Total	Percentage
1	Miscarriage <24 weeks	16	14.4%
2	24–28 weeks	3	2.65%
3	28–30 weeks	7	6.19%
4	31–32 weeks	8	7.07%
5	33–36 weeks	22	19.46%
6	>36 weeks	49	43.36%
7	Ongoing	6	–
8	Lost for follow-up	18	–

Table 3: Comparison of results of various non-KCL studies.

S. No.		Lee et al.	Mansour et al.	Ibericco et al.	Youseff et al.	Gunasheela
1	Mean GA of FR	7.8 weeks	7.2 weeks	7.8 weeks	7–11 weeks	9.7 weeks
2	Mean age	35.4 years	32.6 years	33 years	32.4 years	29.73 years
3	Pregnancy loss	12.5%	8.8%	7.4 %	6.6%	14.4%
4	Birth weight	2,314 g	2,450 g	2,304 g	2,308 g	2,112 g
5	Mean gestation	36 weeks	36.9 weeks	35.1 weeks	35.3 weeks	34.5 weeks
6	Preterm delivery	35.4%	48.5%	63.6%	32.1%	44.94%
7	Take home baby rate	86.1%	73.1%	90%	79.1%	80.9%

(GA: gestational age).

AMERICAN COLLEGE OF OBSTETRICIANS AND GYNECOLOGISTS RECOMMENDATIONS[24]

On the basis of the principles outlined in this Committee Opinion, the American College of Obstetricians and Gynecologists (ACOG) makes the following recommendations:

- Fertility treatments have contributed significantly to the increase in multifetal pregnancies. Primary prevention strategies to limit multifetal pregnancies, especially higher-order multifetal pregnancies, can help to minimize the need for multifetal pregnancy reduction and should be practiced by all physicians who treat women for infertility.
- Obstetrician-gynecologists should be aware that multifetal pregnancies increase maternal and perinatal morbidity and mortality. Higher-order multifetal pregnancies present higher risks than do twin pregnancies.
- Obstetrician-gynecologists should be knowledgeable about the medical risks of multifetal pregnancy, the potential medical benefits of multifetal pregnancy reduction, and the complex ethical issues inherent in decisions regarding multifetal pregnancy reduction. They should be prepared to respond in a professional and ethical manner to patients who request or decline to receive information, or intervention, or both.
- Non-directive patient counseling should be offered to all women with higher-order multifetal pregnancies and should include a discussion of the risks unique to multifetal pregnancy as well as the option to continue or reduce the pregnancy. Resources for providing such counseling can include maternal-fetal medicine specialists, neonatologists, mental health professionals, child development specialists, support groups, and clinicians with procedural expertise in multifetal pregnancy reduction.
- When a patient's request for information on multifetal pregnancy reduction is discordant with a physician's

values, the physician should refer the patient for consultation in a timely fashion and without judgment, explain to the patient the reason for the consultation, and provide all necessary information to the consultant.

- Obstetrician-gynecologists should respect patients' autonomy regarding whether to continue or reduce a multifetal pregnancy. Only the patient can weigh the relative importance of the medical, ethical, religious, and socioeconomic factors and determine the best course of action for her unique situation.

CONCLUSION

With the advances in infertility techniques and improvements in the laboratory, the pregnancy rates with IVF are increasing and in this enthusiasm, 2–3 embryos are transferred into the uterus during embryo transfer. But multifetal pregnancy is an unwanted and most often preventable complication of infertility treatment. It is preferable to avoid the risk of higher-order multifetal pregnancy by decreasing the number of embryos to be transferred or cancelling an IUI cycle, when there are too many growing follicles.

The obstetrician and gynecologists should have a sound knowledge about the medical risks of multifetal pregnancy, the benefits of multifetal pregnancy reduction and the complex ethical issues that patients are faced with while making a decision on reduction of one or two fetuses.

REFERENCES

1. Martin JA, Hamilton BE, Osterman MJ. Three decades of twin birth in the United States, 1980–2009. NCHS Data Brief. 2012;(80):1-8.
2. Martin JA, Hamilton BE, Osterman MJ, et al. Birth: final data for 2015. NATL Vital Stat Rep. 2017;66:1.
3. Centers for Disease Control and Prevention. National Survey of Family Growth; 2013.
4. Martin JA, Hamilton BE, Ventura SJ, et al. Births: final data for 2011. Natl Vital Stat Rep. 2013;62(1):1-69.
5. Dumez Y, Oury JF. Method for first trimester selective abortion in multiple pregnancy. Contrib Gynecol Obstet. 1986;15: 50-3.
6. Evans MI, Hanft RS. The introduction of new technologies. ACOG Clin Semin. 1997;2:1-3.
7. Luke B, Brown MB. Contemporary risks of maternal morbidity and adverse outcomes with increasing maternal and plurality. Fertil Steril. 2007;88:283-93.
8. Task Force of American College of Obstetricians and Gynecologists. Neonatal Encephalopathy and Cerebral Palsy: Defining the Pathogenesis and Pathophysiology. Washington: ACOG; 2003.
9. Petterson B, Nelson K, Watson L, et al. Twins, triplets, and cerebral palsy in births in Western Australia in the 1980s. BMJ. 1993;307:1239-43.
10. Pharoah PO, Cooke T. Cerebral palsy and multiple births. Arch Dis Child Fetal Neonatal Ed. 1996;75:F174-7.
11. Dimitiiou G, Pharoah PO, Nicolaides KH, et al. Cerebral palsy in triplet pregnancies with and without iatrogenic reduction. Eur J Pediatr. 2004;163:449-51.
12. Collins J. Cost efficiency of reducing multiple births. Reprod Biomed Online. 2007;15(Supp 3):35-9.
13. St John EB, Nelson KG, Oliver SP, et al. Cost of neonatal care according to gestational age at birth and survival status. Am J Obstet Gynecol. 2000;182:170-5.
14. Cuevas KD, Silver DR, Brooten D, et al. The cost of prematurity: hospital charges at birth and frequency of rehospitalizations and acute care visits over the first year of life: a comparison by gestational age and birth weight. Am J Nurs. 2005;105:56-64.
15. Ellison MA, Hotamisligil S, Lee H, et al. Psychological risks associated with multiple birth resulting from assisted reproduction. Fertile Steril. 2005;83:1422-8.
16. Mckay S. The Effects of Twins and Multiple Births on Families and their Living Standards. Surrey (UK): Twins Multiple Birth Association; 2010.
17. Berkowitz RL, Lynch L. Selective reduction: an unfortunate misnomer. Obstet Gynecol. 1990;75:873-4.
18. American College of Obstetricians and Gynecologists. Committee Opinion No. 94: Committee on Ethics, multifetal pregnancy reduction and selective fetal termination, Washington. Obstet Gynecol; 1991.pp.1-3.
19. Roze RJ, Tschupp MJ, Arvis PH. Interruption selective de grossesses et malformations embryonnaires des extremites. J. Gynecol Obstet Biol Reprod. 1989;18:673-7.
20. Iberico G, Navarro J, Blasco L, et al. Embryo reduction of multifetal pregnancies following assisted reproduction treatment: A modification of the trans vaginal ultrasound-guided technique. Hum Reprod. 2000;15(10):2228-33.
21. Mansour RT, Aboulghar MA, Serour GI. Multifetal pregnancy reduction: Modification of the technique and analysis of the outcome. Fertil Steril. 1999;71:380-4.
22. Lee JR, Ku SY, Jee BH, et al. Pregnancy outcomes of different methods for multifetal pregnancy reduction: a comparative study. J Korean Med Sci. 2008;23(1):111-6.
23. Evans MI, Berkowitz R, Wapner R, et al. Multifetal pregnancy reduction (MFPR): improved outcomes with increased experience. Am J Obstet Gynecol. 2001;184:97-103.
24. American College of Obstetricians and Gynecologists. Committee Opinion No. 719: Multifetal pregnancy reduction. Obstet Gynecol. 2017;130:e158-63.

Cryopreservation in ART

66

Hrishikesh D Pai, Nandita Palshetkar, Kinjal Shah, Arnav Pai

INTRODUCTION

The field of assisted reproductive technology (ART) has passed through waves of optimization and innovation. Innumerable developments have occurred since the landmark birth of Louise Brown in 1978 through in vitro fertilization.

The success in ART depends on multiple factors like:

- Etiology of infertility and proper patient selection
- Optimum stimulation protocol
- Improvements in the technique of oocyte retrieval
- Intracytoplasmic sperm injection (ICSI) and other sperm selection methods
- Proper embryological technique with high quality embryos
- Move toward extended embryo culture and blastocyst transfer
- *Efficient cryopreservation program*
- Optimization of laboratory techniques
- Highly receptive endometrium
- Skilled atraumatic embryo transfer
- Adequate luteal support
- Competent antenatal management.

Cryopreservation means preserving cells and tissues in live condition at such low temperatures, that all the cell metabolism comes to a standstill. Today, cryopreservation of surplus embryos has become a routine practice in ART and frozen embryo transfer (FET) has become an integral part of modern ART practice.

The first ever pregnancy derived from a frozen human embryo was reported by Alan Trounson and Linda Mohr in 1983 (although the fetus aborted spontaneously at about 20 weeks of gestation). The first-term pregnancy derived from a frozen embryo was born in 1984.

The last decade has witnessed tremendous increase in the use of FETs and the live births resulting thereof. Earlier, only the "second best" embryos were frozen after the morphologically best embryos were transferred in fresh cycles. But today with improved cryopreservation techniques which reduce embryo cryodamage, the confidence in cryopreservation and FET has substantially increased. Cohort banking is also becoming a routine after the use of a gonadotropin-releasing hormone (GnRH) agonist "trigger" to prevent ovarian hyperstimulation syndrome (OHSS) in high responders. Other reasons for the increased use of FET include an overall decrease in the average number of embryos used in each transfer, thus allowing surplus embryos to be cryopreserved. Also, the increased use of genetic screening increases the use of cryopreservation, because embryos are often frozen while awaiting test results, and transfer of confirmed euploid embryos may contribute to increasing FET success rates.

CRYOPROTECTANTS

They are either permeable or nonpermeable and are used usually in a mixture for slow freezing method or vitrification **(Table 1)**.

They protect the cells from cryoinjuries, stabilize intracellular proteins, lower the intracellular water freezing point, and most importantly, they reduce or eliminate lethal intracellular ice formation.

The strategy to decrease the toxicity of one cryoprotectant (CPA) is to use a mixture of two permeable CPAs. Ethylene

Table 1: Difference between permeable and nonpermeable cryoprotectants.

Permeable (permeating or intracellular) cryoprotectants	*Nonpermeable (nonpermeating or extracellular) cryoprotectants*
▪ Small, nonionic, and highly water soluble at low temperature	▪ Long chain polymers
▪ They have low molecular weight and can penetrate the lipid bilayer of the cell easily	▪ They have high molecular weight and so remain in the extracellular solution
▪ Replace bulk of intracellular water	▪ Increase osmolarity of extracellular space
▪ Solidify at lower temperature than water—reduce intracellular ice formation	▪ Dehydrate cells—decrease intracellular ice formation ▪ Avoids osmotic shock.
▪ For example, glycerol, ethylene glycol (EG), 1,2-propanediol (PROH), dimethyl sulfoxide (DMSO), propylene glycol, acetamide, and raffinose.	▪ Sugars like sucrose, trehalose, and glucose, galactose, polymers like polyvinylpyrrolidone, polyethylene glycol, Ficoll, dextran, hydroxypropyl cellulose, polyvinyl alcohol, and proteins like egg yolk.

glycol and dimethyl sulfoxide (DMSO) combination are the most frequently used. Ethylene glycol is an almost indispensable component of all CPAs due to low toxicity, high permeability, and excellent prevention of ice crystal formation. Recently, sucrose has become a standard component in vitrification solutions.

In this chapter, we will discuss the following in detail:

- Cryopreservation of sperms
- Cryopreservation of oocyte, embryo, and blastocyst by slow freezing method
- Cryopreservation of oocyte, embryo, and blastocyst by vitrification method.

CRYOPRESERVATION OF SPERMS

Cryopreservation of human spermatozoa was introduced in 1954. It involves exposure of the spermatozoa to CPAs and then cooling them to subzero temperature.

It is used as:

- In cases of male infertility prior to the treatment for malignant diseases or vasectomy
- Prior to ART storage of partner's semen in case of his unavailability on the day of oocyte retrieval
- In case of severe male factor infertility when the ejaculate contains even a small number of sperms, they can be used for a later date.

There are two methods of semen freezing:

1. Noncontrolled rate cryopreservation, and
2. Controlled rate cryopreservation.

Procedure

Non-controlled Rate Cryopreservation

- Check the blood reports of the couple to screen for human immunodeficiency virus (HIV), hepatitis B virus surface antigen (HBsAg), hepatitis C virus (HCV), and venereal disease research laboratory (VDRL).
- Take the semen freezing consent from the couple.
- Send the husband for collection of semen sample by masturbation in a sterile container.
- After collection of the sample, allow the sample to liquefy at room temperature for 20–30 minutes.
- Take a drop of semen sample on the Makler's chamber and check the sperm count.
- Take 1.5 mL of semen sample in a 14-mL round bottom tube labeled with patient's name.
- Add equal volume, 1:1 in proportion (i.e. 1.5 mL) of CPA media, drop wise to the sample. Mix well for 10 minutes.
- Label the cryovials with patient's name and add the sample to it.
- Write patient's name on the aluminum cane.
- Attach the cryovials to the aluminum cane with cello tape and keep it in the chiller (4°C) for 20 minutes.
- Then, keep on liquid nitrogen vapors (–70°C) poured in the thermocol box (1 ft × 1 ft × 1 ft) for 20 minutes.
- Plunge it in the liquid nitrogen cryocans for storage at –196°C.

All storage containers should be stored in a secure room. Liquid nitrogen levels in the storage units should be checked regularly. At –196°C storage of sperms, even for a long period does not affect the survival rates, as there is virtually no movement of atoms or molecules.

Controlled Rate Cryopreservation

- The vials are placed in a controlled rate freezer and the following preprogrammed, freezing cycle is initiated. The start temperature of which is 20°C. At first, it cools at –5°C/min to 4°C/min. Subsequently, at 10°C to –70°C.
- The samples are held for 10 minutes.

Table 2: The proportion of sperm pellet + media + semen freezing (sf) media is in the ratio of 2:1.

Calculate dilution based on the following table

Sperm count/2 mL ejaculate	***Volume of medium + pellet to be left in tube***	***Addition of sperm freezing media to pellet***
<100	0.8 mL	0.4 mL
100–150	0.8 mL	0.4 mL
151–200	1.1 mL	0.55 mL

- The vials are snapped into aluminum canes.
- They are plunged into liquid nitrogen storage tank.
- The position of the cane is noted and recorded.

Semen Cryopreservation for Intrauterine Insemination Ready Sample

- Sample is collected.
- It is allowed to liquefy.
- Check the sperm count and motility calculated per mL using Makler's chamber. The semen is subjected to density gradient or swim-up method. The volume of the pellet + media is calculated based here in **Table 2**.
- Sperm freeze media is added to pellet based on the following **Table 2**.
- The final mixture is placed in cryovials.
- Vials are frozen as described earlier.
- The vials are snapped into aluminum canes.
- They are plunged into liquid nitrogen storage tank.
- The position of the cane is noted and recorded.

Thawing of the Frozen Semen Sample

- Remove the correct vial and allow it to thaw at room temperature for 20 minutes in the laminar flow hood. Alternately, they can be thawed at 37°C in the water bath for 5–7 minutes.
- Clean the external surface with absolute alcohol and allow the alcohol to vaporize.
- Take 2 mL flushing media in a sterile 5 mL test tube.
- Add the contents of the vial drop wise to the flushing media and mixed well.
- This is further subjected to either the swim-up or density gradient method.

OOCYTE AND EMBRYO CRYOPRESERVATION

There are two techniques:

1. Slow freezing method
2. Vitrification method.

Slow Freezing Method (Equilibrium Cooling)

This is a slow-rate freezing method. Here, extracellular ice formation drives cellular dehydration through an equilibrium process.

Embryos are exposed to 1–2 mol/L solutions of permeable and nonpermeable CPAs, and then loaded into straws, sealed, and cooled rapidly to -6°C by placing the straws into a controlled-rate freezer. With this low concentration of CPAs, no spontaneous ice crystal formation occurs at this temperature. But ice nucleation is induced by "seeding", i.e. touching the straw with forceps that has previously been immersed into liquid nitrogen which is performed far away from the embryo and this ice grows stepwise toward the embryo. The controlled-rate freezer is adjusted to make a very slow cooling (usually 0.3°C/min, to around -30°C/min) after which the straws are immersed into liquid nitrogen for a final cooling and storage. The slow rate of this procedure permits solution exchange between the extracellular and intracellular fluids without any serious osmotic effects (this fact is reflected in the other method called vitrification).

Procedure

Embryo Freezing Pack:
Instructions for use:

- Zygotes or embryos at 2–4 cell development stage are placed in medium from vial one for 5 minutes at room temperature.
- Zygotes or embryos are placed in medium from vial two for 10 minutes and in medium from vial three for 15 minutes, still at room temperature.
- Medium from vial three is used to load the zygotes or embryos in the straws. Freezing is carried out according to the cooling program here.
- Cool from room temperature to -7°C in steps of -2°C/min.
- Hold for 5 minutes, manual seeding.
- Cool from -7°C to -30°C in steps of 0.3°C/min.

- Cool from –30°C to –190°C in steps of 50°C/min.
- Transfer the three straws into liquid nitrogen and store at –196°C.

Embryo Thawing Pack

Instructions for use:

- Remove straws from liquid nitrogen and keep at room temperature for 30 seconds. Then, place the straws in water at 30°C for 1 minute.
- Place zygotes or embryos in medium from vial one at room temperature for 5 minutes.
- Place zygotes or embryos in medium from vial two at room temperature for 5 minutes and then medium from vial three also at room temperature for 10 minutes.
- The zygotes and embryos are then washed in a culture medium and placed in the culture using the same medium to wait for transfer selection **(Figs. 1A to D)**.

Problems with slow freezing are:

- Intracellular ice crystal formation
- Too slow procedure may cause increased exposure to CPA
- Too much dehydration can cause abnormal concentration of intracellular solutes
- Ice crystal formation during thawing
- Long procedure time and costly equipment.

Vitrification Method (Nonequilibrium Cooling)

It is a form of rapid cooling which utilizes very high concentrations of CPA that solidify without forming ice crystals **(Fig. 2)**.

Procedure

The main purpose of this method is complete elimination of ice crystal formation in the whole solution containing the oocytes and embryos. So, how can the ice crystal formation rate be reduced? This can be done by either increasing the concentration of CPAs or by increasing the cooling and the warming rates. If the cooling rate is higher, then lower concentration of CPA is required and vice versa. Recent

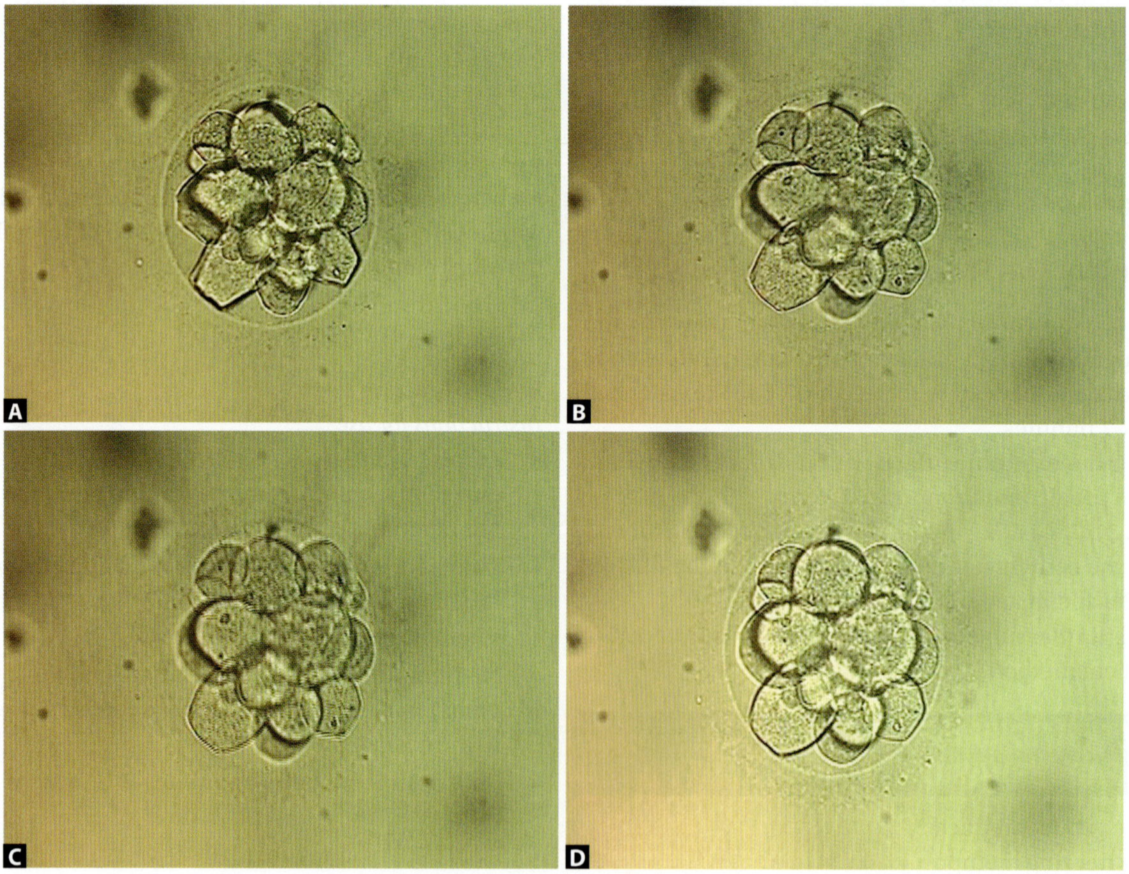

Figs. 1A to D: Thawing of embryos.

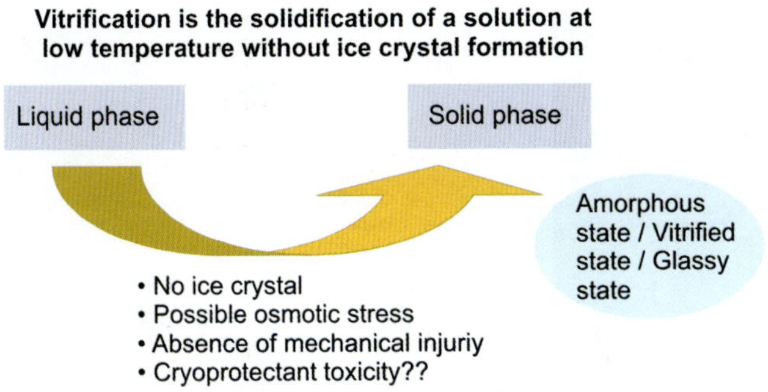

Fig. 2: Process of vitrification.

vitrification methods have focused on increasing the cooling and warming rates to decrease the potential osmotic and toxic damage caused by the high concentration of CPAs.

VITRIFICATION PROCESS

Materials

Tissue culture dish, BD syringe, 140 µm, 170 µm, and 300 µm diameter Flexipets holder, Cryotop, Cryocane, and marker.

Equipment

Pipetting devices, laminar flow hood, dissecting microscope with lighted base, labeling device, timer, heat sealer, forceps, liquid nitrogen Dewar, liquid nitrogen storage canister with lock and alarm, safety goggles, and cryogloves.

Cryosolutions

- *Equilibration solution (ES)*: ES is a 4-(2-hydroxyethyl)-1-piperazineethanesulfonic acid (HEPES)-buffered medium, 7.5% (v/v) of each DMSO and ethylene glycol and 20% (v/v) serum protein substitute.
- *Vitrification solution (VS)*: VS is a HEPES-buffered medium, 15% (v/v) of each DMSO and ethylene glycol and 20% (v/v) serum protein substitutes and 0.5 M sucrose.

Types

Vitrification method is further divided into two types depending on the carrier used as:

1. Open system freezing (carrier: Cryotop, Cryotech, Cryolock, and Cryoloop), and
2. Closed system freezing [carrier: high security vitrification (HSV) straw, Cryotip].

Procedure

- Bring one vial each of ES and VS to room temperature (24–25°C) for at least 30 minutes prior to freezing oocytes/embryos/blastocysts.
- Fill the liquid nitrogen reservoir with liquid nitrogen.
- Determine the number of oocytes/embryos/blastocysts to be vitrified.
- Label the Cryotop/HSV straw with patient's name and date.
- Prepare a tissue culture dish with 40 µL droplet of ES and 20 µL four droplets of VS below it.
- Transfer the oocytes/embryos/blastocysts to ES for approximately 12 minutes for embryos and approximately 15 minutes for oocytes and blastocysts **(Figs. 3 to 5)**.
- Then, transfer the oocytes/embryos/blastocysts to the four droplets of VS serially washing them for approximately 90 seconds.
- In case of open system vitrification, load the oocytes/embryos/blastocysts on the Cryotop with minimal volume.
- Plunge the Cryotop into liquid nitrogen and slightly swirling it.
- Move the plunged Cryotop to the liquid nitrogen container with the Cryotop placed in a goblet, for long-term storage.
- In case of closed system vitrification, oocytes/embryos/blastocysts are loaded on to the cutoff end of the microcapillary tube of HSV straw. The oocytes/embryos/blastocysts are placed in the gutter close to the open end of the tube in a miniscule amount of fluid (<0.5 µL). The capillary tube is then inserted into a straw. The open end of the straw is then closed using a heat sealer. The straw with oocytes/embryos/blastocysts is then plunged in liquid nitrogen (LN2) **(Figs. 6A to D)**.

WARMING PROCESS

Warming Solutions

- *Thawing solution (TS)*: TS is a HEPES-buffered medium, 1.0 M sucrose, and 20% (v/v) serum protein substitute.
- *Dilution solution (DS)*: DS is a HEPES-buffered medium, 0.5 M sucrose, and 20% (v/v) serum protein substitute.
- *Washing solution (WS)*: WS is a HEPES-buffered medium and 20% (v/v) serum protein substitute.

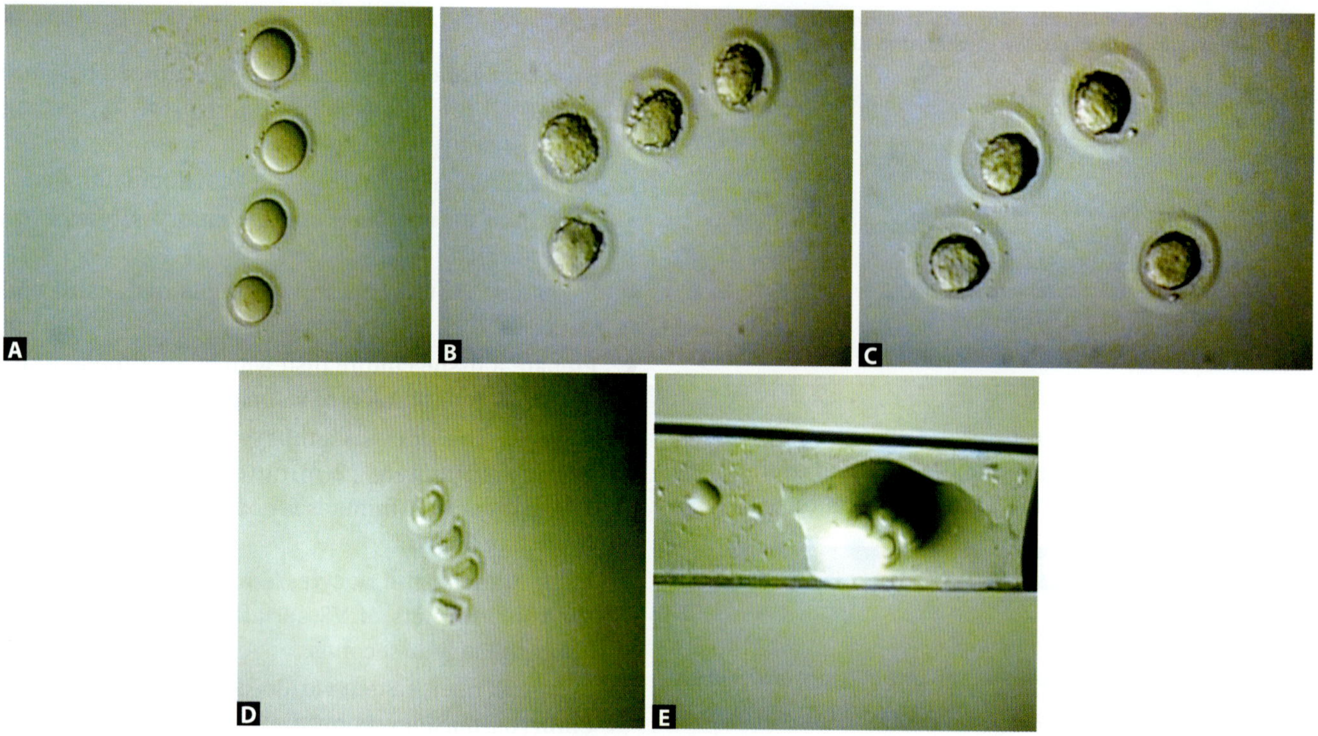

Figs. 3A to E: Vitrification of oocytes in open system—showing initial shrinkage followed by recovery of oocytes in equilibration solution (ES) and loading on Cryotop.

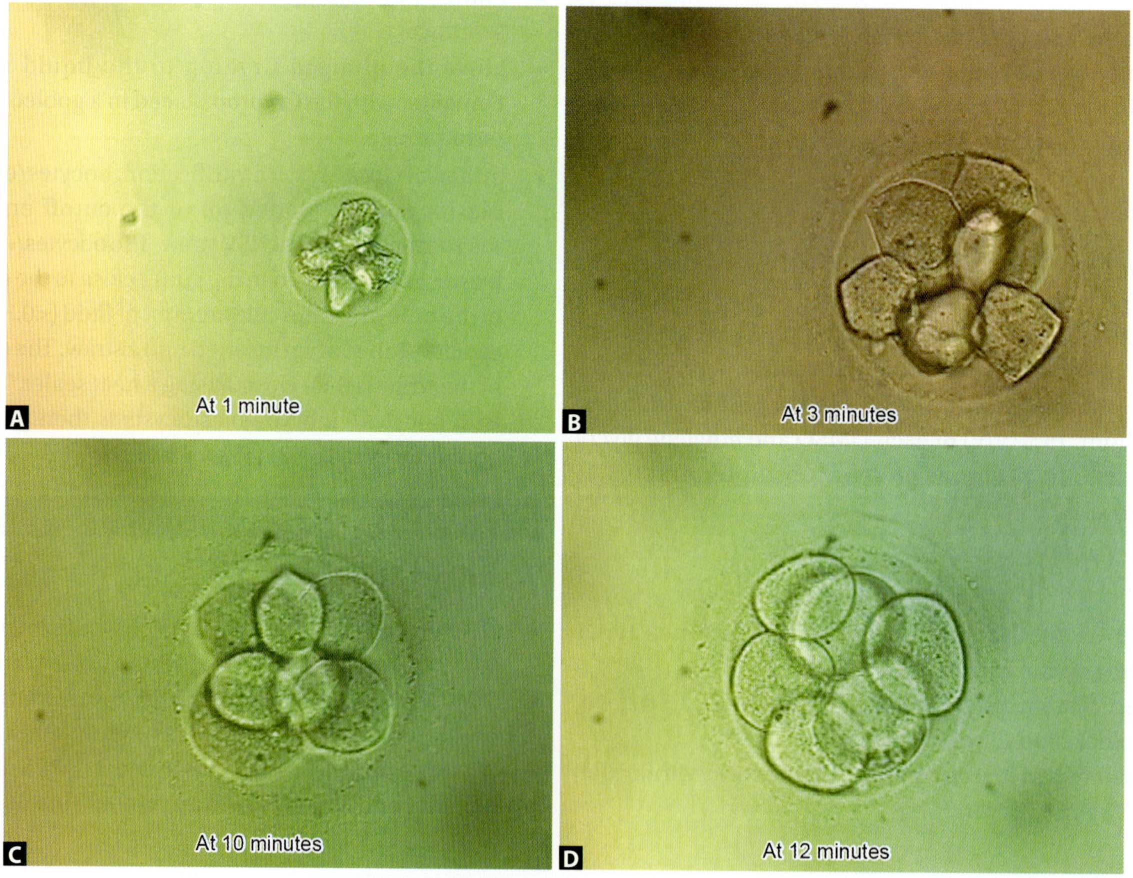

Figs. 4A to D: Vitrification of embryos—showing initial shrinkage and recovery of embryos in equilibration solution (ES).

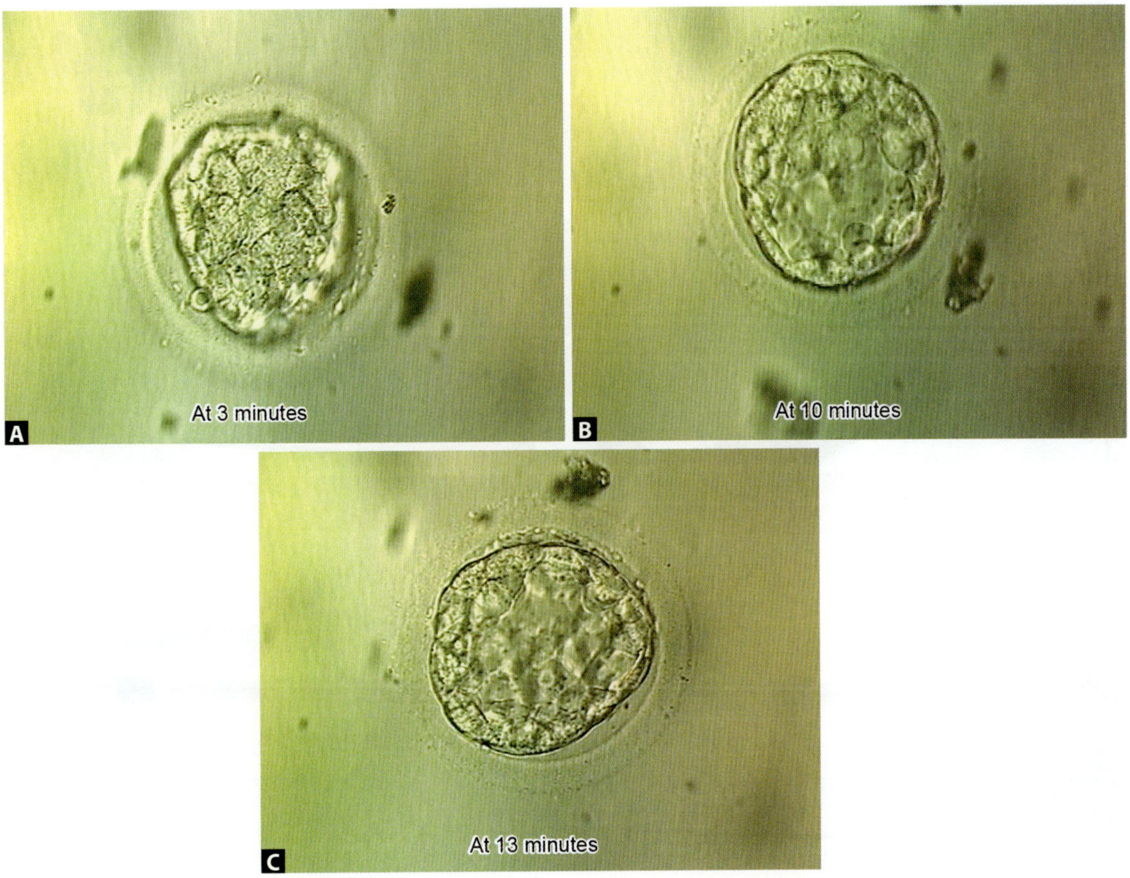

Figs. 5A to C: Vitrification of blastocyst—showing initial shrinkage and recovery of blastocysts in equilibration solution (ES).

Procedure

- Bring one vial of each TS, DS, and WS to room temperature (24–25°C) for at least 30 minutes prior to thawing oocytes/embryos/blastocysts.
- Fill the liquid nitrogen reservoir with liquid nitrogen.
- Determine the number of oocytes/embryos/blastocysts to be thawed with correct patient detail.
- Take the Cryotop out of the liquid nitrogen and quickly transfer the oocytes/embryos/blastocysts into TS (0.8 mL in center well dish at 37°C) for 1 minute.
- Transfer the oocytes/embryos/blastocysts to 0.3 mL of DS for 3 minutes at room temperature.
- Transfer the oocytes/embryos/blastocysts to 0.3 mL of WS 1 for 5 minutes at room temperature.
- Transfer the oocytes/embryos/blastocysts to 0.3 mL of WS 2 for 5 minutes at room temperature.
- Transfer the oocytes/embryos/blastocysts to pre-equilibrated culture medium layered with liquid paraffin and place in the incubator.

Cryoinjuries

Mammalian cells are never exposed to subzero temperatures under physiological conditions. Therefore, injuries may occur at all phases of the procedure **(Table 3)**.[1-3]

There is increasing concern about possible disease transmission between the stored samples mediated by LN2, even though there are no reported cases in literature involving embryos.

Embryos subjected to cryopreservation may undergo a considerable damage during cooling and warming. Fortunately, these embryos have the ability to repair fully or partially this damage and thus, continue with normal development.

COMPARISON OF THE TWO METHODS (TABLE 4)[4-6]

The main difference between the earlier two is that in vitrification, the oocyte/embryo and also the surrounding

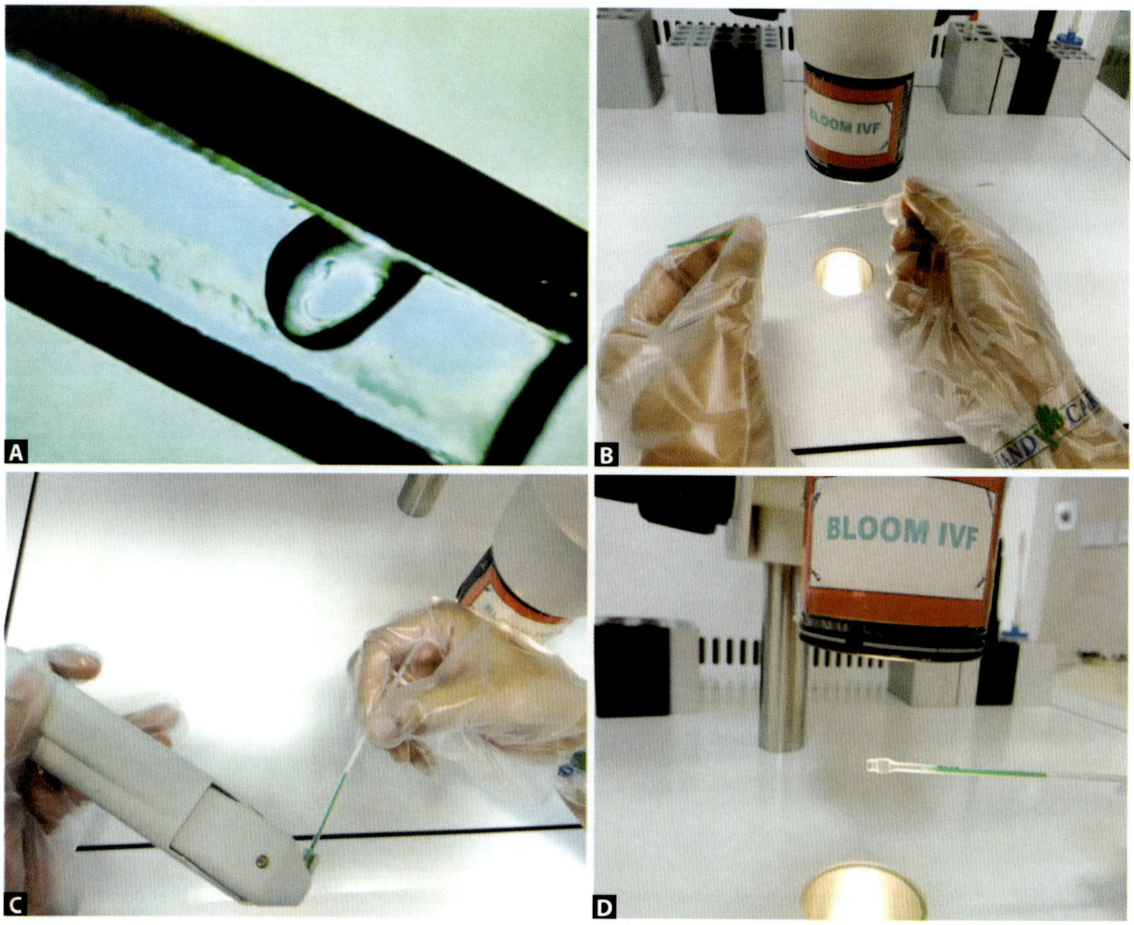

Figs. 6A to D: Vitrification of oocytes in closed system—showing loading on high security vitrification (HSV) straw and heat sealing.

Table 3: Cryoinjuries at different set of temperatures.

At high temperatures between +15°C and –5°C	Chilling injury is the most important type of injury. This may damage the cytoplasmic lipid droplets (irreversible damage leading to death of cryopreserved lipid-rich oocytes and embryos) and the microtubules including the meiotic spindle (reversible damage)[1-3]
Between –5°C and –80°C	Main source of injury is the extracellular or predominantly intracellular ice crystal formation
Between –50°C and –150°C	Fracture damage to the zona pellucida or cytoplasm may occur. But it is unlikely that zona fracture could occur as a simple consequence of osmotic stress
Below –150°C (especially in liquid nitrogen at –196°C)	This is the least dangerous phase in the cryopreservation procedure
Accidental warming	This is the most frequent form of injury

solution solidify in an amorphous structure similar to glass, but without ice crystal formation.

In a meta-analysis of four randomized controlled trials (RCTs) by Loutradi KE et al.,[7] which summarizes information from 8,824 cryopreserved human cleavage stage embryos/blastocysts (vitrification: n = 7,482; slow freezing: n = 1,342), the survival rate of cleavage stage embryos was significantly higher after vitrification as compared with slow freezing (odds ratio 15.57, 95% confidence interval 3.68–65.82). Also, the survival rate of vitrified blastocysts was significantly higher as compared with that observed with slow freezing (odds ratio 2.20, 95% confidence interval 1.53–3.16).

SLOW FREEZING: POST-THAW OUTCOMES

The slow freezing: postthaw outcomes are given in **Table 5**.

Table 4: Difference between slow freezing and vitrification.

	Slow freezing	*Vitrification*
Incubation time	Slow (approximately 3–5 hours)	Fast (few minutes)
Programmable freezing equipment	Required	Not required
Skill	Less skill required	Technically demanding
Cooling rate	–0.3°C/min to –1°C/min to between –30°C and –80°C, then > 200°C/min	–200°C/min to 20,000°C/min
Warming rate	–4°C/min to 100°C/min	–300°C/min to >12,000°C/min
Cryoprotectant (CPA)	Dimethyl sulfoxide (DMSO)/ethylene glycol/propanediol	DMSO/ethylene glycol
Concentration of cryoprotectant	Low (1.5 mol/L)	High (2–5 mol/L). In spite of exposure of high concentration of CPA, it was shown that intracellular concentration of CPAs are actually lower in vitrification as compared to slow freezing[4]
Cryoprotectant injury	Less	More
Seeding	Done	Not done
Ice formation	Yes	No
Osmotic stress	Yes	Limited
Toxic stress	Yes	Yes
Mechanical stress (ice crystal formation)	Yes	No
Chilling injury	Yes	Limited
Carrier	Ampule/straw ("closed")	Electron microscopy grid/open pulled straw (OPS), Cryoloop/Cryotip/Cryotop (semi-closed)/high security straw ("closed")/Cryolock/Cryotec/VitMaster, Gavi system[5,6]/Cryopette, Rapid-I, etc.
Direct contact with liquid nitrogen	No	Yes/no (in case of high security straw)

Table 5: Slow freezing: postthaw outcomes.

Authors	*Method*	*n/N*	*Survival rate*	*Pregnancy rate per transfer*
Zheng (2005)	Slow freezing	8/52	15.4%	Embryo transfer (ET) is not done
Rama Raju (2005)	Slow freezing	72/120	60.0%	17.4%
Kuwayama (2005)	Slow freezing	857/942	91.0%	32.1%

VITRIFICATION: POST-THAW SURVIVAL RATES

The vitrification: postthaw survival rates are described in **Table 6**.

Thus, the meta-analysis proved that vitrification was associated with higher postthaw survival rate than slow freezing.

There are certain controversial areas with cryopreservation:

- Toxicity and long-term effects of the CPAs used
- Chances of viral transmission in open systems
- Higher miscarriage rate.

But today, vitrification as a method to cryopreserve oocytes and embryos has achieved remarkable success due to its multiple advantages like being rapid, simple, inexpensive, and higher survival and developmental rates. Potential sources of contamination include:

- Within the freezing apparatus
- During storage
- From LN2.

Table 6: Vitrification: postthaw survival rates.

Authors	*Method*	*n/N*	*Survival rate*	*Pregnancy rate per transfer*
Zheng et al. (2005)	Vitrification	46/49	93.8%	–
Rama Raju et al. (2005)	Vitrification	121/127	95.3%	35%
Kuwayama et al. (2005)	Vitrification	4,650/4,745	98.0%	53%
Pai et al. (2014)	Vitrification	1,650/1,758	98%	63%

The European Union directive dictates that cooling and storage of embryos must be performed in a way that minimizes the risk of contamination. Basic recommendations [Human Fertilisation and Embryology Authority (HFEA), 1998] for safe storage are:

- Patient screening for hepatitis B, hepatitis C, and HIV
- Careful hygiene throughout
- Double containment of storage straws
- Use of sealed ampules.

Regarding the safety of vitrification, no currently available data indicates a higher incidence of malformation which is reassuring but needs to be confirmed on large scale. Theoretical risk of disease transmission with the open system is there which can be taken care of by the closed system.

There is no doubt that closed system should be preferred, provided the outcome is comparable with open system. Results achieved by using closed system for cleavage stage embryos and blastocysts are promising.[8,9] Studies have shown that open systems are more likely to produce superior results when oocytes are vitrified and to preserve original physiological cell condition.[10,11]

Different methods to avoid cross-contamination are:

- Using closed vitrification systems
- To use vapor storage systems in which oocytes or embryos do not directly contact the LN2.
- While using open vitrification system, to sterilize liquid nitrogen with ultraviolet (UV) radiation as described by Parmegiani et al. They did not find any contamination after irradiation, thus concluding that this method might be used in combination with open carriers.[12]

RELEVANCE OF EMBRYO CRYOPRESERVATION

The relevance of embryo cryopreservation is described in **Box 1**.

Box 1: Relevance of embryo cryopreservation.

- Permits to do a single embryo transfer
- Excess cryopreserved embryos can be used for future pregnancies
- Increases cumulative pregnancy rate from one fresh cycle
- Can help to achieve an OHSS free clinic.
- Can help to avoid embryo transfer in hostile conditions like on the day of embryo transfer if the following is present:
  - Endometrial thickness < 7 mm or > 14 mm
  - Fluid collection in the uterine cavity
  - Spotting or bleeding
  - Serum progesterone > 1.5 ng/mL in normoresponders on the day of trigger
  - Difficult embryo transfer
  - Applebaum scoring < 14.
- Patients undergoing PGS using blastocyst biopsy—in patients undergoing genetic screening, there is increased use of cryopreservation because embryos are usually frozen till test results are obtained and transfer of confirmed euploid embryos may contribute to increased FET success rates.
- Allows for freeze all and embryo transfer in the next cycle.
- In treating recurrent implantation failure due to poor endometrium.

(FET: frozen embryo transfer; OHSS: ovarian hyperstimulation syndrome; PGS: preimplantation genetic screening)

SUMMARY

Vitrification/warming gives a significantly higher survival, fertilization, embryo cleavage, and development and clinical pregnancy rates when compared with slow freezing.

With the introduction of vitrification, cryopreservation techniques have significantly improved.[13,14]

Also, the postwarming survival rates have increased not only for human embryos, but also for human oocytes.[15]

Although preclinical data suggest an inverse relationship between controlled ovarian stimulation and endometrial receptivity, clinical data are controversial. Benefits of elective FET are likely limited to women with hyperovarian response. Clinical evidence is against elective FET for women with poor/suboptimal ovarian response. Current data regarding ART or obstetric outcome do not support a universal freeze-all strategy.[16]

REFERENCES

1. Aman RR, Parks JE. Effects of cooling and rewarming on the meiotic spindle and chromosomes of in vitro matured bovine oocytes. Biol Reprod. 1994;50(1):103-10.
2. Martino A, Pollard JW, Leibo SP. Effect of chilling bovine oocytes on their developmental competence. Mol Reprod Dev. 1996;45(4):503-12.
3. Zenzes MT, Bielecki R, Casper RF, et al. Effects of chilling to 0 degrees C on the morphology of meiotic spindles in human metaphase II oocytes. Fertil Steril. 2001;75(4):769-77.
4. Vanderzwalmen P, Connan D, Grobet L, et al. Lower intracellular concentration of cryoprotectants after vitrification than after slow freezing despite exposure to higher concentration of cryoprotectant solutions. Hum Reprod. 2013;28(8):2101-10.
5. Cuello C, Gil MA, Parrilla I, et al. Vitrification of porcine embryos at various developmental stages using different ultra-rapid cooling procedures. Theriogenology. 2004;62(1-2):353-61.
6. Liu WX, Lu H, Luo MJ, et al. Effects of different cryoprotectants and cryopreservation protocols on the development of 2-4 cell mouse embryos. Cryo Letters. 2011;32(3):240-7.
7. Loutradi KE, Kolibianakis EM, Venetis CA, et al. Cryopreservation of human embryos by vitrification or slow freezing: a systematic review and meta-analysis. Fertil Steril. 2008;90(1):186-93.
8. Van Landuyt L, Stoop D, Verheyen G, et al. Outcome of closed blastocyst vitrification in relation to blastocyst quality: evaluation of 759 warming cycles in a single-embryo transfer policy. Hum Reprod. 2011;26(3):527-34.
9. Liebermann J. Vitrification of human blastocysts: an update. Reprod Biomed Online. 2009;19 Suppl 4:4328.
10. Bonetti A, Cervi M, Tomei F, et al. Ultrastructural evaluation of human metaphase II oocytes after vitrification: closed versus open devices. Fertil Steril. 2011;95(3):928-35.
11. Papatheodorou A, Vanderzwalmen P, Panagiotidis Y, et al. Open versus closed oocyte vitrification system: a prospective randomized sibling-oocyte study. Reprod Biomed Online. 2013;26(6):595-602.
12. Herrero L, Martínez M, Garcia-Velasco JA. Current status of human oocyte and embryo cryopreservation. Curr Opin Obstet Gynecol. 2011;23(4):245-50.
13. Balaban B, Urman B, Ata B, et al. A randomized controlled study of human Day 3 embryo cryopreservation by slow freezing or vitrification: vitrification is associated with higher survival, metabolism and blastocyst formation. Hum Reprod. 2008;23(9):1976-82.
14. Loutradi KE, Kolibianakis EM, Venetis CA, et al. Cryopreservation of human embryos by vitrification or slow freezing: a systematic review and meta-analysis. Fertil Steril. 2008;90(1):186-93.
15. Levi Setti PE, Porcu E, Patrizio P, et al. Human oocyte cryopreservation with slow freezing versus vitrification. Results from the National Italian Registry data, 2007-2011. Fertil Steril. 2014;102(1):90-5.e2.
16. Ata B, Seli E. A universal freeze all strategy: why it is not warranted. Curr Opin Obstet Gynecol. 2017;29(3):136-45.

Semen Banking

67

Milind Shah, Jayshree Pattnaik, Unnati Mamtora, Charumati Pekhale

INTRODUCTION

Semen bank is a facility available for the storage, supply or reserve of the human sperm/semen for future use in assisted reproductive techniques. The alternative terminologies used for semen banking are sperm cryopreservation and semen freezing. It forms an important part of fertility preservation program. Advances in reproductive technologies help to provide childless couples the opportunity to embrace parenthood despite significant limitation of infertility. Cryopreservation is among one of those advancements in the field of assisted reproduction that has made the treatment more effective as well as more flexible. There has been much advancement in equipment, disposables, and the technology of cryopreservation in the last few years.

HISTORICAL SYNOPSIS

The first report of effects of freezing temperature on human spermatozoa was made by Spallanzani in 1776. In 1866, Mantegazza suggested banks for frozen human semen. From 1938 to 1945, Jahnel and Shettles observed that human sperms can withstand freezing temperatures as low as –269°C. Polge et al. discovered the cryoprotective properties of glycerol in 1949 and this laid the foundation for cryopreservation of human sperm. In 1953, human sperm equilibrated with 10% glycerol on dry ice were cryopreserved by Sherman and Bunge and they observed a 67% survival rate.[1] Shortly thereafter, the same authors reported three pregnancies by artificial insemination of frozen-thawed sperms. Many groups like Keettel et al. and Sawada et al. reported pregnancies following insemination with frozen-thawed sperms after this successful pregnancy report. Sherman discovered that storing human sperm at liquid nitrogen (LN_2) temperature (–196°C) was much superior than storage at –75°C.[2] In 1964, Perloff et al. had reported pregnancies from insemination with frozen-thawed sperm after storage for 1–5.5 months.[3]

INDICATIONS

Semen banking provides an opportunity to men to store their semen sample for future use. It may be autologous where the semen sample is stored for use by the person himself or may be for a donor purpose. This can be for various indications and the list has been increasing over a period of years. The indications are listed here:

- *Donor insemination*: Cryopreservation provides sufficient time to screen the donors for infectious agents. It is essential to quarantine a semen sample for 6 months before it is used for insemination according to the Indian Council of Medical Research (ICMR) 2010. It also helps in the ready availability of a wide range of donor phenotypes for insemination according to the patient's choice.
- *Fertility preservation*: Cancer treatment (surgical procedure or chemotherapy or radiotherapy) can have deleterious effect on future fertility. Semen cryopreservation in such males allows them to have their own biological child.

  Radiotherapy or chemotherapy: Semen freezing is done before starting radiotherapy or chemotherapy as spermatogonia are especially sensitive to these treatments. The effect is usually dose-dependent and it might not be permanent unless the spermatogonial stem cell (SSC) population is fully depleted.

Vasectomy—in case of a desire for more children in the future or in cases where there is change in the marital status.

In countries where posthumous procreation is acceptable, it can be done for men in dangerous occupation, e.g. in military forces.

- *Assisted reproductive technology (ART) procedures*: In patients with severe oligozoospermia or intermittent presence of sperms in the semen sample, the cryopreserved sample can be used for various treatment procedures such as artificial insemination (AIH), intrauterine insemination (IUI), in vitro fertilization (IVF) or intracytoplasmic sperm injection (ICSI).
- Cryopreservation is a boon in males with spinal cord injury needing assisted ejaculation, patients with retrograde ejaculation where spermatozoa are collected from urine; patients with stress-related ejaculatory (emotional states or other issues or commitments at the time of oocyte retrieval).[4,5]
- To avoid repeated biopsies in azoospermia—in patients who have undergone testicular sperm aspiration (TESA)/percutaneous epididymal sperm aspiration (PESA)/microdissection TESA, cryopreservation is used to avoid repeated procedures.
- Some chronic disorders such as diabetes and autoimmune diseases can also lead to testicular damage and it is advisable to cryopreserve semen sample in patients suffering from these conditions.[6]
- *Gender reassignment procedures*: Removal of testicles or use of feminizing medicines has a deleterious effect on future fertility. Counseling about fertility preservation as well as fertility treatment options should be given before the surgical procedure or starting the hormonal.

METHODS OF SPERM COLLECTION

The sperms can be collected by the following methods depending on the underlying conditions:

- Masturbation
- Vibratory penile stimulation
- Electroejaculation
- Surgical sperm retrieval—PESA, microsurgical epididymal sperm aspiration (MESA), TESA or testicular sperm extraction (TESE) (testicular tissue).

PRINCIPLES OF CRYOPRESERVATION

The objective of cryopreservation is to remove intracellular water before freezing to reduce the extent of intercellular ice formation to the point where it halts to constitute a threat to the viability of the cell. However, removal of excessive amounts of water can also cause cellular injury and possible death through the effect of highly concentrated intracellular environment on intracellular components, particularly their membranes.

CRYOPROTECTANTS

Cryoprotectants are low-molecular weight substances that are protective to the cell membranes. As the name suggests these cryoprotectants protect the spermatozoa from the deleterious effects of the freezing process. Cryoprotectants act by reduction in the salts and solutes, lowering the freezing point and by reducing intracellular ice formation within the spermatozoa.[7]

The cryoprotectants may be permeating or nonpermeating. Glycerol, ethylene glycol, dimethyl sulfoxide (DMSO), 2-propanediol are the common permeating cryoprotectants used. Raffinose, sucrose and glycine are the nonpermeating cryoprotectants. The permeating cryoprotectants readily move across the cell membranes depending on the osmolarity gradient. They prevent crystallization by forming hydrogen bonds with the water molecules and prevent ice formation. The time interaction between the cells and the cryoprotectants decides the effectiveness of the procedure.[4]

Glycerol is a most commonly used permeating cryoprotectant and also the cryoprotectant of choice. Glycerol counters the harmful effects through its colligative properties and by lowering the freezing point. It causes change in the lipid packing and electrolyte concentration in the cell membrane, thus protecting it from the harmful effects of the freezing process per se.[8] Glycerol is better in comparison to other cryoprotectants like DMSO and ethylene glycol. DMSO has deleterious effect on the sperms at 4°C.[4]

The nonpermeating cryoprotectants are large molecules that remain extracellular and act by causing intracellular dehydration. They are used in combination with the permeating cryoprotectants to prevent cellular toxic effects. These are sucrose, raffinose and glycine.

Cryoprotectant solution also contains other compounds called extenders (for example, citrate, egg yolk and zwitterionic buffers), which also have preservative effects on the cells during freezing and thawing. Measured amounts of these compounds are added to physiological solutions similar to gamete and embryo culture media, to form the cryoprotectant. N-(2-hydroxyethyl)-piperazine-N'-2-ethanesulfonic acid (HEPES) or phosphate buffers are used to maintain the pH of the cryoprotectant solution. The most commonly used extender is the egg yolk. Studies have shown that the various lipid constituents of the egg yolk bind to the spermatozoa membrane.[9] Commonly used media are glycerol egg yolk citrate (GEYC), human sperm preserving medium (HPSM) is a modified Tyrode's medium containing glycerol (5–7.5% v/v final volume), sucrose, glucose and glycine as cryoprotective agents, human serum albumin as stabilizing agent and HEPES as the buffering agent.

TECHNIQUE

Freezing

The cryoprotectant is first warmed to the room temperature. Sperm freezing media and semen sample are then mixed in either equal ratio or in ratio of 1:2, by pipetting up and down gently or drop by drop or by gradual addition with mixing over 10 minutes at room temperature. The mixture is then incubated for 5 minutes at 30–35°. The mixture is then placed in cryovials or straws after proper marking of identification of the patient. In the lower part of the straw, some air space is left. The straw is then sealed. Vials should not be filled more than 90% of the capacity. Semen cryopreservation can be further accomplished by two methods:

1. *Controlled rate cryopreservation in programmable freezers*: These programmable freezers control the injection of LN_2 vapor into the freezing chamber. The straws or cryovials are placed in the programmable freezer. A common program is to cool the straws or cryovials at 1.5°C per minute from 20°C to –6°C and then at 6°C per minute to –100°C. This generally takes about 40 minutes. The straws are then held –100°C for 30 minutes to allow for delays and then they are transferred to LN_2.
2. *Noncontrolled rate cryopreservation*: Though manual method is less controllable than programmable freezers, it gives equally good results. The straws or the vials are placed in a refrigerator freezer (–20°C) for 30 minutes and then transferred on dry ice (–20°C) for 30 minutes before plunging into the LN_2 (–196°C). Alternatively the straws are moved from the –20°C freezer into another freezer at –70°C or kept on LN_2 vapor at (–70°C) for 10–15 minutes before placing into LN_2 (WHO Manual 2010).

Thawing

After identifying the required semen sample, vials or straws are removed from LN_2 and allowed to reach the room temperature. Cryovials generally take about 10–20 minutes and straws take about 6 minutes to reach this temperature. Within 10 minutes the semen sample is withdrawn from the vial or straw. The motility can be checked after thawing. The cryoprotectant is then removed by washing in culture medium and centrifugation (WHO Manual 2010).

Storage

The cryovials are transferred to precooled aluminum canes/goblets for storage into the LN_2 storage tanks. The aluminum canes/goblets, labeled with proper numbering and color code system for proper patient identification are placed in predetermined locations within the cryostorage vessel and a record is kept of the same. All storage containers should be stored in a secured room. There should be regular monitoring of the LN_2 levels in the tanks and these should be refilled at regular intervals.

There is a risk of cross-infection during storage and hence it is of utmost importance to screen for infectious disease before storage. In cases of malignancy, there may not be sufficient time to screen before sample storage. In such cases, quarantine tanks should be used till the screening is completed and reports obtained. The samples of patients with chronic viral diseases should be stored separately to avoid cross-contamination of other samples. A separate tank has to be maintained for each infective pathogenic organism.

Transport of Frozen Semen

The frozen spermatozoa can be transported from one place to another in commercially available cryoshippers. The cryoshippers can hold the samples for days to weeks depending upon its size. However, before any such transfer of samples; local, national and international regulations on shipping LN_2 and human biological samples should be complied with.

EFFECTS OF CRYOPRESERVATION ON THE SPERMS

The success of any cryopreservation protocol is determined by the post-thaw sperm viability. The cryopreservation procedure has a less deleterious effect on the sperms as compared to oocytes and embryos. It affects the sperms to a lesser extent mainly due to the low water content and high fluidity. Despite this, cryopreservation may affect the sperm structural integrity and its motility and viability.[10] Most common effects are the thermal shock, the intracellular and extracellular ice formation and osmotic shock.[11] The rate of cooling plays a very important role. The ice crystals formed can affect the cell survival by causing damage to the membranes and other organelles. The slower the freezing process, higher the cellular concentration of the solutes causing osmotic damage. In case of faster cooling, there is danger of ice formation.[12] The process of freezing can cause damage to the plasma membranes affecting their structure and integrity.[13,14] Studies have reported the detrimental effect on the glycocalyx content of the membrane, which in turn affects the transport of ions and solutes across the membranes, affecting the fertilizing ability.[14] The reactive oxygen species (ROS) can result in peroxidative damage along with damage to the sperm plasma membrane and impairment of the axonemal structure.[15] The high content of ROS can cause cellular apoptosis which in turn is associated with deoxyribonucleic acid (DNA) fragmentation.[16]

EFFECT ON REPRODUCTIVE OUTCOME

Cryopreservation induces reduction in the power of sperm fertilization (decrease in the sperm motility due to harmful effect on the cell membrane and acrosomal structure) and hence the pregnancy rates are reported to be lower in the IVF with frozen-thawed semen samples as compared to fresh semen samples used.[1] Hence cryopreserved semen samples are not recommended for use in IVF/IUI. The considerations are different for ICSI as only a few motile sperms are required for successful fertilization procedure. A large number of studies have been conducted to understand the effect on the outcome of ICSI procedure and they are controversial.[17-26]

ICMR GUIDELINES FOR SEMEN BANKS

The ICMR has set guidelines for all the ART clinics throughout the country.

- All the semen banks require accreditation.
- The donors are screened for sexually transmitted diseases (STDs) such as human immunodeficiency virus (HIV), hepatitis B, hepatitis C, human T-cell lymphotropic virus (HTLV)-I and II and syphilis. They are again screened after 6 months to prevent missing out any positive case if the sample was collected in the window period.
- The sample collection is done in a secluded area assigned for semen collection so that the sample collected is not exchanged by another sample.
- Donor records are to be kept and coding system is to be followed strictly.
- According to the ICMR guidelines, one semen sample should not be supplied to achieve more than 10 successful pregnancies. Sample of a single donor should not be used for more than 75 times.
- It is mandatory for the banks to keep the records for all the samples received, stored and supplied.
- The couple bearing a child through donor insemination is not obliged to give information of the individual's personal identity of the donor whose semen sample was used. However, they cannot hide the information after the child turns 18 years old and the child holds the right to this information.
- Sperm donor can be between 21 years and 45 years of age.
- Spouse consent is must for any ART/IUI procedure.
- Sperm donated by the known relative/friend of either of the couple is not permitted.
- Semen from two separate individuals should not be mixed before use, under any circumstance.
- Semen analysis should be carried out after the donor sample is received using the WHO Manual for semen analysis and should be normal for future use into ART.
- Relevant information of the donor in term of height, weight, skin color, color of eyes, educational qualification, profession, blood group, ethnic background, and history of diabetes, hypertension, psychiatric illness, and genetic disorders like thalassemia is mandatory.
- The semen samples are stored for 6 months before they are used, where the donor is screened again for HIV, hepatitis B and C.
- Suitable record of all the donors needs to be maintained for 10 years. In case an ART bank closes before 10 years, all the records should be transferred to the central database of the Department of Health Research, Government of India. Strict confidentiality should be maintained about the clients and the donors and that information about gamete donation shall not be disclosed to anyone other than the central database of the Department of Health Research, or only if by a court of competent jurisdiction.
- The sample cannot be discarded or used for donation unless proper consent given by the couple. In case of failure of payment of renewal charges, the bank holds the right to discard the sample or use it for research purposes if the charges are not paid after two reminders sent by the bank to the address provided by the couple through registered post.

- In situations where there is death of the donor, the semen sample becomes the property of the legal heir or the nominee mentioned in the register at the time of freezing of the semen sample.
- The sale, transfer or use of gametes, zygotes and embryos, or any part thereof or information related thereto, directly or indirectly to any party outside India is prohibited and shall be deemed to be an offense except in the case of transfer of own gametes and embryos for personal use with the permission of the National Board. The sale of gametes, except for use by an ART clinic for treating infertility, and the sale of zygotes and embryos, or of any information related to gametes, zygotes or embryos, within India, is prohibited and shall be deemed to be an offense under this Act.

CONCLUSION

Semen banking holds a very important role in the fertility treatment. Cryopreservation and subsequent thaw of semen multiple pregnancies have been reported after use of cryopreserved semen sample, cryopreserved for as long as 2–3 decades.[27,28] Till date semen banking has been a commonly used procedure for autologous as well as for donor purpose. The impact of cryopreservation on the sperm structural membrane, its integrity and the DNA integrity is controversial and randomized controlled trails and meta-analysis are required to study its effect on the reproductive outcome. Nevertheless, it has proved to be boon in the era of modernization helping childless couples to embrace parenthood. Semen banking has become an accepted modality for fertility preservation and childless couples.

REFERENCES

1. Sherman JK. Synopsis of the use of frozen human semen since 1964: state of the art of human semen banking. Fertil Steril. 1973;24(5):397-412.
2. Sherman JK. Research on frozen human semen: past, present, and future. Fertil Steril. 1964;15:485-99.
3. Walters EM, Benson JD, Woods EJ, et al. The history of sperm cryopreservation. In: Pacey AA, Tomlinson MJ (Eds). Sperm Banking: Theory and Practice. Cambridge, UK: Cambridge University Press; 2009. pp. 1-10.
4. Fabbri R, Ciotti P, Tommaso BD, et al. Tecniche di crioconservazione riproduttiva. Riv It Ost Gin. 2004;3:33-41.
5. Donnelly ET, McClure N, Lewis SE. Cryopreservation of human semen and prepared sperm: effects on motility parameters and DNA integrity. Fertil Steril. 2001;76(5):892-900.
6. Anger JT, Gilbert BR, Goldstein M. Cryopreservation of sperm: indications, methods and results. J Urol. 2003;170:1079-84.
7. Royere D, Barthelemy C, Hamamah S, et al. Cryopreservation of spermatozoa: a 1996 review. Hum Reprod Update. 1996;2(6):553-9.
8. Mahadevan M, Trounson AO. Effects of cryoprotective media and dilution methods on the preservation of human spermatozoa. Andrologia. 1983;15:355-66.
9. Ramirez JP, Carreras A, Mendoza C. Sperm plasma membrane integrity in fertile and infertile men. Andrologia. 1992;24:141-4.
10. Watson PF. The causes of reduced fertility with cryopreserved semen. Anim Reprod Sci. 2000;60-61:481-92.
11. Stanic P, Tandara M, Sonicki Z, et al. Comparison of protective media and freezing techniques for cryopreservation of human semen. Eur J Obstet Gynecol Reprod Biol. 2000;91(1):65-70.
12. Said TM, Gaglani A, Agarwal A. Implication of apoptosis in sperm cryoinjury. Reprod Biomed Online. 2010;21:456-62.
13. Arav A, Zeron Y, Leslie SB, et al. Phase transition temperature and chilling sensitivity of bovine oocytes. Cryobiology. 1996;33:589-99.
14. Zeron Y, Pearl M, Borochov A, et al. Kinetic and temporal factors influence chilling injury to germinal vesicle and mature bovine oocytes. Cryobiology. 1999;38:35-42.
15. Benoff S. Carbohydrates and fertilization: an overview. Mol Hum Reprod. 1997;3:599-637.
16. Saleh RA, Agarwal A. Oxidative stress and male infertility: from research bench to clinical practice. J Androl. 2002;23:737-52.
17. Ben Rhouma K, Marrakchi H, Khouja H, et al. Outcome of intracytoplasmic injection of fresh and frozen-thawed testicular spermatozoa. A comparative study. J Reprod Med. 2003;48:349-54.
18. Habermann H, Seo R, Cieslak J, et al. In vitro fertilization outcomes after intracytoplasmic sperm injection with fresh or frozen-thawed testicular spermatozoa. Fertil Steril. 2000;73:955-60.
19. Huang FJ, Chang SY, Tsai MY, et al. Clinical implications of intracytoplasmic sperm injection using cryopreserved testicular spermatozoa from men with azoospermia. J Reprod Med. 2000;45:310-6.
20. De Croo I, Van der Elst J, Everaert K, et al. Fertilization, pregnancy and embryo implantation rates after ICSI with fresh or frozen-thawed testicular spermatozoa. Hum Reprod. 1998;13(7):1893-7.
21. Tournaye H, Merdad T, Silber S, et al. No differences in outcome after intracytoplasmic sperm injection with fresh or with frozen-thawed epididymal spermatozoa. Hum Reprod. 1999;14:90-5.
22. Sukcharoen N, Sithipravej T, Promviengchai S, et al. Comparison of the outcome of intracytoplasmic sperm injection using fresh and frozen-thawed epididymal spermatozoa obtained by percutaneous epididymal sperm aspiration. J Med Assoc Thai. 2001;84:S331-7.
23. Cayan S, Lee D, Conaghan J, et al. A comparison of ICSI outcomes with fresh and cryopreserved epididymal

spermatozoa from the same couples. Hum Reprod. 2001;16(3):495-9.
24. Shibahara H, Hamada Y, Hasegawa A, et al. Correlation between the motility of frozen-thawed epididymal spermatozoa and the outcome of intracytoplasmic sperm injection. Int J Androl. 1999;22(5):324-8.
25. Kuczynski W, Dhont M, Grygoruk C, et al. The outcome of intracytoplasmic injection of fresh and cryopreserved ejaculated spermatozoa—a prospective randomized study. Hum Reprod. 2001;16(10):2109-13.
26. Ragni G, Caccamo AM, Dalla Serra A, et al. Computerized slow-staged freezing of semen from men with testicular tumors or Hodgkin's disease preserves sperm better than standard vapor freezing. Fertil Steril. 1990;53(6):1072-5.
27. Evenson DP, Darzynkiewicz Z, Melamed MR. Comparison of human and mouse sperm chromatin structure by flow cytometry. Chromosoma. 1980;78(2):225-38.
28. Evenson DP, Melamed MR. Rapid analysis of normal and abnormal cell types in human semen and testis biopsies by flow cytometry. J Histochem Cytochem. 1983;31:248-53.

Oocyte Banking

68

Nandita Palshetkar, Hrishikesh D Pai, Rohan Palshetkar, Jiteeka Thakkar

INTRODUCTION

Since the inception of assisted reproductive technique (ART), there has always been advancement in technology, which has allowed infertile couples to embrace parenthood. Oocyte banking is one of these advancements which has allowed women to control their parenthood without compromising on oocyte age. With the current generation, parenthood tends to be delayed due to various reasons—careers, waiting for the right partner, and not ready for parenthood. Oocyte freezing gives women the ability to delay child bearing without having the age barrier on their eggs.

Sperm and embryo cryopreservation have been an integral part of in vitro fertilization (IVF) since quite a few years, however there are several problems associated with freezing of oocytes. It has taken over 2 decades for accepting the oocyte cryopreservation as a successful technique with acceptable clinical outcomes. This delay in acceptance can be contributed to several factors affecting survival of oocytes post cryopreservation such as the structure of oocyte, maturation or by biophysical factors, as a result of the technique employed.

Oocyte cryopreservation has become an essential part of ART and since the first reported live birth following oocyte freezing in 1986,[1] this method is being used for various legal, social, and medical reasons.

With new advances in the technique of vitrification, it has superior conception rates than the slow freezing technique. This has opened up new avenues for vitrification.

American Society of Reproductive Medicine (ASRM) and the Society for Assisted Reproductive Technology (SART) have suggested that mature oocyte vitrification, and warming should not be considered as experimental procedures.[2]

TECHNIQUES OF OOCYTE FREEZING

There are 2 techniques of freezing oocytes. They can be divided into vitrification or slow freezing according to the cooling rates as well as the cryoprotective agents used.

In slow freezing technique, extracellular ice formation through an equilibrium process causes dehydration. Therefore, a slow long controlled cooling is required prior to the oocytes are placed in liquid nitrogen (LN).

However in vitrification, cryoprotectants are present in higher concentrations which solidify without forming ice crystals and this allows us to rapidly cool the oocytes by directly plunging them in LN.

Even though there are differences in the freezing technique, the primary principal is similar which is to protect the oocytes from intracellular ice crystal formation, cellular dehydration and abrupt modification in the solute concentrations at high and low temperatures.

Slow Freezing

Oocytes are placed in 1–2 mol/L cryoprotectants which are dissolved in a physiological solution, ice-seeded, cooled in a slow manner. Due to this freezing technique, water is precipitated into ice. This precipitation leads to the separation of water from the dissolved substances. Intracellular ice crystals and a high solute concentration can be fatal to the oocytes. Hence, a slow cooling rate has been proposed to balance the crystallization, osmotic and freezing damages. This causes the intracellular substance to end up, concentrated by slow dehydration in light of the concentration of extracellular unfrozen division amid the development of extracellular ice. The slow freezing method has the following steps:[3]

- Solutions are placed at room temperature before use (22°–24°C).
- Oocytes, 0.6 mL of equilibration solution (ES) is dispensed in well 1 and 0.6 mL of loading solution (LS) is dispensed in well 2 of a four well plate.
- Denuded mature oocytes are transferred from culture media to ES and incubated for 10 mins.
- After this, oocytes are shifted to the LS beginning with first incubated cycle.
- The sample is slowly cooled from +20°C to –7°C at a rate of –2°C/min. Ice crystallization is induced by a process called seeding. Seeding occurs at –5°C to –7°C which results in a heterogeneous ice nucleation that is more stable than super cooling or homogenous nucleation.
- The temperature decreases to –30°C at a rate of –0.3°C/min and then rapidly decreases to –150°C at a rate of –50°C/min.
- Finally the straws are stored in LN.

Vitrification

Vitrification is the process by which a solution is transformed into a stable amorphous glass by rapidly cooling the solution. With vitrification, ice crystal formation is bypassed while as yet keeping up the properties of liquid in solid state.

Vitrification uses a high concentration of cryoprotectant and fast cooling and warming rate to pass through the glass transition temperature and prevent ice formation. Vitrification method has the following steps:[4]

- The oocytes are exposed at room temperature to a high concentration of a cryoprotectant until equilibrium is reached between the cryoprotectant solution and the oocytes.
- Oocytes are then exposed for a very brief period to a high concentration of cryoprotectants.
- Loading of oocytes in carrier devices followed by plunging into LN2 (–196°C) for storage.

In vitrification, 2 types of storage systems are used: open and closed. Closed system alludes to the oocytes that don't interact with fluid nitrogen during storage and open system alludes to the ones that interact with LN.

CRYOPROTECTANTS FOR OOCYTE FREEZING

These are specific molecules which are mixed in freezing solutions to prevent any injury to oocytes during freezing and thawing to maximize quality and outcome. These compounds:

- Increase survival rates of oocytes
- Lowers freezing point of intracellular water
- Decreases or prevents formation of ice crystals
- Increases osmolarity of solutions to which it is added.

Types

- *Permeating*: Small, nonionic, and water soluble compounds. These include ethylene glycol (EG), propylene glycol, dimethyl sulfide (DMSO) and glycerol
- *Nonpermeating cryoprotectants:* They are long chain polymers which include sugars like galactose, glucose, sucrose and proteins.

Permeating cryoprotectants minimize crystallization by replacing intracellular water osmotically. This occurs because solidification occurs at a lower temperature. However, nonpermeating cryoprotectants dehydrate cells before cooling. This increases the osmolarity of extracellular space which reduces ice crystal formation.

APPLICATIONS OF OOCYTE CRYOPRESERVATION

With the advent of oocyte cryopreservation, there are many fields in which cryopreservation would be beneficial to patients:

- *Fertility preservation in malignant and pre-malignant conditions:* Female patients having malignant or pre-malignant conditions, with a good survival rate post chemo or radiotherapy, oocyte freezing is a promising option. Besides malignant conditions, women who are *BRCA1* and *BRCA2* positive, oocyte freezing can be a viable option. These patients may undergo prophylactic salpingo-oophorectomy at an early age as they are predisposed to ovarian cancer. Oocyte freezing in such patients would still maintain their fertility even though their ovaries are removed. Other genetic conditions which may lead to premature ovarian failure (Turner's, fragile X, deletion of X chromosome) can benefit from oocyte cryopreservation

- *Egg donor program:* Women with decreased ovarian reserve or advanced age have difficulty in conceiving with their own oocytes. However, with donor oocytes, their chances of conception increases. But without oocyte freezing, IVF clinics face difficulties like synchronization of the donor and recipients menstrual cycle, lack of quarantine period and large number of supernumerary embryos. With an efficient vitrification technique, the need for synchronization is eliminated. In addition with the establishment of egg banks, the logistics of coordinating the donors with the recipients is no longer required. Furthermore, with freezing of oocytes, testing of donors can be done during and after the quarantine period to prevent the transmission of any diseases.[5]
- *Delaying motherhood*: Women pursuing their professional careers wish to delay their childbearing. The impact of ageing on female fertility is well recognized.[6] Delay in motherhood results in decreased fertility, as the ovarian reserve and egg quality decrease. Besides this there is an increase in spontaneous abortion rates as a woman's age increases. Oocyte vitrification due to "social" reasons could be a viable option for women who wish to preserve their reproductive potential.
- *Accumulation of oocytes in poor responders*: It is a novel application in women with poor ovarian response. Women with poor ovarian response require multiple stimulation cycles when oocyte pooling is decided. Egg banking and vitrification provides a practical option in these patients. Post pooling, all the oocytes are thawed together and intracytoplasmic sperm injection (ICSI) is performed creating embryos, thus mimicking a similar situation to a normal responder.[7]
- *Avoids legal and ethical restrictions of embryo cryopreservation:* In certain countries, there is a restriction of freezing embryos due to moral or religious beliefs. In such countries, oocyte freezing could benefit the couples. As a matter of fact, countries where embryo freezing is forbidden by law, cryopreservation of oocytes is one of the leading options of female infertility.
- *Nonavailability of sperms during oocyte retrieval*: Sometimes on the day of oocyte retrieval, the male partner is unable to give a seen sample due to unexpected problems or failure in yielding sperms during testicular biopsy. In such cases, oocyte cryopreservation provides a practical option.

OBSTETRIC AND LONG-TERM OUTCOMES WITH VITRIFIED OOCYTES

Multiple studies have reported successful clinical outcomes with oocyte cryopreservation. Vitrification has gained more popularity in freezing because of its superiority over the slow freezing method, in terms of having a better oocyte survival rate, fertilization rate, and development of embryo in vitro.

Cobo et al.,[8] published a prospective randomized study in 2016 which evaluated and compared the outcome off vitrification using Cryotop method, in an oocyte donation program with fresh oocytes coming from the same stimulated cycle. Cobo et al., observed that in both groups there was no significant difference in fertilization rates, day 2 cleavage rates, and blastocyst formation in both groups. Therefore, with the use of vitrification technology for oocyte donation programs, excellent clinical outcomes can be achieved. This study also indicates a high potential for setting up oocyte banks. It has been seen that there is a rapid increase in the number of live births over the past decade with cryopreserved oocytes. However there are concerns regarding the obstetric and perinatal outcomes. Besides this, there is also concern regarding long term development evaluation of the infants. This concern can be attributed to the possible increase in risk of chromosomal abnormalities in children born through this technique due to alteration meiotic spindle integrity. However, studies are reassuring regarding this concern.

A study published in 2009[9] analyzed 58 reports from 1986 to 2008 which included 936 live births (308 from slow freezing, 616 from vitrification and 12 from both methods). The study came to a conclusion that 1.3% of the births had anomalies, which is comparable to the prevalence of major birth defects with spontaneous conception which is 0.2–2%.

However, there is limited data available and the question still remains to be addressed whether oocyte vitrification can ensure adequate safety especially for long term development of infants.

CONCERNS RELATED TO OOCYTE CRYOPRESERVATION

Besides obstetric and long term effect on infants, there are other concerns regarding frozen oocytes. One of the primary concerns is the undesirable biological and metabolic changes which occur in the ooplasm following storage in LN. However it is believed that at –192°C, all biological activities of the cell cease completely. Therefore in theory, storage in LN is relatively safe.[10-12]

Another concern is contamination during the open vitrification method. There can be contamination from bacteria and fungi during the storage in direct contact with LN. However there has been no observation of contamination in reproductive tissues from this technique.[13]

PROS AND CONS OF OOCYTE CRYOPRESERVATION

It has been observed that there is a high pregnancy and implantation rate post oocyte cryopreservation. Thus it is an efficient treatment protocol in reproductive medicine. With the era of oocyte cryopreservation, the oocyte donor program has become much easier. There is no need for the synchronization of donor and recipient cycles and therefor reducing the expenditure as well as the inconvenience. In addition to this, any surplus oocytes that are retrieved are not lost. Most importantly, oocyte banking empowers women by preserving their fertility against threat of age or disease.

However the option of oocyte freezing may provide false hope to women/couples who are planning on delaying their pregnancy. Another drawback of oocyte cryopreservation is that the patient needs to go through a surgical procedure for oocyte retrieval. Besides this, the oocytes need to undergo ICSI for fertilization.[14]

FACTORS AFFECTING OUTCOMES OF OOCYTE CRYOPRESERVATION

Oocyte survival post freezing can be affected by several factors such as:

- Stage of maturation
- Size and quality of oocytes
- Biophysical factors from the procedure used
- Stimulation protocols
- Freezing methods
- Devices.

Patient related factors are:

- Age
- Cause of fertility (endometriosis)
- Donor/non-donor cycle
- Number of oocytes available.[15]

RECOMMENDATIONS OF ASRM FOR OOCYTE CRYOPRESERVATION

The practice committee of the ASRM has suggested that there is a requirement for long term studies on congenital anomalies and health risks that may be associated with oocyte cryopreservation. As stated in ASRM-SART guideline "there are not yet sufficient data to recommend oocyte cryopreservation for the sole purpose of circumventing reproductive aging in healthy women because there are no data to support the safety, efficacy, ethics, emotional risks, and cost-effectiveness of oocyte cryopreservation for this indication and more widespread clinic-specific data on the safety and efficacy of oocyte cryopreservation in this population are needed before universal donor oocyte banking can be recommended".[2]

Following recommendations are given by ASRM in collaboration with the SART:[2]

- In patients facing infertility because chemo or other therapies which may affect the gonads, oocyte cryopreservation is advocated with proper counseling (Level B).
- Before oocyte banking can be advocated, there needs to be a larger clinic-specific data on the efficiency as well as safety of oocyte freezing in oocyte donors (Level B).
- Adequate information to suggest oocyte cryopreservation for the sole reason of preventing reproductive ageing in healthy women (Level B).
- More information is required before this technique ought to be utilized routinely in lieu of embryo cryopreservation (Level B).

CONCLUSION

There have been major advances in oocyte freezing over the last few years. Vitrification itself has progressed a lot and has opened a brand new avenue in reproductive medicine. Previously the only indication for cryopreservation was various premalignant or malignant conditions. But now the role of vitrification has expanded to newer horizons. With vitrification gaining popularity, oocyte cryopreservation is a viable alternative to freezing embryos. With proven results of vitrification, oocyte banking will play an integral role in infertility treatments.

REFERENCES

1. Parmegiani L, Cognigni GE, Bernardi S, et al. Freezing within 2 h from oocyte retrieval increases the efficiency of human oocyte cryopreservation when using a slow freezing/rapid

thawing protocol with high sucrose concentration. Hum Reprod. 2008;23:1771-7.
2. Practice committee of American society of reproductive medicine, Society for Assisted Reproductive Technology. Mature Oocyte Cryopresrevation: a guideline. Fertil Steril. 2013;99:37-43.
3. Zacà C, Borini A. The human oocyte: controlled rate-cooling. In Gardner DK, Weissman A, Howles CM, Shoham Z (Eds). Textbook of Assisted Reproductive Techniques, 5th edition. Florida: CRC Press; 2017. pp.269-70.
4. Glujovsky D, Riestra B, Sueldo C, et al. Vitrification versus slow freezing for women undergoing oocyte cryopreservation. Cochrane Database Syst Rev. 2014;(9):CD010047.
5. Chian RC, Wang Y, Li YR. Oocyte vitrification: advances, progress and future goals. J Assist Reprod Genet. 2014;31: 411-20.
6. Lockwood GM. Social egg freezing: the prospect of reproductive 'immortality' or a dangerous delusion? Reprod Biomed Online. 2011;23:334-40.
7. HD Pai, Palshetkar N, Talreja D, et al. Clinical Perspective to Oocyte Cryopreservation. Acta Sci Med Sci. 2017;1:38-40.
8. Cobo A, García-Velasco JA, Coello A. Oocyte vitrification as an efficient option for elective fertility preservation. Fertil Steril. 2016;105:755-64.
9. Noyes N, Porcu E, Borini A. Over 900 oocyte cryopreservation babies born with no apparent increase in congenital anomalies. Reprod Biomed Online. 2009;18:769-76.
10. Whittingham DG, Lyon MF, Glenister PH. Long-term storage of mouse embryos at -196 degrees C: the effect of background radiation. Genet Res. 1977;29:171-81.
11. Glenister PH, Whittingham DG, Lyon MF. Further studies on the effect of radiation during the storage of frozen 8-cell mouse embryos at –196 degrees C. J Reprod Fertil. 1984;70:229-34.
12. Glenister PH, Lyon MF. Long-term storage of eight-cell mouse embryos at - 196 degrees C. J In Vitro Fert Embryo Transf. 1986;3:20-7.
13. Yan J, Suzuki J, Yu XM, et al. Effects of duration of cryo-storage of mouse oocytes on cryo-survival, fertilization and embryonic development following vitrification. J Assist Reprod Genet. 2011;28:643-9.
14. Pai HD, Palshetkar N, Talreja D, et al. Oocyte Cryopreservation. Ann Reprod Med Treat. 2017;2:1016.
15. Cil AP, Seli E. Current trends and progress in clinical applications of oocyte cryopreservation. Curr Opin Obstet Gynecol. 2013;25:247-54.

Ovarian Tissue Freezing

69

Pankaj Talwar, Pooja Awasthi

INTRODUCTION

Non-renewable ovarian reserve of females restricts their freedom to motherhood. Ovarian reserve which at fetal mid-gestational period is around 6–8 million, reduces to 1–2 million at birth and further falls to 300,000 by the onset of puberty and further drops to 25,000 by the age of 37–38 years and are left with only 1,000 or less by the stage of menopause.

The rate of cure of numerous diseases that strike children and young adults, have improved drastically due to the advancements in various fields of medical science and technology. Increased survival rate post-cancer treatment especially, in young women impacts the ovarian reserve leading to premature ovarian failure (POF) and premature ovarian insufficiency (POI). However, to deal with this iatrogenic infertility, various fertility preservation techniques like oophoropexy, assisted reproductive treatment (ART), oocyte freezing, in vitro maturation and follicle culture are available to the reproductive biologists. Cryopreservation of the ovarian cortex is a technique which facilitates the preservation of gonadal function in cancer patients of reproductive ages. Associated risk of cancer therapy including radiotherapy and chemotherapy have detrimental effects on the reproductive health.

HISTORICAL BACKGROUND

Number of cancer patients are on increasing side according to National Cancer Registry of India. Data shows that every year number is increasing about 9.79 lakhs to 11.4 lakhs in 10 years (2010–2020).

Hovatta did the initial work in ovarian tissue cryopreservation on humans. He validated that human ovary is cryo-resistant to frozen-thaw protocol, because the primordial follicles present in cortex are immature, dormant, less differentiated and without zona. Lack of zona and cortical granule make these immature oocytes tolerant to cryoprotectant. Time line contains the name of scientist with their scientific presentations **(Flowchart 1)**.

INDICATION FOR OVARIAN TISSUE CRYOPRESERVATION

Ovarian tissue cryopreservation is an option for patients who require immediate gonadotoxic treatment for aggressive malignancies when there is insufficient time to allow the woman to undergo ovulation induction, oocyte retrieval, and cryopreservation of oocytes and/or embryos. The only option available for fertility preservation in prepubertal girls or in women who have hormone-sensitive malignancies is ovarian tissue cryopreservation. Decrease in both antral follicle count (AFC) and ovarian volume with chemotherapy have been documented by Andersen et al. Rapid fall in AMH and inhibin B were also reported by them during chemotherapy although E2 levels remains same **(Flowchart 2)**.

RECOMMENDED GUIDELINES FOR OVARIAN TISSUE BANKING

- Age (<37).
- Status of the ovarian reserve and function (anti-Mullerian hormone (AMH) level, AFC, premenopausal by follicle stimulating hormone (FSH)).

Flowchart 1: Time line.

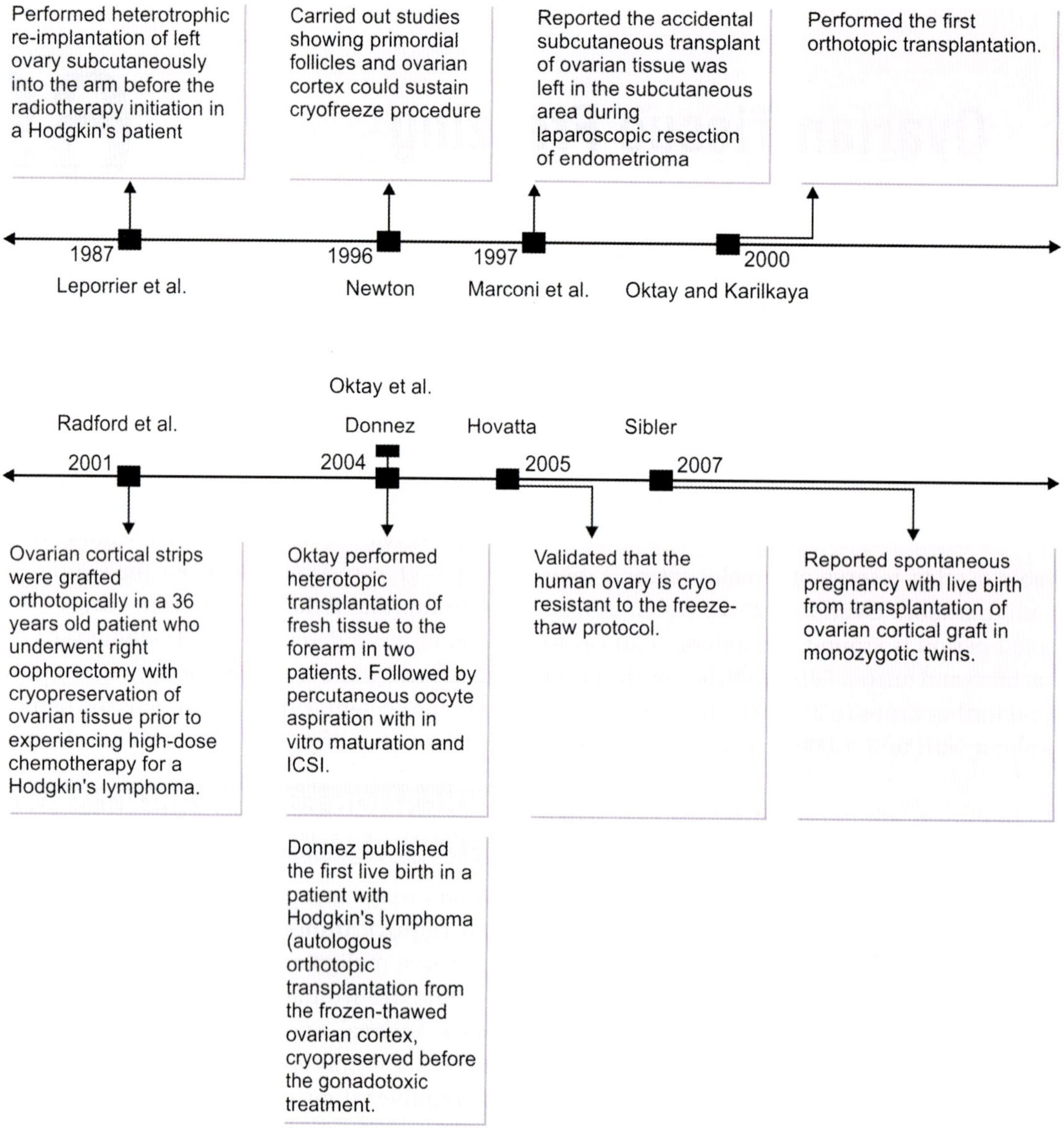

- Detailed discussion between oncologist and patient about cancer treatment plan and prognosis.
- Informed consent from the adult patients should be taken.
- Ovarian transposition: Ovarian transposition (oophoropexy) can be offered when pelvic radiation is performed as cancer treatment.
- Oocyte cryopreservation should be performed when embryo cryopreservation is not possible.
- The experimental nature and potential risks of cancer cell transmission should be explained to the patient.
- Through patient counseling.
- Desire to have children in future (before 50).
- High risk of POF.
- Prepubertal girls, who do not have any other option.
- When embryo and oocyte freezing is not indicated (sensitive to hormonal stimulation and ATR is not allowed).

OVARIAN DAMAGE DUE TO CANCER TREATMENT

At any age, ovarian follicles are vulnerable to agents that lead to deoxyribonucleic acid (DNA) damage, including

Flowchart 2: Time line contains the name of scientist with their scientific presentations.

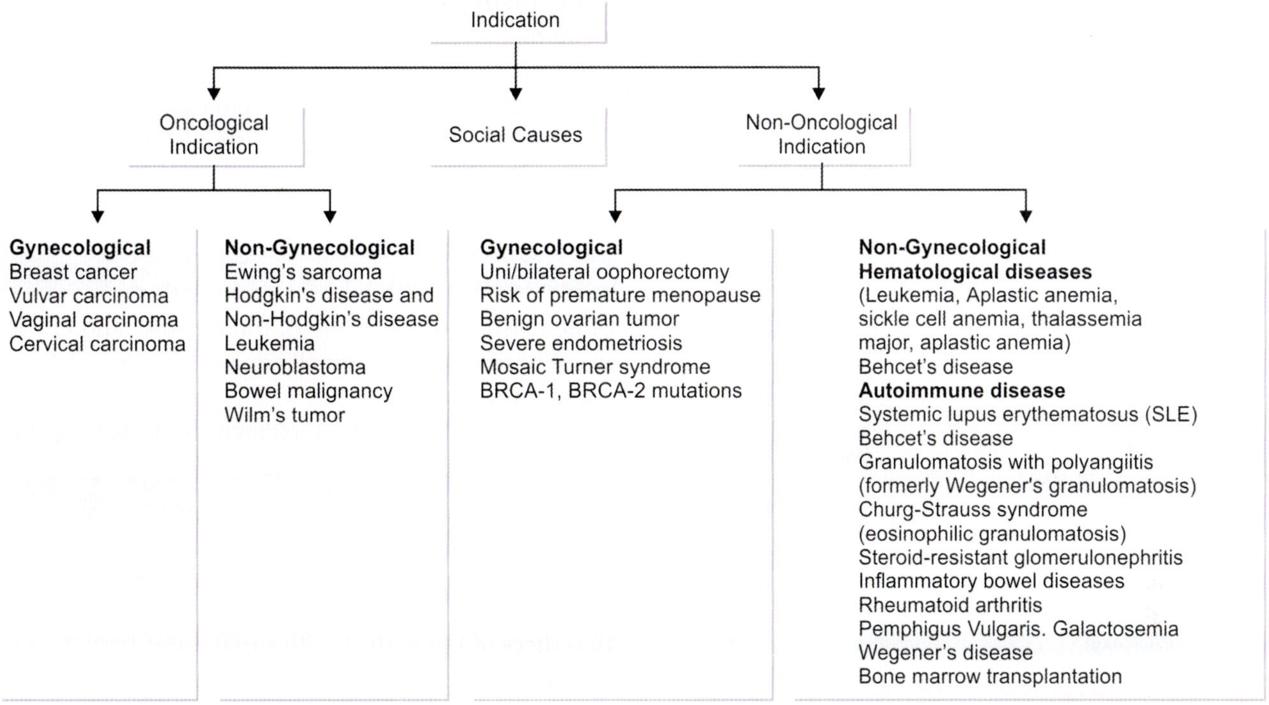

ionizing radiation and chemotherapy. Such anticancer treatments affect the ovarian follicle reserve in a dose-dependent manner, and can eventually cause amenorrhea and premature ovarian failure.

RADIOTHERAPY AND OVARIAN DAMAGE

Cancer patients, who are scheduled to undergo abdominal, pelvic, and total body irradiation is at risk for infertility, reduced gonadal age, and premature ovarian failure due to the loss of primordial follicles. Elderly women are at greater risk of ovarian failure as the degree of ovarian damage is determined by the total irradiation dose, location, fractionation schedule, and age at the time of treatment **(Table 1)**. Radio sensitivity of the human ovary that leads to the loss of 50% of primordial follicles (LD50) is estimated to be 2 Gy.

CHEMOTHERAPY AND OVARIAN DAMAGE

Most of the drugs used in chemotherapy work in a more or less similar fashion, that is, creating DNA cross-links, which in turn cause DNA breaks, eventually triggering apoptosis. Only the taxanes are microtubule-stabilizing agents, and different from DNA-damaging drugs **(Flowchart 3)**.[28-32]

Table 1: Age-related effective sterilizing dose (ESD)

Age	*Effective sterilizing dose*
At birth	20.3 Gy
At 10 years	18.4 Gy
At 20 years	16.5 Gy
At 30 years	14.3 Gy

TECHNIQUES OF OVARIAN TISSUE CRYOPRESERVATION

Follicular viability and integrity of tissue compartments and cell-to-cell contacts must be indemnified by the cryopreservation techniques **(Table 2)** Thus, studies investigating the most favorable cooling rates and dehydration times have been conducted. It is now well established that for obtaining satisfactory results, adequate penetration of cryoprotectant through the stroma and granulosa cells to the oocytes is required. Choosing optimal freezing must minimize ice-crystal formation.

COLLECTION OF OVARIAN TISSUE

Early follicular phase is the best time for the tissue collection in order to avoid large ovarian follicles/cyst or corpus luteum. Being hyper vascular and space occupying, these causes anatomic distortion. The tissues should be

Flowchart 3: Summarizes the most and less toxic effect of chemotherapeutic drugs.

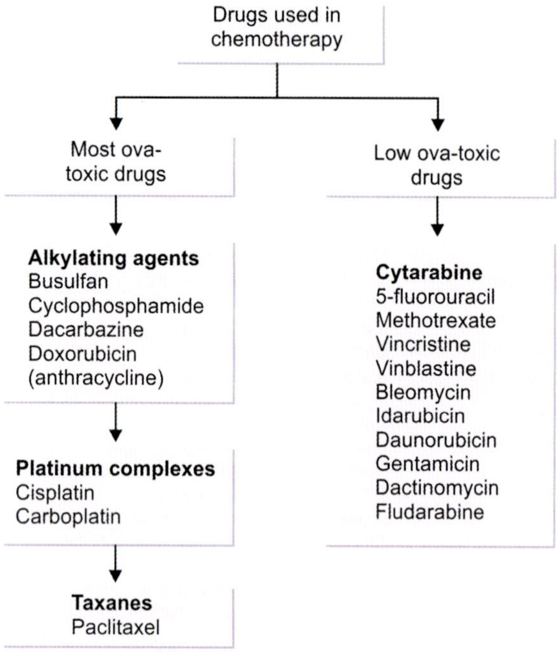

transported to the laboratory on ice, in a 4-(2-hydroxyethyl)-1-piperazineethane-sulfonic acid (HEPES)-buffered medium.

Ovarian tissue is collected by laparoscopy under general anesthesia since it has better and early recovery. Electrocoagulation of the ovary should be avoided as it can lead to thermal damage to primordial follicles in the ovarian cortex.

CRYOPROTECTANT PREPARATION

Dimethylsulphoxide (DMSO), propanediol and ethylene glycol-based solutions are all equally effective for human ovarian tissue freezing.

We do not add protein supplement due to its antigenicity.

PREPARATION OF REQUIRED CRYOPROTECTANTS (TABLE 3)

Thickness of Cortical Slices

Thin slices of 1 mm, thick with surface area from 2 × 2 mm to 5 × 5 mm, tissue is preferred to facilitate equilibration of the cryoprotectant.[25,34,36]

Table 2: Summarizes the various fertility preservation methods in females with cancer fertility preservation techniques in females with cancer[25]

Fertility preservation techniques	***Requirement of ovarian stimulation***	***Does the procedure delay the definitive cancer therapy***	***Requirement of the male partner***	***Success rates***	***Special considerations***
Use of long activity of GnRH agonist	Does not require	Does not delay	Not required	Not documented	Controversial
Oocyte cryopreservation	Required	Yes, it delays	Not required	Pregnancy rate per cycle of 50.2% or per embryo transfer 55.4%	Nil
Embryo freezing	Required	Yes, it delays (advent)	Yes	Cumulative pregnancy rate of 66% among women with cancer	Nil
In vitro maturation	Does not require	Does not delay	Not required	Not documented	Nil
Ovarian cortex cryopreservation	Does not require	Does not delay	Not required	Pregnancy rate of 25% among women with cancer	No indication when high risk of ovarian metastases

Table 3: Preparation of required cryoprotectants.

1. To DMSO 1.06 mL, Sucrose 0. 1M solution 1 mL and patients serum 1 mL add 6.94 mL of bicarbonate media to a final volume of 10 mL.
2. This is then filter-sterilized through a 0.22 µm filter and cocktail is refrigerated.
3. Pour 4 mL of cryoprotective solution in 60 mm dish and place it on the ice at least 30 min so that the solution is ice-cooled before the specimen is put in it for equilibration.
4. Put 1 mL of the solution in cryovial and ice cool it.

HISTOLOGICAL ANALYSIS

Randomly chosen one representative sample of the ovarian cortex, for every patient, should be sent for histopathological examination. The specimens should be fixed in formaldehyde and embedded in paraffin.

Sections (5 μm) are cut perpendicularly to the ovarian surface and stained with hematoxylin-eosin. All follicles are systematically counted. Serial sections are useful for follicle classification.

FREEZING PROTOCOLS (FLOWCHART 4 TO 7)

Flowchart 4

Slow freezing (equilibration procedure)

↓

Tissue slices of 1 mm thickness should be placed in the ice-cold Cryoprotectant solution

↓

Place the slices in 60 mm falcon dish filled with cold cryoprotectant solution

↓

Every 5–10 min swirl the dish so that all pieces become exposed to the cryoprotectant

↓

After 15–20 minutes takes out the cortical slices and immerses them in the pre-cooled cryoprotectant solution in the vials
The cryo-vials must be labeled before freezing commences

↓

Keep the cryo-vials on the ice for 30–45 minutes on the ice and wait

↓

Cooling program and Seeding protocol
Meanwhile, run ovarian tissue freezing program on the cryologic machine. Initially cooling at a rate of 2°C per min to -7°C

↓

After 10 minutes of soakage of the specimen in the cryo chamber at -7°C, manually seed the vials using a cotton wick or pair of pre-cooled forceps

↓

After the ice formation at the meniscus is confirmed put back the cryo-vials in the chamber immediately.
The further cooling rate should be 0.3°C/ min to - 40 °C

↓

Now cooling at a faster rate of 10°C/Min to -140°C and hold for 10 min. The vials can be plunged into liquid nitrogen, and placed on labeled canes for storage

Flowchart 5:

Thawing (slow freezing)

↓

The cryo-vials are removed from the liquid nitrogen
Thaw the vials at room temperature for 30 seconds

↓

The cryo-vials are removed from the liquid nitrogen
Thaw the vials at room temperature for 30 seconds

↓

Wash tissue in progressively lower concentrations of sucrose

↓

Perform the last wash in 10% autologous serum

↓

Cortex is ready for transplantation

Flowchart 6

Vitrification

↓

Ultra-thin slices of the tissue are required for the cryopreservation, as well as rapid revascularization after grafting.

↓

Bring ES and VS to room temperature (25~27°C). Pour the full contents of ES vial (15 mL) into a 60 mm dish.

↓

Place the extracted tissue on the dish and wait for 25 minutes

↓

Pour the full contents of VS vial (15 mL) into a 60-mm dish
Transfer the tissue in ES to the surface of VS using tweezers

↓

Wait for 15 minutes

↓

After the equilibration to VS, place the tissue on the Cryo M device.
Plunge the Cryo M device into fresh liquid nitrogen quickly.

↓

Check whether the tissue is translucent
Insert the Cryo M device into the cap and twist it
Make sure if it is completely sealed

↓

The cortical bits equilibrate in the media for 5 min each and then loaded on the Cryo device and then

Source: Kitazato ovarian cortex Vitrification manual

Flowchart 7

Warming (vitrification)

↓

Take out the tissue from liquid nitrogen, quickly immerse it into Thawing Solution warmed to 37°C within 1 second

↓

Leave the tissue in Thawing solutions for 1 minute after immersing

↓

Pour the DS (15 mL) into a 60 mm dish,
Pour the TS with the tissue into a 90-mm dish

↓

Transfer the tissue in TS to DS using tweezers.
Wait for 3 minutes

↓

Pour the WS1 (15 mL) and WS2 (15 ml) into 60 mm dishes
Do this preparation while waiting for dilution is done

↓

Transfer the tissue from DS to WS1. Wait for 5 minutes

↓

Transfer the tissue in WS1 to WS2. Wait for 5 minutes

↓

After 5 minutes in WS2, immediately transplant or culture the tissues

Note: Refer to Related Picture for Vitrification in Appendix 1
Source: Kitazato ovarian cortex Vitrification manual

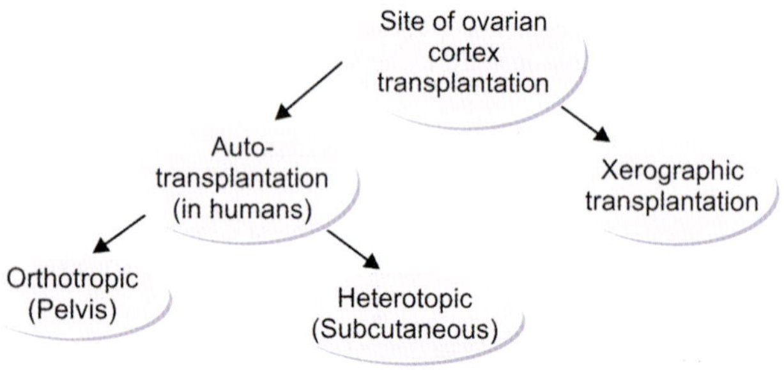

Fig. 1: Transplantation.

TRANSPLANTATION

Each site has distinct advantages and disadvantages. Although both orthotopic and heterotopic sites for transplantation of frozen-thawed ovarian tissue were studied but the remaining menopausal ovary has been the popular site (in orthotopic studies) **(Fig. 1)**.

Ovarian function and spontaneous pregnancy in a 29-year-old female, previously treated with bone marrow transplantation were reported in 2006 by Demeestere I et al., after ovarian tissue transplantation at combined heterotopic and orthotopic sites.

The primary objective of ovarian tissue storage is to re-implant a few thawed cortical strips into the patient (i.e. auto-transplantation) once the patient has completed cancer treatment, is disease free, and desires pregnancy. Re-implantation of frozen-thawed ovarian tissue in the pelvic cavity is usually carried out by laparoscopy. The surgical technique is contingent on the presence (or not) of at least one ovary.

A female, menopausal for 2.5 years, resulted in spontaneous pregnancy and live birth after 3 months of autologous heterotopic transplantation of ovarian tissue to a suprapubic site. It has also been demonstrated in some patients that OTC during childhood was feasible and safe.

Nevertheless, in that case, left oophorectomy should be performed because of the small size of the ovaries. Otherwise, in adults, 4–5 ovarian cortical biopsies (1 cm L, 0.5 mm W, 1.5 mm T) are usually taken.

There are mainly two techniques of orthotopic re-implantation. If at least one ovary is present, slices of thawed ovarian tissue are either fixed on the decorticated medullaor pushed by a small incision under the cortical capsule. If the ovary is absent, the ovarian pieces could be placed in a peritoneal window. The advantages of ovarian tissue re-implantation at orthotopic sites are:

- Natural conception; and
- The favorable condition for follicular development (oxygenation, pressure, the presence of peritoneal fluid).

OUTCOMES OF OVARIAN TISSUE GRAFTING (TABLE 4)

Table 4: Outcomes of ovarian tissue grafting.

Scientist name	***Year***	***Study***
	Restoration of ovarian activity	
Oktay and Karlikaya	2000	Documented orthotopic transplantation of ovarian tissue resulted in follicular development in response to menopausal gonadotropin stimulation
Oktay et al.	2004	Reported heterotopic transplantation of the ovarian cortex to the forearm, after stimulation with gonadotropins, yields three oocytes
Dunlop et al.	2016	Reported the re-implantation of cryopreserved ovarian cortex resulting in restoration of ovarian function, natural conception and successful pregnancy after hematopoietic

Contd...

Contd...

Scientist name	***Year***	***Study***
		stem cell transplantation for Wilms' tumor in a 32-year-old woman, whose ovarian cortex was preserved 10 years before treatment of a high dose of chemotherapy. The patient underwent laparoscopic orthotropic transplantation of cryopreserved ovarian cortex to the original site of biopsy, on the left ovary. She ovulated 15 and 29 weeks post re-implantation with anti-Mullerian hormone (AMH) detectable and conceived naturally following the second ovulation and gave birth to a healthy male infant
	Live birth	
Roux et al.	2010	Reported the live birth after ovarian tissue autograft in a patient with sickle cell anemia disease treated by allogeneic bone marrow transplantation. This case opens up the new perspective in case of non-malignant diseases
Muller	2012	Reported first live birth in Germany from re-transplantation of cryopreserved ovarian tissue in January 2012
Revelli et al.	2013	Reported the live birth after orthopic grafting of the autologous cryopreserved ovarian issue and spontaneous conception in Italy
Prasath et al.	2014	Reported first pregnancy and live birth achieved in 2014 from cryopreserved embryos obtained from in vitro matured oocyte after oophorectomy in an ovarian cancer patient
Jensen et al.	2017	Reported approximately 86 live birth and 9 ongoing pregnancies 95 children have been born or will get birth in the near future worldwide in women transplanted with frozen-thawed ovarian tissue
	Animal studies	
Godsen et al.	1994	Reported the live births of young animals after autographic frozen-thawed ovarian tissue in sheep
Bruno sale	2002	Documented four pregnancies (two singleton and two twin) after transplantation (autografting) of frozen-thawed hemiovary into the hilum of previously removed ovary before grafting (three of six lambs died just after birth)
Lillu et al.	2008	Showed that restoration of fertility is possible in mice after orthotopic grafting of frozen-thawed ovarian tissue

Contd...

FUTURE OF OVARIAN CORTEX PRESERVATION

The successful live births after transplant from both orthotopic and heterotopic sites along with newer methods of in vitro maturation (IVM), culture of primordial follicles and the chances of in vitro activation (IVA) suggests more fertility alternatives for many girls and women. Several pregnancies and few live births have also documented through Vitrification of ovarian tissue as it is a more cost-effective technique with minimal tissue injury. Further, various methods of transplantation have demonstrated important advancements in fertility preservation like transplantation via the artificial ovary with an extracellular tissue matrix (ECTM) scaffolding, as well as the effects of sphingosine-1-phosphate (SIP) and a vascular endothelial growth factor (VEGF) and fibrin modified with heparin-binding peptide (HBP), heparin.

Primordial follicles are remarkably less vulnerable to cryo-injury compared to oocytes due to: (a) smaller size, (b) slow metabolic rates, (c) lack of the zona.

Currently practiced approaches for cryopreservation of ovarian tissues are:

- Ovarian cortical strips cryopreservation.
- Whole ovary cryopreservation.
- IVM.
- Follicle culture.

Whole Ovary Cryopreservation

Recently, whole ovary cryopreservation using multi-gradient freezing device has been reported. With the help of this device unidirectional solidification has been achieve by slowly decreasing the temperature of freezing tubes to 40°C by 0.3°C/min.

After thawing, all ovaries showed normal histologic architecture and follicle counts comparable to the contralateral ovaries which were not frozen.

While these outcomes are encouraging, confirmed restoration of fertility by whole ovary transplantation in human is yet to be reported. Although, the risk of reintroduction of malignancy is also associated with this technique.

In Vitro Maturation

The combination of OTC with immature oocyte collection from the tissue followed by oocyte vitrification via IVM represents another promising approach to fertility preservation in young women with cancer. Abir R, Grynberg M et al. and Prasath reported successful live births through IVM.

Follicular Culture

Apart from ovarian tissue cryopreservation, follicle culture can also be considered as the promising method in preserving fertility.

- Especially for young patients without partners; or
- Patients who cannot undergo ovarian stimulation for oocyte/embryo cryopreservation; and
- Patients for whom the risk for reintroduction of malignant cells precludes transplantation.

CONCLUSION

In case of malignancy, ovarian tissue freezing can be the most appropriate fertility preservation method as cryopreservation of primordial follicles within the cortex have several advantages over oocyte and embryo freezing. Thus, delay in cancer treatment can be avoided. Embryo and oocyte cryopreservation are first-line FP methods in post-pubertal women; however, they have their limitations. Ovarian tissue cryopreservation (OTC) is a controlled ovarian stimulation (COS) independent experimental technique and has a wider application and advantages of keeping the fertility window open for a long time, and it also allows immediate cancer treatment and is currently the only FP option in pediatric patients and hormone-dependent diseases.

Appendix 1

Vitrification

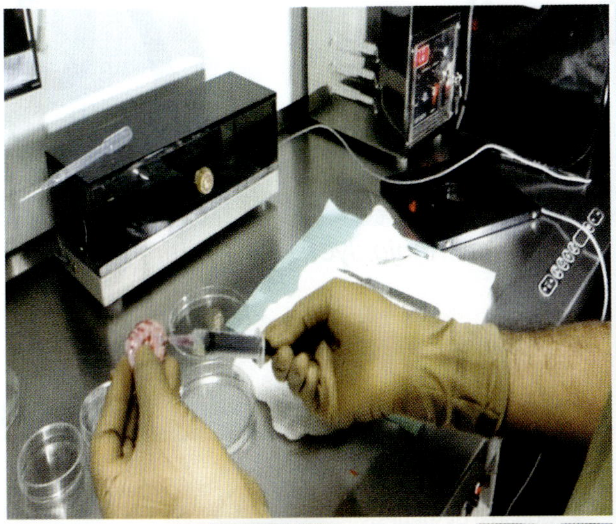
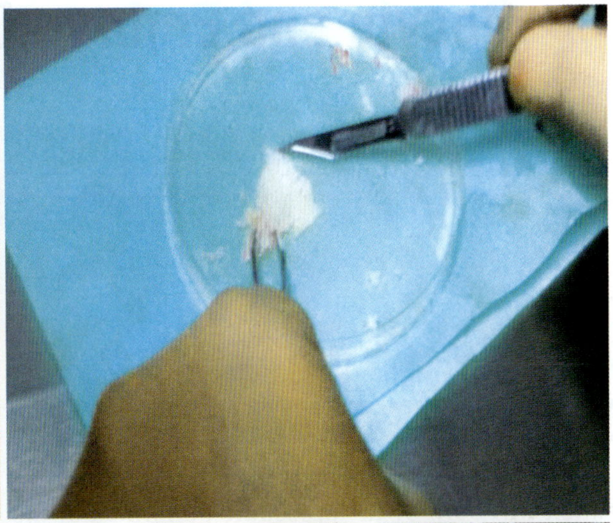
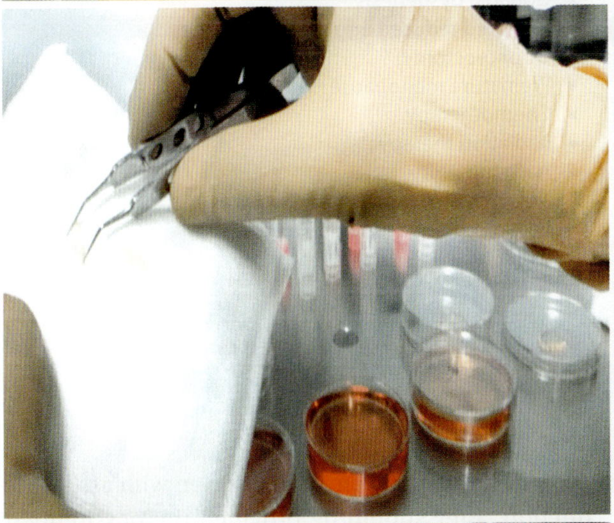
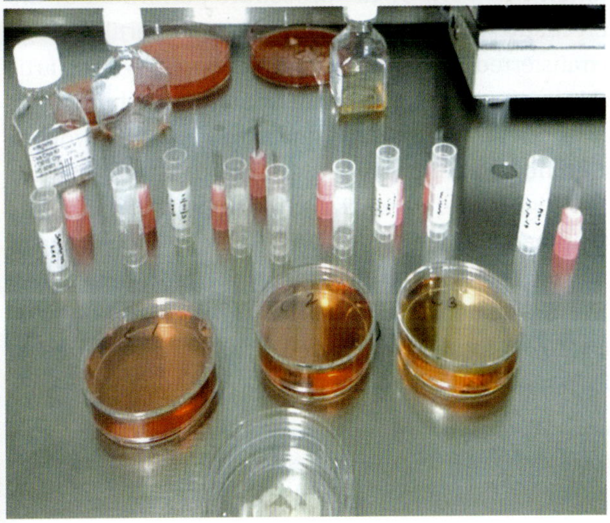
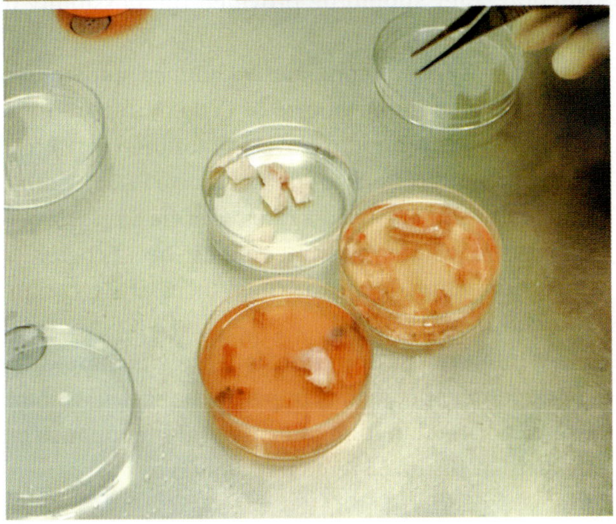

Oocyte and Embryo Donation

70

Maninder Ahuja, Jyoti Malik, Pritimala Gangnurde

HISTORY

In the year 1984, on 3rd February, the first child from egg donation was born by the procedure performed at the UCLA Medical Center in Harbor. Here the fertilized egg was transferred from a woman who has conceived by artificial insemination to a recipient by uterine washing.[1,2]

This scientific procedure opened avenues for women who could not conceive due to ovarian failure or who were at high risk of transmission of genetic disorders. This development formed the technical basis for clinical use of human egg and embryo donation, which has evolved over the years. The oocyte and embryo donation accounts for almost 18% of the births registered in the in vitro fertilization (IVF) in the United States.[3,4]

Box 1: Indications of oocyte donation.

- Congenital absence of eggs
- Turner's syndrome
- Gonadal dysgenesis
- Acquired reduced egg quantity/quality
- Oophorectomy
- Premature menopause
- Chemotherapy
- Radiation therapy
- Autoimmunity
- Advanced maternal age
- Compromised ovarian reserve
- Others
- Disease of X-sex linkage
- Repetitive fertilization or pregnancy failure
- Ovaries inaccessible for egg retrieval

INDICATION FOR THE DONATION OF OOCYTES AND EMBRYOS

Premature Ovarian Failure

Premature ovarian failure is the primary indication for use of donor oocyte, which could be either, primary or secondary. The causes of early ovarian failure where oocyte donation is indicated include; surgical ovariectomy, irreversible gonadal damage after chemotherapy or radiotherapy, Turner's syndrome and other chromosomal disorders that cause gonadal dysgenesis.

Oocyte donation also can be chosen, if there is a risk of transmission of a genetic disease and carrier status of both partners is known **(Box 1)**.

Women having significantly reduced ovarian reserve need to be informed about their limited conception possibilities using their gametes even with assisted reproduction. They should be provided the possibility of egg donation or adoption.[5]

A retrospective comparative clinical study compared the efficacy of donor oocyte in IVF-embryo transfer (ET) patients with premature ovarian failure (POF) to those with other indications for donor oocyte IVF-ET (non POF) and found similar success rates. (Fertile Steril 1996, 65) In about 1% of women early menopause occurs before age 40 and oocyte donation is the most successful technique for these women.[6]

While oocyte donation is widely accepted for the production of pregnancy in perimenopausal women,[7] the use of oocyte donation after natural menopause among the ages of 45 and 55 remains debatable.

Turner's Syndrome

There is a high risk of miscarriage and trisomy 21 in children of women suffering from Turner syndrome, who had spontaneous conception.[8,9]

In women with Turner syndrome, pregnancy rate (PR) after oocyte donation was comparable to those of women with other causes of primary ovarian failure.[10]

An observational study stated a 46% clinical pregnancy rate for the transfer of fresh embryos among women, similar to rates among oocyte recipients with primary impairment in general. But in these cases, the rate of miscarriage was 40% high. The risk of cardiovascular complications, hypertension and preeclampsia was also higher in these women. Therefore, a careful evaluation is suggested before and during pregnancy.[11]

Ovarian Failure after Chemotherapy or Radiotherapy

Cryopreservation of oocytes still has limited success. Embryo cryopreservation remains the option chosen with oocyte donation followed by IVF in women with ovarian failure after cancer treatment.[12]

In Vitro Fertilization Failure

Egg donation is recommended in some cases of repeated failures of fertilization, in which the quality of the oocytes is compromised. In an observational study (n = 32 couples, 119 cycles) in women with previously failed IVF treatment, a pregnancy rate of 24.5% per cycle was reported after oocyte donation.[13]

Genetic Disorders

The use of donor oocytes can be successfully used in the prevention of genetic hereditary diseases.[14]

SCREENING OF OOCYTE DONORS

Oocyte donors are chosen from assisted reproductive technology (ART) banks based on their profile or from clinical database. The donors may also be considered by the treating doctor of infertile couple. After being chosen, the donor undergoes the following screenings:

- *Medical:* Pelvic examination, ultrasonography (USG) (uterine and ovarian assessment for follicles), blood investigations for baseline ovarian hormone levels, biochemical tests and test for infectious ailments

Table 1: Genetic screening form for oocyte donors.

Pregnancy history		
Ethnic background (cystic fibrosis, sickle cell anemia)		
Family genetic history in self/mother/father/siblings		
Familial conditions	***Malformations***	***Mendelian disorder***
High blood pressure	Cleft lip/palate	Color blindness
Heart disease	Heart defect	Cystic fibrosis
Deafness, blindness	Club foot	Hemophilia
Arthritis	Spina bifida	Muscular dystrophy
Juvenile diabetes		Sickle cell anemia
Epilepsy		Glaucoma
Depression		Muscular dystrophy
Alzheimer's		

- *Genetic:* To rule out any mutation (cystic fibrosis) **(Table 1)**
- Psychological assessment by a psychologist.

11% of voluntary oocyte donors were not appropriate for donation due to genetic test results as reported in a cross-sectional study (n = 73). Mutations in cystic fibrosis were identified in 7%, abnormal karyotype in 3.5% and autosomal dominant skeletal dysplasia in 1.4%.[15]

In an analysis of 98 female donors and 1,609 male donors, 2% of female donors were excluded after the discussion on genetic selection and 2% after the karyotype.[16]

Higher pregnancy success rates for recipients were obtained where oocyte donors were young, signifying that age should be a critical factor in selecting potential donors. The pregnancy success rate is 59.1% for donors aged 20–22 years, 45.9% for 26–28 years and 30.9% for 32–34 years.[17]

Hence proved that oocyte donation gives pregnancy rates in older women as good as in younger women. Success of ART depends on the age of the egg donor rather than age of recipient **(Box 2)**.

A retrospective study analyzed 445 donor cycles for the number of recovered oocytes, gravidity, parity, donor age and pregnancy out come in recipients. Pregnancy and prior parity were not associated with successful pregnancy in recipients. The number of oocytes recovered is positively correlated with pregnancy, but the age of the ovum donor is a significant predictor of pregnancy success.[17]

In the sisters of patients with premature ovarian failure (POF), a decreased ovarian response to the stimulation of

Box 2: Tests for screening of egg donor.

- Hormonal tests: AMH, TSH, FSH, LH, E2
- Complete blood count with platelets
- Blood type
- Hepatitis screen
- VDRL
- HIV-1,HTLV-1
- Cervical cultures for *Gonorrhea* and *Chlamydia*
- PAP smear
- Transvaginal ultrasound of pelvis and AFC count
- Appropriate genetic tests

(AFC: antral follicle count; AMH: anti-Müllerian hormone; E2: estradiol; FSH: follicle stimulating hormone; HTLV-1: human T-lymphotropic virus-1; LH: luteinizing hormone; PAP: papanicolaou; TSH: thyroid stimulating hormone; VDRL: venereal disease research laboratory)

Box 3: Tests for screening of oocyte recipients.

- CBC, ABO Rh, LFT, KFT, glucose tolerance test (GTT) urine analysis and C/S
- TSH, serum cholesterol, lipid profile
- Hepatitis and Rubella screen
- HIV, VDRL, HBs
- Transvaginal ultrasound (TVS)
- ECG, Chest X-ray, 2D-echo (if age is more than 40)
- Mammogram
- PAP, Cervical culture for *Gonorrhea* and *Chlamydia*
- Uterine cavity evaluation (by hysteroscopy)

(CBC: complete blood count; HBs: hemoglobin; LFT: liver function test; KFT: kidney function test; TSH: thyroid-stimulating hormone; PAP: papanicolaou; VDRL: venereal disease research laboratory)

gonadotropin and a higher rate of cancellation were found although implantation rates and PR of the derived embryos were similar to anonymous donors. It is recommended to advise that sisters of women with POF may not be ideal egg donors.[18]

According to the recent American Society for Reproductive Medicine (ASRM) guidelines, embryos must be quarantined for a minimum period of 6 months before potential donors are evaluated and analyzed or submitted to a new test, as indicated in the documentation of the negative results. Medical and genetic history must be taken from embryo donors.

In cases of unavailability of donors for assessment or refusal for undergoing testing, embryo should not be rejected as suggested by Food and Drug Administration (FDA). But in such instances, the supplementary documentation needs to be done with proper leveling like: "*Not evaluated for infectious substances and Warning: Inform the recipient about the risks of contagious diseases*". However, the ASRM recommends careful advice regarding the risks of the transfer of these embryos.

SCREENING OF RECIPIENTS

The recipient is screened for infectious diseases **(Box 3)** such as syphilis, gonorrhea, chlamydia, viral hepatitis and human immunodeficiency virus (HIV). In addition, the receiving partner is interviewed by a psychologist to explore the irsopinion on egg donation, expectations and possible implications for the preparation of a baby conceived through egg donation.

Recipients of advanced reproductive age (>45 years) need further examination by the doctor, as pregnancy may precipitate preexisting medical disorders such as hypertension, diabetes mellitus, heart disease and kidney disease, by putting additional stress on heart, liver, kidney and other vital organs.

SYNCHRONIZATION OF THE DONOR AND THE RECIPIENT

In menstruating patients (having their periods) gonadotropin releasing hormone (GnRH) analog injection, such as Suprefact, Lupride or Nasaral spray is started from day 21st of the previous cycle. Once the patient gets their period, 2 mg estradiol valerate tablet is started on the 2nd day of the period. On the 10th day, an ultrasound is performed to evaluate the endometrial receptivity by measuring the thickness of endometrium.

An endometrial thickness of over 7 mm is good for pregnancy. Once this has ensued, good quality embryos are transferred in the uterine cavity under USG guidance. One can wait up to 35 days after starting the estradiol valerate, for a transfer of embryos.

In the case of the menopausal women, cyclic hormones are administered for 3–6 months, until the patient begins to have her menstrual periods. Subsequently, the procedure is the same, starting estradiol valerate tablets from the 2nd day of the period. In these women, it is not necessary to provide GnRH analogues.

Progesterone begins on the 15th day of the receptor cycle and embryo transfer is done 2–4 days after the start of progesterone, i.e. on day 17–19 of recipient cycle in embryo at 2–12 cells stage.[19]

The progesterone dose is 100 mg intramuscularly (IM)/day or 200–600 mg transvaginal/day. Estrogen support is continued in the progestational period, although a study has shown that estrogen continuation is not required.[20]

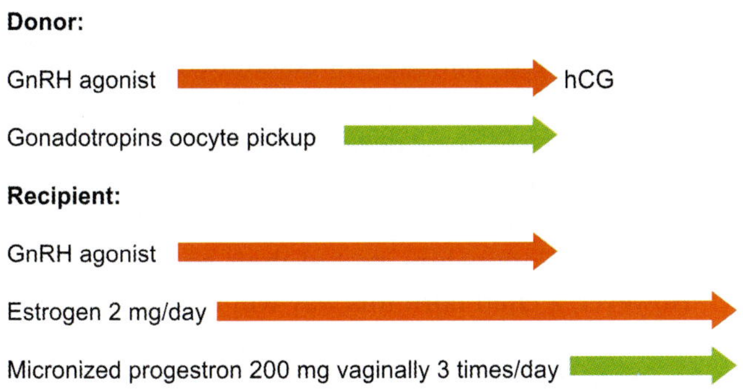

Fig. 1: Endometrial stimulation and synchronization.

Endometrial stimulation and synchronization has been discussed in **Figure 1**.

TYPES OF DONORS

Donors are of the following types:

- *Donors not related to the recipient (Altruistic and/or Monetary):* In the United States, they can be anonymous or semi anonymous, recruited by donor agencies of ova or IVF clinics.
- *Designated donors*: A friend or relative brought by the patient.
- *Shared oocyte donor*: Women who are undergoing IVF treatment may donate their unused eggs to another recipient who will partially help them by paying the cost of their in vitro fertilization treatment. The pregnancy rate with the use of shared oocytes is similar to that of altruistic donors.

EMBRYO SOURCES

Studies have shown that up to 98% of couples choose to cryopreserve their embryos.[21]

Cryopreservation is a turning point in the field of in vitro fertilization. It offers the opportunity to decide the number of embryos that will be transferred in one cycle and to preserve the remaining number for future use. It also helps reduce the risk of multiple gestations and saves the woman multiple attempts at ovarian stimulation and oocyte recovery.

With the increasing success rate of the in vitro fertilization procedure, most couples complete their families and stop the treatment. Furthermore, the laws enacted in some countries limit the number of embryos to be transferred add to the excess embryos available for embryo donation.

Above all, it is profitable for both the donor and the recipient. The donor pair need not take the charges for the continuation of cryopreservation and the receiving couple gets the good quality embryo at an affordable cost.

Many ART programs require the couple to make decisions about the fate of surplus embryos before the ART procedure begins.

The options offered are:

- Continue with cryopreservation indefinitely until the final decision
- Make a donation for an approved research
- To destroy
- Donate to needy couples (elderly couple, couple with poor oocytes and sperm parameters).

Hounshell and colleagues, in a retrospective review, found that 72.4% of couples chose to undergo an autologous transfer. Approximately 4.1% chose to donate embryos to another pair, 17.4% opted for destruction and 6.1% choose to continue with storage.[22]

Other studies conducted by Laurelle C et al. and Lornage J et al. found a higher percentage of couples between 12–39%, they chose embryo donation.[21,23]

About 7–19% of couples chose the option to donate additional embryos for the approved research and 19–34% chose the destruction.

The attitudes and views of couples have not had a significant impact on the decision on the fate of cryopreserved embryos. The woman's parity surprisingly did not represent the problem at all, since the women with multiple gestations were as likely to donate the embryos as those who did not conceive with multiple gestations.

Klipstein et al. in a retrospective analysis studied the couple's attitude towards embryo donation. In the event of death, 22% of the couples of female partners opted for the donation, 59% chose to discard it and 18% chose to cryopreserve the embryos and give them to the new partner of the male.[24]

The embryo quality plays a vital part in the decision-making process of the ART center and of the receiving couple. Embryos of younger women will not be fragmented and will be of better quality than women over the age of 40 and will result in a better pregnancy rate.[25,26]

Younger women will tend to have a relatively larger number of embryos for cryopreservation than older counterparts, since most ART centers will generally only freeze high-quality embryos. The embryos of the younger group are more likely to be accepted for embryo donation, as this would result in higher pregnancy rates.

Many ART centers are faced with the growing problem of the accumulation of a large number of embryos in their storage. This also adds to their financial and legal burdens. The main contributors to this problem are couples who have completed family, but could not decide about their remaining embryos.

For research: Donated embryos provide a major source of stem cells for research, which can help in curing diseases such as Alzheimer's, cancer and Parkinson's disease. Views suggest that the people who have donated embryos for research, report feelings of contribution towards medicine. They feel it's an opportunity to help improve the IVF technology. Whereas the people who refrain from embryo donation lack information on research projects and feel the sense of belonging to their embryos.

ICMR GUIDELINES[27,28]

Requirements for an Oocyte Donor

- The individual must be immune from HIV infections and hepatitis B and C, hypertension, diabetes, sexually transmitted diseases and identifiable and common genetic diseases such as thalassemia
- The blood group and the Rh state of the individual must be determined and recorded
- Other relevant information should be recorded of the donor, such as height, weight, age, educational qualifications, profession, skin and eye color and history of any family disorder
- The age of the donor should be between 21–35 years.

Sourcing of Oocytes and Surrogate Mothers

Law firms and sperm banks can obtain oocyte donors and surrogate mothers through advertisements. These organizations can charge the couple against the provision of an oocyte donor or surrogate mother. The ovum donor will be compensated financially by the law firm or the semen bank against the oocyte donation. However, negotiations between a couple and the surrogate mother must be carried out independently.

Rights of a Child Born through ART

- It is assumed that a child born through ART is the legitimate child of the couple, having been born within the marriage. Therefore, the child will have the legal rights to maintain the parents inheritance and all other rights of a child born of a couple through a sexual relationship.
- Children born through the use of donor gametes and their "adopted" parents will be entitled to genetic or medical information available on genetic parents that may be relevant to the health of the child.
- Children born through the use of donor gametes will not have the right to know the identity (such as name, address, relationship, etc.) of their genetic parents. However, a child born this way will be provided with all other information about the donor when the child wants it, on becoming an adult. Although the couple is not obligated to provide the "other" information on its own, the couple or other interested persons will not deliberately attempt to hide this information from the child when the child requests it.

Responsibility of the Clinic

Keep all information about donors, recipients and partners confidential and secure. Information about the donor (including a copy of the donor's DNA fingerprint, if available, but excluding information about the name and address, or the individual identity of the individual) must be disclosed by the ART clinic after appropriate identification, only for offspring and only if he/she requires it after age 18, or as specified and required for legal purposes, and never to the parents (except when indicated by a court).

To maintain detailed record of all donor oocytes, sperm, or embryos used. It need to be maintained for 10 years after which, there cords should be transferred to central depository for maintenance by the ICMR.

Possible Misuse of ART

- *Sale of embryos and stem cells:* Due to the possibility of embryo been commercially exploited and sold to foreign countries the sale or transfer of gamete/embryo in any form to any place out of country is prohibited. Within the country gametes/embryo, may be provided for their search purpose without any commercial interest.

Box 4: Medical screening in male partner of recipient.

- Blood Rh and Type
- Hepatitis screen
- VDRL
- HIV-1, HTLV-1
- Semen analysis and culture

(HTLV-1: human T-lymphotropic virus-1; VDRL: venereal disease research laboratory)

REFERENCES

1. Friedrich O (1984). Medicine: A Legal, Moral, Social Nightmare. [online] Available from http://content.time.com/time/magazine/article/0,9171,952517,00.html [Last Accessed February 2019].
2. Claudia W.(1984). The New Origins of Life. [online] Available from http://content.time.com/time/magazine/article/0,9171,952514,00.html [Last Accessed February 2019].
3. SART. Clinic Summary Report. [online] Available from Sartcorsonline.com. [Last Accessed February 2019].
4. Richards SE (2013). Get Used to Embryo Adoption. [online] Available from http://ideas.time.com/2013/08/24/get-used-to-embryo-adoption/ [Last Accessed February 2019].
5. Sharara FI, Seifer DB. Testing the ovarian reserve in infertile women. Endocrinologist. 1998;8:279-83.
6. Aubard Y, Teissier MP, Grandjean MH, et al. Early menopause. J Gynecol Obstet Biol Reprod (Paris). 1997;26:231-7.
7. Weiss G. Fertility in the older woman. Clin Consult Obs Gyn.1996;8:56-9
8. Nielsen J, Sillesen I, Hansen KB. Fertility in women with Turner's syndrome. Case report and review of literature. Br J Obstet Gynaecol.1979;86:833-5.
9. Swapp GH, Johnston AW, Watt JL, et al. A fertile woman with non-mosaic Turner's syndrome. Case report and review of the literature. Br J Obstet Gynaecol. 1989;96:876-80.
10. Press F, Shapiro HM, Cowell CA, et al. Outcome of ovum donation in Turner's syndrome patients. Fertil Steril. 1995;64:995-8.
11. Foudila T, Soderstrom-Anttila V, Hovatta O. Turner's syndrome and pregnancies after oocyte donation. Hum Reprod. 1999;14:532-5.
12. Abir R, Fisch B, Raz A, et al. Preservation of fertility in women undergoing chemotherapy: current approach and future prospects. J Assist Reprod Genet. 1998;15:469-77.
13. Burton G, Abdalla HI, Kirkland A, et al. The role of oocyte donation in women who are unsuccessful with in-vitro fertilization treatment. Hum Reprod. 1992;7:1103-5.
14. Van Voorhis BJ, Williamson RA, Gerard JL, et al. Use of oocytes from anonymous, matched, fertile donors for prevention of heritable genetic diseases. J Med Genet.1992;29:398-9.
15. Wallerstein R, Jansen V, Grifo JA, et al. Genetic screening of prospective oocyte donors. FertilSteril. 1998;70:52-5.
16. Selva J. The female donor–the male donor. A genetic control programme developed by the CECOS federation. Contracept Fertil Sex. 1990;18:510-2.
17. Cohen MA, Lindheim SR, Sauer MV. Donor age is paramount to success in oocyte donation. Hum Reprod. 1999;14:2755-8.
18. Sung L, Bustillo M, Mukherjee T, et al. Sisters of women with premature ovarian failure may not be ideal ovum donors. Fertil Steril. 1997;67:912-6.
19. Navot D, Scott RT, Droesch K, et al. The window for embryo transfer and the efficiency of human conception in vitro. Fertil Steril. 1991;55:114-8.
20. Lewin A, Benshushan A, Mezker E, et al. The role of estrogen support during the luteal phase of in vitro fertilization-embryo transplant cycles: a comparative study between progesterone alone and estrogen and progesterone support. Fertil Steril. 1994;62:121-5.
21. Laurelle C, Englert Y. Psychological study of in vitro fertilization embryo transfer participant's attitude toward the destiny of their supernumerary embryos. Fertil Steril. 1995;63:1047-50.
22. Hounshell CV, Chetkowski RJ. Donation of frozen embryos after in vitro fertilization is uncommon. Fertil Steril. 1996; 66:837-38.
23. FDA. Vaccines, Blood and Biologics. [online] Available from https://www.fda.gov/biologicsBloodVaccines/default.htm [Last Accessed February 2019].
24. Klipstein S, Reindollar RH, Regan MM, et al. Gender bias in the disposition of frozen embryos. Fertil Steril. 2001;76: 1181-4.
25. Society for Assisted Reproductive Technology, American Society for Reproductive Medicine. Assisted reproductive technology in United States: 1999 results generated from the American Society For Reproductive Medicine/Society for Assisted Reproductive Technology Registry. Fertil Steril. 2002;77:18-31.
26. Assisted reproductive technology in United States: 1997 results generated from the American Society for Reproductive Medicine/Society for Assisted Reproductive Technology Registry. Fertil Steril. 2000;74:641-53.
27. ICMR (2010). The assisted reproductive technologies (regulation) rules–2010. [online] Available from https://www.icmr.nic.in/sites/default/files/guidelines/ART%20REGULATION%20Draft%20Rules%201.pdf [Last Accessed February 2019].

Surrogacy

71

Nayana H Patel, Shivani Sachdev, Gajendrakant Tripathi

INTRODUCTION

As per Draft ART Bill, 2014, "Surrogacy" means an arrangement in which a woman agrees to a pregnancy, achieved through assisted reproductive technology, in which neither of the gametes belongs to her or her husband, with the intention to carry it and hand over the child to the commissioning couple for whom she is acting as a surrogate. However, the word "surrogate", is emerged from Latin word "Subrogare" (to substitute), which means "appointed to act in the place of". The concept of surrogacy is also rooted in Hindu mythology, as despite of taking birth from the womb of Rohini, Balraam, was regarded as son of mother Devaki and elder brother of Lord Krishna.

Surrogacy is of two types, *Traditional* and *Gestational.*

Traditional surrogacy is the result of artificial insemination of the surrogate mother with the intended father's sperm. This makes surrogate and intended father genetic parents of the baby. On the other hand, gestational (IVF/host/full) surrogacy, is an arrangement where an embryo from the intended parents, or from a donated oocyte or sperm, is transferred to the surrogate's uterus. The gestational carrier has no genetic connection to the child in procedure of gestational surrogacy.

On the basis of monetary arrangement involved, surrogacy may be classified as *commercial (compensated) or altruistic*. In commercial surrogacy, medical costs are reimbursed to surrogate mother and surrogate is paid for her gestational services. In altruistic surrogacy, friend or acquaintances or relative can be a surrogate mother and compensated for pregnancy-related medical cost and for loss of income during pregnancy.

INDICATIONS FOR SURROGACY

- *Congenital or acquired absence of a functioning uterus*: Mayer-Rokitansky-Küster-Hauser (MRKH) syndrome.
- Hysterectomy for various reasons.
- Significant *structural abnormalities*, presence of *multiple fibroids*.
- *Severe adenomyosis.*
- *Persistently thin endometrium due to endometrial tuberculosis (TB).*
- *Asherman's syndrome.*
- *Repeated miscarriages*, repeated *unexplained in vitro fertilization (IVF) failures* despite of good-quality embryos.
- *Repeated IVF failure*: Due to nonreceptive uterus.
- *Medical conditions*, which might be life-threatening for a woman during pregnancy.
- Same-sex male couples or single men.

STEPS INVOLVED IN SURROGACY PROCESS

- Patient selection.
- Source of surrogate [Assisted Reproductive Technology (ART) Bank].
- Selection and screening of prospective surrogate.
- Counseling of patients and surrogate.
- Legal requirements, financial contracts and transparency of arrangement.
- Controlled ovarian stimulation and IVF technique.
- Preparing the surrogate.
- Synchronizing the cycles of the surrogate and the genetic mother or donor.

- Window period for embryo transfer.
- Obstetric care of surrogate.

Selection of Patient

- Patients with medical indication only are considered for surrogacy. While selecting the patient, consultation and counseling on all aspects of the treatment are carried out.
- Couples and individuals who want to consider surrogacy, should research and study surrogacy laws and shall even consult surrogacy professionals to truly understand surrogacy.

Source of Surrogate

For compensated arrangement, surrogate can be selected from the National Registry of ART Banks of the Indian Council of Medical Research. A woman from family or a known person to the couple may act as a surrogate mother in altruistic arrangement. However, she should be of similar age group as the woman desiring her as a surrogate.

Selection and Screening of Prospective Surrogates

A thorough medical, obstetrical and psychological screening is done.

- *Age of surrogate*: Surrogates are generally 21–35 years old (25–35 years as per Surrogacy Bill, 2016).
- Surrogate shall be a married woman having at least one child of her own and of minimum 3 years old.
- To become a surrogate mother, consent of spouse is must.
- An extensive medical and psychological assessment is mandatory along with thorough criminal and financial background checks.
- Routine tests include a hysteroscopy, pelvic and abdominal ultrasonography, tests like complete blood count (CBC), fasting blood sugar (FBS), hemoglobin A1c (HbA1c), Hb electrophoresis, human immunodeficiency virus (HIV), hepatitis B virus surface antigen (HBsAg), hepatitis C virus (HCV).
- Electrocardiography (ECG), pap smear and mammogram are also recommended.
- Medical fitness from physician is necessary.

Counseling

Counseling is very crucial part of surrogacy arrangement. All the parties must counsel enough that they can develop trust in each other and can enter in the agreement with comfort and confidence.

Genetic couple should be counseled for alternative treatment options other than surrogacy along with practical difficulty and cost of treatment legality involved in gestational surrogacy, psychological risk involved and possibility of birth of abnormal child.

On the other hand, surrogate must be counseled for detailed treatment by IVF surrogacy, possibility of multiple pregnancies, oppose by family and friends, risks associated with pregnancy and the possibility of cesarean section and possibility of sense of bereavement while giving baby to the genetic parents.

Proper Controlled Ovarian Stimulation and IVF Technique

If women requesting treatment by gestational surrogacy are perfectly normal with regard to their ovarian function, the management of their IVF treatment cycle is simple. Ovarian follicular stimulation, monitoring and oocyte recovery methods practiced as previously described.

Preparing the Surrogate

Estrogen (4 mg/day to 6 mg/day) is started from D2 or D3 of the recipient's cycle after confirming a thin endometrium (< 5 mm) on the scan. On 10th day, growth of endometrium is checked, a minimum of 8 mm (triple line) is ideal before starting progesterone. 5 days/3 days of progesterone is required either intramuscular (50 mg/100 mg a day) or intravaginal (400 mg/day) before a transfer.

The other popular protocol for surrogate preparation is the leuprolide protocol due to its feasibility and its flexibility. Suppression with leuprolide is done along with previously mentioned endometrial preparation method. Either starting from Day 21 of previous cycle agonist injection for down regulation or stopping it at one-fourth dose their own till the day of progesterone. Luteal phase support has to be accordingly decided.

Synchronizing the Cycles of the Surrogate and the Genetic Mother

The surrogate embryo transfer could be fresh or frozen transfer and subject to availability of the gestational carrier. For a fresh surrogate transfer, the surrogate and the intended mother cycle may be synchronized with oral contraceptive (OC) pills or progesterone pills or surrogate may be put on agonist injection for flexibility of transfer dates.

The surrogate is started on estrogen tablets from the third day of her cycle for around 10 days before her endometrium is assessed. On reaching of minimum 8 mm she is put on progesterone supplementation for 3/5 days before a planned cleavage or blastocyst transfer.

Obstetrics Care of Surrogate

Once a pregnancy is confirmed in the gestational carrier depending on the facility of the ART clinic, she either stays in the surrogate house or at her home. The intended couple are sent regular updates regarding the surrogate's pregnancy in form of her weight gain, vitals, fetal growth and antenatal investigation reports and scans. Postdelivery, the surrogate is kept under observation for minimum 15 days before discharge.

Surrogate House

The concept of "surrogate house", sometimes also referred as "Surrogate Hostel" came into existence with the request of many surrogates to provide shelter during period of surrogacy as they wished to hide their surrogacy pregnancy from relatives and society due to the stigma in society. Extensive obstetrics care is taken. In surrogate house, surrogates stay under the supervision of 24-hour nursing staff along with dietician, physiotherapist, counselors and gynecologist for her medical care. Surrogates get complete rest and healthy, nutritionally complete meals which turn out to be beneficial for their health during pregnancy. As they stay in a group, they get lot of emotional, moral and psychological support from other surrogates. Also, they are allowed to meet their family and kids and be in constant touch with their families via phone. They can go to their place as and when they want, also, young kids of surrogates are allowed to stay at surrogate house during weekends and school holidays. It is voluntary for surrogates to stay in the surrogate house. Any surrogate who wishes to stay at her home can always do that.

In surrogate house, she has to undergo obstetrics assessment every 20 days till the date of delivery, obstetrics scans at 6–8 weeks, 11–13 weeks anomaly scan, at 20–22 weeks (anomaly scan 3D-4D), 28-week and 34–36 weeks (growth scan). Any additional scan is subject to the obstetrics need.

ISSUES RELATED TO SURROGACY

- *Ethical aspects*: Surrogacy has raised large ethical debate in the past. Opponents of surrogacy consider it as exploitation of poor women by rich and commodification of motherhood as women are given monetary benefit to be pregnant and deliver babies. In past, surrogates were even compared with prostitutes. The other major argument against womb commodification is that rich people can take advantage of the willingness of poor women to perform any job as long as they are able to get compensation. Due to all these misconception, there is stigma in society about surrogacy and surrogates.
- *Religious aspects and issues*: Various religions around the world take different stance with regard to surrogacy practice. In Christianity, sperm or ovum donation and surrogacy are considered gravely immoral. Islam also has similar approach regarding their chastity. Jewish religious establishments have now accepted gestational surrogacy only if both intended parents' gametes included in IVF. However, all oppose for surrogacy in religious stands were for traditional surrogacy. Now with advent of IVF and gestational surrogacy the relevance of these beliefs is being questioned.
- *Psychological impact with surrogacy*: Despite increasing success rates surrogacy poses complexity on psychological aspects which require multidisciplinary approach to deal with. Surrogacy creates a cobweb of possible relationships which could sometimes be emotionally taxing. Unlike the donor egg programs where the intended parents do not share a relationship with donor and know only nonidentifying information about her where as intended parents working with a gestational surrogate typically share a personal relationship with her that will last throughout the pregnancy and often beyond. In some cases, surrogate gets depressed while giving the baby to its parents, however this feeling gets diluted with time.

SURROGACY IN INDIA AND GUIDELINES FOR SURROGACY

Commercial surrogacy has been legal in India since 2002. Till the implementation of ART Bill 2015, when surrogacy was allowed for foreigners, Overseas Citizenship of India (OCI), Person of India Origin (PIO) and others, India was emerging as a leader in international surrogacy and as a destination in surrogacy-related fertility tourism because of good medical skills, infrastructure, transparency of procedure, favorable guidelines, and relatively low cost. Here, Surrogacy was found to be symbiotic arrangement as infertile couple gets baby which completes their family and needy surrogate gets compensation which helps for betterment of entire her family. However, one after other regulations from regulatory authority of India is pushing surrogacy practice almost to a halt. The proposed ART Bill, 2015 bans foreign national from commencing surrogacy in India while after that overnight notification in November, 2015 had restricted OCIs and PIOs. The effect of such approach of government toward surrogacy practice had evidently affected the industry negatively. Furthermore, 24th August, 2016 has to be considered a Black Day for surrogacy in India, when the Surrogacy (Regulation) Bill 2016, received the cabinet approval. The Bill bans commercial form of surrogacy, allowing only altruistic arrangement with many other constraints on this practice.

Guidelines as per ART Bill, 2014

- Surrogate mother shall be an ever *married Indian woman.*
- *Age: 23–35 years of age.*
- Shall have *at least one live child* of her own with *minimum age of 3 years.*
- Woman shall act as a surrogate for *only one successful live birth* in her life and with not less than 2 years interval between two deliveries.
- Surrogate mother shall be subjected to *maximum three cycles of medications* while she is acting as surrogate mother.
- Surrogate shall be medically tested for HIV/AIDS and all other communicable diseases and conditions such as cardiovascular disease, thyroid problem, etc.
- She must not have received a blood transfusion or a blood product in the *last six months.*
- *No surrogate* shall undergo *embryo transfer more than three times* for the same couple.
- The *written consent of surrogate mother's spouse* is mandatory before she may act as surrogate.
- The spouse of the surrogate mother shall certify in his written that he will *take care of the well-being of the existing child/children of their own* during the surrogacy period.
- A surrogate shall *relinquish all parental rights over the child* or children.
- The couple and the surrogate, shall enter into a surrogacy agreement or contract.
- All medical expenses, including insurance of the surrogate should be given by commissioning couple.
- Complications arise during pregnancy (i.e. gestational diabetes, chronic hypertension, etc.), which are likely to continue for the rest of her life, shall be covered under insurance.
- The birth certificate of a baby born through surrogacy shall bear the name of couple who commissioned the surrogacy, as parents.
- Surrogacy shall not be allowed for foreigners but permissible to OCIs, PIOs, Non Resident Indians (NRIs) and foreigner married to an Indian citizen (prohibited for OCIs and PIOs, as per notification on 3rd November, 2015 from Ministry of Health and Family Welfare).
- If abnormalities are detected in the child or children during the gestation period, then the commissioning parent shall ensure that the defected/disabled child/children are appropriately insured and compensation to be used for the development and growth of the child/children by the next in the family, in case of accidental death of the commissioning parents during delivery or in the process of delivery of the surrogate child.
- All records and documents shall be preserved for a *period of 10 years* and after which the records shall be transferred to the National Registry of ART Clinics and Banks in India of the Indian Council of Medical Research.
- *For more detail please refer ART Bill, 2014.*

Guidelines as per Surrogacy (Regulation) Bill, 2016

- The intending couple needs certificate of proven infertility from a District Medical Board.
- The surrogate mother needs an eligibility certificate issued by the appropriate authority.
- Surrogate should be between 25 years and 35 years of age, married, having a child of her own.
- Only close relative of the intending couple, shall act as a surrogate mother.
- Surrogacy can be done only once in lifetime.
- The age of the intending couple shall be between 23 years and 50 years in case of female and between 26 years and 55 years in case of male on the day of certification.
- The intending couple must be Indian citizens and married for at least 5 years.
- The intending couple have not had any surviving child biologically or through adoption or through surrogacy earlier.
- *Registration of surrogacy clinics*: Every certificate of registration shall be valid for a period of 3 years and shall be renewed.

- Any intending couple or any person who seeks the aid of any surrogacy clinic, laboratory or of a registered medical practitioner, gynecologist, pediatrician, human embryologist or any other person for commercial surrogacy or for conducting surrogacy procedures for commercial purposes shall be punishable with imprisonment for a term which shall not be less than 5 years and with fine which may extend to five lakh rupees for the first offence and for any subsequent offence with imprisonment which may extend to 10 years and with fine which may extend to ten lakh rupees.
- *For more detail please refer surrogacy (Regulation) Bill, 2016.*

SUGGESTED READING

1. Aittomaki K, Eroila H, Kajanoja P. A population-based study of the incidence of Mullerian aplasia in Finland. Fertil Steril. 2001;76(3):624-5.
2. Aramesh K. Iran's experience with surrogate motherhood: An Islamic view and ethical concerns. J Med Ethics. 2009;35: 320-2.
3. Brinsden PR. IVF surrogacy. In: Brinsden PR (Ed). A Textbook of In Vitro Fertilization and Assisted Reproduction. London: Taylor & Francis; 2005. pp. 393-404.
4. Brunet L, Carruthers J, Davaki K, et al. (2013). A Comparative Study on the Regime of Surrogacy in EU Member States. [online]. Available from http://www.europarl.europa.eu/studies, http://www.europarl.europa.eu/studies [Accessed February, 2019].
5. Deomampo D. Defining parents, making citizens: nationality and citizenship in transnational surrogacy. Med Anthropol. 2015;34:210-25.
6. Draft Assisted Reproductive Technology (Regulation) Bill. Ministry of Health and Family Welfare, Government of India; New Delhi: Indian Council of Medical Research; 2014.
7. Golombok S, Blake L, Casey P, et al. Children born through reproductive donation: a longitudinal study of psychological adjustment. J Child Psychol Psychiatry. 2013;54(6): 653-60.
8. Golombok S, Murray C, Jadva V, et al. Non-genetic and non-gestational parenthood: consequences for parent-child relationships and the psychological well-being of mothers, fathers and children at age 3. Hum Reprod. 2006;21(7): 1918-24.
9. Honjo S, Arai S, Keneko H, et al. Antenatal depression and maternal-fetal attachment. Psychopathology. 2003;36(6): 304-11.
10. Inhorn MC, Patrizio P. Rethinking reproductive "tourism" as reproductive "exile". Fertil Steril. 2009;92(3):904-6.
11. Jadva V, Murray C, Lycett E, et al. Surrogacy: the experiences of surrogate mothers. Hum Reprod. 2003;18(10):2196-204.
12. Kimbrell. The Human Body Shop: The Engineering and Marketing of Life. New York: Harper San Francisco; 1993. p. 101.
13. Lindenman E, Shepard MK, Pescovitz OH. Mullerian agenesis: an update. Obstet Gynecol. 1997;90:307-12.
14. Lindenman E, Shepard MK, Pescovitz OH. Mullerian agenesis: an update. Obstet Gynecol. 1997;90:307-12.
15. MacCallum F, Lycett E, Murray C, et al. Surrogacy: the experience of commissioning couples. Hum Reprod. 2003;18(6):1334-42.
16. Pennings G. Reply: reproductive exile versus reproductive tourism. Hum Reprod. 2005;20:3571-2.
17. Shenfield F, Pennings G, Cohen J, et al. ESHRE Task Force on Ethics and Law 10: surrogacy. Hum Reprod. 2005;20(10): 2705-7.
18. Surrogacy (Regulation) Bill, 2016.
19. Wikland M, Enk L, Hamberger L. Transvesical and transvaginal approaches for the aspiration of follicles by the use of ultrasound. Ann N Y Acad Sci. 1985;442;182-94.
20. "Paragraph 2376". Catechism of the Catholic Church.

Uterus Transplantation

72

Taswin Kaur, Kamini A Rao

INTRODUCTION

A child—is most; if not all married couples dream; rather a family bridge. Infertility, the disease, on the coming century is taking a leap in this era. Almost 48.5 million couples worldwide are silently suffering with the hope of having an offspring, and this number is dwindling yearly.[1,2]

Arrays of causes have been outlined to be the underlying cause of infertility. Absolute uterine factor infertility (UFI) is a catastrophic cause of infertility affecting 3–5% of the general population.[3] Most of the married women dream of carrying a fetus in their own womb. It is devastating for the family, more so over for the woman herself to not be able to carry and deliver her own child. The society and environment make the situation worst where a woman's capability is judged based on her ability to carry and deliver her own child. Infertility due to the inability to carry a pregnancy remains as one of the darkest and perplexing unresolved issues in the infertility dictionary. Till date, adoption or surrogacy was the only option for these women with absolute UFI. The dawn of uterus transplantation has given a ray of hope to this group of couples to bear their babies in themselves.

UTERINE FACTOR INFERTILITY: CAUSES

With the cutting edge fertility technology and treatment available, a third alternative is now available for females with absolute UFI—the first two being adoption and surrogacy. The option of a uterus transplant will allow women to receive the uterus from an allogeneic donor to restore her gestational ability.

The legal and ethical prohibitions to use surrogacy are certainly a boon for uterus transplant.[4-6]

Mayer-Rokitansky-Küster-Hauser (MRKH) syndrome commonly known as Müllerian agenesis is the most common indication for uterus transplant. MRKH affects 1 per 4,500 women.[7,8] It is characterized by the absence of uterus, cervix, and upper one-third of the vagina in an otherwise phenotypically normal 46XX female. The fallopian tubes and ovaries are present. There are two subtypes of MRKH: I and II. Subtype I affecting approximately 44% of MRKH cohort, represents the classical MRKH where there is agenesis of the caudal part of the Müllerian duct (upper vagina, cervix, uterus) without any associated malformations.[7] The atypical type or MRKH type II is the more common type and is associated with malformations, usually affecting the skeletal or the renal system (multiorgan). The subtype MURCS (Mullerian duct aplasia, unilateral renal agenesis, and cervico-thoracic somite anomalies) although nonlethal, is the most severe type of MRKH and has been classified under MRKH type II.

Congenital uterine malformations (other than MRKH) have a prevalence of around 4.3–6.7% in the general population.[9] Here, malformations or aberrations occurring at any step of the development process will arise to congenital malformation. The incidence of congenital malformation is increased in the infertile population, more so in females with recurrent pregnancy losses were as high as 17% of patients in this subgroup can be affected.[10] Common malformations like uterine septum can be surgically corrected with an excellent post procedure prognosis.[11-13] However, women with congenital uterine anomalies have been consistently found to have lower pregnancy rates and increased abortion rates.[12]

Acquired cause of UFI is severe endometrial distortion due to Asherman Syndrome or hysterectomy, with the latter being more common. Hysterectomy was performed due to malignant uterine tumor or benign causes like leiomyoma, and peripartum hysterectomy due to intractable hemorrhage.

The embryo-endometrial dialogue is essential for a successful implantation. Asherman syndrome is characterized by scarring of the endometrium leading to partial or complete endometrial dysfunction with fibrotic tissue adhesions.[14] Endometrial receptivity, the phase where the endometrium is rendered suitable for blastocyst attachment, is hampered, thus leading to a declining fertility.[15]

Although the incidence of invasive carcinomas in the reproductive age group accounts for only 2% of the total cancer population, the incidence of cancer in this younger age group is on the rise.[16,17] With the advent of good chemotherapy, radiotherapy, and state of the art surgical skills and protocols, the cancer survival rates have increased.[18] Gynecological cancer 5-year survival rates have improved over the years—breast cancer 66–90%,[19] cervical cancer 70%, and ovarian cancer 40%.[20] This is in concordance with the goal of the Union for International Cancer Control's World Cancer Declaration 2013: "there will be major reductions in premature deaths from cancer and improvements in quality of life and cancer survival". Although the live expectancy is improved, the fertility preservation technology is still in the fetal stages.[21,22] Effect of radiation on the ovaries leading to premature ovarian failure is widely known. Radiation causes scarring and uterine shrinkage finally resulting in failure to carry a pregnancy.[23,24] This observation has been reiterated in the Childhood Cancer Survivor Study 2009 where female survivors receiving an ovarian or uterine radiation dose of more than 5 Gy are very less likely to ever achieve a pregnancy.[25] In a nutshell, adults with childhood or reproductive age cancers receiving chemo-radiotherapy have a poorer reproductive and obstetrical outcome compared to the unexposed general population.[26]

Fertility preservation and sparing surgeries have come a long way in giving a ray of hope to cancer survivors. Reproductive age cancer patients detected at the early stage, who want to preserve their child bearing capacity, are the ideal candidates for fertility preservation and sparing techniques. Unfortunately, in the advanced stages, due to complications or when expertise for fertility preservation or sparing are unavailable, these patients have no option left other than to undergo an radical hysterectomy. Cervical cancer is now the fourth most common gynecological cancer worldwide.[27] It is caused by present or previous infection with an oncogenic Human Papilloma Virus (HPV) strain.[28] Due to the increased awareness, majority of cervical cancers today are detected in women less than 45 years of age.[27,29] Surgery for cervical carcinoma (radical hysterectomy) is presently limited to Stage IIA, although fertility sparing surgery (trachelectomy) is now an option for early stage cervical cancers. Endometrial carcinoma or sarcomas rarely affect women in the reproductive age group.

To save the life of the mother in situations of torrential hemorrhage (due to adherent placentation/uterine atony/uterine rupture), postpartum hysterectomy is performed. In a recent meta-analysis where 128 studies were included, the incidence of peripartum hysterectomy was 1 per 1,000 deliveries.[30]

Arrays of causes have been attributed to the need of the hour for uterus transplant. Currently, uterus transplant has been done for mainly MRKH syndrome **(Flowchart 1)**.

HISTORY OF UTERINE TRANSPLANT

Like research in any other field of medicine, the preclinical studies and researches were first carried out on animal models where most of the aspects of transplantation were explored and fine-tuned. Attempt of uterus transplantation in animals dates back in 1970s where Richard Mattingly et al. performed auto-transplantation in dogs with successful pregnancies.[31] This publication lighted the spark for more extensive research. In the last decade, a number of animals have been used as experimental models—rats,[32,33] mice,[34,35] pigs,[36] rabbits,[37] sheep,[38] baboon,[39,40] and monkeys,[41] with pregnancies being achieved in some of them. Experiments in animals were done in a step-by-step approach to master the important checkpoints in the transplantation process to develop an effective, safe and practical approach for human use.[42] Transplantation was habituated on nonhuman primates, and after gaining confidence and ethical clearance, it was experimented in humans.[43,44]

In 2000, the first uterine transplant was reported in Saudi Arabia, involving a 26-year-old woman having UFI who had undergone hysterectomy in view of postpartum hemorrhage. The donor was a 46-year-old female undergoing hysterectomy for benign indication. However, this transplant lasted for only 99 days where the uterus had to be removed due to acute thrombosis and necrosis.[45]

Thereafter, for almost a decade, till 2011, there were no further attempts of uterine transplantation. During this period, extensive research on animals was performed to demonstrate possibilities and anastomosis techniques with good graft-host survival rates. In 2011, the second attempt of human uterus transplant was done by a Turkish team

Flowchart 1: Causes of uterine factor infertility and indications of uterine transplant.

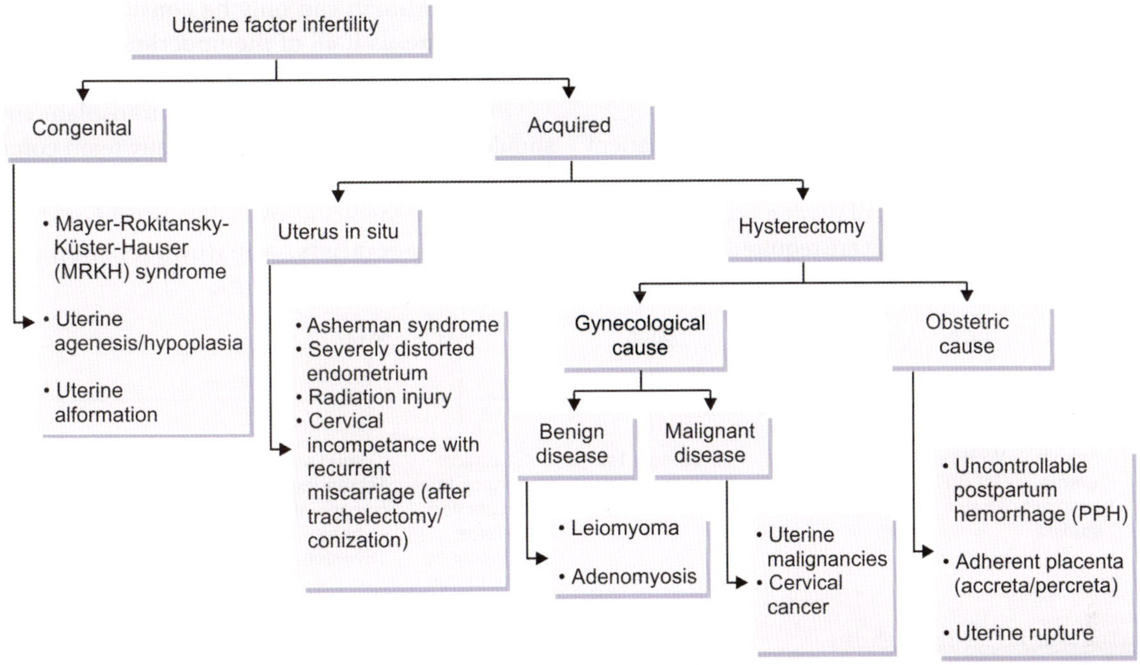

and was novel in using a deceased donor. The recipient was a 21-year-old female with MRKH syndrome who received uterus from a brain dead woman of the same age. Recipient had successful menstruation cycles soon after the transplant. Two attempts of embryo transfer were attempted where both failed—first resulted in a biochemical pregnancy and the second resulted in a spontaneous abortion at around 6 weeks of gestation.[46,47] This is perhaps the longest surviving uterus transplant till date.

In Sweden; Dr Matt Brannstrom and his team experimented for years on various animal models to understand and attempt a successful outcome of uterus transplant—a live birth.[48] His team performed extensive research before attempting their first human transplantation, in contrast to other prior attempts which were not preceded by formal animal attempts. The Swedish Uterine Transplant Trial included nine absolute uterine infertility patients (eight MRKH syndrome) and live donors. Majority of the donors were blood relatives of the recipients with their mean age being 53 ± 7 years. Of the nine attempted transplants, seven were successful. Two transplanted uterus had to be removed within months of transplant due to complications—one due to thrombosis, the other due to severe graft-host rejection (persistent uterine rejection). One year after the successful transplants, embryo transfers were performed. Two women became pregnant at the first embryo transfer attempt. The first live birth after uterus transplant worldwide took place at 31 weeks of gestation due to obstetrical complications by cesarean section on September 4th, 2014.[49,50] The birth of baby Vincent established the end point—proof of concept regarding human uterus transplant.

Following the successful live birth, many countries have attempted uterus transplant—a hopeful solution for absolute UFI. Recently, in 2017, a Chinese group has attempted robotic assisted uterine retrieval **(Figs. 1 and 2)**.[51]

Hence, with the recent advances in surgery and transplant immunology perhaps uterine transplant is here now to stay!

PROCEDURE

Uterine transplant is a technically challenging endeavor for diverse reasons. Endless explorations are ongoing to develop surgical techniques that are harmless for both the recipient and the live donor. Uterus transplantation is a complex treatment procedure that combines the principles of assisted reproduction and solid organ transplantation. Overall, the process of uterus transplant encompasses three main steps:

1. Oocyte retrieval (recipient)—ovarian stimulation followed by oocyte retrieval done as per standard protocol. In vitro fertilization-intracytoplasmic sperm injection (IVF-ICSI) is performed; embryos obtained are cryopreserved before the actual uterus transplant procedure (embryo transfer is done at least a year after successful uterine transplant).

2. Uterus transplant surgery (donor and recipient)-involves harvesting uterus from the donor and transplantation with meticulous vascular anastomosis in the recipient.
3. Immunosuppressant (recipient)—until childbearing process is completed and hysterectomy is done.

Prior to performing uterus transplant, both the patient and the donor selection is of importance. The Montreal Criteria for the Ethical Feasibility of Uterine Transplantation has laid down a set of criteria that are required for a woman to be ethically considered as a candidate for uterine transplantation—donor and recipient. According to these criteria, a woman can only be considered to donate or receive a uterus if all of the underlined criteria are met **(Table 1)**.

Prior to the transplant, a local transplant committee should be set up. It is a multispecialty team composed of transplant surgeons, reconstructive surgeons, gynecologist, reproductive medicine specialist, psychiatrist, infectious diseases specialists, anesthetists, nephrologists, immunologist, and counselors.

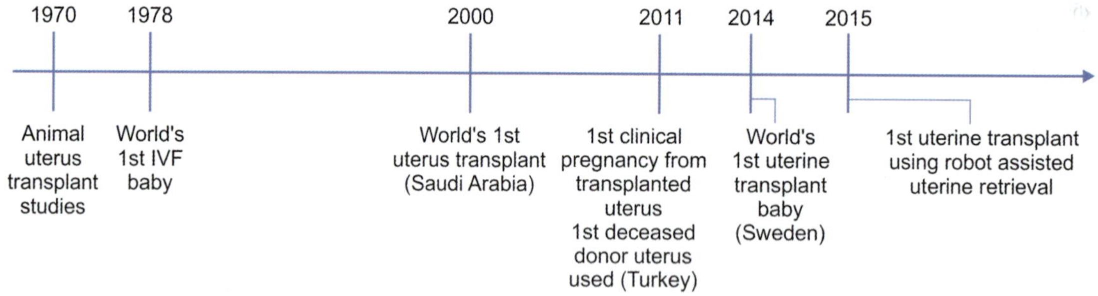

Fig. 1: Timeline of uterus transplant till date.

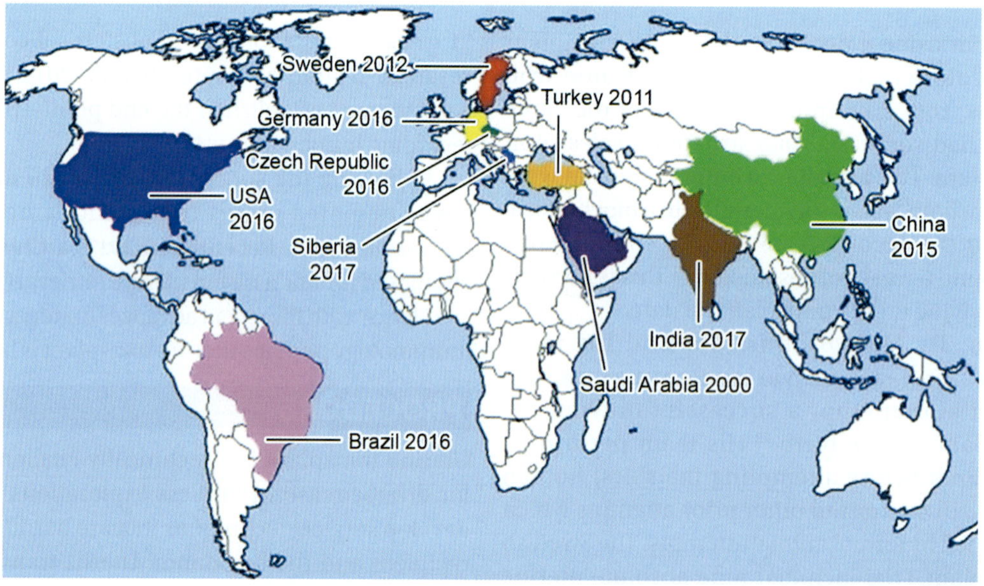

Fig. 2: The World map depicting the countries performing uterus transplantation around the World and the year it was first initiated.[52,53]

Table 1: Montreal Criteria for the Ethical Feasibility of Uterine Transplantation.[54]

Recipient	***Donor***	***Healthcare team***
Reproductive age, genetic female with no medical contraindication for transplantation	Reproductive age female with no medical contraindication to donation	Is part of an institution that meets Moore's third criteria as it pertains to institutional stability
Has documented uterine factor infertility (congenital or acquired) which has failed all current gold standard and conservative therapy	Has repeatedly attested to her conclusion of parity *or* has signed an advanced directive for postmortem organ donation	Provided adequate consent to both parties regarding risks, potential sequel and chances of success and failure

Contd...

Contd...

Recipient	***Donor***	***Healthcare team***
Has personal or legal contraindication to surrogacy and adoption measures *or* seeks the uterus transplant as a sole measure to experience gestation, with an understanding of the limitations provided by the transplant	No history of uterine damage or disease	No conflict of interest independently or with either party
Has not had her decision to undergo uterus transplant as irrational expert psychological evaluation	Is responsible enough to consent, informed enough to make a responsible decision	Has duty to preserve anonymity, i.e. the donor or the recipient do not explicitly waive this right
Does not exhibit frank unsuitability for motherhood		
Is responsible enough to consent, informed enough to make a responsible decision		
Is likely to take antirejection medication and follow up with the treating team in a responsible manner (Revised Montreal criteria)[55]		

Source: Adapted from the Montreal Criteria 2012

Recipient and Donor Screening[56]

Radiology	MRI Chest X-ray Vaginal ultrasound scan
Clinical	ECG Exercise ECG (for donor) Pap smear
Blood chemistry ▪ Liver function	Blood group Alanine transaminase (ALT) Aspartate transaminase (AST) Alkaline phosphatase (ALP) Albumin Total protein Bilirubin
▪ Kidney function	Serum creatinine Blood urea
▪ Electrolytes	Sodium Potassium Chloride
▪ Hemogram	Hemoglobin Platelets White blood cells C-reactive protein
▪ Coagulation profile	Prothrombin time (PT) Activated partial thromboplastin time (APTT)

Contd...

Contd...

Microbiology	Cytomegalovirus (CMV) Epstein-Barr virus (EBV) HIV Hepatitis A, B, C *Chlamydia* Human Papillomavirus (HPV) Gonorrhea
Immunology	Syphilis HLA Grade of matching cross tests
Assessment by specialist in	Gynecology Transplantation Surgery Psychology Clinical Immunology Anesthesiology Internal Medicine Radiology

(ECG: electrocardiography; HLA: human leukocyte antigen; MRI: magnetic resonance imaging)

In concordance with the guidelines of the Montreal criteria, the appropriate recipient selection is done. The recipient should have a good ovarian reserve [basal follicle-stimulating hormone (FSH), *luteinizing hormone* (LH), estradiol, anti-Müllerian hormone (AMH), and a satisfactory antral follicle count], normal female karyotype (46XX), blood parameters in the normal range [hemogram, renal function test (RFT), liver function test (LFT)], blood group and a matching human leukocyte antigen (HLA) typing with the donor, good general health condition with a normal range BMI, and stable psychological health.

The recipient and their families have to be extensively counseled regarding the procedure details, risks, and complications—related to the transplant, immunosuppressant, and anesthesia. The experimental nature of the transplant as worldwide, human uterus transplant is still in its fetal stages and all the alternatives available (surrogacy or adoption) should be documented. It is important that patient is made aware regarding the prolonged immunosuppression required post procedure and the long-term effects of which have not been clearly documented.[3] A realistic picture of pregnancy should be portrayed—the need for IVF, potential inability to achieve a pregnancy or live birth, reduced sensations during pregnancy, absent labor, the absolute indication of undergoing a cesarean delivery, and also the probability of a subsequent hysterectomy (peripartum or postpartum).

Donor Screening

The donor must give consent for organ donation. Routine screening procedure is carried out—blood group, hemogram, RFT, LFT, general health status, and psychological evaluation. In addition, donors HLA typing is done; detail examination for uterine pathology or infections are done by ultrasonography, Pap smear, and HPV testing.

All known medical and surgical risks, and potential complications relating both to the donor or the recipient should be outlined and documented prior to the procedure as uterus transplant involves four parties—the donor, recipient, recipient's partner, and the future child. Hence, it is a subject of ethical controversies!

Surgery of uterus transplant involves both retrieval and transplantation. Uterus retrieval may be from a multiorgan brain dead donor or from a living donor. The principles of uterus transplant are as follows:

- Surgery and vascular anastomosis
- Fixation of the transplanted uterus
- Avoiding ischemic-reperfusion injury
- Immunosuppression and maintenance of rejection

Donor Surgery Procedure[57,58]

It is shown in **Box 1**.

Recipient Surgery Procedure[57,58]

It is given in **Box 2**.

Surgical Challenges

Uterus transplant is still evolving. Numerous surgical challenges are encountered and measures to minimize them are being studied. The main pitfalls for a successful uterus transplant are necrosis and graft host rejection of the transplanted uterus.[45] An adequate blood supply after anastomosis into and out of the uterus is essential to prevent necrosis and vascular thrombosis. The use of deceased brain dead donor is one of the solutions to overcome the challenges during uterine vessels dissection. Second, studies have shown an increasing vascularity especially in the upper portion of the uterus by using utero-ovarian vein.[59] The utero-ovarian vein can be dissected more easily than the uterine vein.

Ischemic time is another important success determining factor in both the living and the deceased donor. Since uterus is not a life-saving organ, in brain dead donors, it is usually recovered after removal of other essential organs. This in turn increases the initial ischemia time. Till date, the minimal or optimal cold ischemia time for uterus is not known.[45,59] However, what is known and believed is that a longer ischemia time may be associated with graft rejection or decreased function.

Box 1: Donor surgery procedure.

Donor: Living or deceased
Anesthesia: General anesthesia
Incision: Infraumbilical midline incision

Procedure
↓
Dissect uterus and vascular pedicles
(uterine vessels and segment of the internal iliac vessels bilaterally)
↓
Remove parts of the round ligament, uterosacral ligament, the peritoneum
(for better fixation in recipients pelvis)
↓
Dissect lateral pelvic wall. Separate ureter from the uterine vessels and cervix
↓
Dissect vagina 10–15 cm distal to vaginal fornix
↓
Clamp vessels (to interrupt blood supply)
↓
Remove uterus and transport to back-end-table
↓
Flush uterus with heparinized solution and then with cold
↓
preservation solution (till time of transplant)

Box 2: Recipient surgery procedure.

Anesthesia: General anesthesia
Incision: Subumbilical midline incision

Procedure
↓
Separate vaginal wall from bladder and rectum
↓
Attach sutures to round ligament, uterosacral ligament, and paravaginal remnant or uterus remnant (for later fixation)
↓
Dissect bilateral external iliac vessels
↓
Place uterus (donor's) in anatomical position
↓
End-to-side anastomosis of external iliac vessels and graft vessels
↓
Release external iliac vein clamp
↓
Mannitol IV bolus (systolic BP maintained above 100 mm Hg)
↓
Release arterial clamp
↓
Use Doppler to quantify blood flow in uterine vessels (probe at uterine artery)
↓
4 cm longitudinal incision on vaginal wall
↓
Anastomose vaginal part of graft it Pouch of Douglas
↓
Fix uterus by binding the prepositioned sutures to the respective ligaments
(structural support, avoiding uterus displacement)
↓
Superimpose graft peritoneum on recipient bladder

(BP: blood pressure; IV: intravenous)

Follow-up

Postprocedure, all recipients are closely monitored for graft rejection with regular clinical visits and laboratory examinations. Initially for the 1st month, recipients are reviewed twice a week, and then two weeks once for the first 6 months; thereafter, patients are reviewed monthly. At each visit, the graft acceptance analysis is made indirectly by macroscopic examination of the cervix and the vaginal rim as well as regular cervical smears and biopsy. It is important to document a two-dimensional ultrasonography preferably by the transabdominal and the transvaginal route to assess the uterus and its vascularity (uterine artery Doppler bilaterally).

Difference between Live and Deceased Donors[60,61]

Table 2 shows difference between live and deceased donors.

IMMUNOSUPPRESSION

Uterus transplant like any other organ transplant relies on immunosuppression maintenance to minimize graft rejection. The challenge is to maintain a balanced drug level in the most favorable immunosuppression range between preventing rejection and having adverse reactions of immunosuppression. In contrast to other solid organs, a successful uterus transplant is only determined after a live birth post-transplant. Thus, immunosuppressant is given for years together; in pregnancy, lactation; until childbearing is completed and the uterus is removed.

There is no constant level of immunosuppression. Initially in the perioperative period, high doses of immunosuppressive drugs are given to attain high circulating blood levels—to prevent an acute rejection episode. Thereafter, drugs are tapered down to a maintenance level where therapy is usually initiated with a combination of three or more drugs, with different mechanisms of action in order to minimize the potential toxicity and side effects. Various combinations of immunosuppression drugs have been tried; however, the principle remains constant.

Immunosuppressant Drugs Commonly Used in Uterus Transplant[62-64]

These drugs are given in **Table 3**.

Episodes of mild rejection are usually treated with short course of high-dose corticosteroids. Immunosuppression is maintained throughout pregnancy and delivery. Thousands of births among women with solid organ transplants have been reported and the congenital malformation rate is almost similar as the general population.[65,66]

ETHICAL ISSUES

Uterus transplant is still in its clinical experimental stages and being a nonvital organ transplant, ethical analysis is essential. The transplant process is a complex one thus requiring a detail risk benefit analysis. Four parties are involved in a case of uterus transplant—the donor, recipient, recipient's partner, and the future child. Hence, it is a

Table 2: Difference between live and deceased donors.

	Living	***Deceased (brain dead-heart beating donor)***
Advantages	Detailed history can be taken	Surgical risk not imposed onto the donor
	Planned, well-designed surgery, scheduling convenience	Possibility of removal of longer vascular pedicles (more radical dissection)
	Easier preoperative assessment—complete infection assessment	Possible to remove a longer vaginal cuff (decreases ascending infections)
	Structural diseases of the uterus (leiomyoma, polyp) and diagnosis of infection (HPV) can be done and treated	May obtain potentially younger donors
	Proximity (decreases cold ischemia time)	Shorter surgical time
	Lower risk of rejection	
	Better histocompatibility	
Disadvantages	Higher surgical risks (urethral injury, risk of mortality)	Less comprehensive assessment—unverified history
	Psychological risks	Higher chances of graft rejection
	Increased average age	Increased ischemia time, greater distance from recipient
	Longer surgical time	Systemic inflammatory changes occur at brain death that affect graft survival
	May not obtain sufficient graft pedicle length	Less convenient scheduling of procedure—may have to be done as an emergency procedure, difficult logistic organization at a short time span
	Ethical issue-risking life of a healthy donor	Consent from kin may be difficult to obtain scarcity of appropriate donors

Table 3: Immunosuppressant drugs commonly used in uterus transplant.

Phase	***Drug***	***Dose/desired level***	***Mechanism of action***	***FDA category***	***Observations***
Induction	Corticosteroid	500 mg IV		B	No evidence of teratogenicity
	Antithymoglobulin or thymoglobulin	5 mg/kg BW or 2.5 mg/kg BW	Depletes peripheral T cells	C	Limited knowledge available on use in pregnant women
Maintenance	Tacrolimus	Dose—0.2 mg/kg/day Desired level 7–15 ng/mL	Calcineurin inhibitor	C	Preterm births, renal impairment, high doses cause transient hyperkalemia
	Mycophenolate mofetil (MMF)	Area under curve trough level maintained 40–60 mg/H/L	Decrease guanine synthesis which is important for T and B cell function	D	▪ To be stopped before pregnancy ▪ Strictly contraindicated in pregnancy ▪ Miscarriage, wide spectrum of congenital malformation
	Azathioprine	Dose < 2 mg/kg/day	Antimetabolites—inhibits nucleotide synthesis preventing mitosis of rapidly dividing cells	D	Preterm births, low birth weight
	Corticosteroids	Dose < 15 mg/day			

priority to weigh the need of the transplant in concordance with principles of bioethics—respect for autonomy, nonmaleficence, beneficence, and justice to ensure the best possible fair outcome.[67]

- Nonlife saving procedure: Uterus transplant is not considered a solid organ vital transplant. Procurement of a donor uterus is considered vital for the recipient couple in terms of having the possibility of pregnancy. Therefore, like the transplant of nonvital organs, uterus transplant maybe considered a life-enhancing procedure.
- Risks or surgery both to the recipient and the donor: Several ethical questions have been made regarding subjecting an otherwise healthy individual through a surgical procedure for a transplant procedure. Recipient not only undergoes the transplant surgery, but will have to undergo repeated surgeries for delivery (cesarean section) and a hysterectomy once her child bearing desire is completed. Each surgical procedure carries a risk of infection, thrombosis, graft rejection, bowel or bladder injury, and anesthesia complications that may cause prolonged morbidity or even mortality. The healthy live donor is also subjected to surgical and anesthetic risks due to extensive dissection.
- Informed consent: Both the donor and the recipient couple should be made aware of the potential risks and the benefits of the procedure. An informed documented consent is essential. It should be made clear of what this transplant procedure may offer and what the expectations of the recipient from the procedure are.
- Choice of donor or recipient: The basic principles of human ethics of respect for autonomy, nonmaleficence, beneficence, and justice.[68]
- Physical and mental risks: Uterus transplant is not a tried and tested procedure. Patients are aware regarding the experimental nature of the procedure. Adequate support and counseling is required to alleviate their worries and mental burden.
- Prolonged immunosuppression in a healthy individual: Uterus transplant is carried out in an otherwise healthy individual. Ethical concerns have been raised regarding prolonged immunosuppression in these patients. Most immunosuppressants cross the placental barrier and the long-term effects of these drugs are not known. Aim of uterus transplant was to achieve a healthy baby. These drugs have been associated with preterm births and low birth weight. Uterus is a unique organ that behaves marvelously in pregnancy to accept the fetus. In case of graft rejection by the body during pregnancy, the only solution is to remove the uterus along with the fetus in situ. Failing to remove the necrotic uterus may lead to a loss of two lives—the mother and the fetus. Hence, with prolonged immunosuppression, the main objective of the transplant process is in question and the prospect of double death is the worst possible outcome for the family.
- Alternative options: Options of surrogacy and adoption should be discussed. Both uterus transplant and surrogacy are done to fulfill the desires of a woman to have their own genetic child. Surrogacy however does not allow the infertile woman an emotional bond of carrying a pregnancy and the magical experience of childbirth and motherhood. Adoption does not allow a genetic link between the child and the parents and the adoption process is not guaranteed. In addition, many countries are banning the use of surrogates and the scarcity of surrogate mothers perhaps is going in favor of uterus transplant.[69]
- Welfare of the newborn: In uterus transplant, the woman who delivers the child is the mother, therefore the legal status of the child is established. Gametes of both the parents are used and hence the problem of right to know about birth does not arise which is of concern in gamete donation. The emotional bond between the mother and the fetus develops. Problems of breach of contract by the surrogate, refusing to return the newborn, rejecting the newborn by the commissioning couple, and compensation for the surrogate will be solved with uterus transplant.

MEDICAL, ETHICAL, AND SOCIAL PROBLEMS ASSOCIATED WITH UTERUS TRANSPLANT[70]

The problems associated with uterus transplant are shown in **Table 4**.

Difference of Uterus Transplant Compared to Other Solid Organ Transplant

- Uterus is a nonvital organ.
- *Ephemeral transplantation:* Transplanted uterus removed after objectives, i.e. childbearing desires are complete
- Nerve innervations are not present: No pain sensation, will not appreciate labor pains.
- Absolute indication for cesarean section
- Still experimental
- Long-term clinical outcomes not known

Table 4: Medical, ethical, and social problems associated with uterus transplant.

Medical	***Ethical***	***Social***
Surgical procedure: Uterus retrieval, ischemia perfusion injury, vascular anastomosis	Nonessential organ transplant	*Social need*: For uterine factor infertility patients
Prolonged immunosuppression	Risks to healthy live donor and recipient	*Financial costs*: Presently in the experimental stage, hence decreased cost
Frequent follow-up: Evaluation for blood flow in the uterus	Prolonged immunosuppression and teratogenicity	
Diagnosis of rejection is difficult: Recognized usually after it is full blown	Physical and mental risks Welfare of the newborn child	
	Alternative option: Surrogate and adoption	

CONCLUSION

Reproductive endocrinology and infertility is constantly an expanding discipline. Four decades have passed since the birth of Louise Brown, and the *assisted reproductive* technology (ART) fraternity has come a long way since trying to culture an embryo in vitro to transplanting uterus. Uterus transplants are an excellent solution for many absolute infertility couples who otherwise cannot conceive their desired child by other treatments. Although clinical application of uterus transplant has just begun, it seems to have a positive outcome. Let us see if it can stand the test of time and become a surrogate for the surrogates!

REFERENCES

1. Mascarenhas M, Flaxman S, Boerma T, et al. National, regional, and global trends in infertility prevalence since 1990: A systematic analysis of 277 health surveys. PLoS Med. 2012;9(12):p.e1001356.
2. Inhorn M, Patrizio P. Infertility around the globe: new thinking on gender, reproductive technologies and global movements in the 21st century. Hum Reprod Update. 2015;21(4):411-26.
3. Milliez J. Uterine transplantation. Int J Gynecol Obstet. 2009;106(3):270-70.
4. Fenton R. Catholic Doctrine Versus Women's Rights: The New Italian Law on Assisted Reproduction. Med Law Rev. 2005;14(1):73-107.
5. Armour K. An overview of surrogacy around the World: Trends, questions and ethical issues. Nurs Women's Health. 2012;16(3):231-36.
6. Fenton-Glynn C. Outsourcing ethical dilemmas: Regulating International Surrogacy Arrangements. Med Law Rev. 2016;24(1):59-75.
7. Fontana L, Gentilin B, Fedele L, et al. Genetics of Mayer-Rokitansky-Küster-Hauser (MRKH) syndrome. Clin Gen. 2016;91(2):233-46.
8. Choussein S, Nasioudis D, Schizas D, et al. Mullerian dysgenesis: a critical review of the literature. Arch Gynecol Obstet. 2017;295(6):1369-81.
9. Chan Y, Jayaprakasan K, Zamora J, et al. The prevalence of congenital uterine anomalies in unselected and high-risk populations: a systematic review. Hum Reprod Update. 2011;17(6):761-71.
10. Saravelos S, Cocksedge K, Li T. The pattern of pregnancy loss in women with congenital uterine anomalies and recurrent miscarriage. Reprod BioMed Online. 2010;20(3):416-22.
11. Ludwin A, Ludwin I, Pityński K, et al. Are the ESHRE/ESGE criteria of female genital anomalies for diagnosis of septate uterus appropriate? Hum Reprod. 2014;29(4):867-68.
12. Venetis C, Papadopoulos S, Campo R, et al. Clinical implications of congenital uterine anomalies: a meta-analysis of comparative studies. Reprod BioMed Online. 2014;29(6):665-83.
13. Pfeifer S, Butts S, Dumesic D, et al. Uterine septum: a guideline. Fertil Steril. 2016;106(3):530-40.
14. Johnson M, Schlaff W. Diagnosis and treatment of Asherman syndrome. Postgrad Obstet Gynecol. 2006; 26(6):1-6.
15. Yu D, Wong Y, Cheong Y, et al. Asherman syndrome: one century later. Fertil Steril. 2008;89(4):759-79.
16. Bleyer A. Cancer in 15- to 29-year-olds by primary site. Oncologist. 2006;11(6):590-601.
17. Xie L, Semenciw R, Mery L. Cancer incidence in Canada: trends and projections (1983-2032). Heal Prom Chron Dis Prev Can. 2015;35(Suppl 1):2-186.
18. Prat J. Ovarian, fallopian tube and peritoneal cancer staging: Rationale and explanation of new FIGO staging 2013. Best Pract Res Clin Obstet Gynaecol. 2015;29(6):858-69.
19. Claudia A, Matsuda T, Di Carlo V, et al. Global Surveillance of Trends in Cancer Survival 2000–14 (CONCORD-3): Analysis of individual records for 37 513 025 patients diagnosed with one of 18 cancers from 322 population-based registries in 71 countries. Lancet. 2018;391(10125):1023-75.
20. Allemani C, Weir H, Carreira H, et al. Global surveillance of cancer survival 1995–2009: analysis of individual data for 25 676 887 patients from 279 population-based registries in 67 countries (CONCORD-2). Lancet. 2015;385(9972):977-1010.
21. Lee S, Schover L, Partridge A, et al. American Society of Clinical Oncology Recommendations on fertility preservation in cancer patients. J Clin Oncol. 2006;24(18):2917-31.
22. Martinez F. Update on fertility preservation from the Barcelona International Society for Fertility Preservation–ESHRE–ASRM

2015 expert meeting: indications, results and future perspectives. Hum Reprod. 2017;32(9):1802-11.
23. Ogilvy-Stuart A, Shalet S. Effect of radiation on the human reproductive system. Environ Heal Perspect. 1993;101:109.
24. Meirow D, Biederman H, Anderson R, et al. Toxicity of chemotherapy and radiation on female reproduction. Clin Obstet Gynecol. 2010;53(4):727-39.
25. Green D, Kawashima T, Stovall M, et al. Fertility of female survivors of childhood cancer: A report from the Childhood Cancer Survivor Study. J Clin Oncol. 2009;27(16):2677-85.
26. Oktem O, Kim S, Selek U, et al. Ovarian and uterine functions in female survivors of childhood cancers. Oncologist. 2017;23(2):214-24.
27. Bermudez A, Bhatla N, Leung E. Cancer of the cervix uteri. Int J Gynecol Obstet. 2015;131:S88-S95.
28. Raab S. American Cancer Society, American Society for Colposcopy and Cervical Pathology, and American Society for Clinical Pathology Screening Guidelines for the Prevention and Early Detection of Cervical Cancer. Yearbook Pathol Lab Med. 2013;2013:273-5.
29. Torre L, Bray F, Siegel R, et al. Global cancer statistics, 2012. CA: Can J Clin. 2015;65(2):87-108.
30. van den Akker T, Brobbel C, Dekkers O, et al. Prevalence, indications, risk indicators, and outcomes of emergency peripartum hysterectomy worldwide. Obstet Gynecol. 2016;128(6):1281-94.
31. Mattingly RF, Clark DO, Lutsky II, et al. Ovarian function in-utero ovarian homotransplantation. Am J Obstet Gynecol. 1970;5:773-94.
32. Wranning CA, Akhi SN, Kurlberg G, et al. Uterus transplantation in the rat: model development, surgical learning and morphological evaluation. Acta Obstet Gynecol Scand. 2008;87:1239-47.
33. Akhi SN, Diaz-Garcia C, El-Akouri RR, et al. Uterine rejection after allogeneic uterus transplantation in the rat is effectively suppressed by tacrolimus. Fertil Steril. 2013;99:862-70.
34. Racho El-Akouri R, Kurlberg G, Brännström M. Successful uterine transplantation in the mouse: pregnancy and postnatal development of offspring. Hum Reprod. 2003;18:2018-23.
35. Racho El-Akouri R, Kurlberg G, Dindelegan G, et al. Heterotopic uterine transplantation by vascular anastomosis in the mouse. J Endocrinol. 2002;174:157-66.
36. Avison DL, DeFaria W, Tryphonopoulos P, et al. Heterotopic uterus transplantation in a swine model. Transplantation. 2009;88:465-9.
37. Saso S, Petts G, David AL, et al. Achieving an early pregnancy following allogeneic uterine transplantation in a rabbit model. Eur J Obstet Gynecol Reprod Biol. 2015;185:164-9.
38. Ramirez ER, Ramirez-Nessetti DK, Nessetti MB, et al. Pregnancy and outcome of uterine allotransplantation and assisted reproduction in sheep. J Minim Invasive Gynecol. 2011;18:238-45.
39. Enskog A, Johannesson L, Chai DC, et al. Uterus transplantation in the baboon: methodology and long-term function after auto-transplantation. Hum Reprod. 2010;25:1980–1987
40. Johannesson L, Enskog A, Dahm-Kähler P, et al. Uterus transplantation in a non-human primate: long-term follow up after autologous transplantation. Hum Reprod. 2012;27: 1640-8.
41. Kisu I, Mihara M, Banno K, et al. A new surgical technique of uterine auto-transplantation in cynomolgus monkey: preliminary report about two cases. Arch Gynecol Obstet. 2012;285:129-37.
42. Castellón L, Amador M, González R, et al. The history behind successful uterine transplantation in humans. JBRA Assisted Reproduction. 2017;21(2):126-34.
43. Brännström M, Diaz-Garcia C, Olausson M, et al. Uterus transplantation: animal research and human possibilities. Fertil Steril. 2012;97:169-76.
44. Kisu I, Banno K, Mihara M, et al. Uterine transplantation in primates: A mini-review of the literature. Transplant Proceed. 2014;46(4):1212-6.
45. Fageeh W, Raffa H, Jabbad H, et al. Transplantation of the human uterus. Int J Gynecol Obstet. 2002;76:245-51.
46. Ozkan O, Akar M, Ozkan O, et al. Preliminary results of the first human uterus transplantation from a multiorgan donor. Fertil Steril. 2013;99(2):470-6.
47. Erman Akar M, Ozkan O, Uraz B, et al. Clinical pregnancy following uterus transplantation. Fertil Steril. 2013;100(3):S142.
48. Akouri R, Brännström M. Human uterus transplantation with live births; Outcome of the first clinical trials. Geburtshilfe und Frauenheilkunde. 2016;76(03):43-51.
49. Brännström M, Johannesson L, Dahm-Kähler P, et al. First clinical uterus transplantation trial: a six-month report. Fertil Steril. 2014;101(5):1228-36.
50. Johannesson L, Kvarnström N, Mölne J, et al. Uterus transplantation trial: 1-year outcome. Fertil Steril. 2015;103(1):199-204.
51. Wei L, Xue T, Tao K, et al. Modified human uterus transplantation using ovarian veins for venous drainage: the first report of surgically successful robotic-assisted uterus procurement and follow-up for 12 months. Fertil Steril. 2017;108(2):346-56.e1.
52. Flyckt R, Davis A, Farrell R, et al. Uterine transplantation: Surgical innovation in the treatment of uterine factor infertility. J Obstet Gynaecol Can. 2018;40(1):86-93.
53. Silva A, Carvalho L. A meta-analysis on uterine transplantation: Redefining the limits of reproductive surgery. Revista da Associação Médica Brasileira. 2016;62(5):474-7.
54. Lefkowitz A, Edwards M, Balayla J. The Montreal Criteria for the Ethical Feasibility of Uterine Transplantation. Transplant Int. 2012;25(4):439-47.
55. Lefkowitz A, Edwards M, Balayla J. Ethical considerations in the era of the uterine transplant: an update of the Montreal Criteria for the Ethical Feasibility of Uterine Transplantation. Fertil Steril. 2013;100(4):924-6.
56. Johannesson L, Enskog A. Experimental uterus transplantation. Best Pract Res Clin Obstet Gynaecol. 2014;28(8):1198-210.
57. Brännström M, Diaz-Garcia C, Hanafy A, et al. Uterus transplantation: animal research and human possibilities. Fertil Steril. 2012;97(6):1269-76.
58. Brännström M. Uterus transplantation and beyond. J Mat Sci: Mat Med. 2017;28(5):72.

59. Arnolds K, Gomez N, Berry A, et al. Assessment of an alternative to the uterine vein for venous drainage in human uterine transplantation: a case series following laparoscopic hysterectomy. Gynecol Obstet Invest. 2016;81:436-41.
60. Lavoué V, Vigneau C, Duros S, et al. Which donor for uterus transplants. Transplantation. 2017;101(2):267-73.
61. Kisu I, Mihara M, Banno K, et al. Risks for donors in uterus transplantation. Reprod Sci. 2013;20(12):1406-15.
62. Saso S, Logan K, Abdallah Y, et al. Use of cyclosporine in uterine transplantation. J Transplant. 2012;2012:Article ID 134936.
63. Johannesson L, Kvarnstrom N, Molne J, et al. Human uterus transplantation trial: Monitoring, rejection episodes and immunosuppression during 1 year. Transplantation, 2014;98:14-5.
64. Kisu I, Banno K, Mihara M, et al. Current status of uterus transplantation in primates and issues for clinical application. Fertil Steril. 2013;100(1):280-94.
65. Dahm-Kähler P, Diaz-Garcia C, Brännström M. Human uterus transplantation in focus. British Med Bull. 2016;117(1): 69-78.
66. Ejzenberg D, Mendes L, Haddad L, et al. Uterine transplantation: a systematic review. Clinics. 2016;71(11):679-83.
67. McCulloch P, Altman D, Campbell W, et al. No surgical innovation without evaluation: the IDEAL recommendations. Lancet. 2009;374(9695):1105-12.
68. Daar J, Klipstein S. Refocusing the ethical choices in womb transplantation. J Law Biosci. 2016;3(2):383-8.
69. Del Priore G, Saso S, Meslin E, et al. Uterine transplantation: a real possibility? Indianapolis Consen Hum Reprod. 2012;28(2):288-91.
70. Brosens I, Ghaem-Maghami S, Pijnenborg R. Uterus transplantation in the human: a complex surgical, medical and ethical challenge. Hum Reprod. 2012;28(2):292-3.

Preimplantation Genetic Testing: A Pivotal Component of ART

73

Joe Leigh Simpson, Svetlana Rechitsky, Anver Kuliev

INTRODUCTION

Preimplantation genetic testing (PGT) is an accepted component of not only prenatal genetic diagnosis overall but assisted reproductive technologies (ART). PGT has been performed for over 500 single gene disorders,[1] and the spectrum of monogenic indications continues to expand. PGT to detect chromosomal abnormalities is likewise widely applied with precise age groups and indications now being refined. PGT is integrated with ART to identify and transfer euploid embryos.

Value of PGT in ART has not always been so recognized. First introduced in the late 1980s and early 1990s, PGT was once considered of arcane "boutique" value, more tour de force molecular technology than generalizable to the broader reproductive medicine community.[2] Relevance of PGT to ART seemed scant. Yet the need to improve pregnancy rates in ART has long been a goal for both disciplines. Aneuploid embryos are a major reason for less than optimal ART success in older women and the known explanation for increased miscarriages. Failure to distinguish aneuploid embryos on the basis of morphology has led to multiple embryo transfers, and undesirable preterm births. The desire for euploid ART pregnancies parallels the use of chorionic villus sampling or amniocentesis to avoid offspring with chromosomal abnormalities. At one time, limited technology precluded widespread acceptance of PGT. In 2019, this is no longer the case.

The current state of PGT integrating well with ART required progress in the molecular era. PGT would be fruitless without ability to amplify DNA [polymerase chain reaction (PCR)] to produce samples of normal and mutant DNA. When this became possible by PCR, detection of monogenic disorders became possible.[3,4] It was with further advances and improvements [array comparative genomic hybridization (CGH), next generation sequencing (NGS)] that it has made possible detection of the 500 different monogenic disorders. In our unit, we have performed PGT for monogenic disorders in 6,000 cycles; 600 were for the increasingly attractive indication of heritable adult-onset conditions. We have performed PGT in another 12,000 cycles to exclude chromosomal abnormalities. Again, technological advances have been pivotal. Initially diagnosis of chromosomal abnormalities depended on fluorescent in situ hybridization (FISH), fluorochromes differentially labeled with a specific chromosome. This allowed exclusion of liveborn trisomies but was of limited value in improving ART pregnancy rates because only 5–7 chromosomes could be interrogated. Next generation now enables all 24 chromosomes to be interrogated. ART benefit from only euploid embryos being transferred.

More innovations can be expected in ART and PGT alike. Indeed, advances in reproductive genetics as well as ART have followed parallel tracks, as described by us in the 2019 Fertility and Sterility Celebration of 40 Years of In Vitro Fertilization.[5] It is illustrative that Nobel Laureate Robert Edwards contributed to both fields PGT and was in fact a Past - President of the Preimplantation Genetic Diagnosis International Society (PGDIS). Earlier, Gardener and Edwards performed blastocyst biopsy in a rabbit embryo, using sex chromatin (Barr body) to distinguish XX from XY embryos.[6] The relevance to X-linked recessive disorders in humans was noted. Among the first clinical revelations of the cytogenetic era in the 1960s was that 50% or more of miscarriages were due to chromosomal abnormalities, especially with advanced maternal age. Had this not have been known, miscarriages after ART might reflexly have been attributed to laboratory-based problems or toxicants.

In this commentary, we will explore current policy and clinical recommendations for preimplantation genetic testing for monogenic (PGT-M) and preimplantation genetic testing for aneuploid (PGT-A).

OBTAINING DNA: BLASTOCYST (TROPHECTODERM BIOPSY)

In 2019, the preferred approach for PGT is biopsy of the trophectoderm of a blastocyst, (5–6 days embryo). There are 120 or more cells in the blastocysts; thus, cells can more safely be removed to provide more DNA and facilitate diagnosis. Another advantage is that the biopsied trophectoderm will differentiate into the placenta, not the inner cell mass where cells become destined to result in organs reside.

Ability to cryopreserve a biopsied embryo while its diagnosis is underway greatly facilitates PGT. At present, the recommended ART protocol is to "freeze all" embryos after biopsy. Embryos that are euploid and normal for any tested monogenic disorder can be transferred at a later time. The endometrium should by then be more favorable for implantation because untoward effects of agents required for ovulation stimulation will have dissipated.

STRATEGY FOR PREIMPLANTATION GENETIC TESTING FOR MONOGENIC DISORDERS

The small amount of DNA obtained by embryo biopsy (6 pg/cell) requires amplification to provide an amount sufficient for diagnostic testing. Whole-genome amplification (WGA) is performed using universal primers, providing sufficient DNA for laboratory diagnosis. However, 5–10% of alleles needed for analysis do not amplify sufficiently. It is pivotal to realize that absence of a DNA sequence does not necessarily mean that portion of DNA is absent from the specimen. Strategies must, therefore, be developed to recognize this phenomenon, which is termed allele drop out (ADO).

Linkage Analysis is an Essential Safeguard Against Failure of DNA Amplification

PGT-M should not be performed if the result is based solely on presence or absence of a mutant (or normal) DNA sequence.[1] A lab result reporting lack of a given mutant DNA sequence could mean genuine absence of the DNA sequence in the sample (a deletion), but results could also mean ADO, that is, DNA is actually present but primers have simply failed to anneal with that sequence; therefore, hybridization cannot occur and this is the reason its presence in the sample is not recognized. If ADO is not appreciated, this could result in erroneous transfer of an affected embryo. If ADO involves an autosomal dominant mutant allele, the clinical consequence would be a false negative. If ADO involves the normal allele in an embryo being interrogated for an autosomal recessive condition, an opportunity to transfer a clinically normal embryo would be lost if the partner's transmitted allele were mutant; the embryo would have been considered homozygous affected. This would be false positive with respect to opportunity for pregnancy.

To avoid diagnostic errors due to ADO and to avoid decreasing pregnancy rates, linkage analysis is performed whenever a monogenic disorder is tested by PGT-M. In linkage analysis, one identifies polymorphic DNA markers on either side (5' or 3') of the mutation site. Alleles exist in pairs, one inherited one from each parent. One of the two alleles is linked to the mutation site, whereas the other allele is linked to the normal allele. Assume each marker is biallelic (A or B, C or D, E or F, G or H, I or J, K or L). The chromosome containing the mutant allele will have a specific sequence of informative polymorphic markers. Suppose for alleles A-C-E-(mutation)-H-I-L exists on one chromosome; those linked to the normal allele might be B-D-F-normal-G-J-K. Initially, the two haplotypes will not be known, but the two different haplotypes becomes readily differentiated on the basis of affected and unaffected family members. Embryos suitable for transfer can thus be distinguished from those not transferable. See elsewhere for details.[1,7]

De Novo Mutations

The strategy outlined above cannot be utilized if PGT-M is requested by an individual having no other affected family members. The mutation causing his or her disorder will have arisen as a result of a de novo parental gamete (sperm or oocyte). Testing his parents' blood will not show the mutant allele because the mutation is not germline and therefore will not be present in their blood or tissue other than germ cells.

Nevertheless, PGT-M is achievable.[8] If the affected individual is male and has an autosomal dominant mutation, one can analyze single sperm, of which there will be two (haploid) groups. Half the sperm will show the sequence of markers linked to the mutant allele, which would thus be detectable. The other half will show a different sequence, linked to the normal allele. Affected from unaffected embryos can be distinguished.

TRADITIONAL INDICATIONS FOR PGT-M (SINGLE-GENE DISORDERS)

Testing for monogenic disorders (PGT-M) can be performed whenever the chromosomal location of a gene causing a disorder is known. Approximately 600 different disorders have been tested worldwide. The most frequent have been hemoglobinopathies, cystic fibrosis, breast cancer, fragile X syndrome, spinal muscular atrophy, and Duchenne muscular dystrophy.[1,7] The most commonly performed PGT-M cases vary by region. Thalassemias are common in the Eastern Mediterranean and South East Asia regions, sickle cell anemia in Africa, cystic fibrosis in the United States. Our group has performed approximately 18,000 PGT cycles; 6,000 were for single gene disorders. The strategy of linkage analysis is always applied. Applicability exists even when the causative nucleotide basis is not known.

If PGT-M is desired, the ART team should contact their genetic referral center to learn of potential applicability. Confirmation is first needed of the previously made diagnosis in the ostensibly affected family member. If molecular analysis has not been performed, sequencing may be needed.

Virtually all monogenic disorders are molecularly heterogeneous; thus, many different nucleotide perturbations may exist. Sickle cell anemia is a notable exception for which one particular mutation is responsible for most cases. In other disorders, there may be a "most common" mutation but such a mutation usually explains less than half the cases. Thus, the same molecular alteration is causative in a given family, but not necessarily beyond. Knowing the exact molecular basis is necessary in order to develop the most robust testing strategy employing linkage analysis.

In our own unit, we recommend PGT-M be accompanied by PGT-A. This is technologically feasible and increasing pregnancy rates.

INDICATIONS APPLICABLE ONLY BY PREIMPLANTATION GENETIC TESTING

Preconception Diagnosis

Preconception diagnosis is possible, identifying a normal oocyte to be fertilized for a normal offspring. This is done by testing of the first and second polar body, both extruded before the embryo has formed (syngamy). This option is invaluable in venues (e.g., Germany) where PGT-A is otherwise not possible for regulatory reasons. Preconception diagnosis is restricted to the first polar biopsy. The reason is that the second polar body is not extruded until the mature oocyte is exposed to sperm.

Analysis of the second polar body thus would not be preconceptional. Fertilization with only unaffected oocytes would result in a normal embryo, but genetic analysis could not be finalized prior to pronuclear fusion.

Avoiding Termination of a Clinical Pregnancy

Chorionic villus sampling (CVS) and amniocentesis have been available for years prior to PGT. The strategy was detection of an abnormal fetus in time for clinical termination. This approach remains that of choice for most couples in the general population, often of advanced maternal age and wishing to avoid affected offspring. However, this approach may not be attractive or tolerable for religious or other reasons. PGT is a method of choice for couples wishing not only to avoid an affected liveborn but also to avoid termination of a clinical pregnancy.

Detecting Genotype Without Disclosure (Nondisclosure)

Suppose a person is at risk for, say, an adult-onset disorder because his or her parent is known to have such a disorder. Suppose this younger son or daughter wishes to remain unaware of his or her genotype—affected or not—yet does not wish to transmit a potential mutation to offspring. PGT makes this possible and practical because multiple embryos can be screened, yet results to the patient not disclosed. One can still transfer only embryos whose genotype will not result in offspring with the mutant gene. Pursuing this strategy requires the patient (son or daughter) remains oblivious to results of the process underway. For example, the patient should remain unaware of the number of embryos arising from ovulation stimulation, number of oocytes aspirated, and number successfully cultured. Otherwise deductions could be made concerning whether they inherited or did not inherit the abnormal genotype for which they are at 50% risk. If only 2 of 10 embryos were said to be transferable, for example, presence of the mutation might be suspected. At present, nondisclosure is practical because PGT-A testing could also be revealing aneuploidy as the result for few to zero transfers. A caveat is that this scenario must be repeated in all subsequent cycles, even if the (undisclosed) patient had in a previous cycle been shown not to carry the mutant gene.

Identifying Human Leukocyte Antigen-compatible Embryos for Stem Cell Transplantation Indication

Another indication for PGT is to obtain an embryo whose cord blood can be used for stem cell transplantation. Suppose a couple is at risk for a single gene disorder that deleteriously affects bone marrow (e.g., β-thalassemia). Suppose further that the couple already has and wishes to avoid having another affected child. Added benefit in the context of testing for β-thalassemia would exist if the human-leukocyte antigen (HLA)—type of the embryo selected for transfer were compatible with HLA type of the previously born affected sibling. Successful treatment of the older, moribund sibling would be possible if the newborn's stem cells were used to repopulate his older sibling's bone marrow. Success rates are well over 90% if HLA compatible, but much less if not HLA compatible.[9]

Odds of selecting an unaffected, HLA-identical embryo transfer are low, but achievable with the multiple embryos obtained than in ART. Multiple cycles may be needed with embryos batched. One in four embryos is HLA compatible with the liveborn (affected) sibling. Three of every four embryos are unaffected for an autosomal recessive disorder (1/4 homozygous affected; 2/4 heterozygous; 1/4 homozygous normal). The overall likelihood of the transferred embryo being both genetically normal and HLA identical is ¼ x ¾ = 3/16. (This does not take into account the 7–8% likelihood recombination in the affected case, which would make a perfect HLA-match impossible. As some couples present for such testing when maternal partners cannot produce sufficient number of oocytes for testing, their younger sister could be tested for HLA match. The sister may prove to be an acceptable oocyte donor. This option has in fact been employed in our practice.

In the United States and Turkey, testing for transfer of HLA-compatible embryos in families *not* being at risk for offspring with a genetic disorder is accepted. A family might have an older sibling with "nonmonogenic" condition, such as leukemia of somatic cell origin. While recurrence in the family is low, the affected individual could still benefit from HLA-matched neonate providing cord blood stem cells for transplantation. In Europe, this indication is uncommon.

PGT-M FOR ADULT-ONSET HERITABLE DISORDERS

An increasing indication for PGT is a heritable adult-onset disorder. Until circa 2000, prenatal genetic diagnosis for single gene disorders was considered applicable to the genetic community only for disorders of childhood onset. It was espoused that heritable adult onset disorders, such as breast cancer due to BRCA1/2, were not appropriate indications. Rather, one should wait until the age of maturity to let the at-risk person decide for themselves whether they should undergo genetic testing. A problem was, of course, that many so-called adult onset conditions manifested symptoms prior to the age of maturity. Naturally, it is desirable to detect for early treatment, or by analogy, to select an unaffected embryo for transfer to prevent. In 2001, Reproductive Genetics Innovation (RGI) performed PGT-M for Li-Fraumeni syndrome, a heritable cancer affecting multiple organ systems[10] and often manifested before the age of 18 years. Since then, individuals at risk for many adult-onset disorders have increasingly sought PGT-M for heritable cancers, cardiac disorders, and neurodegenerative disorders.

Heritable Cancers

The most common heritable cancers for which PGT-M is performed are BRCA1, BRCA2, Li-Fraumeni syndrome, multiple endocrine neoplasia (MEN), familial adenomatous polyposis (FAP), retinoblastoma, and Von-Hippel-Lindau syndrome.[1] All are autosomal dominant. At RGI, we have performed PGT-M for heritable cancers in 600 cycles. At present we do so concomitantly with PGT-A. Liveborn rates approximate 50% per blastocyst transfer, reflecting proven fertility, youth, and concomitant PGT-A.

In single gene disorders undergoing PGT-M, the specific mutation in given heritable cancers is ideally known, just as it is for other indications for single gene PGT-M. Breast cancer is the most common cancer indication for PGT-M. In breast cancer, 72% of women with a pathogenic BRCA 1 mutation manifest neoplasia by age 80 years; in BRCA 2 69% do. [12]The risk for ovarian cancer is also increased.[11] In our experience the most common mutation in women with BRCA 1 seeking PGT-M is 187delAG, responsible for 40% of mutations we detected. The most common mutation we encounter in BRCA 2 is 617delT, responsible for 51% of mutations we detected. For BRCA 1 or BRCA 2, there are many other mutations, each individually uncommon. If a mutation is not identified but BRCA 1 or BRCA 2 seems the likely diagnosis clinically, PGT-M can proceed solely on the basis of linkage analysis.

Heritable Cardiac Disorders

Several autosomal dominant adult-onset cardiac disorders are attractive candidates for PGT-M.[12] Some are pleiotropic disorders, such as Marfan syndrome. In others, phenotype is restricted to the cardiac system. Hypertrophic cardiomyopathy and hypotrophic cardiomyopathy are examples. PGT-M has been successful in multiple different conditions. In these conditions, symptoms leading to cardiac failure are usually manifested during the second and third decade, often unexpectedly. Treatment is not always successful. PGT-M is attractive also for long Q-T syndrome. Arrhythmias manifest unexpectedly and may result in sudden death, sometimes in the context of athletic exertion.

Heritable Neurodegenerative Disorders

Neurodegenerative disorders of adult onset can also result from perturbation in a single gene. Huntington disease has long received attention and is a frequent indication for nondisclosure strategy as discussed above. Other heritable neurodegenerative autosomal dominant disorders include early onset Alzheimer syndrome. Age of onset is less than 50 years, differentiated itself from the more typical Alzheimer syndrome in which age of onset is 75–80 years. In later age Alzheimer syndrome, inheritance is polygenetic/multifactorial; PGT-M is thus not possible.

TRADITIONAL PREIMPLANTATION GENETIC TESTING FOR CHROMOSOMAL DISORDERS

Contemporary Methodology

Because it is not practical to obtain a karyotype from a single cell, PGT for chromosomal abnormalities (numerical or structural) has always had to rely on other methods. As previously disclosed,[2] methodology initially utilized FISH with5–7 chromosome-specific probes per hybridization. Superimposed signals in different plains also make diagnosis hazardous. Further, a single chromosome dividing during mitosis could show 2 signals and with its homologue showing one; thus the 3 signals would mimic trisomy. Diagnosis is now robust using array CGH or NGS. All 24 chromosomes are testable, and accuracy very high.

PGT-A Accompanying PGT-M in Couples at Increased Risk for Liveborns with Monogenic Disorders

Excluding aneuploidy in a pregnant woman at risk because of advanced age usually leads to counseling that includes CVS or amniocentesis is recommended for maximum sensitivity. If only fetal autosomal trisomies are of concern, noninvasive cell-free DNA is preferable. However, if a couple is already undergoing ART for PGT-M, or must undergo ART for infertility, PGT-A becomes the logical method to exclude liveborn aneuploidy. There is no additional risk because DNA from the single embryo biopsy suffices for both PGT-A and PGT-M.

PGT for Structural Chromosome Abnormalities (PGT-SR)

In a couple in which one partner has a balanced translocation, the risk is increased for unbalanced gametes. In most balanced translocations only 10–20% of tested embryos are transferable. A very high proportion of gametes are abnormal as result of patterns of meiotic segregation; thus, a majority of embryos are abnormal. Embryos with duplications/deficiencies usually result in miscarriage or anomalous liveborns.

Couples in which one partner has a balanced translocation are not infertile. Indeed the cumulative likelihood of normal offspring is 65–70%, similar to couples without a translocation. However, PGT-SR (structural) is valuable if a couple has a balanced translocation and is of advanced maternal age. The time needed to achieve pregnancy by natural conception can be an impediment. The mean time to achieve a natural liveborn pregnancy is approximately 5 years in translocation couples, clearly longer than that of couples without a translocation.[13-15] PGT-SR can shorten the time to achieve a liveborn delivery for those having a balanced translocation.

One shortcoming in dealing with a balanced translocation is inability of array CGH or NGS to distinguish genetically normal embryos with 46 separate chromosomes from genetically normal embryos having a balanced translocation. In both the normal amount of DNA is present. In translocations, the DNA sequence is rearranged although total amount of DNA is unchanged.

PGT-A TO INCREASE ART PREGNANCY RATES

PGT to Identify Euploid Embryos to Transfer

ART success declines precipitously with advancing maternal age, principally due to aneuploidy in transferred embryos. Correlates validating this reality include pregnancy rates not decreasing with use of donor euploid oocytes until age 42 years.[16] An obvious strategy is to perform PGT-A and transfer only euploid embryos. This approach is performed in 30–40% of ART cycles in the United States.

Controversy that once existed on this strategy has largely dissipated, having been based on technical reasons. During 1995–2010, most biopsies were of a cleavage stage embryo and used FISH. Several randomized controlled trials (RCTs) failed to show benefit. By 2010-2012, the new analytical and biopsy techniques resulted in success: (1) Trophectoderm biopsy became the preferred biopsy method, rather than the technically more difficult cleavage-stage biopsy. (2) At least 5 cells were readily obtained rather than the single blastomere obtained with cleavage-stage biopsy. (3) 24 chromosome testing became routine, rather than 5–7 chromosomes. All this has led to a15–20% improved pregnancy rates with euploid blastocyst-transfer, compared to transfer of morphologically normal but nonbiopsied (nontested) embryo.[17-19]

A major clinical issue that remains unresolved is the precise maternal age at which PGT-A should be routinely recommended.[3] At present this seems to be ages 35–40 years, based on SART registry data[20] and RCT data comparing PGT-A versus no PGT-A.

A second unresolved issue requiring resolution is, paradoxically, pitfalls arising from increased sensitivity of NGS. High-resolution next generation technologies (NGS) unexpectedly have led to detection of mosaic and subchromosomal variants never evident with a less sensitive array. Approximately 8% of embryos have mosaic aneuploidy. The threshold for identification of a mosaic embryo is 20%. Embryos with less than 20% nonmodal DNA are considered euploid; embryos with greater than 80% are considered nonmosaic aneuploid. Embryos between 20% and 80% mosaicism are mosaic embryos; some yield pregnancies.[21,22] Mosaic embryos are not recommended for transfer so long as aneuploid embryo exists in the cohort. It is in fact uncommon (1% of cycles) for the only potentially transferable embryo to be mosaic aneuploid. In this case, the couple may elect to transfer that embryo. However, risks expected must be explained. PGDIS provides guidelines prioritizing for selection which embryo if more than one aneuploidy in present exists.[22]

PGT-A FOR SINGLE EMBRYO TRANSFER AND REDUCTION IN MULTIPLE GESTATIONS

Single embryo transfer (SET) has long been advocated to decrease the high rate of multiple gestations in ART. SET has, however, not always been practical; pregnancy rates have historically been 10% or lower than with double embryo transfer (DET). The DET strategy was pursued on the assumption that not all embryos transferred were capable of viable pregnancies, given aneuploidy rates. Multiple embryos were thus transferred in order to achieve an acceptable pregnancy rate. This unavoidably resulted in twins and higher order multiple gestations, and in turn premature births that brought criticism to the field.

PGT-aneuploidy testing can now reduce multiple gestations in ART without reducing the ART success. In an RCT, Forman and colleagues[23] stratified women of mean age 35 years into two arms: two morphologically normal blastocysts transferred without PGT-A (DET) versus transfer of one morphologically normal blastocyst known to be euploid (SET). Pregnancy rates did not differ statistically (65% vs 61%); however, the number of twin gestations was much higher (55% vs 0%). Given the very high cost of neonatal care for premature infants, this strategy provides favorable cost benefits analysis.

CONCOMITANT PGT-M AND PGT-A

Stated previously, but deserving emphasis is that PGT-A should accompany PGT-M. The "take-home baby rate" is increased 15–20%. No additional embryo damage exists because DNA from one biopsy suffices for PGT-M as well as for PGT-A.

SAFETY OF PREIMPLANTATION GENETIC DIAGNOSIS

Removal of one cell from an embryo, especially a 6–8 cells cleavage-shaped embryo, logically might impede implantation or decrease survival. Pregnancy rates might be decreased. Viability has been once indirectly estimated to be reduced by 10% when a single blastomere is removed from a cleavage stage embryo. Viability aside, the totipotential nature of embryonic cells reassures us that biopsy should not be expected to result in anomalous in liveborn infants. If one or more cells are lost prior to differentiation into an organ-specific pathway, a neighboring cell should have the capacity to subsume that purpose.

Available data indicate no increased rate of birth defects in liveborn infants having been the result of PGT. Differences are not apparent between offspring resulting from PGT-M versus PGT-A are.

REFERENCES

1. Kuliev A, Rechitsky S, Verlinsky O. Atlas of Preimplantation Genetic Diagnosis, 3rd edition. Boca Raton: Taylor & Francis; 2015.
2. Simpson JL, Kuliev A, Rechitsky S. Overview of preimplantation genetic diagnosis (PGD):Historical perspective and future direction. Methods Mol. Biol. 2019;1885:23-43.
3. Strom CM, Verlinsky Y, Milayeva S, et al. Preconception genetic diagnosis of cystic fibrosis. Lancet. 1990;336(8710):306-7.
4. Handyside AH, Lesko JG, Tarin JJ, et al. Birth of a normal girl after in vitro fertilization and preimplantation diagnostic testing for cystic fibrosis. N Engl J Med. 1992;327(13):905-9.
5. Simpson JL. Reproductive genetics paralleling assisted reproductive technology. Fertil Steril. 2018;110(2, theme issue):221-3.
6. Gardner RL, Edwards RG. Control of the sex ratio at full term in the rabbit by transferring sexed blastocysts. Nature. 1968;218(5139):346-9.
7. Kuliev A. Practical Preimplantation Genetic Diagnosis. London, Heidelberg, New York: Springer; 2013.
8. Rechitsky S, Pomerantseva E, Pakhalchuk T, et al. First systematic experience of preimplantation genetic diagnosis for de-novo mutations. Reprod Biome Online. 2011;22(4):350-61.
9. Rechitsky S, Kuliev A, Sharapova T, et al. PGD impact on stem cell transplantation. Reprod Biomed Online. 2009;18(Supplement 3):S-2.
10. Verlinsky Y, Rechitsky S, Verlinsky O, et al. Preimplantation diagnosis for p53 tumor suppressor gene mutations. Reprod biomed Online. 2001;2(2):102-5.
11. Kuchenbacker KB, Hopper JL, Barnes DR, et al. Risks of breast, ovarian and contralateral breast cancer for BRCA1 and BRCA2 mutation carriers. JAMA. 2017;317(23):2402-16.
12. Kuliev A, Pakhalchuk T, Rechitsky S. Preimplantation genetic diagnosis (PGD) for heart disease determined by genetic factors. Arrhythm Open Access. 2015;1(1):103-6.
13. Otani T, Roche M, Mizuike M, et al. Preimplantation genetic diagnosis significantly improves the pregnancy outcome of translocation carriers with a history of recurrent miscarriage and unsuccessful pregnancies. Reprod Biomed Online. 2006;13(6):869-74.
14. Stephense MD, Sierra S. Reproductive outcomes in recurrent pregnancy loss associated with a parental carrier of a structural chromosome rearrangement. Hum Reprod. 2006;21(4):1076-82.
15. Sugiura-Ogasawara M, Ozaki Y, Sato T, et al. Poor prognosis of recurrent aborters with either maternal or paternal reciprocal translocations. Fertil Steril. 2004;81(2):367-73.
16. Harton GL, Munne S, Surrey M, et al. Diminished effect of maternal age on implantation after preimplantation genetic diagnosis with array comparative genomic hybridization. Fertil Steril. 2013;100(6):1695-703.
17. Yang Z, Liu J, Collins GS, et al. Selection of single blastocysts for fresh transfer via standard morphology assessment alone and with array CGH for good prognosis IVF patients: Resultsfrom a randomized pilot study. Mol Cytogenet. 2012;5:24.
18. Scott RT, Upham KM, Forman EJ, et al. Blastocyst biopsy with comprehensive chromosome screening and fresh embryo transfer significantly increases in vitro fertilization implantation and delivery rates: A randomized controlled trial. Fertil Steril. 2013;100:697-703.
19. Dahdouh EM, Balayla J, Garcia-Velasco JA. Comprehensive chromosome screening improves embryo selection: A meta-analysis. Fertil Steril. 2015;104:1503-12.
20. Centers for Disease Control and Prevention.
21. https://www.cdc.gov/reproductivehealth/Data_Stats/index.htm
22. Greco E, Minasi MG, Florentino F. Healthy babies after intrauterine transfer of mosaic aneuploidy blastocysts. N Engl J Med. 2015;373(21):2089-90.
23. PGDIS. (2016). PGDIS position statement on chromosome mosaicism and preimplantation aneuploidy testing at the blastocyst stage. [online] Available from
24. https://www.pgdis.org/docs/newsletter_071816.html [Accessed February 2018].
25. Forman EJ, Hong KH, Franasiak JM, et al. Obstetrical and neonatal outcomes from the BEST Trial: single embryo transfer with aneuploidy screening improves out-comes after in vitro fertilization without compromising delivery rates. Am J Obstet Gynecol. 2014;210(2):157e151-157el156.

Preimplantation Genetic Testing

74

Ritu Hari, C Mohamed Ashraf, Shailaja Gada Saxena, Dhiraj Gada, Alexia Chatziparasidou

INTRODUCTION

Preimplantation genetic testing (PGT) is a relatively recent testing modality for identification of genetic aberrations in embryos generated through in vitro fertilization (IVF), prior to implantation.[1,2] Thus, PGT facilitates or ensures birth of healthy babies by negative selection of the affected embryos at the preimplantation stage. After testing, only the embryos identified as normal for the disease condition being tested are transferred back, thus weaning the risk of inheriting a genetic aberration. PGT provides an alternative to the current post-conception prenatal diagnostic procedures for the detection of genetic aberrations. In case of prenatal diagnosis, the parents can make an informed decision in consultation with the physicians and genetic counselors, on the option of continuation of the pregnancy and birth of the child, or medical termination of the fetus in case of identification of a genetic aberration in the offspring. As against that, PGT helps to eliminate the dilemma of medical termination of pregnancy that may follow prenatal diagnosis of genetic diseases.

As per the European Society of Human Reproduction and Embryology (ESHRE) preimplantation genetic diagnosis (PGD) consortium best practice guidelines, PGT has been classified into two categories including high-risk PGD and the low-risk PGD also known as preimplantation genetic screening (PGS).[3] PGD is usually performed in couples who are at high risk of transmitting a genetic or chromosomal aberration to their offspring as in case of autosomal recessive or dominant single gene defects of X-linked disorders or chromosomal aberration. On the other hand, PGS is carried out for infertile patients to improve the pregnancy rate in women with advanced maternal age, repeated IVF failure, and couples experiencing repeated abortion with known cause and having normal karyotypes.

INDICATIONS OF PGD/PGS

There is wide variety of disorder for which PGT is performed. The most common group for which PGD is performed includes testing in couples with a high risk of transmitting an inherited monogenic disorder including autosomal recessive disorders (like cystic fibrosis, β-thalassemia, and sickle cell disease), autosomal dominant disorders (like myotonic dystrophy and Huntington's disease) or X-linked disorders (like fragile X syndrome, hemophilia A, and Duchene muscular dystrophy) or a structural chromosomal aberration (like balanced reciprocal and Robertsonian translocation, inversion, etc.). Nowadays, PGD is also being offered for mitochondrial disorders. Apart from this, PGD has also been used for varied indications like human leukocyte antigen (HLA) matching for umbilical cord blood stem cell transplant for an affected sibling. Another condition for which PGD has been offered includes late onset disorders like Huntington's disease and for deselecting genes predisposing to hereditary cancer [BRCA (BReast CAncer) gene testing].

Another major indication for PGT is for screening of embryos for chromosomal aneuploidies (PGS) to increase the chances of an ongoing pregnancy as in cases of advanced maternal age, a history of recurrent miscarriages or repeated implantation failure. It has also been proposed for patients with obstructive and nonobstructive azoospermia. PGS is offered for selecting chromosomally normal embryos, i.e. to rule out aneuploidies.

STEPS INVOLVED IN PREIMPLANTATION GENETIC DIAGNOSIS

For PGD, the oocytes are fertilized in vitro through IVF or intracytoplasmic sperm injection (ICSI). The embryos thus generated are cultured in vitro until the diagnosis is established. With advances in the area of cryopreservation and vitrification, in many cases, embryos are frozen postbiopsy and transferred in a subsequent cycle. In either case, for PGD/PGS, the embryos are subjected to single cell biopsy which may be at various stages of embryo development. The commonly used techniques include polar body biopsy from unfertilized and fertilized oocytes,[4-6] blastomere biopsy from day 3 cleavage-stage embryos **(Figs. 1A to D)**,[7,8] and trophectoderm (TE) biopsy from blastocyst-stage embryos.[9,10]

Sources of Obtaining Embryonic Cells (Table 1)

Polar Body Biopsy

Polar body biopsies permissible in few countries like Germany. Only maternal genetic component can be studied. However, it may be helpful in diagnosis of X-linked disorders.[11] For polar body biopsy, several groups advocate sequential removal of the polar bodies, with the first polar body removed from the oocyte on the day of the oocyte collection between 36 hours and 42 hours post- human chorionic gonadotropin (hCG) injection, i.e. on day zero[4] and the second polar body on day one.[11] In contrast, the first and second polar body can also be simultaneously removed from the zygote between 9 hours and 22 hours postinsemination. For the biopsy procedure, the fertilized oocyte is held with the holding pipette with the polar body at 12 o'clock position. The polar body pipette is introduced through the hole in the zona and one and/or both the first and the second polar body are aspirated.

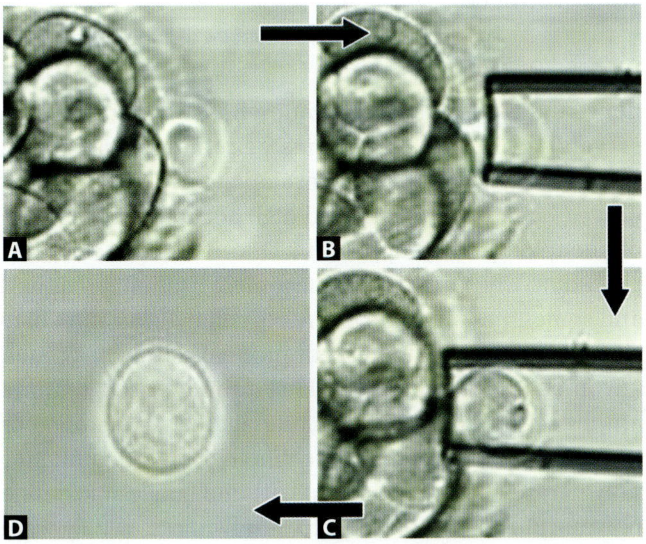

Figs. 1A to D: Cleavage stage embryo biopsy procedure: (A) 8-cell embryo on Day 3 is held with the holding pipette. Hole is drilled in the zona with the laser opposite the cell to be biopsied; (B) The embryo biopsy pipette is introduced through this opening, near the cell to be biopsied; (C) gentle suction is applied to dislodge the blastomere from the embryo; (D) blastomere showing the nucleus.

Blastomere Biopsy

Blastomere biopsy allows analysis of a single blastomere on day 3 of embryo development. It did not prove to be clinically beneficial as was associated with high degree of mosaicism. The zona breaching during cleavage stage is performed using acidified Tyrode's solution, laser or mechanical methods.[12] Cell may be removed from the zona either by aspiration through the hole[13] or extrusion[14] or displacement techniques.[15]

Day 5 Trophectoderm Biopsy

Blastocyst biopsy is gaining more and more popularity for PGD/PGS over the last few years. Several methods of blastocyst biopsy have been reported.[9,10,16-18] These include breaching of the zona on day 3 and removal of the TE on day 5; or zona breaching and TE removal on day 5. The removal of TE cells during blastocyst biopsy, herniation following drilling with laser or mechanical excision have been used.[16,19] Minimum of 5–10 cells removed reduced deoxyribonucleic acid (DNA) amplification failure. In a single biopsy both PGT for aneuploidy (PGT-A) **(Table 2)** and PGT for monogenic diseases (PGT-M) can be performed in the same time on next-generation sequencing (NGS). One of the limiting factors is not all embryos depending on patient factor goes to blast. This hampers the testing strategy in few cases. However, in a well-established IVF setup this can be taken well care of.

Technical Aspects

Since aneuploidy is the major source of adverse outcomes in human reproduction. American College of Obstetricians and Gynecologists and the Society for Maternal-Fetal Medicine now recommend universal screening. Initially PGT involved fluorescence in situ hybridization (FISH) techniques wherein cleavage-stage embryonic cells were

Table 1: Comparison between the different biopsy methods.

	Polar bodies	*Day-3 embryo*	*Day-5 embryo*
Biopsy procedure	▪ Sequential removal of the 1st and the 2nd polar body before and after ICSI. ▪ Simultaneous removal of both polar bodies after ICSI	Removal of 1 blastomere from day-3 embryos with at least 5 cells	▪ Removal of 2-10 TE cells. ▪ Biopsy procedure may need to be repeated several times during day 5 and day 6
Informative	Only for the maternal contribution	For maternal and paternal contribution	For maternal and paternal contribution and mitotic errors
Mosaicism	No	No	Possible
Fresh embryo transfer	Possible	Possible	Often not possible
Negative effect of the biopsy procedure	Not known	There is a potential reduction of embryo viability	Safer than day-3 biopsy, if less than 10 TE cells are removed and inner cell mass remains intact
Limitations	▪ Fragmented polar bodies ▪ Increased error rate ▪ 2 tests for each oocyte ▪ No data for the paternal contribution ▪ Biopsy timing is very crucial	▪ May affect further embryo development and implantation potential. ▪ High mosaicism rate. ▪ High risk for false positive or negative results due to mosaicism	▪ Need for optimized culture conditions ▪ Need for optimized vitrification program ▪ Biopsy efficiency is operator depended
Advantages	▪ Safe, allows time for genetic analysis, and fresh transfer ▪ More accepted from ethical and religious point of view	Allows time for genetic analysis and fresh transfer	▪ ICM remains intact. ▪ More cellular material available for genetic testing
Disadvantages	▪ Labor-intensive ▪ Double biopsy and double tests ▪ Higher cost	▪ One cell may not represent the whole embryo ▪ In some embryos with granular cytoplasm nucleus may not be visible	▪ Only few embryos may progress to blastocyst stage. ▪ Higher rate of cancellation especially for low responders

(ICM: inner cell mass; ICSI: intracytoplasmic sperm injection; TE: trophectoderm)

obtained postbiopsy. This approach did not give promising results in terms of pregnancy rates as minimum number of chromosomes were studied and mosaicism being another limiting factor. However, multiple prospective trials suggested that biopsy of blastomeres followed by embryo selection based out of FISH results led to reduced miscarriage rate and enhanced implantation rate. Technically FISH is the gold standard in prenatal diagnosis in testing aneuploidies for chromosomes 13, 18, 21, and sex chromosomes compatible with life. Past years most of the women undergoing IVF would fall in the category of advanced maternal age or recurrent implantation failures. Hence, a smaller group of patients did benefit post FISH-based PGS. This leads to a rapid growth in the utilization of PGT. Geneticists were continuously working to overcome the limitations so that patients undergoing IVF could benefit from reduced miscarriage rates and increased implantation rates. First-generation PGT failed to produce more benefits; hence there was a need for comprehensive chromosomal screening (CCS). Comparative genomic hybridization (CGH), array one of the first developed techniques for CCS proved beneficial and showed high accuracy of diagnosis of aneuploidy when applied to TE cells. Unlike the FISH procedure where single cell blastomere fixation is required and sometimes multiple rounds of cell hybridization may be required for the fluorescent probe used to check each chromosome, the array CGH required whole genome amplification and then checking against a reference or control sample. Several other technologies like quantitative polymerase chain reaction (qPCR) and single-nucleotide polymorphism (SNP) arrays had drawbacks as they were more expensive and technically challenging.

Now we are in the era of second-generation PGT where NGS technology has taken over and shown to fulfill almost all the technical limitations like mosaicism detection at a good level and subchromosomal segmental changes which

Table 2: Comparison of PGT-A diagnostic test and the different characteristics

	FISH	*qPCR*	*SNPs*	*aCGH*	*NGS*
Result	3 to 12 chromosomes	24 chromosomes	24 chromosomes	24 chromosomes	24 chromosomes
Whole chromosome aneuploidy	No	Yes	Yes	Yes	Yes
Duplications and deletions	No	No	Possible	Yes	Yes
Mosaicism	No	No	Possible	Limited	Yes
Gene mutation	No	Possible	Yes	No	Yes
Duration	6–8 hours	4 hours	30–40 hours	12–15 hours	13–16 hours
Fresh transfer	Possible	Possible	No	Possible	No
Advantages	Quick	Fast and cheap	High Resolution	Cheap and relative fast	Very high resolution/mt DNA copy number
Disadvantages	Not all chromosomes are tested/ signal overlap/ hybridization failure/ high error rate	Low resolution	Not possible in case of consanguinity among the partners	Limited ability to identify mosaicism	High installation cost/ high cost per embryo tested
Polyploidies	Yes	Yes	Limited	No	Yes
Balanced chromosomal rearrangements	Possible	No	Limited	No	Possible
Uniparental disomies	No	No	Yes	No	Yes

(aCGH: array comparative genomic hybridization; FISH: fluorescence in situ hybridization; NGS: next-generation sequencing; qPCR: quantitative polymerase chain reaction; SNP: single nucleotide polymorphism)

can hamper embryo implantation. A latest concept of mitochondrial DNA level quantification is also found to be helpful in selecting an embryo which will have enhancing implantation potential.

A clear benefit to PGT utilizing 23 chromosome pair evaluation at the TE stage has been demonstrated in multiple prospective randomized trials. Additionally, the use of embryo vitrification following PGS biopsy has allowed the process of PGT to be performed with much more flexibility, leading to increased utilization of the technology, particularly in the USA and currently even in India where multiple IVF clinics consider going ahead with the option of setting up an NGS laboratory rather than outsourcing. But in order to set up a PGD clinic it is very essential for the clinic to have a very good blastulation, vitrification rate, and embryo biopsy techniques should be done at an expert level without causing damage to the growing embryo. The clinic should essentially perform large cycles per year in order to overcome the cost associated with PGT. The PGT laboratory should be requiring a controlled environment. Geneticists should be well experienced in handling embryonic cells, processing, and even in providing result interpretation. Making the patient understand the technological limitations forms a very important aspect of counseling. On the other hand embryologist must also have the expertise in giving laser shot during biopsy at the cell junctions. Both tubing and fixing of cells should include biopsying a cell or multiple cells with intact nuclei. Every biopsy should accompany a negative control to rule out contamination. Then only the benefits of offering any PGT would be beneficial. The clinical utilization rate of PGS has dramatically increased in recent years, and this trend is likely to continue for the foreseeable future. There are several advantages of offering NGS-based PGT. NGS analysis provides results in minimum 24 hours facilitating fresh or frozen embryo transfer. Most clinics perform frozen transfers. NGS is hence cost-effective where multiple samples can be multiplexed together. It also has the efficiency to detect partial or segmental ploidies, unbalanced translocations thereby useful in PGT-structural rearrangement (PGT-SR). It is the only technology that can detect mosaicism. It can detect single gene disorder and mitochondrial disorders. CCS along with the detection of single gene disorder can be done in the same NGS chip thereby making it much cost- effective.

Fluorescence in situ Hybridization

Fluorescence in situ hybridization is a molecular cytogenetic method used for recognition of numerical and structural chromosomal aberrations in the embryo. The biopsied cell is fixed onto the glass slide and hybridized to an in situ chromosomal target using fluorescently labeled DNA probe. The probes are targeted to specific regions or genes in the chromosome. Since there are limited sets of fluorophores available, only a few chromosomes can be tested at a given time point. Hence, apart from technical challenges faced with single cell FISH including no hybridization, split signals, overlapping signals, etc. the major drawback is that it is limited to testing of a fixed number of chromosomes. Various probe combinations have been used by different centers with analysis of 5–12 chromosomes on a given blastomere. **Figures 2 and 3** show representative images of FISH on blastomere performed using LSI 13 Spectrum Green/21 Spectrum Orange probe and CEP 18 Spectrum Aqua/X Spectrum Green/Y Spectrum Orange probe, respectively.

Polymerase Chain Reaction

The PCR technique used for detection of single gene disorders is based on in vitro amplification of target DNA in the host cell genome, resulting in a million fold copies of the target region, making it feasible for analysis. It is a highly sensitive and specific technique for single cell analysis for PGD. Precautions to ensure absence of contamination of the host DNA are critical. Another challenge faced is the allele drop out (ADO) due to accidental nonamplification of one of the alleles, compromising the accuracy of the diagnosis. Several PCR techniques have been used for single cell diagnosis including single strand conformation polymorphism (SSCP),[20] denaturing gradient gel electrophoresis (DGGE),[21,22] fluorescent PCR,[23-25] amplification refractory mutation system (ARMS) PCR,[26] etc.

In case of β-thalassemia, if both the parents are the carrier of the same mutation, then the diagnosis in the blastomere is established based on the presence or absence of the normal and the mutant allele using multiplex PCR. The sensitivity of the assay can be improved by using fluorescent primers. Presence of peak representing normal allele and absence of peak for mutant allele demonstrated normal status for β-thalassemia. Presence of peaks representing mutant and normal allele demonstrated β-thalassemia minor status. Presence of peak representing mutant allele and absence of peak for normal allele demonstrated β-thalassemia major status. **Figures 4A and B** demonstrate the results of testing for IVS1-5 (G-C) mutation. The Hex-labeled mutant primer gives green peaks of 285 bp and 384 bp when the mutant allele is present, whereas the TAMRA-labeled normal allele demonstrates black peaks of 285 bp and 384 bp in the presence of the normal allele.

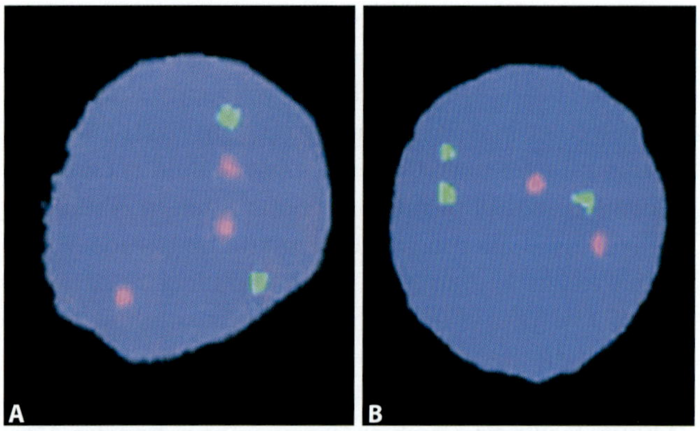

Figs. 2A and B: Fluorescence *in situ* hybridization (FISH) on blastomere using LSI probe for chromosomes 13 and 21. FISH on two representative blastomeres from different embryos for chromosomes 13 (green) and 21 (orange). (A) Presence of two green (Chr. 13) and three orange (Chr. 21) signals indicating trisomy 21; (B) Presence of three green (Chr. 13) and two orange (Chr. 21) signals indicating trisomy 13.

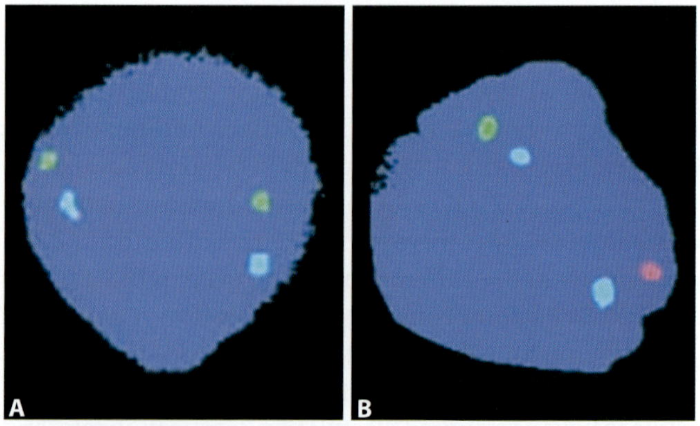

Figs. 3A and B: Fluorescence in situ hybridization (FISH) on blastomere using centromeric-enumeration probe (CEP) probe for chromosomes 18, X and Y. FISH on two representative blastomere samples from individual embryos for chromosomes 18 (aqua), X (green) and Y (orange): (A) presence of two aqua (Chr. 18) and two green (Chr. X) signals indicating normal female; (B) presence of two aqua (Chr. 18), one green (Chr. X) and one orange (Chr. Y) signals indicating normal male.

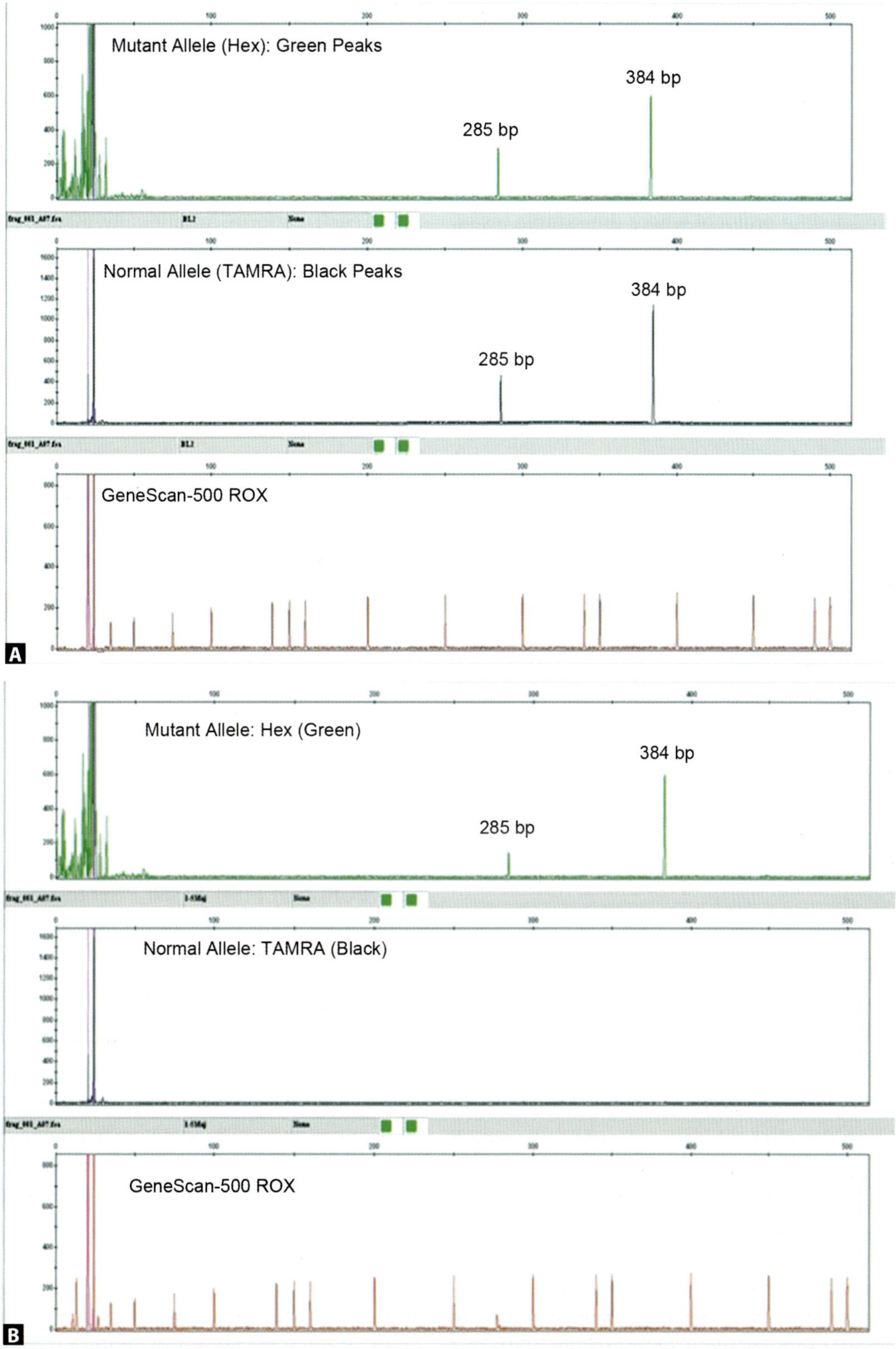

Figs. 4A and B: (A) Fragment analysis results for IVS1-5 (G-C) mutation on blastomere: β-thalassemia minor. β-thalassemia minor status for IVS1-5 (G-C) mutation observed as indicated: (i) Presence of Hex-labeled green peaks for mutant allele at 285 bp and 384 bp size; (ii) Presence of TAMRA-labeled black peak for the normal allele at 285 bp and 384 bp size; (iii) GeneScan-500 Rox marker; (B) Fragment analysis results for IVS1-5 (G-C) mutation on blastomere: β-thalassemia major. β-thalassemia major status for IVS1-5 (G-C) mutation observed as indicated: (i) Presence of Hex-labeled green peaks for mutant allele at 285 bp and 384 bp size; (ii) Absence of TAMRA-labeled black peak for the normal allele at 285 bp and 384 bp size; (iii) GeneScan-500 Rox marker.

Comparative Genomic Hybridization Array-Comparative Genomic Hybridization, and Single Nucleotide Polymorphism

There are two main types of microarrays available for genetic testing. These are *SNP* and *CGH arrays*. For both microarray platforms, the TE cells must be lysed and amplified. Array CGH is a ratio labeling protocol where the sample tested is tagged with a fluorescent dye (green) compared to a normal reference male or female genome usually tagged with a red fluorescent dye. The array CGH chips in use have approximately 4,000 markers spaced throughout the genome. The light emitted from the fluorescent labels is measured and the results are analyzed with the use of specialized software. For the SNP array, approximately 300,000 SNPs (pairs of single nucleotides in genomic DNA that are highly variable within a given species) spaced throughout the genome located in nonexon coding segments of the genome are evaluated. SNP arrays provide a genotype (AA, AB, or BB) for each sample analyzed and compare these results to a human HapMap reference genome. These arrays can identify whole chromosome aneuploidy and can also identify approximately 250 common structural chromosome aberrations throughout the genome.

Real-time quantitative PCR: Real-time quantitative PCR (RT-qPCR) is a PCR-based assay that can identify whole chromosome aneuploidy.[27] For RT-qPCR, DNA from 2–10 TE cells is preamplified using a commercially available preamplification kit and combined with 96 DNA copy number assays (TaqMan), four per chromosome. Preamplified samples are then subjected to quantitative real-time PCR, for the detection of an increase (trisomy) or decrease (monosomy) in chromosome numbers. The whole procedure lasts about 4 hours and can be combined with mutation detection.

Next-generation sequencing: NGS has recently been introduced into the clinics for aneuploidy screening.[28] NGS requires optimized DNA amplification to reduce the introduction of artifacts during the amplification process. After DNA amplification, a barcoding step follows to allow the identification of embryo-specific sequences after which the amplified product is broken down into small sequence-ready fragments. Those fragments are then subjected to massively parallel sequencing. Commercially platforms have been developed for NGS and are currently in use.

All techniques so far used, in the context of PGT-A, from the FISH technique to the latest NGS platform, have significantly contributed to our current understanding of the basic patterns of chromosome abnormalities in early human embryo development. However, there are still important concerns related to their diagnostic accuracy.[29,30] In particular, in the absence of systematic validation processes for each platform and all the steps involved, it has not been possible yet to estimate the expected error rate of each platform. Additionally, there are other concerns about: (1) how accurately the 2–10 TE cells retrieved during blastocyst biopsy represent the genetic status of the inner cell mass (ICM) and (2) the potential impact of the biopsy itself, especially in low-quality blastocyst. All these concerns may explain why as up to date PGT has not yet reached its expected maximum potential and call for action as they imply the presence of a risk of euploid embryos being discarded with the expected negative consequences on the patients' chances for a viable and healthy pregnancy.

PRECAUTION IN PGD/PGS

For the accuracy of results, all steps in case of PGD/PGS need to be performed with utmost care as the diagnosis is based on single to few cells. Since the initial application of PCR-based PGD cycles, marked advances in the reagent quality, better equipment and technology, have enabled development of strong protocols. Despite these advances, correct precautions and skilled expertise is needed for the testing, to avoid misdiagnosis. The errors may be specific to the expertise or test methodology involved, i.e. PCR- or FISH-based tests, or may apply likewise to both PCR- and FISH-based PGD testing. The causes of misdiagnosis affecting both FISH- and PCR-based test results include extraneous DNA contamination because of remaining cumulus cells or extraneous sperm cells.[3] Using ICSI, especially for PCR-based PGD, can help to avoid contamination due to sperm genome and complete removal of cumulus cells before biopsy helps to alleviate errors due to maternal contamination. Other sources of contamination include operator contamination or amplicon carry-over contamination.[31] Adherence to stringent PCR environment helps in avoiding contamination problems. Separate areas for embryo biopsy and pre- and post-PCR procedures help in minimizing contamination. The use of dedicated instruments for PGD-associated procedures and use of stringent quality control at every stage including preparation of reagents and one-use reagent aliquots can help to alleviate these problems.[32] Additionally, inclusion of appropriate negative controls, reagent blanks, and positive controls is essential quality control measure that needs to be implemented. Additional sources of errors include errors in labeling and/or identification of the embryo/ blastomere. Another possible cause of misdiagnosis may be unprotected intercourse during a treatment as the embryos developing in vivo are untested embryos of unknown genotype.[3] Another major cause of misdiagnosis may be inadequate assay validation so that testing methodology is not fully reliable, reproducible or accurate. Hence, before using the method for clinical patient testing, the performance characteristics of the assay need to be validated.

Problems leading to misdiagnosis may be arise at any of the step from collection of cell to the PCR procedure including loss of the cell during cell transfer to the tube, spontaneous cell lysis, and enucleated or degenerate cells. Hence, embryo biopsy, tubing, etc. need to be carried with extreme care, by skilled personnel. Blastomeres from poor grade embryos have inferior amplification efficacies than the high grade embryos.[33] Another source of misdiagnosis, ADO results from selective amplification of one of the two alleles.[34] The magnitude of problem resulting from ADO is dependent on the disorder being tested and its inheritance pattern. In case of autosomal recessive disorders, though ADO results in reduction of net embryos available for transfer, the advantage is that it would at least not result in transfer of an affected embryo. On the other hand, with compound heterozygous or autosomal dominant conditions, ADO may result in misdiagnosis and consequent transfer of affected embryos. Thus, the risk of transferring an affected embryo is approximately 2% for recessive disorders and 11% for dominant disorders.[35]

In case of misdiagnosis, the chance to accomplish root cause analysis, categorize probable process modifications and a strategy for both corrective and preventative action need to be followed. In case of adverse misdiagnosis, resulting either in the birth of a child affected with genetic disorder or requiring termination due to detection of genetic aberration on prenatal diagnosis, the consequences are painful to the patients and the laboratory staff, with severe repercussions to the family and the testing laboratory. The number of cases reported of misdiagnosis are proportionately low, which may be attributed to failure to conceive or carry pregnancy to term, or may be the outcome of absence of indication of misdiagnosis, in the born child who may either by a carrier or may be normal. As a result, it is hard to ascertain precise assessment of the global misdiagnosis rate. The accurate in-house estimates are more reliable. Nevertheless, review of results from various centers worldwide suggest a misdiagnosis rates of less than 1% for PCR-based tests and less than 5% for FISH-based tests.[3]

ETHICAL/LEGAL AND SOCIAL ASPECTS

The increase in the numbers of cases tested and the new indications tested each year, ensures the potential of PGD in biomedical fields. However, like any new technique this field needs to be regulated. Hence, various countries have taken diverse approaches to legislate and regulate PGD based on their ethical, legal, religious, and social belief; thus, allowing it for certain indication and banning it for others. This has given rise to reproductive medicine tourism. PGD is like a double- edged sword which if used judiciously can be put to good use for the benefit of mankind. The science, safety, and efficacy of PGD should be repeatedly assessed as the field develops. However, the notion of misuse or abuse of the technology exists, raising significant ethical concerns, and putting this technique under close ethical, legal and social scrutiny, especially for indications like PGD for susceptibility conditions, late onset disorders, HLA matching for existing child, and perhaps gender selection in sex-based genetic diseases.

Since the first birth reported in 2001 by the Chicago team[36] of PGD for HLA typing of the embryo, so that the child born through PGD can donate umbilical cord blood stem cells to the elder sibling suffering from Fanconi's anemia, many centers have been using PGD for this indication. However, the opponents of PGD ethically challenge the use of this technique with the argument of possible instrumentalization or commodification of the child. PGD is now also being used to detect mutation for susceptibility to cancer, e.g. BRCA1/BRCA2 mutations in early onset breast cancer, and late onset disorders like Alzheimer's disease. These indications come under ethical scrutiny as in many ways we are going toward custom-designed new generation and the ethical dilemma remains on the correctness of offering PGD for a disease condition that would only affect the individual in the fourth decade. The proponent of PGD favors the testing for these conditions as the diagnosis of the affected gene is associated with high probability or certainty of developing the disease condition, which in most cases may not be curable leading to a stressful life and early death. Another indication commonly known as "designer baby" referring to use of PGD for selection of physical traits of offspring is also facing lot of ethic controversy. The opponents of PGD raise objections on the grounds of embryo manipulation, unnecessary utilization of resources, propagations of eugenics, and protection of rights of unborn child.

FUTURE

Early embryo is a unique form of life still very little understood. Higher resolution diagnostic platforms for comprehensive chromosome screening of validated and confirmed accuracy will help us: (1) identify euploid embryos and minimize the risk euploid embryo wastage, (2) estimate the true incidence of mosaicism in the different patient subgroups, and (3) improve understanding of the role of mosaicism in the early preimplantation human embryos.

Moreover, there is an increasing interest towards the development of noninvasive diagnostic techniques for the screening of the embryos via the different molecules released in the culture medium or the blastocoel cavity by the embryo itself. The detailed analysis of the mixture of biomolecules secreted will help us to develop different holistic profiles for viable and nonviable embryos, and eventually reach our ultimately goal to optimize embryo selection and IVF efficiency.

SUMMARY

Preimplantation genetic testing has proved to be a boon to many couples who are either carrier of a genetic disease condition or facing recurrent abortions or recurrent implantation failures. With advances in the field of information technology and biotechnology, application of targeted molecular analysis for assisted reproductive technology has become a feasible proposition. Proper implementation of this technique in the clinical set up requires highly skilled molecular biologists, fully equipped molecular biology laboratory and close collaboration with the clinical geneticist and fertility specialist is essential. The technical breakthroughs in diagnostics are adaptable for PGD, and help ensure accuracy and speed for single cell assays. Improvements in vitrification and cryopreservation protocols have now made it possible to freeze the embryos pre- or post-biopsy, thus enabling transfer in a subsequent cycle. Hence, it is now possible to use more advanced diagnostic techniques such as CGH, α-CGH, SNP arrays, and NGS for better diagnosis. These advances have made PGD possible for many newer indications. Like any new advances, the technique needs to be used judiciously for betterment of the society and mankind.

REFERENCES

1. Egozcue J, Santaló J, Giménez C, et al. Preimplantation genetic diagnosis. Mol Cell Endocrinol. 2000;166(1):21-5.
2. Sermon K, De Rijcke M, Lissens W, et al. Preimplantation genetic diagnosis for Huntington's disease with exclusion testing. Eur J Hum Genet. 2002;10(10):591-8.
3. Thornhill AR, de Die-Smulders CE, Geraedts JP, et al. ESHRE PGD Consortium 'Best practice guidelines for clinical preimplantation genetic diagnosis (PGD) and preimplantation genetic screening (PGS)'. Hum Reprod. 2005;20(1):35-48.
4. Verlinsky Y, Ginsberg N, Lifchez A, et al. Analysis of the first polar body: preconception genetic diagnosis. Hum Reprod. 1990;5(7):826-9.
5. Munné S, Dailey T, Sultan KM, et al. The use of first polar bodies for preimplantation diagnosis of aneuploidy. Hum Reprod. 1995;10(4):1014-20.
6. Montag M, van der Ven K, Dorn C, et al. Outcome of laser-assisted polar body biopsy and aneuploidy testing. Reprod Biomed Online. 2004;9(4):425-9.
7. Grifo JA, Boyle A, Fischer E, et al. Preembryo biopsy and analysis of blastomeres by in situ hybridization. Am J Obstet Gynecol. 1990;163(6 Pt 1):2013-9.
8. Boada M, Carrera M, De La Iglesia C, et al. Successful use of a laser for human embryo biopsy in preimplantation genetic diagnosis: report of two cases. J Assist Reprod Genet. 1998;15(5):302-7.
9. Veiga A, Sandalinas M, Benkhalifa M, et al. Laser blastocyst biopsy for preimplantation diagnosis in the human. Zygote. 1997;5(4):351-4.
10. Kokkali G, Vrettou C, Traeger-Synodinos J, et al. Birth of a healthy infant following trophectoderm biopsy from blastocysts for PGD of beta-thalassaemia major. Hum Reprod. 2005;20(7):1855-9.
11. Strom CM, Ginsberg N, Rechitsky S, et al. Three births after preimplantation genetic diagnosis for cystic fibrosis with sequential first and second polar body analysis. Am J Obstet Gynecol. 1998;178:1298-306.
12. Gianaroli L, Magli MC, Ferraretti AP, et al. The role of preimplantation diagnosis for aneuploidies. Reprod Biomed Online. 2002;4 Suppl 3:31-6.
13. Harper JC, Coonen E, De Rycke M, et al. ESHRE PGD Consortium data collection X: cycles from January to December 2007 with pregnancy follow-up to October 2008. Hum Reprod. 2010;25(11):2685-707.
14. Fallon L, Harton GL, Sisson ME, et al. Preimplantation genetic diagnosis for spinal muscular atrophy type I. Neurology. 1999;53:1087-90.
15. Pierce KE, Michalopoulos J, Kiessling AA, et al. Preimplantation development of mouse and human embryos biopsied at cleavage stages using a modified displacement technique. Hum Reprod. 1997;12(2):351-6.
16. McArthur SJ, Leigh D, Marshall JT, et al. Pregnancies and live births after trophectoderm biopsy and preimplantation genetic testing of human blastocysts. Fertil Steril. 2005;84:1628-36.
17. Kokkali G, Traeger-Synodinos J, Vrettou C, et al. Blastocyst biopsy versus cleavage stage biopsy and blastocyst transfer for preimplantation genetic diagnosis of betathalassaemia: a pilot study. Hum Reprod. 2007;22(5):1443-9.

18. Jones GM, Cram DS, Song B, et al. Novel strategy with potential to identify developmentally competent IVF blastocysts. Hum Reprod. 2008;23(8):1748-59.
19. Dokras A, Sargent IL, Ross C, et al. Trophectoderm biopsy in human blastocysts. Hum Reprod. 1990;5(7):821-5.
20. el-Hashemite N, Wells D, Delhanty JD. Single cell detection of beta-thalassaemia mutations using silver stained SSCP analysis: an application for preimplantation diagnosis. Mol Hum Reprod. 1997;3(8):693-8.
21. Kanavakis E, Vrettou C, Palmer G, et al. Preimplantation genetic diagnosis in 10 couples at risk for transmitting beta-thalassaemia major: clinical experience including the initiation of six singleton pregnancies. Prenat Diagn. 1999;19(13):1217-22.
22. Palmer GA, Traeger-Synodinos J, Davies S, et al. Pregnancies following blastocyst stage transfer in PGD cycles at risk for beta-thalassaemic haemoglobinopathies. Hum Reprod. 2002;17(1):25-31.
23. Van de Velde H, Sermon K, De Vos A, et al. Fluorescent PCR and automated fragment analysis in preimplantation genetic diagnosis for 21-hydroxylase deficiency in congenital adrenal hyperplasia. Mol Hum Reprod. 1999;5(7):691-6.
24. Abou-Sleiman PM, Apessos A, Harper JC, et al. First application of preimplantation genetic diagnosis to neurofibromatosis type 2 (NF2). Prenat Diagn. 2002;22(6):519-24.
25. Harper JC, Wells D, Piyamongkol W, et al. Preimplantation genetic diagnosis for single gene disorders: experience with five single gene disorders. Prenat Diagn. 2002;22(6):525-33.
26. Moutou C, Gardes N, Rongières C, et al. Allele-specific amplification for preimplantation genetic diagnosis (PGD) of spinal muscular atrophy. Prenat Diagn. 2001;21(6):498-503.
27. Treff NR, Tao X, Ferry KM, et al. Development and validation of an accurate quantitative real-time polymerase chain reaction-based assay for human blastocyst comprehensive chromosomal aneuploidy screening. Fertil Steril. 2012;97(4):819-24.
28. Wells D, Kaur K, Grifo J, et al. Clinical utilisation of a rapid low-pass whole genome sequencing technique for the diagnosis of aneuploidy in human embryos prior to implantation. J Med Genet. 2014;51(8):553-62.
29. Paulson RJ. Preimplantation genetic screening: what is the clinical efficiency? Fertil Steril. 2017;108:228-30.
30. Rosenwaks Z, Handyside AH, Fiorentino F, et al. The pros and cons of preimplantation genetic testing for aneuploidy: clinical and laboratory perspectives. Fertil Steril. 2018;110(3):353-61.
31. Lewis CM, Pinêl T, Whittaker JC, et al. Controlling misdiagnosis errors in preimplantation genetic diagnosis: a comprehensive model encompassing extrinsic and intrinsic sources of error. Hum Reprod. 2001;16(1):43-50.
32. Thornhill AR, Snow K. Molecular diagnostics in preimplantation genetic diagnosis. J Mol Diagn. 2002;4:11-29.
33. Ray PF, Ao A, Taylor DM, et al. Assessment of the reliability of single blastomere analysis for preimplantation diagnosis of the delta F508 deletion causing cystic fibrosis in clinical practice. Prenat Diagn. 1998;18(13):1402-12.
34. Hahn S, Garvin AM, Di Naro E, et al. Allele drop-out can occur in alleles differing by a single nucleotide and is not alleviated by preamplification or minor template increments. Genet Test. 1998;2(4):351-5.
35. Navidi W, Arnheim N. Using PCR in preimplantation genetic disease diagnosis. Hum Reprod. 1991;6(6):836-49.
36. Verlinsky Y, Rechitsky S, Schoolcraft W, et al. Preimplantation diagnosis for Fanconi anemia combined with HLA matching. JAMA. 2001;285(24):3130-3.

PGT: Technical Aspects, Biopsy, and Analysis

75

Ritu Hari, C Mohamed Ashraf

INTRODUCTION

Over the recent years, there have been tremendous advancements in assisted reproductive techniques (ARTs), especially after merging with the reproductive genetics in terms of enhancing the live births and prevention of genetic abnormalities. As we know genetic conditions have no cure and diagnosis at an appropriate stage of pregnancy holds an impact. Until now, only option left behind us in avoiding a genetically compromised birth was to make a firm diagnosis at the earliest, say by amniocentesis at 16 weeks or a chorionic villus sampling (CVS) at 12 weeks. From these postconception diagnosis and then aborting these unwanted pregnancies we have moved one step further in diagnosing the same with 100% accuracy even before implantation, that is meant by preimplantation genetic testing (PGT). PGT can be considered as an alternative to prenatal diagnosis for couples at high risk of transmitting a genetic disorder. The detection of genetic disease in the human embryo prior to implantation gives parents the choice to overcome anxiety and be rest assured that pregnancy will be normal, so using this strategy termination of pregnancy can be avoided. For this reason PGT is considered more ethically acceptable among some patients.

All require in vitro fertilization (IVF); biopsy of an embryo, for genetic testing; and then transfer of selected fresh or frozen-thawed embryos into the uterus based on the results of genetic testing.

SOURCES OF OBTAINING EMBRYONIC CELLS

Polar Body Biopsy

Polar body biopsies permissible in few countries like Germany. Only maternal genetic component can be studied. However, it may be helpful in diagnosis of X-linked disorders.

Blastomere Biopsy

Blastomere biopsy allows analysis of a single blastomere on day 3 of embryo development. It did not prove to be clinically beneficial as was associated with high degree of mosaicism. But as a personal experience for cases where either couple being carrier of a balanced translocation. PGT on fluorescence in situ hybridization (FISH) using subtelomere probes on cells post-day 3 biopsy has improved pregnancy rates as in such couples the reason being recurrent pregnancy losses due to unbalanced gametes and advantage of a day 3 biopsy in such cases gives a chance to study more embryos.

Day 5 Trophectoderm Biopsy

It shown great promising effect compared to day 3 biopsy. Removal of few trophectoderm (TE) cells herniating through the zona benefits PGT. Minimum of five to ten cells removed. Reduced deoxyribonucleic acid (DNA) amplification failure.

In a single biopsy, both PGT for aneuploidy (PGT-A) and PGT for monogenic conditions (PGT-M) can be performed in the same time on next-generation sequencing (NGS). One of the limiting factors is not all embryos depending on patient factor goes to blast. This hampers the testing strategy in few cases. However, in a well established IVF setup this can be taken well care of.

Depending on the type of genetic defects ranging from balanced chromosomal translocations in couples to monogenic disorders, few patients opt PGT based on the following reasons: difficult reproductive history, personal ethics, and religious views. Genetic technologies have also evolved over the years and shown to improvise results in terms of success. FISH, reverse transcription polymerase chain reaction (RT-PCR), Sanger sequencing, array comparative genomic hybridization (CGH), NGS, Karyomapping are some of the promising techniques used in the diagnosis of genetic conditions and for aneuploidy. It depends on what indication each one of them has been applied. However, comprehensive chromosome screening for aneuploidies has been shown to benefit elective single embryo transfer.

TECHNICAL ASPECTS

Since aneuploidy is the major source of adverse outcomes in human reproduction. American College of Obstetricians and Gynecologists and the Society for Maternal-Fetal Medicine now recommend universal screening. Initially PGT involved FISH techniques wherein cleavage stage embryonic cells were obtained postbiopsy. This approach did not give promising results in terms of pregnancy rates as minimum number of chromosomes were studied and mosaicism being another limiting factor. However, multiple prospective trials suggested that biopsy of blastomeres followed by embryo selection based out of FISH results led to reduced miscarriage rate and enhanced implantation rate. Technically FISH is the gold standard in prenatal diagnosis in testing aneuploidies for chromosomes 13, 18, 21, and sex chromosomes compatible with life. Past years most of the women undergoing IVF would fall in the category of advanced maternal age or recurrent implantation failures. Hence, a smaller group of patients did benefit post FISH-based preimplantation genetic screening (PGS). This leads to a rapid growth in the utilization of PGT. Geneticists were continuously working to overcome the limitations so that patients undergoing IVF could benefit from reduced miscarriage rates and increased implantation rates. First-generation PGT failed to produce more benefits; hence there was a need for comprehensive chromosomal screening (CCS). CGH array, one of the first developed techniques for CCS, proved beneficial and showed high accuracy of diagnosis of aneuploidy when applied to TE cells. Unlike the FISH procedure where single cell blastomere fixation is required and sometimes multiple rounds of cell hybridization may be required for the fluorescent probe used to check each chromosome, the array CGH required whole genome amplification and then checking against a reference or control sample. Several other technologies like quantitative PCR (qPCR) and single nucleotide polymorphism (SNP) arrays had drawbacks as they were more expensive and technically challenging.

Now we are in the era of second-generation PGT where NGS technology has taken over and shown to fulfill almost all the technical limitations like mosaicism detection at a good level and subchromosomal segmental changes which can hamper embryo implantation. A latest concept of mitochondrial DNA level quantification is also found to be helpful in selecting an embryo which will have enhancing implantation potential.

A clear benefit to PGT utilizing 23 chromosome pair evaluation at the TE stage has been demonstrated in multiple prospective randomized trials. Additionally, the use of embryo vitrification following PGS biopsy has allowed the process of PGT to be performed with much more flexibility, leading to increased utilization of the technology, particularly in the USA and currently even in India where multiple IVF clinics consider going ahead with the option of setting up an NGS laboratory rather than outsourcing. But in order to set up a preimplantation genetic diagnosis (PGD) clinic it is very essential for the clinic to have a very good blastulation, vitrification rate, and embryo biopsy techniques should be done at an expert level without causing damage to the growing embryo. The clinic should essentially perform large cycles per year in order to overcome the cost associated with PGT. The PGT laboratory should be requiring a controlled environment. Geneticists should be well experienced in handling embryonic cells, processing, and even in providing result interpretation. Making the patient understand the technological limitations forms a very important aspect of counseling. On the other hand embryologist must also have the expertise in giving laser shot during biopsy at the cell junctions. Both tubing and fixing of cells should include biopsying a cell or multiple cells with intact nuclei. Every biopsy should accompany a negative control to rule out contamination. Then only the benefits of offering any PGT would be beneficial. The clinical utilization rate of PGS has dramatically increased in recent years, and this trend is likely to continue for the foreseeable future. There are several advantages of offering NGS-based PGT. NGS analysis provides results in minimum 24 hours facilitating fresh or frozen embryo transfer. Most clinics perform frozen transfers. NGS is hence cost-effective where multiple samples can be multiplexed together. It also has the efficiency to detect partial or segmental ploidies, unbalanced translocations thereby useful in PGT-structural rearrangement (PGT-SR). It is the only technology that can detect mosaicism. It can detect single gene disorder and mitochondrial disorders. CCS along with the detection of single gene disorder can be done in the same NGS chip thereby making it much cost-effective.

WHO CAN BENEFIT FROM PREIMPLANTATION GENETIC TESTING?

When PGT was first devised it was thought to be of much use in diagnosing single gene disorders (PGT-M) in embryos for couple who were at risk of carrying the genetic

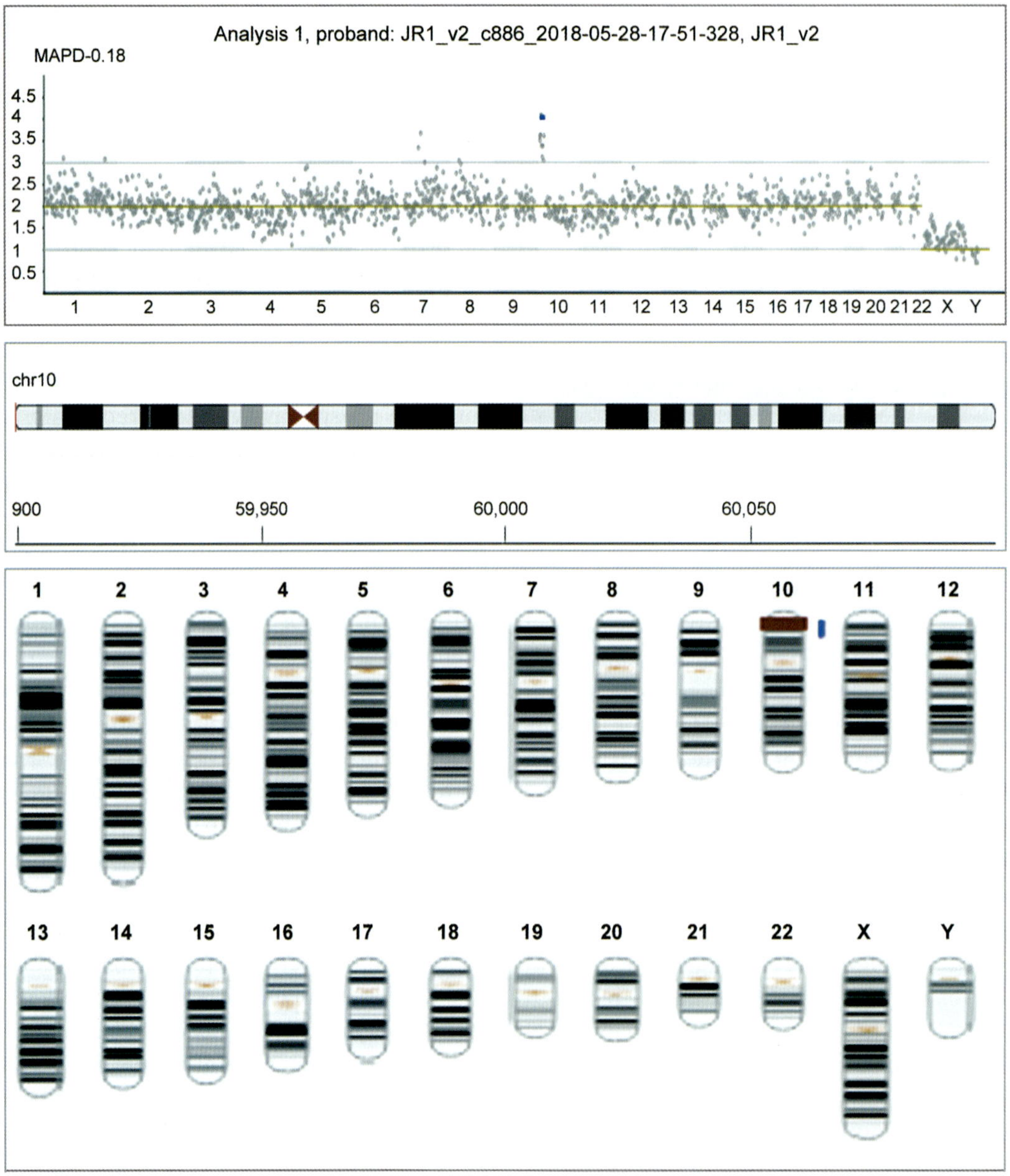

Next-generation sequencing data from Ion Reporter Software shows a segmental ploidy in chromosome 10. This is from an embryo of a patient where the male partner had a karyotype 46,XY t (5p: 11q). CCS hence is necessary in all patient groups opting for PGT.

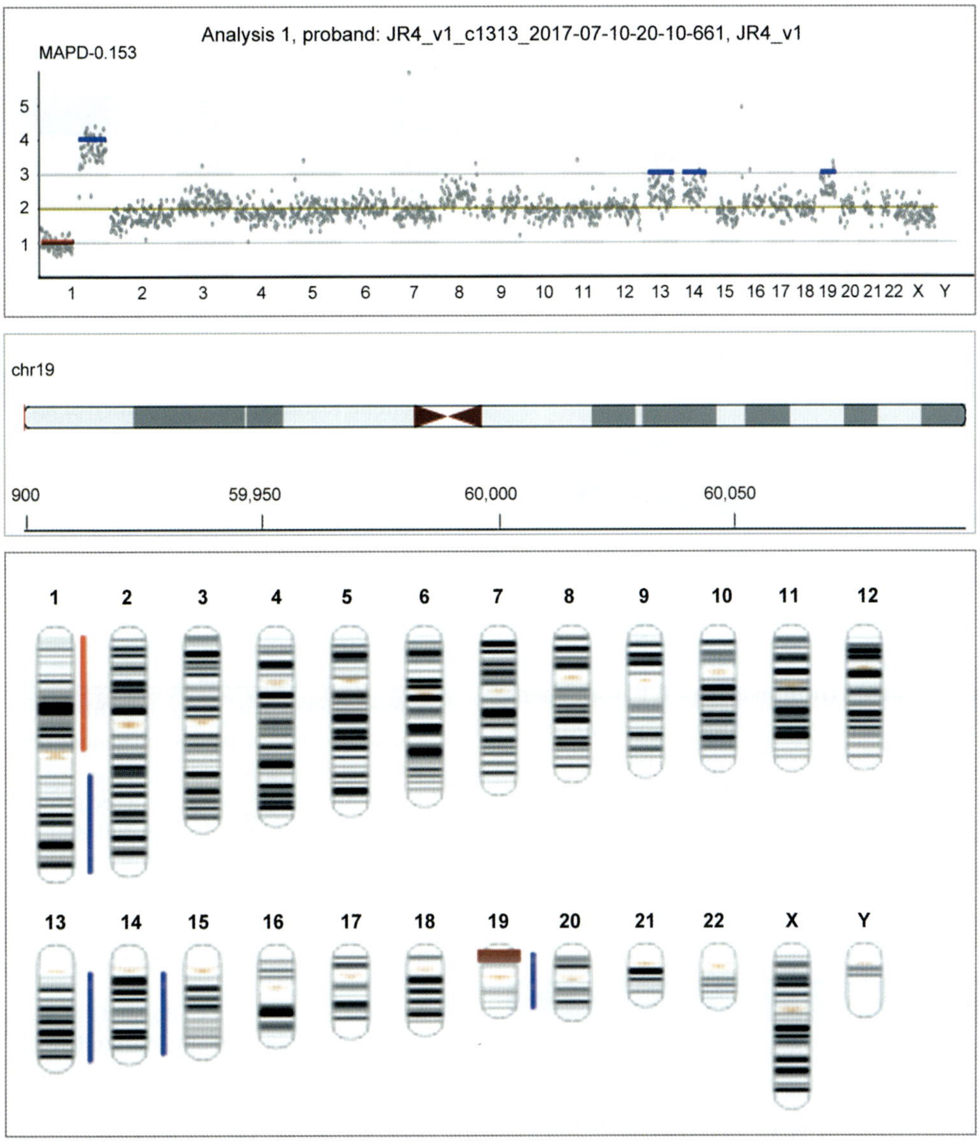

Next-generation sequencing data from a female karyotype 46,XX rob(13:14), a Robertsonian translocation carrier. Embryo showing various ploidies like trisomy 13, 14. Monosomy of 1p, and trisomy of 1q as an example of segmental ploidy.

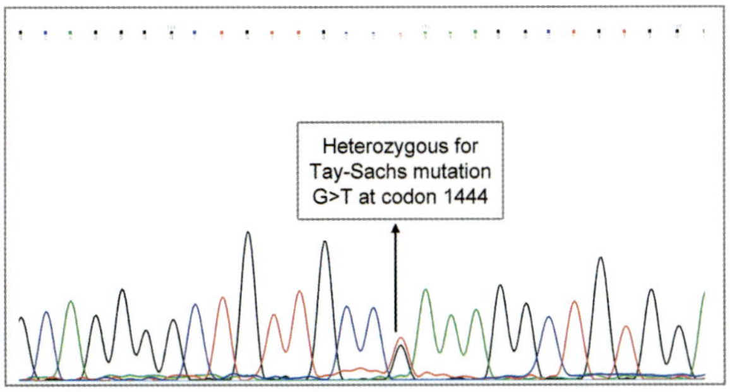

A successful case of a Tay-Sachs carrier embryo transferred and resulted in a delivery of a healthy baby girl. Here the couple were carriers of the Tay-Sachs mutation in the HEXA gene and had previously lost three babies.

abnormality gene or for couples who were carriers of a balanced translocation carrier (PGT-SR). However, its use is much expanded now and adopted in clinical practice in improving IVF outcomes. The regular indications of PGT-A were for advanced maternal age, recurrent pregnancy loss, and recurrent implantation failures. Now the latest trend of single embryo transfer coupled with PGT-A on NGS have shown several benefits like reduced miscarriage rates, improved implantation rates, less complications due to singleton pregnancy, and reduced time to achieving pregnancy. PGT-A can be offered to women under 35 years as they produce several blastocysts. Literature has already shown that one-third of blasts from young women show high aneuploidy. Modern techniques in PGT has definitely taken a leap forward, but the main reason for this evolution is the positive number of cases attempted by experienced geneticists using the classic method of the PGT-M and PGT-SR. Very few clinics in India have proved years back that PGT works wonders by contributing babies free from genetic disorders like Tay-Sachs disease, achondroplasia, and many balanced/Robertsonian translocation couples have given birth to normal babies. This has facilitated the acceptance of PGT more in our country.

FUTURE OF PREIMPLANTATION GENETIC TESTING

The number of patients undergoing PGT continues to increase each year. One of the concerns in this area is getting good number of blastocysts in some poor responders and in some group of advanced age women. In such cases the latest technology involving (noninvasive PGT from spent media) NIPGT-A might serve the purpose, which requires spent media for testing without the need of blastocyst biopsy. Future certainly holds strong for genetic testing as infertility is also raising. NGS-based genetic testing has now made at affordable prices, but still some patients fail to afford it. Indian government should make genetic testing under insurance coverage.

CONCLUSION

Preimplantation genetic testing has overcome all the limitations in terms of technology and process and is now offered routinely. It should not be an only option for couples having genetic issues, but also for those who opt IVF and PGT should be considered as an option to boost pregnancy rates. Patients should never be devoid of giving PGT as an option. PGT is clinically beneficial and cost-effective.

SUGGESTED READING

1. Dahdouh EM, Balayla J1, Audibert F, et al. Technical Update: Preimplantation Genetic Diagnosis and Screening. J Obstet Gynaecol Can. 2015;37(5):451-63.
2. Destouni A, Dimitriadou E, Masset H, et al. Genome-wide haplotyping embryos developing from 0PN and 1PN zygotes increases transferrable embryos in PGT-M. Hum Reprod. 2018;33(12):2302-11.
3. Farra C, Choucair F, Awwad J. Non-invasive pre-implantation genetic testing of human embryos: an emerging concept. Hum Reprod. 2018;33(12):2162-7.
4. Irani M, Zaninovic N, Canon C, et al. A rationale for biopsying embryos reaching the morula stage on Day 6 in women undergoing pre implantation genetic testing for aneuploidy. Hum Reprod. 2018;33(5):935-41.
5. Neal SA, Werner MD. Quest for a less invasive approach to preimplantation genetic testing remains ongoing. Fertil Steril. 2018;110(5):845-6.
6. Popovic M, Dheedene A, Christodoulou C, et al. Chromosomal mosaicism in human blastocysts: the ultimate challenge of Preimplantation genetic testing? Hum Reprod. 2018;33(7):1342-54.
7. Ritu Hari, PGD by *FISH for* a reciprocal translocation-first baby from South India. Reprod Biomed Online. 2018;36: e37-8.
8. Rosenwaks Z, Handyside AH, Fiorentino F, et al. The pros and cons of preimplantation genetic testing for aneuploidy: clinical and laboratory perspectives. Fertil Steril. 2018;110(3):353-61.
9. Verpoest W, Staessen C, Bossuyt PM, et al. Preimplantation genetic testing for aneuploidy by microarray analysis of polar bodies in advanced maternal age: a randomized clinical trial. Hum Reprod. 2018;33(9):1767-76.
10. Wu MY, Chao KH, Chen CD, et al. Current status of comprehensive chromosome screening for elective single-embryo transfer. Obstet Gynecol Int. 2014;2014:581783.

Genetic Analysis: FISH/CGH/ Microarray/NGS

76

Alexia Chatziparasidou

SUMMARY

Preimplantation Genetic Testing (PGT) is one of the most dynamic scientific fields which brought together, for the first time, geneticists, molecular biologists, clinical embryologist and reproductive specialists. Its multidiscipline nature combined with crucial developments in cryobiology, human embryo culture and genetic diagnostics, transformed, radically, the evolution of reproductive medicine. Today an increasing number of in vitro fertilization (IVF) centers offer PGT for aneuploidies (PGT-A) to their patients as a way to improve prognosis. A variety of different genetic tests is available while new ones are underway. In this chapter, a brief history of the available diagnostic tests used in PGT-A from the early days up to date, is presented together with the challenges they present.

INTRODUCTION

In 1990, Alan Handyside and colleagues[1] reported the delivery of healthy babies' after preimplantation genetic screening, for couples with a family history of a sex-linked disease. The couples underwent IVF and the embryos produced were subjected to blastomere biopsy on day 3. All blastomeres removed were tested for the presence of Y chromosome and the male embryos were excluded from uterine transfer. This was the first step of the new and very dynamic scientific field initially known as preimplantation genetic diagnosis (PGD) and more recently renamed to preimplantation genetic testing (PGT). PGT created a unique opportunity for testing the in vitro cultured embryos produced via IVF for couples carriers of monogenic diseases (PGT-M) or at risk of producing aneuploid embryos (PGT-A).

By 1990, it was already known that aneuploidy is the most common cause of reproductive failure throughout nature and IVF. As a result, scientists focused on the development of methods for single cell chromosome screening, aiming to identify aneuploid embryos and exclude them from transfer, as a way to improve prognosis for a viable and healthy pregnancy after IVF. For the first almost 20 years, the most commonly used biopsy method was day 3 biopsy and the main method used for chromosome screening was fluorescence in situ hybridization (FISH). Polar body biopsy reported by Y Verlisky[2] was used to a lesser degree, while blastocyst biopsy was only rarely used **(Table 1)**.

Over the years, the scenery of PGT-A has gradually changed. The accumulated data and experience, combined with important developments such as vitrification, brought PGT-A to its current more advanced level. In PGT-A cycles today, the vast majority of embryo biopsies are performed at the blastocyst stage, the embryos are vitrified post biopsy while the PGT-A practitioners have a variety of diagnostic platforms for chromosome screening to choose from.

HISTORY

For the first 10–15 years of PGT-A, the main genetic tests used for single cell chromosome screening was the FISH technique. Initially 2–3 chromosomes were identified with the use of chromosome-specific fluorescence-labeled probes, later the method was further developed and it became possible to screen 12 or even more chromosomes. However, despite the progress the diagnostic efficiency of the FISH method for PGT-A remained low. The need to screen all 24 chromosomes became apparent especially after the reports which failed to show any benefit in overall prognosis of its use and led multiple major professional

Table 1: Comparison between the different biopsy methods.

	Polar bodies	*Day 3 embryo*	*Day 5 embryo*
Biopsy procedure	▪ Sequential removal of the 1st and the 2nd polar body before and after ICSI ▪ Simultaneous removal of both polar bodies after ICSI	Removal of 1 blastomeres from day 3 embryos with at least 5 cells	▪ Removal of 2–10 TE cells ▪ Biopsy procedure may need to be repeated several times during day 5 and day 6
Informative	Only for the maternal contribution	For maternal and paternal contribution	For maternal paternal contribution and mitotic errors
Mosaicism	No	No	Possible
Fresh embryo transfer	Possible	Possible	Often not possible
Negative effect of the biopsy procedure	Not known	There is a potential reduction of embryo viability	Safer than day 3 biopsy, if less than 10 TE cells are removed and inner cell mass remain intact
Limitations	▪ Fragmented polar bodies ▪ Increased error rate ▪ 2 tests for each oocyte ▪ No data for the paternal contribution ▪ Biopsy timing is very crucial	▪ May affect further embryo development and implantation potential ▪ High mosaicism rate ▪ High risk for false positives or negative results due to mosaicism	▪ Need for optimized culture conditions ▪ Need for optimized vitrification program ▪ Biopsy efficiency is operator depended
Advantages	▪ Safe, allows time for genetic analysis and fresh transfer ▪ More accepted from ethical and religious point of view	Allows time for genetic analysis and fresh transfer	▪ ICM remain intact ▪ More cellular material available for genetic testing
Disadvantages	▪ Labor intensive ▪ Double biopsy and double tests ▪ Higher cost	▪ One cell may not represent the whole embryo ▪ In some embryos with granular cytoplasm nucleus may not be visible	▪ Only few embryos may progress to blastocyst stage ▪ Higher rate of cancellation especially for low responders

(ICM: inner cell mass, ICSI: intracytoplasmic sperm injection, TE: trophectoderm cells)

societies such as the American Society for Reproductive Medicine (ASRM), to release opinions discouraging the general use of PGT-A.[3]

Scientists attributed the lower than expected efficiency of PGT-A mainly to the limitations of the FISH technique and tried to develop other more informative diagnostic tools for comprehensive chromosome screening. Soon, new techniques were introduced including quantitative polymerase chain reaction (qPCR), single nucleotide polymorphism arrays (SNP arrays), and array comparative genomic hybridization (aCGH), while in the most recent years, the Next Generation Sequencing (NGS) platform started to gain increasing attention and use.

The use of the new more advanced diagnostic platforms was combined with blastocyst biopsy, during which 2–10 trophectoderm cells (TE) are removed and vitrification of the biopsied blastocysts instead of a fresh transfer. A number of reports demonstrated an increased efficiency of this new and more advanced PGT-A approach and led to the ASRM Practice Committee statement in 2018: "Several studies demonstrate higher birth rates after aneuploidy testing and elective single-embryo transfer, suggesting the potential for this testing to decrease the risk of multiple gestations".[4] For the first time, PGT-A seemed to be closer than before in fulfilling its primary purpose, to optimize embryo selection and chances for a viable and healthy pregnancy after IVF.

PRESENT

Today the clinical utilization rate of PGT-A has dramatically increased. The diagnostic testing platforms currently in use are capable of testing for all 23 chromosome pairs and have comparable efficacy in identifying whole chromosome aneuploidy but differ widely in their ability to simultaneously identify other structural chromosome abnormalities, single gene mutations or mitochondrial deoxyribonucleic acid (mtDNA) copy number.[5,6]

There are two main types of microarrays available for genetic testing. These are *single-nucleotide polymorphism (SNP) and comparative genomic hybridization (CGH) arrays*. For both microarray platforms, the TE cells must be lysed and amplified. Array CGH is a ratio labeling protocol where the sample tested is tagged with a fluorescent dye (green) compared to a normal reference male or female genome usually tagged with a red fluorescent dye. The array CGH chips in use have approximately 4,000 markers spaced throughout the genome. The light emitted from the fluorescent labels is measured and the results are analyzed with the use of specialized software. For the SNP array, approximately 300,000 SNPs (pairs of single nucleotides in genomic DNA that are highly variable within a given species) spaced throughout the genome located in non-exon coding segments of the genome, are evaluated. SNP arrays provide a genotype (AA, AB, or BB) for each sample analyzed and compare these results to a human hapmap reference genome. These arrays can identify whole chromosome aneuploidy and can also identify approximately 250 common structural chromosome aberrations throughout the genome.

REAL-TIME QUANTITATIVE PCR

Real-time quantitative polymerase chain reaction (RT-qPCR) is a polymerase chain reaction based assay that can identify whole chromosome aneuploidy.[7] For RT-qPCR, DNA from 2–10 TE cells is preamplified using a commercially available preamplification kit and combined with 96 DNA copy number assays (Taq-Man), 4 per chromosome. Preamplified samples are then subjected to quantitative real-time PCR, for the detection of an increase (trisomy) or decrease (monosomy) in chromosome numbers. The whole procedure lasts about 4 h and can be combined with mutation detection.

Next-generation Sequencing

Next-generation sequencing (NGS) has recently been introduced into the clinics for aneuploidy screening.[8] NGS requires optimized DNA amplification to reduce the introduction of artifacts during the amplification process. After DNA amplification, a barcoding step follows to allow the identification of embryo-specific sequences after which the amplified product is broken down into small sequence-ready fragments. Those fragments are then subjected to massively parallel sequencing. Commercially platforms have been developed for NGS and are currently in use.

All techniques so far used, in the context of PGT-A, from the FISH technique to the latest NGS platform, have significantly contributed to our current understanding of the basic patterns of chromosome abnormalities in early human embryo development. However, there are still important concerns related to their diagnostic accuracy.[9,10] In particular, in the absence of systematic validation processes for each platform and all the steps involved in it, has not been possible yet to estimate the expected error rate of each platform. Additionally, there are other concerns about:

- How accurately the 2–10 TE cells retrieved during blastocyst biopsy represent the genetic status of the inner cell mass (ICM)
- The potential impact of the biopsy itself especially in low quality blastocyst.

All these concerns may explain why, as up to date PGT-A has not yet reached its expected maximum potential and call for action, as they imply the presence of a risk of euploid embryos being discarded with the expected negative consequences on the patients' chances for a viable and healthy pregnancy.

It is very important for the PGT-A practitioners to understand the different characteristics and the diagnostic limitations of each platform **(Table 2)**, before selecting the one that meets best for each patient's needs. Moreover, practitioners need to be able to convey the diagnostic limitations of the selected platform to the PGT-A couple prior to treatment in order for them to adjust their expectations accordingly and acknowledge the potential risk of discarding a euploid embryo or replacing an aneuploid embryo.

FUTURE

Early embryo is a unique form of life, still very little understood. Higher resolution diagnostic platforms for comprehensive chromosome screening, of validated and confirmed accuracy will help us to:

- Identify euploid embryos and minimize the risk of euploid embryo wastage
- Estimate the true incidence of mosaicism, in the different patient subgroups
- Improve the understanding of the role of mosaicim in the early preimplantation human embryos.

Moreover, there is an increasing interest towards the development of non-invasive diagnostic techniques for the screening of the embryos via the different molecules released in the culture medium or the blastocoel cavity

Table 2: Comparison of PGT-A diagnostic test and the different characteristics of each test.

	FISH	*qPCR*	*SNPs*	*aCGH*	*NGS*
Result	3–12 chromosomes	24 chromosomes	24 chromosomes	24 chromosomes	24 chromosomes
Whole chromosome aneuploidy	No	Yes	Yes	Yes	Yes
Duplications and deletions	No	No	Possible	Yes	Yes
Mosaicism	No	No	Possible	Limited	Yes
Gene mutation	No	Possible	Yes	No	Yes
Duration	6–8 hr	4 hr	30–40 hr	12–15 hr	13–16 hr
Fresh transfer	Possible	Possible	No	Possible	No
Advantages	Quick	Fast and cheap	High resolution	Cheap and relative fast	Very high resolution/mtDNA copy number
Disadvantages	Not all chromosomes are tested/signal overlap/hybridization failure/high error rate	Low resolution	Not possible in case of consanguinity among the partners	Limited ability to identify mosaicim	High installation cost/high cost per embryo tested
Polyploidies	Yes	Yes	Limited	No	Yes
Balanced chromosomal rearrangements	Possible	No	Limited	No	Possible
Uniparental disomies	No	No	Yes	No	Yes

(aCGH: array comparative genomic hybridization, FISH: Fluorescence in situ hybridization; mtDNA: mitochondrial deoxyribonucleic acid, NGS: next-generation sequencing, qPCR: quantitative polymerase chain reaction, SNPs: single nucleotide polymorphism arrays)

by the embryo itself. The detailed analysis of the mixture of biomolecules secreted will help us to develop different holistic profiles for viable and nonviable embryos and eventually, reach our ultimately goal, to optimize embryo selection and IVF efficiency.

CONCLUSION

Today, despite the immense developments, PGT-A still needs to prove itself as the available data and studies do not show the expected benefit in implantation and delivery rates. Its beneficial role, for the moment, seems to be mainly restricted to lower miscarriage rates and reduced time to pregnancy observed after the transfer of euploid blastocysts.

With the increasing use of PGT-A, there is an urgent need for:

- More randomized control trial (RCT) studies in order to assess the risks and benefits of PGT-A in the different patient subgroups
- Well-designed non selection studies to compare and confirm the PGT-A results
- Systematic validation and reporting of all the available platforms.

REFERENCES

1. Handyside A, Kontogianni E, Hardy K, et al. Pregnancies from biopsied human preimplantation embryos sexed by Y-specific DNA amplification. Nature. 1990;344(6268):768-70.
2. Verlinsky Y, Ginsberg N, Lifchez A, et al. Analysis of the first polar body: preconception genetic diagnosis. Hum Reprod. 1990;5(7):826-9.
3. Practice Committee of Society for Assisted Reproductive Technology, Practice Committee of American Society for Reproductive Medicine. Preimplantation genetic testing: a Practice Committee opinion. Fertil Steril. 2008;90(5): S136-43.
4. Practice Committee of Society for Assisted Reproductive Technology, Practice Committee of American Society for

Reproductive Medicine. The use of preimplantation genetic testing for aneuploidy (PGT-A): a committee opinion. Fertil Steril. 2018;109(3):429-36.
5. Brezina P, Anchan R, Kearns W. Preimplantation genetic testing for aneuploidy: what technology should you use and what are the differences? J Assist Reprod Genet. 2016;33(7):823-32
6. Griffin D, Ogur C. Chromosomal analysis in IVF: just how useful is it? Reproduction. 2018;156(1):F29-50.
7. Treff NR, Tao X, Ferry KM, et al. Development and validation of an accurate quantitative real-time polymerase chain reaction-based assay for human blastocyst comprehensive chromosomal aneuploidy screening. Fertil Steril. 2012; 97(4):819-24.
8. Wells D, Kaur K, Grifo J, et al. Clinical utilization of a rapid low-pass whole genome sequencing technique for the diagnosis of aneuploidy in human embryos prior to implantation. J Med Genet. 2014;51(8):553-62.
9. Paulson RJ. Preimplantation genetic screening: what is the clinical efficiency? Fertil Steril. 2017;108(2):228-30.
10. Rosenwaks Z, Handyside AH, Fiorentino F, et al. The pros and cons of preimplantation genetic testing for aneuploidy: clinical and laboratory perspectives. Fertil Steril. 2018;110(3):353-61.

Guidelines of Assisted Reproductive Technologies and Surrogacy

77

Roya Rozati, RS Sharma

INTRODUCTION

Infertility is the major concern for all the singles who are suffering with it. The main reason for the infertility is psychological and social problems. Infertility leads to the major issues between the couples.

Assisted reproductive technology (ART) refers to technologies where sperms, eggs, and embryos are controlled outside the body. The first and the most common procedure is in vitro fertilization (IVF), but there is an ever increasing list.

ASSISTED REPRODUCTIVE TECHNOLOGY GUIDELINES

Since its beginning, improvements in ART have aided the achievement in pregnancy worldwide for thousands of people. ART plays an imperative role in supporting people to propagate their families and shrink the load of psychological distress related with infertility. Nevertheless, the practice of ART is not without debate and their continue imperative ethical considerations in both the research and clinical circumstances.

Ethical Guidelines

Ethical guidelines deliver a predominant background for the department of ART in both research and clinical practice. These ethical guidelines similarly support the right to fair and reasonable access to healthcare, including ART. These ethical guidelines have been established primarily for Human Research Ethics Committees (HRECs), ART clinicians, embryologists, clinic nurses, administrators, counselors, and researchers. Recognizing the guiding principles should inform the researchers and clinicians to develop the procedures at their facilities. The ethical guidelines protect all events associated with ART as they happen in clinical practice and research.

Primary Infertility Clinics

In primary infertility clinic, preliminary investigations need to be performed to identify the cause and type of infertility in couples. Sperms, egg, and embryo are not to be handled in primary infertility clinic. Couple can be treated at primary infertility clinic, but couples need to consult the secondary and tertiary infertility clinic based on severity of infertility. Consulting doctor and physician at primary infertility clinic should have appropriate degree. All the members at primary infertility clinic must be aware of all the above mentioned responsibilities. Primary infertility clinic does not require any registration.

Secondary Infertility Clinics

Secondary infertility clinic should have set-up for further in-depth investigation and prolonged treatment of infertility. Some of the treatment and investigations facilities that secondary infertility clinics should maintain:

- Facilities for investigations.
- Treatment facilities.

Tertiary Infertility Clinics

Tertiary infertility clinics should be registered and they will have three different purposes to achieve, such as diagnostic processes for female and male infertility, and therapeutic processes at the maximum level of specialization and with the finest facilities and research. If any of the facilities does not exist in the clinic, the clinic should have collaboration with other accredited ART bank, clinic, or laboratory.

NECESSITIES FOR AN ART CLINIC

The achievement of any ART program depends on its IVF laboratory. The chief purpose of an ART laboratory is to offer an ideal environment for embryos and gametes. To establish an ART laboratory, there are three main areas to focus, such as:

1. Location or place of the laboratory.
2. The embryologists.
3. The protocols, quality control, and the laboratory design.

ART layout, consumables, and equipment used in IVF laboratory are an important part in establishing IVF laboratory for any fertility clinic.

Location of the IVF Laboratory

Location of laboratory plays a vital role during setting up an IVF laboratory with high standards. The IVF laboratory should be free from pathogens and provide a non-toxic, safe, and stable environment. Therefore, care must be taken before choosing the location. Laboratory settings are of paramount importance in upholding constant success rates. The laboratory should be far away from polluted areas such as industries or areas where there is high volume of traffic. Locations of IVF laboratories should not be near to gasoline service stations and parking lots. To limit the adverse impacts of pollutants to cell tissue culture, construction areas should also be avoided.

Design to Establish the IVF Laboratory

Before starting an IVF facility, laboratory should be designed after considering the workload. In an IVF facility, design of laboratory is of vital importance to meet the structural and the environmental aspects. Structural design aspects cover specifications related to laboratory layout like flooring, height, lighting, wall paint, etc. Whereas, environmental design is to assure that the eminence of ambient air is favorable for all procedures. It broadly covers material selection and appropriate engineering aspects to reduce contamination which arises due to air handling systems and laboratory structure which can ultimately affect air composition.[1] Laboratory must be constructed adjoining to the operating theater or procedure room.[2] In planning IVF facility, suggestions of clean room experts are highly recommended in order to get rid of chemical air contaminants (CAC) and volatile organic compounds (VOCs) in the laboratory.

The well-designed ART laboratory should have four major parts: andrology section, embryology section, cryopreservation section, and micromanipulation section.

1. *Andrology section:* Here semen assessment, sperm preparation, and surgical sperm retrieval is done.
2. *Embryology section:* The processes related to oocyte retrieval, embryo culture, and transfer are carried out.
3. *Cryopreservation section:* This section mainly deals with vitrification or freezing of oocytes, sperm, embryos, testicular, and ovarian tissues in liquid nitrogen.
4. *Micromanipulation section:* Deals with assisted hatching; intracytoplasmic sperm injection (ICSI), embryo, blastocyst, and polar body biopsy are done.

Air Quality

The ambient air in the laboratory should be highly sterile. This can be provided by the arrangement of heating, ventilation air conditioning (HVAC) system, and an air handling unit that supplies only to the ART laboratory. Pre-filters should be placed on the roof at the fresh air supply inlet. Inlet should be provided with the potassium permanganate filters and activated carbon filters to suck up contaminants and these filters should be changed at regular time intervals to assure highly purified air circulation in the laboratory. The ceiling should be provided with ultra-low penetration air or high efficiency particulate air (HEPA) filters.[3] Care should be taken in such a way that in an hour there should be at least 18 air exchanges in laboratory. The laboratory should be pressurized to prevent air from adjacent rooms entering the laboratory. There should be activated carbon filters placed within the laboratory to absorb VOCs emitted from electrical equipment, new furniture, etc.[1]

Building Material

In painting laboratory walls, it is highly recommended to use non-toxic, non-odor emitting, non-vaporizing, glossy paint. Ceiling should be solid. Flooring should be slip proof preferably vinyl which is easy to clean. Cupboards and tabletops should be laminated with matt finish that is washable and made of heat-resistant material. Furniture should be of normal working height and should be ergonomically designed to reduce fatigue for staff. Lighting should be adjustable by dimmer. There should be enough electrical outlets. The power supply should be maintained without any interruption along with trigger alarm feature for all major equipment such as micromanipulator, incubators, freezing machine, refrigerator, etc.[4] Laboratory should be equipped with a wall-mounted data logger to display laboratory ambient temperature and humidity levels.

Equipment and Maintenance

Incubators are the most crucial equipment in the ART laboratory. The incubators are maintained at 37°C. Embryo culture media are buffered by bicarbonate and therefore, in order to maintain correct pH of the culture medium, the commonly used gas phases are 5% or 6% CO_2 in air or triple gas that consists of 5% O_2, 6% CO_2, and 89% N_2. Low oxygen tension has proven to be the preferred choice.[5] Accuracy of the temperature can be checked by using calibrated thermometer or thermocouple. It is important to check bicarbonate buffered culture medium pH in the incubator maintained by CO_2 by a pH meter regularly. The incubators are used for pre-equilibration of culture medium, sperm incubation, and oocyte and embryo culture. There should be enough incubators in the laboratory. Incubators with 4–6 compartments are preferred. Frequent closing and opening incubator doors should be avoided as this leads to fluctuation of temperature, pH, and osmolarity.[6] Temperature control during ART procedures is extremely important when handling oocytes and embryos. It has been shown that brief exposure of human oocytes to room temperature results in spindle disruption and microtubule disassembly.[7] Therefore, all precursors should be taken to avoid power and temperature fluctuation during handling of embryos or oocytes and the temperature should be maintained at 37°C. For handling oocytes and embryos, a laminar flow hood provided with HEPA filters and with an inbuilt stereo microscope is need. It is also required to maintain temperatures at 37°C in the laminar flow cabinet which can be achieved by heating the tabletop. For micromanipulation and embryo monitoring, inverted microscopes are used as these microscopes can provide a larger working distance and for sperm evaluation upright microscopes are used. For assessment and teaching purposes, these microscopes should be attached with video camera system. An isolated area free from all other laboratory activities is needed to set-up micromanipulator systems.

The entire system consists of an inverted microscope, micromanipulator arms, and microinjector. Inverted microscopes used for micromanipulation should be equipped with 4X, 10X, and 20X objectives with a heated stage and the entire microscope should be mounted on a vibration free platform. Two identical micromanipulator arms are mounted on both sides of the microscope. These arms are capable of three-dimensional movements where in the right side consists injection pipette and the left site is provided with holding pipette. The microinjector consists of a syringe and silicone tubing connected to the microtool at the end of the tubing. These microtools for holding the oocyte and for sperm injection are commercially available. These systems are used for procedures like ICSI, embryo biopsy, etc.

Centrifuge is required to prepare sperm for IVF insemination or intracytoplasmic spermatozoa injection. Centrifuge needs to be regularly cleaned and maintained. A medical refrigerator is crucial for storage of culture medium. The temperature of the refrigerator and freezer is normally charted on the temperature chart. The laboratory should be equipped with a source of ultrapure water purification system. This ultrapure water is required in ART laboratory for preparation of media and essential in cleaning of glassware (principally glass Pasteur pipettes) that is used for handling gametes and embryos.[8] The glass pipettes are soaked in ultrapure water before they are washed, packed, and sterilized. These systems are very expensive and require regular maintenance and regular replacement of various filters.

Nowadays, disposable consumables are used in ART. Dry heat sterilization oven is used while preparing glass Pasteur pipettes. After soaking in ultrapure water, the pipettes are washed, packed, and then sterilized in the dry heat oven. Metal blocks, stainless steel test tube racks, and silicon tubings are sterilized daily in the oven at the end of the day. Ovens need to be checked routinely for accuracy of temperature. There is a need to maintain follicular aspirates' temperature present in test tubes at 37°C, in order to meet these criteria, test tube warmers are required. Suction pumps, though used in the procedure room for follicular fluid aspiration, are the responsibility of the ART laboratory staff. They should be serviced routinely and sent for recalibration to ensure that the suction levels are accurate.

Slow freezing is achieved by the freezing machine where there is a very gradual drop in temperature. The whole freezing program takes about 2–2.5 hours. This method of freezing can be used for cleavage stage embryos, blastocysts, and ovarian tissue. These machines are very expensive and need to be serviced regularly. However, with recent breakthroughs in vitrification, freezing protocols requiring these sophisticated machines may be replaced by vitrification protocols.[9] For cryopreservation of embryos, ovarian tissue, and gametes, liquid nitrogen tankers are needed. These samples can be preserved either in the vapor phase or liquid phase. These tanks are topped up regularly with liquid nitrogen and are fitted with probes that trigger alarm if low levels of liquid nitrogen are detected.

The most crucial step in establishing a new laboratory is purchase of the equipment. It is always advisable to purchase well-reputed models that are in use since a long time in other established recognized centers. Purchase of equipment should be done based on the criteria of reliability, quality, safety, and completion of tests regarding electrical leakage by biomedical engineers. Equipment must be provided with reliable breakdown service and maintenance support. Once equipment have been purchased, maintenance and regular servicing should be carried out. It is important that the suppliers have spare equipment as backup in the event of any malfunction of equipment. Equipment must be provided with a backup power supply with a trigger alarm or call back service to overcome the limitation of problems associated with interrupted power supply.

Minimum Requirement of Staff in Infertility Clinics

The staff necessities given below are compulsory for secondary and tertiary IVF clinics. In the case of small secondary and tertiary IVF clinics, the services of the clinical embryologist, andrologist, and counselor, may be mutual. All newly hired staff should undergo a formal training on all procedures using the murine model. This training should be done simultaneously as the embryology laboratory is being constructed. The training should improve skill sets and give better understanding of procedural and physiological bases of procedures. There should be an emphasis on the strict adherence of the standard operating procedures (SOPs). All the embryologists must attend the various workshops, conferences, and educational programs to increase their knowledge.[10] The entire IVF clinic should have adequate number of staffs to work smoothly in clinic. Less number of staff in IVF clinic may lead to non-adherence to SOP's, staff unhappiness, and confusion in the laboratory.

ROLE OF GYNECOLOGIST IN ART

In a secondary or tertiary IVF clinic, the gynecologist should hold a postgraduate or diploma degree in gynecology and have the adequate knowledge about the ideologies of ovarian stimulation and managing the difficulties ascending thereupon. Gynecologist must be well-versed with all the ART techniques such as artificial insemination with husband's semen (AIH), intrauterine insemination (IUI), artificial insemination with donor semen (AID), IVF, ultrasonographic intervention, ICSI, and other procedures involved in ART. For a tertiary IVF clinic, the gynecologist should have the expertise of ovum pick-up and embryo transfer (ET).

Role of Andrologist in Assisted Reproductive Technology

Male factors are one of the main concerns in the infertility couple. 50% of infertility cases are associated to male factors, numerous of which can be treated by less-invasive procedures and specific ART processes. All andrologists should have adequate knowledge of the infections, occupational hazards, and fever that cause reversible or irreversible forms of infertility. They $must have the knowledge of vasographic and ultrasonographic studies of the male reproductive tract. Andrologist must have the specific knowledge to treat impotence and ejaculatory dysfunction. One single andrologist can work in more than one IVF clinic but he or she should not be disturbed by the work on all IVF clinics and they should be able to take care of their responsibilities without compromising on the quality of service.

Role of Counselors in Assisted Reproductive Technology

Counselor should have at least a degree in psychology, social sciences, medicine or life sciences. He or she should have good information of the numerous reasons of infertility and its social and gender implications. They should have the knowledge about the possibilities offered by the different types of treatment modalities. Single person may act as a counselor for more than one clinic but the counselors must take care of the complete counseling load of all the clinics without cooperating on the excellence of the counseling service.

Role of Co-Coordinator or Director in Assisted Reproductive Technology

Director or program coordinator should be a senior person with significant experience in all facets of ART. The director or programme coordinator must have an appropriate degree in a biological or medical science. The director or programme coordinator should be able to organize the actions of the other team and ensure that stock keeping, staff and administrative matters, finance, statutory requirements, maintenance of patient records, and public dealings are taken care of sufficiently.

Role of Embryologist in Assisted Reproductive Technology

The IVF laboratory should be always maintained and directed by an experienced, qualified, and responsible individual with knowledge in the area of embryology.[4] The embryologists must have a great experience in biological sciences or reproductive biology. They must be well-versed with all the aseptic techniques in IVF laboratory. An embryologist must be maintaining a good relationship with medical staff and should be able to counsel patients. The embryologist should be well-versed in all the facets of embryology which play important role in the establishment of IVF laboratory. Embryologists should ensure that processes and environment in the laboratory are maintained pathogen-free and non-toxic. He or she should be aware of maintenance of parameters for embryos and gametes. It is embryologist's responsibility to check on consumables, equipment, and environmental conditions.

Quality Control and Quality Assurance

After the completion of the new laboratory, there are few important points to be considered. The laboratory should be cleaned and all the equipment should be wiped down before moving into the laboratory. The ventilation rate should be increased and the air pressures should be increased to purge the air in the laboratory to get rid of any irritants or VOCs given out from the new materials, furniture, etc. New clean-room facilities such as ART laboratories undergo a lengthy curing time.[3] The duration depends on the type of construction material used and cleaning regime that is employed, etc. During this burning-in period, there should be no human traffic or activities in the laboratory.

All the consumables which are used in the ART procedure should be from recognized brands which are proven to be safe for the culture of embryos and gametes, and have been used at successful centers. Few plasticwares should be used only for single time such as test tubes, graduated pipettes, Petri dishes, and four-well culture dishes. Some glassware such as holders for ICSI and injection needles should be also used for single time. Oocyte aspiration needles and embryo transfer catheters must be for single use only. In all IVF clinics, powder-free gloves must be used. They should be of tissue culture grade and each lot of supply should have a batch number. Expiration dates should be clearly stated. In ART procedure, different suppliers should be avoided because standardization is crucial.

Culture medium is used to be prepared in the IVF laboratories. Severe quality control is vital in media preparation and is quite laborious. Commercially prepared high-quality culture media are available which are increasingly being used in laboratories all around the world. It is important to use culture media that have been established in the literature as suitable for culture of embryos and human oocytes and are readily obtainable. Only properly registered media should be used for IVF procedures. The entire medium must have a certification of osmolarity, pH sperm survival test, and endotoxin level. All medium must have the date of manufacturing, batch number, and lot number. All the medium containers should be packed properly and temperature should be maintained if it is manufactured in another country. Different companies' medium should not be mixed. Manufacturer's instruction must be followed while using the medium.

Two types of embryo culture systems are used in ART clinic. One is microdroplet culture system with oil overlay and another form of culture system is using normal volume of culture medium without oil overlay.[11] Microdroplet embryo culture with oil overlay must be organized fast as the droplet of culture medium is 10–20 Kl. The main advantage of this system is that it avoids the evaporation of media. This type of system also decreases the variations in pH. Culture of embryos in four-well dishes without oil overlay is other form of system of embryo culture. To reduce variation in pH caused by CO_2 from medium, these dishes can be placed in humidicribs that have an atmosphere of 5% or 6% CO_2 during embryo assessment.

Every laboratory should have a manual detailing of all the procedures done in the laboratory. The procedures should include sperm assessment and preparation for ICSI or IVF insemination, oocyte retrieval, oocyte culture, IVF insemination, ICSI, fertilization check, embryo culture, preparation of embryo culture dishes, embryo selection, embryo transfer, cryopreservation of gametes and embryos, etc. Laboratory protocols have to be transposed into standard operating protocols. All activities performed within the ART laboratory need to be clearly written with sufficient details on the techniques.[12] All SOPs must be signed and dated and all the SOPs must be made accessible to all staff members, so that everyone must be strictly adherent to the SOPs. Non-adherence to SOPs should be dealt with seriously and should not be excused. While doing processes, there must be at least two individuals for patients' specimen. The name and an additional identifier such as an identity number should be used. For all patients, the batch number of culture medium and all consumables of all patients must be documented.

Double witnessing is very important in ART procedures. There must be two different persons confirming, in writing, the identity of the specimen,[13] while transferring sperm samples during the various steps of sperm preparation and during oocyte retrieval. The identity of the embryo transfer patient and the embryos for transfer should be double checked. Double witnessing is also done during gamete and embryo cryopreservation and thawing. While witnessing, both individuals should document the various steps during which the witnessing was done on to the patients' record book.

It is the responsibility of the laboratory to consistently provide a high standard of service. As part of the quality control, it is imperative that there is daily monitoring and recording of the following equipment—the level of CO_2 must be measured daily by CO_2 analyzer; the temperature of the incubator must be maintained and measured daily by calibrated thermocouple; pH of the culture medium should be checked regularly and maintained by pH meter probes. In the incubator, the pH of the medium must also be maintained in regular intervals. The level of CO_2 gas in the cylinder also needs to be checked daily. The temperature of the heated base of the biological safety cabinet and laminar flow hood must be checked in regular basis using a calibrated thermometer. The microscope used in the ART clinic must be calibrated and the temperature of the heated stages must be checked in daily basis and recorded. The temperature of the refrigerator must be recorded every day.[14]

Maintaining sterility is very important in ART clinic as IVF is an extension of the operating theater. Strict SOPs should be followed while hand washing and maintaining the parameters in the ART clinic or laboratory. Laboratory should be cleaned on daily basis before and after use. If there is any type of spillage while doing any procedure, it must be wiped with distilled water followed by dry tissue. While embryos and oocytes are being handled, alcohol should not be used for cleaning. Waste material such follicular fluid, seminal fluid, etc. must be removed as early as the procedure is done. All the important equipment must be maintained and calibrated in the regular intervals. Microscope, incubators, and laminar flow cabinet, which are the most significant equipment in the ART laboratory, must be serviced twice a year. Other types of equipment such as medical refrigerators, oocyte suction pump, centrifuge, and hot air sterilizing oven should be serviced once a year. Maintenance and calibration of all the equipment play important role which is crucial for reproducibility of results.

ASSISTED REPRODUCTIVE TECHNOLOGY PROCEDURES[15,16]

Patient protection is the primary concern for all ART procedures. Another main concern for the ART procedures is the embryos and gametes which form a new entity of life. All ART clinics must follow each and every norm of scientific practices. All patients who are taking the ART treatment must be aware of all the procedures in ART. They must be familiar with significance of all ART procedures.

ART clinic must inform the State Board or National Advisory Board on a continuing basis if there are any novel procedures for ART treatments. There are several procedures used for ART clinic.

ART procedures include:

- Artificial insemination with husband's semen
- Artificial insemination with donor semen
- Intrauterine insemination with either husband's or donor semen (IUI-H or IUI-D)
- In vitro fertilization and embryo transfer
- IVF-associated techniques
- Intracytoplasmic sperm injection with ejaculated, epididymal or testicular spermatozoa:
    - Indications of ICSI with ejaculated spermatozoa
    - Indications of ICSI with surgically extracted sperm (MESA/PESA/TESA/TESE)
    - Indications of ICSI with in vitro matured oocytes.
- Oocyte donation (OD) or embryo donation (ED):
    - Indications for oocyte donation
    - Indications for embryo donation.
- Cryopreservation:
    - Freezing of semen
    - Freezing of embryos
    - Oocyte cryopreservation.
    - Ovarian tissue cryopreservation.

GUIDELINES OF SURROGACY

Surrogacy is a procedure whereby a woman decides to achieve pregnancy by medically inseminated sperm or by implanted embryo. The woman accepts a child for other person, to whom she means to handover the child's care after birth. In return, woman will obtain the reward for carrying and delivering the child **(Fig. 1)**.

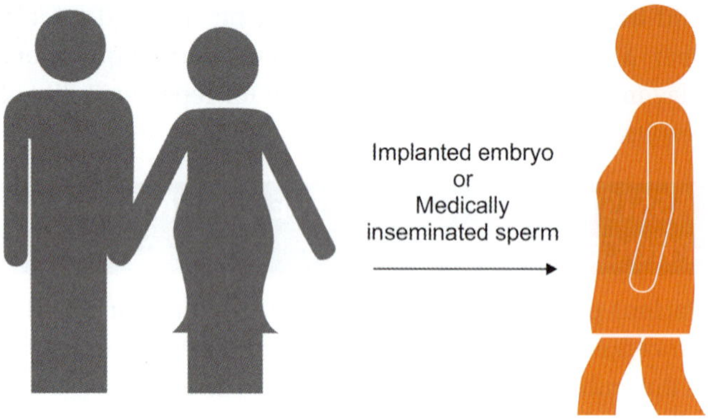

Fig. 1: Surrogacy.

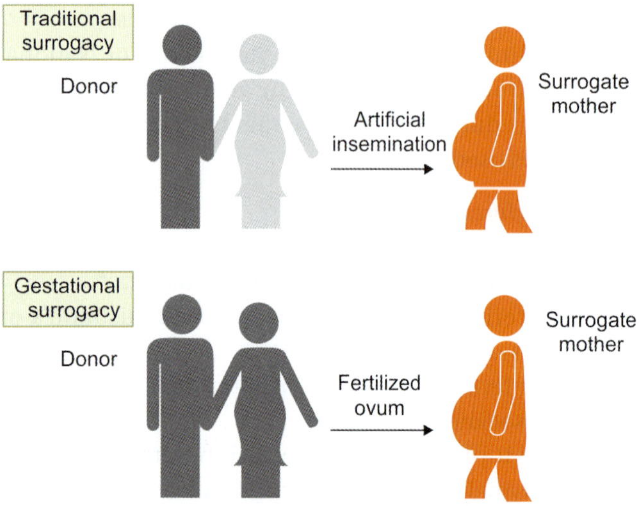

Fig. 2: Types of surrogacies.

Surrogacy is an arrangement in which a woman carries and delivers a child for another couple **(Fig. 2)**.

Surrogacy is an artificial reproductive method which is becoming more common due to upsurge in need of parenthood of infertile couples. India is also being known for commercial country for surrogacy since 2002.

HISTORY OF SURROGACY

- It is an old process since hundreds or thousands of years.
- Abraham and his wife Sarah had child, who were infertile, first known case written in Bible.
- In 1970s, surrogacy became more viable and acceptable process and documented—modern method of child bearing.
- In the mid-1970s, the child who was referred to as Baby M was enacted, it has the first "official" legal surrogacy agreement.
- One infertility center, a company that arranges hundreds of surrogate births every year, was established by the same lawyer, who had braked this agreement.
- In the same time frame, national and international news for world's first "test tube" baby, Louise Joy Brown (technically not a surrogate mother situation) was made by surrogacy.
- It has given the direction for surrogacy now called as gestational surrogacy (implanting process of both sperm and egg in a laboratory to later be placed into the surrogate mother's uterus).
- Past few decades, it has developed as one popular process for surrogacy.
- 2001: The oldest surrogate mother at that time gave birth to her own grandchild.
- 2005: A 58-year-old surrogate mother gave birth to her own twin granddaughters.

Australia

- Legally surrogate mother is considered as mother of child.
- Any surrogacy agreement giving custody to others is void and enforceable by law.
- In the Australian Capital Territory, arranging commercial surrogacy is a criminal offence.
- Northern territory has no legislation governing surrogacy at all. There are no future plans to introduce laws on surrogacy.
- Adoption required in case of surrogacy arrangements.

Canada

- Commercial surrogacy is prohibited by the Canada (under the Assisted Human Reproduction Act, 2004).
- Altruistic surrogacy remains legal.
- In the province of Quebec, contracts that involve surrogacy are unenforceable.

Hungary

Commercial surrogacy is illegal in Hungary.

United Kingdom

- Surrogacy is legal since 2009.
- Illegal in UK to pay more than expenses for surrogacy.
- The relationship can be recognized under Section 30 of Human Fertilization and Embryology Act, 1990.

United States

- State of Florida and California resides most surrogates due to the surrogacy-accommodating laws in these states.
- On the surrogacy, many of the states are having their own laws.
- It is illegal to hire surrogates in New York states.
- It is illegal to hire surrogates in New York. At this point, the laws surrounding surrogacy are well-defined in state of Delaware.

Surrogacy Laws in India

- Commercial surrogacy is legalized in India (The Supreme Court of India by virtue of case, "Baby Manji vs. Union of India").
- India is emerging as a leader in international surrogacy.
- Surrogacy in India is much simpler and cost effective than anywhere else in the world.
- There is no law governing the surrogacy. "Surrogacy Agreement," is the only base which governs the parties to surrogacy.
- Therefore, the commissioning parents are required to be attentive while signing agreement, so that the surrogacy agreement is not held void in court of law.
- Every agreement, should express *purpose* and *situations*, the *need of surrogacy, free will of surrogate, details about the surrogate* and the *terms* on which the surrogate agrees to gestate the child, etc.

Facts on Surrogacy (Fig. 3)

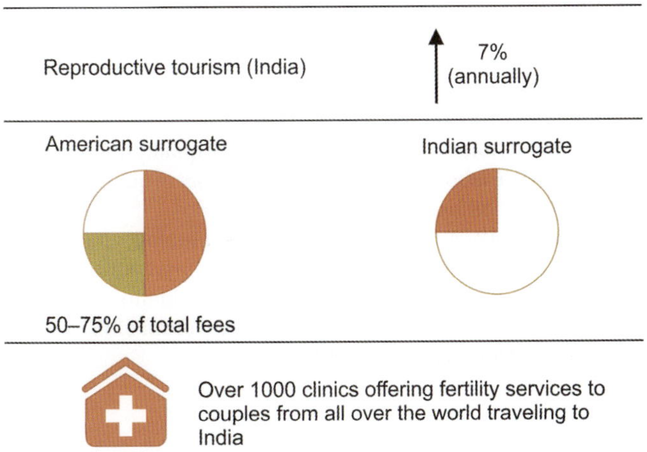

Fig. 3: Facts on surrogacy.

ASSISTED REPRODUCTIVE TECHNOLOGY BILL: OVERVIEW

- Considering the growing number of surrogacy cases, Assisted Reproductive Bill (2010) was made in India.
- The Government of India decided to come up with a law for the challenges that the surrogacy would face in future, which would govern the surrogacy and ART in India.
- A committee of experts was set-up and the said committee has submitted a draft of the proposed bill to the Government of India.
- The said bill is still awaiting with government and has not yet been presented in the parliament.
- The purposed draft namely "Assisted Reproductive Technologies Bill, 2010" has taken into consideration various aspects of surrogacy and has built in safeguards for surrogate mothers.

Salient Features for Assisted Reproductive Technology Bill, 2010

Completely Legal

The process of surrogacy and giving the womb on rent, as it is popularly called, is completely legal in India. Charging financial reimbursement for carrying the baby of an Indian or foreign couple would be absolutely legal.

Couple Defined

The bill defines the term "couple" as two people living together and a sexual relationship that is legal according to Indian legislation. Since court has already given verdict in favor of homosexuality, a gay or lesbian couple can also go for surrogacy and it will be termed legal.

Surrogate Mother

Surrogate mother age has to be 21–35. The maximum "three" number of "live births" are allowed, including her own children.

Single Parent

In the case of single parent opting for surrogacy, the baby will be legitimate child for him or her.

Live in Relationship

In case the intended parents are engaged in live in relationship then the child would be legitimate child of both.

Cost and Remuneration

Complete cost of pregnancy and pay remuneration to the surrogate mother will be bear by intended couple. They may give a contractual obligation under Indian legislation.

Foreign National

In case of foreign national intended couple, they have to submit the surrogacy policy of their country and a certificate regarding nationality of the surrogate child post birth. They also have to nominate a local guardian to take care of surrogate mother during pregnancy.

Assisted Reproductive Technology Banks

Complete details of surrogates and donors will be stored at Government-certified ART banks. State board will give certificate to ART banks. This independent body would have authority to register, maintain, and monitor the functioning.

Sex Determination Illegal

Sex determination of the baby and "selective child birth" through surrogacy is illegal.

CONCLUSION

Establishment of the ART clinic is not an easy task. The ART clinic plays an important role in the treatment of infertile couples. The ART clinic must provide a safe and secure microenvironment to maintain finest parameters for embryonic development. Experienced and highly skilled embryologists should be selected and be able to deliver consistent results. To ensure consistency and reproducibility, quality standards are needed of all methods. Procedures and processes should be clearly written and available. Quality control is main phenomena for the success of ART clinics.

Enacting the laws is important, or else India would be a tourism hub for surrogacy. Surrogacy carries social stigma in the society as it is equated with prostitution and by virtue of that, it is argued that it should be disallowed on moral grounds. Surrogate mothers are set aside in isolation from families and allowed to meet families on weekends, which is against the human rights. Hence, there are number of ethical, social, legal, and psychological issues associated with surrogacy, which require urgent need for framing and implementation of law.

REFERENCES

1. Cohen J, Gilligan A, Willadsen S. Culture and quality control of embryos. Hum Reprod. 1998;13(Suppl.3):137-44.
2. The American Society for Reproductive Medicine. Revised guidelines for human embryology and andrology laboratories. Fertil Steril. 2008;90:S45-59.
3. Boone WR, Johnson JE, Locke AJ, et al. Control of air quality in an assisted reproductive technology laboratory. Fertil Steril.1999;71:150-4.
4. Gianaroli L, Plachot M, Van Kooij R, et al. Guidelines for good practice in IVF laboratories. Hum Reprod. 2000;15:2241-6.
5. Meintjes M, Chantlis SJ, Douglas JD, et al. A controlled randomized trial evaluating the effect of lowered incubator oxygen tension on live births in a predominantly blastocyst transfer program. Hum Reprod. 2009;24(2):300-7.
6. Abramczuk JW, Lopata A. Incubator performance in the clinical in vitro fertilization program: importance of temperature conditions for the fertilization and cleavage of human oocytes. Fertil Steril. 1986;46:132-4.
7. Pickering SJ, Braude PR, Johnson MH, et al. Transient cooling to room temperature can cause irreversible disruption of the meiotic spindle in the human oocyte. Fertil Steril. 1990;54:102-8.
8. Wiemer KE, Anderson A, Stewart B. The importance of water quality for media preparation. Hum Reprod. 1998;13(Suppl. 4):166-72.
9. Balaban B, Urman B, Ata B, et al. A randomized controlled study of human Day 3 embryo cryopreservation by slow freezing or vitrification: vitrification is associated with higher survival, metabolism and blastocyst formation. Hum Reprod. 2008;23(9):1976-82.
10. Alper MM, Brinsden PR, Fischer R, et al. Is your IVF programme good? Hum Reprod. 2002;17:8-10.
11. Lane M, Gardner DK. Effect of incubation volume and embryo density on the development and viability of mouse embryos in vitro. Hum Reprod. 1992;7:558-62.
12. Kastrop P. Quality management in the ART laboratory. Reprod Biomed Online 2003;7:691-4.
13. Pool TB. Practices contributing to quality performance in the embryo laboratory and the status of laboratory regulation in the US. Hum Reprod. 1997;12:2591-3.
14. Mayer JF, Jones EL, Lacey DD, et al. Total quality improvement in the IVF laboratory: choosing indicators of quality. Reprod Biomed Online. 2003;7:695-9.
15. Begum MR. Assisted reproductive technology: techniques and limitations. J Bangladesh Coll Phys Surg. 2008;26:135-41.
16. Jin M, Jin Z, Hyllner SJ, et al. Sensitivity evaluation of a mouse embryo assay (MEA) used for quality control of IVF culture media. Hum Reprod. 1998;13:282.

PCPNDT Act versus IVF/ART: Medicolegal Problems in ART

78

Rajnikant Contractor

INTRODUCTION

The Prenatal Diagnostic Techniques (Regulation and Prevention of Misuse) (PNDT) Act, 1994, was implemented from 1st January 1996, to ensure that the female feticide was kept under check. This Act ensures that there is no determination and disclosure of the sex of the fetus.

The Prenatal Diagnostic Techniques (Regulation and Prevention of Misuse) Act and Rules are constantly being amended to ensure that emerging technologies which may determine the sex of the fetus before and after conception are included in this Act. These amendments have been in place since 14th February, 2003.

"*Prenatal diagnostic techniques*" include all prenatal diagnostic procedures and tests.

"*Prenatal diagnostic procedures*" mean all gynecological or obstetric or medical procedures such as *fetoscopy, ultrasonography (USG), sampling of embryos, chorionic villi, amniotic fluid, blood or any other tissue or fluid of a man or woman* prior or post-conception, that are sent to a genetic laboratory or clinic conducting analysis or pre-natal diagnostic tests for selection of sex prior or post-conception. "*Prenatal diagnostic test*" means *USG or testing or analysis* of chorionic villi, amniotic fluid, blood or any tissue of a pregnant woman to detect the presence of any metabolic disorders, chromosomal abnormalities, genetic disorders or any anomalies or sex-linked diseases.

Definition of "Sex selection" in PCPNDT Act [Section 2(o)]: "Sex selection" encompasses any procedure, technique, test or administration or prescription or provision that *may increase the probability or confirm that the embryo maybe of a particular sex.*

Prohibition of Sex selection [Section 3A]: No person, including a specialist or a team of specialists in the field of infertility, shall conduct or cause to be conducted or aid in conducting by himself or by any other person, sex selection on a woman or man or on both or on any tissue, embryo, conceptus, fluid or gametes derived from either or both of them.

As per *Section 4 (1),* conduct of prenatal diagnostic techniques is allowed only for the detection of:

(*i*) Chromosomal abnormalities

(*ii*) Genetic metabolic diseases

(*iii*) Hemoglobinopathies

(*iv*) Sex-linked genetic diseases

(*v*) Congenital anomalies

(*vi*) Any other abnormalities or diseases as may be specified by the Central Supervisory Board.

Prenatal diagnostic techniques can be used or conducted only when any of the following conditions exist*[Section 4(3)]*:

(*i*) Age of the pregnant woman is above 35 years

(*ii*) The pregnant woman has undergone two or more spontaneous abortions or fetal loss

(*iii*) The pregnant woman had been exposed to potentially teratogenic agents such as drugs, radiation, infection or chemicals

(*iv*) The pregnant woman or her spouse has a family history of mental retardation or physical deformities such as, spasticity or any other genetic disease

(*v*) Any other condition as may be specified by the Board.

As per Section 3A: IVF, ART, surrogacy clinic, and centers are mandatorily registered under PCPNDT Act

1994; depending upon range of the activities performed by the centers. In preimplantation genetic diagnosis (PGD), embryos without any genetic problems being tested and normal embryos are transferred into the uterus. Only in *PGD, there is 100% chance of sex selection possible.* So, Government should only monitor those IVF centers and genetic laboratories which are conducting PGD and demanding all reports why PGD is needed and full family history of those patients undergoing PGD in Form-F (Section C). Fill Form-F (Revised Section A, Section B, Section C, Section D). If you do invasive procedure, then fill Form-G (give one copy to patients).

Q. 1: Is IVF/ART need to be registered under PCPNDT act?

Ans. Yes. All IVF/ART and surrogacy clinics are mandatory to be registered under PCPNDT Act (as per Section 3A).

Q. 2: Which Forms should IVF/ART clinic fill as per PCPNDT act?

Ans. As such no special Form for IVF/ART, but one has to fill revised *Form-F (January 31st 2014). One must fill Form-F (Sections: A, B, C, D) and Form-G, if invasive procedure will be conducted.*

Q. 3: Under which category IVF/ART clinic will be registered as GCC/GC/GL?

Ans. "Genetic Clinic" means clinics, hospitals, institute, nursing homes or any place, by whatever named called, which is used for conducting prenatal diagnostic procedures *[Section 2(d)]. IVF/ART clinic comes under Genetic Clinic.*

Any individual having enough space and being able to or employing:

- A gynecologist who has the experience of performing a minimum of 20 chorionic villi aspiration per vaginum or per abdomen, sampling of chorionic villi, ability to perform an amniocentesis, fetoscopy, cordocentesis, biopsy of fetal skin or organ or fetal blood sampling, etc. under supervision of an experienced gynecologist in the fields mentioned above; or
- A radiologist, sonologist, imaging specialist or a registered medical practitioner possessing a diploma, post-graduate degree or 6 months training or 1-year experience in sonography or image scanning; or
- A medical geneticist can set up an ultrasound clinic/ imaging center/genetic center *[Rule 3 (3)].*

Q. 4: Why not GCC?

Ans. Section 2(c) GCC means a clinic, nursing home, hospital, institute or any place by whatever name called which provides genetic counseling to the patients. IVF/ART clinics are not fit for eligibility criteria as per PNDT Act.

Any individual that is able to or employs:

- A gynecologist or a pediatrician that has 6 months of experience or 4 weeks of training in genetic counselling; or
- A medical geneticist that has enough space and educational charts/models/equipment for carrying out genetic counselling; may set up a center for genetic counselling and get it registered as a genetic counselling center *[Rule 3 (1)].*

Q. 5: Why not under genetic laboratory?

Ans. According to Section 2(e), genetic laboratory includes places where facilities are provided for conducting analysis or test of samples received from GC for PNDT test.

Any person having adequate space and ability or employing:

- *A Medical Geneticist*—includes a person who has a degree or diploma in genetic science in the fields of sex determination and prenatal diagnostic techniques or has experiences of not less than 2 years in any of the above mentioned fields after obtaining any one of medical qualification recognized under the Indian Medical Council Act (102 of 1956), or a postgraduate degree in biological sciences;
- A *Laboratory technician having a Bachelors of Science degree in Biological Sciences* or a diploma or degree in medical laboratory course with a minimum of 1-year experience in conducting appropriate prenatal diagnostic techniques, procedures or tests; may set up a genetic laboratory *[Rule 3 (2a)].*

Such laboratories should have or acquire the following equipment that are necessary for carrying out chromosomal studies, biochemical studies, and molecular studies:

- *Chromosomal studies: 15 equipment*
- *Biochemical studies: 18 equipment*
- *Molecular studies: 18 equipment [Rule 3 (2b)].*

Q. 6: For IUI/Ovulation study/Embryo transfer/Follicular study, do one has to fill Forms?

Ans. Not at all. No need of filling any Forms in OS/ET/FS but if you keep any record of data of such procedure in your computer, you must take a printed copy of record and after it is authenticated by you, you must keep it as a record keeping file as per Rule 9 (7).

Q. 7: Which type of record is to be kept by IVF/ART clinic?

Ans. Same as the one kept as per PCPNDT Act. Maintenance of records of Form-F [Section 29 and Rule 9]. PNDT Register

[Rule 9 (1)] records should be sent to Authority before 5th of next month *[Rule 9 (8)]*.

FOLLOW THE DO'S AND DONT'S IN PCPNDT

Code of conduct to be observed by every Appropriate Authorities (*under rule 18A dated on February 24th, 2014) [Rule 18 A (9)]* PCPNDT Act is Central act; it means all states have to implement uniformly as prescribed in Rules in the Act. Under Section 32 and Section 34 only parliament has power to make Rules and Regulations. So, to avoid any litigation in court of law, every State PCPNDT Authority must follow Central act. No Authority should issue GR or order to implement their own views beyond the Central act.

Do's in PCPNDT Act

1. *Intimation of changes in employees, place or equipment; Apply any changes 30 days in advance:* Registration of place and address is mandatory and any change in place, person, buyback or installation of new USG machine (company name and no.). It is one's duty to inform authorities in writing of which two copies (in official letter head) have to be submitted to authority office *a minimum of 1 month in advance* of expected date of such changes and seek *re-issuance of certificate of registration* from appropriate authority with the changes duly incorporated *[Rule 13]*.
2. *Display board:* Display a board that determination of sex is prohibited at our center at conspicuous place (e.g. OPD) in both in English and local language. (board should include name and address of the clinic and writing "Prenatal sex determination is a punishable offence. Sex determination is not done here") *[Rule 17 (1)]*.

   At least one copy of each of the act and rules shall be available on the premise [Rule 17 (2)].
3. *Reg. Certificate—at the Waiting and Sonography Room:* Keep FORM-B certificate of registration copy, one copy (your registration certificate) in conspicuous place, e.g. waiting area and second in sonography room so the patient can easily read both in OPD and while doing sonography *[Section 19 (4) of PCPNDT Act]*.
4. *Dress code:* Be 100% safe and secure; wear dress code, e.g. white apron with your name and degree on black plate to avoid unnecessary harassment as it happened in Rajasthan (Ganganagar: USG machine were sealed at clinics of 12 doctors) *[Rule 18 (8)]*.
5. *Fill Form-F before USG:* Prior to performing a USG, it is mandatory to fill up *Form-F* with all the details (in detail and declaration by patient and person doing sonography). Always take the signature of the patient prior to performing the USG (If a pregnancy is diagnosed accidentally, while performing USG of the pelvis, then ensure that the *Form-F* is filled out before the patient leaves the clinic).
6. *Always maintain PNDT register [Rule 9(1)]*:
   (i) Serial no.
   (ii) Name and address of the woman and man
   (iii) Name of husband/father
   (iv) Date on which they first reported for counselling, procedure and test.
7. *Record preserve—2 years:* Maintain and preserve of all records (Form-F, consent form, sonography plate, slides, recommendations and letters) for a minimum period of 2 years (In event of any legal proceeding is pending against you , then one has to preserve all records till final disposal of legal proceeding) *[Rule 9 (6) and Section 29 of the PCPNDT Act]*. All such records, at all reasonable times, be made available for inspection to the appropriate authority.
8. *Printed Form-F must be as per provisions of the Act 1994 and New Notification on January 31st, 2014:* One should fill New Revised Form-F and fill all *Sections A, B, C, D* to avoid unnecessary conflict and breach of law *[Section 4(3), Rule 9 (4) and Rule 10 (1A)]*.
9. *Non-use of machine; Surrender Registration Certificate:* In case of *non-use* of machine, change of ownership, management, cessation of function; immediately surrender both copies of PNDT registration certificate to appropriate authority *[Rule 6(6)]*. The certificate of registration shall be nontransferable.
10. As such there is no separate Form-F for IVF/ART clinic but they are mandatorily required to be registered under PCPNDT Act 1994 as per Circular from PNDT Office Government of India on October 9th, 2014 by PNDT Director to all states.
11. *Portable machine-fix:* If you have a small portable machine then fix it to a trolley, table or mount it on a wall or fix it to structure so that it cannot be moved from one place to another (it means outside of your clinic). A portable machine should be readily available during inspection (If you have indoor facilities then you can move it from your consulting room to LR, OT, Ward as per emergency, to attend to patient's condition)—Direction from Dr RK Gupta Director H & FW GOI on February 3rd, 2015.

12. *Renewal/apply 30 days before:* Renewal date of registration should always be remembered and application of renewal should be done 30 days prior to the appropriate authority office on two letter pads (Form-A) with cheque of one half of fee (e.g. ₹12,500 or 17,500) with seal and signature of government staff on receiving copy (Please have acknowledgement of the same from authority). *[Rule 8(1)].* If there is no answer in 90 days of your renewal application, your registration is consider as deemed renewed *[Rule 8 (6)].*
13. *Consult medicolegal advisor before signing:* Always send Form-F monthly report to government authority in PNDT office before the 5th of next month without fail *[Rule 9 (8)].* Always cooperate with government authority whenever they visit for inspection at your clinic. Do not panic if notice is issued against you but *be careful before giving signature or commission of offence on inspection report.* Consult your medicolegal advisor about it.
14. *Keep other government posters:* Keep IEC material from government like *Female Feticide Is Heinous Crime* and *Beti Bachao Beti Padhao* poster at your OPD (supplied by Government authority) just for sensitization and awareness for public.

Don'ts in PCPNDT Act

1. *Do USG—at registered place only:* Never perform a sonography at an unregistered place or where an unregistered sonography machine is there because new *Rule 11 (2)* is now changed and you will be punished under *Section 23.* Never allow any company for demonstration of demo-machine at your clinic without prior written permission of authority.
2. *No to portable USG*: Portable sonography is banned so never do it at any place even on request *[Rule 3].*

   Do not do live demonstration of sonography machine at unregistered place (e.g. at conference in a hotel).

   Do not promote or be afraid to refuse any USG at polyclinic run by unknown, untruthful BHMS, DHMS or unauthorized people. Because in your absence, it is possible that he/she may perform USG for determination of sex by themselves or help of others at that clinic. If the machine is sealed, you are equally liable for the crime. Therefore, it is better to avoid being a visiting sonologist at such clinics.
3. *Take prior permission—USG at two places:* Do not perform USG at more than two places in one district without informing the authorities (time, hours and day).

   Kindly note that there is currently a stay order on this amendment by the High Court of certain states. But this stay only applies in that states (e.g. Delhi). Others states have to follow the new amendment *[Rule 3]. Do not appoint unqualified employees or person at your clinic.*
4. *Do not forget renewal date*: Do not forget date of your renewal of PNDT registration.
5. *Do not encourage* patient or person (agent) for sex determination by you or staff. So if any such enquiry does come, ensure that your OPD staff has strict instructions to not allow such entries into your consulting room.
6. *No change in Form-F:* Do not make any stylish changes in the original prescribed Form-F as per the provision of PNDT Act Section 4 B Rule 9 (4) Rule 10(1 A).

   Do not forget to fill and give one copy of Form-G to patient in case of invasive procedure performed by you.
7. *Do not change USG place without informing.* Do not make any changes in USG unit, place, or management without a written application in duplicate. Ensure that one copy is with you of the permission of authority in writing (prior intimation to appropriate authority before 30 days of expected change).
8. *No sale of USG to unregistered place*: Inform authority. Do not sell or scrapsonography machine to an unregistered place, agent. Do not purchase from an unauthorized agent or person or unregistered center. Inform the proper authority about your selling of machine in prescribed manner.
9. *No advertisement about sex selection:* Do not do sonography without written declaration of patient in Form-F with original signature. Do not publish any advertisement relating to preconceptional sex selection or prenatal sex determination violate *[Section 22].*
10. *Do not ignore government directions*; cooperate with them. Do not ignore any new direction or amendments by the government authority in PCPNDT Act.

    Do not misbehave or be aggressive toward the inspecting authority when they visit for routine inspection at your clinic.

    Do not tamper any records after a notice has been issued by the government authority against you in case of violation of PCPNDT Act.
11. *Do not send biopsy to unregistered place.* Do not send sample of biopsy fluid to an unregistered laboratory in case of invasive procedures (chorionic villous sampling, amniocentesis, etc.). The laboratory should also be registered under the PCPNDT Act

Do not forget to send written report of Form-F—*nil or zero* (even if you do not do single sonography in that particular month).

12. *USG shutdown notice:* Do not forget to inform the government authority in written acknowledgement (two copies with seal and sign of authority) that I will be unable to send monthly Form-F report as I am going on leave for 2–6 months. I will put my sonography machine in safe custody in my premises (locked in my room). Ensure you keep one copy with you.

    It will save you in case of notice issued against you by Authority for not sending report on Form-F.

13. *No staff should sign panchnama*: Never allow your hospital staff to sign in panchnama as a witness in case your sonography machine is being sealed.

    Never confess, admit or sign on panchnama that you have done a mistake but write, e.g. I reserve my Right to Defend my case (Because once you have confessed, it is difficult to prove your innocence in the court of law).

Application of Stem Cells in Infertility 79

Sunita Tandulwadkar, Sejal Naik

"There is such a sweetness in being able to participate in creation"

Pamela S Nadav

INTRODUCTION

The human body is composed of about 200 different types of specialized cells such as blood cells, muscle cells, glandular cells, nerve cells, adipose cells, skin cells, etc. In embryonic phase of life, the stem cells which are undifferentiated or "blank" cells will undergo process of specialization and form tissue or organ. This process of specialization is called differentiation. Additionally, they are self-sustaining and can duplicate for long periods of time. Once a stem cell differentiates, it no longer has the ability to become another type of cell. Unspecialized cells, capable of producing same type of unspecialized cells or into any specialized tissue type depending upon stimulation, sometimes become active after long period of inactivity.

The particular type of physiologic or experimental stimulations can activate and initiate the process of differentiation and stem cells can be coerced into becoming tissue or organ cells with special functional abilities **(Fig. 1)**.

RESEARCH ON STEM CELLS

All over the world, for centuries researches are going on in various fields. It is a known fact that certain species in animal kingdom like reptiles like lizard, earthworm, etc. can regenerate their certain body parts. Human share some of such abilities as our body is constantly regenerating skin, blood, tissues, etc. Cell, the building block of life, was discovered in the mid 1800s. It was also seen that they had the

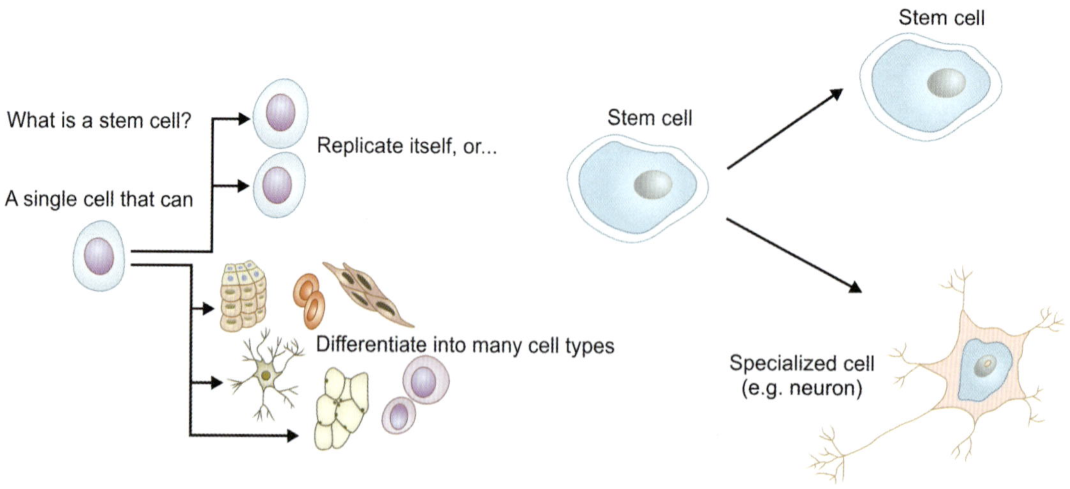

Fig. 1: Stem cells.

ability to produce other cells.[1] There were numerous efforts made to fertilize eggs in vitro. And in the 1900s, it was observed that cells had the capability to generate blood cells. In 1968, two siblings with severe immunodeficiency were treated successfully via bone marrow transplant for the first time.

Attempts were made to fertilize mammalian eggs outside of the human body and in the early 1900s, it was discovered that some cells had the ability to generate blood cells. In 1968, the first bone marrow transplant was performed to successfully to treat two siblings with severe combined immunodeficiency. Other milestones in stem cell research include:[1]

- *1978:* Stem cells were discovered in human cord blood.
- *1981:* First in vitro stem cell line developed from mice.
- *1988:* Embryonic stem cell lines created from a hamster.
- *1995:* First embryonic stem cell line derived from a primate.
- *1997:* Cloned lamb from stem cells.
- *1997:* Leukemia origin found as hematopoietic stem cell, indicating possible proof of cancer stem.[1]

WHY ARE STEM CELLS SPECIAL?

There are some new discoveries in human history which are recognized as milestones. Such milestone discoveries have achieved better diagnosis and treatment of the patients in this modern world of medicine. Stem cells represent one of such a land mark because they have the ability to repair as well as regenerate tissues which are damaged **(Fig. 2)**.

- *Self-renewal:* Stem cells can regenerate themselves almost indefinitely. This phenomenon is called proliferation.[1]
- *Differentiation:* Stem cells have the potential to differentiate into cells which have specific characteristics and functions.[1]

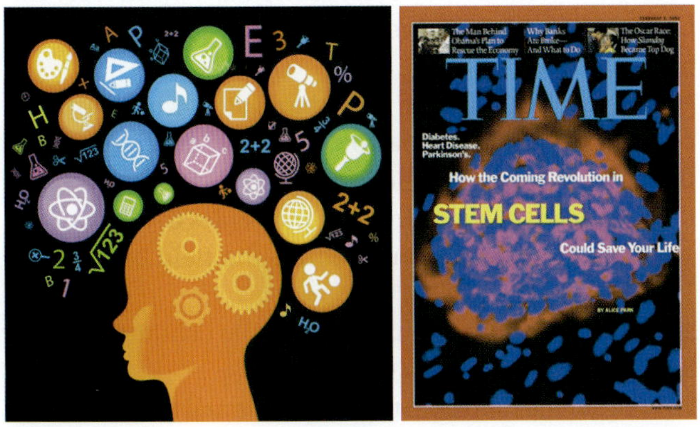

Fig. 2

- *Unspecialized:* Stem cells are unspecialized cells with the ability to become tissue specific.[1]

STEM CELL HARVEST AND INFUSION (OUR BM METHOD)

Stem cells can be isolated from several human organs like bone marrow, umbilical cord, adipose tissue, etc.[2] But, bone marrow is a rich source of stem cells. These stem cells are called autologous hematopoietic stem cells and they are considered to be adult stem cells.[3] These cells can be easily harvested from the bone marrow of hip bone of the patient undergoing the stem cell infusion.[3] With the latest non-touch, digital technology, stem cells can be isolated from the bone marrow of an individual within 30 min in the most sterile conditions. Since there is no hospitalization, no cut and no surgery, immediate mobilization is possible and it becomes patient friendly method of procedure.

ROLE OF STEM CELLS IN INFERTILITY

As can be seen, it is clear that infertility is complex outplay of factors mentioned in decreasing semen parameters and premature ovarian failure (POF) have become a global concern. Treatment options currently rely on the ability of both the male and female partners to develop haploid gametes. Donor gametes are the only option for couples where one or both partners is unable to produce functional gametes. Stem cells are coming up as a miraculous therapy in various conditions, including infertility.

AZOOSPERMIA

Close to 50% of infertile patients is due to the male factor, of which 70–90% is due to impaired spermatogenesis which is clinically seen as either oligo-, azoo- or teratospermia.[4-6] One percent of the male population is azoospermic[4,7] and it is seen in almost 20% of patients with male factor infertility.[4,8] Azoospermia is defined as the complete absence of any sperm in a man's semen.[9] It is found in 20% of men who seek infertility treatment. Normally, man's testicles produce sperms which join with seminal vesicle secretions to become semen.

Types of Azoospermia

- Obstructive (sperm is blocked from exiting the testicle).
- Nonobstructive (sperm is not produced at all).

The testis has both exocrine and endocrine functions. The exocrine function involves the continuous production of spermatozoa, which are released from the testis, transported through the excurrent ducts, and eventually ejaculated. The endocrine activity consists of the secretion of testosterone, which is necessary to maintain secondary sexual characteristics, accessory sex organs and spermatogenesis.

Pilot study of intra-testicular injection of autologous bone marrow mononuclear cells (BMMNCs) at our center on four men with non-obstructive azoospermia.

Inclusion criteria:

- Trial testicular sperm aspiration (TESA) failed to retrieve sperms.
- Genetically normal.

Autologous BMMNCs infused intra-testicular under short propofol. Results of this study will help in changing the perspective of fertility potential in azoospermia patients.

ERECTILE DYSFUNCTION

The inability to obtain or maintain an erection for satisfactory intercourse is known as erectile dysfunction (ED).[10] The cardiovascular disease and neurological problems, e.g. diabetes, trauma from prostatectomy surgery, etc. are common organic cause of impotence. Other causes include hormonal insufficiencies (hypogonadism) or side effects of drugs.

Various large-scale studies (both cross-sectional and longitudinal) estimated the overall prevalence rate of 10–20% worldwide[11] even though there is no uniform definition. There is a strong correlation between age and ED, with the prevalence increasing steadily from 6.5% in men aged 20–39 years to 77.5% in those aged more than or equal to 75 years.

As evaluated by Lin, in 35 published studies, mostly associated with cavernous nerve injury or diabetes. Adipose-derived stem cells used in 18 studies and bone marrow derived in 9. Intra-cavernous injection done. All studies reported improved erectile function, as well as improved muscle, nerve or endothelium in the erectile tissue.[12]

REFRACTORY ENDOMETRIUM

For successful conception, apart from healthy embryo, we need excellent endometrium so as to have healthy dialogue between embryo and endometrium. The cavity of the uterus is lined by the glandular layer known as endometrium. During a woman's reproductive years, there is constant remodeling of the human endometrium. It undergoes regeneration, differentiation and shedding for over 400 cycles. One of the most important factors for the implantation of the embryo and achievement of pregnancy is endometrial thickness.[13] Endometrium grows 0.5–1 mm per day under normal hormonal cycle in response to naturally produced estrogen by developing follicle, and reaches about 8 mm or more in thickness at the time of ovulation. Officially, there is no current cut-off value for thin endometrium, which can result in lower pregnancy rate. The commonly accepted cut-off is less than 7 mm on the day of luteinizing hormone (LH) surge or human chorionic gonadotropin (hCG) administration.[13,14] Incidence of thin endometrium in women undergoing ART is about 0.5%.[15]

Asherman's syndrome is an infrequent disorder which is seen in women. Endometritis and/or repeated or aggressive curettages may cause destruction in the endometrium and lead to this syndrome.[15] Due to this, there is loss of the basal layer of endometrium in many cases and the functionality of the endometrial later is lost. There may be complete obliteration of the uterine cavity dues to intra-uterine adhesions which may lead to amenorrhea, infertility, recurrent pregnancy loss, etc.[15] The small portion of healthy endometrium is left for implantation due to intra-uterine adhesions. Refractory endometrium too, offers very limited treatment options. In absence of normal uterine cavity and endometrial lining, very little scope remains to conceive and to maintain a pregnancy. The only therapeutic modality available for such women is surrogacy.

Endometrial regeneration may be possible with bone marrow stem cells.[16] On the basis of these facts, bone marrow stem cells can be used for regeneration of damaged endometrium.[16] Angiogenesis may occur via recruitment of endothelial cells from a neighboring blood vessels or by the release of endothelial progenitor cells which are released from the bone marrow.[16]

Autologous bone marrow-derived stem cells can be used treat women with severe Asherman's syndrome. This has led to endometrial regeneration as well as successful implantation.[4,6,17]

There is large volume of secretion of growth factors and cytokines by the bone marrow stem cells which result in a therapeutic outcome called "trophic activity."[18] It is known that stem cells secrete bioactive molecules that[18]:

1. Prevent apoptosis and reduce the field of injury or damage **(Fig. 3)**.
2. Inhibit scarring or fibrosis at the site of injury.
3. Promote angiogenesis.
4. Trigger the mitosis of tissue-specific and tissue-intrinsic progenitors.[8,10,18]

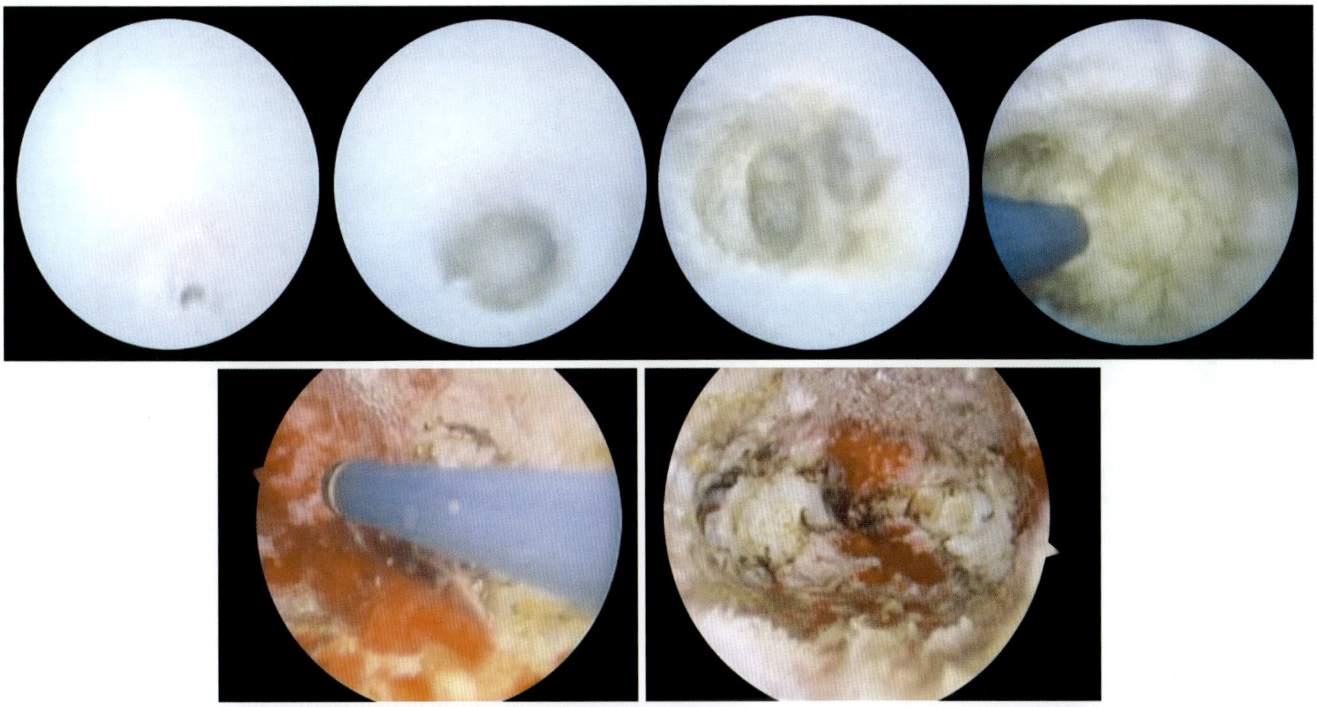

Fig. 3

PREMATURE OVARIAN FAILURE

The fixed amount of oocyte pool is available throughout the lifetime for reproduction. The number of available oocytes declines with advancing age from around 106 at puberty to 0 at menopause. Functional loss of the ovaries prior to the age of 40 is known as premature ovarian failure. It is associated with sex steroid deficiency, amenorrhea, infertility and elevated serum gonadotropins.[11] Majority of the cases underlying cause is not identified.[12] Ten percent of women undergoing IVF show diminished ovarian reserve, though the incidence is increasing by the day. Despite the various treatment options available, the pregnancy rate yet remains low with high pregnancy loss.[19]

Causes include:

1. Genetic aberration which could involve the X chromosome and autosomes.[19]
2. Autoimmune ovarian damage: Antiovarian antibodies are reported in POF by several studies.
3. Iatrogenic following surgical radiotherapeutic or chemotherapeutic interventions as in malignancies.[19]
4. Environmental factors like viral infection and toxins for which no clear mechanism is known.

M. Edessy had injected bone marrow-derived mesenchymal stem cells into the ovaries, via laparoscopically in 10 patients.[20] Endometrial fractional biopsy was histopathologically (HP) and immunohistochemically (IH) stained and evaluated according to Edessy stem cells score (ESS). After transplantation, two cases (20%) (ESS = 5 and 6) resumed menstruation after 3 months, one of them (10%) (Case no. 5) (ESS = 6) got pregnant after 11 months and delivered a healthy full-term baby. The two menstruating cases showed focal secretory changes after being atrophic endometrium in Case 5 and distorted proliferative endometrium in Case 10.[20]

Several researchers in Eunice Kennedy Shriver National Institute of Child Health and Human Development US (January 2017) and Hospital University La Fe (September 2014) have confirmed the presence of ovarian stem cells, as well as bone marrow-derived stem cells that have been able to colonize the ovaries and have folliculogenesis. The first baby of autologous stem cell therapy in POF is a reality and hope. The first stem cell baby "Zein Rajani," is a mature living female, 38 weeks, 3.3 kg.

We, at Ruby Hall IVF Endoscopy Center, have done six cases till now with encouraging results. One of 45 years lady whose anti-Mullerian hormone (AMH) was 0.5, shown improvement with 0.95 in 8 weeks. We could retrieve three eggs and one excellent day 3 frozen embryo transfer gave successful pregnancy, 16 weeks of gestation now (NIPT showing normal karyotyping) **(Fig. 4)**.

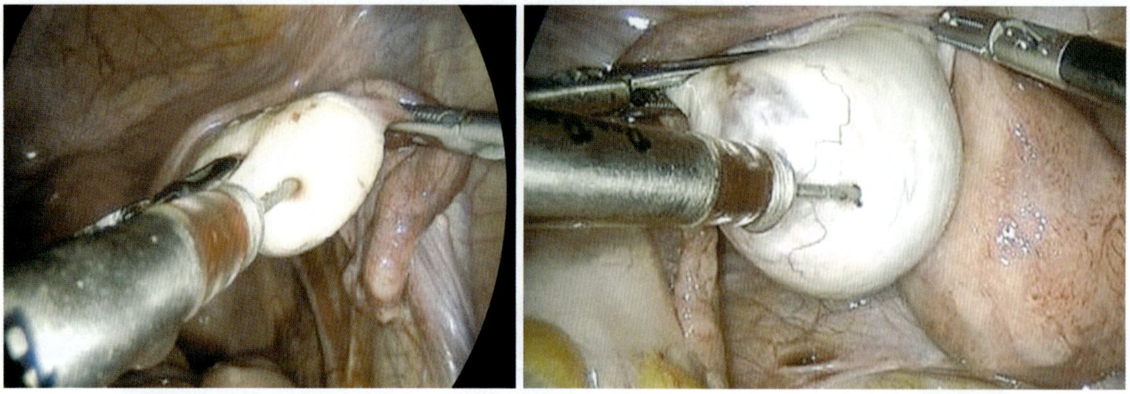

Fig. 4: Instillation of BMMSC in both ovaries.

ETHICAL CONCERNS

Indian Council of Medical Research (ICMR) has approved following guidelines:

- National Guidelines for Stem Cell Research revised by ICMR in November 2017.
- Stem cell use in infertility in India is for investigational purposes at present.
- Approval for clinical trials to be sought from Institutional Ethics Committee (IEC) and National Apex Committee for Stem Cell Research and Therapy (NAC-SCRT).

REFERENCES

1. Source: https://biotechquarter2projectmartens.weebly.com/history.html; http://www.explorestemcells.co.uk/historystemcellresearch.html.
2. Source: https://www.springer.com/in/book/9781617799396.
3. Dabas A, Dabas N, Prabhakar M, et al. A journey from stem cell to a bio-tooth. Ind J Dent Sci. 2013;5(Issue 3):84-7.
4. Greenberg SH, Lipshultz LI, Wein AJ. Experience with 425 subfertile male patients. J Urol. 1978;119:507-10.
5. Ogawa T, Dobrinski I, Avarbock MR, et al. Transplantation of male germ line stem cells restores fertility in infertile mice. Nat Med. 2000;6(1):29-34.
6. Sigman M, Lipshulz LI, Howard SS. In: Lipshulz LI, Howard, SS (Eds). Infertility in the Male, 3rd edition. St. Louis: Mosby; 1997. pp. 173-93.
7. Male Infertility Best Practice Policy Committee of the American Urological Association. Practice Committee of the American Society for Reproductive Medicine (2001). Infertility: Report on Evaluation of the Azoospermic Male (PDF). American Urological Association; American Society for Reproductive Medicine. ISBN 978-0-9649702-8-1.
8. Jarvi K, Lo K, Fischer A, et al. CUA Guideline: The workup of azoospermic males. Can Urol Assoc J. 2010;4(3):163-7. PMC: 2874589 Freely accessible. PMID: 20514278. DOI:10.5489/cuaj.10050.
9. Rönnberg L. The effect of clomiphene citrate on different sperm parameters and serum hormone levels in preselected infertile men: a controlled double-blind cross-over study. Int J Androl. 1980;3(1-6):479-86.
10. NIH Consensus Conference Impotence. NIH consensus development panel on impotence. JAMA. 1993;270: 83-90.
11. Albersen M, Shindel AW, Mwamukonda KB, et al. Emerging drugs for the treatment of erectile dysfunction. Expert Opin Emerg Drugs. 2010;15:467-80.
12. Lin CS. Advances in stem cell therapy for erectile dysfunction. Adv Androl. 2014;2014:20. Article ID: 140618.
13. Zhao J, Zhang Q, Wang Y, et al. Uterine infusion with bone marrow mesenchymal stem cells improves endometrium thickness in a rat model of thin endometrium. Reprod Sci. 2015;22(2):181-8. DOI: 10.1177/1933719114537715
14. Friendler S, Schenker JG, Herman A, et al. The role of ultrasonography in the evaluation of endometrial receptivity following assisted reproductive treatments: a critical review. Hum Reprod Update. 1996;2:323-35.
15. Santamaria X, Cabanillas S, Cervelló I, et al. Autologous cell therapy with CD133+ bone marrow-derived stem cells for refractory Asherman's syndrome and endometrial atrophy: a pilot cohort study. Hum Reprod. 2016;31(Issue 5):1087-96. https://doi.org/10.1093/humrep/dew042.
16. Nagori CB, Panchal SY, Patel H. Endometrial regeneration using autologous adult stem cells followed by conception by in vitro fertilization in a patient of severe Asherman's syndrome. J Hum Reprod Sci. 2011;4(1):43-8.
17. Zhao Y, Wang AM, Tang X, et al. Intrauterine transplantation of autologous bone marrow derived mesenchymal stem cells followed by conception in a patient of severe intrauterine adhesions. Open J Obstetr Gynecol. 2013;03(03):377-80. Article ID: 31293. DOI:10.4236/ojog.2013.33069.
18. Caplan AI. Why are MSCs therapeutic? New data: new insight. J Pathol. 2009;217(2):318-24. DOI:10.1002/path.2469.
19. He X. Microscale biomaterials with bioinspired complexity of early embryo development and in the ovary for tissue engineering and regenerative. ACS Biomater Sci Eng. 2017;3(11):2692-2701. DOI:10.1021/acsbiomaterials.6b00540.
20. Edessy M, Hosni HN, Shady Y, et al. Autologous stem cells therapy, the first baby of idiopathic premature ovarian failure. Acta Med Int. 2016;3(1):19-23.

CatSper Channel

80

Indira Hinduja, Amruta DS Pathare, Kusum Zaveri

INTRODUCTION

Interaction of male sperm and female oocyte is prerequisite to achieve successful mammalian fertilization. It is of paramount importance for spermatozoa to reach the ampulla region of the oviduct where the mature oocyte needs to be fertilized after the ovulation.[1] To accomplish this, the spermatozoa undergoes several processes like priming for fertilization by the mechanism of capacitation, hypermotility of sperm, chemotaxis toward the oocyte followed by acrosomal reaction penetrating the zona pellucida of the oocyte.[2] It has been reported that these physiological processes of sperms have been observed to be associated with calcium ion [Ca^{2+}] concentration changes within the sperm. Although there has been evidence of several voltage-gated Ca^{2+} channels present in testis and even in other organ like brain and heart, cation channel of sperm (CatSper) is the only Ca^{2+} selective channel solely expressed in spermatozoa. It is weakly voltage-dependent, Ca^{2+} permeable, pH sensitive ion channel located in the flagellar membrane of principal piece of the sperm in mice and humans as shown in **Figure 1**.[3]

According to the evidence provided by whole-cell patch-clamp technique, CatSper channel provides the entry of Ca^{2+} ions into the sperm cells activated by intracellular alkaline pH. Influx of Ca^{2+} plays very important role inducing sperm motility and fertility. Also it was observed that, the CatSper channel enables the entry of monovalent cations such as Na and Cs as well as divalent cations like Ba^{2+} in sperm cells in the absence of extracellular Ca^{2+}.[2,4] However, CatSper channel has greatest affinity toward Ca^{2+}.[2,4]

The presence of CatSper channel is directly related to male fertility as reports have been published indicating the inactive CatSper protein in male mice affects the sperm motility, swimming and hyperactivation leading to infertility.[3-5]

THE CATSPER CHANNEL COMPLEX

The CatSper channel is a hereotetrameric comprises of four subunits CatSper 1–4 which are pore-forming α (alpha) subunit and additional three auxiliary subunits, viz. CatSper β (beta), CatSper γ (gamma) and CatSper δ (delta). They are involved in whipping of flagella. The complex is encoded by seven gene.[2,4]

This first pore-forming subunit is exclusively found in spermatozoa and was discovered in 2001 while searching for sequence homology with volatage-gated Ca^{2+} selective channels **(Fig. 1)**. It has shown to have highest homology with Ca^{2+} selective channel with a common signature sequence Thr/Ser-x-Glu/Asp-x-Trp.[1] It has found to play a significant role in sperm motility. The higher expression of CatSper 1 has been observed in "swim-up" selected sperms suggesting their vital role in sperm-swimming. As reported by Carlson and colleagues, CatSper 1 is requisite for evoked Ca^{2+} entry to control sperm hyperactivity and flagellar movement, as no increase in intracellular Ca^{2+} is seen in CatSper-null sperms lacking hyper activation necessary for fertilization.[4,6] It has been reported that, the expression of CatSper 2 is required for the functioning of CatSper 1 and vice versa. As per the previous studies, CatSper 2-lacking mice did not show the expression of CatSper 1 and even no expression of CatSper 2 was found in CatSper 1-lacking mice. However, results indicated that CatSper 1-null mice could express CatSper 3 and CatSper 4 proteins, suggesting that the stable expression of CatSper 3 and 4 is not dependent on the expression of CatSper 1 and 2.[6,7] Moreover, all the subunits of CatSper 1–4 have crucial role in sperm motility, as it was shown that phenotypically CatSper $1^{-/-}$, CatSper $2^{-/-}$, CatSper $3^{-/-}$ and CatSper $4^{-/-}$ mice were found to be similar, lacking the function of sperm hyperactivity due to absence of CatSper current.[8]

Low-sequence homology of four CatSper subunits have been observed in transmembrane region ranging from 16% to 22%.[3,4] Additionally, CatSper channel family shared relatively lower sequence homology among different species. However, Human CatSper is reported to have sequence identity as high as 55%, showing 81% homology in the transmembrane domain whereas 89% in the pore regions.[3]

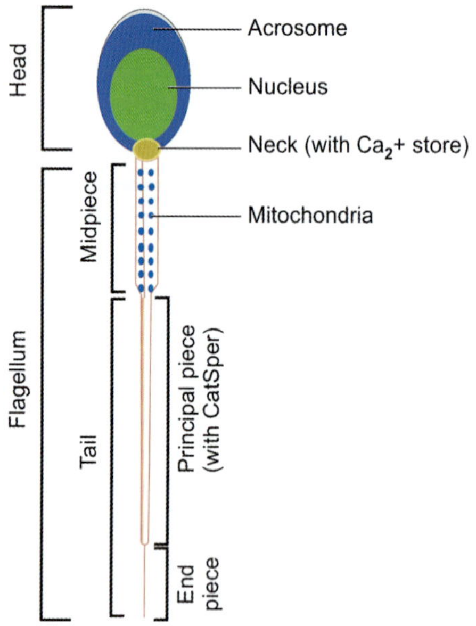

Fig. 1: Localization of CatSper channel.
Source: Reprod Biomed Online. 2015;30(1):28-38.

Each CatSper α subunits of the four separate CatSper subunit 1–4, comprises of six transmembrane segments (S1–S6) forming two distinct functionally active sites, viz. voltage sensor domain (VSD: S1–S4) and the pore-forming domain (S1-P loop-S6). S1–S4 are linked by short cyclic structure, having several positively charged amino acid residues in S4 which functions as a voltage sensor whereas S5–S6 are connected by short hydrophobic cyclic structure having conserved homologues sequence ([T]×[D]×[W]), which is accountable for entry of Ca^{2+} selectively through cell membrane.[1,3] CatSper 1 composed of six positively charged amino acid (lysine/arginine) residues; however, CatSper 2 contains four whereas and CatSper 3 and CatSper 4 possesses only two such residues. The first described auxiliary subunit of CatSper, i.e. CatSper β, comprises of two transmembrane spanning domains. It is relatively less conserved between human and mice and reported to be expressed mainly in testis and sperm tail **(Figs. 2A and B)**. CatSper γ and CatSper δ were reported to encode a subunit having single transmembrane segment.[1,9,10]

EXPRESSION OF CATSPER CHANNEL

Based on multi-tissue Northern blot analysis and gene expression profiling, CatSper 1–CatSper 4 have been reported to be expressed predominantly in mouse and human testis. Also, CatSper subunits have been shown to be transcribed differentially during spermatogenesis. CatSper 1, CatSper 3 and CatSper 4 transcribes at late stage germ line cells, i.e. spermatids whereas CatSper 2 has been reported to be restricted to pachytene spermatocytes in early stages of spermatogenesis. Expression of CatSper β, CatSper γ and CatSper δ are found in spermatids and spermatocytes of testis and localized in principal piece of spermatozoa.[3,11-13]

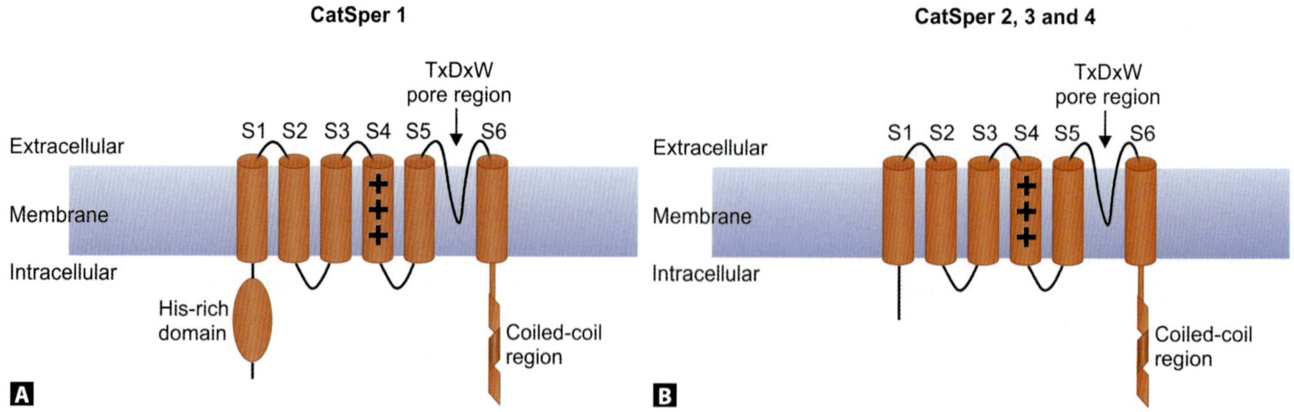

Figs. 2A and B: (A) Structure of CatSper 1. (B) Structure of CatSper 2, 3 and 4.
Source: Reprod Biol Endocrinol. 2003;1:53-67.

pH REGULATION AND CATSPER ION CHANNEL

The pH of sperms is on acidic side around 6.0 or lower when they are stored in epididymis before ejaculation making them quiescent. Higher extracellular pH after ejaculation of sperms enable them to become motile for the first time.[4,5] In female reproductive tract, sperm pH increases by the process of capacitation. To achieve required motility for successful fertilization, the reduction of intracellular $[H^+]$ i and elevation of $[Ca^{2+}]$i is necessary. As per the reported study, Ca^{2+} increase is observed in mice sperm cell in an artificially alkalinized intracellular environment. Though the effect of alkalinization on CatSper channel in sperm is not clearly understood, it is a pH-sensitive ion channel. The CatSper channel is reported to bring about influx of Ca^{2+} into spermatozoa and controls the Ca^{2+} homeostasis. Moreover, Na, K-ATPase (NKA) and Na^+/Ca^{2+} exchanger (NCX) also have effect in milieu of the ion channels in human sperm.[3,14]

FUNCTIONS OF CATSPERS

Out of millions of sperms entering the female reproductive tract, very few sperms arrive at the site of fertilization overcoming obstructions such as immune responses of female, viscous cervical mucus, sticky oviductal epithelium covered with mucus, and epithelial folds and only one will penetrate through the oocyte's cumulus oophorus (CO) and zona pellucida to fertilize the egg. To accomplish this process, the spermatozoa undergoes physiological changes as follows: i) capacitation; ii) after becoming motile for the first time sperm required to achieve hyperactivated motility at the site of fertilization; iii) to use chemotaxis to reach the oocyte; iv) to undergo acrosomal reaction to penetrate the zona pellucida of oocyte.[3-5,10] The influence of CatSper channel in all these process is discussed as below:

Sperm Hyperactivation

Spermatozoa initiate their motility for the first time after ejaculation and mixing with seminal plasma. The increase in sperm intracellular pH and cAMP in extracellular microenvironment is directly correlated with the sperm motility.[5] It is typically characterized by relatively low-amplitude, symmetrical tail bending. However, as sperm reservoir in female reproductive tract migrate to oviduct, it is essential for spermatozoa to achieve hyperactivated motility. This is characterized by large amplitude, whip-like asymmetrical tail beating that effects in higher swimming force than the normal motility. Hyperactivated spermatozoa can swim through the sticky oviductal epithelium covered with mucus and is able to penetrate the protective vestments of the egg, the CO and zona pellucida.[5,15] It is very crucial to have elevated intracellular pH and Ca^{2+} in order to achieve hyperactivation which takes place as a result of process called capacitation. Disruption or mutation in CatSper 1 gene is reported to be markedly reduced sperm motility.[6,13] It has been studied that CatSper null mice sperm showed normal motility but significantly lacked hyperactivated motility with small amplitude, symmetrical and lower curvature of flagella than wild type mice even in the capacitating medium suggesting physiologically defective sperms.[3,6,13,15]

The process of hyperactivity takes place in capacitated sperms. Capacitation is functional maturation of sperm cells in female reproductive tract. Capacitated spermatozoa are able to acquire hyperactive motility, undergo chemotaxis and acrosome reaction.[5] Extracellular Ca^{2+}, bicarbonate and albumin in the oviductal fluid is necessary to increase basal level of $[Ca^{2+}]$i in sperms. These elevated levels of Ca^{2+} and pH are observed to be adequate for sperms to attain the hyperactivation. The further rise in these levels needed for subsequent chemotaxis and acrosome reaction.[5]

Chemotaxis toward Oocyte

The CatSper channel is observed to be activated by the low-nanomolar concentrations of progesterone released by cumulous cell surround the egg, CatSper-mediated Ca^{2+} influx can induce asymmetrical tail beating, enabling the sperm to be moved toward the egg. Thus, the CatSper channel plays important role in hyperactivation and chemotaxis of the sperm.[5,15]

Acrosome Reaction

After locating the oocyte, sperm cells required to penetrate the protective vestment oocyte, i.e the CO, the dense layer of zona pellucida formed by the glycoproteins ZP1, ZP2, ZP3 and ZP4 (secreted by oocyte) formed under the CO.[16] Hyperactivated sperm when penetrated the CO, high concentration of progesterone secreted by cumulus cell stimulated the sperm motility allowing them to reach highest degree of hyperactivation. However, to penetrate the very dense matrix of zona pellucida, after the binding of the sperm head receptor, betal, 4 galactosyltransferase (GalT-1) with glycoproteins of zona pellucida, hydrolytic enzyme is released from the acrosome vesicles located in the sperm head to digest the layer of zona pellucida. This process is called as acrosome reaction.[5] This is reported to be triggered by CatSper channel. It was studied that the contact between sperm head and glycoprotein of ZP, stimulates the extracellular Ca^{2+}-dependent increase in $[Ca^{2+}]i$ in sperm. Experiments using gel purified zona pellucidas reported that, in humans, ZP1 and ZP4 proteins plays role as Ca^{2+} influx inducing protein by elevating the levels of sperm $[Ca^{2+}]i$ and [pH]i.[4] Moreover, Ca^{2+} channel receptor, i.e. transient receptor potential (Trp) protein were found to be activated by ZP3 in mouse, which further stimulates G proteins and phospholipase C to regulate entrance of Ca^{2+}.[1] Furthermore, the progesterone non-genomic receptor in human spermatozoa also reacts with progesterone to stimulate the Ca^{2+} entry in sperm promoting the acrosome reaction.[4]

Though the exact mechanism of involvement of CatSper channel with acrosome reaction remains elusive, the previously performed in vitro fertilization (IVF) assays wherein incubation of superovulated wild type female mature egg with capacitated wild type as well as mutant sperm for 24 h revealed that $CatSper^{-/-}$ sperm could successfully adhere the oocyte but were highly incompetent to penetrate the egg whereas wild type sperm showed 81% fertilization.[1,3,17] This was further confirmed, when the CatSper wild type and mutant sperm was incubated with egg whose zona pellucida was enzymatically removed, found to be penetrate the and fertilized the egg by both wild type as well as mutant sperm.[1,3,17] It suggests that CatSper channel may not be important for egg activation and sperm-egg fusion but it certainly enables the sperm to penetrate the ZP.[3]

CATSPER CHANNEL AND MALE INFERTILITY

Based on the literature reviewed, it is understood that, CatSper plays important role in influx of Ca^{2+} in sperm which is a requisite for sperm hyperactivation, their progressive movement and acrosome reaction. It has been shown that disruption of four alpha subunits of CatSper results in disturbance is CatSper channel resulting in male infertility.[3,8] Mutations in CatSper 1 and CatSper 2 in infertile males have been reported to be associated with asthenozoospermia.[3,18] As reported in the study by Tamburrino and colleagues, CatSper 1 suppressive group showed lower number of sperms with progressive motility and progesterone induced acrosome reaction than the normal sperm. They showed lower CatSper 1 gene expression in patients with asthenozoospermia.[19] As per the report by Avenarius and colleagues, two separate insertion mutations (c.539–540insT and c.948–949insATGGC) in CatSper 1 gene were resulted in male infertility in two consanguineous Iranian families by the autosomal recessive trait.[18] In addition to this, as per the study in mice, inactive CatSper 2 gene leads to immotile sperms and failure in hyperactivity resulting in infertility. In human sperms, homozygous CatSper 2 deletion showed the characteristic severe asthenoteratozoospermia with abnormal motility patterns with very few normal motile sperms.[20] As per the study by Bhilawadikar and colleagues, the lower expression level of CatSper 2 protein was reported in oligoasthenozoospermic than normozoospermic men. Also the CatSper 2 expression was positively correlated with sperm motility.[21] Therefore, CatSper 1 and 2 are observed to be required for normal male fertility, hyperactivated motility of sperms being highly specific flagellar proteins. The studies with knock-out mouse models revealed that there was no significant difference in phenotypic characteristics like weight of body and testis, sperm counts in $CatSper^{-/-}$ mice, but were observed to be impaired in motility. This suggests that CatSper channel has no effect on spermatogenesis but it damages the sperm motility.[3] According to the study by Shu and colleagues, the single nucleotide polymorphism at exonal rs1893316 in CATSPER1 gene was associated with the risk of idiopathic asthenospermia.[22]

Based on the study by Jin and colleagues, CatSper 1 and 2 were localized in sperm flagellum whereas CatSper 3 and 4 were observed to be localized in acrosome of sperm, suggesting the different role than CatSper 1/CatSper 2. The authors have proposed that CatSper 3/CatSper 4 forming heterodimer play a role in acrosome reaction and male fertility as a single channel.[12] However, infertile patients having mutations in CatSper 3 and CatSper 4 were not reported to be associated with male infertility.[3] Moreover, CatSper β and CatSper δ were not reported to be associated with male infertility[4,13] whereas, as per the report by Chung and colleagues in 2010, CatSper δ null mice sperms lack Ca^{2+} current and hyperactivated motility resulted in infertility.[11] In the study by Carkci et al., 150 infertile males evaluated for CatSper channel were divided in four groups such as asthenozoospermia (A), oligozoospermia (B), oligoasthenoteratozoospermia (C), teratozoospermia (D), and their CatSper channel expressions were compared with control group of normozoospermia. The study finding revealed the increased expression of CatSper 1 in B and C groups whereas CatSper 2 showed no significant in these groups.

CatSper 3 was reported to have decreased expression in A, C and D groups. CatSper 4 showed decreased gene expression in A, D whereas increase in B and C. All the CatSper channels were positively correlated with sperm hyperactive motility and sperm morphology.[1]

CATSPER CHANNEL AND ASSISTED REPRODUCTIVE TECHNIQUES

Worldwide, infertility is observed in around 15% of couples. As per the epidemiological study performed in 2015, male factor infertility ranges from 20% to 70% having percentage of infertile men around 2.5–12%.[23] In Asia, male factor infertility is reported to be 37%.[23] Male factor infertility generally characterized by oligo-, astheno-, teratozoospermia, and combination of the three, or even a complete absence of sperm cells.[24] All these types of male infertility lead to poor prognosis even when assisted reproductive techniques are considered. However, with the advent of and advances of intra-cytoplasmic sperm injection (ICSI) technique, the infertility due to male factor has observed to be considerably reduced. The ICSI technique is implemented wherein direct injection of spermatozoa with poor progressive motility and even sperms retrieved microsurgically from epididymis and testis of azospermic men can be employed. According to International Committee for Monitoring Assisted Reproductive Technologies (ICMART), reported that of all the ART cycles, 63.0% used ICSI,[25] of which 58.4% prevalence was from Asia. In spite of advancement in ART, the clinical pregnancy rate remains as low as 30% worldwide.[24] To achieve successful ART, it is crucial to have good quality gametes to develop a good quality embryo. Assessment of male games yet depends up on the semen analysis. However, it is poorly predictive of the success of fertilization and eventually IVF/ICSI cycle. Therefore, there is need for the treatment or therapy or predictive markers to

Table 1: Ca^{2+} channel blocker and activator and their role.

Compound	***Action on Ca^{2+} channel***	***Role***
HC-056456	Blocker	▪ Selectively targets Catsper channel. ▪ Lower Catsper current observed in HC-056456 treated sperm vs. untreated sperm. ▪ Prevents development of hyperactivated motility of capacitated sperms.
Nifedipine and Nimodipine	L-type blockers	▪ Both induce male infertility. ▪ Nifedipine prevents Ca^{2+} entry into sperms which causes alterations in the cholestenone content in sperm membranes leading to membrane disruption.
NNC55–0396 and mibefradil	T-type blockers	▪ Odorants and suppress Ca^{2+} signals under physiological conditions. ▪ Decrease the number of sperm having progressive motility. ▪ No effect on hyperactive motility of sperm.
Quinidine	Blocker	▪ Reversibly blocks the Ca^{2+} channel.
Clofilium	Blocker	▪ Blocks the Ca^{2+} currents irreversibly.
Ketamine	Blocker	▪ Effect on human sperm functions. ▪ Inhibits sperm total motility and progressive motility via decreased sperm Ca^{2+} influx.
Matrine	Blocker	▪ Inhibits sperm total motility, capacitation linear velocity and the progesterone-induced acrosome reaction. ▪ Can be used as a potent contraceptive.
Emodin	Blocker	▪ Inhibits human sperm function. ▪ Decrease in the sperm $[Ca^{2+}]i$ and tyrosine phosphorylation.
Trigonellae semen (TS) and Panax ginseng	Stimulator	▪ Stimulates hyperactivity of sperm by regulating the expression of the Catsper gene. ▪ Could be used as a treatment for oligoasthenospermia.
Cyclamen and Helional	Stimulator	▪ Extracted from plants and bacteria. ▪ Stimulates Ca^{2+} signals. ▪ Can be treated for Catsper-related male infertility.

achieve clinical pregnancy in male infertility with CatSper channel.

As per the recent study by Marchiani and colleagues, the authors have designed a predictive model for the success of ART cycle. In the study, high levels of CatSper 1 gene expression was positively correlated with good quality embryos and the clinical pregnancy rate having cut off of greater than 6.74 median fluorescence intensity (MFI), odds ratio of 14.3 in the females having age less than 35 years. High CatSper gene expression was proposed to be associated with capacitation, hyperactive motility and acrosome reaction to achieve successful fertilization and good quality embryos.[24]

To improve or modify the sperm motility in infertile male by drug discovery could be the most effective treatment option to improve the clinical pregnancy rate. As per the recent study in 2017, development of high-throughput screening (HTS) using intracellular calcium ($[Ca^{2+}]i$) as a surrogate for motility was validated for five compounds by different techniques as computer-assisted sperm assessment (CASA), electrophysiology, liquid chromatography-mass spectrometry showing direct effect on sperm motility and ability of egg penetration. The authors have developed new therapeutic viable approach which could increase $[Ca^{2+}]i$ in human spermatozoa and functionally modify the sperm motility.[26]

CATSPER CHANNEL: PHARMACOLOGICAL APPROACH

Pharmacological targeting of the CatSper channel is based on its agonist or inhibitor compounds. The agonist can be implemented as infertility treatment whereas inhibitors or blockers of CatSper channel serves as efficient compounds to be used as contraceptives as summarized in **Table 1**.[4]

All these compounds are under clinical trials and further research is required to implement them as a targeted therapy for male infertility or as a male contraceptive. As mentioned earlier, HTS has been recently published to be viable treatment option for male infertility.

To summarize, the CatSper channel observed to play important role in male fertility. However, there are limited studies available on mutation and gene expression of CatSper in human subjects. There is a need to detect the most effective mutations in CatSper channel globally and even in Indian population. With the advent of genomic tools like gene editing, in future the defects in CatSper gene can be modified to attain fertility in patients with impaired CatSper channel.

REFERENCES

1. Ren D, Navarro B, Perez G, et al. A sperm ion channel required for sperm motility and male fertility. Nature. 2001;413(6856):603-9.
2. Kirichok Y, Navarro B, Clapham DE. Whole-cell patch-clamp measurements of spermatozoa reveal an alkaline-activated Ca^{2+} channel. Nature. 2006;439(7077):737-40.
3. Singh AP, Rajender S. CatSper channel, sperm function and male fertility. Reprod Biomed Online. 2015;30(1):28-38.
4. Hong SX, Ying ZY, Wang L, et al. The CatSper channel and its roles in male fertility: a systematic review. Reprod Biol Endocrinol. 2017;15(1):1-12.
5. Kirichok Y, Lishko PV. Rediscovering sperm ion channels with the patch-clamp technique. Mol Hum Reprod. 2011;17(8):478-99.
6. Carlson AE, Westenbroek RE, Quill T, et al. CatSper1 required for evoked Ca^{2+} entry and control of flagellar function in sperm. Proc Natl Acad Sci . 2003;100(25):14864-8.
7. Babcock DF. Wrath of the wraiths of CatSper3 and CatSper4. Proc Natl Acad Sci. 2007;104(4):1107-8.
8. Qi H, Moran MM, Navarro B, et al. All four CatSper ion channel proteins are required for male fertility and sperm cell hyperactivated motility. Proc Natl Acad Sci. 2007;104(4):1219-23.
9. Lobley A, Pierron V, Reynolds L, et al. Identification of human and mouse CatSper3 and CatSper4 genes: characterization of a common interaction domain and evidence for expression in testis. Reprod Biol Endocrinol. 2003;1:53-67.
10. Lishko PV, Mannowetz N. CatSper: a unique calcium channel of the sperm flagellum. Curr Opin Physiol. 2018;2:109-13.
11. Chung JJ, Navarro B, Krapivinsky G, et al. A novel gene required for male fertility and functional CATSPER channel formation in spermatozoa. Nat Commun. 2011;2(1):1-25.
12. Jin J-L, O'Doherty AM, Wang S, et al. CatSper3 and CatSper4 encode two cation channel-like proteins exclusively expressed in the testis. Biol Reprod. 2005;73(6):1235-42.
13. Ren D, Xia J. Calcium signaling through CatSper channels in mammalian fertilization. Physiology. 2010;25(3):165-75.
14. Nishigaki T. Intracellular pH in sperm physiology. 2015;450(3):1149-58.
15. Suarez SS, Pacey AA. Sperm transport in the female reproductive tract. Hum Reprod Update. 2006;12(1):23-37.
16. Gupta SK, Bansal P, Ganguly A, et al. Human zona pellucida glycoproteins: functional relevance during fertilization. J Reprod Immunol. 2009;83(1-2):50-5.
17. Quill TA, Sugden SA, Rossi KL, et al. Hyperactivated sperm motility driven by CatSper2 is required for fertilization. Proc Natl Acad Sci. 2003;100(25):14869-74.
18. Avenarius MR, Hildebrand MS, Zhang Y, et al. Human male infertility caused by mutations in the CATSPER1 channel protein. Am J Hum Genet. 2009;84(4):505-10.
19. Tamburrino L, Marchiani S, Minetti F, et al. The CatSper calcium channel in human sperm: relation with motility and

involvement in progesterone-induced acrosome reaction. Hum Reprod. 2014;29(3):418-28.
20. Smith JF, Syritsyna O, Fellous M, et al. Disruption of the principal, progesterone-activated sperm Ca^{2+} channel in a CatSper2-deficient infertile patient. Proc Natl Acad Sci. 2013;110(17):6823-8.
21. Bhilawadikar R, Zaveri K, Mukadam L, et al. Levels of Tektin 2 and CatSper 2 in normozoospermic and oligoasthenozoospermic men and its association with motility, fertilization rate, embryo quality and pregnancy rate. J Assist Reprod Genet. 2013;30(4):513-23.
22. Shu F, Zhou X, Li F, et al. Analysis of the correlation of CATSPER single nucleotide polymorphisms (SNPs) with idiopathic asthenospermia. J Assist Reprod Genet. 2015;32(11):1643-9.
23. Agarwal A, Mulgund A, Hamada A, et al. A unique view on male infertility around the globe. Reprod Biol Endocrinol. 2015;13(1):1-9.
24. Marchiani S, Tamburrino L, Benini F, et al. Chromatin protamination and CatSper expression in spermatozoa predict clinical outcomes after assisted reproduction programs. Sci Rep. 2017;7(1):1-12.
25. Sullivan EA, Zegers-Hochschild F, Mansour R, et al. International Committee for Monitoring Assisted Reproductive Technologies (ICMART) world report: assisted reproductive technology 2004. Hum Reprod. 2013;28(5):1375-90.
26. Martins Da Silva SJ, Brown SG, Sutton K, et al. Drug discovery for male subfertility using high-throughput screening: a new approach to an unsolved problem. Hum Reprod. 2017;32(5):974-84.

81 What is new in Assisted Reproductive Technology?

Dibojyoti, Reeta Mahey, Hrishikesh D Pai, Arnav Pai

INTRODUCTION

Since the birth of Louise Brown in 1978, assisted reproductive technology (ART) has gone way beyond in terms of indications, success rate, and widely available options for couples with different causes of subfertility, recurrent implantation failures, and some genetic disorders.

Latest research in the field of ART is for the couples with genetic disorders. Patients harboring pathogenic mutations causing progressive and lethal diseases with no available cure are often required to make difficult reproductive choices. The available ART options for these couples are gamete/embryo donation, selecting normal embryos or conceptus by genetic testing, or adoption. Latest technologies for these couples, which are being investigated for their clinical application, are mitochondrial replacement therapy (MRT) and gene editing.

MITOCHONDRIAL REPLACEMENT THERAPY

This technique of MRT involves complete replacement of cytoplasm of egg/embryo, thus eliminating the transmission of undesired defective mitochondria in patients with inherited mitochondrial diseases. Mutations can be found both in the nuclear DNA (nDNA) and in mitochondrial DNA (mtDNA) and if pathogenic mutations exist in germline (sperm or oocyte), they would be inherited by the offspring and even passed on to future generations.[1]

Nuclear transfer techniques or MRT are considered to be a potential germline gene therapy for inherited mitochondrial diseases. The same may be used in ART in women with advanced age where clinicians and researchers are considering MRT as technique to solve cytoplasmic defects due to maternal aging.

Mitochondrial Diseases

Mitochondrial disorders affect at least one in 8,000 individuals.[2] While disorders resulting from nDNA mutations follow a Mendelian pattern of autosomal recessive, autosomal dominant, or X-linked inheritance, the inheritance patterns of conditions arising from mtDNA defects are different as follows:

- Affected individuals are usually heteroplasmic, i.e. there is a mixture of normal and mutant mtDNA, the levels of which can differ among tissues. If the mutant load (ratio of mutant to normal mtDNA) exceeds a tissue and individual-specific threshold (60–75%), clinical features become evident.
- Unlike the nuclear genome, mtDNA is transmitted maternally. This is due to significantly higher number of mtDNA molecules in a mature oocyte (200,000–300,000 copies) compared to the sperm (approximately 100 mtDNA copies).[3] In addition, sperm mitochondria that enter via fertilization are eliminated specifically during early embryo development.

At present, there are no widely approved fundamental cures for mitochondrial diseases (Alzheimer's, Parkinson's, and Huntington's diseases, obesity, diabetes, and cancer, etc.) and treatments currently available only alleviate symptoms and slow disease progression. Most of these disorders are dependent on the heteroplasmic state of the mtDNA and associated threshold effects; it is difficult to provide accurate genetic counseling based on preimplantation or prenatal genetic diagnoses.

Different techniques which have been studied for MRT are—cytoplasmic transfer (CT), germinal vesicle transfer (GVT), pronuclear transfer (PNT), polar body nuclear transfer (PBT), and maternal spindle transfer (MST).

Maternal spindle transfer, also referred to as spindle-chromosomal complex transfer (ST), was first reported as a novel revolutionary approach to avoid transmission of inherited mitochondrial disease in 2009.[4] MST is done in mature metaphase II (MII) oocytes where MII spindle-chromosomal complex is isolated as membrane enclosed karyoplast and is transferred into an enucleated (nuclear material free) cytoplast from healthy donor MII oocyte. MST can be considered as a leading technique for MRT and germline gene therapy and has advantages over other techniques.

Advantages of Maternal Spindle Transfer[1]

- Metaphase II spindle-chromosomal complex is relatively smaller than that of GV and PN stage interphase nuclei.
- Metaphase II spindle is devoid of mitochondria so, transmission of unbidden mutated mtDNA can be minimized using MST.
- As compared to GVT, where in vitro maturation (IVM) is required prior to fertilization, reconstructed oocytes via MST are ready for fertilization.
- Maternal spindle transfer may be ethically more acceptable than PNT, where cytoplasts are supplied from fertilized zygotes, and thus, requires destruction of normally fertilized zygotes, not gametes.[5]

In most mitochondrial diseases, a threshold of 60% or higher of mutated mtDNA is required for clinical features to manifest. In this regard, MST would be successful to prevent diseases, as well as sufficient in preventing the transmission of mitochondrial diseases to their offspring.

Despite unresolved issues regarding MRT, Dr J Zhang et al. presented their research on use of MST in birth of a healthy male baby derived from in vitro fertilization (IVF) using a successfully reconstituted human oocyte from a female carrier of mitochondrial disease (Leigh syndrome) with a history of two deceased children from a mutation in mtDNA (8,993 T > G).[6]

Wider Implications of Mitochondrial Replacement Therapy in Assisted Reproductive Technology

- In modern ART, advancing age is one of the major success of limiting factor. It is associated with increased incidence of point mutations and deletions in mtDNA, poor fertilization rates, embryo aneuploidy, poor cleavage and implantation, and increased abortion rates. MRT can be considered as ART technique to solve cytoplasmic defects due to aging.
- Mitochondrial replacement therapy may provide new ART options for young cancer patients by replacing cryopreserved cytoplasm with fresh cytoplasm from young donors.
- It may solve the future problem of availability of oocytes. Unlike spermatogenesis where single spermatocyte produces four sperms, through consecutive meiosis, single oocyte produces only one mature oocyte and three-fourths of the genetic material remains unutilized. But with MRT, polar bodies can be used and two zygotes can be theoretically created using two PB2T (one PB2 from original MII spindle and the other from PB1T spindle), with PN stage zygotes, created with husband's sperm and donor oocytes. This may be beneficial to patients of advanced maternal age, who have a low oocyte yield or are poor responders, commonly observed in ART cycles.[7]

Disadvantages of Mitochondrial Replacement Therapy

- Drastic mitochondrial genetic drifts occur when the mtDNA goes through the female germline, causing a "mitochondrial bottleneck effect". There is a possibility of disease manifestation in future generations of MRT, which will probably become evident after two generations. Limiting MRT to male embryos takes away the fear related to the transmission of mtDNA diseases as well as unexpected side effects of MRT to future generations, since mtDNA inheritance is exclusively maternal.[1]
- Mitochondrial replacement therapy may evoke another side of the ethical argument, with the fear of eventually creating the "designer baby", thus risk of violating the rights of subsequent generation.

GENE EDITING (CRISPR-CAS9)

Genome editing is a type of genetic engineering in which DNA is inserted, deleted, modified, or replaced at specific sites of interest to modify the genome. The technique works by some specific enzymes called endonucleases. The most recent and talked about endonuclease is CRISPR-Cas9, also known as genetic scissors. The endonucleases can make double-stranded breaks (DSBs), which are normally needed in DNA repair pathway to prevent mutation in cases of DNA damage. The DNA repair is done by two pathways—(1) nonhomologous end joining (NHEJ) and (2) homologous recombination (HR).[8]

History

The major breakthrough in gene editing happened with discovery of clustered regularly interspaced short palindromic repeats (CRISPR) which were first identified as classes of repeated DNA sequences at 3' end of alkaline phosphatase gene in *Escherichia coli*. CRISPR works in association with CRISPR-associated (Cas) proteins (Cas9) to provide bacterial immunity against invading phages.[8]

Present Scenario

CRISPR-Cas9 endonucleases were first discovered in prokaryotes like bacteria where they work as an adaptive immune system and cleave infecting DNA to generate short foreign sequences. These sequences are then stored in host bacterium and transcribed into RNA called short CRISPR RNA (crRNA). This fuses with trans-activating crRNA (tracrRNA) to form a single guide RNA (sgRNA) which then interacts with Cas9 endonuclease to generate DSBs in complementary infecting DNA. The DSBs are repaired by either NHEJ resulting in small insertion or deletions (Indels), a class of mutation usually leading to loss of function. In the presence of donor DNA, HR repair mechanism causes precise modification at target site leading to a gain of function.[9] This ability of the CRISPR-Cas9 system to guide an endonuclease to any target sequence with the help of short RNA segment to generate DSBs, makes it most suitable for gene editing. The editing system CRISPR-Cas9 is microinjected into the cytoplasm or pronuclei of zygotes or MII oocytes.[8]

The discovery of CRISPR-based approaches, which is based on RNA-guided nuclease activity, enabled targeted DSBs in eukaryotes with much ease. The ease and speed of designing CRISPR-guided nucleases has made CRISPR/CAS9 system most widely used gene editing tools. *The ultimate therapeutic application of CRISPR/Cas9 system is to repair disease causing alleles by changing DNA sequences at specific sites on chromosomes.* The several applications of gene editing-based approaches are:

- *To cure monogenic diseases (both autosomal dominant and recessive)*: Beta-thalassemia, sickle cell anemia, cystic fibrosis, hemophilia, Huntington's disease, Duchenne muscular dystrophy, lysosomal storage diseases, achondroplasia, polycystic kidney disease, and myotonic dystrophy type 1.[10]
- Chromosomal aberrations like Robertsonian translocations, Turner syndrome (45, X), Klinefelter syndrome (47, XXY), and Y-chromosome deletions (oligozoospermia and azoospermia).
- Viral infections like human immunodeficiency infection and hepatitis B.

In the reproductive field, CRISPR-Cas9 technology can be used to correct mutations in pluripotent stem cells, gametes (oocytes, sperms), and embryos for preventing genetic disorder in offsprings. The pluripotent stem cells can be grown faster and more easily and hence are ideal for research purpose.

Injecting CRISPR-Cas9 components into zygote or early embryo can modify genome in all cells of the organism including the germ cells resulting in permanent change and possibility of eliminating the disease from the entire family.[11]

Future Trends

- Gene editing technologies can also be used to eliminate mitochondrial diseases by removing mtDNA from oocytes or embryos. For the first time, mitochondrial gene editing was used in mammalian oocytes by Juan Carlos and colleagues.[12] They performed gene editing in two mitochondrial diseases—(1) Leber hereditary optic neuropathy and (2) Neurogenic muscle weakness, ataxia, and retinitis pigmentosa (NARP) by fusing patients fibroblasts with mouse oocytes and injecting mitoTALENS. Mutated mtDNA, though still detectable, was reduced sufficiently to prevent phenotypic expression.

Major challenge with this technique is formation of mosaic mutations due to off-target effects at other locations in the genome that share the same sequences as the target area. So, the mutation is repaired in some cells and at the same time in other cells, unwanted off-target mutations or extra mutations are generated in the target gene leading to a mosaic embryo (nonhomologous repair). Hence, the efficiency of genome editing is low in embryos and ranges from 0.5% to 40.9% in mammalian zygotes.[13] For the first time in 2015, the CRISPR-Cas9 gene editing was used in human tripronuclear (3 PN) zygotes by a Chinese group. They found that this technique could effectively cleave the beta-globin gene but the efficiency of HR was low, mosaic embryos were generated, and untoward off-target mutations were identified.[14] Another Chinese group could successfully modify an immune cell gene *CCR5* by introducing engineered CCR5-delta 32 allele into 3 PN zygotes making the cells resistant to human immunodeficiency virus (HIV) infection. However, off-target mutations could not be fully controlled. Recently for the first time, this technique was used in diploid (2 PN) human embryos for correction of point mutation in hemoglobin subunit beta gene and glucose-6-phosphate dehydrogenase (G6PDH) gene, the limitation being mosaic embryos similar to previous studies.[15] In a major breakthrough, Mitalipov and colleagues have greatly improved the precision and safety of gene editing by injecting CRISPR-Cas9 components together with sperms into MII oocytes. This technique and other refinements have addressed the problem of mosaicism to a great extent.[16] Optimization of timing and concentration of CRISPR-CAS9 are needed to reduce the risk of mosaicism to minimum.[17]

CONCLUSION

Mitochondrial replacement therapy and genome editing technology (CRISPR-Cas9) are considered as the most groundbreaking discoveries in the field of science. While the theoretical advantages of these techniques, it is too premature to apply MRT and gene editing for common in fertility treatment at this point and further research is needed. Widespread application of these in the clinical field needs consideration of ethical and social issues as well.

REFERENCES

1. Tachibana M, Kuno T, Yaegashi N. Mitochondrial replacement therapy and assisted reproductive technology: a paradigm shift toward treatment of genetic diseases in gametes or in early embryos. Reprod Med Biol. 2018;17(4):421-33.
2. Chinnery PF, Johnson MA, Wardell TM, et al. The epidemiology of pathogenic mitochondrial DNA mutations. Ann Neurol. 2000;48(2):188-93.
3. Spikings EC, Alderson J, St John JC. Transmission of mitochondrial DNA following assisted reproduction and nuclear transfer. Hum Reprod Update. 2006;12(4): 401-15.
4. Tachibana M, Sparman M, Sritanaudomchai H, et al. Mitochondrial gene replacement in primate offspring and embryonic stem cells. Nature. 2009;461(7262):367-72.
5. Tachibana M, Sparman M, Mitalipov S. Chromosome transfer in mature oocytes. Nat Protoc. 2010;5(6):1138-47.
6. Zhang J, Liu H, Luo S, et al. Live birth derived from oocyte spindle transfer to prevent mitochondrial disease. Reprod Biomed Online. 2017;34(4):361-8.
7. Ma H, O'Neil RC, Marti Gutierrez N, et al. Functional Human Oocytes Generated by Transfer of Polar Body Genomes. Cell Stem Cell. 2017;20(1):112-9.
8. Porteus MH. Towards a new era in medicine: therapeutic genome editing. Genome Biol. 2015;16:286.
9. Sánchez-Rivera FJ, Jacks T. Applications of the CRISPR-Cas9 system in cancer biology. Nat Rev Cancer. 2015;15(7): 387-95.
10. Vassena R, Heindryckx B, Peco R, et al. Genome engineering through CRISPR/Cas9 technology in the human germline and pluripotent stem cells. Hum Reprod Update. 2016;22(4): 411-9.
11. Wang H, Yang H, Shivalila CS, et al. One-step generation of mice carrying mutations in multiple genes by CRISPR/Cas-mediated genome engineering. Cell. 2013;153(4):910-8.
12. Reddy P, Ocampo A, Suzuki K, et al. Selective elimination of mitochondrial mutations in the germline by genome editing. Cell. 2015;161(3):459-69.
13. Tu Z, Yang W, Yan S, et al. Promoting Cas9 degradation reduces mosaic mutations in non-human primate embryos. Sci Rep. 2017;7:42081.
14. Liang P, Xu Y, Zhang X, et al. CRISPR/Cas9-mediated gene editing in human tripronuclear zygotes. Protein Cell. 2015;6(5):363-72.
15. Tang L, Zeng Y, Du H, et al. CRISPR/Cas9-mediated gene editing in human zygotes using Cas9 protein. Mol Genet Genomics. 2017;292(3):525-33.
16. Ma H, Marti-Gutierrez N, Park SW, et al. Correction of a pathogenic gene mutation in human embryos. Nature. 2017;548(7668):413-9.
17. Tanihara F, Hirata M, Nguyen NT, et al. Effects of concentration of CRISPR/Cas9 components on genetic mosaicism in cytoplasmic microinjected porcine embryos. J Reprod Dev. 2019. [Epub ahead of print].

Robotics in Infertility: Technical Aspects and its Present Day Relevance

82

Reem Sabouni, Laurel Stadtmauer

INTRODUCTION

Robotic surgery has revolutionized minimally invasive surgery since its conception in the 1980s when it first emerged in on the scene. As a strategic form of technology, it eliminated many obstacles of conventional laparoscopy allowing the wide spread application of minimally invasive surgery. Physicians across all specialties are turning to the robot as a facilitator in surgery. Particularly in infertility with the growing economic pressure to refer cases to other surgical specialists, the robot has allowed the reproductive surgeon to retain the ability to surgically treat patients through utilizing this intuitive technology with its decreased learning curve in comparison to advanced laparoscopy. In addition, the ability to perform fine suturing for tuboplasty and tubal reanastomosis is improved, as well as closures of the defects in the uterus in multiple layers in cases such as laparoscopic myomectomy. The 3-D visualization allows improved resection of endometriosis and endometriomas with minimal loss of ovarian tissue.

HISTORY

The history of robotic surgery is rooted in with that of minimally invasive surgery. The field of laparoscopic surgery started in the early 1900s with the first laparoscopic procedures performed on dogs in Germany. It then evolved over the years with advancing technology such as the computer chip-based television cameras to the modern form of laparoscopic surgery present today. Prior to the 1990s, gynecologists were the only surgical subspecialists performing laparoscopic surgery with other specialists joining suit in the years that followed. The birth of minimally invasive surgery was a paradigm shift in surgical approach, departing from traditional open procedures and improving patient-centered care.

As minimally invasive surgery took up traction in the 1980s, there was increasing demand for surgical precision, safety and widening the scope and complexity of surgeries that can be accomplished. The limitations of conventional laparoscopy, including two-dimensional visualization, lack of articulation of instruments, ergonomic limitations inflicted on the surgeon and compromised dexterity, gave birth to robotic-assisted surgery.[1] Physical symptoms or discomfort reported by laparoscopic surgeons are as high as 87%, particularly in eye and back complaints that were found to be irrespective of case volume.[2] Robotic surgery technology was originally developed by the US army with the plan of performing remote surgery away from the battlefield. This incorporated the benefits of minimally invasive surgery while solving many of conventional laparoscopy's shortcomings with: three-dimensional visualization, improved dexterity, seven degrees of freedom, elimination of the fulcrum effect, elimination of physiologic tremors, ability to scale motions, ability to perform micro-anastomoses, telesurgery, and ergonomic position.[3] With these allowances offered by robotic surgery, more patients are able to undergo minimally invasive surgery, reaping the benefits, when otherwise a laparotomy would have been necessary. In 2000, the Food and Drug Administration (FDA) approved the da Vinci robotic system for use in intra-abdominal surgery and approval in gynecologic procedures in 2005.

PRESENT SCENARIO

Despite advances in medical management of infertility and improved success in-vitro fertilization (IVF) technology, surgery remains an indispensable tool in the arsenal against infertility and is often done to maximize the success of the IVF procedure. As technology advances surgical approach, modern reproductive surgery is confined to advanced laparoscopy. The reproductive subspecialists, with their unique clinical and surgical perspective on infertility, face a significant obstacle in performing advanced laparoscopic surgeries owing from the time and effort required to achieve and maintain proficiency.[4] Through robotic-assisted surgery, aptitudinal restrictions to the adoption of advanced laparoscopy are minimized due to promoting strategy over technique.[4] These subspecialists predominately utilize robotic surgery as treatment options for tubal anastomosis, myomectomy, adenomyosis, adnexal masses, and other complex laparoscopies for diseases like endometriosis.

Tubal anastomosis was first performed in the 1970s using an open microsurgical technique. With advances in conventional laparoscopy and increasing surgeon experience, utilization of minimally invasive techniques quickly predominated given the advantages in expedited recovery for the patient and the decreased potential for adhesion formation when compared with the open technique. Yet, despite comparable pregnancy rates to the open microsurgical technique, the laparoscopic tubal anastomosis was limited due to an absence of stereoscopic vision, difficulty with intra-abdominal suturing and difficulty handling fine suture with laparoscopic instruments.[5] The utilization of robotic surgery addressed these limitations to conventional laparoscopy, but also eliminates the necessity of a maintaining a unique skill set for an infrequently performed operation.[4] An ongoing debate exists concerning the role of tubal anastomosis in the era of IVF. Despite climbing pregnancy rates with IVF, it too has its drawbacks including expense, time consumption, drug side effects, and risks of multiple gestation. Thus, IVF and tubal anastomosis should be considered complementary and the best therapeutic approach should be individualized for each patient and their reproductive goals.[5]

Myomectomy for surgical treatment in infertility patients is controversial except for submucosal fibroids. Many factors are taken into consideration including the uterine fibroid size, location, number, patient symptoms, age, and obstetrical history. Uterine fibroids are theorized to affect fertility via altering uterine contractility leading to impedance of embryo or sperm transport or they are associated with vascular alterations that hinder embryo implantation.[5] Alternatively, undergoing a myomectomy is not without risks including recurrence of uterine fibroids, endometrial adhesions and pelvic adhesions in addition to the risks of a major abdominal surgery. No differences in fertility and obstetric outcomes are noted after a laparoscopic versus abdominal myomectomy, with significant postoperative outcomes favoring the minimally invasive approach given decreased blood loss, hospital stay and febrile morbidity.[6] Similar to a myomectomy there is adenomyosis resection with its requirement for meticulous suturing in multiple layers and need for enhanced visualization to discern diseased area from healthy myometrium. A significant limitation in the conventional laparoscopic myomectomy or adenomyosis resection is the technical difficulty in laparoscopic suturing to achieve an appropriate closure. This technical challenge is greatly enhanced with robotic surgery's more intrinsic ability for intra-abdominal suturing.

The indications for robotic surgery continues to expand within the field of benign gynecology and infertility. Other advanced laparoscopic cases including surgical treatment of endometriosis and complex adnexal masses have been shown to have similar outcomes compared to conventional laparoscopy, but with longer operative time and higher costs associated with robotic cases.[7,8] Clinically, robotic surgery and conventional laparoscopy are equivalent and require larger randomized control trials to demonstrate this equality.

Figures 1 to 6 show the most common surgical diagnoses requiring robotic surgery.

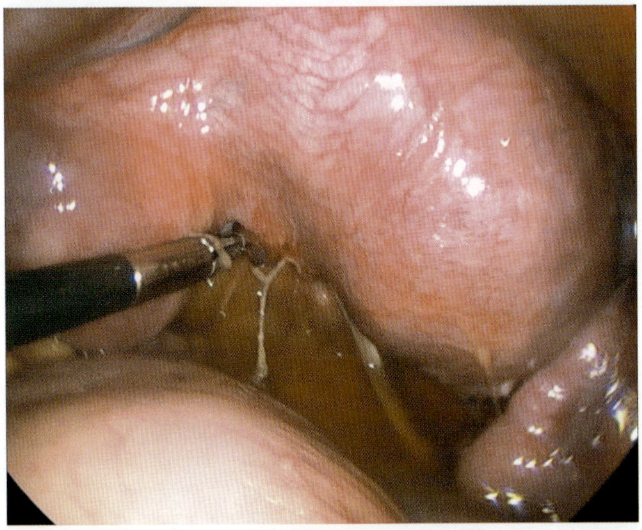

Fig. 1: Unicornuate uterus with a noncommunicating horn.

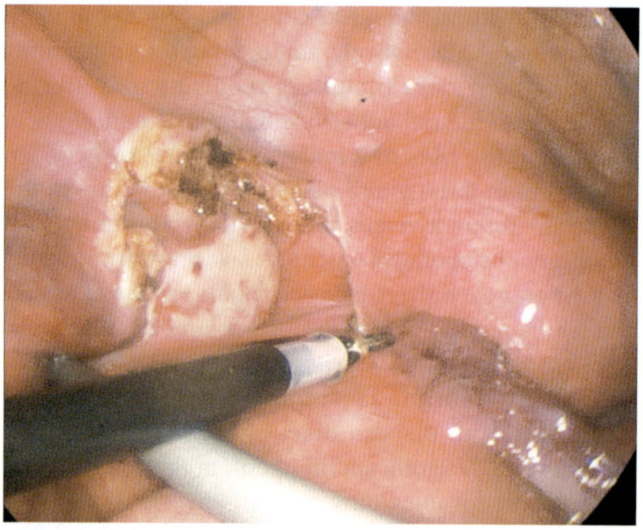

Fig. 2: Resection of noncommunicating horn.

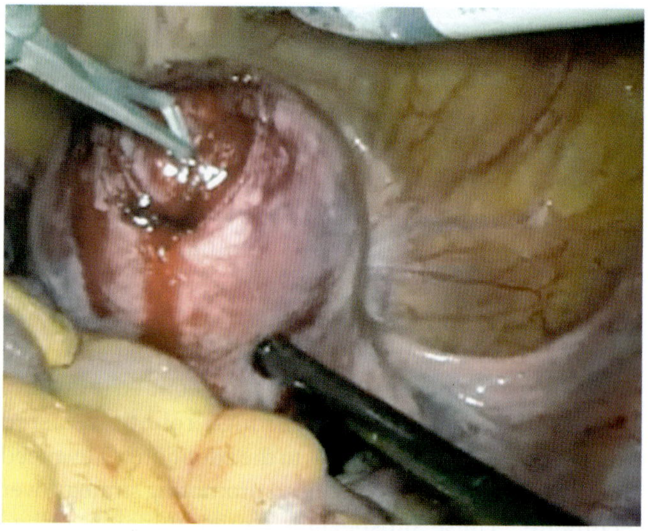

Fig. 3: Uterus with myoma for myomectomy.

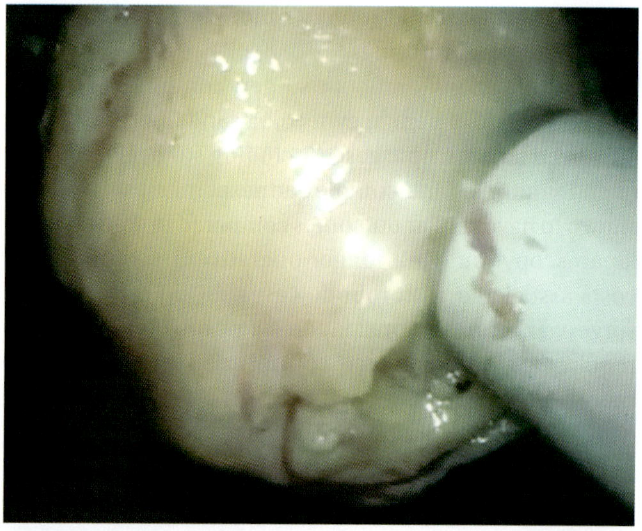

Fig. 4: Morcellation of uterine fibroid.

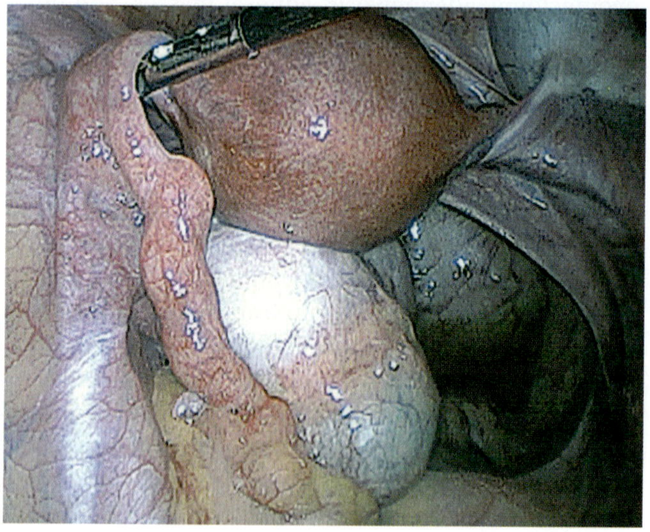

Fig. 5: Dermoid cyst on ovary.

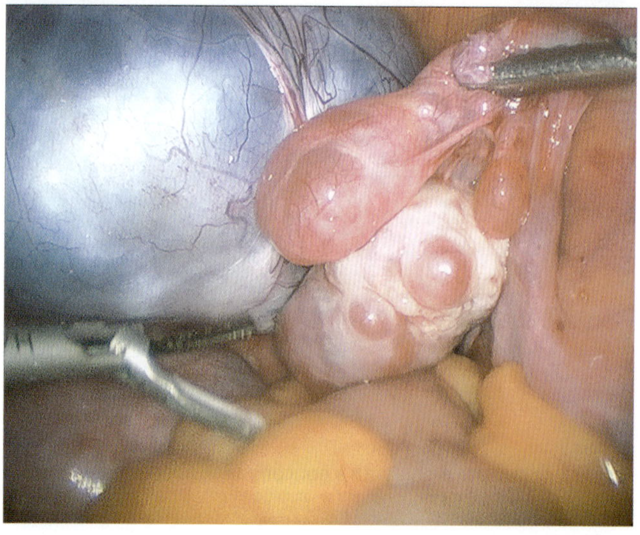

Fig. 6: Hydrosalpinx and urachal cyst.

FUTURE TRENDS

According to Estes et al:

- Uterine transplantation
- Indocyanine green mapping for identifying endometriosis and other procedures
- Additional natural orifice surgery options
- Nanotechnology
- Ovarian tissue transplantation moving from experimental to standard of care
- Telesurgery.

CONCLUSION

Robotic surgery, like most technology, is initially expensive, but with further advancement, it soon will become increasingly economical. With integrated simulator training, innate handling and truncated learning curve, robotic surgery is easier to master and maintain competence.[9] Additionally, it requires less maintenance of particular laparoscopic skill sets, allowing surgeons to focus on the subtleties of the surgery. Through robotic surgery, reproductive specialists have the ability to continue providing comprehensive care to their patients.

SUMMARY

- Robotic surgery has widened capacity for reproductive surgeons to perform advanced laparoscopic surgeries in a minimally invasive fashion.
- Robotic surgery overcomes many of conventional laparoscopy's shortcomings: three-dimensional visualization, improved dexterity, seven degrees of freedom, elimination of the fulcrum effect, elimination of physiologic tremors, ability to scale motions, ability to perform micro-anastomoses, telesurgery, and ergonomic position.
- Aptitudinal restrictions to the adoption of advanced laparoscopy for the reproductive surgeon are minimized through employment of robotic surgery due to promoting strategy over technique.

REFERENCES

1. Ashrafian H, Clancy O, Grover V, et al. The evolution of robotic surgery: surgical and anaesthetic aspects. Br J Anaesth. 2017;119:i72-i84.
2. Park A, Lee G, Seagull FJ, et al. Patients benefit while surgeons suffer: an impending epidemic. J Am Coll Sug. 2010;210(3):306-13.
3. Lanfranco AR Castellanos AE, Desai JP, et al. Robotic Surgery: A Current Perspective. Ann Surg. 2004;239(1):14-21.
4. Antonio RG. Computer-assisted reproductive surgery: why it matters to reproductive endocrinoloyg and infertility subspecialists. Fertil Steril. 2014;102(4):911-21.
5. Sroga J, Patel SD. Robotic Applications in Reproductive Endocrinology and Infertility. J Robotic Surg. 2008;2:3-10.
6. Seracchioli R, Rossi S, Govoni F, et al. Fertility and obstetric outcome after laparoscopic myomectomy or large myomata: a randomized comparison with abdominal myomectomy. Hum Reprod. 2000;15(12):2663-8.
7. Kim S, Luu TH, Llarena N, et al. Role of robotic surgery in treating fibroids and benign uterine mass. Best Pract Res Clin Obstet Gynaecol. 2017;45:48-59.
8. Nezhat CR, Stevens A, Balassiano E, et al. Robotic-assisted Laparoscopy vs. Conventional Laparoscopy for the Treatment of Advanced Stage Endometriosis. J Minim Invasive Gynecol. 2015;22(1):40-4.
9. Choussein S, Srouji SS, Farland LV, et al. Robotic Assistance Confers Ambidexterity to Laparoscopic Surgeons. J Minim Invasive Gynecol. 2017;25(1):76-83.

Index

Page numbers followed by *b* refer to box, *f* refer to figure, *fc* refer to flowchart, and *t* refer to table.

A

Aborters
- primary 438
- secondary 438

Abortion
- rates 192
- risk of 453

Accreditation 277
- main purpose of 277

Achondroplasia 568
Acid-fast bacilli 48
Acidic aniline blue stain 147
Acridine orange assay 148
Acrosin 291
Acrosomal cap 291
Acrosomal membrane, outer 291
Acrosomal reaction 330
Acrosome 292*f*
- reaction 292*f*, 561, 562

Activated partial thromboplastin time 448
Adalimumab 442
Adenomyoma 67, 115, 156*t*
- excision 71

Adenomyosis 66, 68, 73, 113, 115, 253
- after endometriosis surgery, effects of 73
- cystic 67
  - adult 67
- diffuse 67
- focal 67
- histological classification of 67
- penetrating vessels in 156*f*
- posterior 165*f*
- resection 571
- surgical classification of 67
- uteri 66

Adherens 234
Adhesiolysis, hysteroscopic 231
Adhesion 84, 390
- molecules 234

Adipose cells 554
Adipose tissue 40
Adjunctive therapy 178
Adnexal masses 124
Air conditioning system 261, 280
Air quality 280, 286, 541
- considerations 364*t*

Air warming system 361
Airborne particulates 273
Alanine 284
Alanylglutamine 284
Alarm
- state 273
- system 263

Albumin 411
Alopecia 450
Alpha fetoprotein 432, 433, 435
Aluminum cane 460, 461
Alzheimer's disease 566
Amenorrhea 9, 11, 29, 45, 82*f*
American Association of Gynecological Laparoscopists 109
American Board of Bioanalysis 267
American College of Obstetricians and Gynecologists 91, 94, 435, 457, 521
American Society of Clinical Oncologists 224
American Society of Reproductive Medicine 91, 94, 104, 145, 216, 224, 265, 278, 414, 438, 476
- Classification 60, 61*f*
- Guidelines 268, 492

Amino acid 284, 341, 355
- disorders 432

Ammonium, lower levels of 284
Amniocentesis 433
Amniotic fluid abnormalities 433
Amoxicillin, combination of 254
Analgesics 69
Anastrozole 132, 179
Anderson's protocol 217, 217*f*
Androgens 223
- deficiency 141
- Excess Society Criteria 81
- modulating agents 207

Anesthesia 84
- general 372
- local 372
- types of 372

Anesthetic gases 439
Aneuploid embryos 249
- ratios of 250

Aneuploid gametes 248
Aneuploidy 340, 432, 433
- analysis 354
- detection rates 435
- embryonic 249
- interpretation 432*t*
- prenatal diagnosis of 433
- studies, role of 249

Angiogenesis 109
Anovulation
- chronic 82
- classification of 173*b*

Antagonist 85, 200
- protocol 205, 206*f*

Anti-androgenic fashion 128
Anti-angiogenic agents 70
Anti-angiogenic drugs 69
Antibiotics 417
Anti-D prophylaxis 450
Antidepressants 36
Antiepileptic drugs 219
Antiestrogen 131, 175, 176
- indications of 178

Anti-hepatitis B surface antibody titer 93
Anti-inflammatory 418
- agents 69
- therapy 131

Anti-Müllerian hormone 11, 12, 41, 81, 82*f*, 204, 205*f*, 207, 207*f*, 216, 222, 410, 422, 481, 492, 505, 557
Antioxidant 132, 230, 284
- administration 139
- role of 150

Antiphospholipid
- antibodies 254
- syndrome
  - primary 439
  - secondary 439

Antiprogestins 69, 70
Antisperm antibody 19
Antithymoglobulin 508
Antitubercular treatment, history of 118
Antivibration, form of 312
Antral follicle 223
- count 11, 12, 82, 154, 157, 205*f*, 207, 207*f*, 216, 414, 492

Apoptosis, markers of 307
Apoptotic sperm 149*f*
Appetite suppressant 83
Aromatase 179
- activity 222
- enzyme 218
- inhibitors 60, 69, 71, 84, 131-133, 139, 144, 175, 179, 198
  - classification of 179, 179*t*

Array comparative genomic hybridization 513, 523, 536, 538
Artificial insemination 471, 543
Ascites 412

Ascitic fluid 409
Asherman's syndrome 45, 50, 89, 231, 496, 501, 502, 556
recurrence of 231
severe 556
Asoprisnil 77
Asparagine 284
Aspartate 284
Aspiration, vacuum 447
Aspirin 208, 223, 237, 238, 240, 389, 418
dosage of 418
Assisted hatching 108, 330, 331, 352
clinical application of 332
disadvantages of 333
efficacy of 352
mechanism of 331
techniques 331
Assisted human reproduction Act 265
Assisted reproductive technology 3, 42, 43, 56, 58, 66, 73, 92, 93, 113, 126, 134, 154, 248, 261, 264, 277, 278, 305, 315, 330, 351, 363, 368, 377, 394, 402, 411, 416, 422, 423*f*, 438, 444, 453, 459, 476, 510, 530, 543, 563, 566, 567
adjuvant therapies in 416
banks 548
bill 547
clinic 278, 541
management systems 266
cryopreservation in 459
guidelines of 540
in endometriosis 63
in seropositive couples 91
laboratory, setting of 261
misuse of 494
obstetric complications after 428
outcome of 229
pivotal component of 513
pregnancy rates 513, 518
procedures 471, 545
role of
andrologist in 543
counselors in 543
embryologist in 543, 544
team 279
treatment 394
Asthenozoospermia 304, 319
Ataxia 568
Atosiban 380
Atresia, esophageal 433
Atretic oocyte 317*f*
Atypical polypoid adenomyomas 67
Australia, Reproductive Technology Accreditation Committee 278
Autocrine factor 287
Autoimmune ovarian damage 557
Autoimmunity 490
Autosomal dominant 566, 568
disorders 520
skeletal dysplasia 491
Autosomal recessive
disorders 520
Mendelian pattern of 566
Auto-transplantation 486
Auxiliary subunits 559
Azathioprine 508
Azoospermia 19, 21, 31, 125, 136, 137, 319, 555, 568
classification of 136
diagnosis of 136
etiology of 136
factor 125, 126
management of 138
nonobstructive 138, 139
obstructive 137, 138
post-testicular causes of 137
severe 125
testicular 136
types of 555
Azoospermic male, evaluation of 137

B

Bacterial vaginosis 54, 441
treatment of 441
Barcode-based systems 369, 369*t*
Basal body temperature 177
serial 10
Benchtop incubators 280*f*
Benzene 287
Beta-human chorionic gonadotropin, positive 266
Beta-thalassemia 221, 432, 568
Bettocchi hysteroscope based
on 2 mm telescope 104*f*
on 29 mm telescope 104*f*
Bettocchi integrated office hysteroscope 104, 105*f*
Bettocchi system 104
Bicarbonate media, equilibrate 289
Bicornuate uterus 13
Bigatti shaver 106*f*
Bilateral uterine arteries, laparoscopic transient occlusion of 72
Biopsy
methods 522*t*, 536*t*
procedure 522, 536
negative effect of 522, 536
testicular 23, 138
Bipolar
generator 106*f*
needle 105, 105*f*
radiofrequency 71
resectoscope 106*f*, 111
use of 109
Birefringence imaging 352
Birth
defects 431
weight, low 388
Bisphenol A 128
Blank cells 554
Blastocele 301
Blastocyst 283, 301, 460, 514
breaks 301
culture 340, 341, 352, 378
and transfer strategy 341
program 339
development 108, 301, 355
euploidy 424*f*
expanded 339*f*
expansion grade 301*t*
formation, predictors of 339
group 342
implants 337
number of 342
quality 301
stage 340
embryos 353, 354
transfer 337, 339, 341, 342, 498
programs 340
vitrification of 465*f*
with inner cell mass 302*f*
Blastomere 301*f*, 333
biopsy of 354, 521, 530
compaction of 338
fragmentation of 339
fusion, presence of 340
number of 299
premature hatching of 333
symmetry of 299
Blastulation rates 266
Bleeding 219
Blood
cells 554
chemistry 505
count, complete 497
disorders 448
estradiol level, assessment of 185
group 448
pressure 507
transfusion in laparotomy group 446
tumor, presence of 239
Body mass index 9, 10, 40, 190, 207, 222
low 82
Bone marrow
autologous 556
stem cells 556
transplantation 486
Brain 559

Breast tissue, antiestrogenic effect of 218
Breastfeeding 448
Bromocriptine 38
Bronchiectasis 137
Brucellosis 439
Bubble migration analysis 383
Bubble motion, gravity related 383

C

Cabergoline 38
Cadherins 234
Cadmium 129
Caffeine consumption 127
Calcium 411
Canadian Fertility and Andrology Society 265
Cancer 429
effects of 216
fertility preservation techniques 484*t*
gynecological 502
heritable 516
related medical conditions 219
survival 502
treatment 216
Cansort method 151*f*
Capitulum 293
Capnography, use of 122
Carbohydrates 284
Carbon dioxide 273, 285
Carboxylic acid pyruvate 283
Carcinoma, endometrial 502
Cardiovascular disease 176
Carnitines 132
Caseous nodules 45
Catheter
insertion, depth of 382
transfer 379
types of 380, 381*f*
Catsper channel 559, 561-564
complex 559
expression of 560
involvement of 562
localization of 560*f*
Catsper null sperms 559
Catsper subunits 560
Cavity, abdominal 121, 445
Ceftriaxone 229, 254
Cell
free fetal DNA, discovery of 434
gonadotropin system 5
numbers 299
types 356
undergoing apoptosis 251
Center well dish 316
Centers for disease control 94
and preventions guidelines 92
Central air handling unit 286
Centromeric-enumeration probe 524*f*
Cephalosporins 230
Cerebral palsy 394
rate of 453
Certolizumab 442
Cervical
incompetence 395
insufficiency 440
manipulation 382
mucus 84, 155*f*, 382
quality of 97
removal of 382
represents 382
pregnancy 446
sonographic surveillance, serial 440
stenosis 111
Cervix 46, 155, 501
Cesarean scar pregnancy 447, 450
Cesarean section 96, 99, 509
scar, complications of 96
Cetrolizumab 442
Chemical
air contaminants 261, 279
hatching 352
techniques 332
Chemotaxis 561
toward oocyte 561
Chemotherapy 470, 490
Child born, rights of 494
Chlamydia 363, 492
antibody test 13
cervical cultures for 492
trachomatis 54, 55, 131
attributes 444
bacteria 55
Chorioamnionitis 454
Chorionic gonadotropin injection, post-human 521
Chorionic villus sampling 433, 515, 530
Chorionicity 454, 456
Chromomycin A3 assay 147
Chromopertubation 13
laparoscopic 89
Chromosomal
abnormalities 429, 432, 549
anomaly 433
constitution 330
disorders 517
organizations 295
Chromosome aneuploidy, whole 523, 538
Chronic low-dose step-up protocol 182*fc*
Ciliary dyskinesia, primary 126
Circulating hot water 71
Clavulanate 254
Cleavage rate, stimulation of 284
Cleavage stage embryo 299, 341
biopsy procedure 521*f*
Clindamycin 229
Clofilium 563
Clomiphene 84, 131, 144, 177, 180*t*, 403
antiestrogenic effect of 177
citrate 83, 84, 176, 180, 187, 198, 200, 212, 214
advantages over 180
adverse effects 180
challenge test 11
effects of 199*t*
failure 178
isomers of 177, 177*t*
resistance 178
Cloning, concept of 356
Closed system
freezing 463
vitrification 463
Coenzyme 132, 416
Collin's knife 105
and electrodes 106*f*
Colloid therapy 413
Color Doppler 154
in infertility, role of 160
studies 69
Color flow Doppler ultrasonography 237
Combined therapy 84
Comet assay 148
Committee of Society of Assisted Reproductive Technology 278
Communication failure 122
Comparative genome hybridization 354, 526, 531
Complete genomic hybridization 441
Complex etiopathogenetic therapy 229
Comprehensive chromosomal screening 390, 522, 531
Computer assisted scoring system 378
Computer-aided analysis, virtual organ 187*f*, 193*f*
Computerized tomography scan 88
Conception, mode of 457*t*
Congenital anomalies 253, 549
Contingent sequential screen 434, 435
Contraceptives, use of 16
Controlled ovarian
hyperstimulation 27, 235, 389, 394, 402, 403
stimulation 174, 216, 218, 219, 388
individualization of 204
Controlled rate cryopreservation 460, 472
Corifollitropin alpha 223
Corona
cumulus complex 294
radiata 295

Coronal cells removed 321*f*
Corpus luteum 8
  degeneration of 6
  life span of 402
Cortical slices, thickness of 484
Corticosteroids 84, 418, 508
  high dose 507
Cryocycles 231
Cryoinjuries 465, 466*t*
Cryopreservation 94
  cycles 273
  indication for 479
  noncontrolled rate 460, 472
  objective of 471
  oocyte, techniques of 353
  principles of 471
  procedure 472
  section 541
  technique, advances in 353
  technology of 470
  use of 459
Cryoprotectant 459, 471
  concentration of 353
  nonpermeable 460*t*
  nonpermeating 471, 477
  penetration of 483
  preparation 484
    of required 484, 484*t*
  solution 471
Cryotherapy 71
Cryptorchidism 141
  bilateral 17
Cryptozoospermia 136, 319
Crystalloid therapy 413
Culture media 267, 280, 283
Culture system 285
Cumulus 188
  cells 256
  oocyte complex 294, 316, 361
  oophorus 158*f*, 188*f*
Cumulus-oocyte complex
  expanded 295*f*
  method for 295*b*
Cyst
  adenomyotic 67
  rupture of 414
Cystic
  adenomyosis, juvenile 67
  fibrosis 520, 568
    transmembrane conductance regulator 125, 138
Cytokine 234, 253, 556
  abnormalities 439
  factors 76
Cytomegalovirus 93, 94, 440
Cytoplasm
  amount of 299
  homogenous 297*f*
Cytoplasmic anomalies 300
Cytoplasmic structure 330
Cytoplasmic transfer 567

D

Danazol 60, 69, 70
D-Chiro inositol 83
De Novo mutations 514
Degenerative diseases 356
Dehydroepiandrosterone 30, 178, 416
  sulfate 84
Density 304
  gradient centrifugation 251
Deoxyribonucleic acid 7, 293, 312, 530
  amplification 514
  damage 482
  fragmentation 473
Depression 491
  maternal 454
Designing in vitro fertilization laboratory 261
Dexamethasone 178
Diabetes 395, 556
  gestational 429
  insulin dependent 398
  juvenile 491
  mellitus 221
Dichlorodiphenyldichloroethylene 129
Dienogest 60, 70
Diethyl phthalate 128
Diiodotyrosine 25, 25*f*
Dimeric inhibin 435
  alpha 435
Dimethyl sulfide 477
Dimethyl sulfoxide 460, 471, 484
Di-N-butyl phthalate 128
Dipeptide 284
Direct androgen supplementation 417
Direct stimulatory theory 131
Distal tubal
  block 118
  disease 118
Distension device 102
Distension media 101
  electrolyte properties of 102*t*
  features of 102*t*
Distorted pelvic anatomy 59
Doer's syndrome 432
Dominant follicle selection 8
Donor
  embryo transfer 456, 457
  gametes 256
  intrauterine insemination 93, 118, 470
  oocytes 312
  recipient transfer cycle 406
  screening 506
  sperm 3
  surgery procedure 506, 506*b*
  types of 493
Dopamine 35
  agonists 38, 175, 182, 411
    dosage and risks 182
    mechanism of action 182
DOTS treatment 50
Double embryo transfer 396*t*, 397, 397*t*, 518
Double ovarian stimulation protocol 218
Down syndrome 354, 432, 434, 435
  screening for 434
Doxycycline 229
Drastic mitochondrial genetic drifts 567
Droplet method 318
Duchenne muscular dystrophy 432, 568
Ductal obstruction, acquired causes of 137
Duodenal atresia 433
Duostim protocol 217
Dydrogesterone 405, 406
Dynein protein extends 293
Dysmenorrhea 59, 68, 96, 99
Dyspareunia 68, 96

E

Ealoxifene 70
Early embryo 528, 537
  visibility test 347*f*
Ebola 94
  virus 94
Echogenicity 170
Eclampsia 395
Ectopic comprising, ruptured 446
Ectopic gestation 414, 446
Ectopic pregnancy 266, 382, 390, 429, 444, 445, 447, 450
  diagnosis 444
  management, effects of 450
  medical management of 448, 450
  persistent 449
  post-medical management of 450
  rate, lower 391
  resolution of 449
  risk factor for 444
  surgical
    management of 450
    procedures 446
    treatment 445
  treatment of persistent 449
Ectopic tissue left, persistent 450
Edwards syndrome 432, 434
Eevatm test 347
Egg
  banks, establishment of 478
  congenital absence of 490

donor
program 478
screening of 492*b*
quantity/quality, acquired reduced 490
Eight cell embryo 300*f*
Ejaculatory duct
dysfunction 137
trans-urethral resection of 138
Elastography 168
Elective single embryo transfer 341, 351, 394, 395, 397, 398
Electric probe 110
Electrical system 262
Electroacupuncture 237, 239
Electrocardiography 505
Electroejaculation 471
Electrolytes 505
Electron microscopy, scanning 332
Electronic witness system 269
Embryo 219, 280, 286, 287, 311, 312*t*, 370, 389, 460, 474, 514, 542, 556
accumulation 392
assessment 544
capacity 330
cryodamage 459
cryopreservation 231, 411, 414, 461, 476, 482
ethical restrictions of 478
relevance of 468, 468*b*
culture 318, 542
day two 300*f*
development 298, 299, 338*f*
disruption of 360
stage of 243
donation 545
energy production 283
epigenetic modifications of 439
expansion of 301
freezing 371, 390, 484, 545
pack 461
genetic competence 426
grading 108, 349*t*
implantation 379, 381, 416
in vitro 288
morphokinetic analysis of 345
morphology 298
multinucleated 340
nonviable 528
protective immunomodulation 404*fc*
quality 59, 397, 417
and selection 377
evaluation 299
selection 338
algorithm 348, 349*fc*
sources 493
techniques of 204
thawing of 462, 462*f*
transfer 56, 214, 318, 337, 351, 361, 377, 382, 503, 543, 545
catheter 378, 544
clinical part of 379
depth of 382
number of 398
optimize 377
part of 377
personalized 244, 246
procedure 383
process 383
pump-regulated 383
selective single 378
simulations 378
single 214, 283, 349, 377, 394, 396*t*, 397, 397*t*, 398, 518, 533
skilled atraumatic 459
technique 255, 379
transport 6
utilization rate 266
vitrification of 464*f*
Embryoendometrial
dialogue 234, 502
dyssynchronization 254
Embryology 265
Embryonic cells 521
sources of obtaining 530
Embryonic genome 251, 284
activation 338
Embryonic implantation potential 355
Embryonic stem cells, use of 356
Embryoscope 346, 346*f*
Embryoslide dish 346
Emodin 563
Emotional stress, reduced 213
Empiric medical therapy, types of 133
Enclomiphene 177, 198
Endocervical mucus 434
Endocervical type, adenomyoma of 67
Endocrine 204
abnormalities 59
disrupters 439
disrupting chemicals 128
neoplasia, multiple 516
Endocrinopathy, subclinical 132
Endogenous organisms 55
Endometrial ablation 71
Endometrial abnormalities 97
Endometrial angiogenic stem cells, autologous 240
Endometrial basalis, invagination of 66
Endometrial biopsy 48, 244
and histology 10
Endometrial cavity 337
Endometrial cycle 6
phase of 7
Endometrial cytokine leukemia inhibitory factor 255
Endometrial echogenicity 156*f*
Endometrial epithelium 234, 256, 337
Endometrial evaluation 190
Endometrial events 6
phases of 7*f*
Endometrial folds 159*f*
Endometrial hyperplasia 243
Endometrial midline 157*f*
Endometrial morphofunctional potential 229
Endometrial myometrial interface 190, 190*f*
Endometrial nitric oxide synthase 403
Endometrial polyps 13, 231, 235, 252, 390
Endometrial preparation and biopsy 244
Endometrial receptivity 243, 248
analysis 243, 244, 245*f*
clinical outcome 244
indications 244
test 243, 245*t*, 246
array 254
biomarkers of 234
defective 254
Endometrial receptors, activity of 229
Endometrial regeneration 556
Endometrial responsiveness 240
Endometrial scratching 230, 231, 253, 418
Endometrial stimulation 493
Endometrial thickness 177, 199, 230, 236, 237*f*, 240
higher 180
measurement of 156*f*
Endometrial transcriptomics 243
Endometrial vascularity
pulse Doppler of 192*f*
zones 192*f*
Endometrial volume 193
calculating 193*f*
Endometriosis 14, 58, 59, 62, 113, 116, 198, 235, 373, 389, 479
classification 60
concomitant 68
diagnosis 59
incidence 58
possible sites of 58
signs 59
symptoms 59
with infertility, management of 60
Endometriotic cystectomy 116
effects of 116
Endometritis 243
chronic 229, 254
Endometrium 6, 45, 84, 155, 170, 171, 180, 229, 230, 240, 253, 342, 380, 390, 556
affects implantation 236
basalis layer of 7

B-mode features of 190
causes thin 235
changes in 161
Doppler features of 191
functional 97
grade A 191*f*
grade B 191*f*
highly receptive 459
hormonal support of 6
maternal 337, 339
morphology of 190
physiology of 234
receptive 177
refractory 556
thickness of 492
thin 234, 389
three-dimensional imaging of 237
transcervical resection of 106
treatment options thin 237
volume ultrasound assessment of 193
Endomyometrial
functional zone 76
junction 167*f*, 168*f*, 171
Endosalpingitis 54
Endoscopy 49, 123
medicolegal aspects of 121
Endothelial growth factor, vascular 209, 409, 419, 487
Endothelial progenitor cells 556
Endotoxin level testing 280
Energy source, primary 283
Environmental sensors 273
Enzyme
acrosin 7
hydrolytic 291, 561
thyroid peroxidase 25
use of 252
Epidermal growth factor 418
Epididymal sperm aspiration, microsurgical 471
Epididymis 251, 561
examination of 17
Epididymo-orchitis, chronic 131
Epilepsy 491
Equilibration solution 463, 477
Equilibrium cooling 461
Erectile dysfunction 556
Escherichia coli 568
Estradiol 11, 244, 492, 505
levels 174
remove 8
progesterone, exogenous 389
valerate, administration of 389
Estrogen 230, 402, 406, 409
exogenous 238
receptor
inhibitor 69, 71
modulator, selective 69, 70, 133, 176
secretion resumes 179
sensitive
cancers 218
tumors 218
Estrogenic stimulation 253
Etanercept 442
Ethambutol 50
Ethylene glycol 471, 484
Ethylenediaminetetraacetic acid 284
Ethylnorgestrienone 70
Euploid embryos, selecting 340
European Society for Gynaecological Endoscopy 75, 166
European Society of Human Reproduction and Embryology 197, 224, 265, 278, 426, 520
European Union Tissue and Cells Directive 278
Extracellular ice formation 473
Extracytoplasmic
defects 297
deformities 297
structures, absence of 294
Extrauterine sac 450

F

Facility monitoring system 273
Fallopian tube 45, 50, 56, 88, 252, 283, 338*f*, 444
patency, assessment of 88
right 48*f*
transports 88
Falloposcopy 89
Familial adenomatous polyposis 516
Fatspers, functions of 561
Female genital tuberculosis 45, 47*b*, 49*f*, 50, 50*f*, 51*t*
clinical features 46
diagnosis 46
endometrial factors 46
epidemiology of 45
medical treatment 50
pathogenesis 45
pathology 45
treatment 50
Female infertility 540
causes of 10*f*
Female reproductive tract 561
Fertility 29, 40
causes of 479
enhancing
hysteroscopic surgery 108
laparoscopic surgeries 113
preservation 353, 470, 477, 502
counseling about 471
methods 484*t*
techniques 484
restoration 40
treatment 3, 457
Fertilization 8, 337, 559, 561
failed oocytes 369
failure 318, 319
rates 266
repetitive 490
Fertilize mammalian 555
Fertilized egg implants 444
Fetal
cells 434
chromosomal abnormalities 354
DNA sequences, paternally-inherited 435
extraembryonic membranes 302
growth restriction, severe symmetrical 433
heartbeat 456
reduction 453, 454, 457*t*
different methods of 456
perform 454
routes and methods of 455
stem cells 356
tendency 431
Fibrinolytics 229
Fibroblast endometrial stromal cells 234
Fibroids 75, 76, 109, 155*f*, 156*t*, 159*t*, 235, 243, 252, 253, 373
and adenomyosis on ultrasound 165*f*
classification of 166
diagnosis 109
FIGO classification of 166, 166*f*
large submucous 167*f*
mapping 168
steps for 169
measurement of 170
on fertility 109
posterior wall 165*f*
relationship of 170
typical ultrasonography features of 165
ultrasound mapping of 164
Fibronectin 234
FIGO leiomyoma subclassification system 76*f*
Fimbrial block 118
First embryo transfer attempt 503
First trimester
blood loss 398
reduction 454
screening 431, 434, 435
Fitz-Hugh-Curtis syndrome 50*f*, 55*f*
Fixed multiple dose
protocol 449
regimen 449
Flap method, triple 72
Fluconazole 230
Fluorescence in situ hybridization 250, 354, 390, 521, 523, 524, 524*f*, 530, 535, 538
Fluoxetine 36

Fluvoxamine 36
Follicle
atresia of smaller 179
culture 481, 487, 488
Doppler parameters of 189
multiple 185
number per ovary 158
selection, single dominant 212*f*
stimulating hormone 5, 12, 30, 35, 131, 133, 138, 139, 142, 173, 174, 175*f*, 182, 185, 197, 205*f*, 207, 207*f*, 207*t*, 211, 212*f*, 216, 388, 417, 425, 481, 492, 505
basal serum 221
elevated 352
high 331
recombinant 204, 209
Follicular antrum 294
Follicular aspiration 411
Follicular assessment 188
volume ultrasound for 187
Follicular characteristics assessment 162
Follicular culture 488
Follicular development 158, 417, 486
Follicular fluid 373
concentrations 188
contents of 321
Follicular growth 222
moment of 316
Follicular monitoring 185, 214
Follicular number 223
Follicular phase 5, 6, 6*f*
early 222, 483
Follicular quality 188
Follicular start, late 217
Follicular viability 483
Follicular volume 187
calculation of 187*f*
Follicular wall 294
Folliculogenesis 5, 175*f*
optimal 416
Formaldehydes 286
Four-cell embryo 299*f*
Fragile X syndrome 520
Fragmentation, amount of 299
Freezing
methods 479
protocols 485
technique 472
temperature, effects of 470
Fresh embryo transfer 388, 522, 536
Frozen
assisted reproductive treatment 397*t*
embryo transfer 388, 404, 428, 456, 457, 459, 468, 557
human embryo 353, 459
semen
sample, thawing of 461
transport of 472
thawed embryo 332, 530
transfer cycles 73
thawed ovarian
cortex 354
tissue, re-implantation of 486
Fully equipped mobile cart 101*f*
Fundal
adenomyoma, large 115*f*
myoma 114*f*
subserosal fibroid 170*f*

G

Gamete
abnormal 6
and embryo morphology 291
intrafallopian transfer 283, 305
morphology 294
use of 474
Gametogenesis 5
Gardnerella vaginalis 54
Gas
composition 345
environment, triple 108
storage room 262
Gastrointestinal tract 58
Gel over capsules, advantages of 405
Gene
disorders, single 432, 515
editing 567
future trends 568
present scenario 568
technologies 568
mutation 523, 538
Genetic
aberration 557
abnormalities 429
analysis 535
counseling 432
couple 497
defect 141
diagnosis, safety of preimplantation 518
diseases 520
at birth, prevalence of 432*t*
sex-linked 549
disorders 432, 491
etiologies 129
examination 138
factors 76
information 293
laboratory 550
metabolic diseases 549
service, components of 432
testing 21
strategy for preimplantation 514
traditional preimplantation 517
Genital
bacterial vaginosis 439
examination 137
injuries 141
tract
infections 131
inflammation of upper 54
tuberculosis 48*f*, 49*f*
and infertility 46
Genome, maternal 284
Genomic hybridization 250, 537
Gentamicin 229
Gentle atraumatic transfer 379, 380
Germ cell aplasia 136
Germinal vesicle 175*f*, 316, 317, 321
breakdown 175*f*
oocyte 296*f*
transfer 312, 567
Gestation, heterotopic 414
Gestational age 457
Gestational sac development 266
Gestrinone 70
Glandular cells 554
Glandular epithelium 6
Glass pipette delivering ultraviolet 332
Globozoospermia 126, 319
Glucocorticoids 418
Glucose
6-phosphate dehydrogenase deficiency 432, 569
concentration of 283, 284
metabolism, abnormal 440
tolerance, impaired 395
Glutamate 284
Glutaraldehydes 286
Glycemic control 440
Glycerol 471
egg yolk citrate 472
Glycine 284, 471
Glycolysis, suppressing 284
Glycoproteins 330
matrix 352
Gonadal dysgenesis 490
Gonadal stromal cells 6
Gonadotropin 85*f*, 132, 175, 180, 181, 198, 199, 200, 202, 206, 218, 222, 403, 411, 425
administration 139
disadvantages 199
dose of 181, 199, 200*t*, 217
exogenous 181, 422
indications 199
long-acting 221

low dose of 212
preparations 198, 204
reducing doses of 208
releasing hormone 12, 30, 75, 173, 138, 141, 160, 175, 182, 205*f*, 207, 207*f*, 211, 221, 389, 459, 492
agonists 60, 69, 71, 77, 174, 175, 208, 253, 406
analogs 183
antagonist 77, 85, 175, 208, 223, 410
secretion 6
stimulates follicular growth, release of 179
stimulation 119, 217
treatment period 132
types of 219
Gonorrhea 492
cervical cultures for 492
Graafian follicle 6
Gradient method 307*f*
Graft-host rejection 503
Granulocyte colony stimulating factor 231, 239, 389, 442
use of 230
Granulosa cells 5, 6, 294, 295, 483
Graves' disease 29
Growth
factor 284, 556
transforming 420
hormone 35, 223, 416, 417
supplementation 207
Gynecomastia 37

H

Hemorrhage
postpartum 43, 111
torrential 502
Halloween sign 98*f*
Hamou endomat 102, 103*f*
Hamper embryo development 370
Handling media and buffers 288
Hashimoto's thyroiditis 25, 29
Hatching blastocyst 302*f*, 333
Headache 141
Heart 559
disease 395, 398, 439
Heating 261
Hegar's dilator 455
Hematospermia 138
Hematuria 138
Hemochromatosis 141
Hemoconcentration 409, 412
Hemodilution, gradual 413
Hemoglobin 239, 448
glycosylated 433
subunit beta gene 569
Hemoglobinopathies 549
Hemogram 505
Hemolytic disease, risk of 434
Hemophilia 520, 568
Hemorrhage
accidental 388
antepartum 453
Hemostasis 446
Heparin 389, 418, 487
binding peptide 487
sulfate 234
Hepatic disease, chronic 448
Hepatitis
A virus 93
B 91, 93, 363, 473
virus 93, 373, 460, 497
C 91, 93, 363, 473
virus 93, 373, 460, 497
Hepatoprotectors 230
Herbicides 128
Heritable cardiac disorders 517
Heritable neurodegenerative disorders 517
Herpes simplex virus 94
High efficiency particulate air 261, 312, 313*f*, 541
filters 280
High performance liquid chromatography 147
High resolution next generation technologies 518
High security straws 94
High anti-Müllerian hormone 388
Histamine 409
Hormonal cycle, normal 556
Hormonal hyperstimulation 341
Hormonal therapy 69, 70
Hormone 35
analysis 21*t*
replacement therapy
cycle 234
protocol 245*f*
Hormonogenesis 5
Human albumin eliminates, recombinant 284
Human Andrology and Embryology Laboratories, guidelines for 278
Human chorionic gonadotropin 6, 36, 133, 159, 182, 209, 218*f*, 244, 253, 361, 375, 389, 406, 410, 418, 432, 433, 434, 449
secreting tumors 29
supplementation 139
Human embryo
culture 535
implantation of 337
metabolism, study of 355
Human embryonic
secretome 356
stem cells 356
Human fertilization 468
and Embryology Authority 264, 368
Human herpes viruses 94
Human immunodeficiency
infection 568
virus 91, 92, 363, 373, 473, 492, 497, 569
infection 45
screen for 460
Human leukocyte antigen 505, 516
Human menopausal gonadotropin 133, 175*f*, 211
Human menotropin, highly purified 223
Human oocyte
biopsy of 312*t*
cryopreservation 353
fertilization of 312*t*
mature 294
Human papilloma virus 93
strain 502
Human placental lactogen 35
Human Preimplantation Embryo Development 284
Human reproduction and embryology 248
Human Research Ethics Committees 540
Human sperm
foundation for cryopreservation of 470
preserving medium 472
Human spermatozoa, cryopreservation of 460
Human T-cell lymphotropic virus 473, 492
Human tripronuclear zygotes 568
Human uterus transplant 506
Huntington's disease 520, 566, 568
Hyalobarrier gel 231
Hyaluronan 284, 285
enriched medium 284
Hyaluronic acid 150, 308
dynamic secretion of 294
Hyaluronidase 291
enzyme 295
assists 291
Hydrocele 141
Hydroflotation 117*f*
Hydrosalpinx 118, 119, 157*f*, 243, 373, 572*f*
Hydroxyethyl cellulose 13
Hygroma, cystic 433
Hyperandrogenemia 82
Hyperandrogenic state 235
Hyperandrogenism 439
Hyperemia 45
Hyperestrogenic endometrium 191
Hyperfunctioning ovarian teratomas 29
Hyperkinesis 29
Hyperosmolar glucose, local injection of 450
Hyperprolactinemia 35, 36, 38, 439
causes of 36
clinical manifestations of 36

diagnosis of 37, 38*fc*
drug-induced 36, 37
management of 37, 38*fc*
Hyper-responders, treatment strategy for 208
Hyperstimulation syndrome 426
Hypertension 388, 395, 439
essential 398
Hyperthyroidism 29, 29*b*, 30, 439
causes of 29*b*
correction of 30
hormonal changes in 30*t*
signs in 29*b*
subclinical 29
Hypogonadism 556
hypogonadotropic 130, 141
Hypogonadotropic hypogonadism, congenital 125
Hyponatremia 412
Hypopituitarism, risk of 38
Hypoproteinemia 409
Hypospermatogenesis 319
Hypothalamic dysfunction 178
Hypothalamic pituitary
gonadal axis 40
lesions 36
ovarian axis 173, 234
testicular axis 125
testis axis, sex steroid suppression of 141
Hypothalamus 37*fc*
pituitary ovary axis 8
produces 7
Hypothyroidism 25, 27, 36, 37, 439
causes of 26*t*
clinical evaluation in 28*fc*
hormonal changes in 26*t*
signs of 26*t*
subclinical 25, 27
symptoms of 26*t*
Hypovolemia, intravascular 409
Hysterectomy 69, 446
Hysterosalpingo-contrast sonography 13, 89
Hysterosalpingogram 450
Hysterosalpingography 12, 13, 48*f*, 88, 92, 108, 158
Hysteroscope
matching cervical OS, oval shape of 104*f*
modified 103
Hysteroscopic
morcellation device 107
polypectomy, operative 110
procedures 71
resection 71
tubal cannulation under laparoscopic guidance 118
Hysteroscopy 92, 101, 447
glycine in 121
role of 108
routine 108
virtual 166*f*

I

Ideal ovarian reserve test 11*b*
Imatinib 219
Immune cell 333
compartments 234
Immune modulators 253
Immunoglobulin 234
intravenous 255, 441
Immunosuppressant drugs 508*t*
Immunosuppression 507
level of 507
prolonged 509
Impaired implantation 59
Implantation 162, 252
personalized window of 243
window of 243
Impotence 37
In situ hybridization 513
In vitro activation, chances of 487
In vitro fertilization 1, 19, 50, 56, 68, 88, 92, 108, 133, 134, 142, 154, 197, 204, 211, 243, 246, 248, 264, 270, 283, 295, 305, 315, 318, 332, 345, 360, 361*t*, 368, 369, 372, 377, 388, 422, 428, 447, 453, 457, 471, 490, 503, 520, 530, 535, 562
and embryo transfer 394
baby 351
color Doppler in 162
conventional 316
cycle of 46, 218
development of 1
efficiency 528
embryo transfer 384
failure 332, 491
repeated 496
integral part of 476
laboratory 261, 278, 279, 368, 371
location of 541
natural cycle 223, 315
pretreatment of 416
program 277
sperm preparation for 316
treatment 402
In vitro maturation 86, 457, 481, 484, 488
newer methods of 487
selected group for 353
Incubators 280, 285
time lapse 273
Indemnity insurance, role of 123
Indian Council for Medical Research 2, 278, 470
Indian Society for Assisted Reproduction 3
Indocyanine green mapping 573
Indomethacin 212
Infections 219, 440
control 363
Infertile
couples 173
evaluation of 16
Infertility 9, 25, 26, 31, 35, 40, 58, 59, 68, 75, 96, 140, 154, 211, 402, 501, 540
anovulatory 42
baseline scan in 154
branch of 368
clinics
minimum requirement of staff in 543
primary 540
secondary 540
tertiary 540
etiology of 459
immunological 131
management of 134*f*
mechanism of 76
robotics in 570
treatment
integral role in 479
rate of 355
unexplained 178, 197, 198, 354
Inflammation, immunohistochemical signs of 229
Inflammatory bowel disease, severe 442
Infliximab 442
Inhibin
A 174, 434
B 21
Inner cell mass 301, 330, 339*f*, 522, 536
grade 301*t*
infolding of 158*f*
large 302*f*
morphology 301
quality of 345
Insemination 3, 318, 371
duration of 318
media for 318
method of 318
time of 318
Insulin
like growth factor 417
sensitizers 42, 175, 180
sensitizing agents 83, 178
Integrins 234
Intensive luteal phase support 208
Interferon, ratio of 442
Interleukin 404, 409
Internal quality control 267
International Committee for Monitoring Assisted Reproductive Technology 3
International Federation of Fertility Societies 3

International Federation of Gynaecology and Obstetrics 76, 166
International normalized ratio 448
Intervention, minimal surgical 69
Intracellular
  components, intracellular environment on 471
  homeostasis 271
  ice crystal formation 462
Intracytoplasmic morphologically selected sperm injection 251, 308, 325, 351
Intracytoplasmic sperm injection 18, 28, 132-134, 197, 214, 246, 250, 270, 280, 283, 295, 305, 312, 315, 319, 320*f*, 326*f*, 346, 351, 361, 363*f*, 364, 365, 365*f*, 370, 416, 424, 457, 459, 471, 478, 503, 521, 522, 536, 545
  manipulators 362*f*
  technique 319, 322, 326
    physiological 310
Intralipid 419, 441
  infusion 256
Intramural fibroids 253
Intrauterine
  adhesions 101, 111, 231, 253
  Bigatti shaver 106
  contraceptive device 440
  death 433
  device 231
  fibroids 101
  granulocyte-colony stimulating factor 253
  insemination 63, 92, 110, 133, 134, 154, 187, 189, 197, 198, 200, 201, 417, 456, 457, 471, 543
    complications 201
    factors for 197
    indications 197
    lab, setting up of 202
    semen cryopreservation for 461
    timing 200
    variables affecting 197
  instillation 389
  pregnancy 240, 420, 448
    presence of 448
  pressure 103
  system 69
Intravaginal progesterone, types of 404
Intravascular volume, symptoms of 412
Intrinsic embryonic lysine 331
Invasive techniques 22, 354
Iodine administration, exogenous 29
Ischemic time 506
Isoechoic homogeneous grade C endometrium 191*f*
Isoniazid 50
Isopropanol 287
Isthmocele 96, 97*f*, 98*f*, 111
  diagnosis 96
  future pregnancy 98
  future trends 99
  intraoperative laparoscopic excision and repair of 98*f*
  investigations 97
  pathophysiology 97
  presentation 96
  prevalence 96
  risk factors 97
  treatment 97

K

Kallmann's syndromes 17, 125, 136
Karman's cannula 455
Kartagener's syndrome 17
Karyotypes, normal 520
Ketamine 563
Keyhole surgery 121
Kidney
  absent 433
  functions 413, 505
  problem 395, 398
Kinetic markers 348, 348*t*
Kinetic parameters 346, 348
Klinefelter's syndrome 17, 137, 139, 143*f*, 568
Koninckx and Martin classification 60

L

Lactate 283
Laminar air flow 280*f*
Laparoscopic
  adenomyomectomy, steps of 115*f*
  dye test 13
  myomectomy 78, 114, 571
    preoperative evaluation before 113
    steps of 114*f*
  surgery 447, 570
    for recurrent endometriosis 116
Laparoscopy 13, 98*f*, 283, 446
  advantages of 446
  operative 447
Laparotomy 446, 447
L-arginine 208, 237, 238
Laser
  ablation 78
  assisted hatching 252, 332, 351, 352
Lasmars score 167*f*
Lectin-biofunctionalized polysilicon 369
Leiomyoma 75, 113, 502
  concomitant 68
  distorting endometrial cavity 113
Lethal embryos 333
Letrozole 84, 132, 179, 180, 180*t*, 198-200, 208, 213, 218, 219, 219*f*, 403
  effects of 199*t*
Leukemia inhibitory factor 234, 418
Leukocytosis, degree of 412
Leukocytospermia 131
  refractory 131
Levofloxacin 229
Levonorgestrel intrauterine system 69, 77
Levothyroxine 440
Li-Fraumeni syndrome 516
Light electron microscopy 332
Lipoprotein
  high density 41
  low density 41
Liquid nitrogen 273, 463, 470, 476
  reservoir 463
Live
  and deceased donors 508*t*
  birth rate 377, 410
  dysfunction 178
  enzymes, transient elevation of 450
  failure 178
  function 413, 505
    test 505
Living oocytes 296
Local hemodynamics, restoration of 229
Loop electrode 105, 110
Low birth weight 429
Low molecular weight 389, 418
  heparin 255
    use of 255
Low vitamin D levels, correction of 441
Luteal halt 217, 217*f*
Luteal phase 6
  defect 162, 439
  deficiency 178, 402, 440
  reflects 402
  start 218*f*
  support 402, 403
    modified 208
Luteinization 6
Luteinized unruptured follicle 162
Luteinizing hormone 5, 30, 41, 138, 142, 175*f*, 218*f*, 222, 426, 492, 505, 556
  addition of 207
  concentrations of 298
  concept of 176*b*
  premature 217
  recombinant 204
  secretion of 35
Luteum deteriorates 6
Lyme's disease 439
Lymphocyte immune therapy 441
Lysosomal storage diseases 568

M

Macrolides 230
Macroprolactinemia 36, 141
Macrosomia, risk of 391
Magnetic activated cell sorting 307, 308*f*
procedure 307
Magnetic microspheres 307
Magnetic resonance imaging 14, 36, 38, 67, 69, 88, 445, 505
guided focused ultrasound surgery 73, 78
Makler's chamber 460, 461
Male factor infertility, severe 354
Male fertility 43, 126*t*, 128, 128*t*, 130, 140, 460, 540, 562
genetic of 125
lifestyle factors in 126
management of 133*f*
medical management of 130, 134*f*
mild 197
severe 311
Male partner evaluation 178
Male reproductive
system 7
tract 144*f*
Mammalian development, stages of 356
Mammalian fertilization 559
Mapping fibroids, methods of 168
Masturbation 471
Maternal age 432
advanced 354, 490
Maternal circulation 434
Maternal diabetes, uncontrolled 433
Maternal risk factors 433
Maternal spindle transfer, advantages of 567
Maternal weight, low 433
Matrine 563
Maturation, stage of 479
Mature follicle, B-mode features of 185
Mayer-Rokitansky-Küster-Hauser syndrome 501
Mechanical hatching 352
Mechanical techniques 331
Medical geneticist 550
Medical organizations, role of 123
Medical termination of pregnancy 520
Medical therapy 62
Medicolegal defense, strategize 121
Medicolegal safety 122
Meiotic spindle 295
Menopause, premature 490
Menstrual cycles, irregular 40
Menstrual disturbance 99
Menstrual history 10
Menstrual phase 6
Mesterolone 131
Metabolic disease 432
Metabolic profile 178, 355
Metabolic syndrome 126, 127
Metabolomics 108, 355
techniques of 355
Metal
cannula 455
catheter 201
Metastatic disease 239
Metformin 83, 84, 180, 181, 411
role of 209
usage, indications for 83
Methotrexate 448, 449
administering single dose 449
pharmacokinetics of 448
postoperative 447
regimens in practice 449
single dose 447
therapy 448
adverse effects of 450
treatment protocols 449
Methylenetetrahydrofolate reductase mutations 254
Metronidazole 229, 230
Mibefradil 563
Michael Wolff's protocol 217
Microarrays, types of 526
Microbes, malignant 286
Microbial air
monitoring, passive 272
sampling 270
Microbial biocenosis, recurrence of 230
Microdose flare protocol 206, 213
Microflare protocol 206*f*
Microfluidics 150
chamber 150*f*
Micromanipulation
general principles of 311
history 311
section 541
technique 312
chronological development of 312*t*
of zona drilling 312
Micromanipulators 312, 314, 319
Micropipettes 314
alignment of 320*f*
Microribonucleic acids 284
Microtubule organization 286
Microwave 71
Mifepristone 77
Mild stimulation
basis of 211
benefits of 212
protocols, limitations of 214
Miliary tubercles 45
Minimally invasive surgery 121, 570
Miscarriage 40
rates 382
higher 383
recurrent 438, 439*b*, 440*f*
repeated 496
risk of 439*t*
reduced 417
unexplained recurrent 441
Miscarried developed chorioamnionitis 456
Mitochondria 7, 128
Mitochondrial deoxyribonucleic acid 126, 536, 538, 566
Mitochondrial diseases 566, 568
Mitochondrial genetic defects 125
Mitochondrial replacement therapy 312, 566, 567
disadvantages of 567
Mitochondrial sheath 293
Mock embryo transfer 380
Molecular biologists 535
Molecular technology 513
Monitoring system, time-lapse 351
Monochorionicity 454
Monochorionic-monoamniotic twins, frequency of 429
Monofollicular
growth 179
selection, permits 174
Monogenic disorders 514
Monoiodotyrosine 25*f*
Monopolar resectoscope 111
Monopolar surgery 106
Monozygotic twinning
incidence of 342
risk of 333
Monozygotic twins 341
formation of 333
Mood swings 178
Morphokinetic 340
Mosaic embryos 518
Mosaicism 523, 536
detection 531
problem of 569
Mother-to-child transmission 93
Motile sperm
count 305
organelle morphology examination 308, 352
Motile spermatozoa, isolated 326
Mouse embryo assay 280, 286
Moxifloxacin 230
Mucins 234
Mucolytic enzymes 55
Müllerian abnormalities 439
Mullerian anomalies 110, 252
Müllerian duct 501
aplasia 501
cysts 137
Müllerian remnants 66

Multicentric promise study, randomized 440
Multidrug resistant tuberculosis 45
Multifactorial conditions 432
Multifetal pregnancy 429, 457, 458
higher order 457
medical risks of 457
reduction 454, 455
benefits of 458
Multigravida 432
Multinucleation, presence of 299
Multiorgan 501
Multiple gestations, reduction in 518
Multiple oocytes develop 394
Multiple pregnancy 84, 178, 200, 266, 382, 395, 398, 433, 453
consequence of 398
contraindications for 399
higher order 394
problems with 453
rate, high 397
reduction 341
risk of 84, 394, 395
Multiple vaginal punctures 374
Multiple-doses regimen 449
Multizygotic gestations 429
Muscle cells 554
Mycobacteria 45
growth indicator 48
Mycobacterial smear and culture 48
Mycobacterium
bovis 45
tuberculosis 45, 48
Mycophenolate mofetil 508
Mycoplasma 54
genitalium 54, 230
Myoma 77, 165*f*
ablation 221
bulge 114*f*
transcervical resection of 106
Myomectomy 77, 109
abdominal 78
hysteroscopic 78, 109, 167*f*
Myometrial cysts 69
Myometrial mass 167*f*
Myometrial reduction 72
Myometrium 167*f*, 447
Myosure morcellator 107
Myosure system hysteroscope 107*f*
Myosure tissue removal system 107*f*
Myotonic dystrophy 520

N

Nandrolone 142
Nanotechnology 573
Narishige scientific instrument laboratory 311
National ART Registry of India 3
National Cancer Registry of India 481
National Health System 398
National Institute for Health and Care Excellence guidelines 252
National Institute of Standards and Technology 270
Natural conception 417, 430, 486
Natural cycle, modified 206
Natural fertility and obesity 42
Natural killer cell 76
activity 418
cytotoxicity 419
suppresses 109
Natural micronized progesterone, use of 404
Nausea 178
Neighboring blood vessels 556
Neisseria gonorrhoeae 54, 55
Neonatal intensive care 429
unit 453
Nerve cells 554
Neural tube defects 433
Neurodegenerative disorders 517
Neurogenic muscle weakness 568
Neurological diagnosis, risk of 394
Neurological problems 556
risk of 394
Neutropenia 219
Newborn
intensive care unit 43
welfare of 509
Next generation sequencing 243, 250, 441, 523, 526, 536-538
data 533
Nifedipine 563
Nitrogen dioxide 363
Non-apoptotic sperm 149*f*
selection 309
Noncommunicable disease 40
Noncommunicating horn, resection of 572*f*
Noncompliances, types of 268
Nonembryo-toxic gel 13
Nonequilibrium cooling 462
Nonhomologous end joining 568
Nonhormonal therapy 69
Noninvasive methods, newer 434
Noninvasive prenatal
diagnostic methods 433
testing 434
Nonlife saving procedure 509
Nonselective estrogen receptor 176
Non-sperm cells, products of 304
Nonsteroidal anti-inflammatory drugs 69, 77
Nonsteroidal triphenylethylene derivative 176
Nontubal ectopics, surgery for 446
Normosmic hypogonadotropic hypogonadism 125
Nuclear genome 566
Nuclear magnetic resonance spectroscopy 355
Nuclear membrane 291
Nucleation 300
Nuclei, multiple 299
Nucleotide polymorphism
arrays, single 536, 538
single 354, 523, 526, 531

O

Obesity 40, 42, 43, 127, 144, 566
anatomic 41
android 41
classification of 40, 40*t*
deleterious effects of 43
endocrine changes in 41
exercise in 43
gynecoid 41
types of 41*f*
Obstetric management 432
Obsti bag 103*f*
Obstruction, reversal of 138
Office operative hysteroscopy 103
Ofloxacin 229, 230
Oligoanovulation 82
Oligoasthenoteratozoospermia 130, 134, 134*f*
Oligoasthenozoospermic sperm samples 306
Oligomenorrhea 9, 42
Oligospermia 319
mild 140
moderate 140
severe 140
Oligozoospermia 125, 130, 140-142, 568
evaluation of 142
idiopathic 144
laboratory testing in 143
risk factors 140
severe 304
Oocyte 59, 188, 219, 298*f*, 311, 323*f*, 324*f*, 356, 370, 425, 461, 487, 542, 562
accumulation of 478
activation 322
and embryo
donation 490
indication for donation of 490
and surrogate mothers, sourcing of 494
aspiration, transabdominal 375
banking 476, 479
empowers 479
center of 324*f*
cryopreservation 224, 354, 460, 476, 478, 478, 479, 481, 482, 484, 545
application of 477

cost-effectiveness of 479
drawback of 479
efficacy of 479
era of 479
pros and cons of 479
culture 320
dish 316
cumulus
complexes 321*f*
oophorus 561
cytoplasmic quality of 311
denudation, partial 318
donation 73, 399, 490, 545
indications of 490*b*
donor
genetic screening form for 491*t*
program 479
requirements for 494
screening of 491
female 559
fertilized 299, 354
freezing 481
cryoprotectant for 477
in oocyte donors, safety of 479
techniques of 476
types, cryoprotectant for 477
grading of 316, 321
identification of 321
in vitro maturation of 353
luteinized 317*f*
maturation 411, 416
mature 6, 297*f*
metaphase II 296*f*, 323*f*
retrieved 424
maturity
grading of 295*t*, 309*t*
studies grade 295
metaphase I 296*f*
metaphase II 296*f*, 297*f*
morphology 298
nuclear
maturation 295
maturity 295
number of 12, 219, 422, 491
mature 424
partially denuded 318, 321*f*
pick-up 361
postmature 317*f*
pronucleate 283
quality of 294, 298
measure 352
recipients, screening of 492*b*
retrieval 372, 372*f*, 375, 419, 479, 503
technique 372
scanning of 321
dish 316
secreted by 561
size and quality of 479
techniques of 204
terms of 221
use of cryopreserved 353
vitrification of 464*f*, 466*f*, 478, 488
vitrified 478
with granular cytoplasm 297*f*
yield, optimal 422
Oogenesis 175*f*
Oolemma 324*f*
apparent 323*f*
binding 19
Oophorectomy 490
Oophoropexy 482
techniques like 481
Ooplasm 295, 296
Ooplasmic penetration 325
Ooplasmic transfer 312
Ophthalmoplegia 36
Optic 365
neuropathy 568
Oral contraceptive 69
pills 70, 178
Oral dydrogesterone 405
Oral estrogen 406
Oral micronized progesterone 404
Oral moxifloxacin 229
Oral ofloxacin 229
Oral ovulogens 182
Oral steroids 131
Orthotopic reimplantation, techniques of 486
Orthotopic sites 486
Osmotic shock 473
Ovarian activity, restoration of 486
Ovarian biomarkers 422
Ovarian cancer 178
Ovarian cortex
cryopreservation of 481, 484
preservation, future of 487
Ovarian cortical biopsies 486
Ovarian cortical strips cryopreservation 487
Ovarian cycle 5
physiology 8
Ovarian cysts, functional 178
Ovarian displacement 375
Ovarian drilling, laparoscopic 84, 85, 116, 117*f*, 183
Ovarian failure
after chemotherapy 491
after radiotherapy 491
premature 481, 490, 491, 555, 557
Ovarian follicle
development of 174
reserve 483
Ovarian function 486
and fertility 175
Ovarian hormone 240
production 219
Ovarian hyperstimulation 27, 181
aspirin in 410
critical 413
protocols 367
random-start controlled 217
risk of 410
syndrome 11, 82, 159, 178, 199, 204, 205*f*, 207*f*, 219, 266, 353, 373, 388, 409, 410, 412, 412*fc*, 468
classification of 410*t*
high risk of 410
lower risk of 212
pathogenesis of 409, 409*fc*, 412
prevention 410
risk of 353
treatment of 412, 413
types of 410
Ovarian pathologies 158
Ovarian pregnancy 447
Ovarian reserve 116
and function, status of 481
compromised 490
markers 12*t*
of females restricts, non-renewable 481
tests 11, 206, 216
abnormality 221
Ovarian responders, poor 205
Ovarian response 216
prediction of 204, 204*b*, 221
Ovarian stimulation 173, 207*f*, 217, 298, 503
conventional 213, 217, 217*f*, 411
initially 341
protocol 217
mild 211
Ovarian tissue 484
banking 481
collection of 483
cryopreservation of 354, 481, 487, 488, 545
indication for 481
techniques of 483
freezing 481
grafting 486, 486*t*
reimplantation, advantages of 486
transplantation of 353, 486, 573
vitrification of 487
Ovarian torsion 414
Ovarian transposition 482
Ovariectomy, bilateral 354
Ovary 46, 157
changes in 160
cryopreservation, whole 487
dermoid cyst on 572*f*
inaccessible for egg retrieval 490
Overt hyperthyroidism 29
Ovulation 556
confirmation of 158

inducing drugs, doses of 175
induction 83, 85*f*, 173, 175, 200, 315, 403
complication of 409
drugs 198
evolution of 174
mechanism of 6
physiology of 174
rate 84
stimulation 162
tests of 10
trigger 185, 208
Ovulatory abnormalities 59
Ovulatory dysfunction 197
Ovulatory function 10
Ovum pick up 286, 316, 372
difficult 374
trolley 373*f*
preparation of 373
Ovum quality 186
Oxygen 273, 285
Oxygenation 486

P

Pain, abdominal 450
Parkinson's disease 20, 566
Paroxetine 36
Patau syndrome 432
Patency of distal segment, confirmation of 119
Patent ductus arteriosus 395
Peak systolic velocity 161
Peculiar pharmacokinetics 223
Peginterferon-alpha 93
Pelvic infection, high risk of 375
Pelvic inflammatory disease 54, 56, 113, 444
clinical manifestation 55
diagnostic procedures 56
etiology 54
pathogenesis 54
prevention 56
risk factors 54
signs 55
treatment 56
Pelvic pain 96, 99
Pelvic pathology 373
Pelvic venous system, bilateral 48*f*
Penetration air, ultra-low 280
Penis, examination of 137
Pentane 287
Pentoxifylline 231, 237, 238, 240
Peptic ulcer disease 448
Percutaneous epididymal sperm aspiration 138, 319, 471
Performing micromanipulation, concept of 314
Periconceptional period 433
Perifollicular blood flow 162*f*
Perifollicular resistance index 186
Perihepatic adhesions 50*f*
Perimenopausal women, production of pregnancy in 490
Perinatal mortality, higher 398
Peripartum hysterectomy 502
Peritoneal factors 14
Peritoneal fluid, presence of 486
Peritoneal function 59
Peritoneum 46
Perivitelline space 294, 297
of oocyte 311
Permeable cryoprotectants 460, 460*t*
minimize crystallization 477
Pesticides 128
Petri dish containing culture medium 315
Phenotypes, different types of 82*t*
Phosphate buffered saline 147
Phosphatidylserine 151
Phospholipid phosphatidylserine 307
Phthalate 128
compounds 128
Physical and mental risks 509
Piezo micromanipulation 252
Piezo technology 332
Pills 497
Pioglitazone 83
Pipette, microinjection 322*f*, 324*f*
Pituitary
adenoma 36, 141
dysfunction 178
tumors 36, 37
Placenta
accreta 96
previa 96, 395, 429
Placental abruption 395
Placental formation 234
Placentation, abnormal 388
Plasma
electrolytes 413
membrane 291
Platelet activate 419
Platelet-rich plasma 239, 420
infusion, autologous 230, 231
treatment 239*f*
Plumbing system 262
Pluripotent stem cells 356
Pneumonitis 450
Polar body
biopsy 521, 530
nuclear transfer 567
Polar nuclei 361
Polarization microscopy 352
Pollution 129
Poloscope, use of 352
Polychlorinated biphenyls 128
Polycystic kidney 433
disease 568
Polycystic ovarian morphology 82
Polycystic ovarian syndrome 1, 36, 37, 40, 42, 80, 81, 82*t*, 113, 173, 174, 180, 197, 353, 388, 416, 439
clinical presentation of 81
different phenotypes of 81
etiology of 81*f*
etiopathogenesis of 80
evolutionary
advantages of 80*f*
disadvantages of 80*f*
management plan of 83*f*
Polycystic ovary 388
Polyethylene oxide-sodium carboxymethylcellulose gel 231
Polymerase chain reaction 49, 92, 125, 126, 513, 524, 531
analysis 354
quantitative 523, 538
real-time quantitative 526, 537
Polymorphism, single-nucleotide 522
Polypectomy 231
hysteroscopic 110
Polypoid adenomyoma 67
Polypoid adenomyosis 67
Polyps 101, 109, 159*t*
adenomyomatous 67
hysteroscopic polypectomy of 110
large 106
Pomeroy's technique 120
Poor ovarian response, Bologna criteria for 222
Poor responders, benefits in 213
Poseidon-based stratification 426
Postacrosomal region 293
Postcompaction embryo 284, 284*t*
Postejaculate urine examination 20
Postfertilization 291
Postintrauterine insemination supplementation 202
Postmenstrual spotting 96
Postthaw survival rates 468*t*
Potassium
chloride 454, 455
injection 450
Precompaction embryo 284, 284*t*
Preconception counseling 430
Preconception diagnosis 515
Predinisolone 131
Preeclampsia 395, 429, 453
risk of 428
Pregnancy 43, 123
abdominal 447

after assisted reproductive technology 428
associated plasma protein A 434
biochemical 390, 391
complete loss of 454
cumulative 177
early 390
failure 490
heterotopic 447, 450
induced diabetes 395
induced hypertension 394, 395
interstitial 445, 446
loss 221
complete 456
early 68, 429
recurrent 402, 433, 441*t*
repetitive spontaneous 354
role of infection in recurrent 440
maintenance of 419
multifetal 457
of unknown location 445
outcome 64, 428
rate 84, 192, 342, 396*t*, 397*t*
biochemical 346
clinical 346
higher 383
low 389
reported high 352
screening in 431
spontaneous 486
termination, previous 68
test 410
Preimplantation development 330
stages of 355
Preimplantation genetic
diagnosis 248, 340, 351, 354, 521, 531, 535, 550
screening 108, 249, 339, 351, 354, 468, 520, 531
testing 311, 354, 513, 515, 520, 532, 534, 535
future of 534
Preimplantation human embryo 283
Prelabor rupture of membranes, premature 454
Premature birth, risk of 395
Premature delivery 395
Prenatal diagnosis 433
Prenatal diagnostic techniques 549
Prenatal screening in pregnancy 431
Prenatal sex determination 551
Prenatal testing, indications for 433
Preovulatory follicle 158, 186*f*, 188*f*
Preovulatory uterine artery waveform 193*f*
Prepubertal girls 481
Pressure symptoms 68
Preterm birth 429, 395
incidence of 429
Preterm deliveries 453
spontaneous 429
Preterm labor 454
incidence of 429
Preterm prelabor rupture of membrane 398, 453
Pretesticular azoospermia 136
acquired causes of 136
congenital causes of 136
Primigravida 432
Primitive cells types 356
Primordial follicles 483, 487
culture of 487
Progestational agents 69
Progesterone 402, 403, 406
administration of 405, 405*f*
routes of 404
capsules 405
depot injection 455
dose 492
exogenous 406
gel 405
in oil 404
natural 405
nongenomic receptor 562
pills 497
preparation 404
receptor 70
modulators, selective 69, 70
rise, premature 389
supplementation, duration of 405
Progestins 69, 70
Programmable freezers 472
Progressive motility 130, 140
Prolactin 35, 37, 138, 142
functions 35
release-inhibiting factor 35
secreting pituitary adenoma 36
Prolactinomas 38
Proline 284
Pronase 352
Pronuclear transfer 312, 567
Pronucleus formation 19
Propanediol 484
Prophylactic antibiotics 454
Prophylactic tocolysis 455
Propylthiouracil 30
Prostaglandin 409
Prostate, examination of 17
Prostatectomy surgery 556
Protein
crispr-associated 568
supplementation 284
Proteoglycan 234
Proteomics 355
application of 355
Prototype micromanipulators 311
Proximal tubal block 118
Pseudo blocks 89
Psychological distress related with infertility 540
Psychology 431
Psychosis 29
Pulmonary disease
active 448
chronic 439
Pulmonary tuberculosis 45
Pulsatile gonadotropin-releasing hormone therapy 182
Pulse Doppler 186*f*
analysis 193
Pyrazinamide 50
Pyridostigmine 208
Pyruvate, concentration of 283

Q

Quadruple test 434
Qualitative defects 126*t*
Quality assurance 264, 544
Quality control 264, 265, 544
Quality management 266
culture 265
programs, total 264, 265
system 277
Quantitative defects 125*t*
Quartz fiber delivering infrared 332
Quinidine 563

R

Radiation therapy 490
Radical procedures 69
Radioactive iodine 31
Radiofrequency identification 369, 370
based systems 370*t*
system 369, 370*f*
technology 269
Radioiodine 31
Radiotherapy 141, 470
and ovarian damage 483
Raffinose 471
Raloxifene 179
Randomized controlled trial 214, 250
Random-start protocol 217
Reactive oxygen species 132, 473
estimation 20
Rebound theory 131
Recipient and donor screening 505
Recipient surgery procedure 506, 507*b*
Rectovaginal endometriosis 67
Rectovaginal lesions 62
Recurrent implantation failure 230, 243, 245*t*, 248, 249, 419

etiology 249
incidence 249
Recurrent miscarriage 403, 438
etiology 438
incidence 438
recurrence risk 438
treatment 439
Regimen
single-dose 449
two-dose 449
Regulation and Prevention of Misuse Act 549
Remote monitoring systems 272*t*
Renal agenesis, unilateral 501
Renal and liver function tests 448
Renal anomalies 433
Renal disease, chronic 439
Renal function test 505
Renal system 501
Renin angiotensin system 409
Reproductive
disorders 35
endocrinology 173
history 16
medicine 1
bills 3
tourism 527
outcome 73
physiology, role in 35
tissues 479
tract 58
Resectoscope 105, 106*f*
working element of 106*f*
Resectoscopic surgery, different settings for 103
Residual trophoblastic disease 445
Respiratory distress syndrome 398
active 413
Retinitis pigmentosa 568
Retinoblastoma 516
Retrograde ejaculation 137
evaluation of 20
Retroperitoneal adenomyosis 67
RhD-negative women 450
Rhesus sensitization, severe 439
Ribavirin 93
Ribonucleic acid transcripts, maternal 251
Rifampicin 50
therapy of 50
Robertsonian translocations 249
chromosomal aberrations like 568
Robotic assisted adenomyoma excision 73
Robotic surgery 570, 573
history of 570
Rosiglitazone 83
Ru 486 77
Rubella 440
Rudimentary horn pregnancy 447

S

Sacrococcygeal teratoma 433
Saline infusion
sonography 13
sonohysterography 109
Salpingectomy 119, 445, 446
bilateral 119
laparoscopic 446, 450
laparotomy for 446
partial 446
total 446
Scar
dehiscence 96
ectopic 96
surgical 58
Screening strategies, types of 435
Screening, pyramid of 431
Scrotal color Doppler 22, 22*f*
Scrotal fungal dermatitis, chronic 130
Scrotal palpation 137
Scrotal ultrasound 22
Scrotum
clinical examination of 17*f*
transillumination of 17
Second trimester
reduction 454
screening 431, 434-436
Secretory phase 6, 7
Selectins 234
Self-blood glucose monitoring 440
Semen
analysis 18, 92, 142, 142*f*, 142*fc*, 143
classification based on 18
normal 140
parameters, normal 19*t*
standard 145
banking 470
indications 470
banks 473
classification 143*t*
culture 20
examination 137
factors 439
freezing of 545
fructose in 19, 138
parameter 129
pH 138
preparation
methods of 202
techniques 200
quality 140
sample, use of cryopreserved 474
volume 130, 137
Seminal plasma 304, 308, 561
like prostaglandins 304
Seminal vesicles, normal ultrasound anatomy of 23*f*
Septate 13
Septum 390
Sequential culture media 287
Sequential screening 435
Serine 284
Serotonin reuptake inhibitors 36
Sertoli cell only syndrome 136, 319
Serum
albumin 284
alpha fetoprotein, maternal 433, 434
anti-Müllerian hormone level 11
concentration 404
follicle-stimulating hormone 11
gonadotropin 128
growth hormone 178
progesterone 10
levels 177, 389
prolactin levels, normal 37
thyroid-stimulating hormone 440
Sex chromatin 513
Sex determination illegal 548
Sex hormone binding globulin 30, 82, 141
Sex selection 549
prohibition of 549
Sex steroid
levels 128
production, endogenous 142
Sexual characteristics, maintain secondary 556
Sexual dysfunction 16, 37
Sexually transmitted disease
complications of 54
organisms 55
screened for 473
Sexually transmitted infections, incidence of 1
Sexually transmitted viruses 93
Shanghai protocol 217, 218
Sibutramine 83
Sickle cell
anemia 356, 568
disease 520, 432
Sildenafil 231, 239
Single cell 249
Singleton
pregnancies 394
proportion of 429
rates of 429
Sinusitis, triad of 137
Sion test 158
Skin cells 554
Slow freezing 467*t*, 476
method 460, 461
Smoking amongst women 444
Smooth cavity 159*f*

Social and economic implications 454
Society for Assisted Reproductive Technologies 265, 476
Society for maternal-fetal medicine 521, 531
Sodium chloride 454
Solid organ transplant 509
Somatic cell nucleus, transfer of 351, 356
Sono-based automated volume calculation 161*f*
Sonography-based automated volume count 160
Sonohysterography 14, 14*f*, 92, 159, 168
  cavity lesion on 160*f*
  nomenclature 159*f*
Sonosalpingography 158
Sperm 92, 323*f*, 555, 559
  acrosome 128
  axonemal structure 294*f*
  birefringence 308
  cells 561
  charge selection 308
  chromatin
    dispersion assay 145, 149
    structure assay 145, 149
  collection, methods of 471
  components of 292*f*
  concentration 130, 140, 318
  counts 129
  cryopreservation of 460
  deposition 325
  DNA fragmentation 20, 145
    causes of 146
    clinical consequences of 146
  DNA organization 146*f*
  during oocyte retrieval, nonavailability of 478
  egg membrane fusion 293
  factor 250
  flagella, multiple morphological abnormalities of 126
  function and semen, specialized test of 20
  head 291
    ultrastructure of 291
    vacuolated 326*f*
  hyperactivation 561
  immobilized 322*f*
  incubation 542
  injection 326*f*
    morphologically selected 150, 351
    technique 326
  low number of 130
  macrocephaly 126
  mitochondria 566
  morphology 291
    and vacuoles 327
  neck, ultrastructure of 293
  number, total 140
  optimization of 133*f*
  parameters 130*t*
  pH increases 561
  preparation
    advanced methods for 308
    method 150
  preparation techniques 304, 305
    choice of method 304
    general principles 305
  production 144
  promoting 562
  retrieval, surgical 471
  selection
    and immobilization 322
    approach 309
    mature 309
    method 150
  separation 151*f*, 304
    efficiency of 304
  shape, abnormal 130
  sorting using magnetic separator 151
  survival test 280
  transfer, microinjection 311
  ultrastructure of 291
  viability 97
  vitalizers 132
  wash technique 92
Spermatocyte produces four sperms, single 567
Spermatogenesis 7, 30, 125*t*, 126*t*
  inhibition of 129
  transient suppression of 31
Spermatozoa 125, 148*f*, 322, 330
  defects 125
  manipulate 311
Spermatozoon 293
Spinal anesthesia, under 456
Spinal muscular atrophy 432
Spindle transfer 312
  maternal 567
Spongiosum 6
Sporadic miscarriages 438
Standard operating
  procedure 281, 543
  protocols 264
Standard scoring system 378
Standardized Training Programs 267
Stem cell 356, 554*f*, 555
  adult 555
  application of 554
  embryonic 356
  enriched cord blood 356
  harvest and infusion 555
  hematopoietic 356, 555
  in infertility, role of 555
  infusion 555
  research on 554
  special 555
  therapy 239
  transplantation
    indication 516
    therapies 356
Sterile transfer pipette 321
Sterilization reversal 119
Sterilization surgery, laparoscopic 122
Stimulation protocols 216, 479
  minimal 206
Storage technique 472
Streptococcus fecalis 131
Stress 126
Stromal cells 256
Structure of Catsper 560*f*
Structure of sperm 291*f*
Styrene 286
Subfertility 1, 4, 40
  treatment options for 1
Submucous
  fibroid 13, 109
  myoma 109, 166, 166*f*
    classification of 166, 167*t*
  polyps 243
Subrogare 496
Subzonal insemination 312, 319
Sucrose 471
Superovulation 173
Surgery
  complications of 30
  risk of 84
Surgical therapy 62
Surrogacy 256, 496, 498, 546*f*
  arrangement, part of 497
  clinics, registration of 499
  commercial 498
  facts on 547, 547*f*
  guidelines of 540, 545
  history of 546
  indications for 496
  issues related to 498
  Laws in India 547
  pregnancy 498
  process 496
  professionals 497
  psychological impact with 498
  traditional 496
  types of 546*f*
Surrogate 497
  age of 497
  and genetic mother, synchronizing cycles of 497
  embryo transfer 497
  house 498
  mother 547
  obstetrics care of 498

preparing 497
prospective 497
source of 497
Swim-up
and density-gradient centrifugation 304
method 305, 305*f*
Synechiae 13
Syphilis 492
Syringe-catheter complex 379
Systemic conditions 439
Systemic syphilis 439
Systolic hypertension 29

T

T helper cell, proinflammatory 234
Tacrolimus 508
Tamoxifen 70, 131, 176, 179, 218
based protocol 218
citrate 131
therapy 68
T-cell lymphotropic viruses 93
Technologies evaluating embryos 354, 355
Telescopes 103
small diameter 103
Telesurgery 573
Temperature 273, 280, 286
Teratozoospermia 130, 304, 319
Testicular examination 137
Testicular failure, secondary 141
Testicular sperm 251
aspiration 138, 251, 471, 556
extraction 138, 319, 471
Testicular weights 129
Testis, bilateral 137
Testosterone 138
gel 417
Tetracyclines 230
Thawing 472
solution 463
Theca cells 6
Thermal balloon 71
Thermochrons 270
Thermosafe warm air system 313
Thiazolidinediones 83
Thioamides 30
Threatened miscarriage 403
Thromboembolic events 219
Thrombophilia 254
acquired 243
inherited 439
Thymoglobulin 508
Thyroid 25
autoantibody-positive euthyroid 28
autoimmunity 26
carcinoma, metastatic differentiated 29
disorders 25
dysfunction 440
follicular cell against electrochemical gradient 25
function 27
hormones, formation of 25*f*
peroxidase 25*f*
antibody 28
profile 138
stimulating hormone 25, 25*f*, 28, 31, 38, 198, 492
secreting tumors 29
Thyroiditis, acute 29
Thyrotoxicosis
evaluation of 31*fc*
factitia 29
Thyrotropin-releasing hormone 35, 37
Thyroxine 25*f*
Tissue 356
compartments, integrity of 483
culture dish 463
injuries, acute 356
matrix, extracellular 487
TNF-alpha blockers 442
Tocopherol 237
Toluidine blue 147
Topography 160, 167
Toxic
multinodular goiter 29
nodule, solitary 29
Toxicity of one cryoprotectant 459
Toxins, environmental 439
Toxoplasmosis 439, 440
Trachelectomy 502
Transabdominal reduction 455
disadvantages 455
procedure 455
Transabdominal ultrasound 168
Transcervical aspiration 455
disadvantages 455
procedure 455
Transcervical method 455
Transcriptome, characterization of 356
Transcutaneous electrical acupoint stimulation 384
Transdermal form 230
Transplantation, ephemeral 509
Transrectal ultrasonography 138
Transsphenoidal surgery 38
Transvaginal sonography 14, 108, 154, 449
technical aspects of 154
Transvaginal technique 455
Transvaginal ultrasonography 10
Transvaginal ultrasound
three-dimensional 14, 69
volume measurement, two-dimensional 69
Trauma 141
endometrial 68
Tri-gas incubators 273
Trigonellae semen 563
Triiodothyronine 25, 25*f*
Trilaminar endometrium 244
Trisomy 21 detection 435
Trophectoderm 301, 345, 522, 530
biopsy 354, 424*f*, 514
day five 521, 530
cells 536
grade 301*t*
morphology 302
Trophic activity 556
Trophoblastic activity 450
Trophoblastic invasion 234, 337
Trophy scope-campo compact hysteroscope 105*f*
Troubleshooting 360, 375
exercise 366
in procedures 364
Truclear hysteroscope 107
Truclear hysteroscopic morcellator 107
Truclear reciprocating blade 107
Truclear rotating cutting blade 107
Tubal cornua 445
Tubal epithelium 256
Tubal evaluation 12
hysteroscopic guided 89
tests for 13*t*
Tubal factor infertility 88, 117, 429
Tubal inflammation 55
Tubal occlusion 119
Tubal patency 120
ultrasonography evaluation of 158
Tubal pathology 255, 256
Tubal reanastomosis, advantages of 119
Tubal recanalization 119, 119*f*
laparoscopic 118*f*
Tuberculosis 45, 89, 439
endometrial 496
Tuberculous peritonitis 46
Tubes 156
Tubo-ovarian
abscess 55
masses 48*f*
bilateral 47*f*
Tumor, benign 14*f*
Tunel assay 148
Turner's syndrome 395, 432, 434, 490, 491, 568
Twin phenomenon, vanishing 429
Twin transfusion syndrome 342
Two cell
embryo 299*f*
gonadotropin system 5*f*
Two embryo transfer policy 398

Tyrode's medium, modified 472
Tyrode's solution 252, 521

U

Ulterus, evaluation of 13
Ultramorphology, selection based on 309
Ultrarapid vitrification technique 351
Ultrasonic antral follicle count 222
Ultrasonography 88, 448
guided procedures 160
monitoring, role of 159
Ultrasound 68, 154
abdominal 22
role of 154
Umbilicus 58
Unconjugated estriol 433, 434
Unfertilized oocytes, cryopreservation of 353
Unicornuate 13
Urachal cyst 572*f*
Ureaplasma urealyticum 131
Urethra, inflammation in 141
Urinary luteinizing hormone 10
levels 177
Urinary tract 58
infection 138
Urine and vaginal swab cultures 454
Uterine artery 191
Doppler 193
bilaterally 507
embolization 72, 78, 447
waveform 162*f*
Uterine blood flow 403
Uterine cavity 13, 14*f*, 166*f*, 380, 384
evaluation 159
routine 379
irregular 48*f*
Uterine cervix 380
Uterine contraction 194, 380, 382
alteration of 76
initiation of 380
minimal 384
Uterine cornua, multilayer suturing of 447
Uterine factor 252
infertility 501
causes of 503*fc*
Uterine fibroid, morcellation of 572*f*
Uterine fluid contains low levels of pyruvate 283
Uterine malformations 395
congenital 501
Uterine natural killer cells 234, 439
Uterine perfusion 161
Uterine rejection, persistent 503
Uterine scar 445
Uterine septae 101
Uterine surgery, previous 68
Uterine synechiae and polyps 439
Uterine transfer, embryo for 352
Uterine transplant 503
history of 502
indications of 503*fc*
Uterine transplantation 573
ethical feasibility of 504*t*
Uterine vessels, vasoconstriction of 7
Uterine wall 14*f*
Uterine washing 490
Uterocervix angle 201
Uterotubal transport 59
Uterus 45, 155, 164, 169, 201, 501
chronic inflammatory disease of 229
hypoplastic 395
rendered image of 167*f*
sagittal section of 165*f*
transplant 501, 503, 504, 507, 508*t*, 509, 510*t*
surgery of 506
transplantation 501, 504*f*
with myoma for myomectomy 572*f*

V

Vagina 46
upper 501
Vaginal entry 169
Vaginal gel 406
Vaginal hemorrhage 375
Vaginal irrigation 373
Vaginal progesterone 214, 404
Vaginal secretions 441
Vaginal sildenafil 240, 389
citrate 237
Vaginal wall 373
Varicocele 137, 138, 141
associated nonobstructive azoospermia, management of 139
detection of 22
examination of 17, 18*f*
Vas deferens
absent 141
congenital bilateral absence of 19, 125, 137
obstruction in 141
Vasa deferentia 23*f*
Vascularity, zones of 192*t*
Vasoepididymostomy 138
Vasography 22
Vasopressin
injection 114*f*, 115*f*
solution 446
Vasovasostomy 138
Venereal disease research 492
laboratory 363, 373, 460
Venous thromboembolism, prevention of 122
Ventilation 261, 280
air conditioning 541
Vibratory penile stimulation 471
Viral
hepatitis 492
infections 568
markers 449
Virus
positive female 93
positive male 92, 93
specific management 92
Vision
blurred 178
deteriorate 365
Visual disorders 179
Visual disturbances 178
Visual field defects 141
Vitamin 230
E 238
Vitrification 467*t*, 468*t*, 477, 489
method 460, 462, 463
process 463, 463*f*
cryosolutions 463
equipment 463
materials 463
procedure 463
types 463
solution 463
technique of 476
Volatile organic compound 261, 273, 279, 541
levels 271
presence of 286
Volume contrast imaging 171
von-Hippel-Lindau syndrome 516
Vulva 46

W

Warming process 463
Washing solution 463
Waterfall sign 89
Weight loss 29
White blood cell 412
Wolffian duct cysts 137
World Health Organization 130, 173, 315
guidelines 16

X

X chromosome, deletion of 477
Xiltrix laboratory monitoring system 272
X-linked inheritance 566
X-sex linkage, disease of 490

Y

Y-chromosome
 deletions 125, 568
 microdeletion 136
  testing 129
 sequences 435
Young's syndrome 17, 137

Z

Ziehl-Neelsen staining 48
Zika virus 94
Zinc 304
Zona
 binding 19
 dissection 331
  partial 319
 drilling 319
Zona pellucida 8, 252, 294, 295, 297, 298*f*, 323*f*, 330, 333, 338*f*
 glycoproteins of 561
 intracytoplasmic sperm injection, barcodes in 371*f*
 layer of 561
 matrix of 561
 mechanical technique, expansion of 332
 of oocyte 561
 purified 562
 softening of 352
 thicker 297*f*
Zona penetration 19
Zuclomiphene 177, 198
Zwitterionic buffers 471
Zygote 298, 299, 397, 461, 474, 567, 568
 genetic constitution of 291
 intrafallopian transfer 283, 429
 morphology 298
 place 462
 pronuclei of 568
 scoring system 298